TOTAL HIP
ARTHROPLASTY

VOLUME I

TOTAL HIP ARTHROPLASTY

Nas S. Eftekhar, M.D.
Professor of Orthopaedic Surgery
College of Physicians and Surgeons,
Columbia University, New York;
Attending Orthopaedic Surgeon and Chief of Hip and Implant Service,
New York Orthopaedic Hospital at Columbia Presbyterian Hospital, New York

**Art coordinator and
medical illustrator**

Robert J. Demarest
Director of Medical Illustration
College of Physicians and Surgeons
Columbia University, New York

With 2363 illustrations

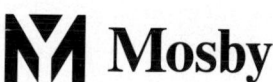 Mosby

St. Louis Baltimore Boston Chicago London Philadelphia Sydney Toronto

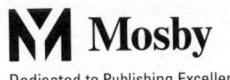

Publisher: George Stamathis
Developmental Editors: Kathryn H. Falk/Eugenia A. Klein
Project Manager: Carol Sullivan Wiseman
Production Editor: Shannon Canty
Designer: David Zielinski
Manufacturing Supervisor: Kathy Grone
Cover art: Robert J. Demarest

Printed in the United States of America
Composition by Graphic World, Inc.
Printing/binding by Maple Vail Press

Mosby–Year Book, Inc.
11830 Westline Industrial Drive
St. Louis, Missouri 63146

International Standard Book Number 08016-1669-7

93 94 95 96 97 GW/MV 9 8 7 6 5 4 3 2 1

To my wife, Barbara,
and my children, Kim and Kirt

. . . and in memory of my teacher, Sir John Charnley, for his outstanding contributions to orthopaedic surgery

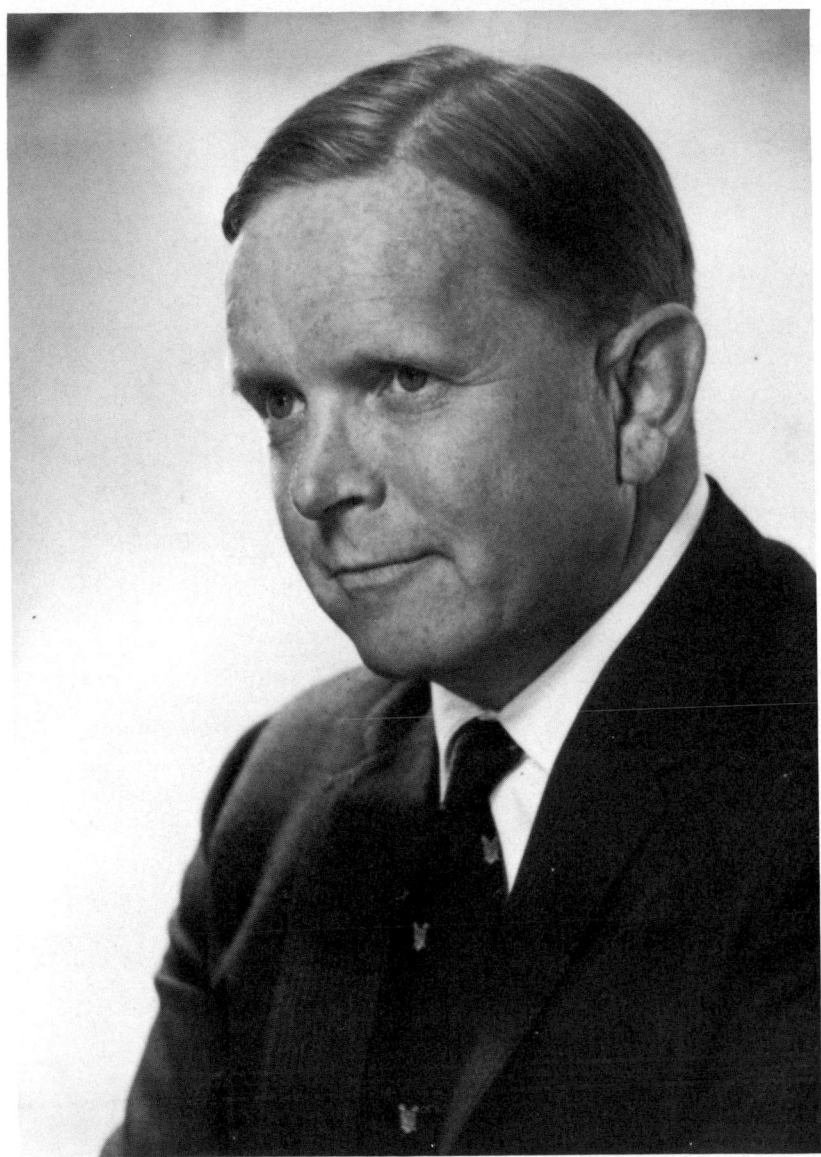

August 29, 1911 – August 5, 1982

Foreword

When I accepted Dr. Nas Eftekhar's invitation to write a foreword for his new book on total hip replacement arthroplasty, I had no idea that I was being given the unique opportunity to comment on a text against which past and future books on total hip surgery would be compared. This book is truly a masterpiece. It represents a formidable undertaking, likely to have long term significance and importance to students and practitioners of hip surgery.

Much has been said about the greatness of Sir John Charnley; of his understanding of hip disease and his unique and lasting contributions to hip surgery. Dr. Eftekhar's book is a superb testimony to him because it brings into focus, more than any other book, the enormous significance of Sir John's philosophy, his penetrating insight, the depth of his thinking, his appreciation for the limitations of the operation he developed, his logical approach to investigation and education, and his impeccable integrity.

Dr. Eftekhar points out the errors that surgeons often make when trying to improve on someone else's original contributions before truly understanding the fundamentals of those contributions and before in a serious and mature way testing their premises. I, personally, admit that at one time I thought that I could improve upon the original stainless steel Charnley prosthesis by making it of a more flexible titanium alloy. Though my actions were based on what I thought were logical and physiological reasons, they proved to be wrong. After 18 years of using the titanium prosthesis, I have returned to the original Charnley design.

History will probably prove that the problems that we are seeing today with new total hip implants are, to a great extent, due to the hasty implementation of inadvertently ill-conceived concepts aimed at improving surgical results. I have surmised that if our efforts over the past 25 years had been focused solely upon improving the wear properties of polyethylene, many of the complications we are now confronting would never have taken place. The addition of metal backing to the cemented polyethylene component to improve the performance of the cemented acetabula proved to be erroneous. Not only did those metal reinforcements fail to reduce the incidence of bone-cement interface loosening, but created an environment where the fall of the plasma sprayed metal from the cup into the acetabulum, aggravated the wear damage of the polyethylene, and resulted in new complications. The value of some other so called "improved modern cementing techniques" and the design of different prostheses have not improved the final results. In many instances, it has made them worse.

The mistaken belief that cement could produce a "disease" led to the development of porous uncemented implants. The concept is, needless to say, logical and in some instances the release of those implants has been preceded by serious laboratory research. Up to this point, however, those modular prostheses have demonstrated a complication rate higher than those with the original cemented Charnley arthroplasty. Furthermore, complications with the new uncemented implants appear to be more significant than those encountered with cemented arthroplasty. Progressive lysis of the femur and, to a lesser extent, of the acetabulum is being reported with increasing frequency. I personally believe that the reported data justify our beginning to raise the question of whether or not a moratorium should be imposed on such implants.

Many of the new implants are marketed as being superior, and often the advertisements imply that their effectiveness has been thoroughly documented. However, this is not always the case. Very little research precedes the introduction of many of the new implants that appear to be designed and modified for business reasons. These disingenuous claims have done much to increase confusion and skepticism on the part of orthopaedic surgeons as they observe with great suspicion the "war" fiercely fought between manufacturing concerns, each competing for customers. Orthopaedic surgeons and society as a whole have a responsibility to address these issues and, through dialogue and debate, find the most appropriate answers.

The early good results with noncemented acetabula in combination with cemented femoral components are encouraging. However, we should temper our enthusiasm with this new approach. Early evidence suggests that, though the complications on the acetabular side are very few, the incidence of complications on the femoral side may be greater. Thus far, the inability to firmly and permanently anchor the plastic liner against the metallic cup; the corrosion of metals in the acetabular component; the fretting of the Morse tapered necks and their subsequent fractures are creating complications that cannot be taken lightly.

An important point that should not be missed in the reading of this excellent textbook is the one related to the economics of total hip surgery. Not only the United States, but almost every other country in the world is experiencing major difficulties from the escalating cost of health care. Rationing of health care is now freely discussed at all levels and is actually taking place in different ways in various parts of the world. The increased longevity of man will produce a growth in the number of elderly people with chronic arthritic disorders. Therefore the number of elderly patients in need of total hip replacement arthroplasty will multiply many fold. The cost of care for that large number of patients will be enormous.

Though Dr. Eftekhar has deviated from Charnley's original technique in some regards, he has remained faithful to the sound fundamentals and the basic premises of low-friction arthroplasty. This text will be heralded as a landmark for students of hip surgery for many a decade.

Augusto Sarmiento, M.D.

Foreword

It has been 14 years since the publication of John Charnley's classic text *Low Friction Arthroplasty of the Hip*. In the succeeding years much has been learned as the operation has come into worldwide application and the duration of follow up has increased. Unfortunately, the knowledge derived has been largely anecdotal, retrospective, and based on results achieved by multiple surgeons with differences in skill and technique. Therefore it is refreshing to see this scholarly work by Dr. Eftekhar, representing his 25 years of experience following the principles of John Charnley but modified by time and experience.

Some of the important aspects of Dr. Eftekhar's book are the prospective nature of his documentation of patients, his emphasis on patient selection, as well as surgical technique and careful analysis of results over time. While adhering to the principles espoused by John Charnley, Dr. Eftekhar has shown a flexible approach to modification of technique where information has come to light suggesting such alteration. An example would be his conversion from routine transtrochanteric approach to routine posterolateral approach, reserving transtrochanteric approach for difficult primary and revision situations.

The organization of the book is excellent; it is divided into 9 sections in 2 volumes, containing 37 chapters. One third of the chapters are devoted to surgical technique with important sections on indications and contraindications and prevention of complications, such as deep venous thrombosis and infection. In addition, Dr. Eftekhar emphasizes the importance of careful preoperative planning—the "sweat equity" of the orthopaedic surgeon. He emphasizes quite correctly that most problems encountered during the surgical procedure can be avoided by the anticipation resulting from careful preoperative planning and templating. There is an old adage that the amount of preoperative worry and planning is inversely proportional to the frequency of complications; this text gives some excellent examples.

A particularly useful aspect of the organization of this text is the construction of a concise summary of each chapter with the salient features emphasized. Although this is a technique found in most scientific papers, it is too infrequently used in texts and Dr. Eftekhar illustrates how useful it can be.

Beautiful illustrations and clear text combine to produce an outstanding contribution to the orthopaedic literature. Representing the concepts, techniques, and results of a single, skilled, and experienced surgeon, the book stands as testimony to what can be achieved by total hip arthroplasty using cemented implants. It will stand as a standard against which other approaches must be compared.

Clement B. Sledge, M.D.

Preface

This text appears at a most propitious time, three decades after the introduction by Sir John Charnley of low-friction arthroplasty using acrylic cement for fixation. By using 22 mm as the smallest outer diameter for the femoral component it was possible to use a thick wall socket, offering both the possibility of retaining 2 to 3 mm of cement, as well as a rate of energy absorption not possible with thin-walled designs. The work presented in this book includes long-term follow-up studies on this technique reported during a period when large femoral heads, curved stems, thin plastic cups, metal-backed acetabular components, double cups, and cementless devices dominated the field. However, much energy, time, and interest has been generated recently in developing total hip arthroplasty procedures *eliminating* the use of acrylic cement for fixation. While this trend discredits the use of cement because of its failures, there seems to be no universal agreement as to whether or not the failure of cement is due to its biological incompatibility, biochemical instability, or even improper patient selection or a poor surgical technique. Significantly, tissue reaction to particles of high-density polyethylene and its long-term potentially harmful effects on bone have been vastly overshadowed by the so-called failure or weakness of cement and even the term *cement disease* has been used to implicate cement as a pathogen. This unfortunate scenario has resulted in a generation of orthopaedic surgeons who have not been taught nor ever seen the proper use of cement but have only been introduced to its failures.

Paradoxically, the orthopaedic community has become disillusioned by a lack of consensus on the efficacy and reproducibility of newer cementless techniques. New techniques are continually being modified and occasionally abandoned and replaced by even newer ones. Ironically, many surgeons are still ready to change their methods for the most "recent idea" and will do so although no fundamental principles may be involved and even though new hazards may lie ahead with unpredictable problems in the long run. To expect that the new "solution(s)" will be free from their own problems is the triumph of hope over logic and an eternal dream for a magical operation that anyone can do.

This author and many colleagues who have precisely followed Charnley's principles in performing low-friction arthroplasty of the hip, support and are in accordance with Charnley's dogma that A) acrylic cement is well tolerated by osseous tissue over a long period of time; B) outstanding clinical long-term results can be achieved in a large majority of patients; and C) the results of low-friction arthroplasty are consistently reproduced as long as minor details related to patient selection and surgical technique are observed.

This book is based on the extensive experience of one surgeon at one institution over a period of 25 years. The clinical examples presented throughout the text are from patients I have seen, treated, or consulted including some patients with prior surgery. Similar work by others and modifications including newer ideas have not been ignored as evidenced by the many references at the end of each chapter that are cited within the text. Undoubtedly controversies exist among the reports and between the reports and the author's view on certain issues. However, this should not distract the reader from the facts presented in this text. With the newer technology developing and unforeseen problems arising in the clinical situation, innovative solutions are continually being sought. With this in mind, undoubtedly, some of the opinions expressed in this text may have to be revised in the future. No clinical situation is presented or exemplified that did not in fact occur.

The writing of this text by one individual surgeon became possible as the author initiated a prospective documentation of the clinical and radiographic records of all patients who subsequently had a total hip replacement. These were kept in an area separate from the general hospital records resulting in an accumulation of data for analysis. Conclusions reported in this text are derived largely from operations performed by the author and from patients who have remained continually under surveillance. Good results obtained from total hip arthroplasty are cited throughout the text, but there are also failures that often can be traced to a common cause, that is, poor surgical technique, improper selection of patients, patient's lack of compliance, excess wear of high density polyethylene, and occasional infection. Despite the common belief and pessimism regarding the use of acrylic cement, the result of low-friction arthroplasty in young patients has been very favorable in the femur as evidenced by this author's own experience and others. The main concern is the rapid wear of a high density polyethylene socket with resultant osteolysis, which may remain a permanent obstacle in the success of total hip arthroplasty in young and active individuals.

It is not the aim of this author to be entirely complacent or to undermine the significance of a mass of useful information which has been gathered during the past 15 years and since the publication of this author's earlier work on the subject in 1978. (Eftekhar, NS, *Principles of total hip arthroplasty*, St Louis, 1978, Mosby–Year Book). During this period there have been problems including socket wear and resultant osteolysis leading to loosening and late dislocation. It may be said that excess medialization of the socket by deepening and loss of strong load-bearing bone of the acetabulum was unnecessary as shown by this author's own studies. It may also be argued that because a successful union of the greater trochanter cannot be guaranteed in all cases, the notion of a routine osteotomy of the greater trochanter must give way to selective osteotomy reserved for revision and difficult anatomical situations.

Because development of cementless, porous, ingrown prostheses, newer press fit devices, and ceramics are recent (less than 10 years) and lack long-term follow-up studies, their biomechanical properties are only briefly mentioned. In most instances review of the literature concerning the various designs is anecdotal and, with some exception, most series follow up include only 5 year results.

In assembling this book I have learned a great deal by reading the literature, and I trust that the reader will also. With newer technology developing and unforeseen problems arising in clinical situations innovative solutions are being sought that will undoubtedly necessitate a revision of this text in the future. It is my hope that this book will in some way help those who are interested in the medical and surgical management of suffering patients afflicted with and handicapped by hip disorders.

Nas S. Eftekhar, M.D.

Acknowledgments

As in all endeavors in life, usually many hands must work together to accomplish a given task. Much help comes from those whose contributions are not visible to receive credit for their efforts.

Foremost among my colleagues, I thank my teachers in orthopaedics: Thomas Hunter, F.R.C.S., Douglas Freebody, F.R.C.S.; late Professor Robert A. Robinson, M.D.; Professor Robert D. Ray, M.D., Ph.D.; and the late Professor Sir John Charnley, C.B.E., F.R.C.S., F.A.C.S. I would like to acknowledge Sir John's contributions especially, because his work was the single source of inspiration in writing this text. It is hoped it will be a lasting tribute and a testimony to his wisdom, ingenuity, and dedication to orthopaedics.

With warmest regards and fond memories, I wish to recognize and remember my good friend and senior colleague, late Dr. Frank E. Stinchfield, former chief of orthopaedics at the New York Orthopaedic Hospital at Columbia Presbyterian Medical Center, who invited me to join the staff at his institution in 1968 where I spent my subsequent 25 years of professional life. With Dr. Stinchfield's support, not only was I able to introduce the philosophy and practice of Charnley's low-friction arthroplasty but also develop a hip and implant unit by establishing a fellowship in hip surgery. Dr. Stinchfield's leadership of the department was legendary, and his impact in the field of orthopaedics was extraordinary. Dr. Stinchfield will be long remembered as the founder of the Hip Society (USA) and the International Hip Society, both significant organizations in advancing the surgery of the hip during the past two decades.

Indeed, it is my privilege to offer my special thanks to Dr. Clement Sledge and Dr. Augusto Sarmiento for responding positively to my request to write a foreword for this book. I chose them because they are among the most respected and recognized orthopaedic surgeons and educators of our time. Their highest standards in professionalism and their intellectual and scientific honesty are uniquely exemplary. Both men, despite their enormous workload as leaders in American orthopaedics, reviewed the manuscripts of this text and made a valuable contribution by their forewords. For their efforts, I am indebted.

Among the positive features of this book are the outstanding illustrations by my good friend, Robert J. Demarest. It has been my good fortune to know Bob over 25 years, and I have worked with him on many projects, including several scientific exhibits and articles, as well as three books. It is my special privilege to thank him for his talent and patience during the long, tireless, 3 years of work that he put into preparation and rendering of the illustrations for this text. He patiently watched, photographed, and sketched many operations and used his extra time in rendering the final product by his unique and innovative transparent air-brush technique. Bob (RJD) never compromised, nor did he begin to illustrate before defining the problem and mastering the subject; as such, he never released the work that was not considered correct or communicative of a message. I thank him for his significant contribution to this text. (See About the Artist.)

Although the presentation is the work of one author, a number of individuals must be recognized for their time, their efforts, and their excellent work in making this production possible. At Mosby, special thanks to Kathy Falk and Eugenia Klein for their assistance in developing the original idea for this text and the continuous support as developmental editors that included critical reviews and revisions of the manuscripts as many times as was necessary to make the text correct and lucid. Thanks also to Shannon Canty for her efforts as the production editor, Jim Ryan as executive editor, and Anne Patterson, the editor in chief.

I would like to express my special thanks to my personal secretary, Michelle Griffin, who helped me organize our documentation center initially and has updated the records and follow up of my patients throughout the years. The statistical analysis of personal experience and case presentations throughout the book would not have been possible without her loyalty. I thank her for her dedication and hard work. I am also deeply appreciative of part-time editorial assistance by Peter Ferrara, Susan Wensley, and Dr. Babek Sheikh. Dr. Sheikh proofread the entire book.

Typing and retyping of the manuscripts was carried out patiently and with care by Susan Davis and Marie Brown. I am deeply appreciative of their excellent work.

Special thanks to Renald Von Muchow, Virgil Sweden, Kirt Eftekhar, and Dr. Seneki Kobayashi for their black and white photography of patients, specimens, instruments, and prostheses used in this book. For their fine work and cooperation, I am grateful.

I am grateful also to all colleagues in orthopaedics and other fields of surgery and medicine who showed their trust and confidence in me by referring their patients for treatment. Among them, special thanks to my personal physician, Ralph Blume, M.D., who also evaluated and cared for a large number of my patients with dedication — especially in those patients who were at high risk for complications from anesthesia and surgery. For his dedication to patients and care, I am grateful. I am equally grateful to our fellows; all of whom have been personally associated with some part of my work during their one year of fellowship and residents for their hard work and care given to my patients during the past 25 years. I am indebted to two of our most recent fellows in hip surgery (1991-1992), Seneki Kobayashi, M.D., Ph.D., of Shinshu University, Japan, and Richard Iorio, M.D., currently at the Lahey Clinic in Massachusetts, USA. They reviewed and analyzed the data that is presented in Chapters 28 and 29.

I wish to express my appreciation to the orthopaedic nursing staff for their excellence of care given to the patient, both on the floor and in the operating room. Without their dedication and care there would not have been any successful surgery. I am also grateful to the orthopaedic attending staff at New York Orthopaedic Hospital and the chief of the service, Dr. Harold Dick, for his continuous support and encouragement during the preparation of this book. I am especially indebted to Dr. Ronald Grelsamer and Ohannes Nercessian for the support they have given me. They have collaborated with me on a number of clinical projects, reviewed a few chapters of this book, and graciously covered my service while I was temporarily absent from my office. My special thanks also goes to Mr. Rudolph Gand for his assistance, execution, and fabrication of all my surgical instruments and prototypes (total hip and total knee prostheses [Author's design]). None of these ideas could have been realized without his unusual skill and hard work as a designer-machinist.

I acknowledge with sincere thanks Professor Joseph Mulier, Dr. Michael Mulier, and Dr. Louis Brady of Orlando, Florida for their generosity in sharing their knowledge and their advice during a 2 year clinical trial of intraoperative prosthetic stem manufacturing at New York Orthopaedic Hospital. Equally, special thanks is due to James Boyd, John Engelhart, Vickie Wallace, Glen Richardson, and Xavier Falcones for their technical assistance during that period.

I am indebted to the following colleagues for their contribution of illustrations: A.G. Rosenberg, M.D.; C.A. Engh, M.D.; E.A. Salvati, M.D.; Professor B.M. Wroblewski, F.R.C.S.; J.D. Bobyn, M.S.; J. Pugh, PhD; Professor R. Pawluk, M.S.; A.J. Malcolm, M.D.; W. Head, M.D.; C.A.L. Bassett, M.D.; Mr. Hugh Howorth, Mr. E.F. Di Carlo, John P. Collier, DE; and Dr. H. Dick.

Last but not least, I deeply appreciate the genuine love, understanding, and support from my wife, Barbara, and my children, Kim and Kirt, during the period of writing of this text and to whom I have dedicated this work.

About the Artist

■ "...the soul never thinks without an image."
Aristotle

I am honored to introduce Robert J. Demarest, a personal friend of more than a quarter century, the most talented and seminal medical illustrator of our time, and a co-worker on this work. Robert J. Demarest's ancestral roots can be traced back to the town of Demarest in New Jersey, a few miles from Paterson, (America's first industrial city), where RJD was born. He has lived all of his life in New Jersey and has been associated with the College of Physicians and Surgeons since 1954. His career has spanned over three decades as medical illustrator at the College starting as a part-time illustrator in the Anatomy Department and going on to become Director of the newly founded Center for Biomedical Communications in 1979.

Bob's contributions to his field and the Association of Medical Illustrators are well known. He is an Association of Medical Illustrators Fellow and served as a member of its board of governors from 1963 to 1969 and as its chairman in 1967. He was president of the Association for two terms, the first from 1968 to 1969 and the second from 1988 to 1989. The Association has recognized Bob's talents with five Ralph Sweet Awards (Best of Show), the Outstanding Illustrated Medical Book Award, The Federation of Biocommunications Society's award, a first place award in medical exhibit design and many first place awards in all categories of medical illustration and graphic design.

Bob's work has appeared in *Life, Time, Newsweek, Reader's Digest, Modern Medicine, Geriatrics, World Book Encyclopedia, National Geographic Books,* and countless other books, magazines, and journals. His career and illustrations were the subject of a special feature in *Science-1983* and in the *World Book Health Annual* in 1987. The Harvard Library of Medicine includes his work in its permanent archives.

Indeed, the best introduction to Bob may be found in the *Journal of Biocommunication* (Vol 17, no. 4, 1990) which reported that the Association of Medical Illustrators at their fall meeting awarded RJD their highest honor, the AMI Lifetime Achievement Award. This award is voted on by past presidents and chairmen of the Association. The criteria for this award are: 1) long term consistent excellence in the profession of medical illustration; 2) meaningful contributions to the field of medicine; 3) service to the Association of Medical Illustrators; 4) inspiration to fellow illustrators and; 5) demonstrated humanity.

Bob's career as a medical illustrator began with the late Emanuel Kaplan's book, *Surgical Approaches to the Back, Neck and Upper Extremity.* He has been involved in many illustration projects but prefers illustrating books, saying that their diversity, challenges, and permanence make for a very satisfying experience.

One of the most impressive aspects of working with Bob has been his systematic approach to his illustrations. He believes in extensive research and preparation in order to understand the objectives of each illustration. He has said that working with the author on a book is like entering into a marriage.... the relationship continues as a lasting friendship or it ends acrimoniously. During the past 25 years that I have known Bob, his clear mind, acute awareness, and intellectual curiosity have helped me clarify my thoughts about surgical techniques and enhanced my ability to teach and convey a message. His suggestions for the design of the entire book (including the covers) are examples of his meticulous attention to detail. This has enriched the quality of this book, for which I am most grateful.

Contents

VOLUME II

xxviii Contents

Color Plates

Color Plates 1 through 3 are located after page 160 in Chapter 4.
Color Plate 4 is located after page 192 in Chapter 5.
Color Plate 5 is located after page 1474 in Chapter 31.

Introduction

This two-volume text is organized in nine parts to facilitate access to the groups of chapters related to a set of topics. The first volume begins with a brief history of arthroplasty followed by related basic sciences, general surgical principles, and perioperative care of the patient and ends with five chapters on techniques for primary total hip arthroplasty. The second volume opens with four chapters relating to specific pathologic conditions requiring deviation from standard technique, followed by sections on conversion and revision, early and long-term results, and postoperative complications.

A certain degree of repetition in the same and between the two volumes, including duplications of a few illustrations has been unavoidable to facilitate access to the material. This deliberate effort obviates the need for frequent reference from one section to another and from one volume to the other, but in some instances tends to stress the importance of a topic under discussion.

Because the results of total hip arthroplasty depend largely on a sound surgical technique, this author has devoted one third of this book to the surgical technique; primary and revision procedures. In some instances, more than one alternative technique has been offered from which the surgeon may choose the one most suitable under the circumstances and based on his/her training. The choice of surgical approach is very important, therefore a detailed discussion comparing the various surgical approaches has been advanced in Chapter 3.

Infection and thromboembolic complications (which are mostly preventable) following total hip arthroplasty have an emotional, physical, and economical impact on the unfortunate patient and the surgeon attempting to treat them. Because of their devastating impact, prevention has been emphasized. Prevention of infection and thromboembolic complications (Chapters 8 and 9) are a must for those undertaking primary and revision total hip arthroplasty. Diagnosis, management, and the results of infected total hip arthroplasties are discussed in Chapters 26, 27, and 31 respectively.

The importance of preoperative planning and perioperative management of patients undergoing total hip arthroplasty cannot be overemphasized. This has been covered in Part IV, Chapters 10 to 14. The principles of bone preparation and bone grafting for bone deficient acetabulum and femur have been outlined in Chapter 14.

To avoid repeating the steps that are common to all surgical techniques and approaches, as well as prostheses, Chapter 15 details principles common to all surgical approaches. It should be studied before reviewing any other chapters related to technique.

The surgical technique for the anterolateral, posterolateral, direct lateral, and transtrochanteric approaches are described in Chapters 16 to 19. In this author's experience the most effective and versatile approach in performing total hip arthroplasty is the transtrochanteric approach with which all hip surgeons must become familiar (Chapters 18 and 19). However, as experience is gained, most routine total hip arthroplasties can be performed with safety and effectiveness without detaching the greater trochanter. This author has adopted the posterolateral approach (Chapter 16) for a routine and uncomplicated total hip arthroplasty, whereas a transtrochanteric approach is reserved for all anatomically difficult primary and revision surgery (Chapters 18 and 19).

Variations of technique for specific anatomical situations such as congenital dysplasia and dislocation of the hip, inflammatory arthritis, protrusio acetabuli, tumors, and tumorous conditions have been detailed in Part VI (Chapters 20 to 23). Because total hip arthroplasty is being performed on younger and younger patients, much space and time is dedicated to revision and conversion procedures that include previously inserted prosthetic components (Chapters 24 to 27).

Undoubtedly, the objective value of any surgical procedure is judged by resultant clinical outcome. Without objective, impersonal methods or organized and meticulously planned prospective documentation of all cases, the long-term efficacy of a procedure or a device cannot be tested. The clinical results (Part VIII) and Chapter 26 are a reflection of results following total hip arthroplasty using acrylic cement. Cementless devices are a relatively new development (specifically in view of many modifications of the original designs) and cannot be compared with the long-term results of total hip arthroplasty using acrylic cement. No discussion of resurfacing procedures (double cup) has been offered because this procedure, due to early clinical failures when compared with the conventional hip replacements, is considered obsolete by the author and most orthopaedic surgeons. Similarly, because of early failures of nonbonded stems and the smooth, threaded acetabular cups, these results have not been included.

The choice of cemented vs cementless total hip arthroplasty continues to be a subject of controversy in the orthopaedic community. It is this author's impression that the debate is based on a lack of consistency and reproducibility in cementless femoral components to relieve pain (with customization and with or without porous coated provisions) and potential for stress shielding and difficulty in the removal. Because the role of modular cementless components, over 10 to 15

years, remains unknown and many modifications have been made, these techniques are only mentioned for interest at this time. The age of arthroplasty (time elapsed since the index operation) is recorded on the radiographs, which should provide the reader a quick reference for the length of follow up in years. Finally, each chapter in this book begins with a word of wisdom and a brief introduction, followed by the text and a summary of essentials. The summary provides a quick overview of the content of each chapter. I recommend reading the summary of each chapter before reviewing the entire text. The extensive reference list, although not all inclusive by computer search, has been reviewed during the preparation of this text and should be a stimulus to the orthopaedic residents in training for future research and further review of the subject.

PART ONE

HISTORY

CHAPTER ONE

History and Development

■ We must welcome the Future, remembering that soon it will be the Past; and we must respect the Past, remembering that once it was all that was humanly possible.
George Santayana

Preserved skeletons show that osteoarthritis and rheumatoid disease have afflicted man since earliest times. Half a million years ago, Java man suffered from osteoarthritis of the hip.[46] Although a complete citation of historical milestones in the development of hip joint surgery is beyond the scope of this book and can be found in other sources,[83] this section briefly explores the groundwork that led to the concept of a movable hip joint and the development of total hip arthroplasty. The history of hip arthroplasty may be considered in five major steps: osteotomy arthroplasty, interpositioning arthroplasty, reconstructive arthroplasty, partial replacement arthroplasty, and total arthroplasty (bicompartmental replacement) (Table 1-1).

OSTEOTOMY ARTHROPLASTY

For centuries the problem of rendering an ankylosed hip mobile captured the imagination of surgeons. Charles White,[100] a famous physician in Manchester, England, who had treated a patient whose proximal humerus had been destroyed by infection, also performed experimental resection arthroplasty on the cadaver hip joint. However, he never was credited with performing the procedure on a living subject.[9] Anthony White[89] also was credited with an osteotomy and subsequent excision of a femoral head diseased by tuberculosis in a young lad, who survived for 12 years after the operation. A clearly planned osteotomy of the upper femur with the objective of gaining motion (arthroplasty) has been credited to John Rhea Barton. Barton performed an osteotomy on an ankylosed hip in 1826.[8] By intertrochanteric osteotomy, he devised an artificial joint that he manipulated for 20 days after surgery to maintain mobility. After 6 weeks the hip joint

was mobile, and 3 months later the patient walked with a cane and had functional mobility at the site of the osteotomy. However, 6 years later the hip lost full range of motion. The patient died of pulmonary tuberculosis 10 years later, but it was said that he enjoyed a pain-free functional joint until his death (Fig. 1-1, *A*).[83]

In 1863, Sayre[78-80] reported an osteotomy for an ankylosed hip after resection of a bone fragment, which was a modification of Barton's operation.

INTERPOSITIONAL ARTHROPLASTY

A New York general surgeon named Carnochan used a wooden block between the surfaces of a resected neck of a mandible in 1840,[18] and Verneuil used soft tissue for interpositional arthroplasty in 1860. It was Ollier's work in 1885,[69] however, that created immense interest in this procedure. By that time, surgeons were using interpositioning materials such as muscle, fibrous tissue, celluloid, silver plates, rubber sheets, magnesium, zinc, and decalcified bone. The interpositioning of these materials between the articulating surfaces helped maintain motion at the site of osteotomy and prevent recurrence of bone growth. However, continuous motion usually led to ankylosis at the site of arthroplasty.

In the early 1900s, Murphy,[66,67] Lexer,[52] and Payr[71] advocated the use of tensor fascia lata muscle for interpositioning arthroplasty. Foedral found that pig's bladder was sufficiently strong to withstand the stress of weight-bearing and intraarticular pressure. In 1919, Baer[7] popularized pig's-bladder arthroplasty at the Johns Hopkins Hospital.

Skin was used as an interpositioning material in the first decade of this century by Loewe[53] and later by

Table 1-1 Hip Arthroplasty: a Historical Summary

A. OSTEOTOMY ARTHROPLASTY			
A White	1822	Gant	1872
JR Barton	1826	Pauwell	1935
Bouvier	1835	McMurray	1936
Langenbeck	1854	Blount	1943
Sayre	1863	Moore	1944
Brodhurst	1865	Dickson	1947
W Adams	1869		

B. INTERPOSITIONAL ARTHROPLASTY

I. Tissue Interpositioning Arthroplasty

Ollier	1885	
Murphy	1902	Soft tissue
Lexer	1908	
Payr	1910	Fascia
Loewe	1913	
Baer	1918	Skin
Putti	1921	
Campbell	1926	
McAusland	1929	
Kallio	1957	

II. Mold (Cup) Arthroplasty

Smith-Petersen	1923	Glass
Smith-Petersen	1933	Pyrex
Smith-Petersen	1937	Bakelite
Smith-Petersen	1938	Vitallium
Aufranc	1957	Vitallium

C. RECONSTRUCTIVE ARTHROPLASTY

Brackett	1917
Whitman	1921
Jones	1921

C. RECONSTRUCTIVE ARTHROPLASTY—CONT'D

Magnuson	1932
Colonna	1935
Girdlestone	1945

D. FEMORAL REPLACEMENT ARTHROPLASTY

Delbet	1919	Reinforced rubber
Hey-Groves	1927	Ivory
Bohlman & Moore	1940	Metallic
Judet & Judet	1943	Acrylic
Thompson	1950	Metallic
AT Moore	1952	Metallic (fenestrated stem)

E. TOTAL HIP ARTHROPLASTY

I. Early Contributors

Gluck	1890
Wiles	1938
Haboush	1951
McKee	1951
Wiltse	1952
Ring	1964
Müller	1966

II. Charnley's Contributions (1958–1982)

a. Basic research into the lubrication of animal joints
b. Use of acrylic cement for fixation of prosthesis
c. Principles of low-friction arthroplasty using plastic bearing Teflon
d. Use of HDP-bearing material
e. Aseptic techniques and development of clean air technology
f. Long-term safety studies including the histology against cement

From Hip Surgery "Then and Now." Based on a lecture delivered before an AAOS 50th anniversary meeting, Anaheim, CA, 1983, AAOS Bulletin.

Kallio.[50] During this period, Sir Robert Jones[47] of Liverpool used gold foil to cover a reconstructed femoral head in femoral arthroplasty.

The popularity of interpositional arthroplasty eventually spread to Italy and Germany. In Italy, Putti[74] used every feasible material available in a large number of patients (Fig. 1-1, *B*).

In 1923, Smith-Petersen placed a glass mold in a patient's hip.[84-86] Although it proved too fragile, as did Pyrex and available plastics, the concept of a mold prosthesis proved to be a major contribution in the development of hip arthroplasty. In 1938, Smith-Petersen, at the suggestion of his dentist, John Cooke, used Vitallium, a cobalt-chromium alloy, as an interpositioning material.[86] This proved to be clinically successful, and the Smith-Petersen mold became a valuable tool in the orthopaedic surgeon's armamentarium. Thus after half a century of other experimental work, Smith-Petersen must be given credit for proving that the acetabulum will tolerate a foreign body performing a weight-bearing function (Fig. 1-1, *C*).

RECONSTRUCTIVE ARTHROPLASTY

Credit for popularizing resection joint arthroplasty in practice must go to James Syme of Edinburgh. In his famous book, *Excision of Diseased Joints*, he detailed many resection arthroplasties.[9,88] Among others, Henry Jacob Bigelow also excised a hip joint in 1852.[10] Foch[28] reportedly resected the femoral head for degenerative osteoarthritis. In his report about 78 cases of femoral head excision, 26 patients "failed to survive" the operation. Presumably this means they died from the operation!

Brackett[11] and Whitman[101,102] described the concept of arthroplasty of the hip joint by reconstruction of the upper femur (Fig. 1-2, *A*). Among others, Magnusen,[56] Colonna,[25] Luck,[55] and Wilson[104] modified these reconstructive procedures to suit each individual problem.

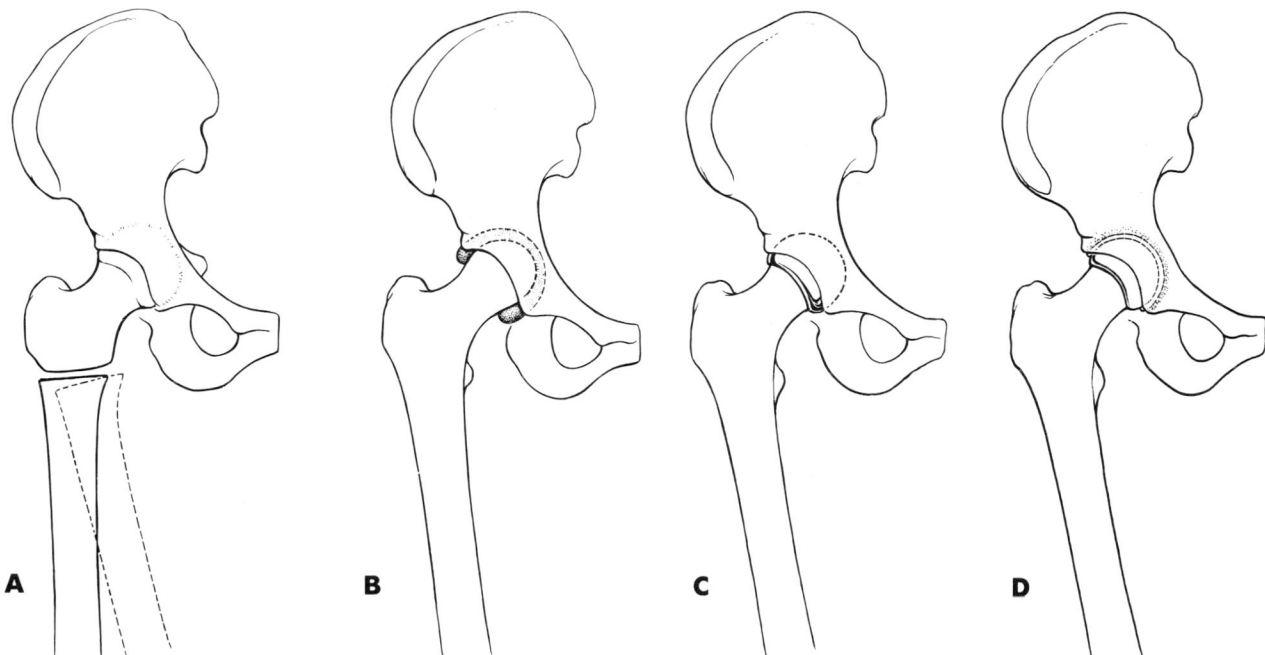

Fig. 1-1. A, Osteotomy arthroplasty as first performed by John Rhea Barton, who performed an osteotomy on an ankylosed hip in 1826 to maintain motion at osteotomy site. **B,** Example of interpositional arthroplasty performed by Ollier and others in 1885. Numerous interpositioning materials such as muscle, fibrous tissue, celluloid, silver plates, and rubber sheets were used. **C,** First formal Vitallium mold *(cup)* arthroplasty was performed by Smith-Petersen in 1937. **D,** Resurfacing *(double-cup)* arthroplasty was introduced by John Charnley in early 1950s.

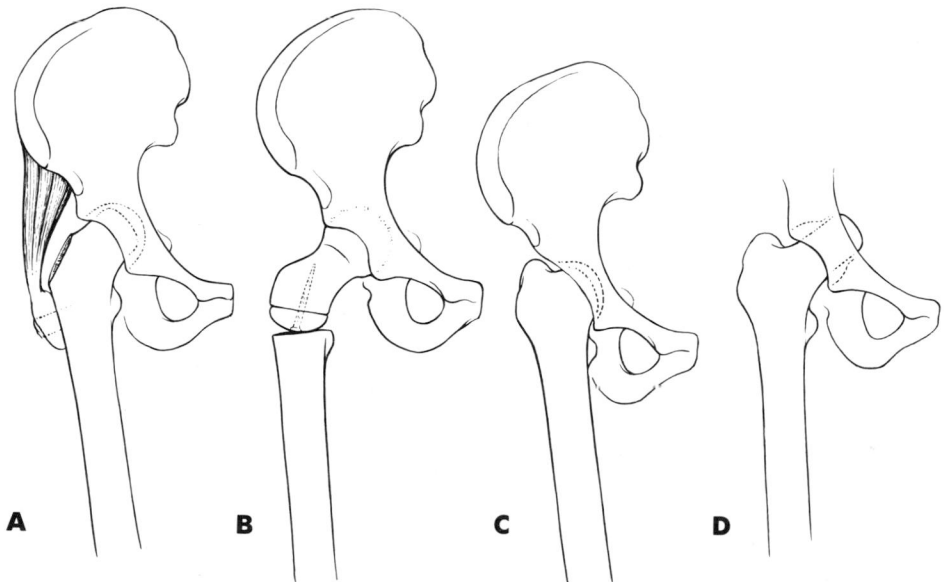

Fig. 1-2. A, Whitman arthroplasty by reconstruction of acetabulum and transfer of abductor muscles. **B,** Type of arthroplasty proposed by Jones using osteotomy of neck and retaining motion at site of osteotomy. **C,** Example of Girdlestone operation. Head and neck are resected, and superior portion of acetabulum is removed. **D,** Charnley's central dislocation-stabilization operation proved of great value in certain patients by producing motion and mechanical improvement for hip.

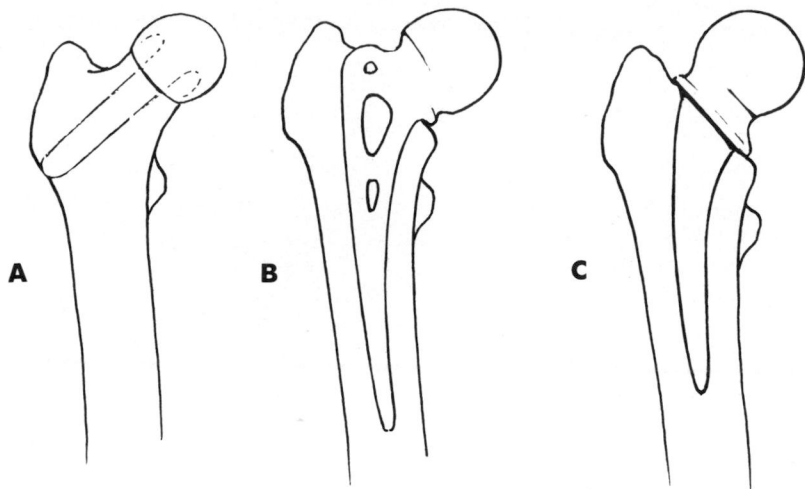

Fig. 1-3. Hemiarthroplasty prostheses: **A,** Acrylic Judet; **B,** self-locking Moore; **C,** Thompson.

Sir Robert Jones[47] popularized a neck osteotomy known as Jones's pseudarthrosis (Fig. 1-2, *B*), and Girdlestone[36,37] used resection of the hip joint to maintain motion (Fig. 1-2, *C*). Charnley's central dislocation-stabilization operation helped create a pain-free and stable hip during the pre–total hip era (Fig. 1-2, *D*).[19] In some patients, this operation was the product of a failed arthrodesis procedure.

Resection of the femoral head combined with an osteotomy of the upper femur has a recent origin. It was introduced by Henry Milch in the United States as a salvage operation for degenerative disease associated with congenital dislocation of the hip.[60]

REPLACEMENT ARTHROPLASTY

Hey-Groves[43–45] in England used a prosthetic replacement of the femoral head in 1927 with limited success. It was made of ivory, never functioned well, and finally failed. In 1919, Delbet[26] in France used a rubber prosthesis.

In 1940, Bohlman and Moore removed a tumor from the upper end of a femur and inserted the first metallic prosthesis. They published an original case report in the *Reporter* of the Columbia Medical Society in South Carolina in 1942 and in the *Journal of Bone and Joint Surgery* a year later.[63] This operation is the first known metallic replacement hemiarthroplasty.

Credit for the widespread use of the femoral head replacement belongs to the Judet brothers, who received much acclaim for their plastic (methyl methacrylate) prosthesis in 1948 (Fig. 1-3, *A*).[48] However, breakage and loosening of the prosthesis and absorption of bone often called for secondary intervention, and the celebrated original results eventually fell into

disrepute. The Judet prosthesis was subsequently made of nylon and other synthetics. The Judets' contribution is significant because it proved that mechanical replacement of the hip using plastic material can be tolerated in the human body with minimum tissue reaction.

In 1951, Peterson[73] devised a short-stemmed steel prosthesis, which was fixed to the femoral shaft by screws. Other innovations were MacBride's "doorknob" and JEM Thompson's "light-bulb" prostheses.[93]

Throughout the 1950s, more than 50 types of prostheses were introduced; the short-stem type was replaced by the intramedullary long-stem type, which gave more stability, and the nonmetallic type was replaced by the metallic type, which provided greater durability. Numerous designs used here and abroad today share common features of the two types developed by FR Thompson[90–92] in 1950 (Fig. 1-3, *C*), and Moore[61] in 1952 (Fig. 1-3, *B*). The acetabular replacement by a fixed cup was introduced by Urist[97] and others. However, failure usually resulted from the bipolar nature of arthritis and the loosening of these devices.

TOTAL REPLACEMENT ARTHROPLASTY

In a series of lectures in Berlin in the 1890s, Themistocle Glück[39,40] described a system of operations that included both articular replacements (acetabulum and femur) using ivory and a cement made of colophony, pumice, and gypsum. Indeed, using the cement as a "filler" he performed the first total hip arthroplasty by a ball-and-socket design made of ivory.[76] According to descriptions by Pean,[72] these prostheses failed because of absorption. It is of historical interest to note that attempts have been made to fixate a prosthesis date

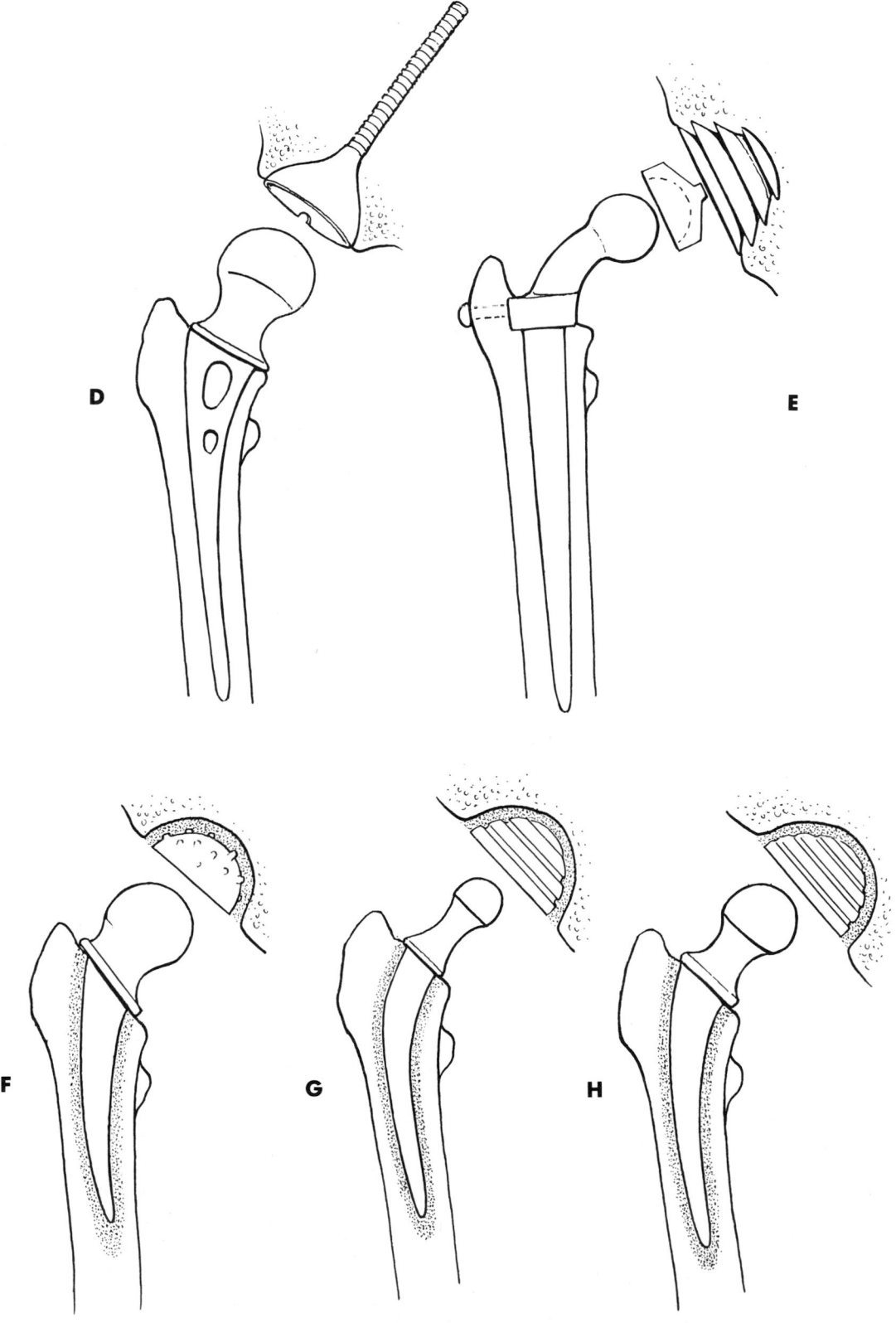

Fig. 1-3—cont'd. Total arthroplasty (bipolar) prostheses: **D,** Ring; **E,** Sivash; **F,** McKee-Farrar; **G,** Charnley; **H,** Müller. NOTE: No cement was used in **D** and **E,** but acrylic cement was used in **F, G,** and **H.**

back to 1890 when Glück,[38,40] in a lecture to the German Medical Society, discussed the use of bone glue or cement to fasten ivory devices.[81] At that time, cement was composed of colophony, pumice powder, and plaster of Paris. It was apparently well tolerated and became walled off in the marrow cavity.[82]

In the English literature, as far as we can determine, total hip arthroplasty was first introduced by Wiles[46,103] in 1938 at Middlesex Hospital in London. He used stainless steel parts that fit into one another precisely. The acetabular component was anchored to a buttressed plate by screws, and the femoral component was secured to the neck of the femur by a bolt. He placed this total hip joint into six patients with severe rheumatoid arthritis but reported in 1950 that the procedure was not totally satisfactory. No other work appears to have been recorded until 1951, when Haboush[41] published his experiences with self-curing acrylic cement in total hip arthroplasty at the Hospital for Joint Diseases in New York City. In 1952, Haboush used a Vitallium prosthesis, but because he did not apply the principles of arthroplasty (equalization of forces) and because he used cement only for fitting and not for the transmission of the load, the results were poor. A similar prosthesis was used in 1951 by McKee and Watson-Farrar,[59] who later used acrylic cement with improved results.

McKee[57] states that he developed a series of models of total hip arthroplasties but did not insert these into a human until 1951, when the first artificial lag-screw joint was introduced. From 1956 to 1960, he had a 54% success rate; revision was required mainly because of loss of fixation. His success rate increased with the use of methyl methacrylate introduced by Charnley[58] (Fig. 1-3, *F*).

From 1952 to 1957, Wiltse and his associates[105] conducted extensive experiments with acrylic cement, and Henrichson and his associates[42] experimented on pigs to test tissue reaction to acrylic cement. Since then, researchers have undertaken many laboratory experiments to determine the safety and mechanical properties of cement and its biological compatibility in humans.

After trying a number of prostheses, Müller[64] developed a plastic acetabular cup with a 32-mm chromium-cobalt-molybdenum femoral head, which he has used extensively in his clinic since 1966 (Fig. 1-3, *H*). Peter Ring[77] began his clinical experience with total joint arthroplasty by metallic components (metal against metal) without cement in 1964 (Fig. 1-3, *D*). It was somewhat parallel to the work of Russian surgeons who originally developed a metal-to-metal "single unit" prosthesis but subsequently used an interpositioning high-density polyethylene surface (Fig. 1-3, *E*).

Since the original work by the British surgeons,

numerous other devices of metal against metal and metal against plastic have been introduced in the United States and abroad. As most of these are in the experimental stage, the future will reveal their merits and shortcomings.

Dr. Frank E. Stinchfield of New York must be recognized as one of the most outstanding of the orthopaedic surgeons who have contributed to the advancement and better understanding of problems related to hip joint surgery. His scientific contributions in mold arthroplasty, hip arthrodesis, femoral head replacement, and total hip arthroplasty span years of detailed studies. Under the leadership of Dr. Stinchfield, American surgeons anticipated the extraordinary demand by the public for total hip arthroplasty and established The Hip Society in 1968. The express primary purpose of The Hip Society is to study improvements, benefits, risks, and long-term clinical results of operations such as total hip arthroplasty. In addition to founding The Hip Society in the United States, Dr. Stinchfield has been instrumental in establishing The International Hip Society for the better understanding of problems related to hip joint surgery throughout the world.

RESURFACING ARTHROPLASTY

Resurfacing arthroplasty, also known as *double-cup arthroplasty*, was introduced and used by Charnley in the early 1950s.[20,21,24] He used polytetrafluoroethylene (Teflon).* The cups were hemispherical and were shaped to be press-fitted into the acetabulum and over the refashioned femoral head. Charnley abandoned the procedure because of early failures (Fig. 1-1, *D*). Haboush[41] reported two resurfacing procedures using a double cup made of metal and fixed by acrylic cement. Townley[94,95] experimented with a combination of polyurethane cup against a metal cup. Müller and Boltzy[65] also experimented with a double-cup procedure using uncemented metal-to-metal components. With early failures, they also abandoned this procedure. Among others, Gerard,[31,32] Paltinieri and Trentani,[70] Furuya,[32] Freeman,[29–31] Capello and associates,[16,17] Amstutz,[1–6] and Wagner[98] experimented and reported on various early results with their own modifications of the surgical principles and the prosthesis. In most cases, both components were metal against plastic and were fixed by acrylic cement. Because of a high rate of early failures and at times severe acetabular damage, this procedure, although originally received enthusiastically, fell into disrepute within 5 years after its introduction as an alternative to the stemmed total hip prosthesis.[68]

---

* Nonproprietary name and trademarks of drug: Polytef – PTFE paste for injection and Teflon.

CHARNLEY'S CONTRIBUTIONS TO MODERN SURGERY OF THE HIP

In 1958, John Charnley first reported his clinical experiences with the replacement of a human joint using steel femoral components and Teflon. In 1960, he described fixation of the components with acrylic. In November 1962, the acetabular component was replaced by a more wear-resistant plastic, high-density polyethylene (Fig. 1-3, G).

Charnley's development of low-friction arthroplasty (LFA) and the introduction of self-curing acrylic cement represent this century's most significant developments in orthopaedic surgery. His work from 1954 to 1974 is best described in his own account of the evolution of LFA at his clinic at Wrightington Hospital.[23] In this paper, presented at the College of Physicians and Surgeons of Columbia University at the time he received the honorary Lasker Award in recognition of his achievement, Professor Charnley divides his work into six basic phases of development.

Basic Research into the Lubrication of Normal Animal Joints

Squeaking in an artificial joint indicates friction at the site, which does not occur naturally in joints. Charnley observed this in 1954 and began to investigate the phenomenon of lubrication that produces low friction. The only direct experimental work he found was by Dr. E Shirley Jones, who had reported a very low friction coefficient of 0.02 in animal joints, based on work with a homemade contraption duplicating joint action. Dr. Jones concluded that lack of friction was caused by hydrodynamic lubrication; that is, in a ball-bearing situation, fluid enters the zone of contact and lubricates it. Charnley further speculated that oscillation on load bearing prevents this hydrodynamic action; he decided that synovial fluid could not be the crucial factor contributing to low friction in normal joints, since cartilage remained smooth even after it was wiped clean. He concluded that "boundary" lubrication was a specific feature of intraarticular cartilage and was responsible for low frictional resistance. He then assumed that a material such as polytetrafluoroethylene (Polytef), which was self-lubricating, would be an appropriate substitute for the damaged cartilage and proceeded to use it with excellent temporary results.

Use of Polytetrafluoroethylene (PTFE) or Polytef Teflon

In the first Polytef arthroplasty, both sliding surfaces were made of Polytef replacements for the damaged articular cartilage. Early results were "phenomenal," but after 12 months there was evidence of failure and mechanical loosening. The stump of the neck of the femur lost its blood supply and became necrotic; the assumption that nothing would stick to Polytef was proved false by the accumulation of a brown, sticky material on the sliding surfaces, which prevented sliding and caused movement and wear between the plastic socket and the bone of the acetabulum.

Low-Friction Arthroplasty as a Principle

From this failure, Charnley learned the significance of the principles of LFA: not only must low frictional resistance be maintained within a joint, but the turning force (torque) transmitted from the metal femoral head to the socket must be resisted for a successful arthroplasty. Since torque is the product of frictional force and the length of the lever on which it acts, and since the frictional force between metal and plastic surfaces is constant for a given load, torque can be decreased only by reducing the diameter of the prosthetic head. Likewise, the frictional force and resistance (turning of the plastic socket in the acetabulum) can be augmented by using a socket with a thick wall, thereby increasing the outside diameter of the socket.

Charnley then began to work with a smaller diameter metal head and more efficient bonding of implants to bone.

Bonding of Implant to Living Bone by Quick-Setting Acrylic Cement

Because "the points of direct contact between an implant and bone" that produce a tight fit are "points where the bone would absorb and leave the implant inadequately supported," Charnley felt that using small amounts of acrylic cement only as an adjuvant to a tight mechanical fit was a mistake. He therefore tried making the implant a loose fit, with acrylic used not as an adhesive but as a "grout," and found that this bold and generous use of cement improved the chance for fixation by a factor of 200.[6]

Introduction of High-Density Polyethylene

After the failure of Polytef, a salesman approached Charnley with a new product, high-density polyethylene, which he rejected. However, one of his assistants decided to test it. It proved remarkably wear resistant, and although it lacked Polytef's self-lubricating property, it was capable of being lubricated by synovial fluid. This was a most fortunate coincidence, and after 5 years of testing, the material proved to be highly valuable for the construction of artificial joints. The first high-density acetabular prosthesis was inserted in a human hip joint in November 1962.

Attempt to Identify the Cause of Failures

Chemical rejection of the cement was first suspected as the cause of the 10% failure rate in total hip arthroplasty. The 90% success rate justified the continuation of the procedure but called for further investigation into the problem.

A clean-air operating room was designed, and with its use there were immediate dramatic results. Complications were reduced by more than half, and the consensus was that failure was largely caused by bacterial infection.

Although the clean-air idea has still not been universally adopted, Charnley's statistics and the preceding facts attest to its validity.

Charnley's contribution to the understanding of total hip arthroplasty is indeed a milestone in orthopaedic surgery. A thorough and accurate record of his life and work, *John Charnley: The Man and the Hip,* was published in 1990,[99] and I regard it as a must for the student of orthopaedics interested in the study of the hip joint. Much of the work presented here is based on his biomechanical concepts, which have influenced many surgeons and bioengineers throughout the world. His work and teachings have been the wellspring of inspiration in the writing of this volume.* Charnley's

---

* For further biographical information, see Eftekhar NS: The life and work of John Charnley (Aug. 29, 1911–Aug. 5, 1982), *Clin Orthop* 211:10, 1986.

contributions have been graphically shown, as have many other advances in technology and related sciences in total hip arthroplasty during the past three decades (Fig. 1-4).

BIOLOGICAL FIXATION BY POROUS-SURFACED PROSTHESES

The earliest use of a porous-coated stainless steel stem was by Tronzo[96] although the earliest design of an endoprosthesis demonstrating the possibility of an advantage for biological fixation was developed by Austin Moore in the 1950s.[61–63]

In the late 1960s and early 1970s, Judet[49], Lord,[54] and others developed prostheses with rough and porous surfaces that were used in Europe (Fig. 1-5). Although Rayan[75] first published clinical reports of the use of a porous cobalt-chromium–coated prosthesis of the Austin Moore variety, Cameron and co-workers[13–15] were among the first to use such prostheses. During the 1970s, extensive laboratory investigations were carried out to more fully characterize the morphological, mechanical, and structural properties of titanium-fiber metals and porous chromium-cobalt alloys, as well as Proplast, porous polyethylene, porous polysulfone, plasma-sprayed tita-

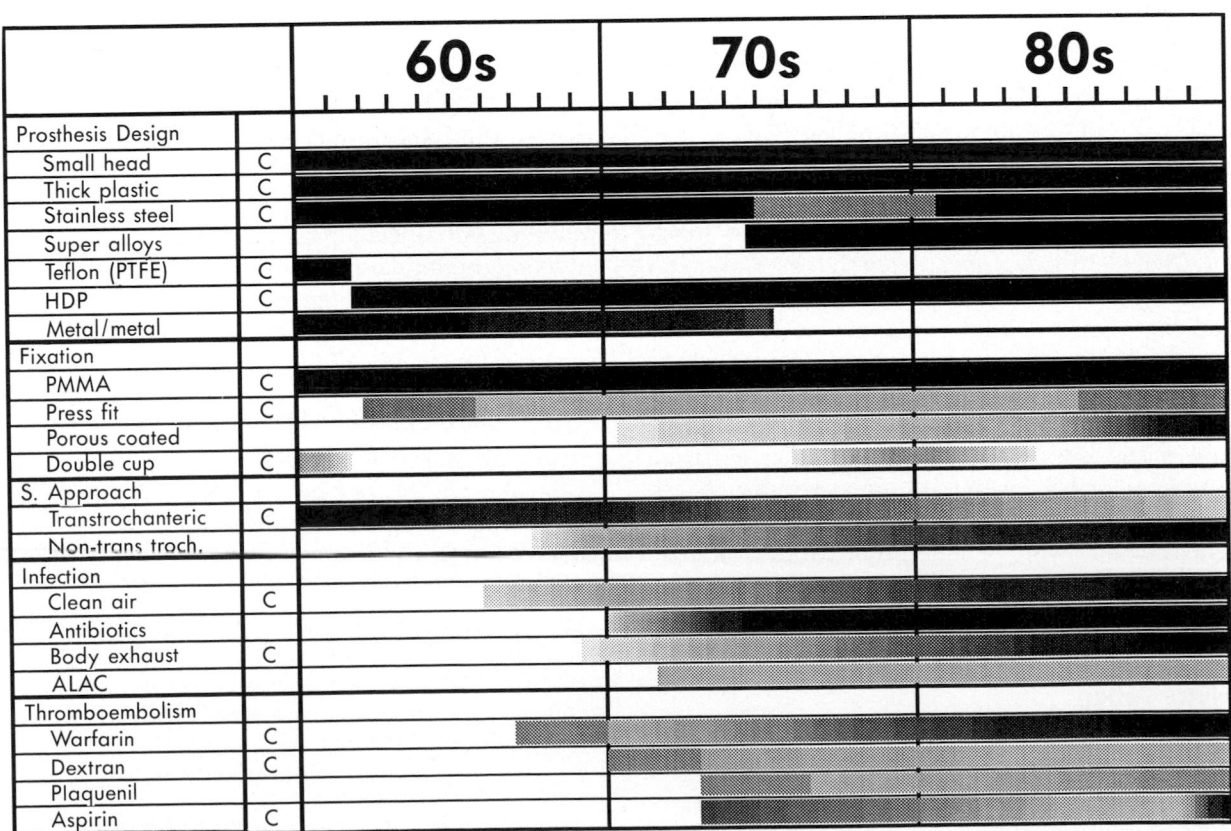

Fig. 1-4. Graphic presentation of advances in total hip arthroplasty technology over past 3 decades. *C,* John Charnley's contributions.

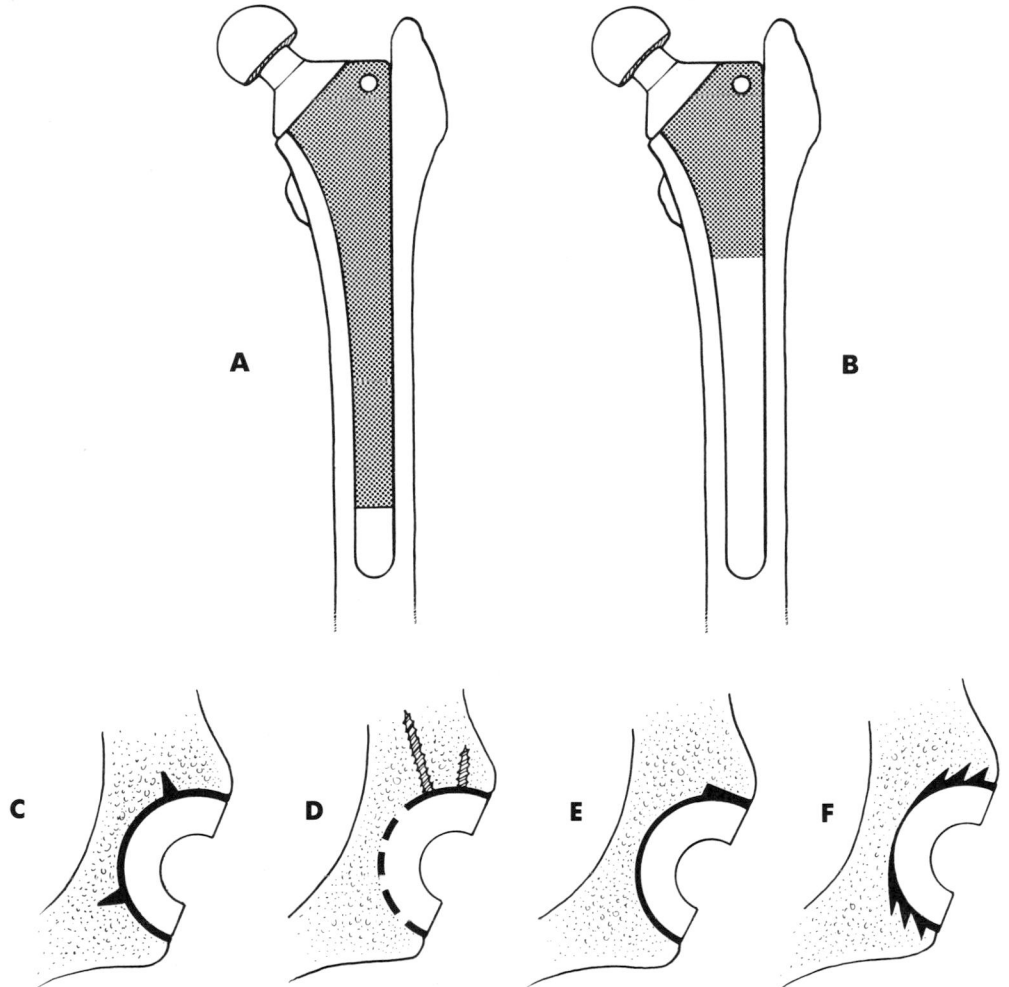

Fig. 1-5. Cementless devices using porous-coated surfaces for biological ingrowth. **A,** Fully porous coated and **B,** one third porous coated AML (T.M.) stems, **C,** Porous-coated AML cup, **D,** Harris-Galante cup, **E,** PCA porous-coated cup, **F,** Threaded (non-porous) cup.

nium, and other materials. Galante and co-workers[33,51] were notable among early investigators of the use of the fiber-metal composite wire mesh. Spector[87] and Engh and Bobyn[27] offer a detailed historical background on porous-coated implants. At present, an exact place for porous-coated devices from a historical perspective cannot be defined because of the continuing controversy related to the biological response produced and affected by these devices. Longer follow-up of clinical case studies is required.

SUMMARY OF ESSENTIALS

- The history of arthroplasty of the hip may be considered in five major historical phases: osteotomy arthroplasty, interpositioning arthroplasty, reconstructive arthroplasty, replacement arthroplasty, and total arthroplasty.

- The history of arthroplasty begins with John Rhea Barton of Lancaster, Pa, who performed an osteotomy on an ankylosed hip in 1826 and maintained motion at the site by manipulation after osteotomy.

- Many surgeons in Europe and the United States attempted interpositioning arthroplasty at the turn of the century by placing a variety of materials between the articulating surfaces of the hip joint. An arthroplasty of this type performed by Smith-Petersen in 1923 led to the clinical success of cup arthroplasty, and he proved that the acetabulum could tolerate a foreign body performing a weight-bearing function as a method for arthroplasty.

- Around the turn of the century, many surgeons used reconstructive procedures involving the acetabulum and the upper femur with the hope of formation of pseudarthrosis. Brackett, Whitman, Magnusen, Colonna, Jones, Girdlestone, and others are responsible for the development of arthroplasty of the hip without any formal interpositioning material.

- The Judet brothers' contribution was significant because it proved that mechanical replacement of the hip can be tolerated, a concept subsequently refined by Frederick Thompson of New York and Austin Moore of South Carolina.

- The concept of total hip arthroplasty is credited to many surgeons; Wiles, Haboush, McKee, and Charnley were among the early pioneers in the field. Charnley's major contributions to the understanding of total hip arthroplasty, milestones in the history of orthopaedic surgery, include the introduction and popularization of acrylic cement for fixation and high-density polyethylene plastic as the bearing material of the socket. Charnley's work has had a worldwide influence on many surgeons and engineers, who are today working to identify the inherent problems in total joint arthroplasty and to improve existing methods and materials.

- Charnley also pioneered the first resurfacing procedure using Teflon for bearing, but he soon abandoned the concept. Among others, Gerard, Paltinieri, Freeman, Amstutz, and Wagner refined this procedure.

- The earliest use of a porous-coated prosthesis was by Tronzo, although Judet, Lord, and Cameron were among the first to popularize such devices.

- Notable among early basic research investigators in the field of porous-coated surfaces for ingrowth of bone were Galante, Spector, Engh, and Bobyn.

- Professor Joseph Mullier of Belgium is the first surgeon on record to introduce the concept of intraoperative manufacturing of the stem for an identical fit of the prosthesis to the patient.

REFERENCES

1. **Amstutz HC:** The THARIES hip resurfacing technique, *Orthop Clin North Am* 13:813, 1982.
2. **Amstutz HC:** Development and nine-year results of THARIES resurfacing arthroplasty. Presentation to International Symposium on the Young Patient with Degenerative Hip Disease. Stockholm, 1984.
3. **Amstutz HC, Clarke IC, Christie J, et al:** Total hip articular replacement by internal eccentric shells: the "tharies" approach to total surface replacement arthroplasty, *Clin Orthop* 128:261, 1977.
4. **Amstutz HC, Graff-Radford A, Gruen TA, et al:** THARIES surface replacements: A review of the first 100 cases, *Clin Orthop* 134:87, 1978.
5. **Amstutz HC, Graff-Radford A, Mai LL, et al:** Surface replacement of the hip with the tharies system. Two- to five-year results. *J Bone Joint Surg* 63:1069, 1981.
6. **Amstutz HC, Thomas BJ, Jinnah R, et al:** Treatment of primary osteoarthritis of the hip. A comparison of total joint and surface replacement arthroplasty, *J Bone Joint Surg* 66:228, 1984.
7. **Baer WS:** Arthroplasty with the aid of animal membrane, *Am J Orthop Surg* 16:1, 1918.
8. **Barton JR:** On the treatment of ankylosis by the formation of artificial joints, *North Am Med Surg J* 3:279, 1827.
9. **Bick EM:** *Source book of orthopaedics,* ed 2, New York, 1968, Haftner Publishing.
10. **Bigelow HJ:** Resection of the head of the femur, *Am J Med Sci* 24:90, 1852.
11. **Brackett EG:** Fractured neck of the femur; operation of transplantation of femoral head to trochanter, *Boston Med Surg J* 192:1118, 1925.
12. **Bohlman HR:** Replacement reconstruction of the hip, *Am J Surg* 84:268, 1952.
13. **Cameron HU, Macnab I, Pilliar RM:** A porous metal system for joint replacement surgery, *Int J Artif Organs* 2:104, 1978.
14. **Cameron HU, Pilliar RM, Macnab I:** The effect of movement on the bonding of porous metal to bone, *J Biomed Mater Res* 7:301, 1973.
15. **Cameron HU, Pilliar RM, Macnab I:** The rate of bone ingrowth into porous metal, *J Biomed Mater Res* 10:295, 1976.
16. **Capello WN, Ireland PH, Trammel TR, et al:** Conservative total hip arthroplasty: a procedure to conserve bone stock. I. Analysis of sixty-six patients. II. Analysis of failures, *Clin Orthop* 134:59, 1978.
17. **Capello WN, Misamore GW, Trancik TM:** Conservative total hip arthroplasty, *Orthop Clin North Am* 13:833, 1982.
18. **Carnochan JM:** Archives of Medicine 284, 1860. Cited in Thompson FR: An essay on the development of arthroplasty of the hip, *Clin Orthop* 44:73, 1966.
19. **Charnley J:** *Compression arthrodesis, including central dislocation as a principle in hip surgery,* Edinburgh and London, 1953, E & S Livingstone.
20. **Charnley JC:** Arthroplasty of the hip: a new operation, *Lancet* 1:1129, 1961.
21. **Charnley J:** Tissue reactions to polytetrafluoroethylene, letters to the editors. *Lancet* 2:1379, 1963.
22. **Charnley J:** A biomechanical analysis of the use of cement to anchor the femoral head prosthesis, *J Bone Joint Surg* 47[Br]:354, 1965.
23. **Charnley J:** Total hip replacement, *JAMA* 230:1025, 1974.
24. **Charnley J:** *Low friction arthroplasty of the hip: theory and practice,* New York, 1979, Springer-Verlag.
25. **Colonna PC:** A new type of reconstruction operation for old ununited fracture of the neck of the femur, *J Bone Joint Surg* 17:110–122, 1935.
26. **Delbet P:** Résultat éloigné d'un vissage pour fracture transcervicale du fémur, *Bull Mem Soc Chir Paris* 45:434, 1919.
27. **Engh CA, Bobyn JD:** *Biological fixation in total hip arthroplasty,* Thorofare, NJ, 1985, Slack.
28. **Foch C:** Bemerkungen und Erfahrungen Hüftgelenk Langenbecks, *Arch Chir* 1:172, 1861.
29. **Freeman MAR, Bradley GW:** ICLH double cup arthroplasty, *Orthop Clin North Am* 13:799, 1982.
30. **Freeman MAR, Cameron HU, Brown GC:** Cemented double cup arthroplasty of the hip: a five-year experience with the ICLH prosthesis, *Clin Orthop* 134:45, 1978.
31. **Freeman MAR, Swanson SAV, Day WH, et al:** Conservative total replacement of the hip. In Proceedings and

reports of universities, colleges, councils, and associations, Great Britain, British Orthopaedic Assoc., *J Bone Joint Surg* 57[Br]:114, 1975.

32. **Furuya K:** Results of socket-cup arthroplasty, *J Jpn Orthop Assoc* 50:721, 1976.

33. **Galante J, Rostoker W, Lueck R, et al:** Sintered fiber metal composites as a basis for attachment of implants to bone, *J Bone Joint Surg* 53:101, 1971.

34. **Gerard Y:** Hip arthroplasty by matching cups, *Clin Orthop* 134:25, 1978.

35. **Gerard Y, Segal PH, Bedoucha JS:** Hip arthroplasty by matching cups, *Rev Chir Orthop* 60(Suppl):281, 1974.

36. **Girdlestone GR:** Arthrodesis and other operations for tuberculosis of the hip. In Girdlestone GR, editor: *The Robert Jones birthday volume,* London, 1928, Oxford University Press.

37. **Girdlestone GR, Watson-Jones R, Stamm T, et al:** Discussion on the treatment of unilateral osteoarthritis of the hip-joint, *Proc R Soc Med* 38:363, 1945.

38. **Glück T:** Autoplastik: transplantation: implantation von Fremdkörpern, *Berl Klin Wochenschr* 27:421, 1890.

39. **Glück T:** Die Invaginationsmethode der Osteound Arthroplastik, *Berl Klin Wochenschr Circulation* 33.752, 1890.

40. **Glück T:** Referat über die durch das moderne chirurgische Experiment gewonnenen positiven Resultate, betreffend die Naht und den Ersatz von Defecten höherer Gewebe, sowie über die Verwerthung resorbirbarer und lebendiger Tampons in der Chirurgie, *Arch Klin Chir* (Berl.) 41:187, 1891.

41. **Haboush EJ:** A new operation for arthroplasty of the hip based on biomechanics, photoelasticity, fast-setting dental acrylic, and other considerations, *Bull Hosp Joint Dis* 14:242, 1953.

42. **Henrichsen E, Jansen K, Krogh-Poulsen W:** Experimental investigation of the tissue reaction to acrylic plastics, *Acta Orthop Scand* 22:141, 1953.

43. **Hey-Groves EW:** Arthroplasty, *Br J Surg* 11:234, 1923.

44. **Hey-Groves EW:** Reconstructive surgery of the hip, *Br J Surg* 14:486, 1927.

45. **Hey-Groves EW:** Surgical treatment of osteoarthritis of the hip, *Br Med J* 1:3–5, 1933.

46. **Javson M,** editor: *Total hip replacement,* Philadelphia, 1972, JB Lippincott.

47. **Jones R,** editor: *Orthopaedic surgery of injuries,* London, 1921, Frowde. 2 vols.

48. **Judet J, Judet R:** The use of an artificial femoral head for arthroplasty of the hip joint, *J Bone Joint Surg* 32[Br]:166, 1950.

49. **Judet R, Siguier M, Brumpt B, et al:** A non-cemented total hip prosthesis, *Clin Orthop* 137:76, 1978.

50. **Kallio KE:** Arthroplastia cutanea. Proceedings of the Nordisk Ortopedisk Forenings Twenty-eighth Assembly in Helsinki. June 1956, *Acta Orthop Scand* 26:327, 1957.

51. **Lembert E, Galante J, Rostoker W:** Fixation of skeletal replacement by fiber metal composites, *Clin Orthop* 87:303, 1972.

52. **Lexer E:** Über Gelenktransplantation, *Med Klin Berlin* 4:817, 1908.

53. **Loewe O:** Über Hautimplantation an Stelle der freien Faszienplastik, *Munch Med Wochenschr* 60:1320, 1913.

54. **Lord GA, Hardy JR, Kummer FJ:** An uncemented total hip replacement: experimental study and review of 300 madreporique arthroplasties, *Clin Orthop* 141:2, 1979.

55. **Luck JV:** A reconstruction operation for pseudarthrosis and resorption of the neck of the femur, *J Iowa Med Soc* 28:620–622, 1938.

56. **Magnuson PB:** The repair of ununited fracture of the neck of the femur, *JAMA* 98:1791, 1932.

57. **McKee GK:** Artificial hip joint, In Proceedings and Reports of Universities, Colleges, Councils, and Associations. Regional Orthopaedic Societies, *J Bone Joint Surg* 33[Br]:465, 1951.

58. **McKee GK:** Development of total prosthetic replacement of the hip, *Clin Orthop* 72:85, 1970.

59. **McKee GK, Watson-Farrar J:** Replacement of arthritic hips by the McKee-Farrar prosthesis, *J Bone Joint Surg* 48[Br]:245, 1966.

60. **Milch H:** The "pelvic support" osteotomy, *J Bone Joint Surg* 23:581, 1941.

61. **Moore AT:** Metal hip joint: new self-locking Vitallium prosthesis, *South Med J* 45:1015, 1952.

62. **Moore AT:** The self-locking metal hip prosthesis, *J Bone Joint Surg* 39:811, 1957.

63. **Moore AT, Bohlman HR:** Metal hip joint. A case report, *J Bone Joint Surg* 25:688, 1943.

64. **Müller ME:** *Die Huftnahen Femurosteotomien,* Stuttgart, 1957, Georg Thieme Verlag.

65. **Müller ME, Boltzy X:** Artificial hip joints made from PROTOSOL, *Bull Assoc Study Problems Internal Fixation,* 1968.

66. **Murphy JB:** Ankylosis. Arthroplasty—clinical and experimental, *JAMA* 44:1573, 1905.

67. **Murphy JB:** Arthroplasty, *Ann Surg* 57:593, 1913.

68. **Murray WR, Van Meter JW:** Surface replacement hip arthroplasty: results of the first seventy-four consecutive cases at the University of California, San Francisco. In *The Hip Society: the hip, proceedings of the tenth open scientific meeting of The Hip Society,* St Louis, 1982, Mosby–Year Book.

69. **Ollier LXEL:** *Traité des résection et des operations conservatrices qu'on peut practiquer sur le systeme osseus,* Paris, 1885, Masson et cie, editeurs.

70. **Paltinieri M, Trentani C:** A modification of the hip arthroprosthesis, *Chir Organi Mov* 60:85, 1971.

71. **Payr E:** Blütige Mobilisierung versteifter Gelenke, *Zentrabl Chir* 37:1227, 1910.

72. **Pean JE:** Des moyens prosthetiques destinés a obtenir la reparation de parties osseuses, *Gaz de Hop, Paris* 67:291, 1894.

73. **Peterson LT:** The use of a metallic femoral head, *J Bone Joint Surg* 33:65, 1951.

74. **Putti V:** Arthroplasty, *J Orthop Surg* 3:421, 1921.

75. **Rayan GM, Booker AF Jr:** Porous-coated endoprosthesis in treatment of subcapital fractures, *Orthopedics* 3:660, 1980.

76. **Riley LH Jr:** The evolution of total knee arthroplasty, *Clin Orthop* 120:7, 1976.

77. **Ring PA:** Complete replacement arthroplasty of the hip by the Ring prosthesis, *J Bone Joint Surg* 50[Br]:720, 1968.

78. **Sayre LA:** A new method for artificial hip joint in bony ankylosis—two cases, *Trans Med Soc NY* pp. 111–127, 1863. Cited in Shands AR: Historical milestones in the development of modern surgery of the hip joint. In Tronzo RG, editor: The surgery of the hip joint, Philadelphia, 1973, Lea & Febiger.

79. **Sayre LA:** Exection of the head of the femur and removal of the upper rim of the acetabulum for morbus coxarius, *NY J Med* 14:70, 1855.

80. **Sayre LA:** Exection of the head of the femur for morbus coxarius, *Med Record* 6:281, 1871–1872.

81. **Scales JT:** Acrylic bone cement—bond or plug? *J Bone Joint Surg* 50[Br]:698, 1968.

82. **Scales JT, Lowe SA:** Some factors influencing bone and joint replacements. In Jayson M, editor: *Total hip replacement,* London, 1971, Sector Publications.

83. **Shands AR:** Historical milestones in the development of modern surgery of the hip joint. In Tronzo RG, editor: *The surgery of the hip joint.* Philadelphia, 1973, Lea & Febiger.

84. **Smith-Petersen MN:** A new supra-articular subperiosteal approach to the hip joint, *Am J Orthop Surg* 15:592, 1917.

85. **Smith-Petersen MN:** Arthroplasty of the hip; a new method, *J Bone Joint Surg* 21:269, 1939.

86. **Smith-Petersen MN:** Evolution of mould arthroplasty of the hip joint, *J Bone Joint Surg* 30[Br]:59, 1948.

87. **Spector M:** Historical review of porous-coated implants, *J Arthrop* 2:163, 1987.

88. **Syme J:** *The excision of diseased joints,* Edinburgh, 1831.

89. **Thompson FR:** An essay on the development of arthroplasty of the hip, *Clin Orthop* 44:73, 1966.

90. **Thompson FR:** Vitallium intramedullary hip prosthesis preliminary report, *NY J Med* 52:3011, 1952.

91. **Thompson FR:** Two and a half years' experience with a Vitallium intramedullary hip prosthesis, *J Bone Joint Surg* 36:489, 1954.

92. **Thompson FR:** An essay on the development of arthroplasty of the hip, *Clin Orthop* 44:73, 1966.

93. **Thompson JEM:** A prosthesis for the femoral head. A preliminary report, *J Bone Joint Surg* 34:175, 1952.

94. **Townley CO:** Intramedullary cup-stem arthroplasty for the hip joint. A 16-mm film. Chicago, AAOS, Audio-Visual Film Library, 1964.

95. **Townley CO:** Conservative total articular replacement arthroplasty (the TARA Procedure) with the fixed femoral cup, *J Bone Joint Surg* 5:3, 1981.

96. **Tronzo RG:** Long-term follow-up of a biologically fixed hip implant. In Weinstein AM, Hedley AK, editors: *Uncemented total joint replacement.* Phoenix, 1984, Harrington Arthritis Research Center.

97. **Urist M:** *Hip arthroplasty,* Baltimore, 1965, Williams & Wilkins.

98. **Wagner H:** Surface replacement arthroplasty of the hip, *Clin Orthop* 134:102, 1978.

99. **Waugh W:** *John Charnley. The man and the hip,* New York, 1990, Springer-Verlag.

100. **White C:** *Phil Trans London,* 59:39, 1769.

101. **Whitman R:** A new treatment for fracture of the neck of the femur, *Med Rec* 65:441, 1904.

102. **Whitman R:** The reconstruction operation for ununited fracture of the neck of the femur, *Surg Gynecol Obstet* 32:479, 1921.

103. **Wiles P:** The surgery of the osteo-arthritic hip, *Br J Surg* 45:488, 1958.

104. **Wilson PD:** Trochanteric arthroplasty in the treatment of ununited fractures of the neck of the femur, *J Bone Joint Surg* 29:313, 1947.

105. **Wiltse LL, Hall RH, Stenehjem JC:** Experimental studies regarding the possible use of self-curing acrylic in orthopaedic surgery, *J Bone Joint Surg* 39:961, 1957.

PART TWO

BASIC SCIENCE

CHAPTER TWO

Applied Surgical Anatomy

■ There is but little room for inexactness in the field of surgery; a deviation of even a centimeter or two from the correct approach may change success into disaster.
Lord Brock

This chapter is intended as a brief review of applied anatomy and describes only those anatomical features relevant to hip surgery. Several later chapters (12, 14, and 22) refer to information given here. The reader interested in anatomical details unrelated to hip replacement may refer to standard texts in anatomy.*

PELVIS

The two coxal or hip bones, also known as *innominate bones,* articulate firmly with the sacrum and with each other at the pubis symphysis; with the sacrum and coccyx they form the bony skeleton of the pelvis. The coxae are tightly bound together with the sacrum and coccyx by ligaments, forming the "pelvic ring." The walls of the pelvis are padded with muscles and other structures from within and without, so the living pelvis is very different from a bony specimen. Orientation of the pelvis on the operating table can be somewhat altered by the position of the soft tissue about the hip. For example, when a patient is supine on the operating table and severe bilateral flexion deformity is present, a forward tilt of the pelvis results. The surgeon can best determine this tilt by assessing the presence and amount of compensatory lumbar lordosis. Attention to the bony surface landmarks of the pelvis and thigh will assist in the proper placement of the incision at surgery (Fig. 2-1).

The ilium, pubis, and ischium all contribute to the formation of the acetabulum, which faces not only outward but also somewhat downward and anterior. A mental visualization of the acetabular origination is

essential when directing the reamers for preparation of the acetabulum. The weight-bearing upper and posterior walls of the acetabulum are especially heavy, whereas the inferior wall is less substantial at the site of the acetabular notch (Fig. 2-2, *A*). The formation of the hemipelvis is of interest (Fig. 2-2, *C*). The iliac and ischial segments are massive and provide major support for muscular attachment and formation of the acetabulum (Fig. 2-2, *B*). The pubic bone (anteriorly) contributes to the acetabulum to a lesser degree.

When preparing the acetabulum for the cup, the surgeon must strive to obtain the maximum fixation from the best available bones, the iliac (superiorly) and the ischium (posteriorly). Although the inferior wall is absent in normal conditions, in protrusion or osteoarthritis a wall may form by fusion of opposing osteophytes extending beyond the intracotyloid notch. The surgeon can use this wall as a supporting structure for fixation of cement or porous-coated acetabular components.

The acetabular notch leads into the "acetabular fossa," a rough area at the center of the articulating portion of the acetabulum; it is the thinnest portion of the floor and a zone that may transilluminate on a dry specimen since the inner and outer tables of cortical bone are fused at this site without interpositioned cancellous bone (Fig. 2-3). It is of paramount importance that the surgeon avoid deepening the socket beyond this zone or breaking through this area; this could lead to failure of fixation of cement and a complete medial migration of the prosthetic device. It is a fortunate coincidence that in most osteoarthritic hips, especially in congenital dysplasia, marked thickening of the floor takes place, which allows further

---

* References 9, 16, 19, 20, 27, 34.

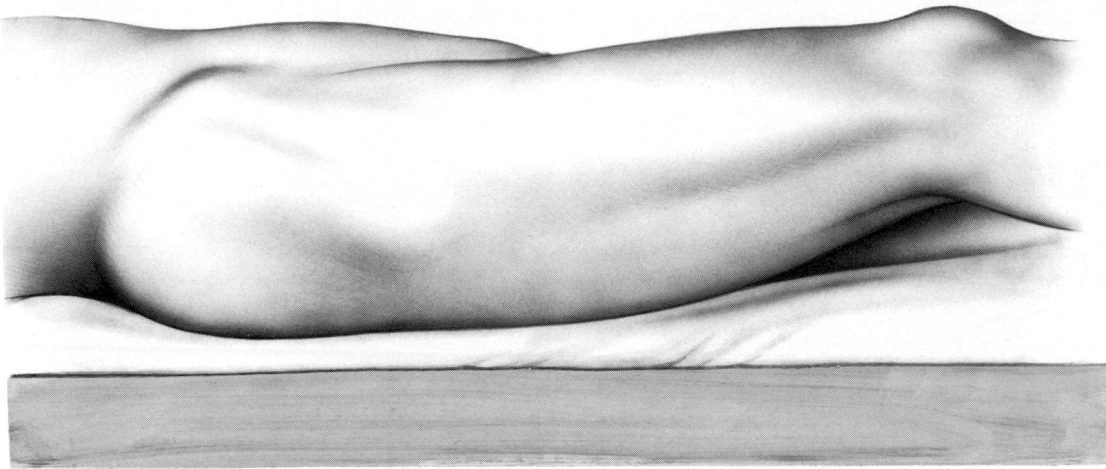

Fig. 2-1. Surface anatomy of hip and thigh as patient lies on operating table. Important landmarks include anterosuperior spine, crest of ilium, greater trochanter, and iliotibial track. NOTE: concavity behind greater trochanter, denoting site of greater trochanter. Also observe prominent tensor fascia femoris and depression between gluteus medius and tensor fascia femoris muscle. These surface landmarks should assist in proper placement of skin incision at surgery.

deepening at this level. This is usually evidenced by radiological "teardrop" widening on anteroposterior views of the pelvis (Fig. 2-4).

The medial wall of the acetabulum, indicated by a "teardrop" figure (inferior is U-shaped), is located inferomedially. This figure represents the extent of the medial wall to the top of the obturator foramen. The lateral border of this figure (radiologically best located on the anteroposterior view of the pelvis) is the external acetabular wall. The medial wall of the acetabulum is the medial border. However, because of the parallax, the relationship between the teardrop figure and the ilioischial line changes for as little as 10 degrees in horizontal obliquity if the radiograph is not a true anteroposterior view of the pelvis. The teardrop sign (unlike the ilioischial line) on x-ray of the pelvis is a constant and reliable point of reference for detecting protrusion and medial wall deficits[8] and proximal migration of the acetabular component of the total hip prosthesis (Fig. 2-4; see Chapter 22).

Ilium

The ilium is the component of the coxa that can be palpated by the examiner approximately 4 to 6 cm inferior to the rib cage. It is somewhat fan-shaped with the hinge of the fan at the acetabular level. The margin of the fan extends from the anterior to the posterior border, with the iliac crest between them, thus separating the abdominal wall from the gluteal region. The hollow area between the rib cage and the crest allows the surgeon to palpate the iliac crest for the level of the pelvis, even through a draped surgical field. The anterior end of the iliac crest ends in an important

landmark, the "anterosuperior spine," which gives origin to the inguinal ligament and may be palpated through the surgical draping. Palpation is best performed with both hands of one examiner at surgery. The two spines denote the transaxis of the pelvis. The acetabular cup is fixed in reference to this line.

A second landmark is an external lip that is prominent 5 to 7 cm above and behind the anterosuperior spine and is known as the *tubercle of the crest.* The examiner should consider these landmarks as points of reference for (1) position of the patient on the operating table, (2) placement of the incision, (3) trochanteric position, and (4) measurements of length of the extremity and orientation of the acetabular component. A fixed abduction or adduction may alter their locations in reference to the axis of the body, a major consideration in orienting the acetabular cup guide at positioning.

The muscles of the lateral and posterior abdominal walls and fascia lata of the thigh are attached to the iliac crest and can be conveniently detached from their insertions to make the ilium accessible for bone grafting if necessary during hip arthroplasty. Surgical draping must not make the iliac crest (from the anterosuperior spine to its posterosuperior spine) inaccessible.

The bony pelvis gives the appearance of having been twisted on itself at the site of the acetabulum (Figs. 2-5 to 2-7). Therefore the two planes cut each other nearly at right angles, the upper one roughly corresponding to the ilium and the lower one corresponding to the

Text continued on p. 23.

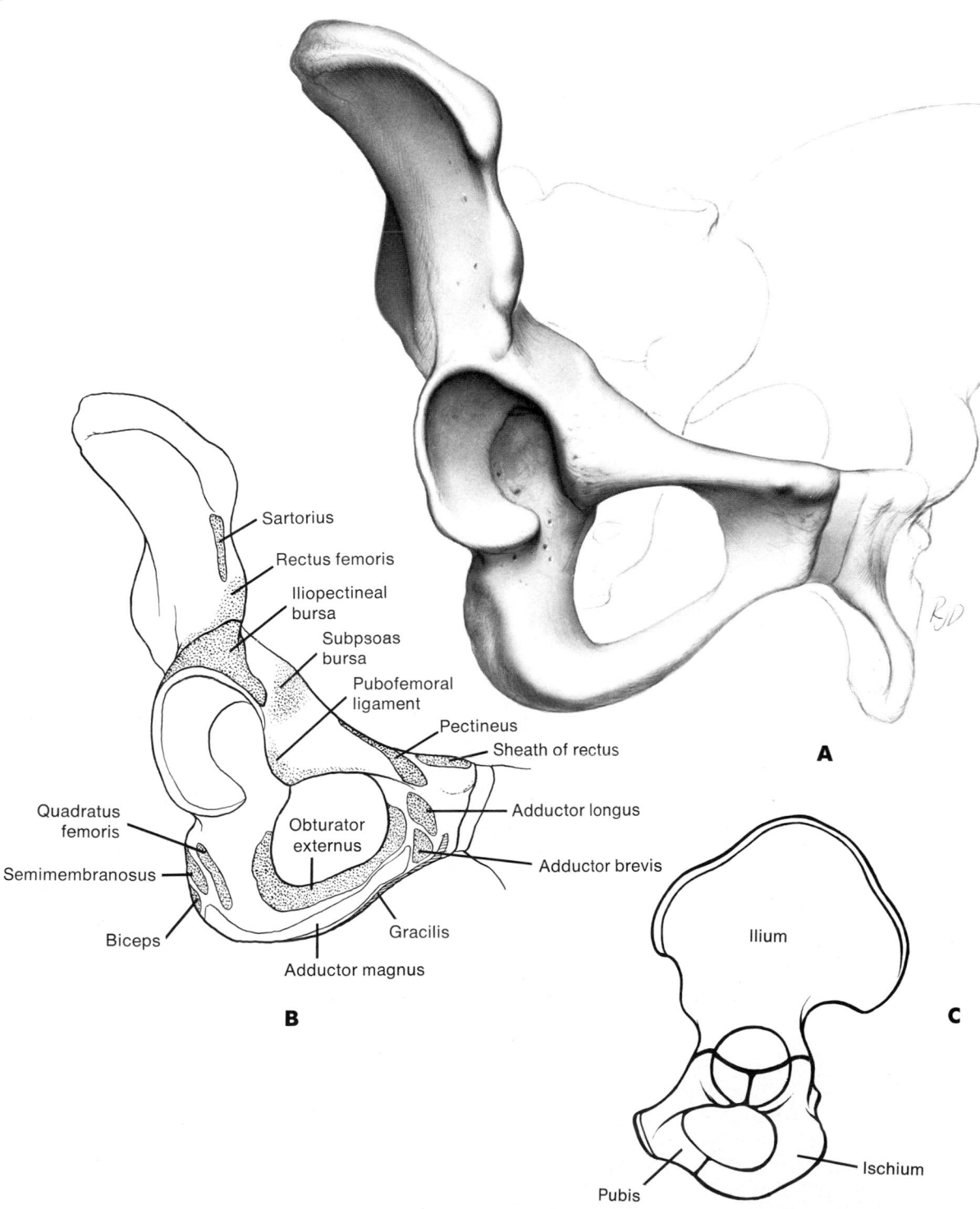

Fig. 2-2. A, Hemipelvis. NOTE: orientation of acetabulum, intracotyloid notch, and zone of acetabulum (acetabular fossa). **B,** Site of insertion *(dotted area)* and origin of muscular attachments about hip joint. **C,** Formation of hemipelvis.

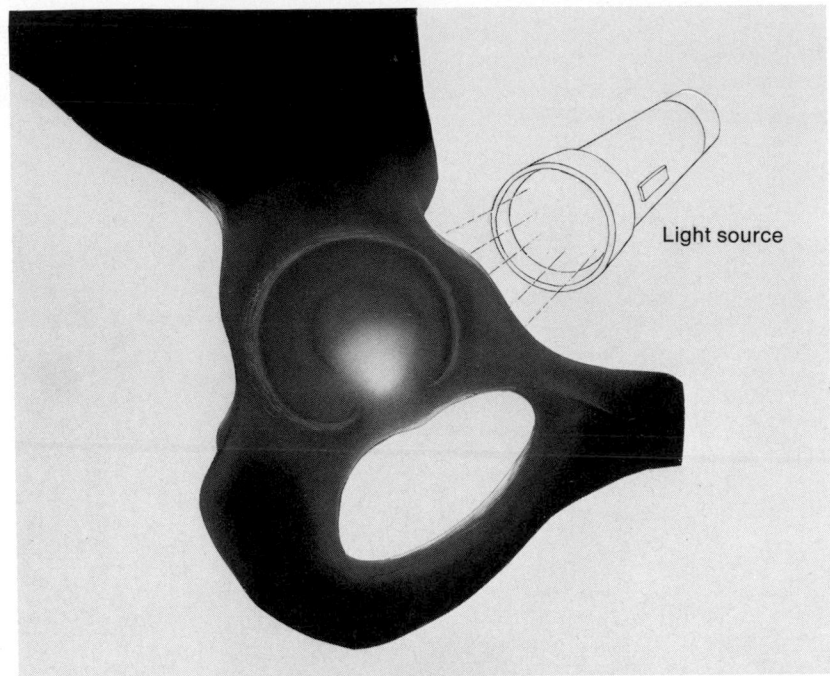

Fig. 2-3. Acetabular fossa may transilluminate on a dry, bony specimen.

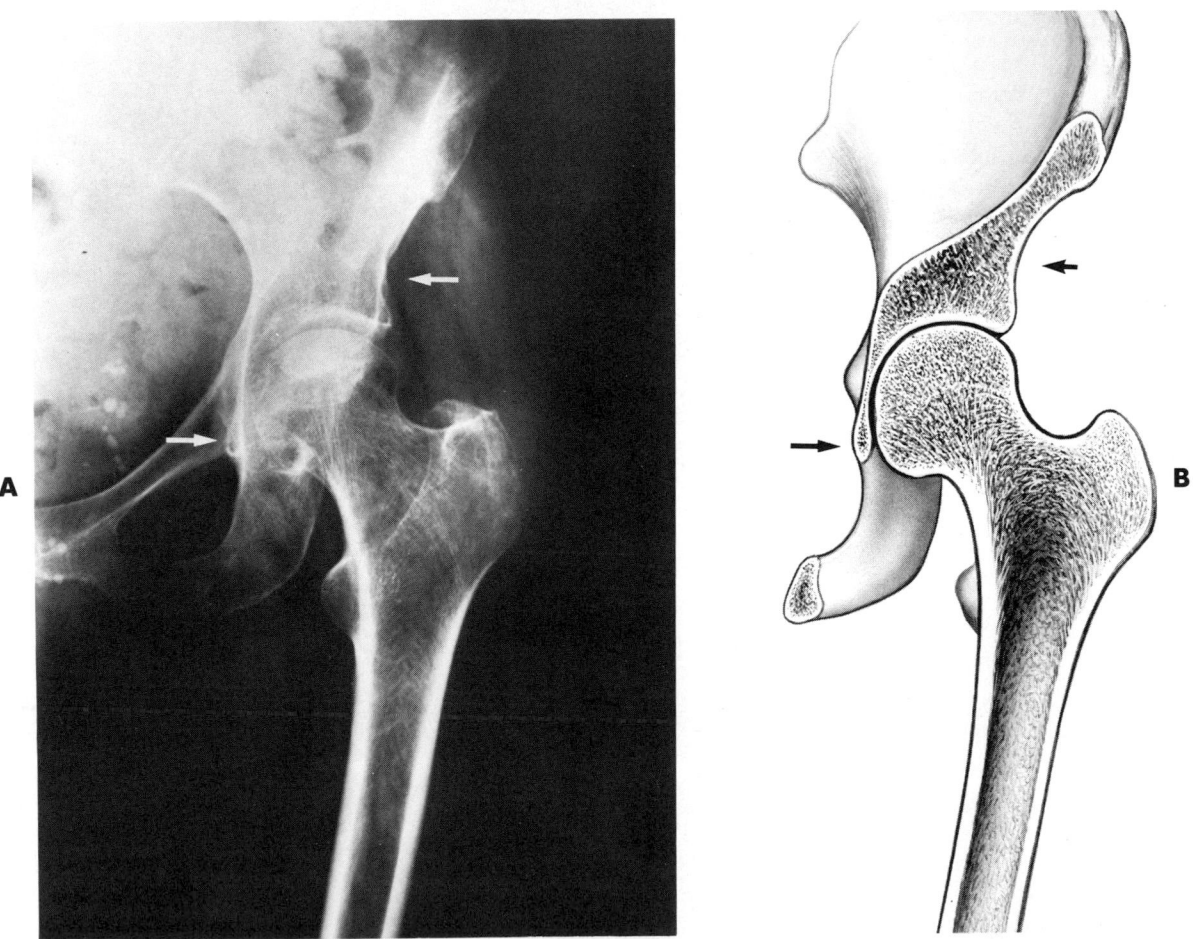

Fig. 2-4. Frontal view of hip joint. **A,** Anteroposterior representation of normal hip joint. Arrows indicate "teardrop" and cancellous zone of weight-bearing portion of acetabulum. **B,** Cross-sectional view of hip in frontal plane at site of "teardrop" illustrates "teardrop" representation and thinnest segment of acetabular floor. Top arrow also indicates superior weight-bearing cancellous zone of hip at level of acetabular roof.

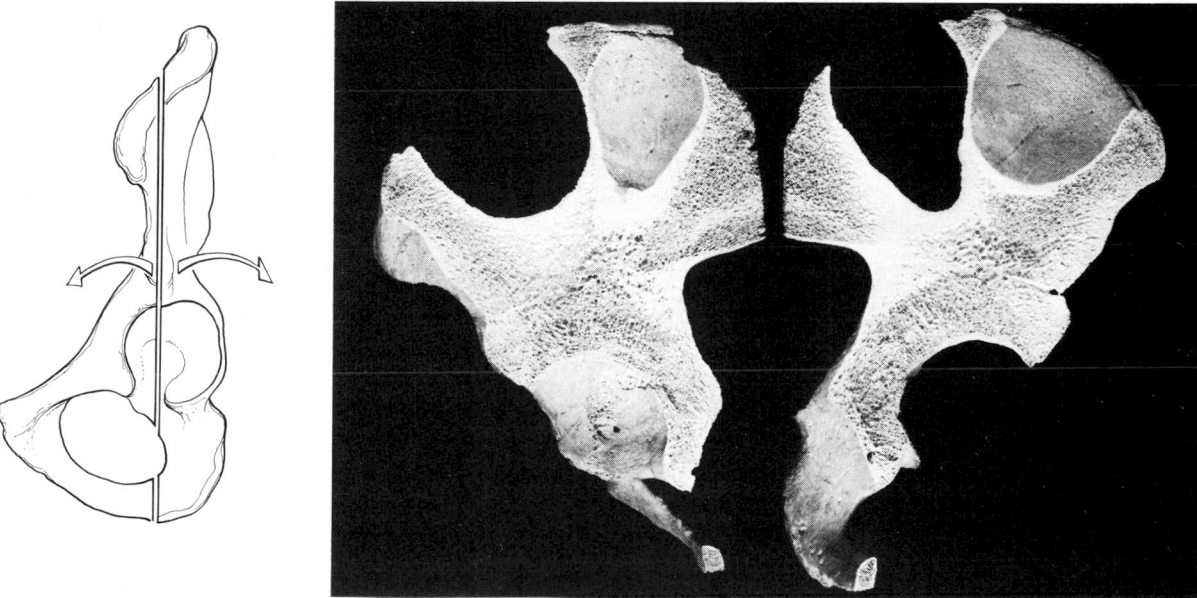

Fig. 2-5. Bony pelvis gives appearance of having been twisted on itself at site of acetabulum. Two planes cut each other nearly at right angles. Upper one roughly corresponds to ilium, and lower one corresponds to ischium and pubis. Photograph illustrates cancellous portions of ilium when pelvis is sectioned in plane of wing of ilium (*drawing*).

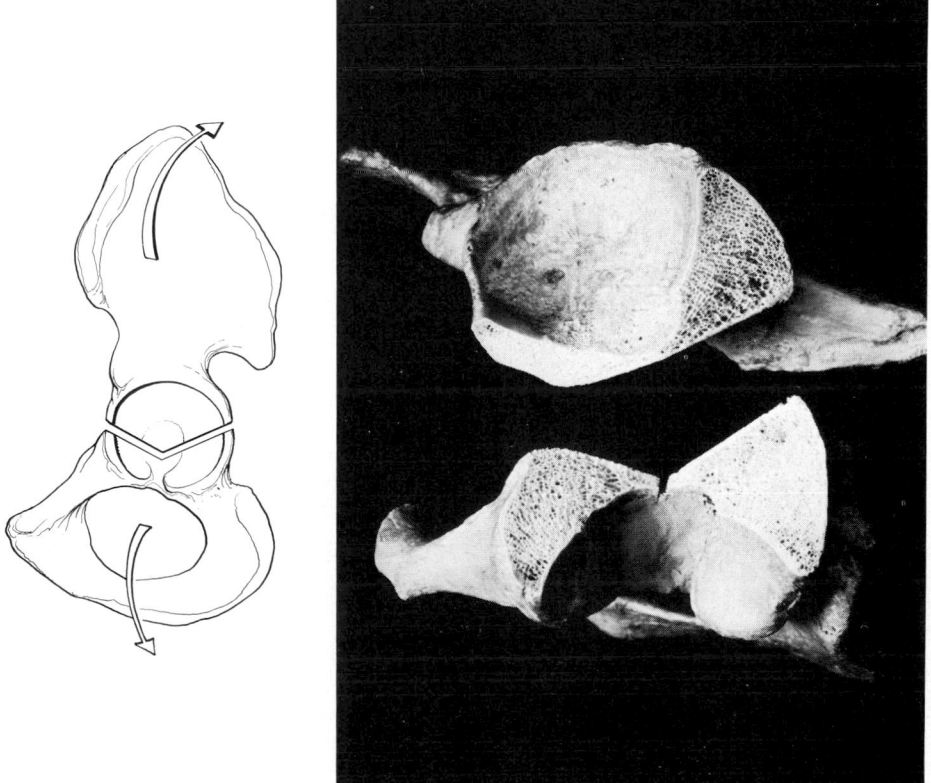

Fig. 2-6. Same as Fig. 2-5, but sectioned pelvis is perpendicular to axis of ischium, and pubis reveals segment of cancellous bone in regions of pubis and ischium. NOTE: posterior segment of ilium is also substantial and rich in cancellous bone. Drawing illustrates plane of sectioning of pelvis.

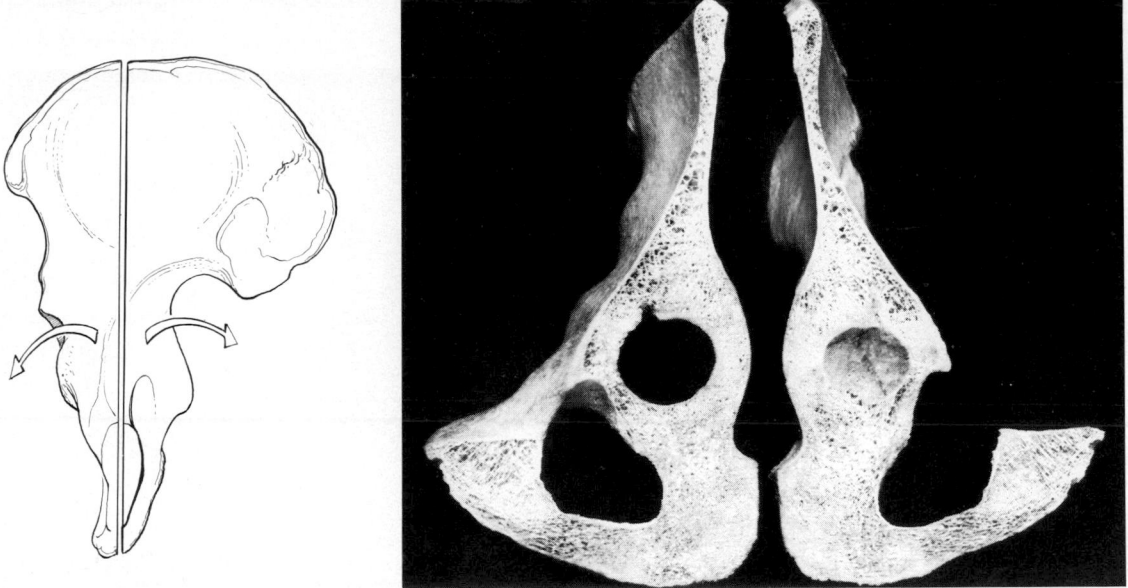

Fig. 2-7. Same as Figs. 2-5 and 2-6, but section of pelvis through ischium and pubis is perpendicular to plane of ilium. Photograph illustrates best available bone for fixation of total prosthesis, principally in region of ischium and ilium. Drawing illustrates plane of section of ilium used for photograph.

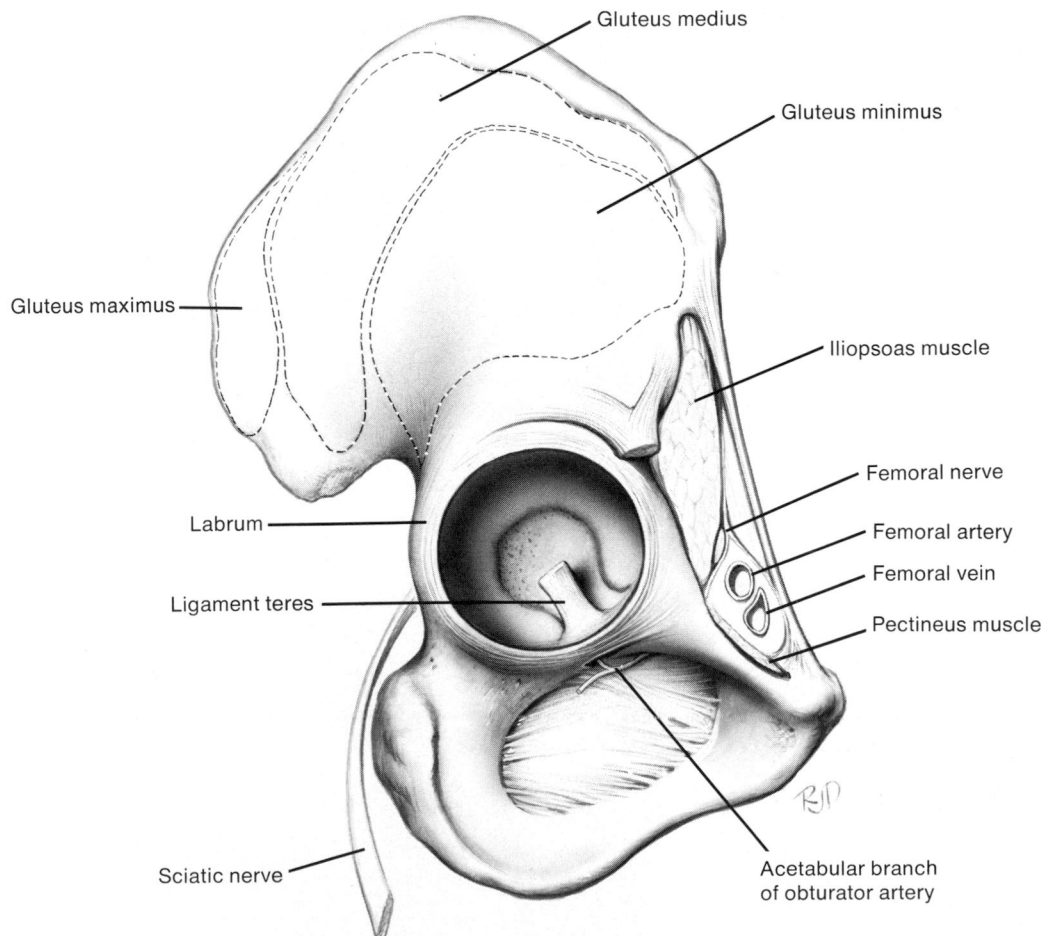

Fig. 2-8. Site of origin of gluteal muscles on ilium is indicated. Relationship of sciatic nerve to acetabulum, acetabular branch of obturator artery, femoral artery and vein, femoral nerve, and iliopsoas in relation to acetabulum should be noted. Acetabular floor is marked by horseshoe articulating zone and acetabular fossa. Ligamentum teres and its synovial folding are supplied by acetabular branch of obturator artery.

ischium and pubis. This is an important consideration in the orientation of the pelvis on the operating table; it also explains the lack of availability of bone in the iliac region despite the anteroposterior view of the radiographs of the pelvis that give a deceptive representation of a flat "iliac fan" as an excellent bony stalk in this region (see Figs. 2-5 to 2-7).

The ilium with its wide gluteal surface is completely covered by glutei. Only in a dissected bone specimen is it marked by anterior, posterior, and inferior gluteal lines (Fig. 2-8). The whole crest of the ilium extends between the anterosuperior and posterosuperior iliac spines. The "anterior gluteal line" marks the posterosuperior border of the margin of the gluteus minimus and the anteroinferior border of the origin of the gluteus medius. The posterior gluteal line separates the origin of the gluteus maximus from the medius. The inferior gluteal line is the inferior boundary of the origin of the gluteus minimus. The inner surface of the wing of the ilium is the iliac fossa; on its posterior portion is the articular surface for the sacrum. Below the anteroinferior spine is an ill-defined notch, the "iliopubic eminence," which marks the junction of ilium and pubis. This landmark is a guide for the insertion of a pointed retractor (Hohmann retractor) to visualize the anterior portion of the acetabulum at the junction of the ilium and the pubis (see Chapters 15 to 19). Below the posteroinferior spine is the deep greater sciatic notch, which the examiner can conveniently palpate through the inner wall of the pelvis by subperiosteal dissection or after exploration of the sciatic nerve in the buttock. For example, with injury to the sciatic nerve after fracture dislocation of the hip joint requiring decompression of the sciatic nerve, the examiner can reach the sciatic notch conveniently by palpating along the sciatic nerve to the point of its exit from the notch. Near the anterior border of the sciatic notch at the base of the wall of the acetabulum is another rounded thickness that marks the junction of the ilium and ischium.

Ischium

The ischium is the most massive contributing element of the posterior acetabular wall; it has facets on its posterolateral aspect for the origin of the hamstring muscles. Above this area is the lesser sciatic notch, which is separated from the greater sciatic notch by a projecting sharp spike known as the *ischial spine*. In front of the ischium lies the body of the pubis. The ischium and the pubis jointly form the obturator foramen, bounded below by the "ischiopubic ramus," and the inferior ramus of the pubis projecting backward from the pubic bone. It is essential to assess the orientation of the body of the ischium with the bone of the pubis so that anchoring holes for cement fixation

are created in the body of the ischium and not in the ilioischial junction or near the obturator foramen, a common error (see Chapters 15 and 18).

Pubis

This area is less developed in size than the ilium and the ischium. The pubic body articulates at the symphysis with the pubic bone of the other side. Its superior ramus runs above the obturator foramen to form part of the acetabular wall, and its inferior ramus curves inferiorly and posteriorly to fuse with the ischium. The examiner must appreciate the direction and size of the pubis on a dry bony specimen and compare this with its radiological magnification to ascertain its orientation, thus avoiding extensive expansion during preparation and removal of bone for anchorage at surgery (Figs. 2-2 and 2-8) (see Chapters 15 and 18). The pubis, which anteriorly forms the boundary of the obturator foramen and inferiorly the ischiopubic ramus, gives origin to the adductor muscles (Fig. 2-2). The upper end of the symphysis pubis at the angle with the crest gives attachment to the rectus abdominis and terminates laterally in the prominent point of the "pubic tubercle," to which the inguinal ligament is attached. Lateral to this the superior ramus extends to the "iliopubic eminence," where it joins the ilium. Its inferior border gives attachment to the "pubofemoral ligament" of the hip joint and overhangs the obturator foramen. From the pubic tubercle, the pectineal line runs along the superior ramus to the "iliopectineal eminence." The pubic tubercle gives origin to the reinforcing capsular ligament—the pubofemoral ligament of the hip joint.

Inner Wall

From the inner side of the pelvis, three contributing areas are recognizable.[5]

1. In the back and upper portion of each coxa, an articular surface shaped like an ear is termed the *auricular surface;* above and behind each auricular surface is a rough tuberosity for the strong interosseous sacroiliac ligament. Behind this area is the expanded posterior part of the crest for the erector spinae muscle. This area is of no interest to us in replacement surgery unless it has been invaded through previous surgery or disease.
2. The second area, however, is of greater concern: the ventral surface of the ilium, which is slightly concave and forms the bony iliac fossa, gives origin to and is covered by the iliacus muscle. Because the ventral surface of the ilium is completely covered by the iliacus muscle, all neurovascular structures are well cushioned within the pelvis. Yet this surface is thin and may be easily penetrated during an attempt to struc-

ture an acetabulum at that level, for example, at the site of a pseudoacetabulum of a congenital dislocation of the hip (Figs. 2-9 and 2-10).

3. The third part, the lower portion, comprises the obturator foramen, which is covered by the obturator internus, which also arises from the periphery of this segment. Entry to the obturator foramen from the outside by deep dissection often leads to damage of the obturator vessels and bleeding, which may be a nuisance to control. Flow of excess cement in this region may cause obturator nerve palsy. The main trunk of the obturator nerve is closely applied to the iliopubic segment of the pelvis before entry to the thigh by the obturator foramen (see Chapter 33).

ACETABULUM

Because of the importance of the acetabulum, knowledge of some details of this territory is essential. Over two fifths of the acetabulum is contributed by the ischium, less than two fifths by the ilium, and only one fifth by the pubis (Figs. 2-5 to 2-7). The so-called *triradiate cartilage*, which is responsible for the formation of the acetabulum (Fig. 2-2, *C*), develops from a variable number of small ossifying centers joined at the floor of the acetabulum and known as *os acetabuli*.[34]

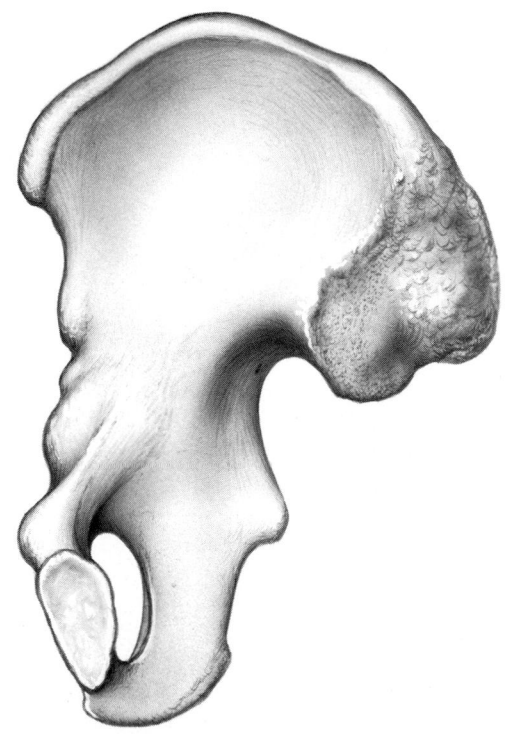

Fig. 2-9. Middle zone of inner wall of pelvis is of greatest concern because it comprises floor of acetabulum and is thinnest segment of pelvis. It is mainly covered by iliacus muscle.

Based on postmortem studies of 10 normal full-term infants and 3 children (age 3 to 9 years), Ponseti[25] concluded that the concavity of the acetabulum is a response to the presence of the spherical femoral head. The increase in depth of the acetabulum during the developmental years results from the interstitial growth of the acetabular cartilage, the oppositional growth at the periphery of this cartilage, and the periosteal new bone formation at the acetabular margin.[25] The acetabular cartilage itself is triradiate medially and cup shaped laterally. This cartilage is located between the three centers of ossifications—the ilium, ischium, and pubis—that form the acetabulum. The expansion of the acetabulum during growth periods is also due to interstitial growth of the triradiate cartilage.

Ultimately, these centers fuse to make a unified floor. The nonarticulating surface, known as the *acetabular fossa* or the *pulvinar*, contains some fibrofatty tissue (haversian fat pad) and opens below toward the obturator foramen at the acetabular notch (see Fig. 2-8). The surgeon can best expose this area by traction on the stump of the ligamentum teres and curettage at its base; more conveniently, the surgeon can excise it with an electric knife to minimize bleeding. The acetabular fossa indicates the innermost and thinnest (transilluminating) zone of the floor. The surgeon should beware of the danger of further deepening toward the midline in this area. The notch is bridged by the "transverse ligament," a tendinous structure continuous with the fibrocartilaginous acetabular labrum, which in turn is attached to the whole periphery of the mouth of the acetabulum (see Fig. 2-8). The surgeon can excise the transverse ligament, but an incision at a line perpendicular to its fibers allows adequate entry to the bottom of the notch, where maximum exposure is necessary. Incision may be anterior or posterior but should be close to the bone. Vascular structures pass through the notch under the transverse ligament to enter the ligamentum teres into the femoral head (see Fig. 2-8).

On careful examination of the "articular lunate" surface of the acetabulum, one sees that the pubic articulating surface is distinct from the surface of the iliac segment, which also bears a small notch on the rim (see Fig. 2-2). This is a common site for the iliopectineal bursa to communicate with the hip joint. The distinction is helpful to appreciate the dividing zones of the acetabulum contributed by the ilium and pubis. The examiner can best visualize the state of the acetabular cartilage of the iliac segment by inserting pin retractors to retract the superior capsule of the joint (see Chapters 18 and 19). The fibrocartilaginous acetabular labrum is attached to the bony rim within the capsule of the joint, adding to the depth of the

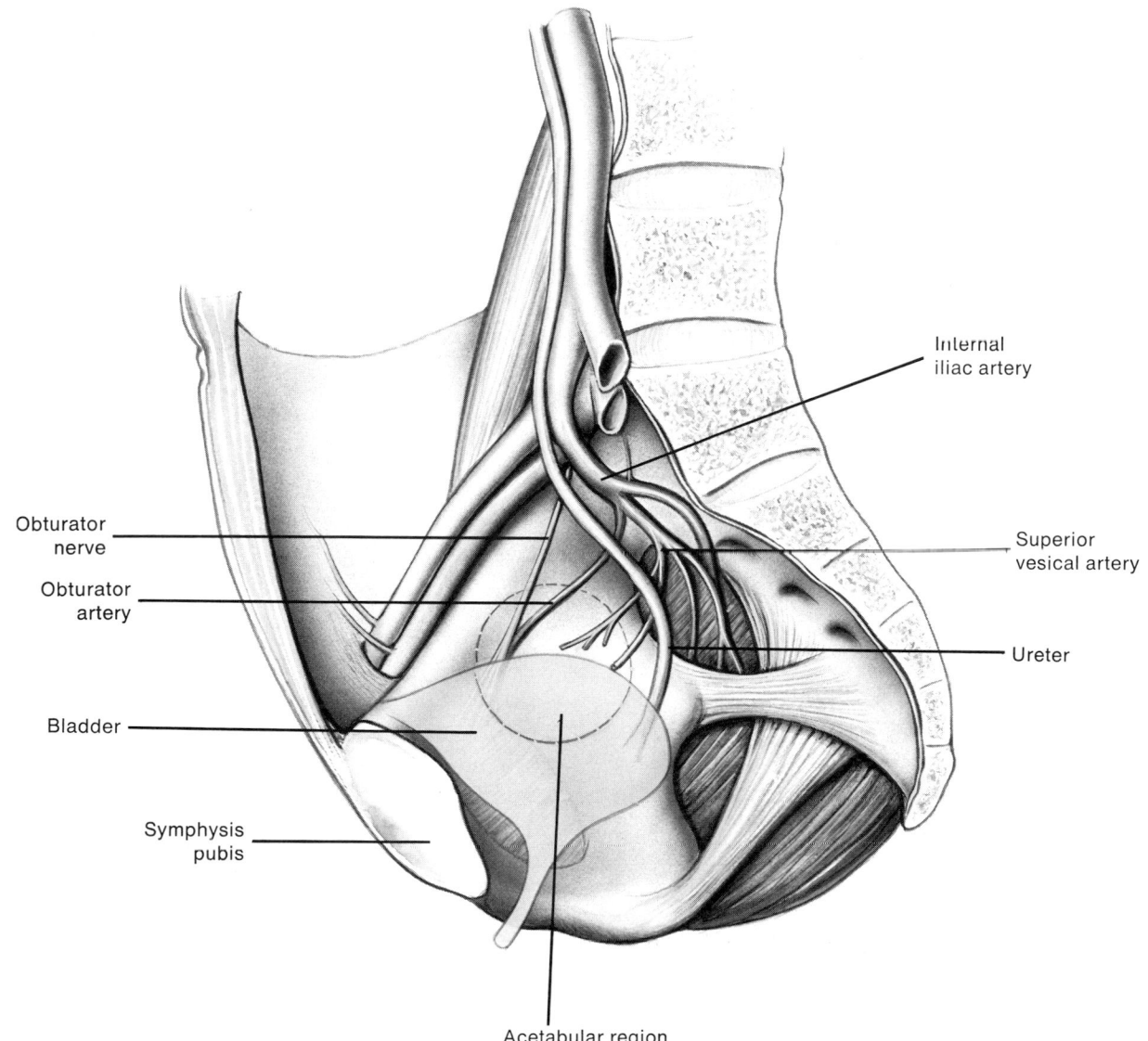

Obturator
nerve

Obturator
artery

Bladder

Symphysis
pubis

Internal
iliac artery

Superior
vesical artery

Ureter

Acetabular region

Fig. 2-10. Bony and ligamentous walls of pelvis minor are shown. Corresponding zone of acetabular floor is traced (*circle*) in background. Position of ureter and bladder in relation to acetabular floor is identified. Obturator nerve and artery and vein traversing behind iliopubic segment and small branches of superior vesical artery are shown. It is a fortunate anatomical coincidence that no major vital structure is present immediately adjacent to bone of inner wall of acetabulum (*circled*). Note position of common iliac artery and vein in relation to lesser bony pelvis.

cavity. At times it is quite hypertrophic and might be taken for the true bony periphery, leading to inadequate deepening. Its routine excision is necessary to provide visualization of the rim. Exposure of the bony rim is perhaps the most important step in preparing the acetabulum and appreciating the relationship of the bony masses and their articulating surfaces. When the surgeon inserts the prosthetic cup, a crescent forms between the cup and the acetabulum, which the surgeon should pack with cement only after a full visualization.

Periacetabular Architecture and Subchondral Bone

The Law of Bone Remodeling describes the relationship between load and bone response.[13,17,35] As with other parts of the skeleton, quantitative correlations exist between the pressure distribution and strength of trabeculae in the pelvis and acetabulum. Periacetabular bony architecture shows that the subchondral bone of the acetabulum is thicker than any of the trabecular bone in the body, suggesting its significance in structural weight bearing. I emphasize the importance of subchondral bone of the acetabulum during total hip arthroplasty (see Chapters 6 and 19). Brand et al[3] have noted two general systems of periacetabular trabecula, one (the more prominent of the two) radial to the center of the acetabulum and the other (less prominent) in somewhat concentric spheres about the acetabulum. Invasion of these structures by overreaming may cause migration of the acetabular component because of a resultant lack of bone support.

In protrusio acetabuli the medial wall is often expanded and thin toward the midline. The very thin cortical bone requires careful preservation at surgery. When a membranous defect is present, the surgeon can reinforce it by bone, graft, or wire mesh (see Chapters 14, 22, and 25). In protrusion the acetabulum is barrel shaped with a narrow opening, as if the acetabulum has been blown out like a balloon.

As the result of disease, such as protrusio acetabuli or rheumatoid disease, the acetabulum may be markedly distorted, with an altered relationship to the osseous and soft tissue of the pelvis. For example, in protrusio acetabuli, the floor of the acetabulum is extremely thin and occasionally membranous, expanded toward the midline; the entrance of the cavity is narrowed like a barrel top, requiring expansion at the rim.

On the other hand, because of extensive inferior marginal osteophyte formation (overgrown), the nonarticular portion of the acetabulum may be completely covered and thus invisible after hip dislocation. Generally, the teardrop sign on x-ray film is markedly widened, and at times thick cortical bone lateral to it indicates a "false floor." Only removal of this new bone reveals the actual pulvinar and its contents (see Chapter 15).

FEMUR

The femur is the longest bone of the skeleton and articulates with the hip bone above and the tibia below; it carries the patella in front of it. The femur consists

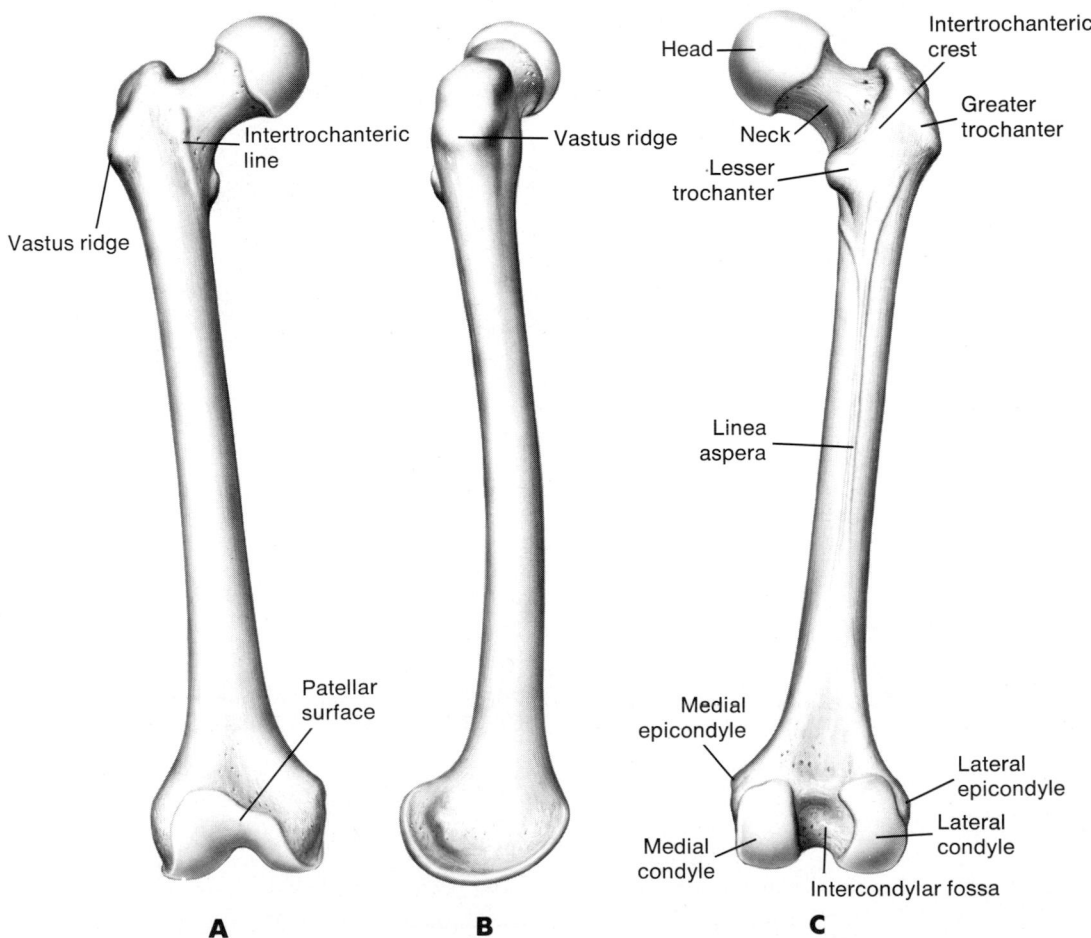

Fig. 2-11. A, Anterior view; **B,** lateral view; and **C,** posterior view. Upper femur consists of head, neck, and trochanters. Prominent greater trochanter at base *(vastus ridge),* lesser trochanter, and bony landmarks are helpful in orientation of osteotomy of greater trochanter as well as orientation of femoral component of prosthesis.

of a shaft that is directed downward medially and slightly forward (Fig. 2-11). The surgeon should fully understand its general curvatures, the details of its ends, and the complex angles of the upper femur in normal as well as pathological states. The shaft of the femur twists on itself (femoral torsion or anteversion). The patella in front of the femur provides an important landmark, a reference point when the limb is positioned for orientation of the reamers during preparation, as well as for insertion of the prosthesis. Therefore the surgeon should ensure the patella is not excessively hidden in the free leg drape.

The upper end of the femur consists of the head, neck, and the trochanters (Fig. 2-12).

Head and Neck

The head has a separate epiphysis; the epiphyseal line practically, but not absolutely, corresponds with the edge of the articular surface.[5] A prolongation of the cartilage covering the surface of the front of the neck, which extends onto the bony ridge, frequently runs along the upper front part of the neck. This ridge is called the *eminence* of the neck. The articular extension underlies the iliopsoas tendon if there is a large bursa opening; otherwise it seems to support the inner part of the iliofemoral ligament. The head of the femur, larger in the male than in the female, forms two thirds of a sphere. (The sphericity of the head has been debated in the past.) The size and shape of the femoral head determine the size and shape of the acetabulum. Thus a small head removed at surgery suggests a small acetabulum, a misshapen head (that is, flattened) denotes a misshapen acetabulum, and so on. The position and size of the fovea vary; one or two small foramina, which represent the entry site of a branch of the obturator artery (the ligamentum teres artery) and the vein, sometimes occur. These are often absent in an arthritic hip. The synovial funnel that surrounds these vessels is attached in the depressed margin of the fovea and terminates at the margin of cartilage covering the head. Numerous vascular foramina originate from the synovial membrane, which covers the entire anterior surface of this bone extending toward the head.

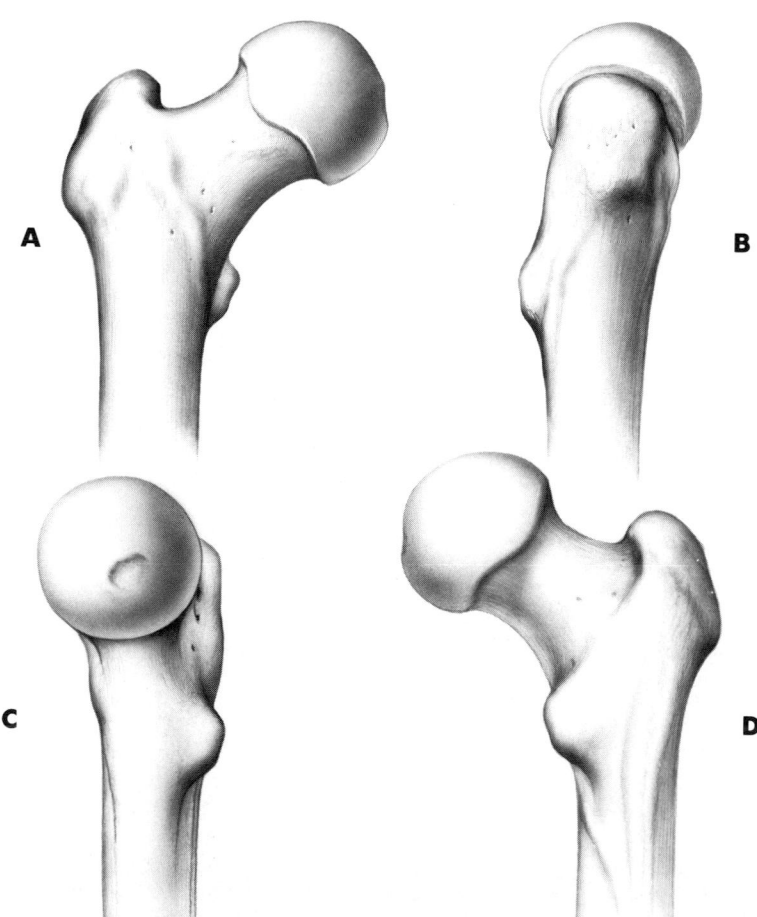

Fig. 2-12. A, Upper femur in frontal view; **B,** lateral view; **C,** lateral view with head in front; **D,** posterior view.

These typical anatomical characteristics are not present in an arthritic hip, in which the head and neck junction is often distorted by osteophytes; therefore the site for amputation at the femoral neck and the opening of the neck may not be clearly identifiable. The posterior aspect of the neck is usually smooth, and the line of reflection of the synovium is about halfway up the neck, continued up from the turned-up lower end of the intertrochanteric line. The obturator externus, obturator internus, and gemelli are closely applied to the upper neck of the femur and the quadratus femoris, posteriorly and inferiorly. The surgeon should appreciate the close relationship of these muscles when mobilization of the upper femur is necessary, requiring disinsertion of these muscles from the upper femur by maximum internal rotation of the limb, thereby facilitating their detachment (Figs. 2-12 and 2-13). The surgeon must consider the neck shaft angle in both the anteroposterior and lateral planes before and during surgery (Figs. 2-11 and 2-14). An excessively anteverted neck in a congenital dislocation of the hip or a displaced osteotomy at the neck shaft angle calls for special preparation of the upper femur. In a variety of conditions the neck length may be shortened and might require a careful evaluation before osteotomy to prevent further shortening. The examiner must carefully evaluate displaced osteotomies or malunion of neck fractures in particular, not only in relation to varus/valgus angles but to rotational deformity (see Chapters 20 and 24).

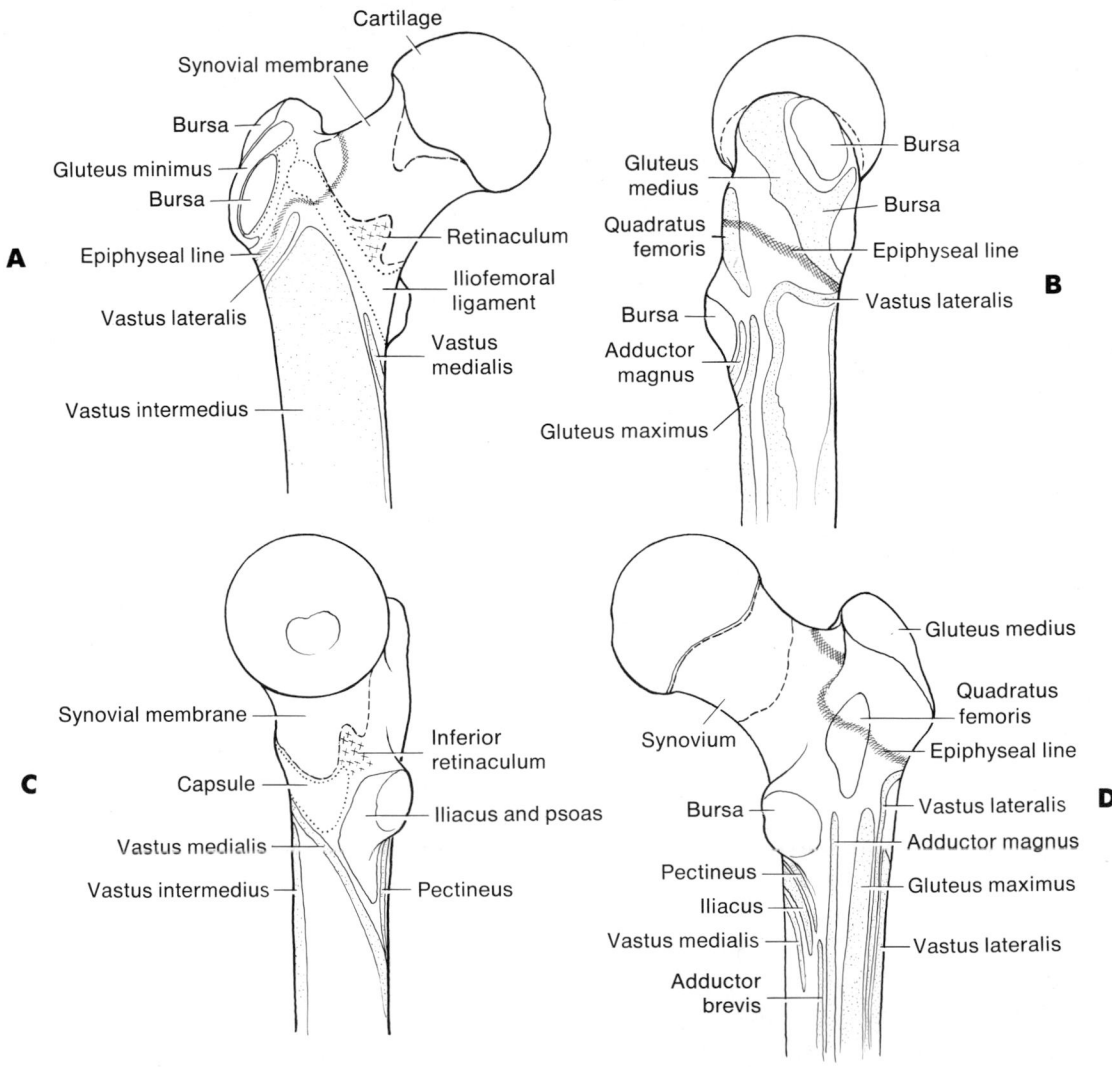

Fig. 2-13. Corresponding to bony landmarks in Fig. 2-12, site of major muscular attachment, capsular attachment, synovial folding attachments, and major ligaments and bursa are illustrated. **A,** Frontal view; **B,** lateral view; **C,** lateral view from front; and **D,** posterior view. (Outline of synovial capsular muscular and ligamentous structure was adopted from Breathnach AS, editor: *Frazer's anatomy of the human skeleton,* ed 6, Boston, 1965, Little, Brown.)

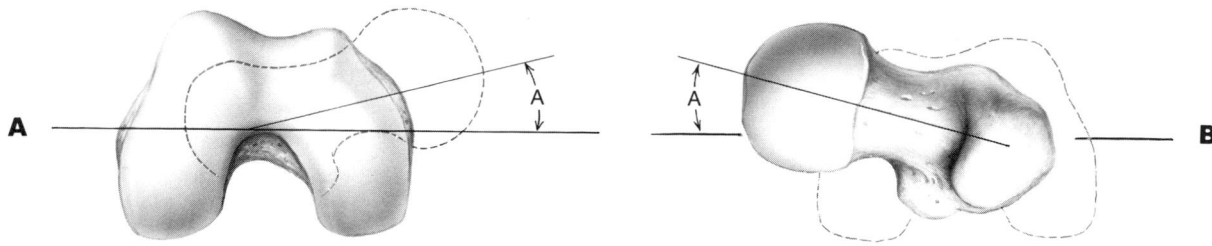

Fig. 2-14. Neck shaft angle both in anteroposterior and lateral planes must be considered before and during surgery. Excessively anteverted neck is common. **A,** Represents anteversion as femur is viewed from femoral condyles. **B,** Illustrates anteversion as femur is viewed from top of neck of femur.

Greater Trochanter

The term *greater trochanter* applies to the mass of bone that stands up at the base of the neck and gives attachment to the gluteal muscles. In situations like coxa vara or "sunken prosthesis" (for example, Moore self-locking prosthesis), the trochanter appears substantial in size since it "stays proud" (projected) in reference to the remainder of the shaft. It normally consists of the whole body at the base of the neck including the femoral tubercle at the top of the intertrochanteric line, the so-called upper aspect of the neck. The gluteus minimus bursa occupies the anterior smooth surface, and the piriformis inserts along the whole length of the upper crest of the trochanter, while the obturator internus and gemelli are inserted medial to and in front of it on the slope of the trochanter. On the lateral surface of the trochanter a well-marked oblique ridge exists for the insertion of the gluteus medius, which occupies the whole breadth of the ridge. Above the oblique ridge, the trochanter is completely covered by the gluteus medius insertion and its intervening bursa. The widened base of the neck is marked anteriorly by a roughened ridge of bone known as the *intertrochanteric line* and posteriorly by the "intertrochanteric crest," the prominent ridge between the two trochanters (see Figs. 2-11 and 2-12). An understanding of the complex shape of the trochanter is important at the time of its removal and reattachment in total hip surgery.

On the lateral surface and at the base of the trochanter is the "vastus lateralis ridge." The examiner can best palpate this landmark at the base of the greater trochanter by placing a finger or thumb against the shaft of the femur over the vastus lateralis and moving upward to appreciate its projection while the vastus lateralis is still undetached from the shaft of the femur. The vastus ridge may be partially covered by a trochanteric bursa and the surgeon often best recognizes it after its removal. The ridge identifies the level of removal of the trochanter; it is also an eminence that is useful for interlocking the trochanter at the reattachment stage. The trochanter proximal to the ridge

is the site of the tendinous insertion of the gluteus medius (see Fig. 2-13). The intertrochanteric line marks the attachment site of the iliofemoral ligament. The strong lateral limb of the ligament goes to the tubercle at the upper end of the line (Fig. 2-15). The

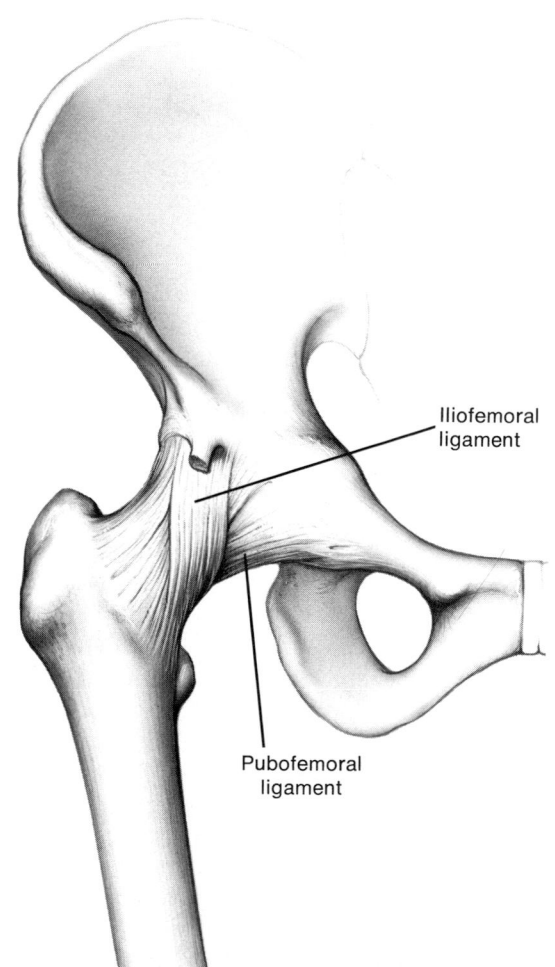

Fig. 2-15. Intertrochanter line marks attachment site of iliofemoral ligament. Strong lateral limb of ligament goes to tubercle at upper end of line, medial band proceeds to lower end of line. Capsular reinforcing ligaments provide anterior stability for hip joint.

medial band proceeds to the lower end of this line with its intermediate band, which goes to the thinner portion of the line in between.[5] The interval between this line and the lesser trochanter offers insertion to the muscular fibers of the iliacus. The examiner can best identify the inner wall of the greater trochanter above the neck after an opening in the capsule. The surgeon should note recession of the digital fossa toward the posterolateral aspect and the posterior ridge of the trochanter. The posterior crest extends medially as far as the lesser trochanter. This asymmetry and the direction of the fossa hamper passing of the clamp from the front to recover the sawband when its direction is not observed. If the limb is fixed in external rotation owing to arthritis, the tip of the clamp naturally enters the fossa, piercing the capsule posteriorly but superficial to the trochanteric crest.

Lesser Trochanter

The lesser trochanter presents two surfaces: a posterior smooth surface related to a bursa at the upper border of the adductor magnus and a rough medial area giving insertion to the psoas major. This insertion continues down on the shaft to just below the trochanter and above the ridge of the linea aspera femoris, which continues the intertrochanteric line over the medial aspect of the bone to its posterior surface. The surgeon can detach the tendon's muscular insertions from the lesser trochanter to free the upper femur. To ensure a safe surgical dissection the surgeon should perform the disinsertion next to the bone of the lesser trochanter, from the front, with the extremity in external rotation.

As stated, the posterior surface is completely free of tendinous insertions and muscle attachments, but it is covered by a well-formed bursa separating it from the adductor magnus. At the site of the lesser trochanter deep within the shaft, the femur is strengthened by a bony bar or column visible at sections extending into the neck and known as the *calcar femorale*.[12] The relationship of the calcar femorale and the lesser trochanter is apparent at surgery after removal of the greater trochanter when the leg is maximally adducted. The lesser trochanter forms an additional landmark to the transcondylar line of the knee joint, which the surgeon should observe in the preparation of the femoral canal. It is particularly important in cases of excessive anteversion of the femoral neck. The surgeon may remove the psoas tendon and the iliacus muscle from the lesser trochanter to mobilize the upper femur in difficult pathological situations. However, beyond this level no other soft tissue structure keeps the femur attached to the pelvis, and careless hyperadduction can cause severe damage to the soft tissue of the medial thigh. The lesser trochanter is an excellent point of

reference on x-ray films of the hip, indicating the degree of hip rotation at the time radiographs were obtained. A prominent lesser trochanter indicates an externally rotated hip joint, whereas the greater trochanter appears less prominent than usual because the rotation causes its apparent "overlapping" by the femur head.

The examiner cannot determine the true diameter of the femoral width required at total hip arthroplasty without obtaining radiographs with known magnification and rotation. As little as 20 degrees of femoral rotation, for example, can cause definite and apparent changes in varus/valgus angulation if the stem is not perfectly centered in the canal. Likewise, a relatively small amount of rotation, that is, 15 degrees, can cause significant changes in proximal femoral dimensions on anteroposterior x-ray films of the hip.

Variations in Shape and Size

For the surgeon concerned with the replacement of the upper femur, two characteristics of the femur are of particular practical interest: (1) external geometry and size, and (2) internal geometry and size. The external geometry, such as neck shaft angle, angle of anteversion, and the offset, provides the basic information governing prosthesis choice. For example, the selected neck length and prosthetic offset (in addition to the position of the center of rotation of the hip) influence the abductor-moment-arm/body-moment-arm ratio and thus the function of the hip and leg length (see Chapter 6) (Fig. 2-16).

On the other hand, the shape and size of the natural architecture of the femur determine the shape and size of the prosthesis. In addition to considering the size of the prosthesis, the surgeon considers its general configuration, such as "tapered angle," metaphysis/diaphysis ratio, length of the stem and valgus, and neck length. In this context, flexibility in selecting the prosthesis becomes extremely limited if no cement is used for fixation and the surgeon relies on the use of a prefabricated prosthesis for the best fit. The following discussion of the variation in geometry and size of the femur emphasizes the difficulties the surgeon may face in replacing the upper femur because of its complex geometry and size variation (Fig. 2-17).

The geometrical shape and size of the upper femur as an anatomical entity (similar to other anatomical features of the human skeleton) are influenced by genetic and environmental factors. Noble examined 200 femoral anatomical specimens of donors (age 22 to 95, with average age of 69.9 years) by two plane radiographs of known magnification (1.5%) (Fig. 2-18) and recorded the average dimensional values (Tables 2-1 to 2-4). Scattered plots of the femoral data showed a great variability in every instance, although a normal

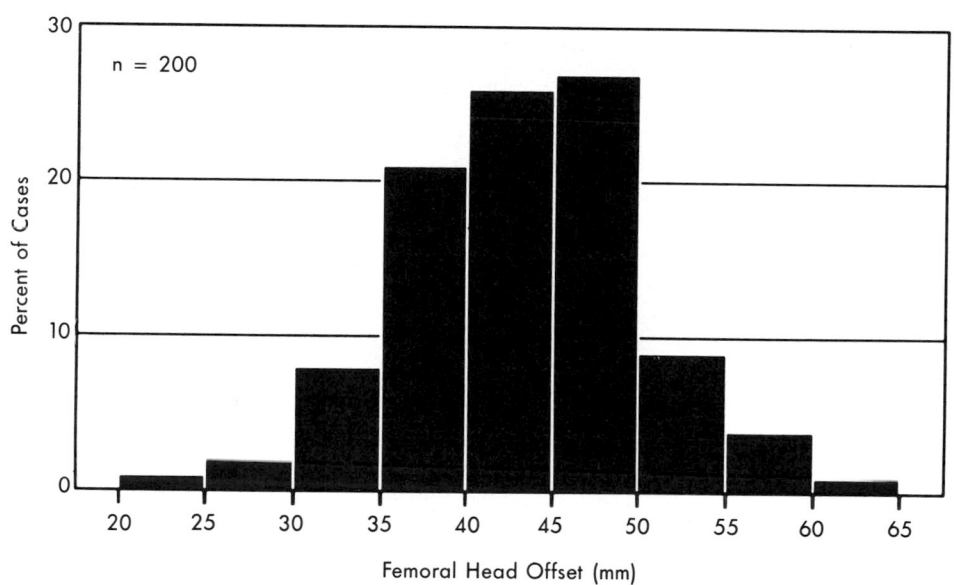

Fig. 2-16. Distribution of values of the femoral head offset (dimension A in Fig. 2-18; n = 200).

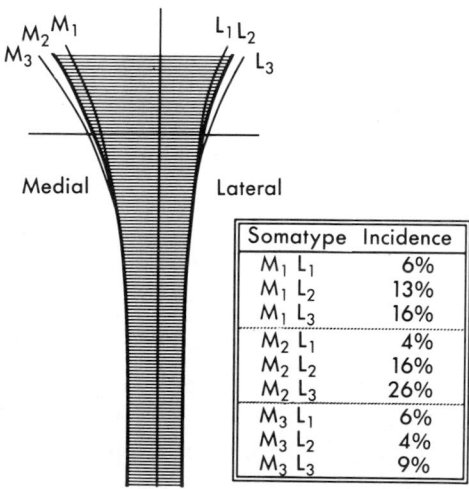

Somatype	Incidence
$M_1 L_1$	6%
$M_1 L_2$	13%
$M_1 L_3$	16%
$M_2 L_1$	4%
$M_2 L_2$	16%
$M_2 L_3$	26%
$M_3 L_1$	6%
$M_3 L_2$	4%
$M_3 L_3$	9%

Fig. 2-17. Diagrammatic representation of one method of derivation of canal somatotypes. Bones of a given distal canal diameter are classified according to their medial and lateral endosteal profiles. The incidence of each combination of medial and lateral contours is a direct indication of the most common shapes of canals occurring in bones of each distal size.

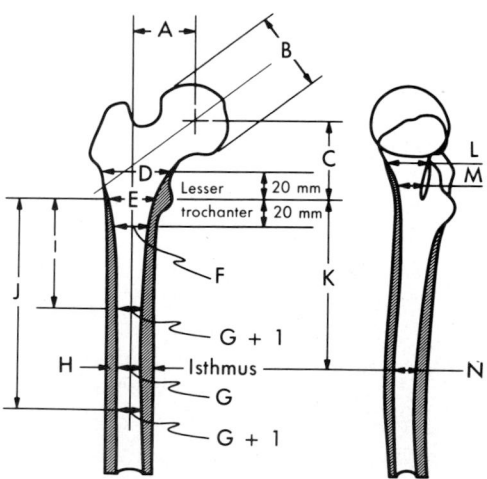

Fig. 2-18. Diagrammatic representation of the standard dimensions of the femur in the anteroposterior and lateral views. See Table 2-1 for a legend describing each lettered dimension. (From Noble PC, Alexander JW, Lindahl LJ, et al: *Clin Orthop* 235:148, 1988.)

Table 2-1 Variables Characterizing the Femoral Specimens

Dimension	Number	Average	Standard deviation	Minimum	Maximum
Femoral head offset	200	43.0 mm	6.8 mm	23.6 mm	61.0 mm
Femoral head diameter	200	46.1 mm	4.8 mm	35.0 mm	58.0 mm
Femoral head position	200	51.6 mm	7.1 mm	32.8 mm	74.3 mm
Canal width (lesser trochanter +20 mm)	200	45.4 mm	5.3 mm	31.0 mm	60.0 mm
Canal width (lesser trochanter)	200	29.4 mm	4.6 mm	17.0 mm	41.9 mm
Canal width (lesser trochanter −20 mm)	200	20.9 mm	3.5 mm	11.0 mm	29.5 mm
Isthmus width (mediolateral)	200	12.3 mm	2.3 mm	8.0 mm	18.5 mm
Extracortical width (mediolateral)	200	27.0 mm	3.1 mm	20.5 mm	36.0 mm
Proximal border of isthmus	200	86.1 mm	17.8 mm	37.0 mm	199.0 mm
Distal border of isthmus	200	145.0 mm	19.4 mm	92.0 mm	205.0 mm
Isthmus position	200	113.4 mm	16.4 mm	63.0 mm	157.0 mm
AP canal width (osteotomy level)	99	24.1 mm	3.1 mm	15.5 mm	31.0 mm
Medical diameter of femoral neck	99	16.5 mm	2.9 mm	10.0 mm	22.5 mm
Isthmus width (AP)	196	16.9 mm	3.5 mm	10.0 mm	27.0 mm
Neck-shaft angle	200	124.7°	7.4°	105./7°	154.5°
Femoral length	132	436.8 mm	35.3 mm	353.0 mm	523.0 mm
Effective neck length	200	35.5 mm	2.6 mm	30.0 mm	41.1 mm
Age (years)	100	79.9	13.0	22.0	95.0

From Noble PC, Alexander JW, Lindall LJ, et al: *Clin Orthop* 235:165, 1988.

Table 2-2 Typical Values of Correlation Coefficients for Pairwise Correlation of Femoral Dimensions

Variables	Correlation coefficient (r)	Statistical significance (p)
(A) Periosteal/Periosteal		
Femoral length *vs.* head diameter	0.76	$p < 0.0001$
Femoral head diameter *vs.* extracortical	0.70	$p < 0.0001$
Femoral length *vs.* femoral neck length	0.70	$p < 0.0001$
Femoral length *vs.* femoral head position (C)	0.52	$p < 0.0001$
Femoral head diameter *vs.* neck-shaft angle	−0.04	$p > 0.05$
(B) Endosteal/Endosteal		
Canal width (LT −20, F) *vs.* isthmus diameter	0.66	$p < 0.0001$
Canal width (LT −20, F) *vs.* canal width (LT +20, D)	0.65	$p < 0.0001$
Canal width (LT +20, D) *vs.* isthmus diameter	0.31	$p < 0.0001$
Isthmus depth (K) *vs.* femoral head position	0.15	$p < 0.05$
(C) Periosteal/Endosteal		
Canal width (LT −20, F) *vs.* femoral head diameter	0.59	$p < 0.0001$
Isthmus diameter *vs.* extracortical width (H)	0.49	$p < 0.0001$
Isthmus depth (K) *vs.* head offset	0.22	$p < 0.005$
Canal width (LT −20, F)	−0.02	$p > 0.05$

From Noble PC, Alexander JW, Lindahl LJ, et al: *Clin Orthop* 235:148, 1988.

Table 2-3 Accuracy of Prediction of Femoral Dimensions

Dimension	Accuracy of prediction (95%) confidence)	Percent of average value
Head offset	± 12.4 mm	± 29%
Femoral head diameter	± 7.6 mm	± 17%
Femoral head position	± 13.1 mm	± 25%
Canal width (LT +20)	± 8.0 mm	± 17%
Canal width (LT)	± 4.4 mm	± 15%
Canal width (LT −20)	± 2.5 mm	± 12%
Isthmus width (mediolateral)	± 3.3 mm	± 27%
Extracortical width	± 5.1 mm	± 19%
Isthmus position	± 30.0 mm	± 27%
AP canal width (osteotomy)	± 5.3 mm	± 22%
Femoral neck diameter	± 5.4 mm	± 33%
Isthmus width (AP)	± 5.6 mm	± 33%

All estimates are based upon femora with canals of average width at a point 20 mm below the lesser trochanter.
From Noble PC, Alexander JW, Lindahl LJ, et al: *Clin Orthop* 235:148, 1988.

Table 2-4 Some Typical Proportionality Indices for Periosteal and Endosteal Dimensions of the Femur

Dimension	Proportionality index
Periosteal	
Femoral head offset	1.13
Extracortical width of diaphysis	1.20
Femoral length	1.22
Femoral head diameter	1.23
Endosteal	
Depth of isthmus from lesser trochanter	1.20
Mediolateral width of isthmus	1.56
Width of canal at osteotomy level	1.65
Width of canal 20 mm distal to lesser trochanter	1.79

From Noble PC, Alexander JW, Lindahl LJ, et al: *Clin Orthop* 235:148, 1988.

bell-shaped curve was also present. This analysis showed that the mediolateral width of the femoral canal at 20 mm distal to the lesser trochanter was the most predictable dimension of the femur for measurements with 95% level of confidence (Table 2-2). Noble,[23] like Averill,[2] Dewey,[7] Ruff,[28] and Sumner,[32] demonstrated a good correlation between the periosteal dimension of the head of the femur and its length (Fig. 2-19).

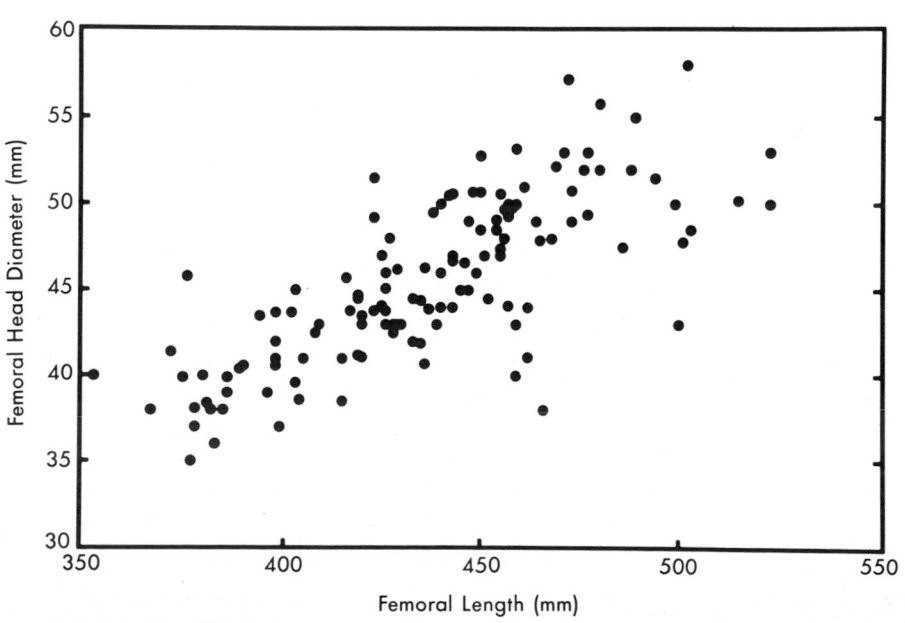

Fig. 2-19. A typical correlation of the periosteal dimensions, in this case between femoral length and the diameter of the femoral head (r = 0.76, n = 100, p < 0.0001). (From Noble PC, Alexander JW, Lindahl LJ, et al: *Clin Orthop* 235:148, 1988.)

Despite a statistically significant correlation between the endosteal mediolateral width of the canal proximally and medullary isthmus measurements (Fig. 2-20), the variation was ± 8 mm and ± 3.3 mm respectively. This wide variation makes the measurements useless for design of the size and shape of the prosthetic stem unless a minimum of 1 to 2 mm mismatch is allowed between the prosthesis and medullary

canal[23] (see Chapter 6). A wide range of "flare index" —the widest opening in mm (A) divided by the narrowest opening at the isthmus (B)—was observed (see Table 2-4 and Figs. 2-21 and 2-22). Noble described three common shapes: stovepipe (with flare index less than 3.0 mm), normal canal shape (with flare index between 3.0 and 4.7 mm), and champagne-fluted canal shape (with flare index between 4.7 and 6.5 mm) with fre-

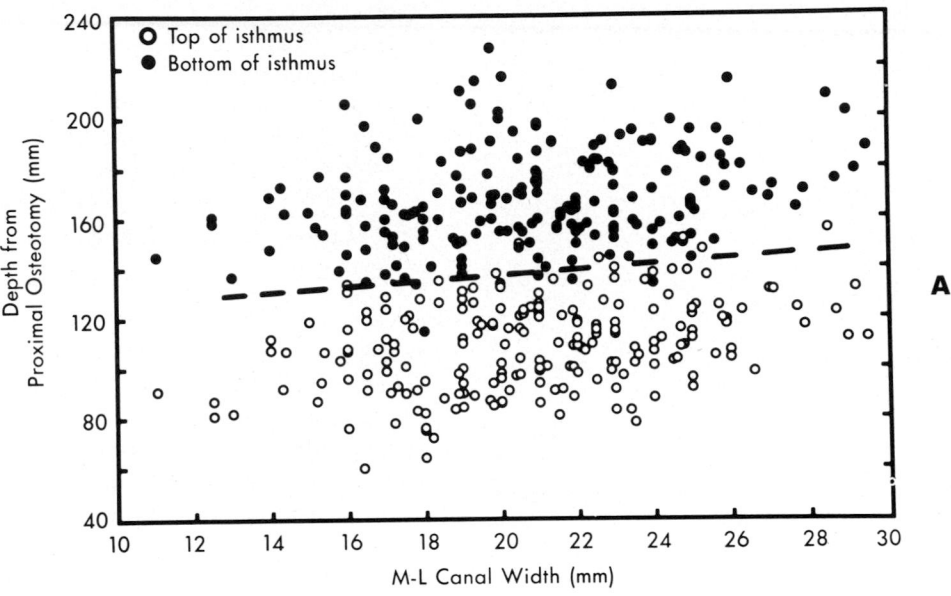

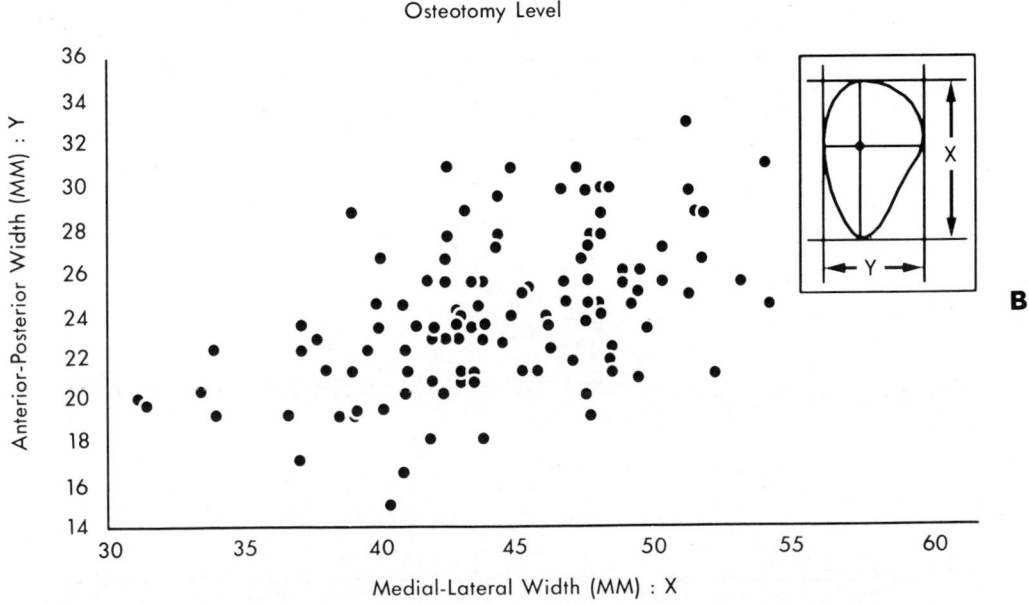

Fig. 2-20. A, The position of the upper and lower borders of the canal isthmus measured from the level of the femoral neck osteotomy. The broken line represents the optimal selection of stem length as a function of canal width. **B,** Correlation of the mediolateral and anteroposterior widths of the metaphysis at the level of the femoral neck osteotomy (13 mm superior to the proximal border of the lesser trochanter; r = 0.40, n = 99, p < 0.0001).

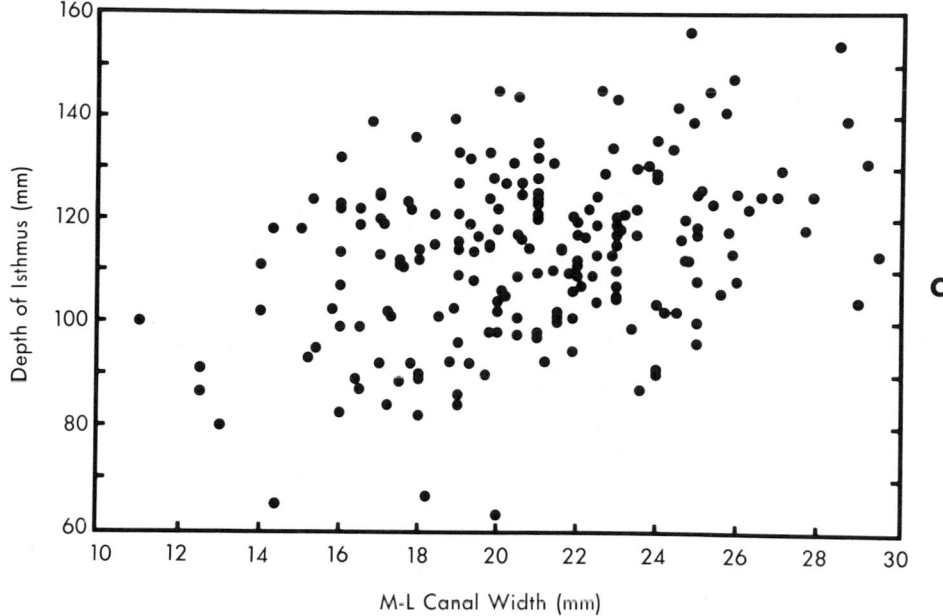

Fig. 2-20—cont'd. C, Correlation between the depth of the isthmus from the center of the lesser trochanter and the mediolateral width of the femoral canal at a point 20 mm distal to the center of the lesser trochanter (r = 0.37, n = 200, p < 0.0001). (From Noble PC, Alexander JW, Lindahl LJ, et al: *Clin Orthop* 235:148, 1988.)

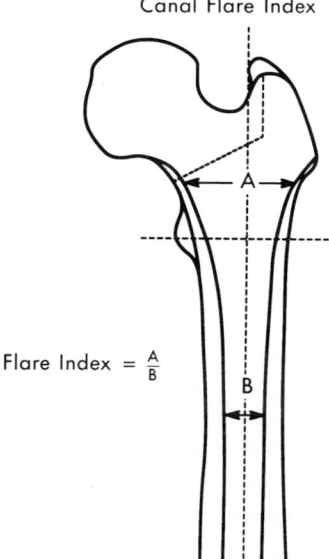

Fig. 2-21. Diagrammatic representation of the canal flare index. (From Noble PC, Alexander JW, Lindahl LJ, et al: *Clin Orthop* 235:148, 1988.

quencies of 9%, 83%, and 8% respectively for 200 specimens studied (Table 2-3 and Fig. 2-22).

As a rule, the femurs with a smaller canal have a champagne-fluted configuration, and the larger medullary canals give a stovepipe shape to the canal. As such, there is an inverse ratio between the canal flare index and the size of the isthmus (Fig. 2-23). Changes in the dimensions of the femur are largely caused by extension of the medullary canal from within. A progressive thinning of the femur results in an expansion of the femur, which occurs in the fourth or fifth decade of life.* In a pathological situation, such as in a mechanically failed total hip arthroplasty, the rate of expansion was twice that of a control patient with successful hip arthroplasty.[15] In Noble's study, almost every femur younger than 55 years of age had a canal flare index of 4.0 or greater. Conversely, every femur older than age 80 years had an index of less than 4.0. The aging thought to occur after age 55 resulted in a widening of the medullary canal estimated to average 1.3 mm per decade (Figs. 2-24 and 2-25).

ASSEMBLED HIP JOINT

The hip is a simple ball-and-socket joint in which the spherical head of the femur fits closely in a deep bony

---

* References 1, 26, 29, 30, 33.

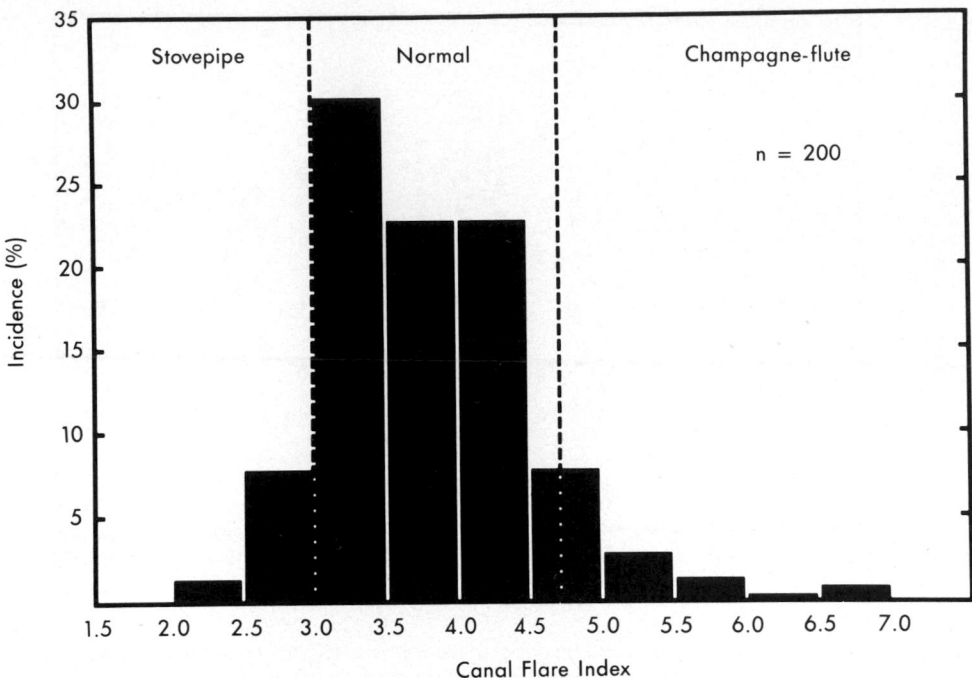

Fig. 2-22. Distribution of values of the canal flare index with corresponding subjective descriptions of canal shape. (From Noble PC, Alexander JW, Lindahl LJ, et al: *Clin Orthop* 235:148, 1988.)

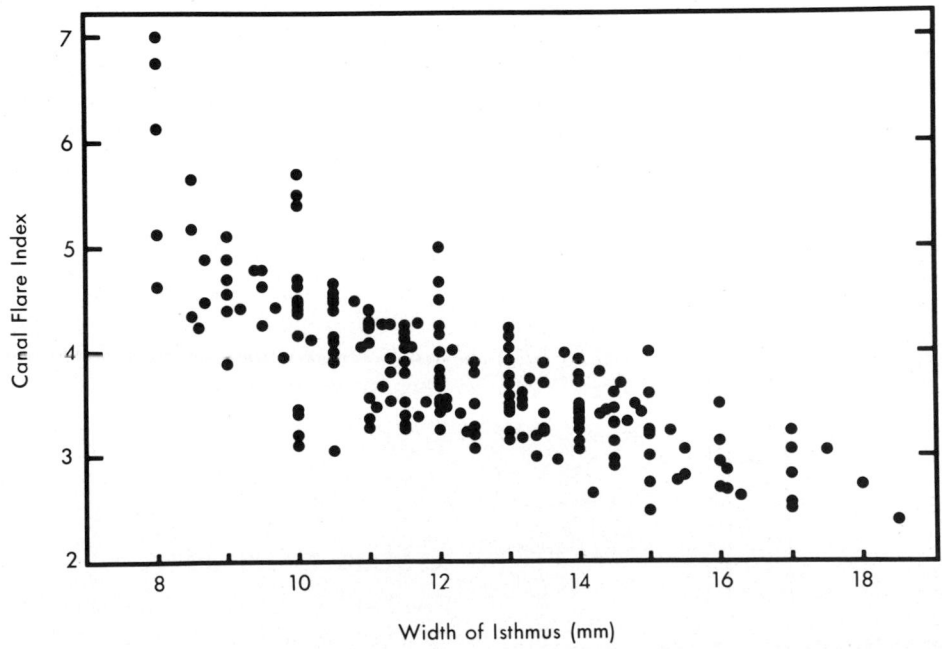

Fig. 2-23. The canal flare index is observed to vary inversely with the mediolateral width of the isthmus ($r = 0.39$, $n = 200$, $p < 0.0001$). (From Noble PC, Alexander JW, Lindahl LJ, et al: *Clin Orthop* 235:148, 1988.)

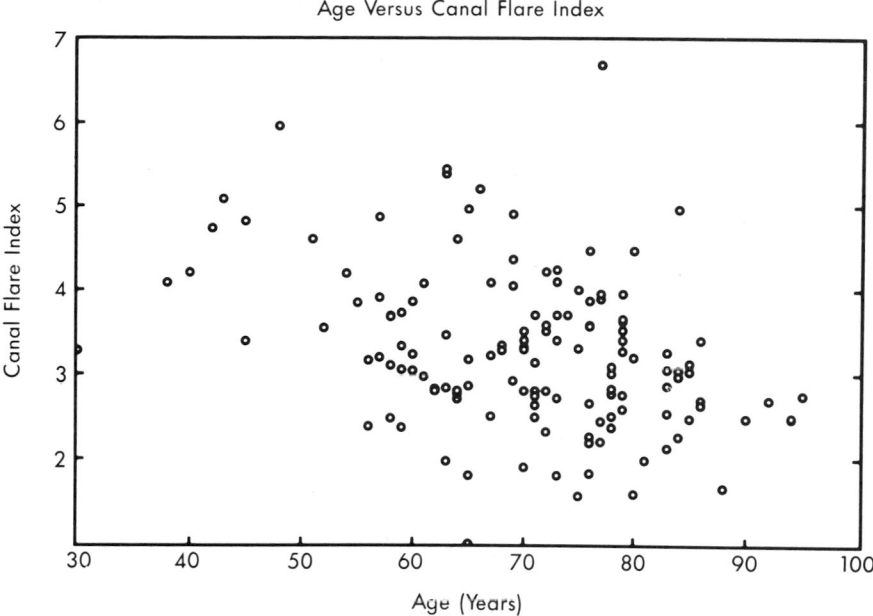

Fig. 2-24. Correlation between the canal flare index and the age of the femur showing a significant change in endosteal shape with aging (r = 0.39, n = 200, p < 0.0001). (From Noble PC, Alexander JW, Lindahl LJ, et al: *Clin Orthop* 235:148, 1988.)

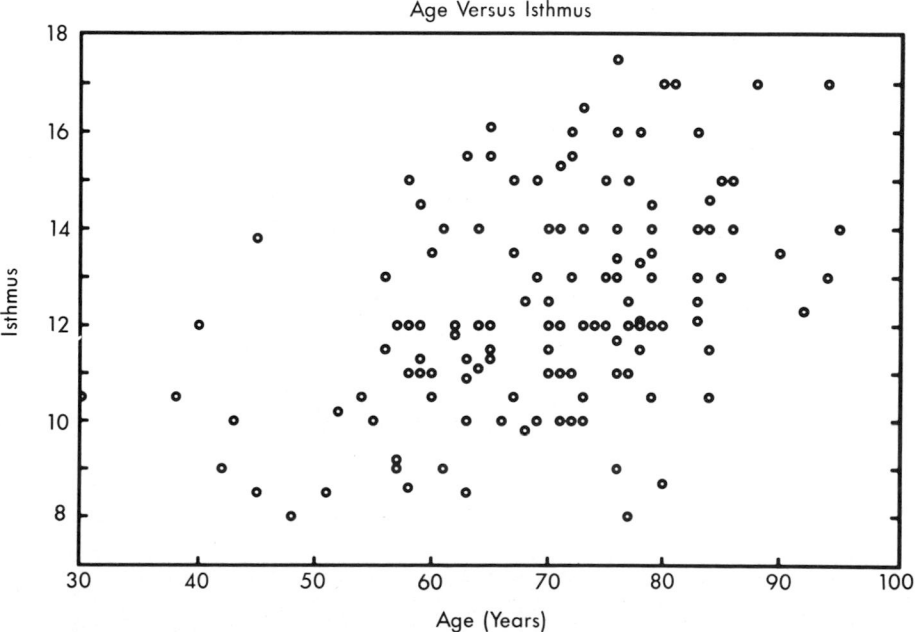

Fig. 2-25. The observed correlation between age and mediolateral width of the isthmus. Overall, the canal expands at a rate of approximately 1.3 mm per decade (r = 0.42, n = 100, p < 0.0001). (From Noble PC, Alexander JW, Lindahl LJ, et al: *Clin Orthop* 235:148, 1988.)

cavity reinforced by a capsule and its strong ligaments. There has been much controversy in the past about the sphericity and the fit of the femur in the acetabulum and its true weight-bearing area. In pathological conditions the bony acetabulum is generally expanded and enlarged by arthritis and often deepened by osteophytes, especially in the superior and posterior portions. While this can be favorable in the replacement of arthritic hips, it is disadvantageous in the fracture of a normal acetabulum; that is, most of these neck fractures require replacement with an extremely small-sized prosthesis. In pathological conditions it is generally defective anteriorly, as in most cases of osteoarthritis. The acetabulum is deepened by the fibrocartilaginous labrum attached to its rim; transverse fibers constituting the acetabular ligament bridge the gap formed by the acetabular notch and act as retaining structures for the head of the femur within the bony acetabulum. At the time of dislocation for replacement, it should be remembered that the constricting fibrocartilaginous labrum should be incised along with the posterior capsule to allow the head to escape from the depth of the acetabulum. (Additionally, a suction or vacuum effect at surgery may prevent the head from dislocating.) Whether the orbicular ligament or a band of the capsule derives some of its fibers from the deep tendons of the gluteal muscula-

ture or from the reflected head of the rectus is only of academic interest. However, at times the hypertrophied "orbicular ligament" may hinder dislocation of the femur head at surgery. The surgeon can best release this structure at the level of the junction of the ilium and ischium at the posterosuperior segment of the acetabulum. At the lower part of the neck, many of these fibers pass into the inferior retinaculum, which closely surrounds the bone, and are closely applied to the femoral head, helping to retain the head of the femur in the socket (Figs. 2-10 and 2-26).

The Y-shaped ligament of the hip joint capsule (Bigelow's ligament) reaches the trochanteric line between a tubercle at its upper end and the medial side of the shaft (see Fig. 2-17). The posterior and slightly medial aspect of the trochanter is marked by a vertical ridge known as the *quadrate tubercle* for the insertion of the quadratus femoris, which covers the bone medially to its insertion. The quadratus femoris attaches to the intertrochanteric crest. The crest is a part of the trochanteric mass removed (along with this muscle insertion) with a large trochanter at surgery. Therefore it is not surprising to find that, despite removal of the trochanter from the femur, it assumes a position posterior to the acetabulum when the external rotators are contracted.

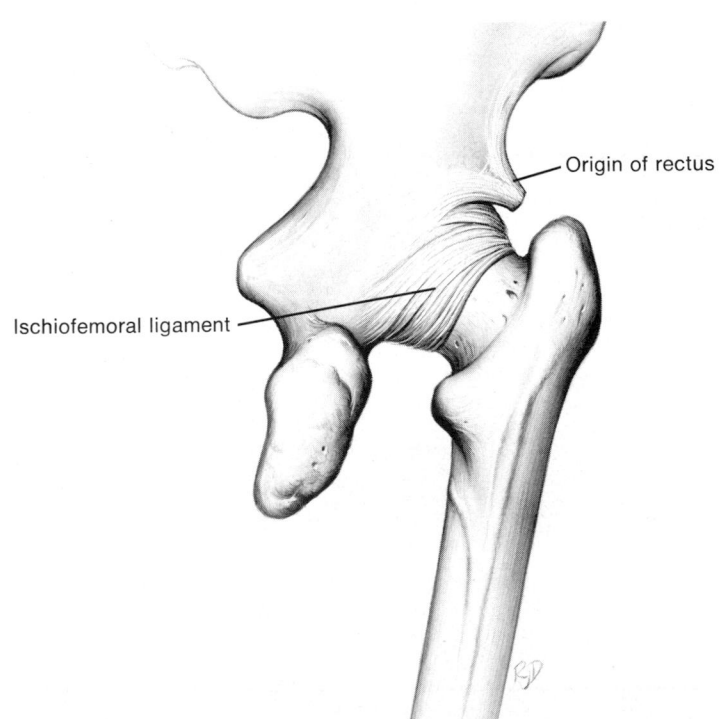

Origin of rectus

Ischiofemoral ligament

Fig. 2-26. Orbicular ligament may hinder dislocation of femoral head at surgery. This structure is best released at junction of ilium and ischium at posterior segment of acetabulum to allow head to escape from depth of acetabulum. Fibers of ischiofemoral ligament are closely applied to femoral head, thus retaining head of femur in socket.

REINFORCING CAPSULAR LIGAMENTS OF THE HIP JOINT

Reinforcing capsular ligaments of the hip provide stability for the joint, and the surgeon should take care to preserve them. The surgeon can prevent anterior dislocation by keeping the fibers tautly extended. The longitudinal fibers that cover the articular zone in front of the hip joint extend in a vertical plane from the anterior margin of the hip bone to the intertrochanteric line of the femur. The fibers attached to the antero-inferior spine are thicker than their counterpart fibers attached to the upper pubic ramus. Both of these ligaments reinforce the anterior capsule in a Y-shaped manner and are known collectively as the *Bigelow's ligament*. The direction and orientation of the contributing iliofemoral and pubofemoral fibers provide stability in maximum external rotation and extension, and both the fibers are tightened when the upright position is assumed. At surgery, when an anterior approach is used, an incision made along the midline of the neck of the femur generally divides the two portions of this ligament without severing either. By preserving both components, the upper portion remains intact and attached to the capsule of the joint and the trochanter, while the inferior portion remains with the inferior capsule. Incision below the neck level preserves both divisions. These ligaments are proportionately shorter in women because of the greater obliquity of the female pelvis and the convexity of the female lumbar spine. The surgeon can better see them at surgery after removing the paraarticular and precapsular fat and transecting blood vessels traversing this zone.

The "ligamentum teres" has little significance in hip replacement surgery except that, when present, it may make surgery for dislocation of the hip more difficult. But it is usually avulsed from the head and retained within the acetabulum at the position of maximum adduction. This ligament has a weaker synovial attachment to the head of the femur than the acetabular fossa and occasionally contains small vessels that bleed after dislocation. The surgeon removes remnants of the ligamentum teres from the acetabular floor before preparing the acetabulum to appreciate the depths of the pulvinar (acetabular fossa). The flattened base of the ligamentum teres is attached by two bands, one into each side of the acetabular notch, and one small strip between the two bands that blends with the transverse ligament.[5] Therefore the surgeon can excise either part of the ligamentum teres base or the base in combination with the transverse ligament to allow access to the inferior portion of the acetabulum and the notch and to provide visualization of the fossa for deepening of the acetabulum. The surgeon should keep in mind that the ligamentum teres is relaxed when the hip is in a semiflexed and abducted position

and is taut when the hip is adducted. For this reason, firm adduction at dislocation allows for easy detachment from its insertion. Generally this ligament is absent in advanced rheumatoid and osteoarthritic hips.

CAPSULE OF THE HIP JOINT

The capsule of the hip joint is a strong and dense fibrous structure. It attaches above the margin of the acetabulum 5 or 6 mm beyond the labrum. The surgeon should take care not to disturb it when excising the labrum from within the capsular cavity. In front of the outer margin of the labrum, opposite the acetabular notch and further down, the capsule attaches to the transverse acetabular ligament and to the edge of the obturator foramen. On the neck in front it attaches to the trochanteric line above, to the base of the neck behind, and to the neck about 1 cm above the trochanteric crest and below to the lower part of the neck close to the lesser trochanter (see Fig. 2-15). The capsule is particularly thickened in the case of osteoarthritis and constitutes an especially heavy fibrous structure in the superior and inferior portions of the neck. It is shortened posteriorly in severe external rotation deformity and anteriorly when severe adduction deformity prevails. It may become expanded if the head has migrated cephalad. In a completely congenitally dislocated hip, the capsule may be divided into two separate segments connected by an isthmus (hourglass type). The surgeon should not disturb the capsule if the exposure of the hip joint is complete, since it enhances the stability of the hip after arthroplasty, and in toto resection will cause undesirable bleeding. On the other hand, if the trochanter is not removed, as in the anterior approach (see Chapter 3), a complete capsulectomy is a necessity for exposure before dislocation of the hip joint. Using a posterior or a posterolateral approach, an anterior capsulectomy must not be done. For fixed flexion deformity a capsulotomy is best performed along the anterior margin of the acetabulum (see Chapter 17). From the front of the neck, retinacular fibers containing blood vessels enter the bone from the capsule at many points. The capsule of the joint is very thin posteriorly. Two sets of circular and longitudinal fibers reinforce it. The longitudinal fibers have been described previously; however, the circular fibers of the "zona orbicularis" are deep, forming a collar around the neck of the femur. These fibers only attach to the capsule, not to the bone. In addition to the longitudinal and circular ligaments, the "ischiofemoral ligament" reinforces the capsule. It has a spiral appearance on the back of the joint from its attachment to the ischium below and behind the acetabulum, and it directs upward and laterally over the back of the neck of the femur. Some of its fibers are continuous with those of the zona orbicularis, while others are fixed to the greater trochanter anteriorly and lead to the iliofemoral ligament.[9] This intricate system of reinforcing ligaments substantiates the complexity of the capsule of the joint as a stabilizing mechanism of the hip that should not be disturbed unnecessarily if severe preexisting deformity of the hip is not present at surgery. Perhaps it is because of the efficiency of this design that a newly formed capsule after hip replacement does not usually give a full range of flexion.

MUSCLES ABOUT THE HIP JOINT

A gross anatomical representation of the muscles of the hip is illustrated in Figs. 2-27 to 2-30. The origins of the muscles and their attachments are shown in Figs. 2-2 and 2-27 to 2-30. The hip joint is covered by muscles on all sides, anteriorly by the lateral fibers of the

pectineus, and lateral to the pectineus, the tendon of the psoas major with the iliacus on its lateral side. The femoral artery is on the psoas tendon, and the femoral nerve lies deep in the groove between the tendon and the iliacus. More laterally, the straight head of the rectus femoris crosses the hip joint, and at the lateral border the deep layer of the iliotibial tract blends with the fibrous capsule. Superiorly, the reflected head of the rectus and the gluteus minimus cover the lateral part. Inferiorly, the lateral fibers of the pectineus lie on the capsule as they incline backward; more posteriorly, the obturator externus crosses obliquely to gain the posterior aspect of the hip joint. Posteriorly, the capsule is covered with the tendons of the obturator externus, which separate it from the quadratus femoris. The latter is accompanied by the ascending branch of the medial circumflex artery. Above the tendon of the obturator internus, the two gemelli are in contact with

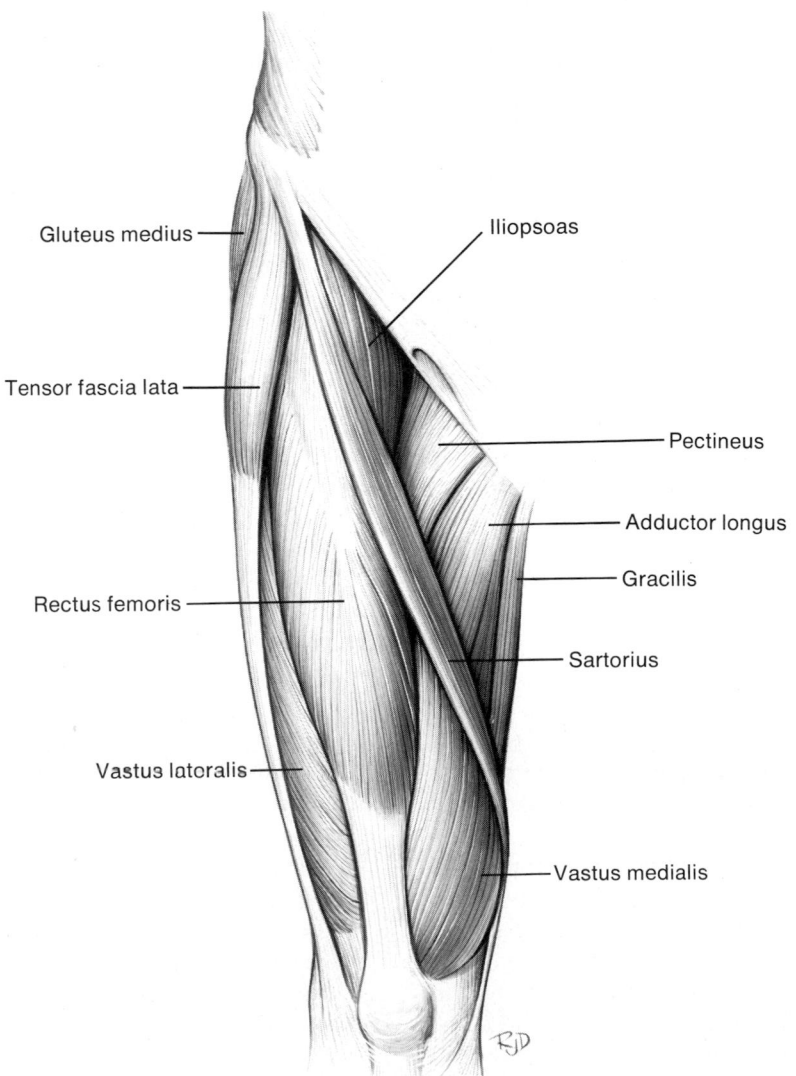

Fig. 2-27. Anterior thigh muscles (flexor group).

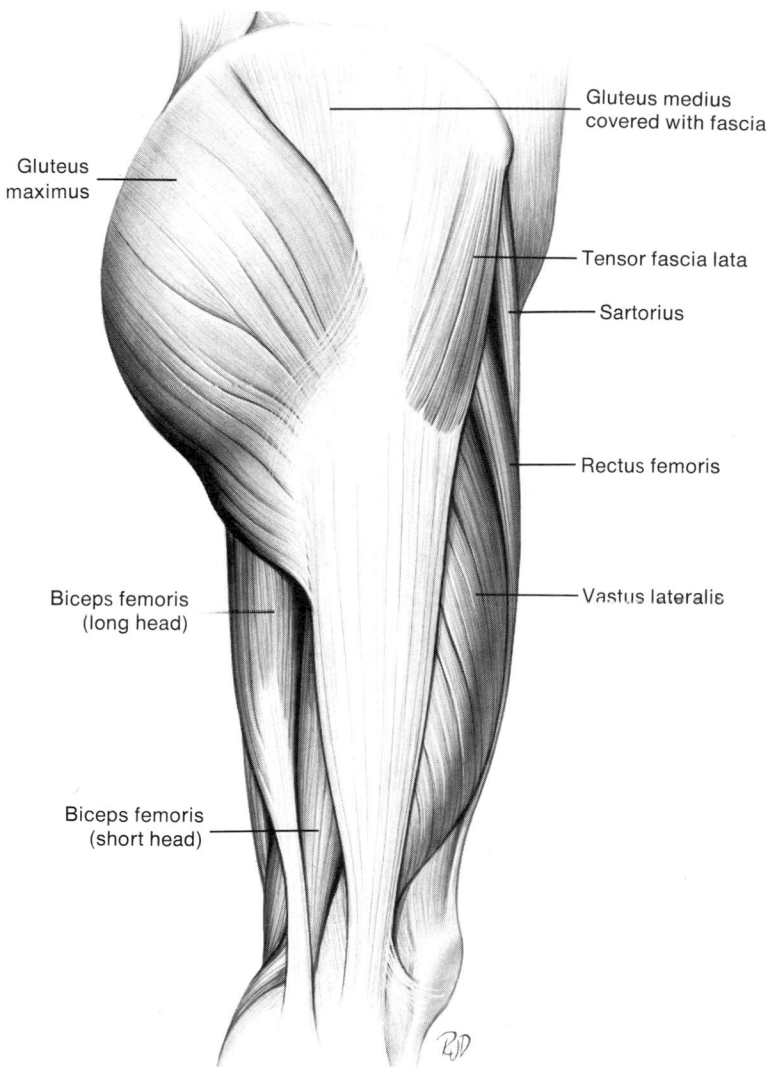

Gluteus medius
covered with fascia

Gluteus
maximus

Tensor fascia lata

Sartorius

Rectus femoris

Biceps femoris
(long head)

Vastus lateralis

Biceps femoris
(short head)

Fig. 2-28. Musculature of lateral thigh. The relationship of three muscles constituting the "pelvic deltoid."

the joint and are separated from the piriformis by the sciatic nerve (see Fig. 2-29).[14] The nerve to the quadratus femoris lies deep to the obturator internus tendon and descends on the most medial part of the capsule. The piriformis crosses the uppermost part of the posterior surface of the articular capsule. When the trochanter is removed intraarticularly and the posterosuperior capsule and piriformis tendon are incised, brisk arterial bleeding at the site of division is a constant anatomical feature.

To the hip surgeon, knowledge of the origin and insertion of all muscles contributing to the movement of the hip is essential. For brevity, Table 2-5 presents the functional anatomy and the sources of innervation of the hip muscles. For details of muscular origins and

insertions, the reader is referred to standard anatomy texts.*

Seven noteworthy musculatures with their tendons traverse the hip joint in the back. From above downward they are: the posterior border of the gluteus medius, the piriformis, the gemellus superior, the tendon of the obturator internus, the gemellus inferior, the quadratus femoris, and the adductor magnus. The vertical muscles, the hamstrings, if apparent at all, are located very close to the ischium. The description of the superficial structures of the hip (pelvic deltoid) by Henry[14] is of special interest. The "key muscle" in this

---

* References 9, 16, 19, 27, 34.

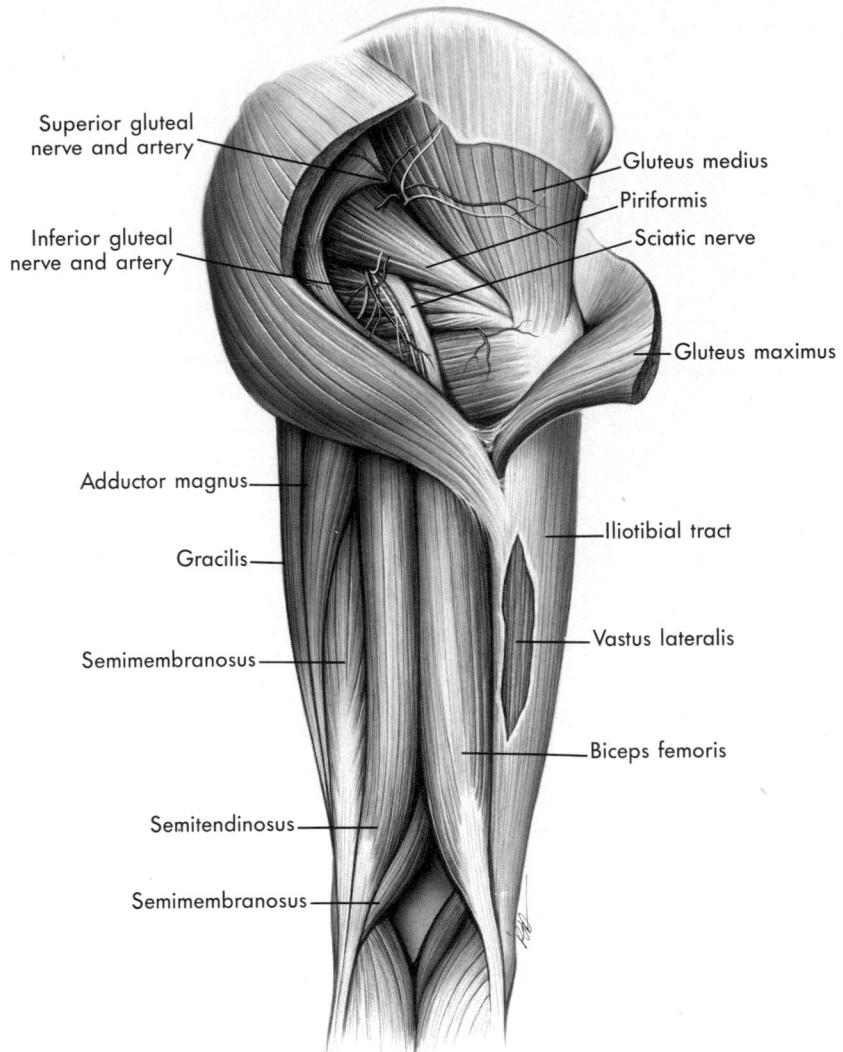

Fig. 2-29. Posterior musculature of thigh and buttock. Gluteus maximus has partially been removed to show deeper layers, which include short rotators, and position of sciatic nerve, superior and inferior gluteal nerves, and arteries; piriformis is "key" muscle.[14]

region of the hip is the piriformis; at its upper edge the examiner can identify the superior gluteal artery and nerve, and at its inferior border the most superficial structure to emerge is the inferior gluteal nerve. Along the posteromedial edge is the great sciatic nerve.[14] At surgery, after releasing the external rotators (for example, detaching the piriformis from its insertion to the greater trochanter and the quadratus femoris from its femoral attachment close to the bone), the surgeon should note that the sciatic nerve is located halfway between the posterior border of the ischial portion of the acetabulum (see Fig. 2-29).

ARTERIES AND NERVES

Major nerves and vessels in the hip region supply local structures as well as the lower extremity with blood and innervation. In the posterior aspect these structures include the sciatic nerve, posterior femoral cutaneous nerve, superior gluteal nerve and vessels, inferior gluteal nerve and vessels, and the nerves to the short rotators and articular branches. Anterior structures include the femoral cutaneous nerve branches, the obturator cutaneous nerve, the lateral femoral cutaneous nerve, and the femoral nerve (cutaneous branches, articular branches, and muscular branches). Femoral vessels include the profunda (the largest branch) and femoral circumflex vessels, medial and lateral—both commonly a branch of the profunda.

The origin, distribution, and location of the major nerves and arteries of the hip joint are illustrated in Figs. 2-8, 2-10, and 2-30 to 2-37. The femoral nerves at the anterior rim of the acetabulum are the most

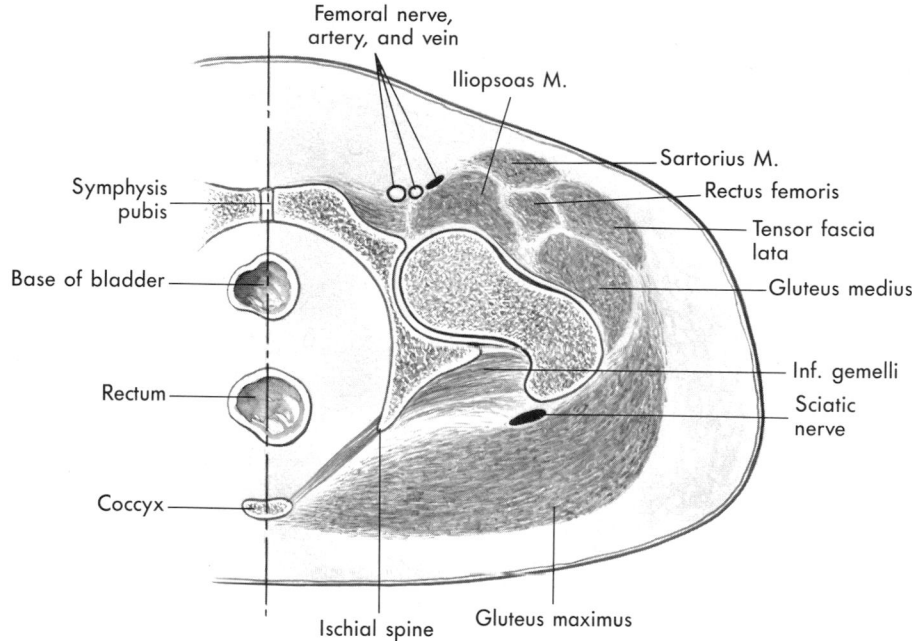

Fig. 2-30. Artist's rendering of MRI of right hip at the hip joint level illustrates the proximity of the neurovascular supply and muscles to the femur and the acetabulum.

Table 2-5 Summary of Functional Anatomy of Hip Muscles

Function	Muscle	Nerve supply
I. Flexors		
A. Primary flexors	Ilipsoas	Nerve to iliopsoas
	Pectineus	Femoral or obturator
	Tensor fascia femoris	Superior gluteal
	Adductor brevis	Obturator
	Sartorius	Femoral
B. Secondary flexors	Adductor longus	Obturator
	Adductor magnus	Obturator
	Gracilis (anterior fibers)	Obturator
	Gluteus medius	Superior gluteal
	Gluteus minimus	Superior gluteal
II. Extensors		
A. Primary extensors	Gluteus maximus	Inferior gluteal
	Adductor magnus (posterior fibers)	Tibial
B. Secondary extensors	Semimembranosus	Tibial
	Semitendinosus	Tibial
	Biceps femoris	Tibial
	Gluteus medius	Superior gluteal
	Gluteus minimus	Superior gluteal
	Piriformis	Nerve to piriformis (L_4–S_2)
III. Adductors		
A. Primary adductors	Adductor brevis	Obturator
	Adductor longus	Obturator
	Adductor magnus	Obturator and tibial
	Gluteus maximus	Inferior gluteal
B. Secondary adductors	Pectineus	Femoral or obturator
	Gracilis	Obturator
	Obturator externus	Obturator
	Iliopsoas	Nerve to iliopsoas
	Hamstrings	Tibial

Continued.

Table 2-5 Summary of Functional Anatomy of Hip Muscles—Cont'd

Function	Muscle	Nerve supply
IV. Abductors		
A. Primary abductors	Gluteus medius	Superior gluteal
	Gluteus minimus	Superior gluteal
B. Secondary abductors	Tensor fascia femoris	Superior gluteal
	Piriformis	Nerve to piriformis
	Sartorius	Femoral
V. Internal rotators		
A. Primary internal rotators	Gluteus medius	Superior gluteal
	Gluteus minimus	Superior gluteal
	Tensor fascia femoris	Superior gluteal
B. Secondary internal rotators	Adductor magnus (posterior part)	Tibial
	Semitendinosus	Tibial
	Semimembranosus	Tibial
VI. External rotators		
A. Primary external rotators	Gluteus maximus	Inferior gluteal
	Piriformis	Nerve to piriformis
	Obturator externus	Obturator
	Obturator internus	Nerve to obturator
	Superior gemellus	Superior gemellus
	Inferior gemellus	Nerve to inferior gemellus and quadratus femoris
	Quadratus femoris	
	Adductor brevis	Obturator
	Adductor longus	Obturator
	Adductor magnus (anterior part)	Obturator
	Pectineus	Femoral or obturator
B. Secondary external rotators	Gluteus medius	Superior gluteal
	Gluteus minimus	Superior gluteal
	Sartorius	Femoral
	Iliopsoas	Nerve to iliopsoas
	Biceps femoris	Tibial

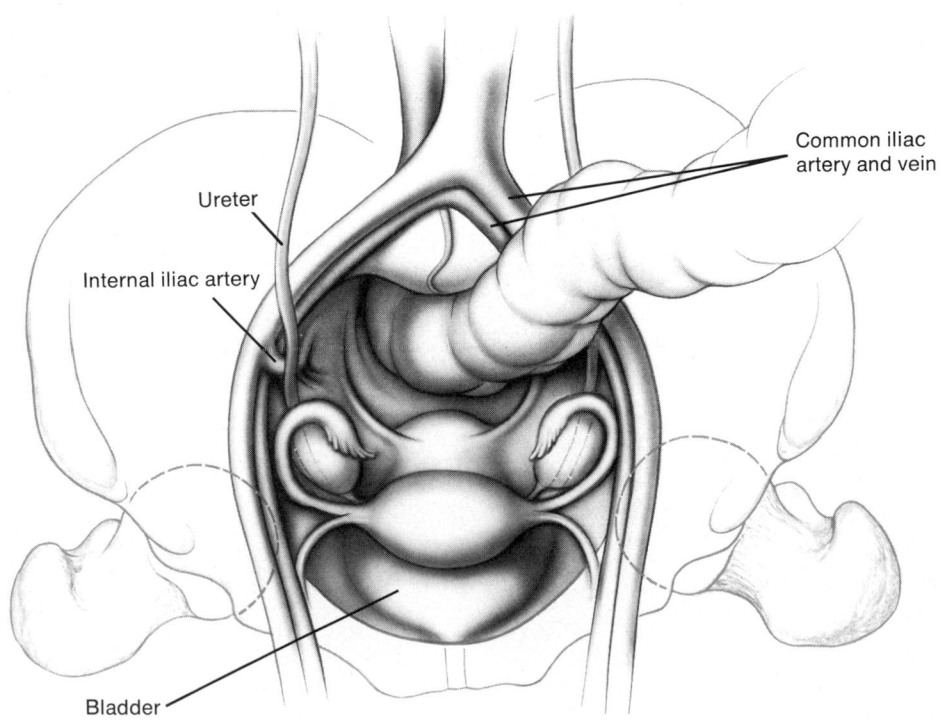

Fig. 2-31. Structures of lesser pelvis in female and proximity of its content to floor of acetabulum are shown. Distended bladder and ureter are closest viscera in addition to internal iliac artery and vein in region of hip joint.

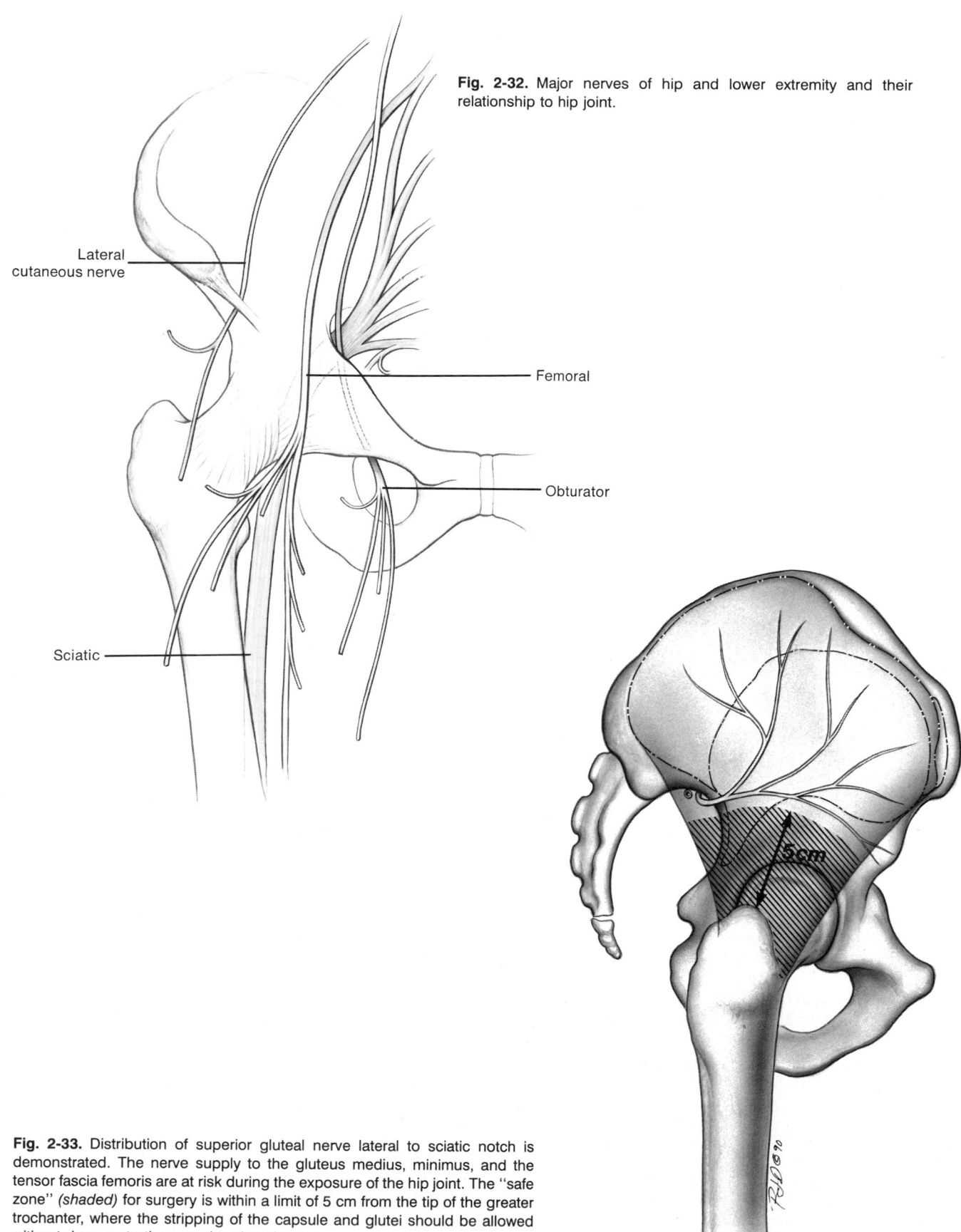

Fig. 2-32. Major nerves of hip and lower extremity and their relationship to hip joint.

Lateral cutaneous nerve

Femoral

Obturator

Sciatic

Fig. 2-33. Distribution of superior gluteal nerve lateral to sciatic notch is demonstrated. The nerve supply to the gluteus medius, minimus, and the tensor fascia femoris are at risk during the exposure of the hip joint. The "safe zone" *(shaded)* for surgery is within a limit of 5 cm from the tip of the greater trochanter, where the stripping of the capsule and glutei should be allowed without damage to the superior gluteal nerve.

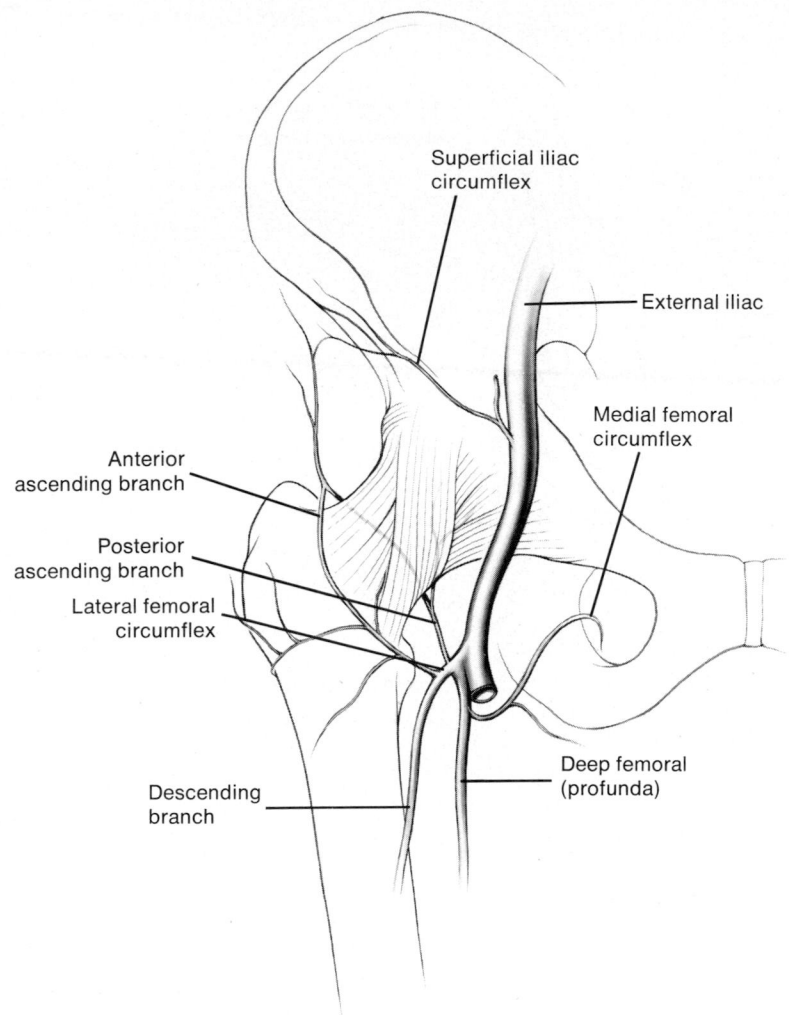

Fig. 2-34. Major arteries of hip and lower extremity and their relationship to hip joint.

vulnerable in the area, especially when this wall is defective, as in congenital dysplasia (see Chapter 20). The sciatic nerve may be injured if the posterior wall is defective, that is, during revision surgery in difficult hip problems. Good exposure of the back of the pelvis and complete visualization of the nerve at this level ensure its safety if bone grafting to the back of the acetabulum is planned. As stated, the surgeon may injure the obturator nerve during excessive preparation of the pubic segment of the acetabulum by anchor holes entering the obturator foramen or the iliopubic ramus and flow of cement into this area. In establishing the anchor holes the surgeon must bear in mind the location of these nerves lest deep penetration of the cement causes damage.

The superior gluteal nerve is important in surgery of the hip joint, since damage to it can result in severe disability from weakness of the abductor mechanism of the hip. Denervation of the abductors will result in an abductor lurch and a positive Trendelenburg.[11,31] All primary abductors of the hip, the gluteus medius and minimis, and the tensor fascia femoris muscles are innervated by the superior gluteal nerve. Anatomical texts vary greatly in their descriptions of the superior

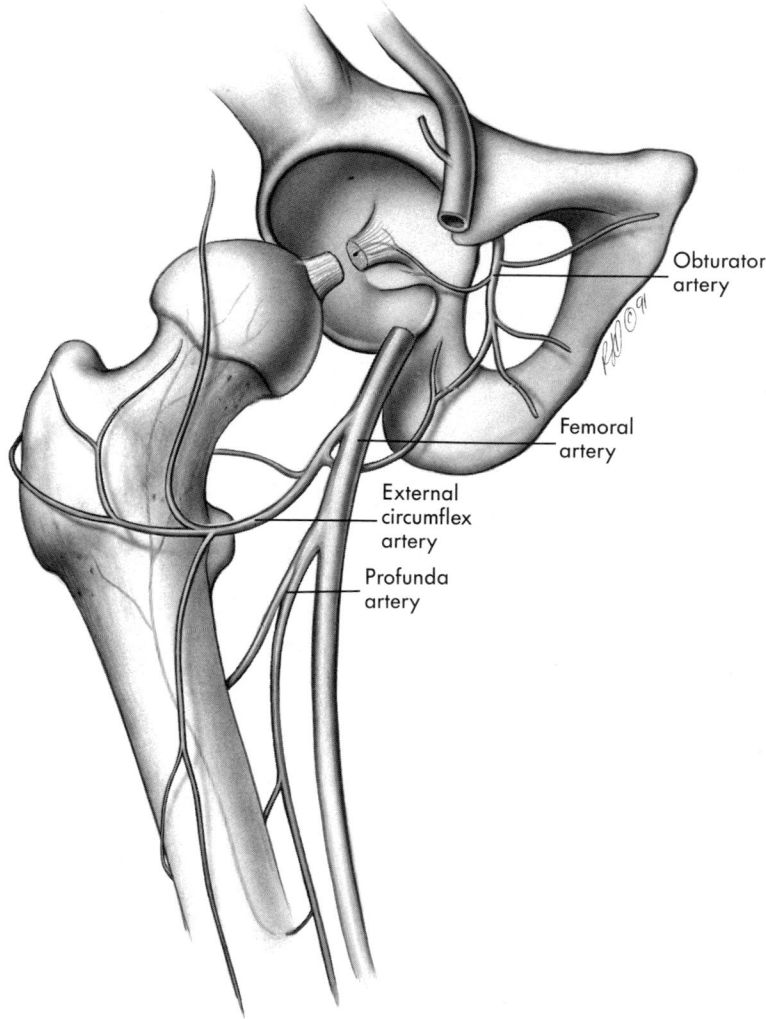

Fig. 2-35. Arterial supply to upper femur.

Obturator
artery

Femoral
artery

External
circumflex
artery

Profunda
artery

gluteal nerve's location and course.[4,22,27,34] This nerve has been redefined for its anatomical location and its vulnerability in a direct lateral approach[6,10,21] or anterolateral approach to the hip joint.

Jacobs and Buxton[18] have found that distribution of terminal branches of this nerve are in two groups, anterior and posterior, the division being an arbitrary line drawn from a midpoint of the superior border of the greater trochanter to the iliac crest in the coronal plane (see Figs. 2-29 and 2-33). The points of termination of all branches form an arcuate pattern along the middle third of the gluteus medius muscle. The "safe zone" for avoidance of nerve injury is a distance of 5 cm from the top of the greater trochanter. The shaded area in Fig. 2-33 indicates the safe zone along the base of the ilium during surgical exposure of the superior acetabular region during hip arthroplasty and bone-grafting procedures.

The relationship of the common iliac and femoral artery and veins to the wall of the pelvis is illustrated in an inlet view of the pelvis in Fig. 2-31. Inadvertent penetration of the pelvis may cause serious damage to these major vessels or to viscera such as the bladder.

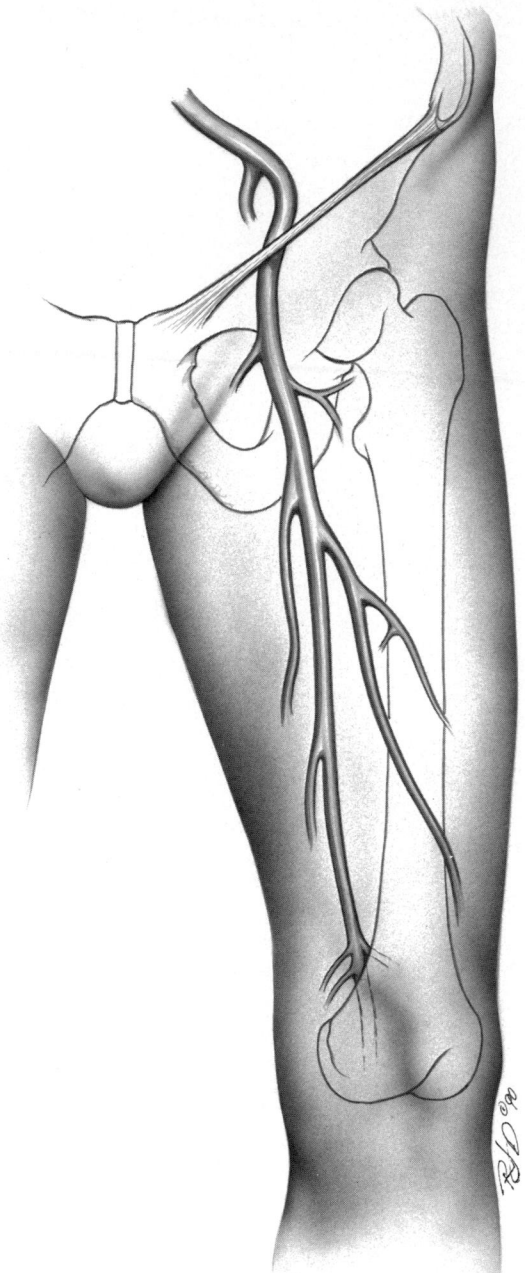

Fig. 2-36. Anatomy of venous system proximal to knee.

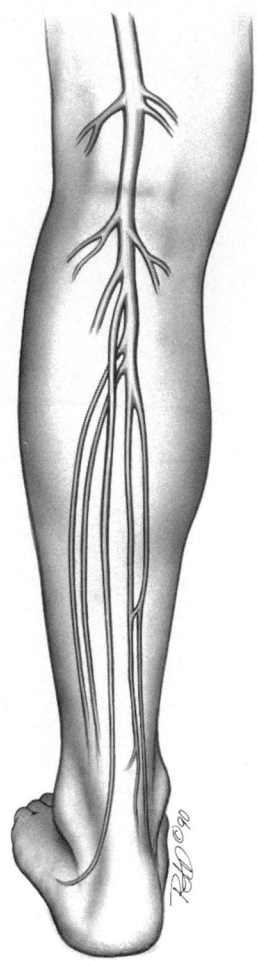

Fig. 2-37. Anatomy of venous system distal to knee joint.

SUMMARY OF ESSENTIALS

■ Knowledge of the applied anatomy of the hip is of paramount importance for the surgical approach and technique in relation to orientation and insertion of prosthetic components. The surgeon performing total hip arthroplasty must study a bony skeleton and review anatomy in detail on a bony cadaveric specimen, dissecting the hip with particular attention to the neurovascular structures of the hip. A simulated hip arthroplasty on a cadaveric specimen will expand the surgeon's comprehension of the gross anatomy of the pelvis and hip and may well prevent future surgical complications.

■ The ilium, pubis, and ischium contribute to the formation of the acetabulum, which faces outward and somewhat downward anteriorly. In addition to structure, the surgeon should know the anatomical orientation of the acetabulum and pelvis. The weight-bearing upper and posterior walls of the acetabulum are especially heavy, whereas the anterior wall is usually less developed. The inferior wall is less substantial at the site of the acetabular notch opening into the obturator foramen.

■ The "acetabular fossa," a rough area located at the center of the articulating portion of the acetabulum, is the thinnest portion of the floor of the acetabulum. At this site the inner and outer tables of the pelvic bone are fused without interpositioned cancellous bone. This zone comprises the thinnest possible area beyond which the surgeon may render damage if he or she deepens the acetabulum. In osteoarthritic hips (especially in congenital dysplasia), this area is thickened, and further deepening of the socket is possible here. This level corresponds with the radiological "teardrop" on an anteroposterior radiograph of the pelvis.

- In pathological anatomy of the acetabulum and during the acetabular reaming and protrusio acetabuli, the surgeon refers to the radiographic teardrop sign in vertical and transverse axes, since it defines the true site of the acetabulum.

- The bony pelvis appears to have been twisted on itself at the site of the acetabulum, creating two planes at right angles to each other. The upper portion roughly corresponds to the ilium and the lower corresponds to the ischium and pubis. This is an important consideration when observing the anteroposterior radiographs of the pelvis, which generally show the pelvis somewhat in a frontal plane and the ischium and pubis in a more sagittal plane. The examiner should keep in mind this deceptive x-ray presentation of a flat "iliac fan" when preparing the acetabulum. The examiner should consider the three-dimensional configuration when orienting the patient's pelvis on the operating table.

- The surgeon can conveniently reach the greater sciatic notch both through the inner wall of the pelvis by subperiosteal dissection or from the outside by exploring the sciatic nerve in the buttocks.

- The ilium and ischium are the major contributors to the formation of the acetabulum. The surgeon must appreciate the direction and the small size of the pubis and iliopubic ramis on a dry bony specimen to avoid damage to this region of the pelvis at surgery. The anterior aspect of the pelvis is especially dysplastic in most hips with osteoarthritis at the zone of the pubic contribution to the formation of the acetabulum.

- Because the ilium and the ischium each provide two fifths of the acetabulum and the remaining one fifth is contributed by the pubis, the pubis particularly requires protection by careful placement of liver-type retractors during the preparation of the acetabulum.

- The acetabular fossa containing fibrofatty tissue is the key in identifying the depth of the floor at that level. By removing the soft tissue from the fossa, the surgeon can appreciate the true depth of the socket. Preparing the rim of the acetabulum involves strong retraction of the capsule superiorly and anteriorly in addition to exposing the acetabular notch.

- The size and shape of the acetabulum are represented by the size and shape of the femoral head. It can be used as a guide to the anatomical size and shape of the acetabulum during reconstruction.

- The best way to assess the angular shape of the femur along its length is by maximum adduction of the hip while observing its relationship with the transcondylar line, patella, and lesser trochanter.

- Successful detachment and reattachment of the greater trochanter include appraisal of its size, shape, and location in relation to the shaft, the neck of the femur, the intertrochanteric line, the intertrochanteric crest, the tip, the digital fossa, the vastus lateralis ridge, and the quadratus femoris tubercle.

- The lesser trochanter provides a reference guide for preparation of the upper femur and also denotes the medial muscular structures and the level of the calcar femoral. Both the lesser and greater trochanter denote degrees of anteversion or retroversion of the upper femur, but the best reference in this regard is the transcondylar line of the femur.

- The upper margin of gluteus maximus tendon attachment to the femur is located at the level of the lesser trochanter (a good landmark), which is intimately applied near the perforating vessels near the femur. The sciatic nerve is located just anterior to this structure, which must be protected during release of this tendon.

- The shape and size of the upper femur vary considerably because of genetic and environmental factors. Accordingly, a large inventory of prostheses should be maintained for the purpose of interference fit (despite allowance for a 1- to 2-mm mismatch between the prosthesis and bone).

- Although a good correlation exists between the periosteal dimensions of the head of the femur and its length, other scattered plots of the femur show great variability in a normal bell-shaped curve that is also present.

- A significant change in shape of the upper femur occurs after age 55 because of progressive enlargement of the diaphyseal portion of the femur. This changes the femur from a "champagne-fluted" shape to a more cylindrical shape known as *stovepipe* shape.

- The capsule of the hip joint is preserved in some techniques of total hip arthroplasty. With its reinforcing ligament, the capsule can augment the stability of the hip joint. The capsular attachment to the periphery of the acetabulum provides an excellent support for retractors to aid visualization during surgery while avoiding major neurovascular injuries.

- To make a safe surgical approach, the surgeon must keep in mind the key anatomical landmarks and their relationship to vital structures.

- The anatomical discussion in this chapter is intended to apply to total hip arthroplasty. Specifics are thus limited to the replacement surgery. The reader is advised to consult standard texts for detailed anatomy of the hip joint.

REFERENCES

1. **Atkinson PJ, Woodhead C:** The development of osteoporosis: a hypothesis based on a study of human bone structure, *Clin Orthop* 90:217, 1973.
2. **Averill RG, Pachtman N, Jaffe WL:** A basic dimensional analysis of normal human proximal femora. In *Proceedings of the Eighth Annual Northeast Bioengineering Conference,* Cambridge, Mass, 1980.
3. **Brand RA, Crowninshield RD, Pedersen DR:** Architecture of the periacetabular trabecular bone, *Orthopedics* 5(3):299, 1982.
4. **Brash JC:** *Neuro-vascular hila of limb muscles: an atlas,* Edinburgh, 1955, E & S Livingstone.
5. **Breathnach AS,** editor: *Frazer's anatomy of the human skeleton,* ed 6, Boston, 1965, Little, Brown.
6. **Dall D:** Exposure of the hip by anterior osteotomy of the greater trochanter. A modified anterolateral approach, *J Bone Joint Surg* 68[Br]:382, 1986.
7. **Dewey JR, Bartley MH Jr, Armelagos GJ:** Rates of femoral cortical bone loss in two Nubian populations: utilizing normalized and non-normalized data, *Clin Orthop* 65:61, 1969.
8. **Goodman SB, Adler SJ, Fyhrie DP, et al:** The acetabular teardrop and its relevance to acetabular migration, *Clin Orthop* 236:199, 1988.
9. **Grant JC:** *An atlas of anatomy,* ed 5, Baltimore, 1962, Williams & Wilkins.
10. **Hardinge K:** The direct lateral approach to the hip, *J Bone Joint Surg* 64[Br]:17, 1982.
11. **Hardy AE, Synek V:** Hip abductor function after the Hardinge approach: brief report, *J Bone Joint Surg* 70[Br]:673, 1988.
12. **Harty M:** The calcar femorale and the femoral neck, *J Bone Joint Surg* 39:625, 1957.
13. **Hayes WC, Snyder B:** Correlations between stress and morphology in travecular bone of the patella, *Trans Orthop Res Soc* 4:88, 1979.
14. **Henry AK:** *Extensile exposure,* ed 2, Baltimore, 1957, Williams & Wilkins.
15. **Hofmann AA, Bigler GT, France ER, et al:** Increased endosteal bone loss after hip arthroplasty, *Trans Orthop Res Soc* 11:470, 1986.
16. **Hollinshead WH:** *Anatomy for surgeons,* vol 3, *The back and limbs,* New York, 1958, Harper & Row.
17. **Jacob HA, Huggler AH, Dietschi C, et al:** Mechanical function of subchondral bone as experimentally determined on the acetabulum of the human pelvis, *J Biomech* 9:625, 1976.
18. **Jacobs LG, Buxton RA:** The course of the superior gluteal nerve in the lateral approach, *J Bone Joint Surg* 71:1239, 1989.
19. **Last RJ:** *Anatomy, regional and applied,* ed 2, London, 1959, J & A Churchill.
20. **Lockhart RD, Hamilton GF, Fyfe FW:** *Anatomy of the human body,* Philadelphia, 1959, JB Lippincott.
21. **McFarland B, Osborne G:** Approach to the hip: a suggested improvement on Kocher's method, *J Bone Joint Surg* 36[Br]:364, 1954.
22. **McMinn RMH, Hutchings RT:** *Color atlas of human anatomy,* Chicago, 1977, Year Book Medical.
23. **Noble PC, Alexander JW, Lindahl LJ, et al:** The anatomic basis of femoral component design, *Clin Orthop* 235:148, 1988.
24. **Oberländer W:** Die Beanspruchung des menschlichen Hüftgelenks V Die Verteilung der Knochendichte im acetabulum, *Z Anat Entwicklungsgesch* 140:367, 1973.
25. **Ponseti IV:** Growth and development of the acetabulum in the normal child. (Anatomical, histological and roentgenographic studies), *J Bone Joint Surg* 60:575, 1978.
26. **Poss R, Staehlin P, Larson M:** Femoral expansion in total hip arthroplasty, *J Arthroplasty* 2(4):1, 1987.
27. **Romanes GJ,** editor: *Cunningham's textbook of anatomy,* ed 12, London, 1981, Oxford University Press.
28. **Ruff CB:** Allometry between length and cross-sectional dimensions of the femur and tibia in homo sapiens sapiens, *Am J Phys Anthropol* 65:347, 1984.
29. **Ruff CB, Hayes WC:** Age changes in geometry and mineral content of the lower limb bones, *Ann Biomed Eng* 12:573, 1984.
30. **Ruff CB, Hayes WC:** Subperiosteal expansion and cortical remodeling of the human femur and tibia with aging, *Science* 217:945, 1982.
31. **Sudlow RA, Roper BA:** The Trendelenberg test after differing approaches to the hip joint. In Proceedings and Reports of Universities, Colleges, Councils, Associations, and Societies. British Orthopaedic Association, *J Bone Joint Surg* 67[Br]:498, 1985.
32. **Sumner DR Jr:** Postembryonic dimensional allometry of the human femur, *Am J Phys Anthropol* 64:69, 1984.
33. **Van Gerven DP, Armelagos GJ, Bartley MH:** Roentgenographic and direct measurement of femoral cortical involution in a prehistoric Mississippian population, *Am J Phys Anthropol* 31:23, 1983.
34. **Williams PL, Warwick R,** editors: *Gray's anatomy,* ed 36 (British), Edinburgh, 1980, Churchill Livingstone.
35. **Wolff J:** *Das Gestez der Transformation der Knochen,* Berlin, 1892, Hirschwald.

See Chapters 6, Biomechanics: Fixation and Loosening; 15, Principles Common to all Surgical Approaches; 18, Transtrochanteric Approach (modified Charnley); 19, Transtrochanteric Approach (author's method); and 22, Protusio Acetabuli for additional information.

CHAPTER THREE

Applied Surgical Approaches

- A mind that understands principles will work out the methods.
  Hugh Owen Thomas

Total hip arthroplasty requires greater exposure than most other hip procedures for complete access to the acetabulum and the upper femur. A complete fascial and muscular release should be considered a prerequisite to the correction of all existing fixed deformities. The surgeon must understand the anatomical basis for each alternative approach to the hip and must critically consider the merits and disadvantages of each. Because the technology of total hip arthroplasty is still evolving and because prosthesis and surgical approach are interrelated, it is reasonable to suggest that each prosthetic design be used with the approach proposed by its originator. The choice, however, also must be based on the functional outcome, which must be reproducible and which achieves maximum accuracy during insertion of the prosthesis with minimal complications, thus maximizing the life and function of the artificial joint.

When surgeons recommend new approaches or modifications they may claim certain merits for the approach itself while disregarding its disadvantages when applied to total hip arthroplasty procedure. Few new approaches are truly original; many are either modifications or rediscoveries of approaches already in use. It is beyond the scope of this text to describe all these approaches, their usefulness, and their disadvantages. For a comprehensive discussion of this topic the reader is referred to surgical texts.*

Reducing operative time and blood loss is of concern to most surgeons to minimize morbidity. Surgical technique also influences the speed of recovery. Whenever possible, the surgeon should approach the hip without detaching muscular insertions, since detachment prolongs recovery time and increases morbidity. The surgeon must weigh the advantages of an approach against significant disadvantages, such as restricted exposure leading to soft tissue damage from

heavy retraction or technical errors, such as malpositioning or compromise fixation of the components and inadequate correction of the deformities. These disadvantages are particularly critical when the patient shows a severe anatomical distortion or scarring from previous operations.

An important consideration in any surgical approach to the hip joint is the positioning of the patient on the operating table, best ascertained when "landmarks," such as both anterosuperior spines and the greater trochanter, can be palpated through the draping for orientation. In the original technique of McKee and Müller, as well as that of Charnley, the patient remains in the supine position. This facilitates positioning the components in reference to the pelvis. However, many surgeons modified these techniques by placing the patient in positions ranging from semiprone to lateral decubitus, and at times tilted a few degrees by elevating the operating side with a sandbag. Regardless of the surgical approach used, if the surgeon disregards the position of the patient on the table, the positioning of the components may be compromised. In choosing an approach, it is important that the surgeon consider patient position so that the components will be accurately oriented.

Many surgical approaches to the hip have been described for specific operations, but some are not necessarily suitable for total hip arthroplasty. For example, Moore's "southern exposure" was designed for the insertion of the Moore self-locking prosthesis,[66,67] and while it is quite sufficient for this purpose, it is inadequate for total hip arthroplasty when acrylic cement is used. This surgical approach produces a deep wound with inadequate access to the stump of the femur or the acetabulum; correcting the deformity may be difficult, particularly if extensive capsular release and mobilization of the upper femur are necessary.

Because more exposure is required for unrestricted access to the soft tissue and bone in total hip

---

* References 1, 7, 12, 13, 27, 47.

arthroplasty, the incision must be extensive to avoid injury to the skin and soft tissue. The incision must be versatile so that the surgeon can obtain additional exposure of deep anatomical planes if difficulties are encountered during the operation. The incision must be away from the perineum to avoid contamination and pressure on the suture line during recovery. To spare operative time, it must not be excessively complicated, involving tedious dissection and potential violation of neurovascular structures.

COMMON SURGICAL APPROACHES

Approaches commonly used in hip surgery are categorized according to anatomical planes of exposure, as follows: anterior, anterolateral, direct lateral, lateral (transtrochanteric), posterolateral, posterior, and combined anterolateral and posterolateral.

Anterior Approach

Fahey[34], Heuter-Schade,[86] Jergenson and Abbott,[50] Luck,[58] and Smith-Petersen[6,83,84] described and popularized common anterior approaches.

Despite extensive use of Smith-Petersen cup arthroplasty in the United States and Europe, the anterior approach has not gained popularity in total hip arthroplasty because extensive time and intervention with muscle attachments are usually necessary to provide complete exposure. Further, as with most anterior approaches, the Smith-Petersen approach requires extensive detachment of tendinous insertions and retraction of muscle, with potential for heterotopic ossification and damage to vital structures such as the femoral nerve. Disturbance of the lateral cutaneous

nerve of the thigh, with resultant numbness and "meralgia paresthetica," is another common complication of this approach. However, a limited anterior approach using only a segment of the Smith-Petersen approach is quite suitable for procedures such as biopsy.

Light[56] has claimed that an anterior approach involving tensor fascia lata splitting has produced a satisfactory exposure with minimum morbidity for primary total hip arthroplasty. This approach, similar to other modifications of the Smith-Petersen approach,[57,59] may produce adequate access to the acetabulum. However, it impedes access to the femur because of the bulk of the abductors, a handicap similar to those produced by other anterior or anterolateral approaches such as the Watson-Jones approach.

Anterolateral Approaches

The anterolateral approach without trochanteric osteotomy was popularized for total hip arthroplasty by McKee[63] and Müller.[73]

Müller,[74] one of the proponents of surgery without osteotomy of the greater trochanter, believes that adequate instrumentation and an incision adequate for the exposure of the acetabular cavity and femoral neck produce results as good as those of osteotomy in more than 90% of primary operations. He believes that osteotomy is required in only about 10% of all cases, in which it will diminish the risk of breakage of the femoral shaft in severe osteoporotic or obese patients or when ankylosis is present. Müller has stated that the only reason he sees for osteotomy of the greater trochanter in any case is that after osteotomy it is easier to push the prosthesis down the femoral shaft into the

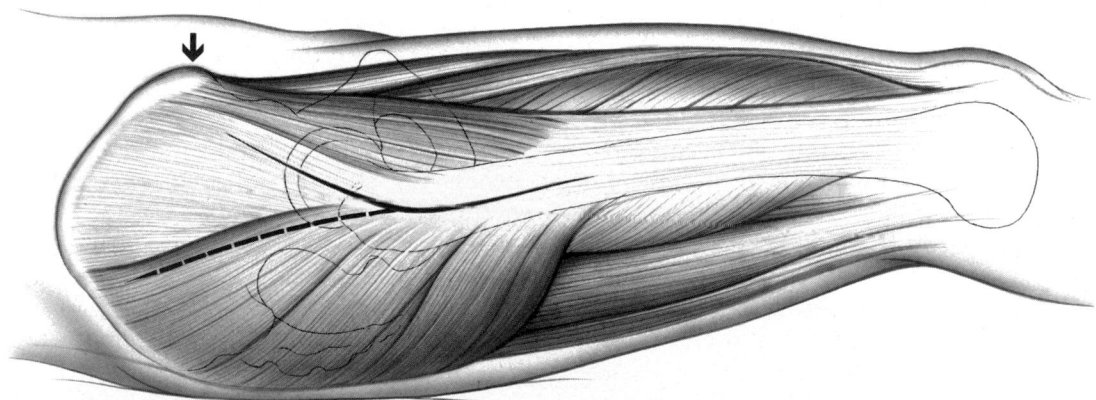

Fig. 3-1. With the anterolateral approach, the patient must be in supine position. The original incision described by Watson-Jones is curved toward the anterior superior iliac spine. For total hip replacement the proximal limb of the incision should extend toward the posterior superior iliac spine *(dotted line)* for approximately 2 to 3 cm beyond the level of the anterior superior iliac spine.

correct valgus position, giving a better headward expansion of the cement and thus a better bond between bone and cement. In his vast experience with total hip arthroplasty, Müller used an anterolateral exposure. Originally described by Watson-Jones,[91] this approach is versatile and provides good exposure of the neck of the femur and hip joint. The incision begins 1 inch distal and 1 inch posterior to the anterosuperior iliac spine, curves distally and laterally to the tip of the greater trochanter, and extends toward the lateral surface of the femoral shaft to 2 inches distal to the base of the trochanter (Fig. 3-1). The anatomical plane for this approach is between the glutei laterally and the tensor fascia femoris medially (Fig. 3-2).

To allow anterior dislocation of the femoral head, a complete capsulectomy is performed, including the fibers of the reflected head of the rectus femoris (anteriorly) and the vastus lateralis (inferiorly) (Fig. 3-3). The branch of superior gluteal nerve to the tensor fascia femoris is found at the interval between the gluteus medius and tensor fascia femoris; this nerve may inadvertently be damaged when exposing the capsule of the joint (Fig. 3-4). Dislocation is sometimes possible after complete capsulectomy and removal of osteophytes as well. The surgeon dislocates the head by traction, external rotation, and adduction, and cuts the neck at the desired level with a reciprocating or oscillating saw. The head is removed in a retrograde fashion, and exposure of the acetabulum is completed with the aid of Hohmann-type retractors (placed anteriorly, posteriorly, and occasionally one inferiorly). During insertion of pointed Hohmann retractors or preparation of the acetabulum with reamers, injury to the neurovascular structures at the acetabular level can occur. Care must be taken to keep the retractors close to the bone and to use the reamers judiciously to avoid the serious neurovascular complications associated with this approach (Fig. 3-5).

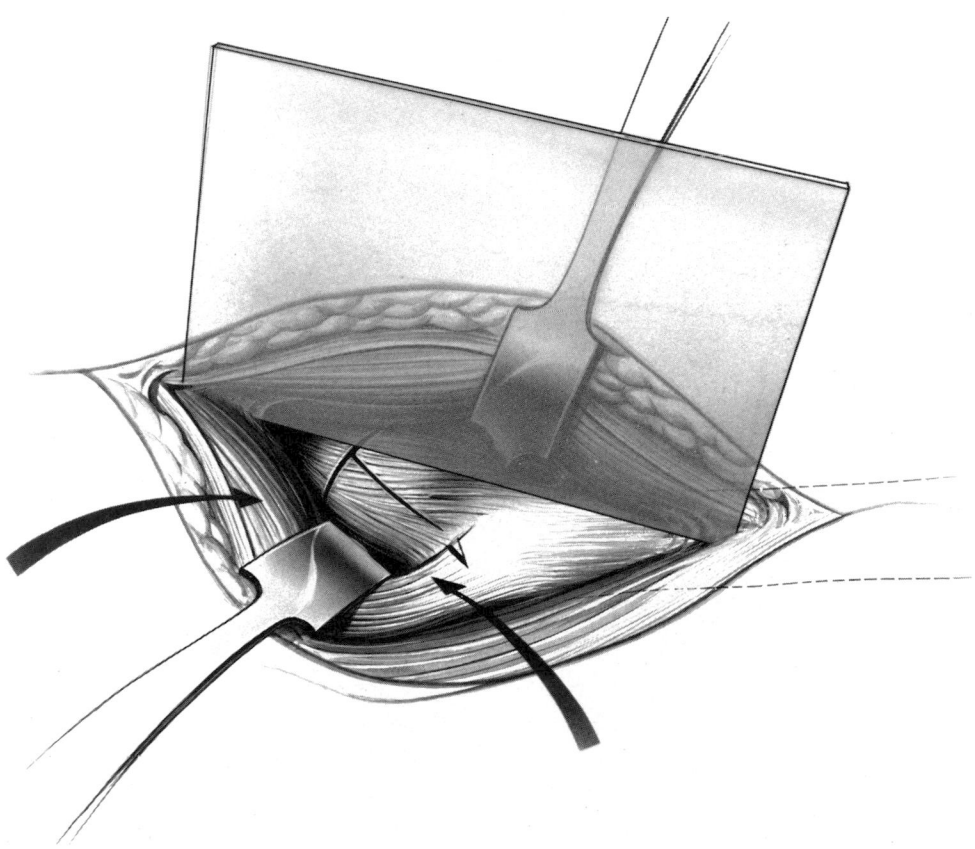

Fig. 3-2. The anatomical plane for anterolateral approach. The anterior capsule is exposed by retraction of the gluteus medius posteriorly and the tensor fascia femoris anteriorly. Heavy retraction of the gluteus medius and minimus is necessary to visualize the width of the neck and the periphery of capsule. A portion of the gluteus medius and minimus tendon may have to be detached to provide exposure. T-shaped incision of the capsule facilitates complete capsulectomy, which is necessary for this exposure. Arrows indicate excess tension on the muscle requiring release from the femur to avoid avulsion.

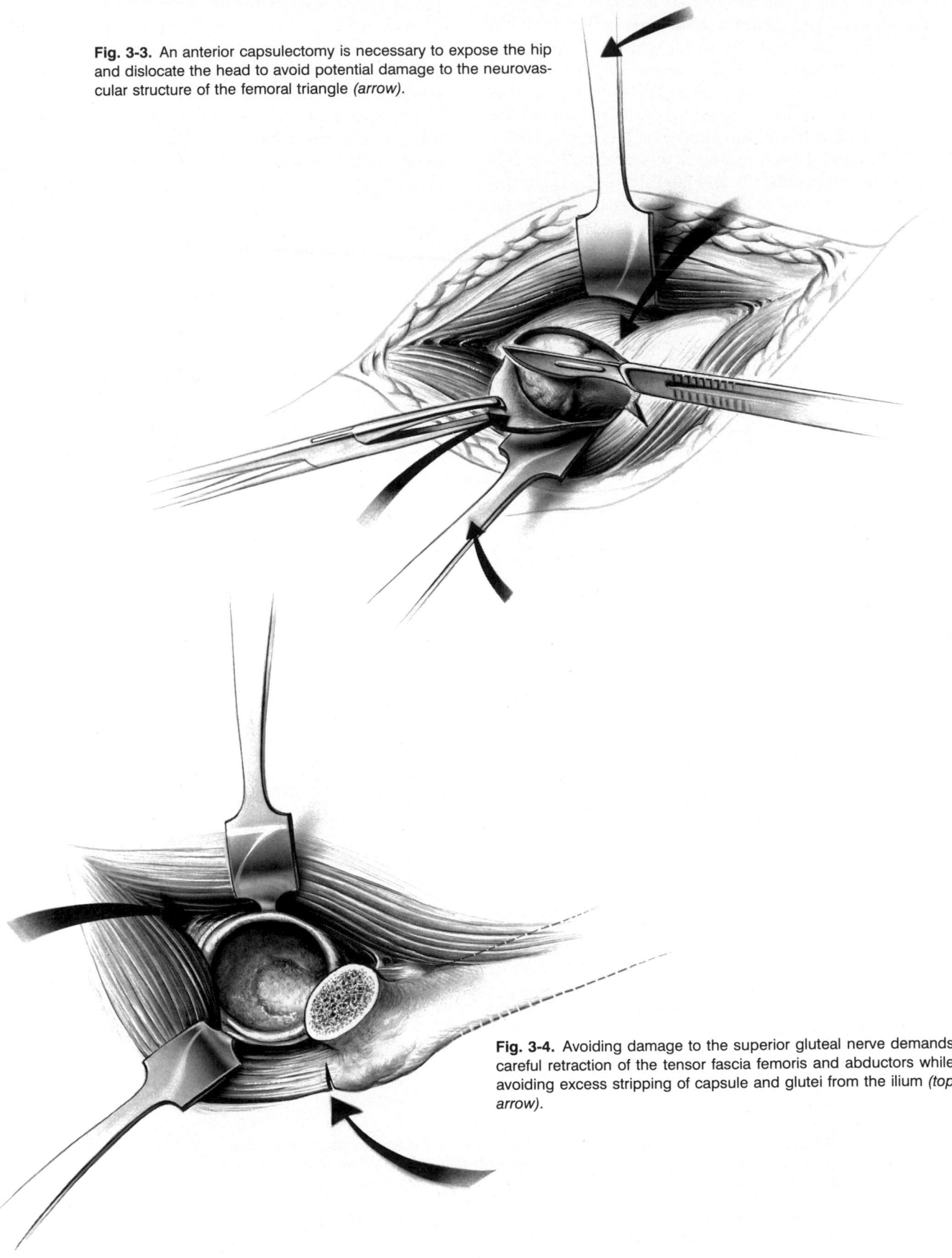

Fig. 3-3. An anterior capsulectomy is necessary to expose the hip and dislocate the head to avoid potential damage to the neurovascular structure of the femoral triangle *(arrow)*.

Fig. 3-4. Avoiding damage to the superior gluteal nerve demands careful retraction of the tensor fascia femoris and abductors while avoiding excess stripping of capsule and glutei from the ilium *(top arrow)*.

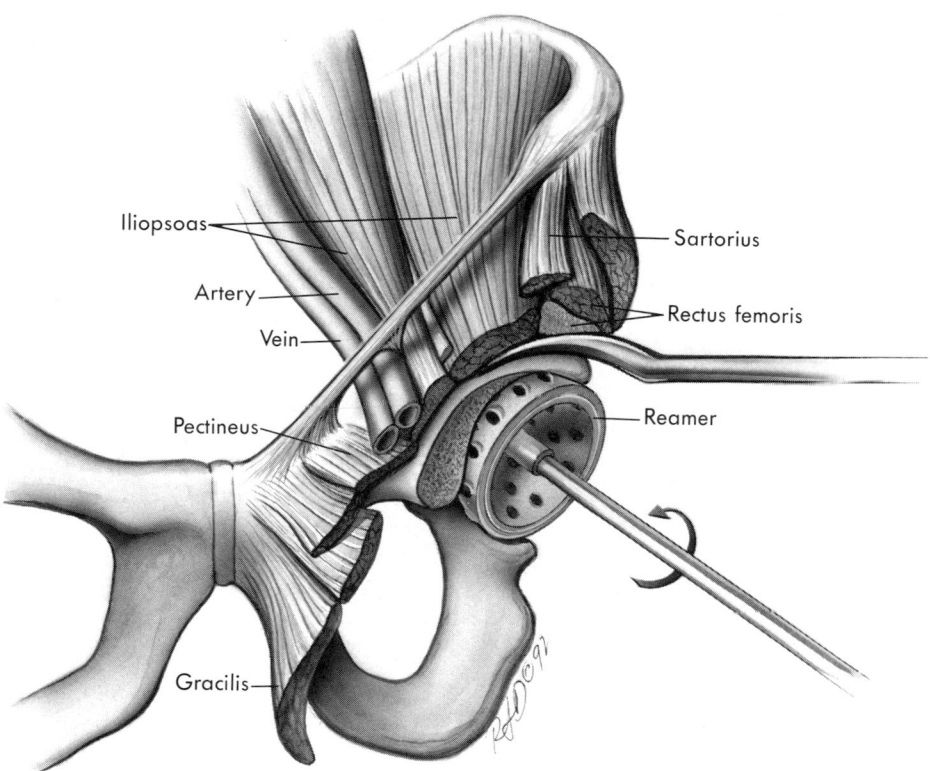

Fig. 3-5. Correct insertion of the anterior retractor and reamer. Because of the proximity of the femoral nerve, artery, and vein to the anterior rim of the acetabulum, pointed Hohmann retractors must be kept as close to the bone as possible. Excess damage to a deficient anterior wall of the acetabulum (iliopubic ramus) by reamers may also damage these structures.

With this approach, the short external rotators may be divided by placing the limb in external rotation; in particular, the piriformis should be placed under tension, pulled forward on a bone hook, and cut with a knife. During preparation of the medullary canal, a wide retractor with narrow points is placed under the greater trochanter to lift the femur forward. The glutei are protected by a second small retractor, and the third retractor is hooked under the psoas muscle. Insertion of broaches should provide anteversion of no more than 10 degrees. The transcondylar axis of the knee serves as a reference. To expose the opening of the neck of the femur, considerable external rotation is necessary. To improve access, a portion of the gluteal tendon may be detached from the trochanter. Müller has emphasized the proper insertion of Hohmann retractors for better exposure in conjunction with this approach.[73] Figs. 3-3 through 3-5 demonstrate the site of application of these retractors during the exposure of the hip.

A complication associated with the anterolateral approach is potential damage to the femoral shaft and malpositioning of the femoral stem. During preparation of the femur, the curved broaches must be inserted as lateral as possible to avoid damage (perforation of the femoral shaft). To lateralize insertion of the broaches, some damage to the abductors is unavoidable because a major portion of the abductors lies anterior to the femur and trochanter (Fig. 3-6).

For further details of the Müller techniques and their anterolateral approach, see Chapter 17.[62,73]

Direct Lateral Approach (Transgluteal)

The direct lateral approach is based on an anatomical observation by McFarland and Osborne that the gluteus medius and minimus and the vastus lateralis are in functional continuity.[62] This approach, which is considered an improvement over Kocher's method, bisects the thick and firm periosteum covering the greater trochanter while preserving continuity of the conjoined tendinoperiosteal attachment of the two muscles, the gluteus minimus and medius proximally and the vastus lateralis distally (Fig. 3-7). Hardinge first popularized this approach for total hip arthroplasty and termed it a "direct lateral approach to the hip."[41] The obvious advantage of this approach is to obviate osteotomy of the greater trochanter and to allow, by the incision's midlateral position, access to the

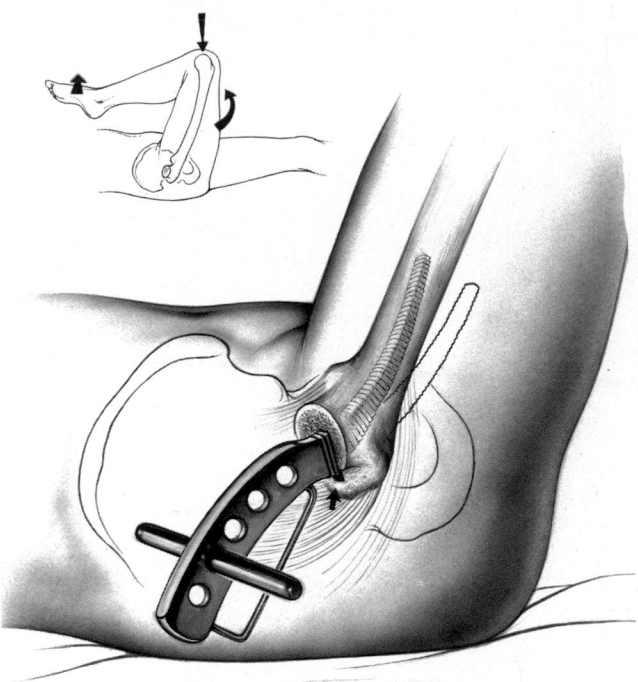

Fig. 3-6. Forceful external rotation, flexion, and abduction of the lower extremity are required during preparation of the femur. Broaches must be inserted as lateral as possible to avoid perforation of the femur shaft or a varus orientation of the stem. Lower arrow indicates the site of injury to abductors as the broach is being inserted.

front and back of the hip joint. This approach has been modified and described by Bauer and co-workers,[8] McLaughlin,[65] Hungerford,[49] Hardinge,[41] and Head.[46] Preferably the patient should be positioned supine (as described by Hardinge) but at the surgeon's preference may also be positioned in a lateral decubitus position. The surgeon makes the incision in the midlateral position along the shaft of the femur. The fascia is opened along the entire length of the incision, which is also midlateral, allowing a good view of the greater trochanter at the center of the wound. The deeper layer of the approach is "nonanatomical" in that the gluteus medius muscle and tendon are incised by electric knife (Fig. 3-8). The surgeon continues the incision distally through the fibers of the vastus lateralis near the anterior surface of the femur. Sharp dissection separates the anterior position of the gluteus minimus and the anterior capsular reinforcing ligament, revealing the capsule of the joint, which is incised circumferentially. The continuity of the strong tendon of the gluteus medius (located posteriorly) attached to the femur and the vastus lateralis is essential in this approach. Repair of the abductor tendons and muscle and vastus lateralis muscle is also essential to provide a good functional result. Hardinge recommends closure in three layers, the first consisting of the iliofemoral ligament, the second of the

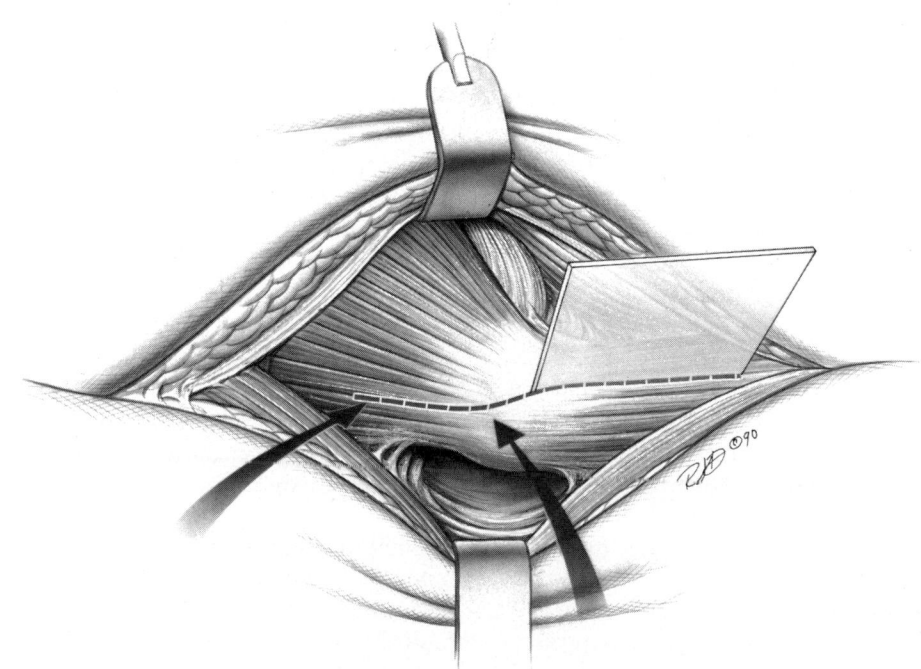

Fig. 3-7. The direct lateral approach as a "nonanatomical" route to the hips *(dotted line)*. The vastus lateralis is split down to the femur (one third medially and two thirds laterally), then the incision is swung backwards as it splits the gluteus medius one third posteriorly, two thirds anteriorly. The superior gluteal nerve is located within 5 cm of the tip of the greater trochanter *(arrows)*.

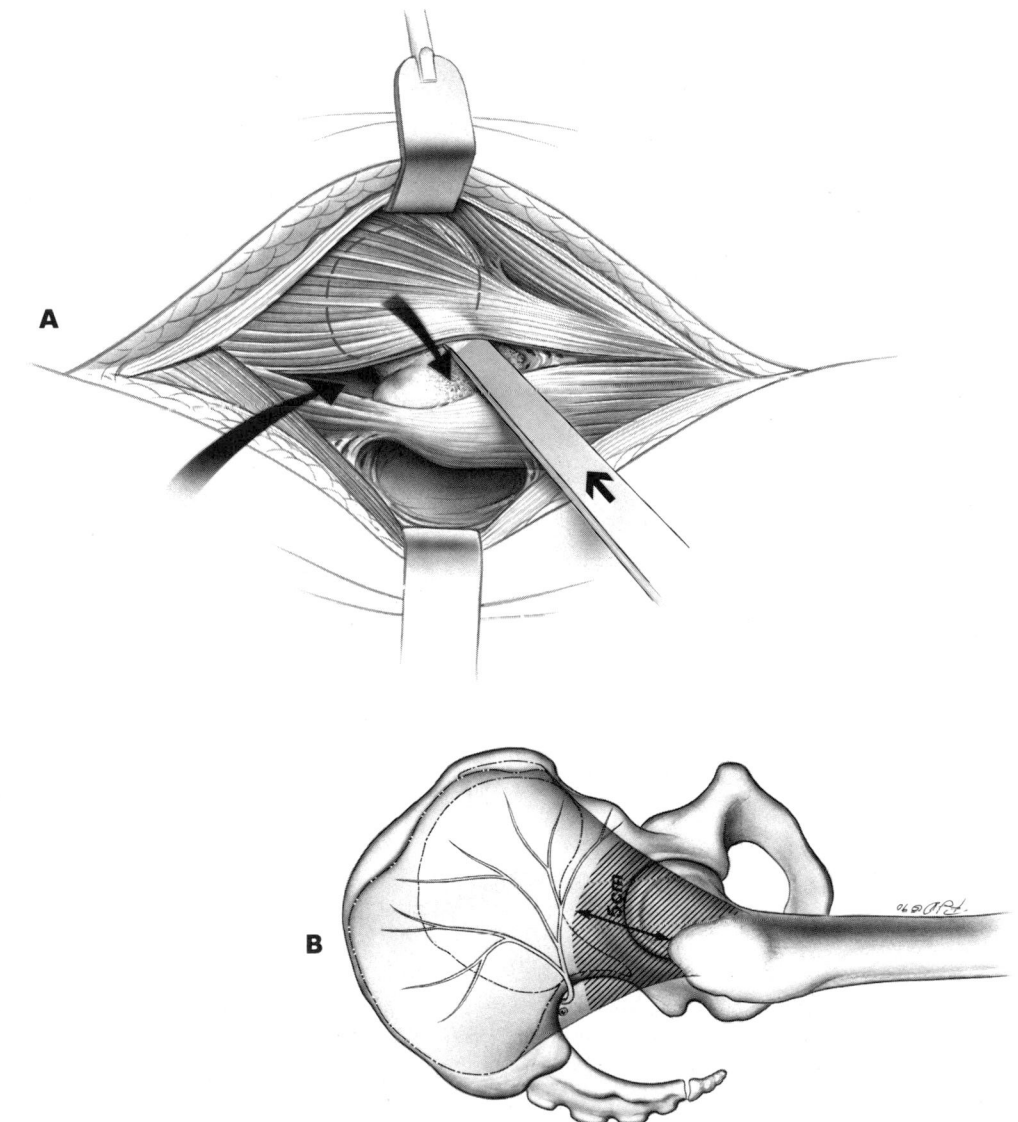

Fig. 3-8. A, Deeper dissection for the direct lateral approach includes sharp detachment of the insertion of the gluteus minimus, medius, and vastus from the femur while avoiding injury to the superior gluteal nerve. **B,** Location of superior gluteal nerve and its relationship to the acetabulum and the tip of the greater trochanter. Shaded area is considered the "safe zone" for surgery.

tendon of the gluteus medius, and the third of the iliotibial band and gluteal fascia.

Others have recommended an "osteoperiosteal" flap consisting of the capsule and gluteus minimus for subsequent repair of the anterior aspect of the hip joint.[35,46] Also, the length of the incision is extended with a further extensile development of the tissue for dealing with complex reconstructions and revisions.[46]

In addition to the inevitable damage to the abductors, a significant disadvantage of the direct lateral approach is the limitations on the proximal limb of the incision in the acetabular region; the incision can damage the superior gluteal nerve if it is extended too far proximally (see Chapter 2). The superior gluteal nerve exits

the pelvis above the piriformis muscle and runs transversely, laterally, and forward between the gluteus medius and gluteus minimus as it branches off to give innervation to both of these muscles. It also supplies a terminal branch to the tensor fascia femoris muscle. According to Brash, the branches to the gluteus medius enter deep, while innervation to the gluteus minimus is on the superficial surface at about midposition.[15] Hardy evaluated seven patients clinically and electromyographically for neuropraxis, axonotmesis, or neurotmesis of branches of the superior gluteal nerve after a direct lateral approach for total hip arthroplasty.[42] All patients had undergone primary total hip arthroplasty for osteoarthritis of the hip; they were randomly selected. Six of the seven patients were asymptomatic, but one required revision surgery. One patient (a fit woman) exhibited electromyogram (EMG) changes suggestive of mild neurological changes in the tensor fascia lata and gluteus medius on the affected side but none on the opposite side. Another patient also showed bilateral EMG evidence suggestive of mild bilateral nerve root irritation (without any symptom of a lumbar nerve root problem). Others did not seem to show any clinical or EMG evidence of detectable disturbances in the function of the gluteus medius or tensor fascia lata.

This approach also imposes limitations by an ability to distract the hip joint for lengthening the limb or accommodating the prosthesis if the head of the femur has preoperatively been displaced proximally (Shenton's lines broken) or in patients with severe deformity, such as flexion and adduction.

Lateral Transtrochanteric Approach

No approach can be considered truly lateral unless the greater trochanter is removed or the abductor tendons are disinserted or removed from it.[16,26] For this reason, the transgluteal, lateral transtrochanteric, and anterolateral or posterolateral approaches are distinguished. The lateral transtrochanteric approach, as originally described by Ollier in 1881, was made with a U-shaped skin incision at the trochanteric level.[27] This approach, which included trochanteric osteotomy, has been modified by many surgeons. Murphy, for instance, added a longitudinal extension at the midpoint ("goblet" incision).[27] Charnley remained faithful to this surgical approach, using a straight midline incision. He used it for central stabilization and central dislocation arthrodesis of the hip joint. I have used a modified oblique incision and, like Brady, find that it further improves exposure.[14] Aufranc and Stinchfield used a modification of Charnley's skin incision extensively in their work with mold arthroplasty.[6] In describing this approach, Harris[43,44] recommended it only for operations requiring extensive exposure.

Charnley uncompromisingly believed that a transtrochanteric approach was of fundamental importance in performing total hip arthroplasty.[23] He never minimized the disadvantage of failing to achieve bony union after osteotomy of the greater trochanter. He believed that reattachment of the greater trochanter tested the surgeon's natural mechanical instincts.[23,25] From an anatomical standpoint, Charnley's view on the surgical approach for total hip arthroplasty may be best summarized in the following quotation:

> The most gentle way of retracting the gluteus medius and minimus is by detaching the greater trochanter. In a heavy muscled patient a considerable volume of gluteus medius lies anterior to the greater trochanter. How much of this

muscle remains active after anterior exposure without detaching [the] trochanter is unknown. To the damage that retraction may inflict on the gluteal muscles may be added the danger of damaging the nerve supply of the tensor fasciae femoris.

While trochanteric problems were almost entirely eliminated under Charnley's hand, a 5% radiological failure of trochanteric union persisted.[10] Among residents in postgraduate training, the incidence of this complication was 2.3 times higher (11.5%). Methods of detachment and reattachment of the trochanter are discussed in Chapters 18 and 19. Among these methods, no technique is 100% perfect.

This author believes that transtrochanteric lateral approach is the safest approach in total hip arthroplasty; it is more physiologically sound when the greater trochanter is detached, providing that the union of the greater trochanter can be ensured by its subsequent firm reattachment to the lateral aspect of the shaft. While this approach provides wide exposure both anteriorly and posteriorly, it does not interfere with neurovascular structures of the hip, and muscle fibers are spared from damage by avoidance of heavy retraction. Transtrochanteric lateral approach is particularly suitable for total hip arthroplasty because it permits correction of deforming soft tissue structures where difficult anatomical situations are present, and it permits restoration of the tension and functional capacity of the abductor mechanism when the muscle fiber length is restored after transfer of the greater trochanter. The surgeon achieves good visualization of the anterior and posterior aspects of the hip during dislocation, having a full view of the entire acetabulum after dislocation.

Before osteotomy of the greater trochanter, the surgeon can enter the interval between the tensor fascia femoris medially and the anterior border of the gluteus medius and minimus laterally, sparing the nerve to the tensor fascia femoris (Fig. 3-9). The capsule of the joint is incised but may be excised if absolutely necessary. Unlike the anterolateral or posterolateral approaches, dislocation of the hip (even in the most anatomically deformed hips) can be achieved without torsional forces on the femur. With simple adduction of the femur the femoral head escapes the depth of the acetabulum (Fig. 3-10). A complete capsulectomy is not needed to obtain access to the acetabulum. Posteriorly, this approach permits detachment of the short rotators from the upper femur and the piriformis tendon from the greater trochanter as needed. Troublesome bleeding of the posterior shaft after detachment of short rotators can readily be controlled. With this exposure, potential damage to the sciatic nerve and the femoral nerve and artery is very rare. Chapters 18 and 19 details this surgical approach

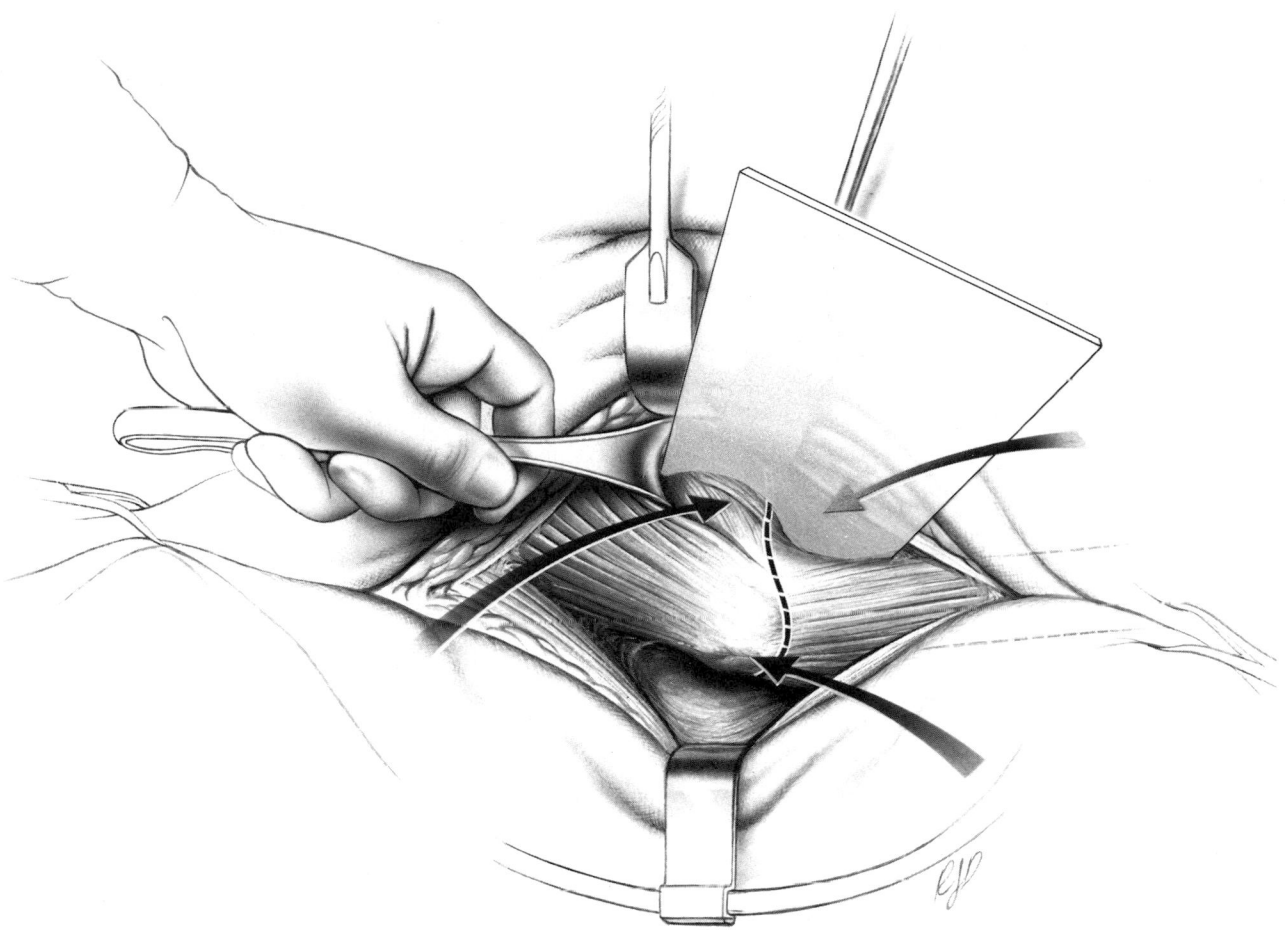

Fig. 3-9. The plane of the interval *(right arrows)* between the tensor fascia femoris muscle and the glutei; the capsule has been revealed *(left arrow)*. The vastus lateralis ridge is the main reference for the level of trochanteric osteotomy on the femur *(lower arrow)*.

as used in total hip arthroplasty.

On the debit side of this approach is the nonunion and migration of the greater trochanter, which can occur in as many as 2% to 5% of cases. This complication is the main concern that caused this author to abandon this approach in favor of other approaches (without osteotomy of the trochanter). This author believes that if the surgeon is experienced in using (and observing) details of the surgical technique, he or she will soon be able to perform up to nearly 90% of total hip arthroplasties without detaching the greater trochanter. Thus transtrochanteric approach must be reserved for revision and difficult anatomical situations. During the 1970s and 1980s, improvements in total hip arthroplasty technology related to the prosthesis and instrumentation led this author to conclude that the posterolateral approach provides the best exposure for nontranstrochanteric exposure of the hip (see Chapter 16). As such, I reserve the transtrochanteric approach for large-muscled in-

dividuals and difficult anatomical deformities, such as congenital dislocation, revision surgery, and so on.

Modifications of the Transtrochanteric Approach

Modifications of the transtrochanteric approach are included with the intention that these modifications will be used for more successful reattachment and bony union. Glassman and Engh introduced and used the first modification.[39] Their approach takes advantage of an intact musculotendinous continuity comprising the gluteus medius and vastus lateralis firmly attached to the trochanter. By keeping the vastus lateralis attached to the trochanter as the trochanter is osteotomized, the stability of the trochanter is ensured, providing a safeguard against its proximal migration.

The second modification of trochanteric osteotomy was based on a direct lateral approach to the hip. Similar to the modification of Glassman and Engh, it depends on the observation that the gluteus medius and vastus lateralis are in direct functional continuity

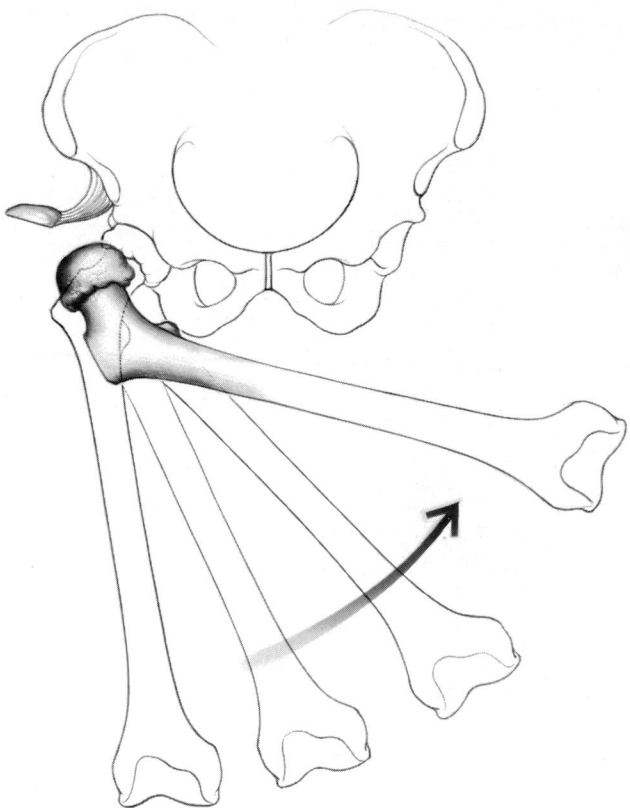

Fig. 3-10. Hip dislocation after transtrochanteric approach is facilitated by capsular release and retraction of the trochanter. Only modest adduction is required (without external or internal rotation) to dislocate the hip.

through their thick covering and insertion to the trochanter.[62] The Stracathro approach, described by McLaughlin,[65] involves splitting the gluteus medius in the line of its fibers and obtaining two rectangular slices of the trochanter, one anteriorly and one posteriorly, with an osteotome. Retraction of the two sections reveals the gluteus minimus, which is split in the line of its fibers. The hip is then dislocated anteriorly. McLaughlin claims that in more than 2000 hips this approach has produced an "excellent result," the only complication being occasional discomfort in the region of the greater trochanter during the first 3 months postoperatively.

The third modification was introduced by Dall,[28] who proposed an anterior osteotomy of the greater trochanter, leaving the major portion of the gluteus medius tendon attachment to the greater trochanter intact. The clear advantages of this technique are that the nerve supply to the gluteus minimus, gluteus medius, and tensor fascia femoris is not compromised, the abductor function remains intact (as a result of continuity of the tendinous junction between the anterior half of the gluteus medius and vastus lateralis), and the remaining abductor muscle and tendon

maintain continuity with the vastus lateralis. With this technique, osteotomy of the greater trochanter can be accomplished intracapsulary or extracapsulary. Reattachment of the greater trochanter frequently is easy because of stability from the continuity of the anterior fibers of the gluteus medius and minimus tendons with the vastus lateralis, and as described by Dall, because the vastus lateralis is supplied by branches of the femoral nerve, which enter it at the deep surface of the proximal and middle third.[15] To avoid denervation, this muscle should be split as posterior as possible. "Half" osteotomy of the anterior trochanter is attractive for its stability, ease of reattachment of the trochanter, and maintenance of abductor function and for avoiding denervation of the superior gluteal nerve to the gluteus minimus and tensor fascia femoris. As stated by Dall, however, this approach may not be adequate if destruction of the joint is necessary to gain length or in revision surgery.

Controversy over the Routine Transtrochanteric Approach

This aspect of total hip arthroplasty technique remains controversial.* Three schools of thought are represented:

- Recommendation of routine trochanteric osteotomy in all cases.
- Advocacy of removal only in difficult anatomical situations.
- Recommendation of total arthroplasty without trochanteric osteotomy.

While controversy over the need for routine osteotomy of the greater trochanter continues, I believe this approach is indispensable in difficult anatomical situations and revision surgery. When adopted as a routine technique by surgeons who devote their careers to the surgery of the hip joint, the advantages are obvious and rewarding. In theory, osteotomy and transfer of the greater trochanter improve the mechanical situation of the hip and increase stability against dislocation. Based on personal clinical and teaching experience, I believe that the abductor muscle is better protected because it remains undamaged when the greater trochanter is removed. Certainly, a less experienced surgeon has a greater margin of safety with the removal of the trochanter. This is particularly true when the surgeon faces an unexpectedly difficult anatomical situation at surgery, but he or she is also less confined when fixed deformity and severe contractures are present.

Disadvantages attributed to trochanteric osteotomy include increased blood loss and operative time, delayed postoperative ambulation, nonunion, symp-

---

* References 53–55, 64, 79, 82, 85, 87, 89.

tomatic nonunion, rupture of wires (used for fixation of the greater trochanter), painful bursitis, and dislocations resulting from separation of the trochanter.[3,32,33,73] These problems, however (see Chapter 37), must be balanced against the advantages, real and theoretical (Table 3-1). Complications of trochanteric osteotomy can be kept to a minimum only when the surgeon masters the technique by routine experience.

The most serious complication resulting from the transtrochanteric approach is a nonunion that accompanies migration, resulting in a limp and a hip that dislocates early or late postoperatively.

The criticism that osteotomy necessitates increased operating time and greater blood loss requires further study under controlled conditions for clarification. The criticism may be valid for surgeons who perform trochanteric osteotomy only in cases of technical difficulty in which extra time and blood loss would be routinely encountered regardless of the technique.

The question remains whether the greater trochanter should be osteotomized routinely or only in difficult cases. Routine osteotomy of the greater trochanter provides the surgeon with unique experience in its handling, proper removal, and reattachment; with familiarity and practice, the surgeon's efficiency increases. During surgery, therefore, the time spent removing and reattaching the trochanter will be regained because ease of exposure and better access

Table 3-1 Advantages and Disadvantages of Trochanteric Osteotomy

Theoretical and practical advantages	Theoretical and practical criticism
Wide and extensive exposure	Increased operating time
Improved mechanics of the hip	Handling of the trochanter at surgery
Protection of anatomical structures	Delayed weight bearing postoperatively
Correction of fixed deformity	Increased blood loss
Ease of dislocation at operation	Trochanteric bursitis
	Trochanteric nonunion
Ease of preparation of acetabulum and femur	Painful nonunion
Ease of insertion of components	Breakages of wire and migration
Improved cement fixation technique	
Improved stability after surgery	
Improved quality of clinical results	
Low incidence of mechanical failure	

facilitate proper surgical implantation of the prosthesis. Regular use of osteotomy by the experienced surgeon reduces the number of technical complications in handling the greater trochanter. This experience is not gained if the surgeon osteotomizes the trochanter only occasionally, that is, in difficult cases. In these surgical situations, trochanteric complications are increased, and it is in these cases in particular that a good reattachment is of paramount importance for stability. Facileness gained from previous trochanteric experience will increase the probability of a straightforward, uncomplicated operation requiring minimum time and effort and ending with good results. Moreover, it is not always feasible to predict the difficulty or ease of a case by x-ray films and clinical examination before surgery and thus plan whether the trochanter should be removed or not.

It is often stated that rehabilitation is slow, and the patient must remain in bed for a longer time when the greater trochanter is removed. This is simply untrue. Rehabilitation after low-friction arthroplasty with routine osteotomy of the greater trochanter is not restricted because of the surgery on the trochanter. In the first 48 to 72 hours the patient is unable to move out of bed because of general recovery from surgery. When the trochanter has been well attached, there should be no difference in postoperative management and rehabilitation between these patients and those operated on without osteotomy of the greater trochanter.

However, even the most experienced surgeon encounters occasional intraoperative problems such as fracture of the trochanter or severe osteopenia of the bone for which a protective cast or brace may be required with additional and extended nonweight bearing. Bursitis resulting from the use of hardware is relatively uncommon, and only a few patients have symptoms severe enough that require wire removal postoperatively (see Chapter 37).

Rationale for Routine Trochanteric Osteotomy

Charnley advocated a routine transtrochanteric approach in total hip arthroplasty.[22,23]

The rationale for routine trochanteric osteotomy may be considered within the framework of three major areas: (1) biomechanical theory, (2) technical aspects, and (3) restoration of function.

BIOMECHANICAL THEORY The biomechanical advantages of trochanteric osteotomy include:

- Reduction of socket load (wear and loosening)
- Reduction of stem load (loosening and fatigue fracture)
- Improved abductor power (excellence of gait)

Pauwels has analyzed the biomechanical principles of the moments of force on the hip joint, and Rydels practically related the load on the joint to muscular function based on analysis of the level arm systems.*

As noted in Chapter 6, the socket load may be reduced by medial displacement of the socket, lateral displacement of the abductor mechanism or both. An elongation of the neck of the femoral prosthesis might have the same result, with limited effect. A limp after total hip arthroplasty may be a "sparing" phenomenon adopted by the patient. It may create a "disadvantageous ratio of leverage" in the hip, with excessive compensatory muscle forces unnecessarily loading the implant. Loading the socket to such an extreme that the abductors do not function to their full capacity might cause future problems, even though short-term results are considered successful.

Equalization of the moments of the lever arms on the hip results in a reduction of the socket load, thus theoretically prolonging survival of the fixation. On the same theoretical basis, wear that is the function of both load and velocity can be minimized[19,21,70] (see Chapter 6).

Excess load on the socket may be detrimental and may cause eventual loosening of the prosthesis.†

Lateral displacement of the greater trochanter is the only means of lever arm equalization when the floor of the acetabulum cannot be deepened because of anatomical restrictions. When medial displacement and the greater trochanteric transfer are both possible, it is advantageous to use the latter for equalization of the lever arms in young patients to avoid excessive damage to the floor of the acetabulum by deepening. Unfortunately, because of the multifactor sources of mechanical failure, the theoretical advantages outlined cannot be proved on clinical documentation alone. However, good judgment indicates the advisability of taking advantage of all possible and theoretical features that might be of long-term value.

Documentation of these theoretical values in regard to wear and loosening is not possible for the following reasons.

1. Unfortunately, no documentation of long-term results is available using a 22-mm prosthetic head without detachment of the greater trochanter.
2. Degrees of deepening of the socket and lateral displacement cannot be independently evaluated in Charnley's operation.
3. Uncontrollable factors such as the patient's degree of activity and batch variations of plastics make comparison impossible.
4. Surgical technique, bone stock, bone pathology,

and so on are almost never compatible in all situations.

5. No comparable data are available from total hip arthroplasty procedures in which trochanteric osteotomy was not performed, but early clinical results seem to be satisfactory. The statistical data on the use of a large femoral head prosthesis without routine trochanteric osteotomy[24] are not conclusively unacceptable (see Chapter 28).
6. Finally, no one knows how much of the abductor muscle volume can be sacrificed by surgical trauma before a limp is produced or before it can be noted on mechanical testing of the abductors.

TECHNICAL ASPECTS

EXPOSURE OF THE ACETABULUM With removal of the greater trochanter, the surgeon can get a direct face-on view of the socket, as if he or she were looking in a tin with the lid off. When the self-retaining retractors are in place and the limb is in maximum adduction with 30 to 40 degrees flexion across the opposite thigh allowing direct access to the acetabulum, its depth is better exposed and deficiencies of the rim or walls or osteophytes are revealed. Heavy retraction of the glutei in muscular or obese patients is obviated. Without trochanteric osteotomy, when unexpected difficulties are encountered, the surgeon may be forced to release the adductor tendons segment by segment from their insertions onto the femur without any formal planning for their subsequent reattachment. By removing the greater trochanter, the surgeon is formally planning for its subsequent reattachment. It must be recognized that an excellent exposure of the acetabulum can also be achieved using periacetabular lever-type retractors. However, because of the required lateral decubitus position of the patient, an "exact" orientation of the cup cannot always be ascertained.

DISLOCATION OF THE HIP In a severely deformed hip accompanied by marked stiffness, attempts to dislocate the hip can fracture the femur.

Dislocation after osteotomy of the greater trochanter requires minimal manipulation of the shaft, a vital issue when severe osteoporosis or weakening of the femur is present as the result of a previously inserted nail and plates or a prosthesis (see Chapter 24). Dislocation is particularly difficult when the head of the femur or prosthesis has sunk into the pelvis and protrusio acetabuli is present (see Chapter 22).

EXPOSURE OF THE UPPER FEMUR During preparation and insertion of the femoral prosthesis the surgeon must be able to deliver the stump of the upper femur out of the depth of the wound. Failure to do this results in misjudgment of the direction of branches and stem, leading to unnecessary damage to the upper femur or malpositioning of the component. Addition-

---

* References 5, 19, 21, 22, 25, 81.

† References 5, 20, 24, 70, 71, 75.

ally, in certain femora, a neutral or slightly vagus orientation of the stem may not be easy to achieve. In an attempt to lateralize broaches and reamers, partial damage to the abductors (without the attachment of the greater trochanter) may be unavoidable.

Unimpeded access to the top of the femur after trochanteric osteotomy also provides an excellent opportunity for the surgeon to deliver and pressurize the cement while avoiding admixture of blood or vendor problems related to the insertion of the stem. Also with detachment of the trochanter, mobilization of the upper femur allows ease of resection of heterotopic ossification, removal of previous hardware and prosthesis, and excision of scar to regain length for the extremity.

Nowhere is the need for mobilization of the upper femur better exemplified than in the case of a frankly congenital dislocation of the hip in which the medial upper femur is bound tightly against the wall of the pelvis, requiring resection of the soft tissue to lower the level of the hip joint. In this way, often as a benefit of the maneuver, considerable length is obtained.

Removal of a previous prosthetic stem without adequate exposure can be dangerous. An intramedullary femoral head prosthesis (cemented or noncemented) requires removal before replacement. After osteotomy of the greater trochanter, it is possible to enter the curve of the upper portion of the prosthesis and gain access to the stem or the bones of fenestration of the Moore self-locking prosthesis. An attempt to remove the prosthesis without removing the trochanter may lead to fracture of the femur. After osteotomy, the bed of the trochanter is the logical site to enter, using a reciprocating saw. A complete mobilization of the upper femur facilitates direct access to the medial aspect of the prosthesis, which allows placement of the chisel over the medial neck of the prosthesis for extractions. Most surgeons agree that in revision surgery (despite increased incidence of trochanteric complications) the transtrochanteric approach is preferred for better exposure and safety. Surgeons advocating a nontranstrochanteric approach in *all cases* of primary or revision are likely to treat major complications such as femoral fractures, nerve palsies, and dislocations as a "tradeoff" for a few nonunions of the trochanter in revision and anatomically difficult hips.[9]

SAFETY OF GLUTEI AND NERVE SUPPLY TO TENSOR FASCIA FEMORIS As stated previously, damage to the abductor system is often unavoidable when these muscles are well developed and the anterior segment is considerably hypertrophied. Paradoxically, very athletic men with a well-developed abductor system are more prone to injury of their hypertrophied muscles than are frail, elderly patients. With the anterior approach, heavy retraction (despite partial release of the abductor tendon from the trochanter) may be necessary for the acetabulum and may damage the anterior fibers of the glutei. At times, the nerve supply to the tensor fascia femoris may also be in jeopardy. Since it is an important abductor muscle and an important stabilizing element, damage to its nerve supply must be avoided. Further, considerable muscle damage may be incurred when lever-type retractors are applied to expose the acetabulum.

MUSCLE TENSION, LEG LENGTH, AND DISLOCATION With fixed flexion and adduction deformity, detachment of the greater trochanter allows a complete capsulectomy and removal of contracted tissues about the hip. Without detachment of the greater trochanter, the only means of stabilizing the hip is by increasing muscle tension across the hip by adding length to the limb using a long-neck prosthesis. Reattachment of the trochanter in a distal and lateral position provides an excellent means of stabilizing the hip while avoiding overlengthening of the extremity. In this author's practice, a low incidence of postoperative dislocation in revision surgery without overlengthening the limb may be attributable to the transtrochanteric approach and a lateral and distal transfer of the abductors (see Chapters 29 and 32).

RESTORATION OF FUNCTION AND ITS RESULTS As stated previously, a severely deformed hip can be restructured only with complete mobilization of the upper femur. In this way the hip joint is mechanically improved, the aim being full functional activity with an intact abductor mechanism (including the gluteus medius and minimus and the tensor fascia femoris). The fascial and muscular structure of the thigh can be compared to a sleeve that incorporates the iliotibial tract, as well as muscular septa of the thigh. Although these structures are somewhat inelastic beyond a given point of traction, nevertheless they function only when the length of the musculature has been placed with the appropriate tension and orientation. Therefore the degrees of advancement of the trochanter may be varied according to the demands in each technical situation. For example, the capsule and abductor muscles are heavily contracted in a high-riding nonunion of the neck of the femur with marked displacement or a failed pseudarthrosis. If the trochanter is not removed in cases of severe deformity, it is impossible to restore the good general alignment necessary for functional abductors.

Charnley[20] attributed the excellence of gait after low-friction arthroplasty to the transposition of the greater trochanter laterally and, to a lesser extent, the center of rotation of the hip medially.

Similarly, in experiences with cup arthroplasty, Johnston and Larson[51] found that shifting the central rotation of the hip medially and the greater trochanter laterally proportionally increased the frequency of negative Trendelenburg's tests. If these principles are applied to total hip arthroplasty, the procedure might more accurately be considered "total hip reconstructive arthroplasty" rather than resurfacing the diseased hip with an artificial hip joint.

In summary, the removal of the trochanter in total hip arthroplasty is not purely the surgeon's option for certain pathological deformities of the hip. It is an essential and intricate part of the procedure to ensure the short- and long-term success of total hip arthroplasty. For a statistical analysis of greater trochanteric complications, see Chapter 37.

Several studies have attempted to compare various surgical approaches for their safety, savings in operative and anesthesia time, savings in blood loss, ease of postoperative rehabilitation, clinical and radiological results, and operative complications. The validity of these studies is often compromised by the many factors that cannot be quantified by nonprospective, nonrandomized (double-blind), and nonquantifiable parameters, such as the surgeon's experience.*

A surgeon should never underestimate functional results. The surgeon should remain objective and truly make a "collective observation" on the overall clinical results, including total absence of pain, absence of limp, and excellent fixation of the prosthesis.[76] Although most reports emphasize a short operative time and less need for blood transfusion resulting from approaches without trochanteric osteotomy, in their comparisons they fail to indicate rates of injury to the neurovascular structures, dislocations, and above all, the long-term functional results of the arthroplasty, which should be the surgeon's prime interest. This author never underestimates loss of function after trochanteric nonunion and migration, postoperative limp, and occasional recurrent dislocation of the hip, all of which can be very damaging to the patient—and to the surgeon's pride.[76]

Additionally, one is struck by the fact that failure of fixation and even postoperative infection may result from an inadequate surgical exposure and excess trauma to the soft tissue, results that have generally been attributed to poor design of the prosthesis, use of acrylic cement, or lack of aseptic conditions in the operating room.

Posterior Approaches

As with anterior and lateral approaches to the hip, several posterior approaches have been described in the past century. Numerous modifications of the posterior approach involve the skin incision and deeper incision, and each has its limitations and advantages.* The posterior approach was first advised by von Langenbeck in 1874.[90] Kocher modified von Langenbeck's approach, as described by Dumont in 1887.[1] Procedures described by MacFarland and Osborne, Zahradnicek, and Moore are basically alterations of the original incision and Kocher's approach, later further modified by Gibson.[36–38] Other posterior approaches were devised by Ober,[77] Osborne,[78] Caldwell,[17] Henry,[47] and Horowitz.[48] Gibson's modification of the posterior approach was described in 1949[36] and further modified by Marcy and Fletcher.[66] I have found this approach and exposure of the hip without removal of the greater trochanter helpful for partial arthroplasty, such as insertion of a femoral head prosthesis, and for noncomplex total hip arthroplasty.[30]

Perhaps the most popular approach is Moore's "southern exposure,"[68,69] which is used extensively throughout the world in prosthetic replacement of the femoral head. Its advantages include relative ease and adequate exposure for insertion of a noncemented prosthesis. In this approach, the incision is begun approximately 4 inches distal to the posterosuperior iliac spine and is extended distally and laterally parallel with the fibers of the gluteus maximus to the posterior margin of the greater trochanter. It is then directed distally 4 or 5 inches parallel with the femoral shaft. In this approach the sciatic nerve is exposed and protected; it is not suitable for total hip arthroplasty because of its depth without easy access to the upper femur.

Posterolateral Approaches

Horowitz in 1952[54] and Marcy and Fletcher in 1954[66] described their modification of Gibson's approach. These modifications constitute a posterolateral approach to the hip joint. I[29,30] have used this modified approach[66] extensively and find it the most suitable approach for adequate exposure and access to the acetabulum and upper femur. It is a useful approach for the insertion of a femoral head prosthesis and total hip arthroplasty when performed without osteotomy of the greater trochanter. It is superior to the anterolateral approach of Watson-Jones as advocated by Müller and McKee. Its advantages include less forceful retraction of the glutei and better access to the upper end of the femur in a bloodless field.

As in the posterior approaches, the patient is placed in the lateral decubitus position (Fig. 3-11). However, the incision is made further anteriorly than in Moore's southern exposure (toward the posterosuperior in-

---

* References 4, 11, 18, 35, 40, 72, 79, 80, 88, 92.

* References 6, 36–38, 62, 66, 68.

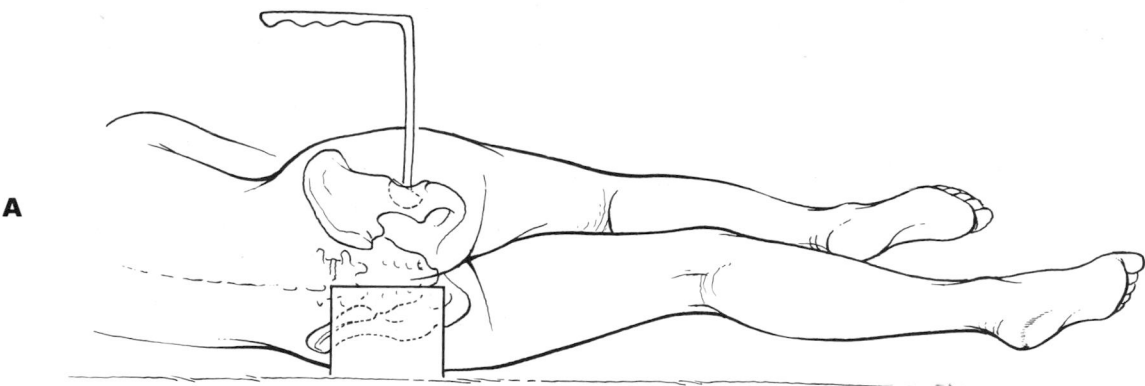

stead of the posteroinferior iliac spine), eliminating the possibilities of contamination of the incision and of the patient lying on the incision. In this surgical exposure there is no need to visualize the sciatic nerve, since the incision is located just behind the femoral shaft and the dividing muscle interval between the posterior border of the gluteus medius and the upper border of the fibers of the gluteus maximus; nevertheless, many surgeons using this approach prefer to visualize the sciatic nerve. There is no vascular structure along this approach line and no disturbance to any muscular attachments. In an obese patient who might require further exposure, however, one third of the posterior attachment of the gluteus medius tendon may be damaged (torn), resulting from heavy retraction or a part of trochanteric fracture.

Unlike the southern exposure, this approach gives the surgeon ready access to the acetabulum, obviating the need for retracting the huge bulk of gluteus maximus muscle fibers. The skin incision begins three fingers anterior to the posterosuperior spine and progresses to the greater trochanter and the second limb. It then extends distally along the femur for approximately 10 to 15 cm (Fig. 3-12). The fascia and gluteofemoral bursa are incised in line with the skin incision, and the interval between the posterior border of the gluteus medius and the anterior border of the gluteus maximus is then entered. By separating the

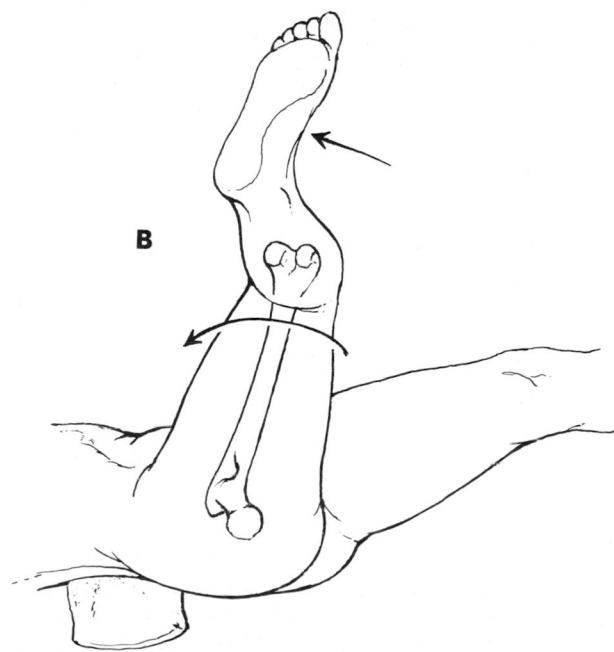

Fig. 3-11. A, Position of the patient on the operating table must be absolutely secured to make orientation of acetabular component possible with any degree of accuracy. **B,** During preparation of the femoral canal, maximum internal rotation of lower extremity is necessary to produce access to the upper end of the femur.

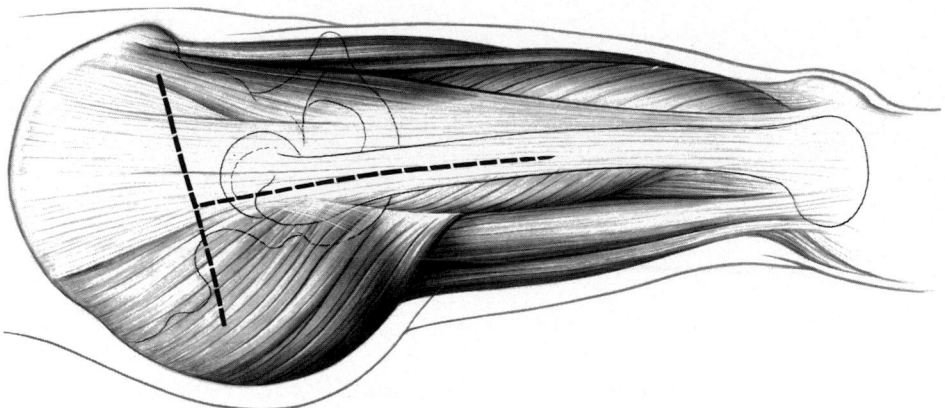

Fig. 3-12. Incision for posterolateral approach includes a midfemoral orientation distally (centered along the parallel fibers of iliotibial band) and is inclined proximally toward the posterior superior iliac spine. The incision will be located along the top bundle of gluteus maximus muscle.

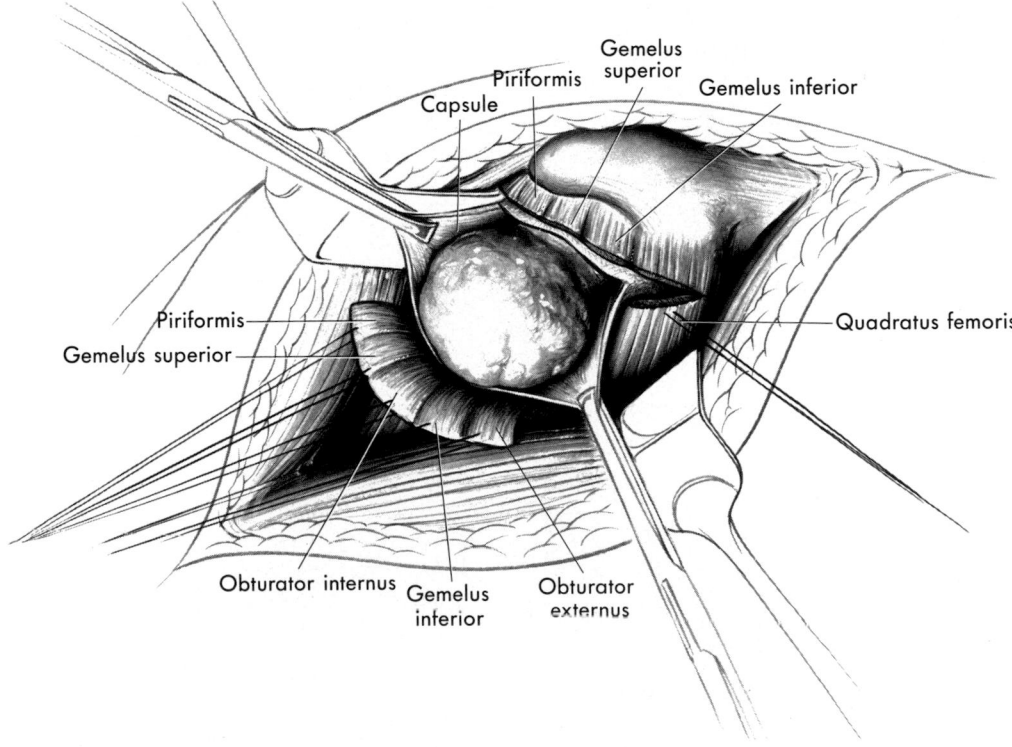

Fig. 3-13. The capsule is incised and retracted and the head is then dislocated by maximum and internal rotation of the hip positioned in flexion. All short rotators must be reattached to the posterior aspect of the femur (the trochanteric crest) with or without repair of the joint capsule.

gluteus minimus from the underlying capsule, this muscle can be retracted anteriorly and superiorly, thus exposing the capsule completely. Short rotators are then detached from the femur. The capsule is incised or excised as indicated to provide maximum exposure, preserving the anterior part but excising as much from the posterior and inferior segments as necessary to allow dislocation by internal rotations of the hip. With excision of the capsule and placement of Hohmann retractors (anteriorly and inferiorly), the acetabular exposure with this approach is complete and adequate. Dislocation of the hip joint is accomplished by maximum internal rotation (Fig. 3-13) (see Chapter 16).

The femur is placed anteriorly and retracted during the exposure of the acetabulum. Both the anterior and the inferior margins of the acetabulum can be conveniently exposed using lever-type retractors.

Preparation of the upper femur is possible by internal rotation of the femur and delivery of the end of the femur by a lever-type retractor. Capsular release may be required for ease of access to the top of the femur. Routine detachment of the gluteus maximus insertion to the femur facilitates the exposure. The gluteus maximus tendon must be reattached to the femur at the completion of the surgery. The transcondylar line of the femur is a guide for orientation of the broaches and the prosthesis. Good access for medullary reaming is possible after mobilization of the upper femur by detachment of the capsule as required.

The major disadvantages of this approach are:
1. The inability of the surgeon to assess the exact position of the pelvis on the table, thus the possibility of malpositioning the acetabular component. To overcome the problem, many methods, including insertion of a guide bar to the pelvis, have been suggested.[2]
2. The potential for sciatic nerve palsy despite efforts to locate, visualize, or protect the nerve during surgery. A higher incidence of sciatic neurapraxia, neurotmesis, and neurolysis has been recorded than with the transtrochanteric approach (see Chapter 15). However, this risk can be minimized by avoiding dissection around the nerve and avoiding placing a retractor near the nerve.
3. An increased incidence of postoperative dislocation of the hip has been recorded, which may be related to (a) malpositioning of the acetabular component, (b) disturbance of the posterior capsule, (c) detachment of the short rotators, and (d) a combination of these factors. These factors can be overcome by careful positioning of the patient and correct component orientation.
4. The possibility of compartment syndrome of the "well" leg, which has been described in the literature. Although rare, this is a serious complication

(see Chapters 15 and 33).
5. An error of orientation can be caused by careless draping of the knee joint during surgery. The transcondylar line of the femur is an important reference for orientation of the femoral component. It should remain accessible.

Combined Anterolateral and Posterolateral Approaches

Aufranc deserves credit for a versatile approach that combines an anterior and posterior capsulectomy of the hip for arthroplasty of the hip.[6] This approach (without osteotomy of the greater trochanter) requires that two intervals be identified: between the tensor fascia femoris and gluteus medius and minimus anteriorly (Watson-Jones approach), and between the posterior border of the gluteus medius and top bundle of the gluteus maximus posteriorly (Marcy and Fletcher's modification of Kocher's). It also requires that anterior/superior and posterior capsulectomy be performed before dislocating the hip. Dislocation can be carried out anteriorly or posteriorly. The patient may be placed in the lateral decubitus or supine position. If supine, the patient is tilted away from the surgeon 30 to 40 degrees by a sandbag, which is removed before reaming of the acetabulum. The incision is straight, similar to the one used for a transtrochanter or posterolateral approach. The distal end of the incision may be curved somewhat posteriorly and beyond the level of the lesser trochanter (which corresponds to the proximal level of the insertion of the gluteus maximus to the linea aspera of the femur). By retracting the posterior border of the gluteus medius tendon anteriorly and with the limb maximally internally rotated as the short rotators are tensioned, the piriformis tendon is detached and marked by a suture as the sciatic nerve is located. After detachment of the remaining short rotators to the quadratus, the posterior capsule is incised or excised. The posterosuperior capsule may also be excised as necessary. The tendinous insertion of the gluteus maximus to the femur may then be detached to allow further mobilization of the femur. Alternatively, the external rotators and the posterior capsule can be detached as a single layer and tagged by sutures for identification and subsequent repair. The hip must remain maximally internally rotated with the knee flexed during this stage of the operation. The anterior portion of this exposure comprises an approach similar to the anterolateral (Watson-Jones) approach. It requires that for this portion of the procedure the limb be placed in slight abduction, with flexion of approximately 45 degrees and maximal external rotation. As the anterior capsule of the joint becomes taut a rectus lever-type retractor is used to expose the anterior capsule. After capsulotomy, capsulectomy, or both, as required, the hip can be dislocated anteriorly or posteriorly. However, during preparation of the acetabulum similar to that of the posterolateral exposure, the femur is reflected anteriorly. As one might expect, this approach can be used in place of a transtrochanteric approach, but neurological and vascular damage still may occur in patients with hips with marked stiffness or deformity and in larger and heavier patients.[61] I agree with Harris, who recommends that the surgeon perform anterior capsulectomy only if the posterior portion of this approach is insufficient in mobilizing the femur.[45] It should be recognized that a complete capsulectomy may render the hip unstable. It then follows that the surgeon may be forced to use a prosthesis with a longer neck that results in overlengthening of the limb.

Utility Incisions

Several utility incisions are useful either to produce a greater exposure or to accommodate some of the old incisions. During early development of the total hip arthroplasty, Charnley routinely used a triradiate incision to enhance exposure of the hip; he used this for arthrodesis and arthroplasty of the hip. The vertical limb of the incision is from the anterosuperior spine toward the ischium, which is crossed at the level of the tip of the greater trochanter by the transverse limb of the incision. The transverse limb of the incision is perpendicular to the line just described. The fascial incision follows the line of the skin incision.

I have used a "goblet-shaped" incision; the proximal limb is curved with the center of the arc just proximal to the level of the tip of the greater trochanter. It travels anteriorly toward the anterosuperior spine and posteriorly toward the ischium. The straight limb of the incision (the stem of the goblet) is parallel to the midshaft of the femur. The combination of the two incisions provides ample access to the back and front of the hip. This incision may be used when an exceptional need exists for added exposure. It can be used with or without trochanteric osteotomy. This author has used this incision, infrequently, for difficult anatomical situations such as infected revisions and for Girdlestone pseudarthrosis procedures for which access to both the front and back of the hip was essential. Recently, Krackow described a modification of this incision with indications for its use similar to those previously mentioned.[52]

When obtaining bone graft from the ilium and performing total hip arthroplasty are indicated, the "Z" incision is a utility incision that allows access to the hip joint, to the ilium, and along the shaft of the femur as long as necessary (Fig. 3-14). It can be used with a transtrochanteric, anterior, or direct lateral approach; the latter locates the distal limb of the incision over the proximal shaft of the femur to the tip of the greater trochanter. The proximal limb extends from this point to 1 cm lateral and proximal to the anterosuperior spine. It then traverses along the lateral border of the iliac crest as far as indicated.

Medial Approaches

Medial approaches to the hip joint are not suitable for performing total hip arthroplasty[31,60] because they provide only limited exposure of the proximal femur and the lesser trochanter. Approaches to the medial

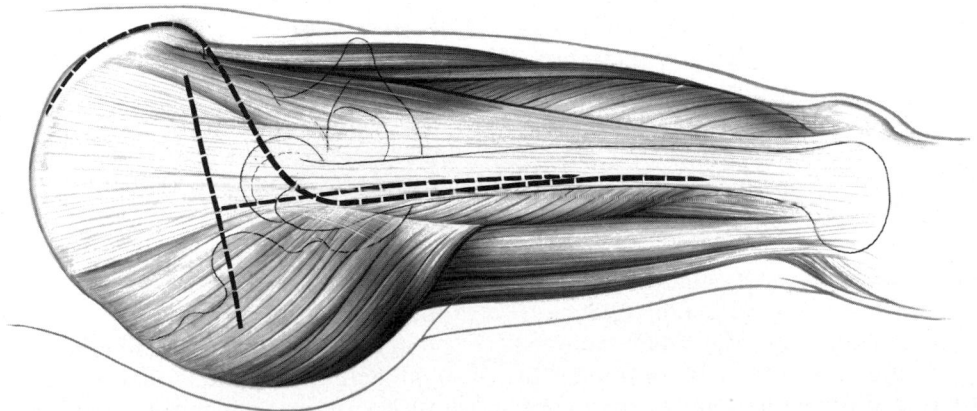

Fig. 3-14. Example of two utilitarian incisions for added exposure. One travels along the crest of the ilium (enabling the surgeon to obtain bone graft), then extends to the tip of the trochanter and finally along the shaft of the femur. In the other, a proximal limb (vertical) may be added to a transverse incision along the shaft to produce greater access to the front and back of the joint. It may be "Mercedes" or goblet-shaped.

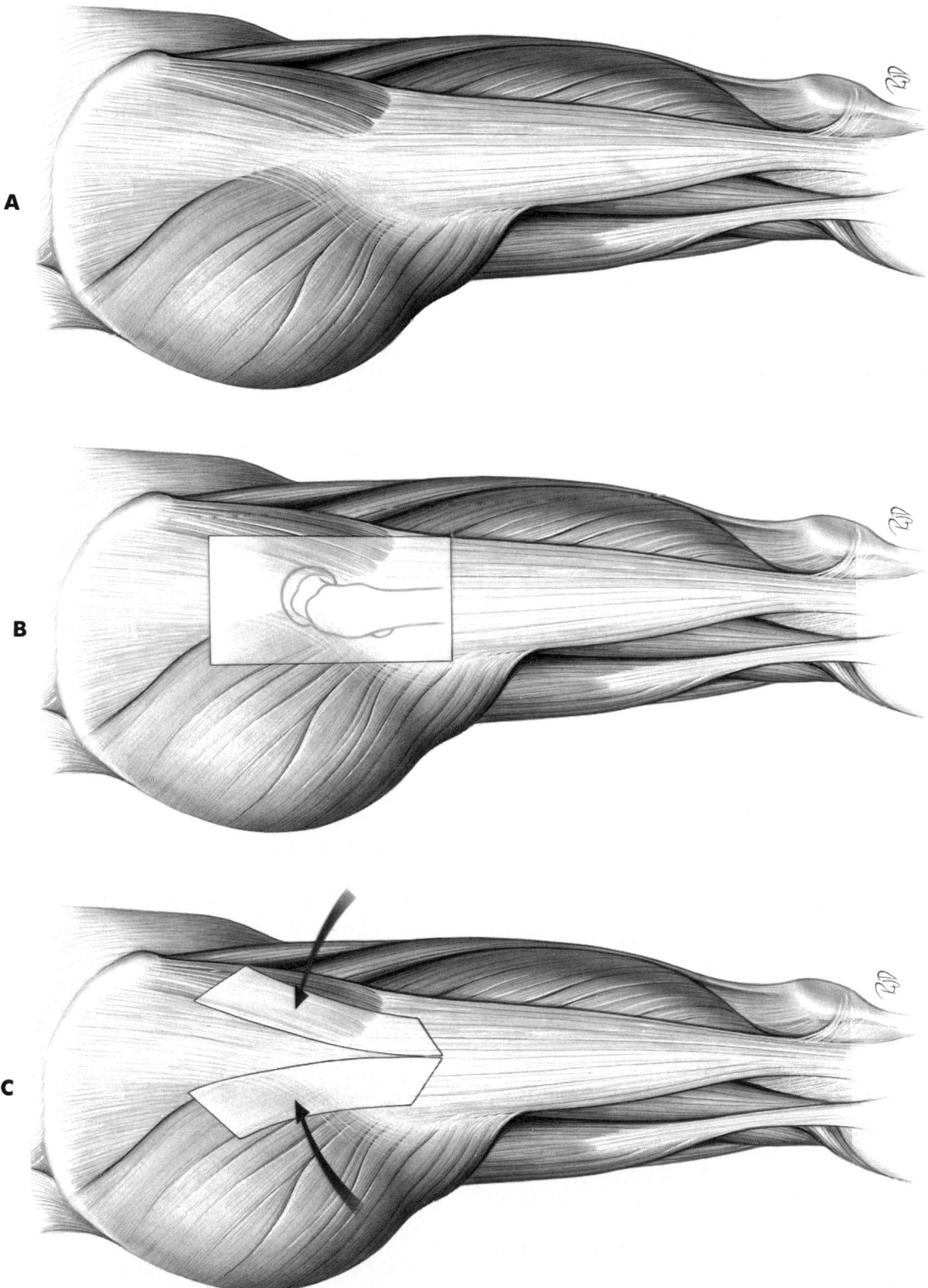

Fig. 3-15. A, The iliotibial band "pelvic deltoid" and "key tendon," is demonstrated as an anatomical guide for anterolateral, lateral, and posterolateral approaches. **B,** The widest exposure is achieved by a transtrochanteric approach (the square zone) because it permits unimpeded access to the hip joint. **C,** Limited access (relative to **B**) is possible anterolaterally (between the abductors and tensor fascia femoris) or posterolaterally (between the gluteus maximus and posterior border of gluteus medius), the front and back "walkways."

Continued.

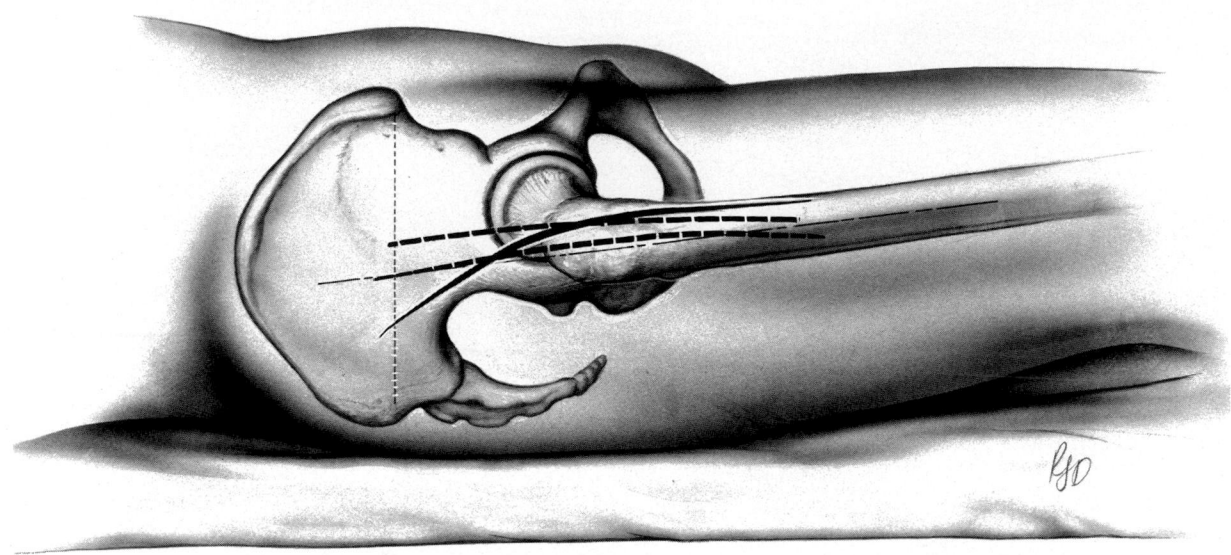

Fig. 3-15—cont'd. D, Three skin incisions for anterolateral, lateral, and posterolateral approaches.

aspect of the hip may have a place in congenital dislocation hip surgery and in myotomy and neurectomy in the region of the adductors.

SUMMARY OF APPROACHES TO THE HIP AND AN ANALOGY

I compare the hip joint to a house and consider the various approaches to it: a main gate at the center, a second "walkway" at the front, and another in the back (Fig. 3-15, A–C). The main entrance or gateway is the largest (the trochanter) and gives the best and easiest access. The other routes, front and back, also allow entrance but are limited if greater traffic demand is placed on them. The "front walkway" (anterolateral approach) is situated between the tensor fascia femoris (anteriorly) and gluteus medius (posteriorly), and the "back walkway" (posterolateral approach) is formed between the gluteus medius anteriorly and the upper border of the gluteus maximus posteriorly. With this analogy, one can readily see that "grand entrances" and major events are best arranged through the main gateway (by lifting up the greater trochanter and thus opening the main gateway), and less important events can take place by the secondary routes. If the main events are staged through the smaller entrances, effect and efficiency are reduced and unavoidable objects block the way and damage the walkways.

For effective surgery, one can theoretically consider all three possible approaches, but the "main gateway" is the most logical and effective course to follow for difficult deformities and major reconstructive procedures. The skin incisions for the three common approaches used for total hip arthroplasty are demonstrated in Fig. 3-15, D.

SUMMARY OF ESSENTIALS

- Total hip arthroplasty requires a greater exposure than most other hip procedures to provide complete access to the acetabulum and upper femur. It should provide access to all anatomical planes for a safe release of contracted tissue, removal of ectopic bone, and correction of fixed deformities. The incision must be located so that it is extensile along the appropriate anatomical planes.

- Full knowledge of all alternative surgical approaches to the hip and evaluation of the advantages and pitfalls of each equip the surgeon to choose the most suitable approach for total hip arthroplasty.

- The best approach for any extensive surgery, including total hip arthroplasty, is one that provides maximum exposure with minimum soft tissue damage. The positioning of the patient at surgery is an intricate part of surgical exposure; the position must allow optimum orientation for inserting the cement and the prosthesis.

- The choice also must be based on the functional outcome, which must be reproducible and achieve maximum accuracy during insertion of the prosthesis with minimum complications, thus maximizing the life function of the artificial joint.

- Approaches using a supine position on the operating table are advantageous since, unlike those requiring a lateral decubitus position, they provide landmarks that enable the surgeon to place the components more accurately and determine the leg length intraoperatively.

- The anterolateral, lateral, and posterolateral approaches are most suitable for performing total hip arthroplasty. The anterior, posterior, and medial approaches to the hip provide inadequate exposure of the upper femur and the acetabulum for this surgery.

- The anterolateral approach without trochanteric osteotomy, that is, Watson-Jones exposure of the hip as used by McKee and Müller and the posterolateral approach modification of Gibson's approach without removal of the greater trochanter, may provide adequate exposure of the acetabulum in a hip with no deformity and a good range of motion. This author prefers the posterolateral approach for the nontranstrochanteric route. However, access to the upper femur may be somewhat limited, and its preparation and the insertion of cement may be difficult. Orientation of the femoral stem prosthesis may be jeopardized when these approaches are used.

- The main criticism of the anterolateral approach is the potential for damage to the anterior portion of the gluteus medius muscle, which is located anterior to the greater trochanter, and for damage to the superior gluteal nerve branch to the tensor fascia femoris. The approach also requires a complete capsulectomy of the hip joint and does not always produce the upper femur out of the depth of the wound without heavy retraction of the gluteus medius and minimus. Routine detachment of the gluteus medius and the tendon of the gluteus minimus cannot be adequately repaired.

- Unlike other approaches, the transgluteal (direct lateral) approach is nonanatomical in that the gluteus medius and minimus are split longitudinally, and retraction can damage the nerve to the superior gluteal nerve. A good repair of conjoint tendon may be required for a good outcome.

- The transtrochanteric approach provides extensive exposure and protects the anatomical integrity of the hip structures. This approach provides access to the front and back of the hip, including the greater trochanter, and requires no muscle release other than removal of the abductors. This approach is considered physiologically sound when the greater trochanter is subsequently firmly reattached to the lateral aspect of the femoral shaft. It spares heavy retraction of the abductor muscles (and is therefore especially suitable for muscular individuals) and

allows good exposure and access to the cement and orientation of the prosthesis.

- Among the many advantages of a transtrochanteric approach to the hip are a wide and extensive exposure, protection of anatomical structures, correction of fixed deformities, ease of dislocation at operation, ease of preparation of the acetabulum, ease of insertion of components, improved cement fixation technique, improved stability after surgery, and above all, improved quality of long-term clinical results.

- Several theoretical and practical criticisms of the transtrochanteric approach exist. They include increased operating time, handling of the trochanter at surgery, delayed weight bearing postoperatively, increased blood loss, trochanteric bursitis, trochanteric nonunion, and breakage of wire and proximal migration of the trochanter. This approach is nevertheless indicated in difficult anatomical situations and revision surgery.

- Choice of a surgical approach must be made within the context of total hip reconstructive arthroplasty (as opposed to simple replacement of articular surfaces). The surgical approach must provide the opportunity to remove all deformity and balance the forces about the hip after reconstruction. The long-term success of arthroplasty depends entirely on excellence of surgical technique, and a good surgical exposure paves the way for good technique. Together they constitute an essential and intricate procedure, parallel in importance to the selection of patients and the choice of prosthesis.

- The posterolateral approach is this author's preferred method for nontranstrochanteric approach in total hip arthroplasty. This approach (unlike the southern exposure) provides good exposure of the acetabulum and femur with minimum damage to the bulk of abductor muscles located anterior to the trochanter. The main disadvantage of this approach is the requirement for lateral positioning of the patient, which makes accuracy of the socket orientation less reliable. A good repair of the short rotators, capsule of the joint, or both is mandatory.

- Most surgeons agree that in revision surgery (despite increased incidence of trochanteric complications), a transtrochanteric approach provides better exposure and safety. Surgeons advocating a nontranstrochanteric approach in all cases of primary or revision surgery are likely to treat major complications such as femoral fractures, nerve palsies, and dislocations as a trade-off for a few nonunions of the trochanter in anatomically difficult hips.

REFERENCES

1. **Acton RK:** Surgical approaches to the hip. In Tronzo RG, editor: *Surgery of the hip joint*, Philadelphia, 1973, Lea & Febiger.
2. **Adler L:** Pelvic stabilization in the lateral decubitus approach to total hip replacement, *Orthop Rev* 4(12):49, 1975.
3. **Amstutz HC:** Complications of total hip replacement, *Clin Orthop* 72:123, 1970.
4. **Amstutz HC, Maki S:** Complications of trochanteric osteotomy in total hip replacement, *J Bone Joint Surg* 60:214, 1978.
5. **Andersson GB, Freeman MA, Swanson SA:** Loosening of the cemented acetabular cup in total hip replacement, *J Bone Joint Surg* 54[Br]:590, 1972.
6. **Aufranc OE:** *Constructive surgery of the hip*, St Louis, 1962, Mosby–Year Book.
7. **Bankes SW, Laufman H:** *An atlas of surgical exposures of the extremities*, Philadelphia, 1968, WB Saunders.
8. **Bauer R, Kerschbaumer F, Poisel S, et al:** The transgluteal approach to the hip joint, *Arch Orthop Trauma Surg* 95:47, 1979.
9. **Berman AT, Salter FL, Koenig T:** Revision total hip replacement without trochanteric osteotomy, *Orthopedics* 10:755, 1987.
10. **Boardman KP, Bocco F, Charnley J:** An evaluation of a method of trochanteric fixation using three wires in the Charnley low-friction arthroplasty, *Clin Orthop* 132:31, 1978.
11. **Borja F, Latta LL, Stinchfield FE, et al:** Abductor muscle performance in total hip arthroplasty with and without trochanteric osteotomy. Radiographic and mechanical analyses, *Clin Orthop* 197:181, 1985.
12. **Bost FC, Schottstaedt ER, Larsen LJ:** Surgical approaches to the hip joint. In *American Academy of Orthopaedic Surgeons: instructional course lectures*, vol 11, Ann Arbor, 1954, JW Edwards.
13. **Brackett EG:** Study of the different approaches to the hip joint with special reference to the operations for curved trochanteric osteotomy and for arthrodesis, *Bost Med Surg J* 166:235, 1912.
14. **Brady JP:** Lateral oblique incision for the Charnley low-friction arthroplasty, *Clin Orthop* 118:7, 1976.
15. **Brash JC:** *Neuro-vascular hila of limb muscles: an atlas*, Edinburgh, 1955, E & S Livingstone.
16. **Burwell HN, Scott D:** A lateral intramuscular approach to the hip joint for replacement of the femoral head by a prosthesis, *J Bone Joint Surg* 36[Br]:104, 1954.
17. **Caldwell JA:** Subtrochanteric fractures of the femur; operative approach for open fixation, *Am J Surg* 59:370, 1943.
18. **Carlson DC, Robinson HJ Jr:** Surgical approaches for primary total hip arthroplasty. A prospective comparison of the Marcy modification of the Gibson and Watson-Jones approach, *Clin Orthop* 222:161, 1987.
19. **Charnley J:** *Comparison of dynamic frictional torque in different total hip implants by a pendulum method*, Internal Publication No. 35, England, Centre for Hip Surgery, Wrightington Hospital.
20. **Charnley J:** Total hip replacement by low-friction arthroplasty, *Clin Orthop* 72:7, 1970.
21. **Charnley J:** Comparison of the lever systems in the low-friction arthroplasty and the McKee-Farrar arthroplasty, England, 1971, Internal Publications, Centre for Hip Surgery, Wrightington Hospital.
22. **Charnley J:** The rationale of low-friction arthroplasty. In *The Hip Society: the hip, proceedings of the first open scientific meeting of The Hip Society*, St Louis, 1973, Mosby–Year Book.
23. **Charnley J:** *Low-friction arthroplasty of the hip: theory and practice*, Berlin, 1979, Springer-Verlag.
24. **Charnley J, Cupic Z:** The nine- and ten-year results of low-friction arthroplasty of the hip, *Clin Orthop* 95:9, 1973.
25. **Charnley J, Ferreira A:** Transplantation of the greater trochanter in arthroplasty of the hip, *J Bone Joint Surg* 46[Br]:191, 1964.
26. **Colonna PC:** The trochanteric reconstruction operation for ununited fractures of the upper end of the femur, *J Bone Joint Surg* 42[Br]:5, 1960.
27. **Crenshaw AM:** *Campbell's operative orthopaedics*, ed 4, St Louis, 1963, Mosby–Year Book.
28. **Dall D:** Exposure of the hip by anterior osteotomy of the greater trochanter. A modified anterolateral approach, *J Bone Joint Surg* 68[Br]:382, 1986.
29. **Eftekhar NS:** Status of femoral head replacement, Part I, *Orthop Rev* 2:19, 1973.
30. **Eftekhar NS:** Status of femoral head replacement, Part II, *Orthop Rev* 2:23, 1973.
31. **Etienne E, LaPeyrie M, Campo A:** The route of internal access to the hip joint, *Int Abst Surg* 84:276, 1947.
32. **Evanski PM, Waugh TR, Orofino CF:** Total hip replacement with the Charnley prosthesis, *Clin Orthop* 95:69, 1973.
33. **Evarts CM, Wilde AH, DeHaven KE:** Total hip joint arthroplasty, proceedings: the American Academy of Orthopedic Surgeons, *J Bone Joint Surg* 54:1562, 1972.
34. **Fahey JJ:** Surgical approaches to bones and joints, *Surg Clin North Am* 29:65, 1949.
35. **Gammer W:** A modified lateroanterior approach in operations for hip arthroplasty, *Clin Orthop* 199:169, 1985.
36. **Gibson A:** Vitallium-cup arthroplasty of the hip joint: review of approximately 100 cases, *J Bone Joint Surg* 31:861, 1949.
37. **Gibson A:** Posterior exposure of the hip joint, *J Bone Joint Surg* 32[Br]:183, 1950.
38. **Gibson A:** The posterolateral approach to the hip joint. In *American Academy of Orthopaedic Surgeons instructional course lectures*, vol 10, Ann Arbor, 1953, JW Edwards.
39. **Glassman AH, Engh CA, Bobyn JD:** A technique of extensile exposure for total hip arthroplasty, *J Arthroplasty* 2(1):11, 1987.
40. **Gore DR, Murray MP, Sepic SB, et al:** Anterolateral compared to posterior approach in total hip arthroplasty: difference in component positioning, hip strength, and hip motion, *Clin Orthop* 165:180, 1982.
41. **Hardinge K:** The direct lateral approach to the hip, *J Bone Joint Surg* 64:17, 1982.
42. **Hardy AE, Synek V:** Hip abductor function after the Hardinge approach: brief report, *J Bone Joint Surg* 70[Br]:673, 1988.
43. **Harris WH:** A new lateral approach to the hip joint, *J Bone Joint Surg* 49:891, 1967.
44. **Harris WH:** Extensive exposure of the hip joint, *Clin Orthop* 91:58, 1973.
45. **Harris WH:** Advances in surgical technique for total hip replacement: without and with osteotomy of the greater trochanter, *Clin Orthop* 146:188, 1980.
46. **Head WC, Mallory TH, Berklacich FM:** Extensile exposure of the hip for revision arthroplasty, *J Arthroplasty* 2:265, 1987.

47. **Henry AK:** *Extensile exposure,* Edinburgh, 1960, E & S Livingstone.

48. **Horowitz T:** The posterolateral approach in the surgical management of the basilar neck, intertrochanteric and subtrochanteric fractures of the femur, *Surg Gynecol Obstet* 95:45, 1952.

49. **Hungerford DS, Hedley A, Habermann E, et al:** Surgical technique for the PCA total hip system. In *Total hip arthroplasty: a new approach,* Baltimore, 1984, University Park Press.

50. **Jergensen F, Abbott LC:** A comprehensive exposure of the hip joint, *J Bone Joint Surg* 36:798, 1955.

51. **Johnston RC, Larson CB:** Biomechanics of cup arthroplasty, *Clin Orthop* 66:56, 1969.

52. **Krackow KA, Steinman H, Cohn BT, et al:** Clinical experience with a triradiate exposure of the hip for a difficult total hip arthroplasty, *J Arthroplasty* 3:267, 1988.

53. **Lazansky MG:** Complications in total hip replacement with the Charnley technic, *Clin Orthop* 72:40, 1970.

54. **Lazansky MG:** Total replacement arthroplasty of the hip: the Charnley low-friction technique, Proceedings: The American Academy of Orthopedic Surgeons 52A:834, 1970.

55. **Lazansky MG:** Trochanteric osteotomy in total hip replacement. In *The Hip Society: the hip, proceedings of the second open scientific meeting of The Hip Society,* St Louis, 1974, Mosby–Year Book.

56. **Light TR, Keggi KJ:** Anterior approach to hip arthroplasty, *Clin Orthop* 152:255, 1980.

57. **Lowell JD, Aufranc OE:** The anterior approach to the hip joint, *Clin Orthop* 61:193, 1968.

58. **Luck JV:** A transverse anterior approach to the hip, *J Bone Joint Surg* 37:534, 1955.

59. **Luck JV:** Surgical approaches for total hip replacement, *Orthop Rev* 6(4):53, 1977.

60. **Ludloff K:** The open reduction of the congenital hip dislocation by an anterior incision, *Am J Orthop Surg* 10:438, 1913.

61. **Lusskin R, Goldman A, Absatz M:** Combined anterior and posterior approach to the hip joint in reconstructive and complex arthroplasty, *J Arthroplasty* 3:313, 1988.

62. **McFarland B, Osborne G:** Approach to the hip: a suggested improvement in Kocher's method, *J Bone Joint Surg* 36[Br]:364, 1954.

63. **McKee GK:** Development of total prosthetic replacement of the hip, *Clin Orthop* 72:85, 1970.

64. **McKee GK, Watson-Farrar J:** Replacement of arthritic hips by the McKee-Farrar prosthesis, *J Bone Joint Surg* 48[Br]:245, 1966.

65. **McLauchlan J:** The Stracathro approach to the hip, *J Bone Joint Surg* 66[Br]:30, 1984.

66. **Marcy GH, Fletcher RS:** Modification of the posterolateral approach to the hip for insertion of femoral-head prosthesis, *J Bone Joint Surg* 36:142, 1954.

67. **Markolf KL, Hirschowitz DL, Amstutz HC:** Mechanical stability of the greater trochanter following osteotomy and reattachment by wiring, *Clin Orthop* 141:111, 1979.

68. **Moore AT:** The self-locking metal hip prosthesis, *J Bone Joint Surg* 39:811, 1957.

69. **Moore AT:** The Moore self-locking Vitallium prosthesis in fresh femoral neck fractures. In *American Academy of Orthopaedic Surgeons instructional course lectures,* vol 16, St Louis, 1959, Mosby–Year Book.

70. **Morris JB:** McKee-Farrar and Charnley total hip replacement arthroplasty. In Proceedings and Reports of Universities, Colleges, Councils and Associations: Australian and New Zealand Orthopaedic Associations, *J Bone Joint Surg* 50[Br]:680, 1968.

71. **Morris JB, Nicholson OR:** Total prosthetic replacement of the hip joint in Auckland, *Clin Orthop* 72:33, 1970.

72. **Mostardi RA, Askew MJ, Gradisar IA, et al:** Comparison of functional outcome of total hip arthroplasties involving four surgical approaches, *J Arthroplasty* 3:279, 1988.

73. **Müller ME:** Total hip prosthesis, *Clin Orthop* 72:46, 1970.

74. **Müller ME:** Total hip replacement without trochanteric osteotomy. In *The Hip Society: the hip, proceedings of the second open scientific meeting of The Hip Society,* St Louis, 1974, Mosby–Year Book.

75. **Nicholson OR:** Total hip replacement. An evaluation of the results and technics, 1967–1972, *Clin Orthop* 95:217, 1973.

76. **Nutton RW, Checketts RG:** The effects of trochanteric osteotomy on abductor power, *J Bone Joint Surg* 66[Br]:180, 1984.

77. **Ober FR:** Posterior arthrotomy of the hip joint, *JAMA* 83:1500, 1924.

78. **Osborne RP:** The approach to the hip-joint: a critical review and suggested new route, *Br J Surg* 18:49, 1930.

79. **Parker HG, Wiesman HG, Ewald FC, et al:** Comparison of preoperative, intraoperative and early postoperative total hip replacements with and without trochanteric osteotomy, *Clin Orthop* 121:44, 1976.

80. **Robinson RP, Robinson HJ Jr, Salvati EA:** Comparison of the transtrochanteric and posterior approaches for total hip replacement, *Clin Orthop* 147:143, 1980.

81. **Rydell NW:** Forces acting on the femoral head-prosthesis. A study on strain gauge supplied prostheses in living persons. *Acta Orthop Scand* 88(37: Suppl):1, 1966.

82. **Sledge CB:** Discussion: osteotomy of the greater trochanter, In *The Hip Society: the hip, proceedings of the second scientific meeting of The Hip Society,* St Louis, 1974, Mosby–Year Book.

83. **Smith-Petersen MN:** Treatment of malum coxae senilis, old slipped upper femoral epiphysis, intrapelvic protrusion of the acetabulum, and coxa plana by means of acetabuloplasty, *J Bone Joint Surg* 18:869, 1936.

84. **Smith-Petersen MN:** Approach to and exposure of the hip joint for mold arthroplasty, *J Bone Joint Surg* 31:40, 1949.

85. **Stinchfield FE, Henry JH, Eftekhar NS, et al:** Total hip replacement. In Ahstrom JP Jr, editor: *Current practice in orthopaedic surgery,* vol 5, St Louis, 1973, Mosby–Year Book.

86. **Sutherland R, Rowe MJ Jr:** Simplified surgical approach to the hip, *Arch Surg* 48:144, 1944.

87. **Thompson RC Jr, Culver JE:** The role of trochanteric osteotomy in total hip replacement, *Clin Orthop* 106:102, 1975.

88. **Vicar AJ, Coleman CR:** A comparison of the anterolateral, transtrochanteric, and posterior surgical approaches in primary total hip arthroplasty, *Clin Orthop* 188:152, 1984.

89. **Volz RG, Mayer DM:** The predictive factors necessitating trochanteric osteotomy in total hip replacement, *Orthop Rev* 5(12):23, 1976.

90. **von Langenbeck B:** Vorstellung cines Falles von geheilter Enterotomie, *Verh Deutsch Ges Chir* 7:40, 1878.

91. **Jones RW:** Fractures of the neck of the femur, *Br J Surg* 23:787, 1936.

92. **Wiesman HJ Jr, Simon SR, Ewald FC, et al:** Total hip replacement with and without osteotomy of the greater trochanter: clinical and biomechanical comparisons in the same patients, *J Bone Joint Surg* 60:203, 1978.

ADDITIONAL READINGS

Clarke RP Jr, Shea WD, Bierbaum BE: Trochanteric osteotomy: analysis of patterns of wire fixation failure and complications, *Clin Orthop* 141:102, 1979.

Cubbins WR, Callahan JJ, Scuderi CS: Fractures of the neck of the femur; open operation and pathologic observations. New incision and new direction for use of simplified flange, *Surg Gynecol Obstet* 68:87, 1939.

Fulkerson JP, Crelin ES, Keggi KJ: Anatomy and osteotomy of the greater trochanter, *Arch Surg* 114:19, 1979.

Harris WH: A new approach to total hip replacement without osteotomy of the greater trochanter, *Clin Orthop* 106:19, 1975.

Harris WH, Crothers OD: Reattachment of the greater trochanter in total hip replacement arthroplasty: a new technique, *J Bone Joint Surg* 60A:211, 1978.

Harris WH, Jones WN: The use of wire mesh in total hip replacement surgery, *Clin Orthop* 106:117, 1975.

Jensen NF, Harris WH: A system for trochanteric osteotomy and reattachment for total hip arthroplasty with a ninety-nine percent union, *Clin Orthop* 208:174, 1986.

Lindgren U, Svenson O: A new transtrochanteric approach to the hip, *Int Orthop* 12:37, 1988.

Mallory TH: Total hip replacement with and without trochanteric osteotomy, *Clin Orthop* 103:133, 1974.

Volz RG, Brown FW: The painful migrated ununited greater trochanter in total hip replacement, *J Bone Joint Surg* 59A:1091, 1977.

Weaver JK: Total hip replacement: a comparison between transtrochanteric and posterior surgical approaches, *Clin Orthop* 112:201, 1975.

Woo RY, Morrey BF: Dislocations after total hip arthroplasty, *J Bone Joint Surg* 64A:1295, 1982.

See Chapters 6, Biomechanics: Fixation and Loosening; 15, Principles Common to all Surgical Approaches; 16, Posterolateral Approach; 17, Anterolateral and Transgluteal Approaches; 18, Transtrochanteric Approach (modified Charnley); 19, Transtrochanteric Approach (author's method); and 37, Trochanteric Osteotomy Complications for additional information.

CHAPTER FOUR

Biomaterials: Compatibility and Wear

■ A "bland" or biologically inert material is "one which does not destroy the viability of adjoining tissues and provokes no inflammatory response beyond that occasioned by trauma accompanying the insertion and by its presence as a physical and nonvital structure, and which does not impede the process of fibrous or osteogenic repair.

E. Clarke

This chapter covers the interrelationship of materials and mechanical aspects of the artificial hip joint. Concepts concerning biomaterials and biomechanics for artificial hip joints are rapidly changing. New developments are based on investigations in biomechanical laboratories and the correlation of these findings to clinical problems as long-term results of hip arthroplasty operations become available. Work is in progress in many areas, but even now, some years will elapse before laboratory investigation of a specific situation can be verified by clinical observations.

Orthopaedic surgeons are concerned with areas of the body that are in continuous movement (after prosthetic structures are applied). Unlike the "stationary devices" used in fracture fixation, hip replacement devices are expected to perform a mechanical function of lifelong duration by transmission of load and motion.

Structures and mechanical functions are usually constructed to serve for a specific length of time, termed the *design life* by engineers. It is possible as an engineering exercise to calculate the magnitude of stresses (applied loads and mechanical properties of materials) and to conceptualize a design with expected behavior. However, it is not realistic to apply such a model to human function and the body environment, expecting behavior comparable with calculated laboratory performances. On this premise, laboratory work has its limitations and can be used only as a guide or for verification of some aspects of clinical application.

In a young patient the magnitude of forces generated in the hip joint from various activities is incredibly difficult to estimate. Examples of extreme conditions are contact sports, jumping, and running. The average load applied to the head of the femur in the stance phase of normal walking (heel strike of a 77 kg person walking 0.9 m/sec) may be around 100 kg/force. If a person walks 1 mile the dynamic intermittent load may increase to as much as four or five times the body weight. If the hip is loaded about 1000 times, in the course of 1 year the bearing may be loaded as many as 1 to 2.5 million times. If we consider that the total hip joint may be required to perform for 50 years, this obviously surpasses most limits of engineering design life* — even barring the hostile environment of the body and the unusual physical demands made (that is, athletic performances). Producing such a prosthesis is the greatest orthopaedic and engineering challenge faced by the surgeon and engineer. At the same time, tissue reaction from by-products of wear and degradation of the material must remain inert to human tissue.

From earliest times, surgeons have tried to replace missing or deformed parts of the body. Crutches were

---

* Under ideal lubricating conditions some ball bearings may last 10^9 to 10^{10} cycles.

among the early ameliorative attempts used by the most primitive men, and as technology grew, more sophisticated appliances were developed.

Efforts to replace tissues in the body are reported throughout early literature with occasional accounts of successful results, principally with metals. A golden nose is said to have been worn by Tycho Brahe 400 years ago to hide a cavity he had acquired in a tavern fight. Early appliances such as gold skull plates and segments of bone have been documented, but it was not until this century that metallurgists developed alloys that were sufficiently mechanically stable and chemically inert to be used for dependable insertion. After more than half a century of development, the orthopaedic surgeon can now use metal safely and predictably for repair and replacement surgery.

Because the development of implantable polymers is relatively recent, the issue of their complete prosthetic acceptability has not been fully resolved. Although some of these plastics have remained implanted in thousands of humans for as long as 30 to 40 years and have been well tolerated, the question of long-term reactivity to them remains unanswered. Questions surrounding short-term results, applicability of animal test results to humans, and degradation of plastics after 30 or 40 years are all facets of the larger issue that concerns the orthopaedic surgeon. Even though it has been suggested that the average cell life span in man and the rat is comparable, other factors do not allow exclusion of the idea that these materials may become harmful to the body over an extended period of time. With emergence of sarcomas reported at the site of metal or plastic joint materials, the questions related to carcinogenicity of these materials when applied to very young patients must be answered only by very careful and prolonged documentation and follow up. Obviously, when new or old materials are used in a different form from previously experienced methods, surgeons should be particularly concerned about the potential harm of ionic release from metal trace elements of various alloys, as well as the generation of particles from metals or plastics. For example, at this time surgeons performing joint arthroplasties using uncemented prostheses with expanded surfaces (porous-coated), especially in younger patients, must be increasingly aware of possible carcinogenic effects of the materials used. Experimental studies have documented that certain varieties of chromium-cobalt alloys, in the form of wear debris, are carcinogenic in rodents,[117] while solid implants of the same material do not cause tumors in rats after 2 years of exposure.[96] This difference might be related to low doses of ion release from solids and not from wear debris.

Electrolytic action in the body usually makes the use of dissimilar metals (alloys) for the two surfaces of a joint impossible; one exception is chromium-cobalt alloys, which have been used in combination for a total hip prosthesis (McKee-Farrar total hip prosthesis). For a metal-against-metal prosthesis to withstand incumbent stresses (such as in the hip joint), it must have a large-diameter head to permit flow of a lubricating film of fluid between the mating parts. A simple ball-and-socket bearing (metal against plastic) exposed to tissue fluid is most effective provided that (1) the plastic is wear resistant and (2) any particulate matter released as the result of wear will not cause tissue reaction in the body. Since the latter presents the most serious problem, the design and choice of materials should be aimed toward inertness of the wear by-product and tissue tolerance.

In-vivo research should be directed toward the selection of biocompatible materials for the bearing joints. Using any new materials clinically must be done judiciously. For example, when polytetrafluorethylene (Teflon) was used for socket material, the procedure was limited to individuals with extreme disability for whom no alternate method of treatment existed at that time (before 1962). Charnley's choice of Teflon as a bearing material was logical for its low coefficient friction properties; yet the wear particles proved to be extremely noxious to osseous tissue with the passage of time, leading to failure of almost all operations in patients who survived for 5 or more years after surgery, despite Teflon's good record for inertness in the body in bulk form.

The total joint prosthesis is a complex and challenging engineering product; it must be problem free to perform a lifetime of service without failure. The material should be adequately fatigue resistant to withstand weight-bearing stresses. Wear must be minimal, with the level of frictional resistance reduced to a minimum to protect the fixation (bond) from excess stress. The material should also withstand corrosion and degradation in the hostile environment of the body; further, the weight-bearing element must be capable of attenuating the forces (absorbing energy), be compliant and, above all, have local and remote biological compatibility. Only then can we safely apply it to young patients without long-term future concern.

A histologically "stable" interface between the implant and the skeleton is of such fundamental importance that no further development in this field can be achieved without appreciation of this stability. Sir John Charnley must be credited not only with the introduction of acrylic cement in orthopaedics and high-density polyethylene (HDP) for material used in joint arthroplasty[43] surgery, but also with his ceaseless efforts in histological studies of response to these materials.[43,47]

Many surgeons have recently abandoned acrylic cement in favor of other methods of fixation of artificial joint stems. Although a stable cellular interface may be achieved between acrylic and bone, there is no agreement as to (1) whether this stability can be maintained permanently and, if it cannot, (2) what set of circumstances alters a histologically stable interface, leading to bone destruction and mechanical loosening. Unfortunately, no authoritative opinion has yet been engendered by the pathologists in this field. Until recently, much of the adverse reaction found in failed prostheses had been attributed to polymethylmethacrylate (PMMA), not to HDP particles that are found together with acrylic cement in most histological specimens.

The reactive membrane between the implant and the host (prosthetic synovitis) can be interpreted from morphological and histochemical standpoints only under physiological load bearing and function in humans (in the absence of infection) to be representative.

INERTNESS OF BIOMATERIALS

Compatibility is a conditio sine qua non for any material to be developed for use in prosthetic implants. According to Clarke, a "bland" or biologically inert material is one "which does not destroy the viability of adjoining tissues and provokes no inflammatory response beyond that occasioned by trauma accompanying the insertion and by its presence as a physical and nonvital structure, and which does not impede the process of fibrous or osteogenic repair."[56]

In addition to its chemical makeup, the physical form of the material may determine the tissue response to implants.* Teflon may be considered a classic example in this regard. Teflon does not cause any severe reaction when used in bulk in humans (that is, plates, sheets, or rods), but considerable tissue reaction is engendered by small particles when present in total hip arthroplasty.

In experimental conditions, most plastics produce severe reaction in their particular forms and also may produce tumors in rats.[190,191] Autogenous bone grafts commonly used in orthopaedic surgery may also produce severe inflammatory and histiocytic reactions when used in powdered form or implanted subperiosteally.

As a general rule, most foreign bodies, regardless of their chemical constituency or physical makeup, will cause a local inflammatory process after implantation and finally become enclosed by a fibrous capsule.[34,175] Authors generally agree that foreign material influences the type of reaction at a cellular level depending on their size and shape and their chemical composition.[57,244,271] The relationship between the size of the

particles released from joint implants and the cellular reaction and the ultimate tissue response largely depends on the volume of the foreign matter present rather than its chemical composition. As previously stated, while general fibrosis encapsulates most materials in the body, histiocytic response and granulomatosis by multinucleated giant cells are caused by smaller particles (released into the surrounding tissue), which may lead to necrosis. Investigators also have implicated the size and shape of the particles in causing neoplastic lesions.[40]

Surface energy and roughness of implants on bone resorption are related to macrophage-release mediators, which stimulate bone resorption.[185] Murray and associates demonstrated that the amount of bone resorption increased by 2.5 to 10 times when macrophages adhered to a foreign surface (material). They concluded that bone absorption depends on physical properties such as surface energy and roughness of the implant, which can cause loosening, rather than the chemical nature of the implant itself. As a corollary to these investigations, Leak and associates and Rich and Harris demonstrated that macrophage migration and spreading were influenced by surface energy and the roughness of the surface on which they were cultured.[136,210]

Ideally, the inertness of plastic and metals should not deteriorate after implantation as a result of attack by body fluids nor from their own chemical changes. The material should not generate a foreign body reaction leading to formation of granulation tissue or hypersensitivity. It should also be able to withstand stresses without structural changes to provide long and enduring service. It must be inexpensive, easily produced and manufactured, and the method of sterilization must be easy, practical, and economical. Quality control and manufacturing methods must be standardized to ensure uniform performance. Most significant of all, the material must not be carcinogenic in humans.

Regarding the chemical makeup of the implant, most established implants used in orthopaedics are chemically inert and do not have a necrotizing effect that alters cellular enzyme function to induce immunological changes or cause significant cellular effects. However, monomer released from polymerizing acrylic cement is toxic at the cellular level and can cause inflammatory response.

The materials commonly used in total hip replacement include the following:

1. Acrylic cement (PMMA)
2. HDP
3. Stainless steel
4. Chromium alloys
5. Titanium

---

* References 47, 48, 106, 107, 244.

Regarding acrylic cement, Chapter 5 details the chemical, physical, and mechanical properties and the biological response in terms of exothermic reactions and toxicity studies, including teratogenicity, fetal toxicity, carcinogenicity, effects on chemotaxis of polymorphonuclear cells, liver function, and other safety and biocompatibility aspects. In this chapter, specific issues of tissue response to PMMA at a cellular level are considered, including the following:

1. Injury and repair after implantation.
2. Tissue response, state of stability.
3. Tissue response in the femur.
4. Tissue response in the acetabulum.
5. Tissue response, state of instability.
6. Prosthetic synovitis.
   a. In presence of bacterial infection.
   b. In absence of bacterial infection.
7. Radiology of prosthetic interface.
8. Histochemistry assays of cemented implants.
9. Micromotion theory of loose cemented implants.
10. Localized invasive osteolysis.
    a. In presence of gross loosening.
    b. In absence of gross loosening.

INJURY AND REPAIR

A classic animal study by Wiltse and co-workers and histological studies of Willert after total hip arthroplasty recognized immediate necrosis that occurred at the interface during the first 3 weeks after the implantation of PMMA.[265,269,270] The authors observed necrotic tissue and fibrin up to 3 mm thick, which they attributed to (1) heat of polymerization, (2) monomeric effect, and (3) loss of blood supply to the injured area. Larger necrosis observed in the trochanteric region and in the medullary cavity was indistinguishable from bone infarcts. Repair of tissue damage at the interface that began after 3 weeks had ended within approximately 2 years. This repair was manifested by peripheral hyperemia, migration of lipophages, ingrowth of fibroblasts, and new capillaries.[265,269] However, the investigators observed occasional focal necrosis even at this stage; these areas were smaller than those occurring within the first 3 weeks. The necrotic bone actually had been repaired by (1) remodeling, (2) reinforcement, and (3) replacement. Repair was mainly by the mechanisms of apposition of new lamellar bone or by osteoblastic metaplasia. In these studies, the investigators found acrylic pearls in most implant beds and in foreign body giant cells and occasionally in nearby connective tissue and lymphatic vessels. Rhinelander and associates, using microangiography techniques, showed severe devascularization and necrosis of large areas of the cortex after reaming, followed by full recovery at 6 months.[209] Repair had not occurred 1 year after introduction of cement after reaming.

In our laboratories at Columbia-Presbyterian Medical Center, to characterize histologically the nature of the interface, we conducted three sets of experiments using 11 adult beagles (7.7 to 13 kg in weight).[132] Our specific objective was to study the effects of monomer leaching and heat liberated from curing methacrylate plugs in situ. We accomplished separation of the two effects in three group experiments: (1) plugs were cured and leached of monomer before plug implantation, thus the absence of heat and monomer; (2) plugs were cured but not leached, thus the absence of heat only; and (3) plugs were implanted 4 minutes after the initiation of cement mixing, thus the presence of heat and monomer.

This experiment illustrated that self-curing methylmethacrylate (MMA) cement (as used in this experiment) was well tolerated by osseous tissue and that the bone did grow in direct apposition to methacrylate without interposition of fibrocartilage. The plugs in these experiments were all rigidly press-fitted into drilled holes (except for those experiments in which cement was allowed to cure in situ).

We could identify no definite noxious effect from the heat or polymerization or from the monomer from the MMA as used in these experiments. Fig. 4-1 compares a typical histological morphology of the interface with the histological changes in a drilled hole without an implant and one with a plug of Teflon, all indicating a direct bone apposition against a stable implant.

Bone Remodeling Against PMMA

In addition to early studies by Charnley and Crawford,[49] Charnley, Follacci, and Hammond,[51] Hendrichsen and associates,[118] and Wiltse,[270] a direct apposition of bone formation was substantiated by electron microscopy studies of Linder and Hansson[143]; they showed that direct, viable bone, without other intervening tissue, can be found as evidence of bone remodeling after insertion of PMMA in vivo. In a study of histomorphology of the bone-cement interface, Draenert evaluated fully developed California rabbits for remodeling of the cortex and revascularization of the medullary canal at the following intervals: at 1, 2, 3, 6, and 8 days; at 2, 3, 4, 6, and 8 weeks; at 3, 6, 9, and 11 months; and at 1½, 2, and 2½ years.[74] The following summary is based on this animal study transposed on histology of retrieved human specimens.

1. Bone cement integration (osteointegration) occurred in the absence of mechanical stress.
2. The existing gap between bone and implant was filled rapidly by newly formed bone (woven bone). Gaps up to 8 μm were filled by lamellar bone. Larger gaps were also bridged by woven bone.
3. Regeneration of the medullary canal occurred,

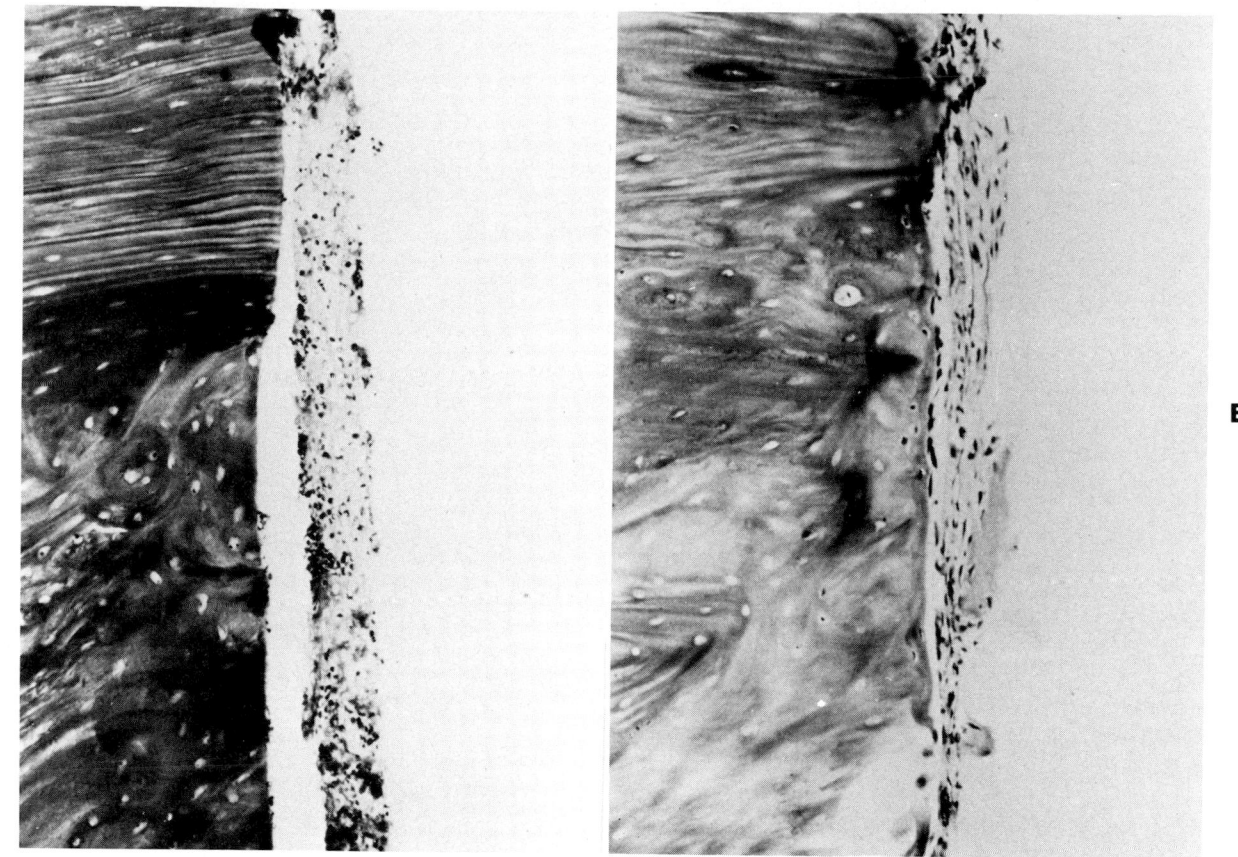

Fig. 4-1. A, 4-day specimen showing layer of coagulum containing acute inflammatory cells interposed between wall of cortical defect and MMA plug that occupied space to right. **B,** At 2 weeks, cement plug was separated from cortical bone within defect by very cellular fibrous tissue oriented perpendicular to long axis of cortex.

Continued.

and the medullary canal was fully revascularized to its original state.

4. New medullarization occurred as a second remodeling process resulting from revascularization of the cortex, replacing partially necrotic bone.

5. The force transmission to bone optimally occurred for compression but not by tension.

6. Intimate contact between bone and cement occurred without interruption by fibrous or molecular connection.

7. While no tissue reaction was observed at 2½ years after implantation, osteoblasts were conveniently deposited directly onto the bone-cement interface.

8. This study again confirms Charnley's original observation that newly formed bone can be seen directly on the surface of the cement on the old cortex and thus the process of new cortex formation.

PMMA Effect on Bone Circulation

The anatomy of the blood supply to the long bones has long been established.[30,204,206] The supply to the bone by the vascular branches is viewed in general as metaphyseal and diaphyseal. The metaphyseal blood supply is from the arteries entering on all sides at the ligamentous attachments. The cancellous structure of the metaphysis is well supplied by many vessels entering it. As a general rule, because of good vascularity, healing of the metaphysis is excellent after fractures. The diaphyseal blood supply is from three sources: (1) nutrient arteries, (2) metaphyseal arteries (anastomosis by proximal and distal supply), and (3) periosteal arterioles, which enter the bone at the fascial attachments to supply one third of the cortex. It must be emphasized that the periosteal source cannot substitute for the medullary arterial supply when the medullary supply is destroyed. The contribution of the periosteal supply to the femoral diaphysis is restricted

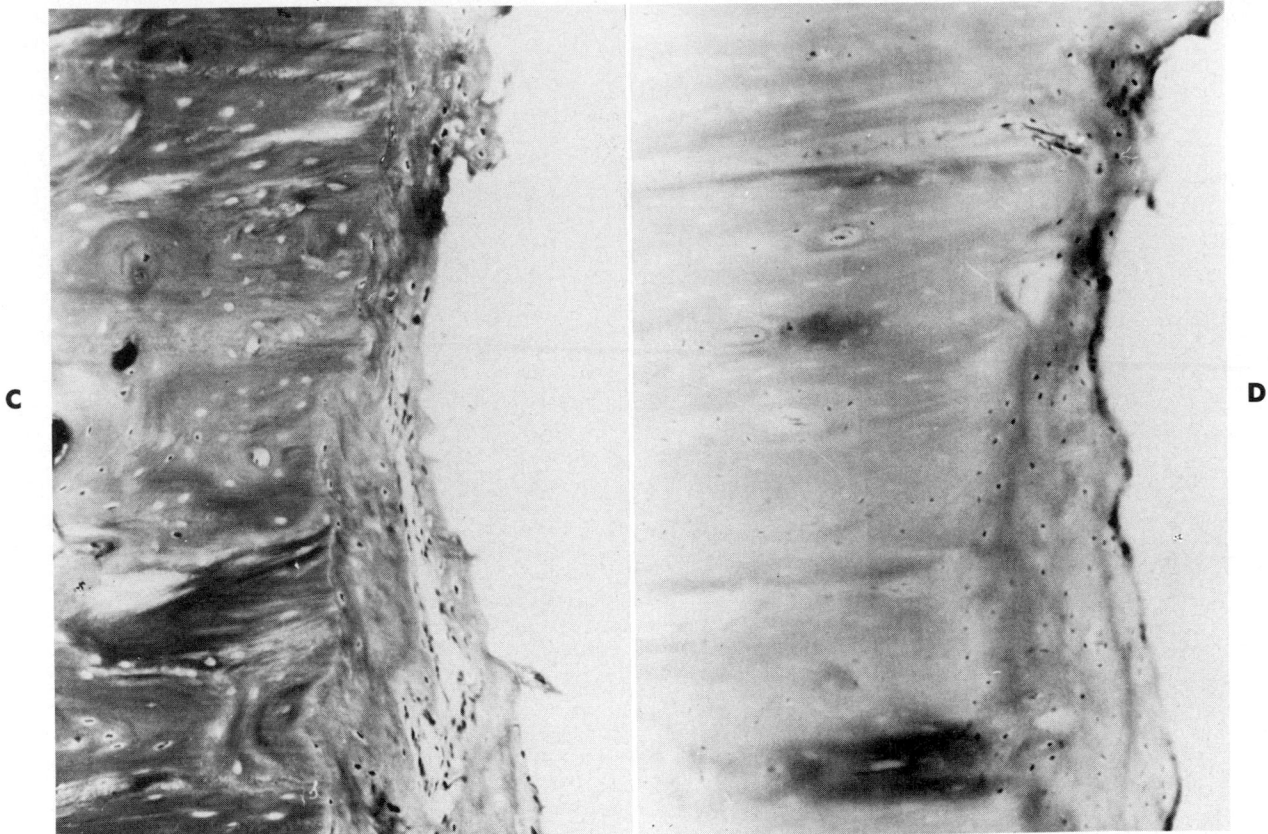

Fig. 4-1—cont'd. C, At 4 weeks, fibrous layer was almost completely replaced by newly formed bone. Defect to right was filled with MMA implant. NOTE: the empty lacunae within original cortical bone. Zone of dead bone is about 300 μ wide. NOTE: in this specimen MMA was inserted similar to operating condition; that is, cement was polymerized in situ. NOTE: presence of giant cell reaction and impressions of cement on surface of fibrous layer now completely replaced by newly formed bone. **D,** 6-month specimen that shows small area of fibrous tissue between MMA plug that occupied space to right and cortical bone. Also note semicircular impressions of cement in bone.

to the small contribution from the periosteum in posterior cortex (linea aspera) since there are no other fascial attachments to the femur. Therefore the entire remainder of the femur is supplied by the medullary source.[205,207–209]

The crucial portion of the blood supply to the femur in relation to replacement is the junction of the metaphysis and diaphysis. In this region the richly blood-supplied cancellous nature of the metaphysis joins the lesser vascularized zone of the medullary source of the diaphysis.

Rhinelander and associates,[205,207,208] using a technique of bone angiography developed by Trueta and others,[12,253] studied in an experimental model the effect of reaming and implantation of acrylic cement (without disturbing the hip joint). The authors reached the following conclusions:[209]

1. The most significant changes occurring after reaming alone were devascularization and apparent necrosis of large areas of the subtrochanteric region and femoral diaphysis. The necrotic region fully recovered within 6 months.
2. Extensive bone necrosis occurred when the medullary canal was reamed and filled with acrylic cement. The necrosis was extensive in the inner layers of the diaphysis. Evidence of necrosis persisted beyond 1 year.
3. A fibrous membrane was found at the cement-bone interface, indicating a lack of osteointegration.
4. After devascularization as a result of PMMA insertion, the cortex revascularized without osteoclasis.
5. Because of damage caused to the intramedullary

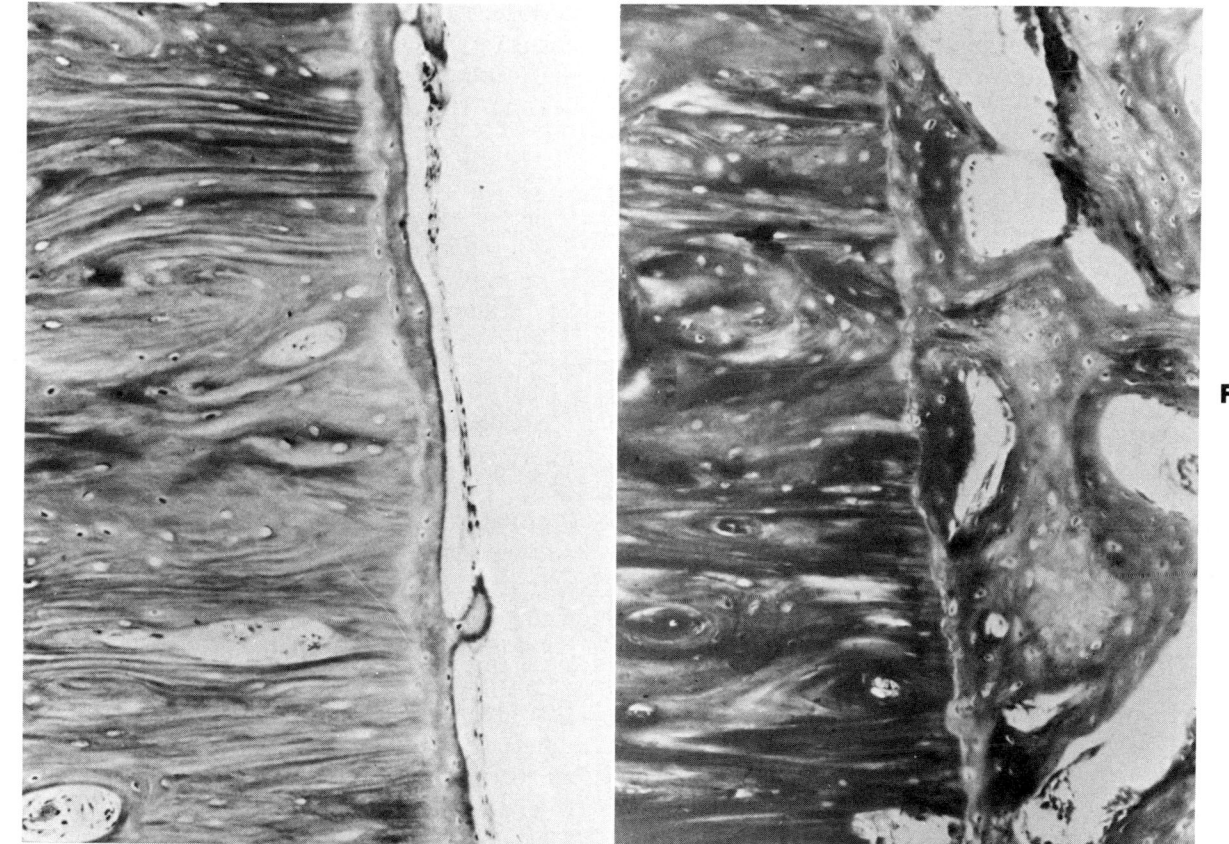

Fig. 4-1—cont'd. E, 4-week specimen that contained Teflon plug zone of dead bone is noted within vicinity of implant presumably from trauma of surgery. **F,** At 4 weeks cortical defect that is allowed to heal without implantation of foreign material also demonstrates zone of cortical necrosis adjacent to defect. Line of demarcation between wall of defect and reactive new bone is clearly shown (**A** to **F** ×40). (Courtesy Pawluk and Bassett.)

blood supply by reaming and the presence of PMMA, bone formation and the remodeling process were dramatically reduced.

In a similar study regarding bone healing in the presence of PMMA, the incidence of nonunion was much higher after reaming and injection of PMMA in dogs as compared with no reaming or with reaming without the use of PMMA.[238] Parallel to these observations, impairment of circulation caused by reaming and the presence of cement was responsible for bone death and poor remodeling rather than the chemical trauma or the heat of polymerization by cement.

Effect of Temperature

Several authors have measured bone surface temperature during total hip arthroplasty and before insertion of cement or prosthesis, demonstrating variations from normally assumed body temperature of 37.5° C. Miller noted surface temperatures varied as much as 6° C (after using irrigating solutions) as a result of the ambient room temperature.[179] Rhinelander and co-workers did not consider temperatures reaching as high as 55° C to be unsafe in terms of damage to tissue in their experimental model after implantation of PMMA,[209] since they observed healthy osteocytes adjacent to the cement in 6-week-old specimens.

Effect of Monomer at Cellular Level

Albrektsson and associates have studied tissue injury resulting from leakage of monomer from polymerizing bone cement using a titanium test chamber and vital microscopy methods.[2–4] With this method, tissue response in the same animal could be studied from the time of cement application to as long as 350 days later. The authors made the following observations:

1. The immediate effects from monomer were vascular flow interference including flow stasis and intravascular hemolysis.
2. The effects on the fatty marrow were widespread but were limited in bone. This appeared to reflect the affinity of monomer to fatty tissue.
3. With further follow-up the authors noted marked resorption of marrow fat cells during the first weeks after injury, but they observed very little bone resorption.
4. In this study there was no indication that the polymerized cement exerted a toxic effect on the tissue.

The affinity for fat-soluble monomer in marrow tissue had been demonstrated previously by Bechtel and others.[15] Hemolysis and vascular effects of monomer were observed by Linder and Romanus, who also noted that hydrated tissues appear to be protected from monomeric action.[144]

Effect of Weight Bearing

The effect of weight-bearing stresses on the nature of the mechanical properties of interface tissue is essentially related to the patient's postoperative care. Several investigators have expressed opinions regarding the effects of weight-bearing on the interface and bone remodeling after total hip arthroplasty. Among those favoring a period of nonweight bearing are Lindwer and Van Den Hooff, who suggest that because of bone necrosis resulting from the heat of polymerization, disruption of blood supply, and toxicity of monomer, osteoclastic absorption of bone may subsequently undergo repair by new bone formation.[145] Therefore during the critical phase of bone resorption and bone replacement, the patient should remain nonweight bearing. Spinelli reached a similar conclusion in an experimental sheep model in which he studied the interface by scanning electronmicroscopy; an intimate bonding between cement and bone resulted without interpositioning fibrous tissue, in contrast to weight-bearing animals that produced a fibrous membrane caused by micromotion.[240] Contrary to the views expressed by those authors, Willert and co-workers presented observations on histological specimens[267] based on five biopsies of patients after early loosening in which they noted an increased turnover of bone; thus they concluded that early weight bearing was desirable to decrease bone turnover and reactive osteoporosis at the junctional tissue. Charnley's observations suggested that fibrous membrane at the junctional tissue between cement and bone responds to weight-bearing stress, and thus fibrocartilage and metaplastic bone can replace the original fibrous tissue resulting from osteoclastic activities.[51] Gitelis and associates, using total hip arthroplasty in male dogs,

performed a knee disarticulation in one group to ensure nonweight-bearing conditions and compared the results to a control group, which had full weight bearing. The authors concluded the following[103]:

1. Osteoclastic resorption of necrotic cortical bone and its replacement by new bone formation was not impeded by early postoperative weight bearing.
2. Muscular activity in amputated animals was similar to muscle activity in a nonweight-bearing situation in humans.
3. Early postoperative weight bearing did not seem to specifically influence biological reaction to PMMA.

The basic influence of mechanical stress on the interface between bone and prosthesis was reviewed by Ling,[147] who coined the term *junctional tissue*. He postulated that one of the barriers to understanding the subject has been the use of the terms *fixed* and *loose* with reference to artificial joint components. It must be a given that there will always be some movement between a prosthesis and bone, even if the amplitude is so small that it cannot be measured or the site of movement cannot be identified. When two materials of different modulus of elasticity are simultaneously subjected to load, motion occurs within the substance of one or in the interface between the two. For this reason alone, the motion between the two elements cannot be eliminated in the living subject. With regard to the effects of weight bearing, the nature of interface tissue must also be considered. Soft tissue is capable of transmitting a considerable amount of compressive stress; thus it is likely that compressive forces are well tolerated. For tensile and sheer forces to be transmitted to bone, osteointegration is essential. It is for this reason that the presence of a soft tissue interface in the acetabulum is better tolerated than in the femur; it may be that the major forces generated in the acetabulum are mainly compressive while in the femur they are tensile, torsional, and compressive. The presence of a fibrous interface in continuum can be regarded as an unsuitable medium for load transmission because of unacceptable levels of tensile and torsional stresses in the femur.

Changes in Bone Mineral Content

Quantitative measurements of bone mineral content have been established after injury and fractures.* The bone mineral content of the distal part of the femoral shaft of the operated leg after total hip arthroplasty was measured at 1 to 2 weeks before surgery and at 4, 8, 16, 36, 48, and 72 weeks after surgery as monitored with single-photon gamma absorptiometry in 46 patients with osteoarthritis. After an initial bone mineral con-

---

* References 6, 7, 19, 153, 186–188, 262.

tent increase (greater in men than in women), a decrease occurred during the first postoperative year to the initial value in men, but in women the final result was a 10% net loss. The loss of bone mineral content was remarkably low compared with the results obtained after injuries of similar or even lesser magnitude.[141]

HISTOLOGY OF IMPLANTED CEMENT IN HUMANS
Histological Studies

Histological evaluation of both animal and human bone and cement has been extensively reported by several authors.* Charnley reported in detail the histological findings of human specimens (37 calcar and 26 acetabulum) after patient death from natural causes; all specimens studied had a successful total hip arthroplasty. The average time after operation was 7.3 years; the longest period was 13 years, and 13 patients were evaluated more than 9 years after operation. All of these cases were 100% successful arthroplasties, an essential feature in the proper interpretation of cement in contact with living tissue.[38,266] In available literature, considerable confusion has occurred when the studies of loose and infected prostheses have been reported along with those of successful cement-fixed implants.[53] Consequently, it is important to consider the histology of bone and cement contact in the absence of infection in two separate situations: (1) state of rigidity, that is, successful arthroplasty, and (2) state of looseness, that is, failure.

In numerous histological reports from both human postmortem studies and animal experimental work, the necrosis of bone, periosteal new bone formation, and reaction to the implanted cement (and in combination with HDP) were interpreted differently. Most authors reported the presence of fibrocartilage or fibrous connective tissue in the interface between bone and cement, and some believed that the implant was encapsulated in connective tissue.†

Tissue Response with Rigidly Fixed Cement

GROSS APPEARANCE Close contact between cement and bone is easily recognized by close observation of a horizontal or vertical cross-section of the femur or the acetabular region (Fig. 4-2). Sometimes a layer of fibrous tissue is visible to the naked eye at the cement-bone junction, especially at the areas of cancellous bone in the acetabular region. On the other hand, this state almost never exists at the interface between cement and femur, which is well fixed. At

times, however, under low-power magnification, it appears that the cement is in direct contact with the bone, but there is a normal amount of fat cells close to the surface of the cement. The molding of the cement injected into the cancellous bone can be appreciated after careful removal of the cement from the bone. The following three important histological features of the gross specimens should be noted:

1. Negative impressions of the cement's forcible injection into the bones that resulted from formation of a mold of the interior surface of the bone, indicating a direct bone-cement contact. This may also represent evidence of osteointegration.
2. Fibrous tissue with no preferred orientation interposed between bone and cement, indicating the absence of direct contact and suggesting possible loosening or inadequate pressure injection. It may also suggest areas of bone absorption and replacement by fibrous tissue.
3. Smooth surface areas of highly organized fibrous tissue or fibrocartilage, suggesting possible soft tissue contact and load transmission zones.

MICROSCOPY To recognize the histology of cement-tissue contact areas, investigators must be aware of the microscopic structure of acrylic cement itself when in contact with the tissue.

The polymer powder consists of spheres ranging from 30 to 80 μm. Because decalcified sections are not satisfactory for the purpose of detailed examination, the cement is usually dissolved out. The impressions left by the granules are easily recognizable as evidence of contact between the cement and the tissue. Fig. 4-3 shows evidence of osteointegration in the femur.

It is essential in a study of the bone-cement interface for specimens to be obtained from patients who are known to have had a successful clinical result and in whom the state of weight bearing and function has been perfect.[45,49,91]

Postoperative tissue damage begins at surgery and leads to bone necrosis at the site of cement insertion. This is related to metaphyseal and intramedullary interference by the trauma of broaching, devascularization of bone, and cell death by monomer or possibly the heat of polymerization. Therefore it is not unusual to find segmental or zonal necrosis in the trochanteric shaft or calcar region of the femur at a later stage. Investigators frequently observe hemispherical cement impressions in direct contact with bone trabecula containing living osteocytes right up to its surface.

Within the first 2 or 3 weeks after insertion of the cement, a coagulum of connective tissue is visible (interposed between cement and bone). The repair is manifested by local hyperemia, migration of lipo-

---

* References 35, 46, 49, 51, 53, 118, 266.
† References 91, 145, 167, 201, 211, 231–233, 256.

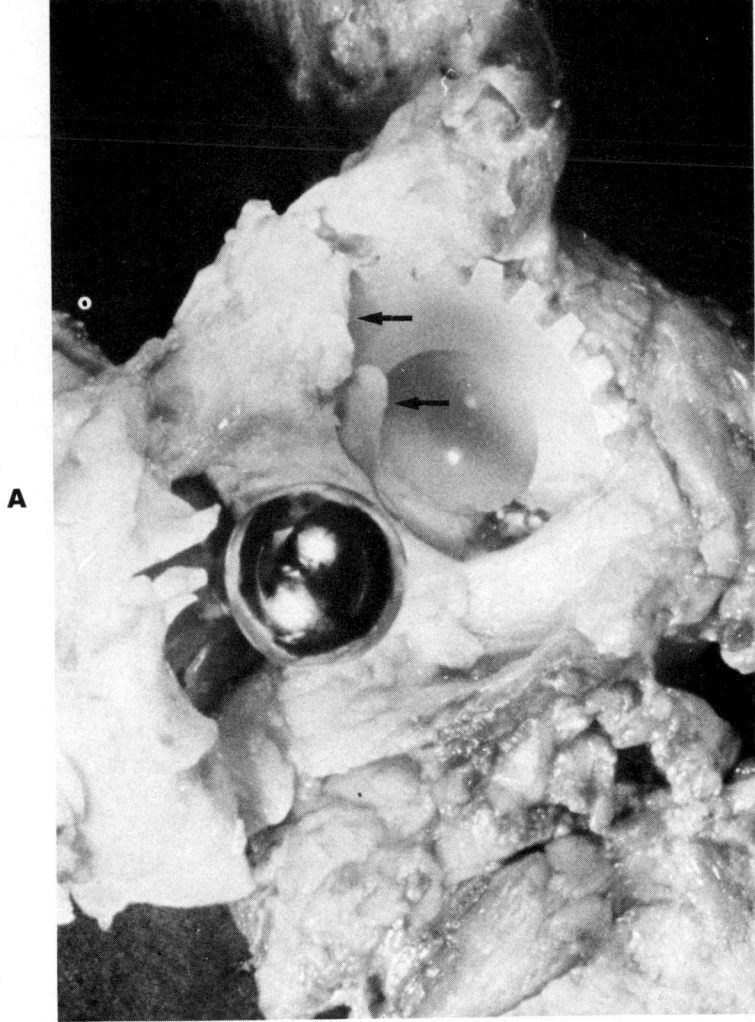

Fig. 4-2. Examination of postmortem specimens of total hip prostheses using HDP against stainless steel has shown minimum tissue reaction. Gross specimen (postmortem) is removed 7 years and 3 months after successful low-friction arthroplasty. NOTE: marked capsular thickening as evidence of capsular repair *(top arrow)*. At certain points thickness reaches more than 1 cm. Only evidence of gross histological tissue reaction was evidence of two small proliferative synovial-type reactions at inferior portion of joint *(bottom arrow)*. Prosthetic components were rigidly fixed to bone by cement. **A,** Low-power photomicrograph taken from capsular lining of joint showing giant cell reaction. **B,** Photomicrograph of portion of synovial lining. Tissue obtained from the same specimen showing small but frequent giant cell reaction. **C,** High-power photomicrograph of giant cells presumably containing particles of HDP. **D** to **G,** Similar to **A** to **C** but under polarized light. NOTE: double refractive material (HDP) within giant cells, evidence of wear particles of HDP.

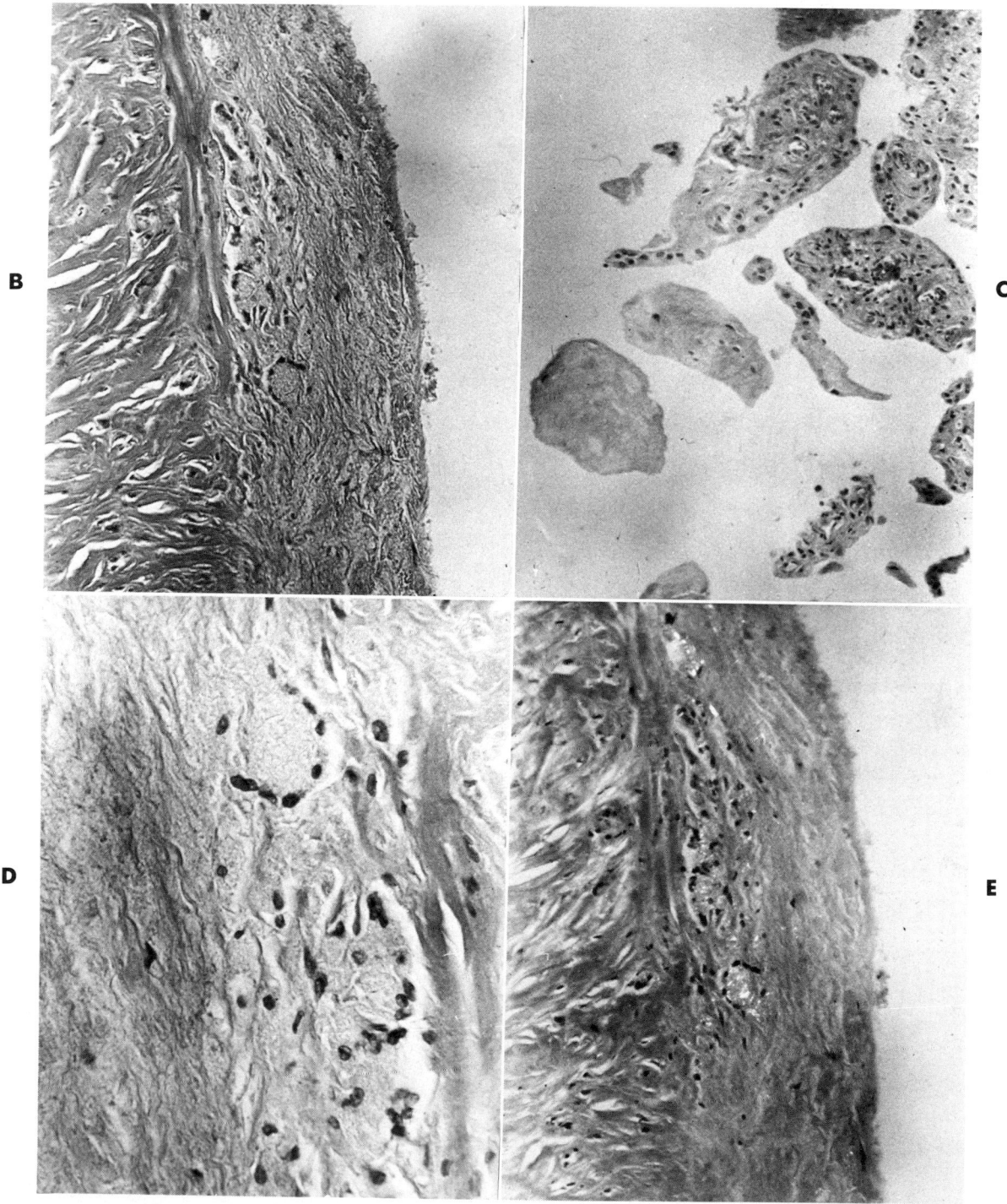

Fig. 4-2—cont'd. See legend on opposite page.

Continued.

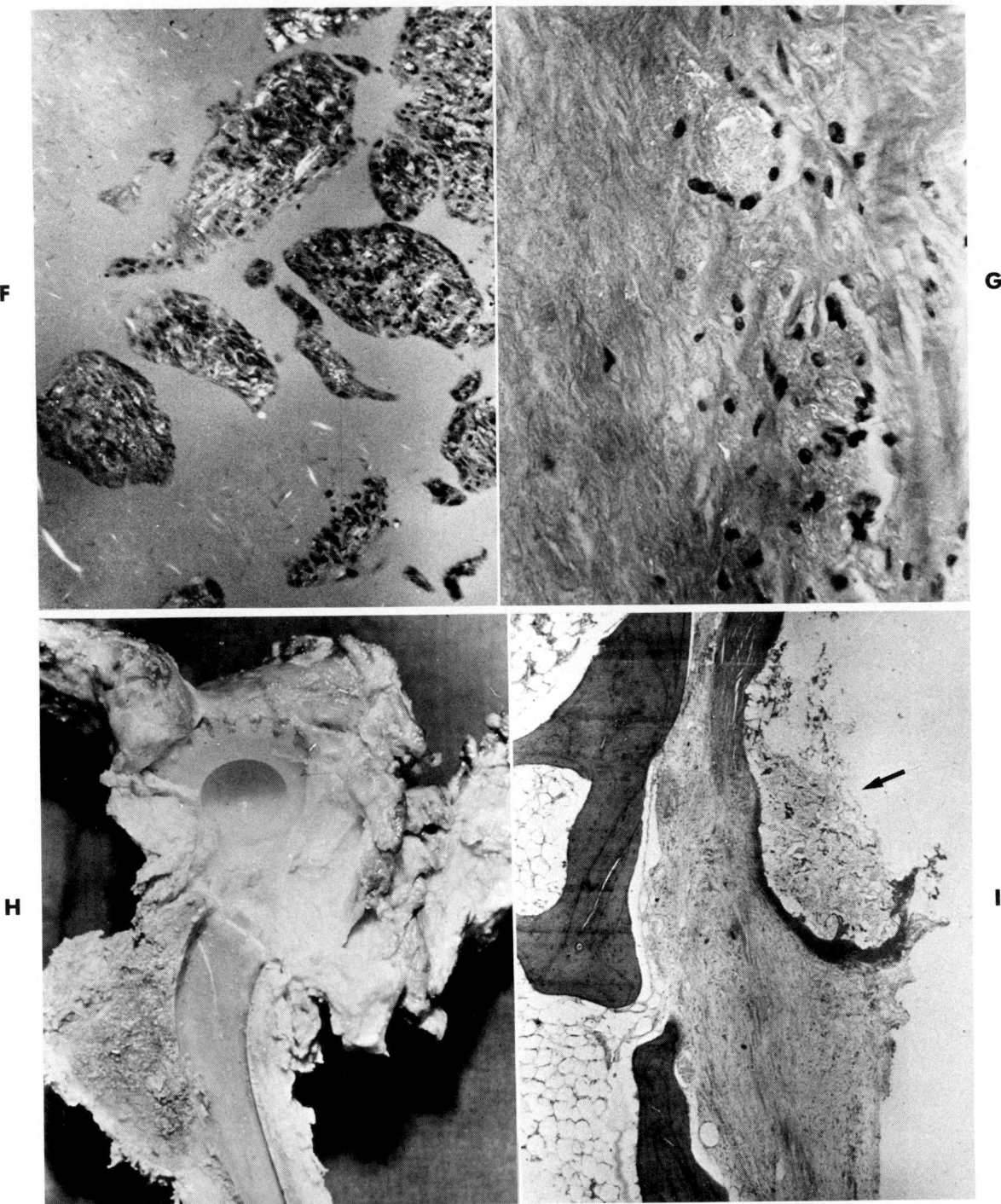

Fig. 4-2—cont'd. D to **G,** Similar to **A** to **C** but under polarized light. NOTE: double refractive material (HDP) within giant cells, evidence of wear particles of HDP. **H,** Specimen after removal of femoral component. Prosthesis was absolutely rigidly fixed in bone. There was no gross fibrous lining between metal and cement, but whitish fibrinoid-like material was smeared throughout length of prosthesis. There was smooth lining of interface between cement and bone without evidence of cavitation or cystic changes. **I** and **J,** Two areas of bone in contact with cement and interposed by fibrous tissue. Fibrous tissue is highly organized and in certain areas suggestive of fibrocartilage containing only occasional giant cells. NOTE: cement contact, **I,** with fibrocartilage and impressions of cement spheres within fibrocartilaginous layer. Portion of cement in this specimen had not been fully dissolved out of specimen *(arrow)*. Healthy marrow is noted.

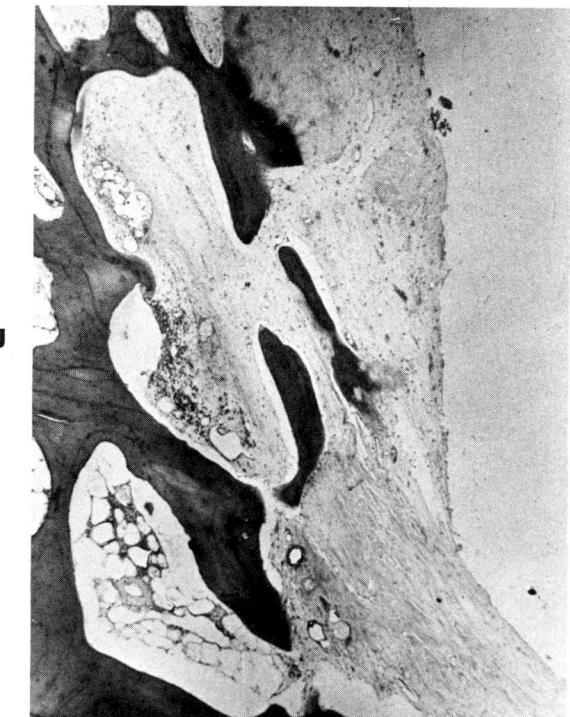

Fig. 4-2—cont'd. See legend on opposite page.

phages, and ingrowth of capillaries and fibroblasts. As time progresses, the interface tissue becomes more organized, with four types of contact between cement and bone generally observable for up to a year.

FEMUR In the femur all histological samples of successful arthroplasty, rigidly fixed femoral components, and specimens obtained at postmortem examination show, at some points, a fibrous membrane between the acrylic cement and bone of the femur. When the specimens were obtained below the level of the lesser trochanter, the interface can best be described as a delicate areolar tissue without continuity. This appearance is somewhat different from that of the specimens obtained at the level of the heavily loaded femoral neck, where the interface is similar to that at the acetabulum. In general, in specimens obtained from the femur, the fibrous interface is usually extremely thin and never completely lines the entire endosteal surface of the femur.[43,47–49] The load bearing appears to take place through "caps" of fibrocartilage or modified bone matrix; thus no tissue of any kind is interposed between the cement and bone (Fig. 4-3, *D* to *F*). These points of contact indicate that a perfect fixation to skeleton is possible through these caps and that load is transmitted only through selected points of the endosteal surface of the femur through the bony trabeculae. The marrow cells are separated from cement by a delicate membrane, which shows no evidence of macrophages or granulation formation.

Absence of radiolucencies after total hip arthroplasty in the femur and often lack of demarcation are the rule rather than the exception and can be interpreted as a positive and favorable response that is maintained in the femur over a long period of time. It is possible that at least three factors favor the use of cement in the femur: (1) the ability to contain the cement within the tube of the femur, (2) the ability to pressurize the cement at surgery, and (3) the ability to resist bleeding pressure in the femur while the cement is being polymerized, conditions that may not prevail at insertion of cement in the acetabulum.

After two decades of controversy, Linder and Hansson, in an electronmicroscopy study of three cases of cement-bone interface, supported Charnley's view that in a perfectly successful case the cement may lie in direct contact with living bone.[143]

ACETABULUM Clinical and radiological findings after cement has been used for acetabular fixation indicate a higher incidence of radiolucencies and demarcation than found in the femur.

Unlike the histology of the interface in the femur, Charnley noted that repair of the acetabulum after 10 years had not reached an endpoint. The presence of histiocytes and a few giant cells suggested an unstable state of repair, which he called "suspended animation," with neither positive repair nor positive destruction even after 10 to 15 years of notable clinical success in life.[48,49] Figs. 4-4 and 4-5 demonstrate a clinically

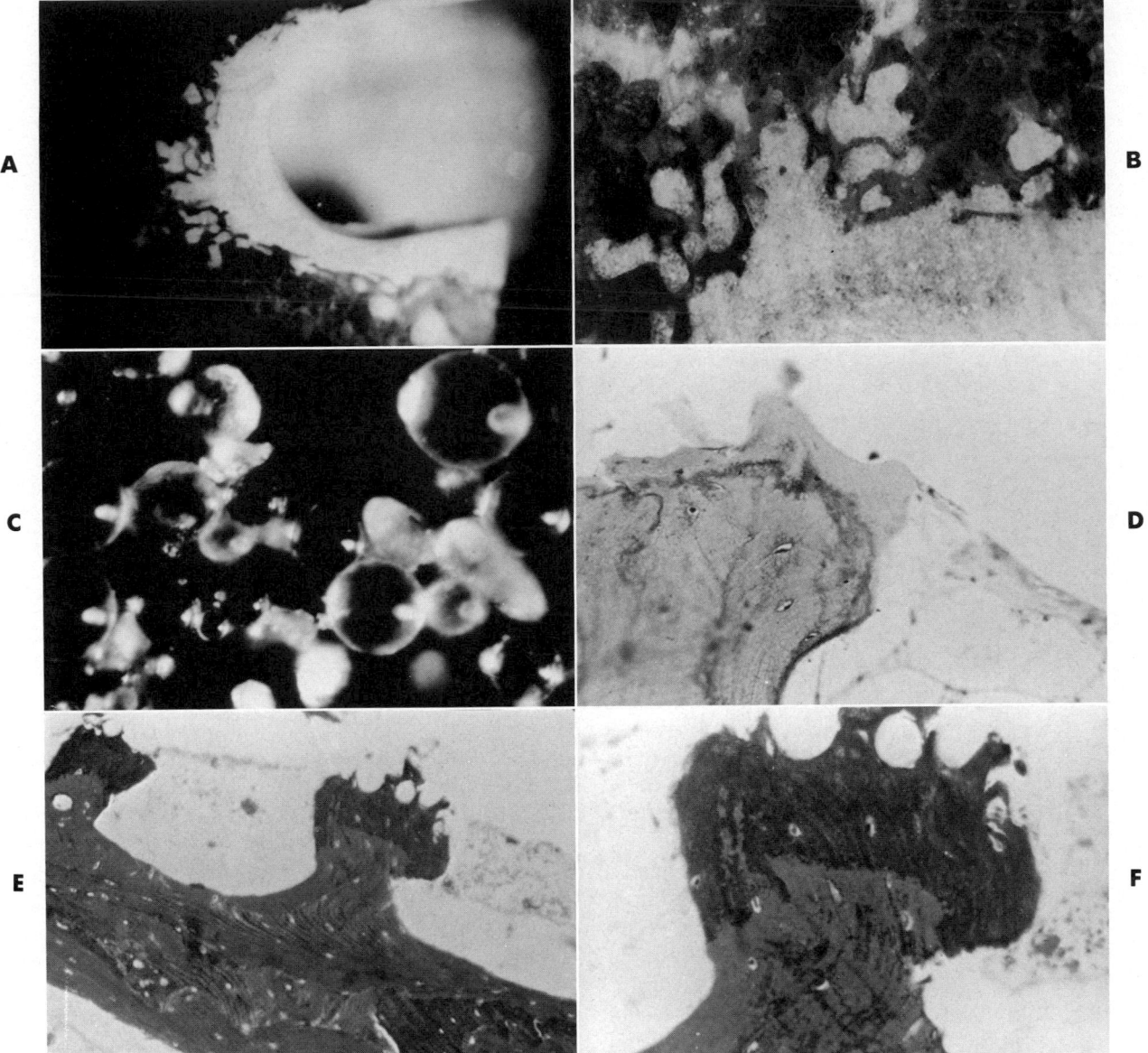

Fig. 4-3. A, Cross section of the femur and cement mantle is shown at 1 cm above the lesser trochanter. The femoral component had been implanted 12 years previously with an excellent result. NOTE: a good bony penetration by cement in the very heavy load area of the femur. **B,** Penetration of cement and direct contact with bone can be seen (at 1.5 cm below the level of the lesser trochanter) over the medial aspect of the femur. **C,** The polymer powder in PMMA mix consists of microspherules ranging from 30 to 80 μm. Identification of the spherules or their histological impressions (on the bone) can be regarded as evidence of osteointegration. **D,** The load-bearing in a cemented femur is demonstrated histologically to occur through newly formed "caps" of fibrocartilage or modified bone matrix without any other interposing tissue. These caps in turn transmit load through selected points of the endosteal surface of the femur through its trabecular system to the cortex. Light microscopy H & E stain shows healthy marrow adjacent to caps after cement has been dissolved. **E** and **F,** Low and high magnification areas of direct cement contact with bone. (**D** to **F** from Charnley J: Low-friction arthroplasty of the hip: theory and practice, Berlin, 1979, Springer-Verlag.)

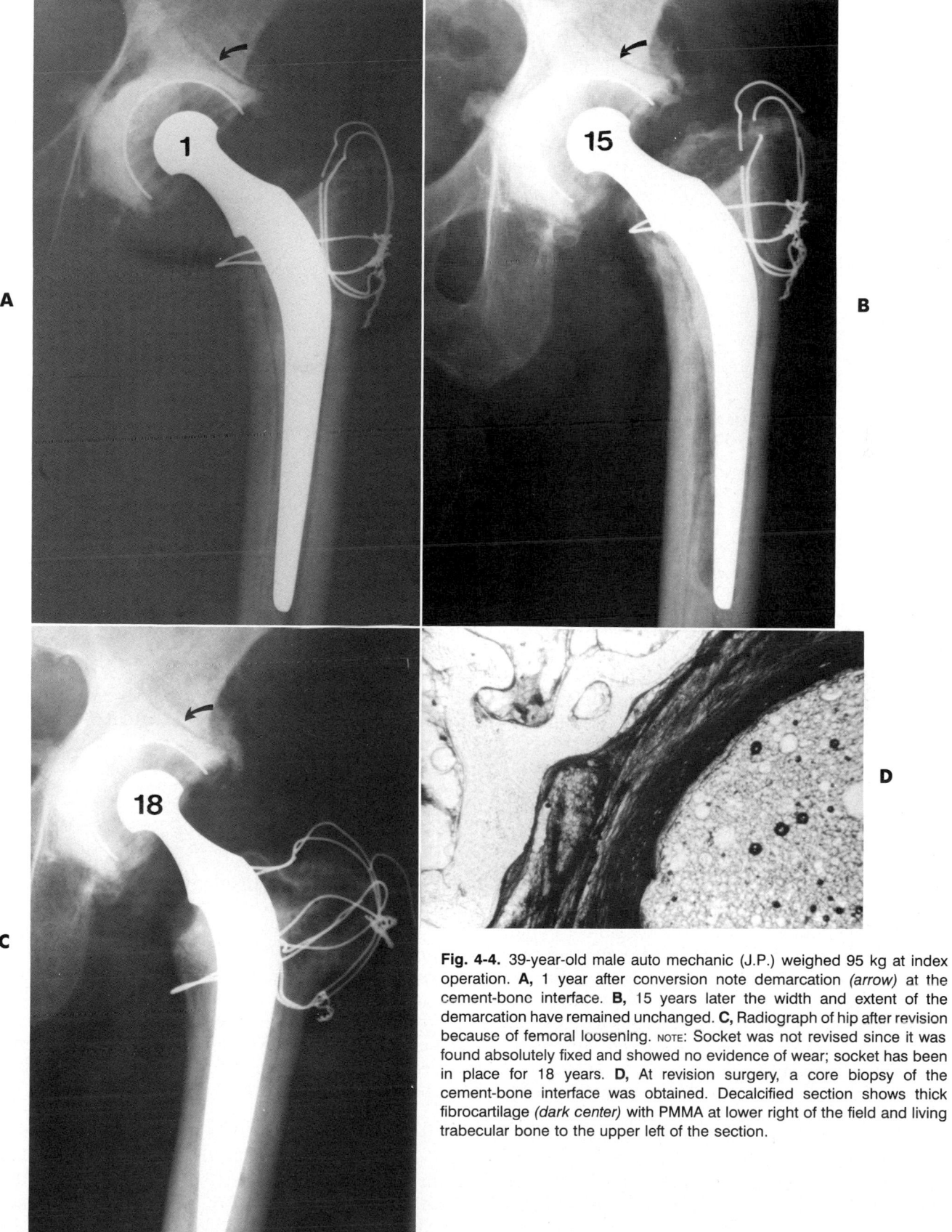

Fig. 4-4. 39-year-old male auto mechanic (J.P.) weighed 95 kg at index operation. **A,** 1 year after conversion note demarcation *(arrow)* at the cement-bone interface. **B,** 15 years later the width and extent of the demarcation have remained unchanged. **C,** Radiograph of hip after revision because of femoral loosening. NOTE: Socket was not revised since it was found absolutely fixed and showed no evidence of wear; socket has been in place for 18 years. **D,** At revision surgery, a core biopsy of the cement-bone interface was obtained. Decalcified section shows thick fibrocartilage *(dark center)* with PMMA at lower right of the field and living trabecular bone to the upper left of the section.

B

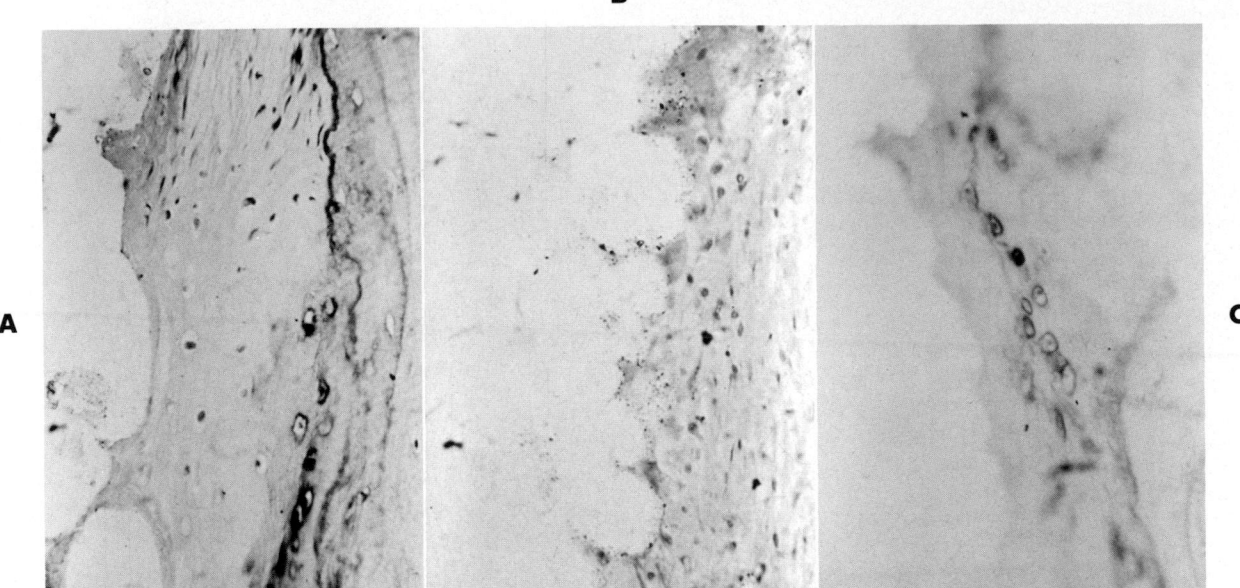

A   C

Fig. 4-5. Same patient as Fig. 4-4. **A** to **C**, Three different areas of the interface resembling cartilage cells. In some areas fibrocartilage is present). Semicircular impressions indicate likelihood of load of transmission via cement because of presence of PMMA polymer spherules.

successful long-term acetabular fixation despite the absence of osteointegration between bone and cement. Fibrocartilage medium was capable of transferring the load adequately for up to 18 years.

The presence of macrophages at the bone-cement interface was described by Charnley and Crawford in 1968 and was considered a direct response to PMMA.[49] Freeman and associates less optimistically interpreted the presence of macrophages at the cement-bone interface as evidence of "tissue response" to PMMA, whether solid or in pearls.[91] They compared such a response with the response to chromium-cobalt alloy that was minimal and that resulted only in a fibrous interface. They concluded that the macrophages were attracted to the minute bands of PMMA similar to the way they were attracted to catgut and chromium-cobalt alloy in its particulate form. The presence of macrophages at the interface is of concern because they are precursors of osteoclasts and thus instigators of bone resorption.[41] These authors considered the mere presence of macrophages to be an indicator of eventual failure of fixation, since stimuli that are known to excite the macrophages are (1) dead cells, (2) bacteria, and (3) foreign debris in minute particles from prosthesis and autogenous bone debris.[18,221,243,244]

In an in-vivo study of cementing the acetabular component in dogs using techniques for pressurization, Paul and Bargar found tissue response differed significantly from that in the femur.[194] They observed new bone formation by 2 weeks, and bone remodeling

continued to be active up to 6 months after operation in the femur. However, they noted little new bone formation by 6 weeks in the acetabulum. The authors interpreted that these differences between the acetabulum and femur are caused by a difference in bone formation and difference in the vascularity of the bone.[193] Certainly, micromotion and stress patterns must play an important role in the histological difference observed between the acetabulum and the femur.

MECHANICAL PROPERTIES OF BONE-CEMENT INTERFACE

The mechanical strength of the interface is largely dependent on the method of applying the cement and the strength of the recipient bone. Because the strength of fixation is achieved by penetration of cement into the microstructures of the cancellous bone, two interrelated variables must be considered: (1) preparation of the cancellous recipient bone by removal of debris and fat marrow using high-pressure lavage and (2) the depth of penetration of cement into the bone by methods to facilitate penetration.[130,162,180]

BIOLOGICAL FIXATION OF IMPLANTS

Considerable experience with cementless total hip arthroplasty has been reported from Europe during the 1970s and 1980s. Most of these prostheses incorporated a porous surface similar to one described by Lord[149] and known as *Madreporique*. In the United States, the most widely used prostheses are based on two principal designs: (1) cobalt-chromium alloy with metallic beads or (2) titanium alloy (Ti-6AL-4VA) coated with a commercially pure titanium bead, wire mesh, or plasma spray. For mature bone to consistently develop uniformly within the pores, the following three criteria must be met:

1. The optimum size should be between 100 and 400 μm.[24,239].
2. Close contact with bone must be present.[25,112]
3. The initial contact achieved must be maintained as ingrown bone matures.[39,112]

Bobyn and others[24,25,39,112,239] have characterized bone ingrowth into porous surface of implants (regardless of the material) as a fracture healing phenomenon that occurs with surface porosities between 50 and 500 μm with the following general observations:

- Pore size less than 50 μm diameter results in fibrous ingrowth.
- Bone ingrowth occurs with equal rates of maturity irrespective of pore size, providing the pore size is between 50 and 500 μm.
- Direct contact with bone and immediate immobilization are essential for successful bone ingrowth.
- Micromotion adversity affects all types and qualities of bony ingrowth. Bone ingrowth does not occur if it exceeds the pore diameter.
- Although bone ingrowth occurs readily in most experimental animals, it occurs with less predictability in humans.
- A substantial bone ingrowth occurs by 3 weeks and can be at a maximum by 6 to 8 weeks after implantation.
- Once the bone healing onto the surface is initiated, it is capable of filling every space that is available to it. There is, however, certain osteoinductive potential for bone ingrowth into a porous implant that is not in actual contact with bone.[25]
- At a distance greater than 2 mm between bone and implant, bone apposition and ingrowth diminish.
- While a maximum incorporation occurs by 12 weeks in animals, secure biological fixation can occur through the surface of the implant.
- Continuous remodeling will occur after resumption of function, resulting in further bone formation or absorption since stress is being transferred to the interface between the bone and implant.

The process of bone ingrowth into two commonly used porous coated implants is shown in Figs. 4-6 to 4-21, representing lab animal experiments and retrieved human specimens.

Tissue Response with Prosthetic Instability

The early literature regarding the compatibility of PMMA is mainly unclear in describing the difference

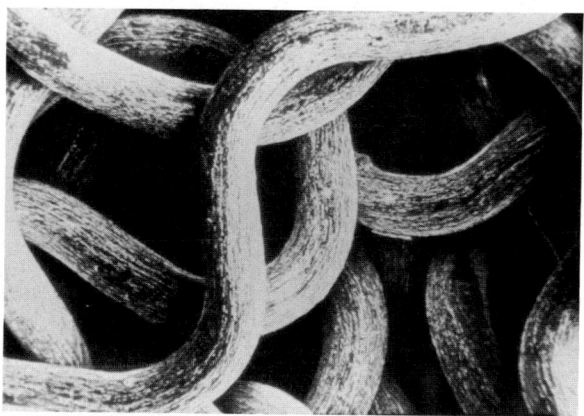

Fig. 4-6. Scanning electron micrograph of a porous titanium fiber metal sample. This material is made with titanium wire that is kinked and then compressed and heated, creating multiple spot welds in the wires. Average pore size and percent porosity are controlled by altering variables in the manufacturing process (×250). (Courtesy AG Rosenberg M.D.)

between the tissue response of failed total hips and infected total hips (where those tissue responses had not previously been identified and the failures were largely attributed to acrylic cement).[35,53,257] For example, loose fragments of cement, along with caseation, cavitation, and necrosis, are frequently reported in a loose cemented prosthesis where motion has been present for some time before surgical intervention. In the presence of infection, reactions are obviously different in that signs of osteitis usually are present and microabscesses are frequently visible at the interface. In addition to infection, mechanical defects occurred in metal-to-metal total hip prostheses, which may suggest sensitivity to metal particles, especially chromium and cobalt particles. It should be emphasized that extensive tissue reaction with giant cell formation and caseation suggests the presence of loosening of cement fragments in the bone for a long time before surgical intervention. Further, it was not clear to some reviewers that cement particles were not birefringent, since birefringent material was related to the particles worn from polyethylene. Unfortunately, since no specific stain technique is available for acrylic cement (MMA), the presence or absence of cement particles accompanying giant cells and macrophages was difficult to verify.

Early loosening must be considered a complication of surgical technique. It is usually related to fragments of cement becoming mobile in a soft tissue bed; the bone shows increased osteoclastic activity and remodeling at the site with sequestered acrylic pearls at the bed of the implant. If loosening is of long standing, a permanent organized tissue bed is produced with movable cement within it. This tissue usually exhibits

Text continued on p. 97.

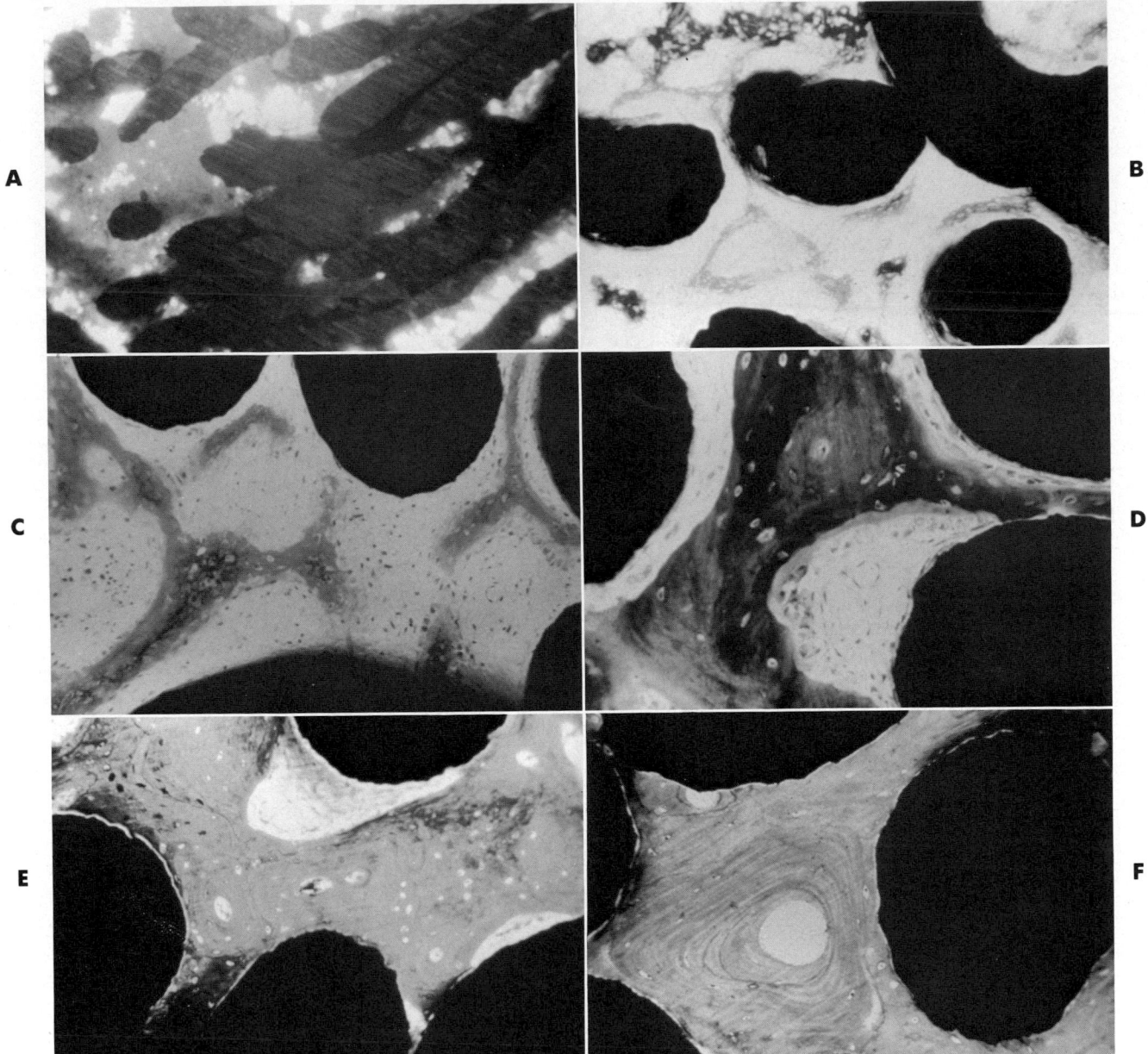

Fig. 4-7. Photomicrographs of the time sequence of bone ingrowth. The black spaces represent cross sections of the titanium wire that makes up the porous substrate for ingrowth. **A,** 1 day after implantation in canine model a post-traumatic hematoma is noted (×200). **B,** 1 week after implantation in canine model, the hematoma is replaced by a cellular pluri-potential mesenchymal infiltrate. Small strands of osteoid are noted (×400). **C,** 2 weeks after implant in canine model, the abundantly cellular mesenchymal tissue continues to produce osteoid. Calcification is beginning to take place (×450). **D,** 6 weeks after implantation in canine model, lamellar bone with haversian systems are seen. Osteoid seams, multinucleated giant cells, and rimming osteoblasts are present. In many areas, a cellular layer remains interposed between bone and the fiber metal (×450). **E,** 6 months after implantation in canine model, mature lamellar bone is noted. A relative paucity of cellular or fibrous tissue is interposed between the new ingrowth bone and the metal surface (×450). **F,** 10 years after implantation in primate model, mature lamellar bone and absence of intervening tissue layer between bone and metal are noted. Osteoid systems are prominent (×450). (Courtesy AG Rosenberg M.D.)

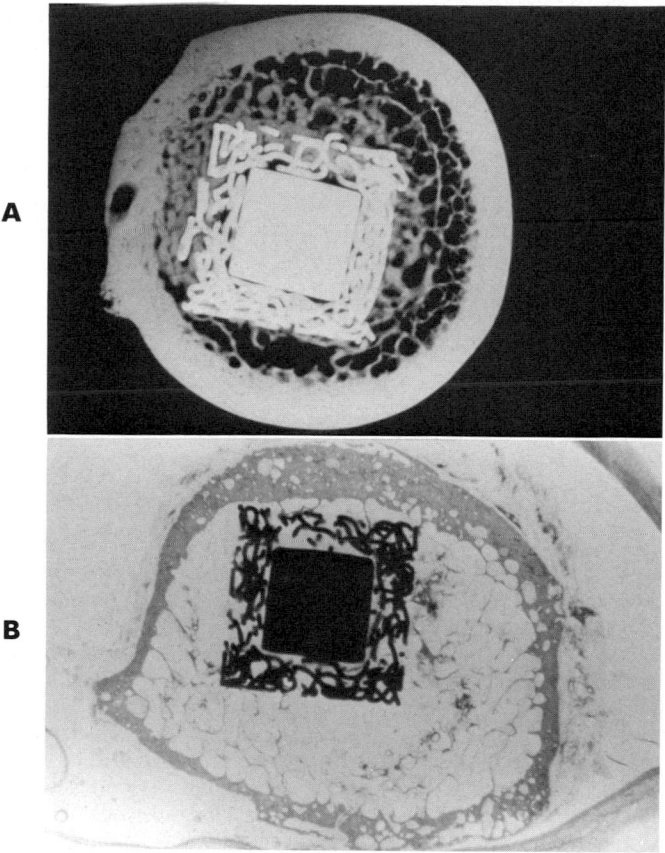

Fig. 4-8. Matched canine femora explanted 6 months after bilateral total hip implantation with fully coated femoral stems. **A,** This hip dislocated in the early postoperative period and rendered the limb nonweight-bearing. **B,** In the weight-bearing limb note the robust trabeculae extending from the cortex to implant and the dense ingrowth in the porous layer extending to the underlying prosthetic substrate. Contrast this to **A** with severe cortical atrophy and scanty trabeculae with minimal ingrowth.
(Courtesy AG Rosenberg M.D.)

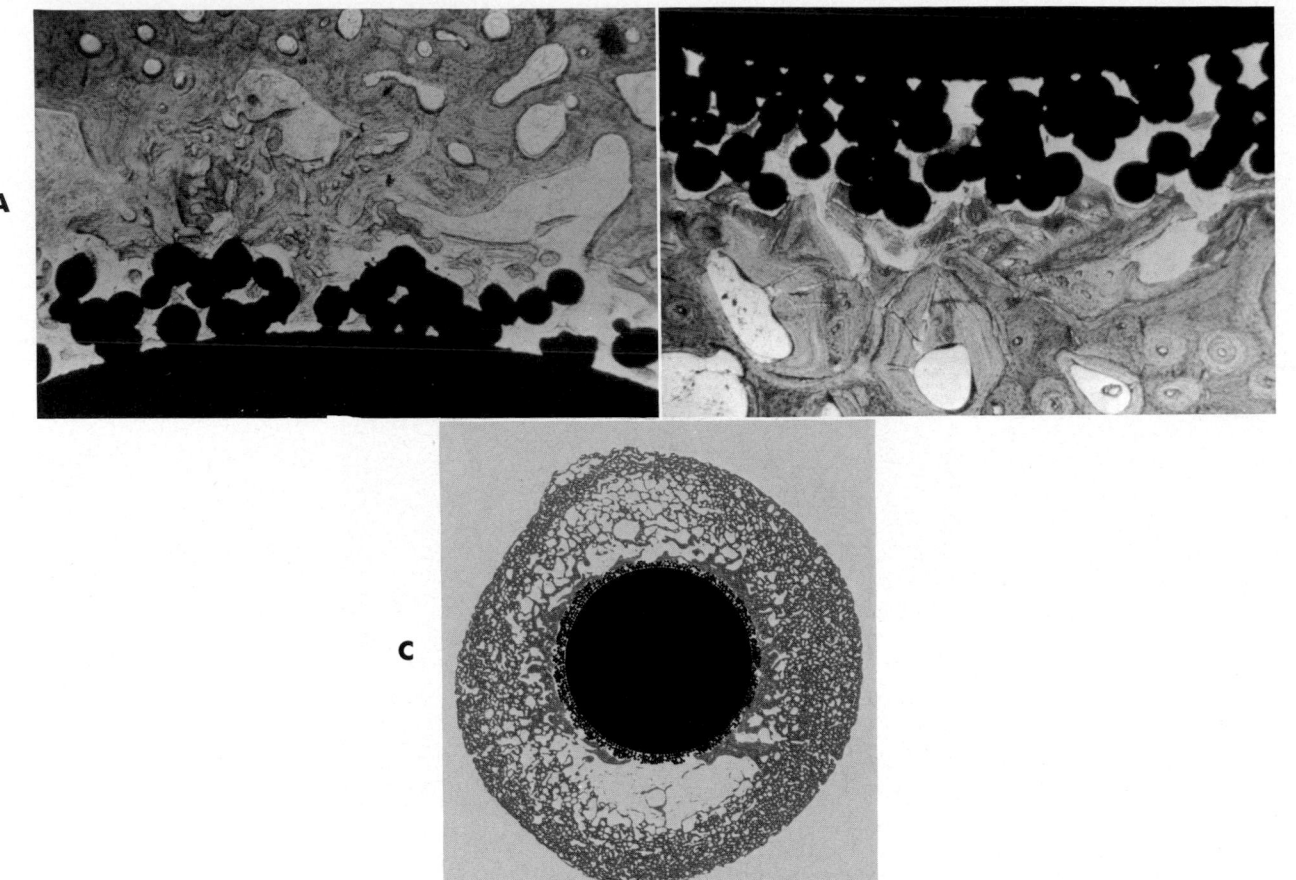

Fig. 4-9. A, Histological photomicrograph of a transverse section through a 10.5 mm diameter fully porous-coated AML stem implanted for 6 weeks in an 87-year-old female (diagnosis: subcapital fracture). In this posterolateral region of near-contact with the endosteum at the isthmus, there is neoformed bone between the endosteum and the implant and also within the implant porosity. Original magnification ×20. **B,** Histological photomicrograph of a transverse section taken at the isthmus through a 15 mm diameter 4/5 porous-coated AML stem implanted for 6 months in an 82-year-old male (diagnosis: osteoarthritis). A small region of shallow bone ingrowth arising from the endosteum is observed. Original magnification ×20. **C,** Histological photograph of a transverse section taken at the isthmus through a 13.5 mm diameter 4/5 porous coated AML stem implanted for 2 years in a 77-year-old male (Diagnosis: osteoarthritis). Note the generalized osteopenia of the cortex and the encapsulation of the implant by a thick, dense shell of bone. The bone has grown extensively into the porous coating, particularly on the lateral side *(right field).* (From Engh CA, Bobyn JD: *Biological fixation in total hip arthroplasty,* Thorofare, NJ, 1985, Slack, Inc.)

Fig. 4-10. Anteroposterior radiographs immediately postoperative, **A** and 3 years, **B** after implantation of fully porous coated 10 mm diameter AML stem in a 73-year-old male (Diagnosis: osteoarthritis). **C,** Histological photomicrograph of a region of bone ingrowth on the posterior side just under the collar (×20). Note the lacunae and nutrient vessels deep within the porous coating. **D,** Histological photograph of a transverse section prepared about 1.5 cm distal to the collar. Note the bone ingrowth medially *(left field)* and laterally *(right field).* **E,** Histological photograph of a transverse section prepared just distal to the lesser trochanter. There is new endosteal bone formation and bone ingrowth (possessing slightly different characteristics than original bone) around half of the implant circumference. The posterior aspect of the porous coating *(top field)* is void of bone and fibrous tissue. (From Engh CA, Bobyn JD: *Biological fixation in total hip arthroplasty,* Thorofare, NJ, 1985, Slack, Inc.)

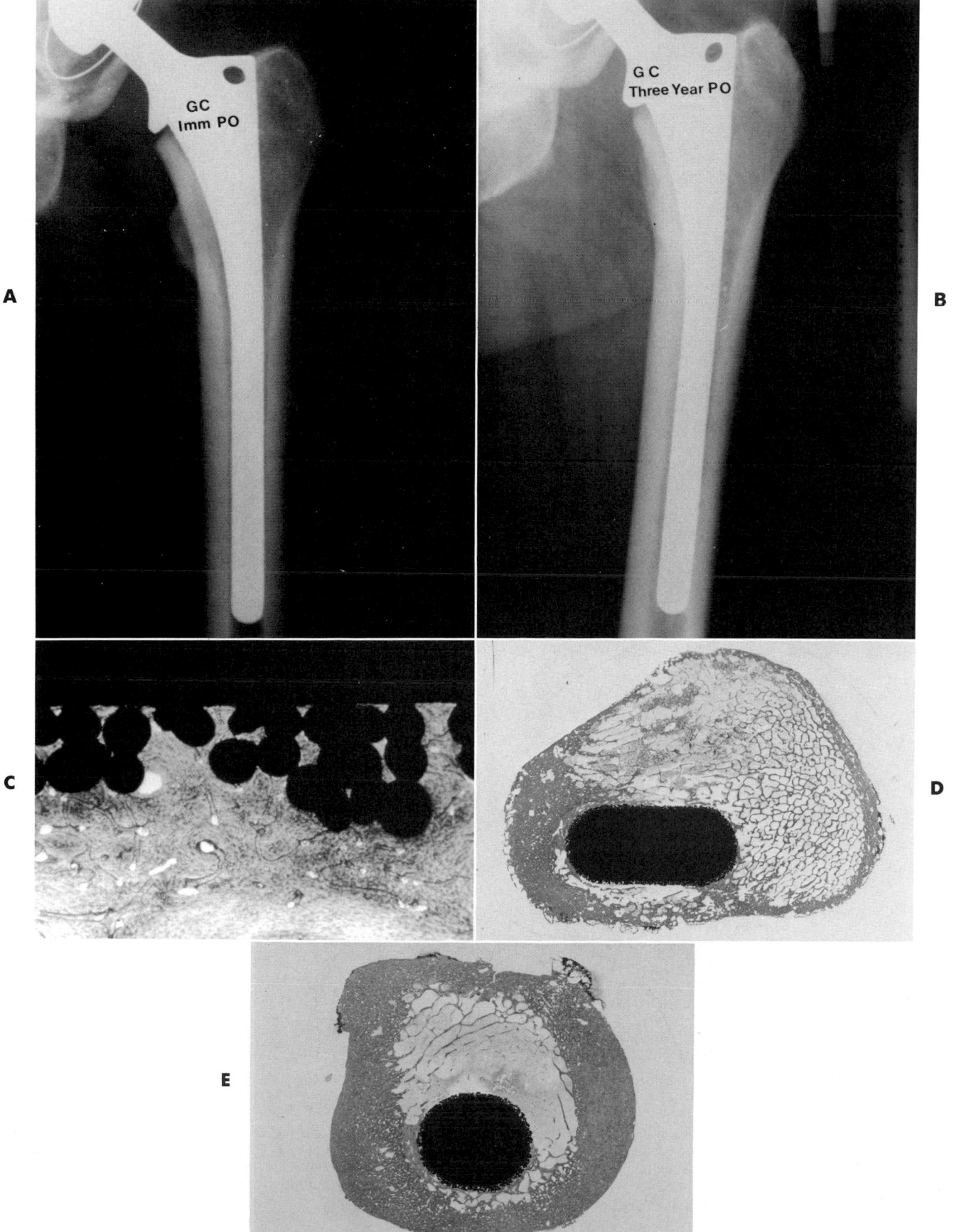

Fig. 4-10—cont'd. See legend on opposite page.

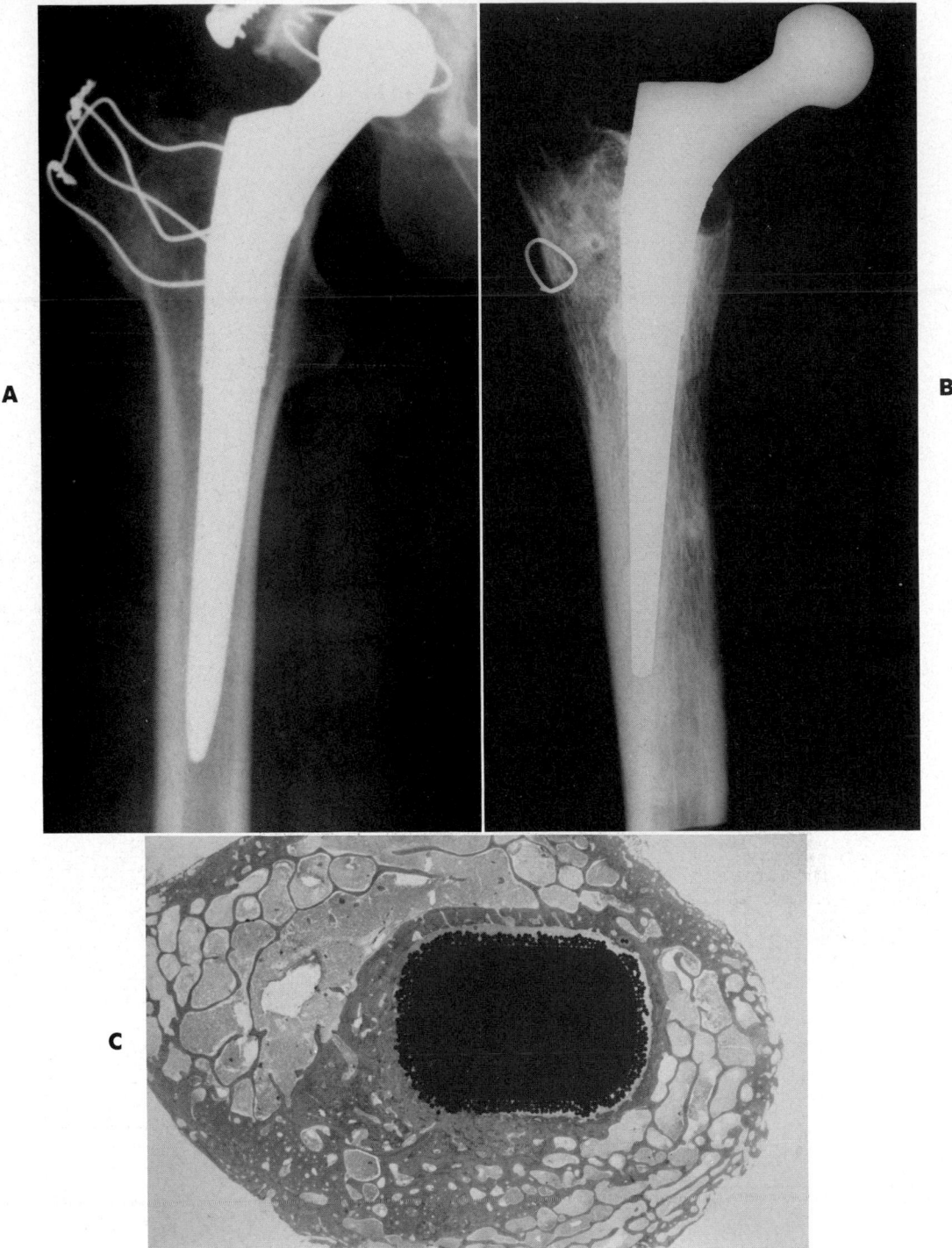

Fig. 4-11. A, Immediately postoperative and **B,** postmortem AP radiographs of a proximally porous-coated custom stem implanted for 5 years in a 17-year-old male (diagnosis: CDH). Extensive bone resorption occurred medially along the entire implant length. Note also the endosteal bone hypertrophy at the junction of the porous and smooth implant surfaces, suggestive of focused load transfer. **C,** Transverse histological section prepared near the junction of porous and smooth implant surfaces shows a new endosteal cortex, an osteopenic original cortex, and both bone ingrowth and fibrous encapsulation at the porous interface (×20). (From Collier JP, Bauer TW, Bloebaum RD, et al: *Clin Orthop* 274:97, 1992.)

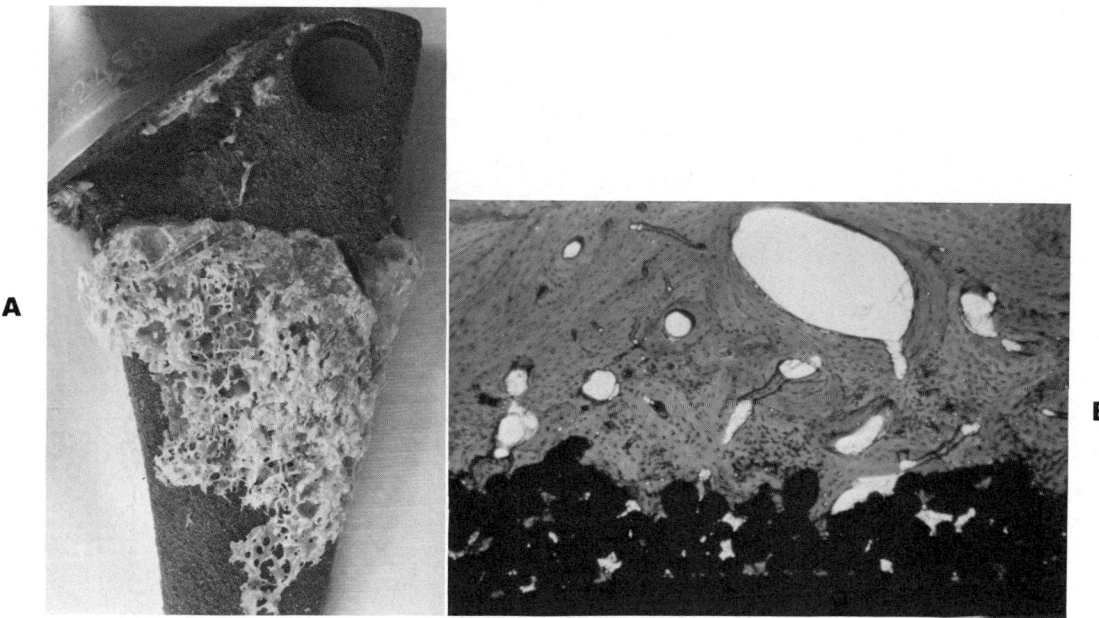

Fig. 4-12. **A,** Photograph of proximal region of fully porous coated 10.5 mm diameter AML prosthesis implanted for 7 years in a 58-year-old male (diagnosis: AVN). The prosthesis was stable but grossly undersized and removed at the same time as a loosened cemented cup. A large plaque of bone was firmly adherent to the anterior and posterior aspects of the proximal stem. **B,** Transverse histological section through the bony plaque illustrating bony apposition and ingrowth down to the implant substrate. This is particularly remarkable since the implant was of the original AML design, possessing only a 100 μm pore size. (Courtesy Engh CA, Bobyn JD, Glassman AH)

tears accompanied by a fibrous exudate and an occasional zone of necrosis (see Fig. 4-2, *G* to *I*). Willert and associates have also suggested that excessive load applied early during the repair stage is detrimental to fixation.[267] The greatest risk in securing a good fixation comes from insufficient immediate contact between cement and bone (microinterlock), leading to early motion and damage to both tissue and cement.

Cystic erosions in the calcar region of the femur after a successful arthroplasty of many years may be attributed to microfractures in the cement and minor loosening at this heavily loaded zone. Occasional extensive bone absorption and cystic changes along the shaft may also be related to motion between the cement and the bone. When amplitude motion is not severe, the patient may be asymptomatic, but with the passage of time and further loosening, clinical failure will result. Cracks and cleavage planes within the cement cone may allow pumping of minute cement or high-density polyethylene particles to occur, causing erosive changes in the bone; the macrophagic response is usually proportional to the amount and size of these particles. Usually there are three types of foreign body giant cells: large giant cells, small giant cells, and

histiocytes. Perhaps these types of cells are all manifestations of the same phenomenon, but the reactions to the different sizes and shapes of the particles result in different kinds of cells. The large, hollow spaces associated with foreign body giant cells are large particles of acrylic cement, and most of the small giant cells contain particles of HDP. Areas pertaining to the sheets of histiocytes are related to the formation of small particles of HDP (produced by wear).[46]

In summary, the histology of tissue contact with cement that is rigidly fixed in the bone is entirely benign, and the occasional giant cells revealed in nonweight-bearing zones of the interface (unique to acetabular fixation) are the only suggestion of tissue response to cement. Any evidence of severe tissue response, such as giant cell reaction and caseous formation leading to bone cavitation, must elicit a suspicion of mechanical loosening of the cement in the bone. Acrylic cement is not birefringent, and histological evidence of birefringent material is indicative of wear debris from HDP (Fig. 4-22). Where severe bone necrosis accompanies focal cell infiltration and fibrinous necrosis, the possibility of infection (see Chapter 32) must also be considered.

Text continued on p. 105.

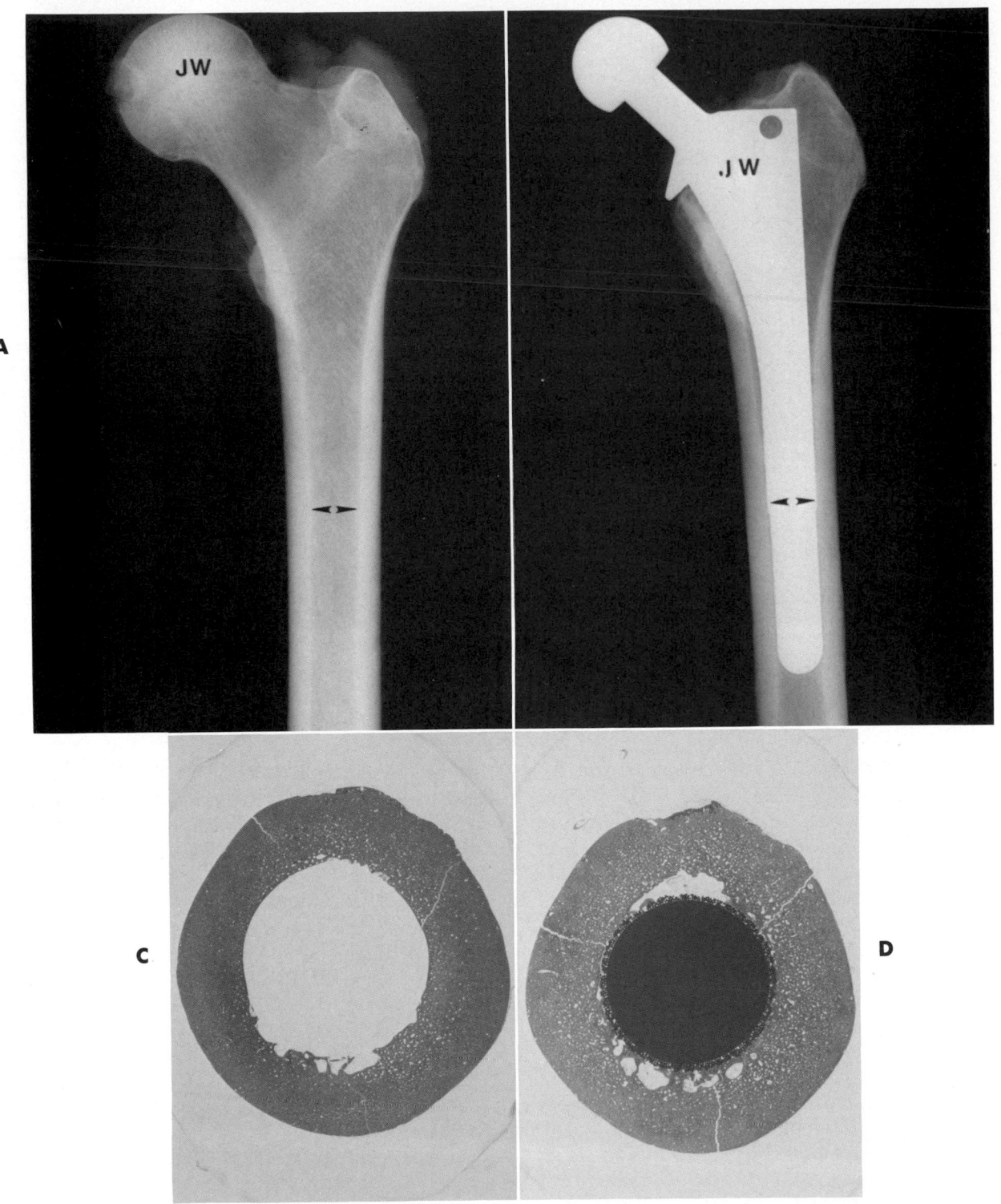

Fig. 4-13. Postmortem radiographs, **A** and **B,** and histological sections, **C** and **D,** of a pair of femora retrieved 7 months after operation. The 16.5 mm stem had been implanted with a press fit. The cortical thickness and density of both femora are similar. The transverse sections were taken at a level marked by arrows in **A** and **B.** The cracks are artifacts. Bone ingrowth fixation is evident, and there is more cortical osteopenia on the implanted side. (Courtesy CA Engh, MD.)

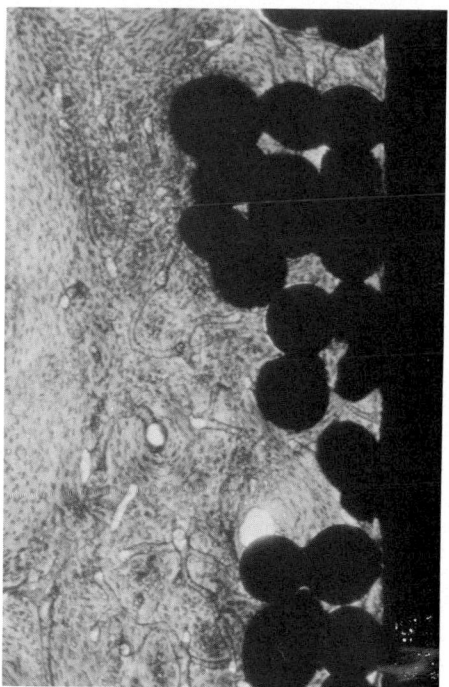

Fig. 4-14. Higher magnification shows the cortical-type bone ingrowth typically found. Nutrient vessels and osteocyte lacunae are visible deep with the porosities. (Courtesy CA Engh, MD.)

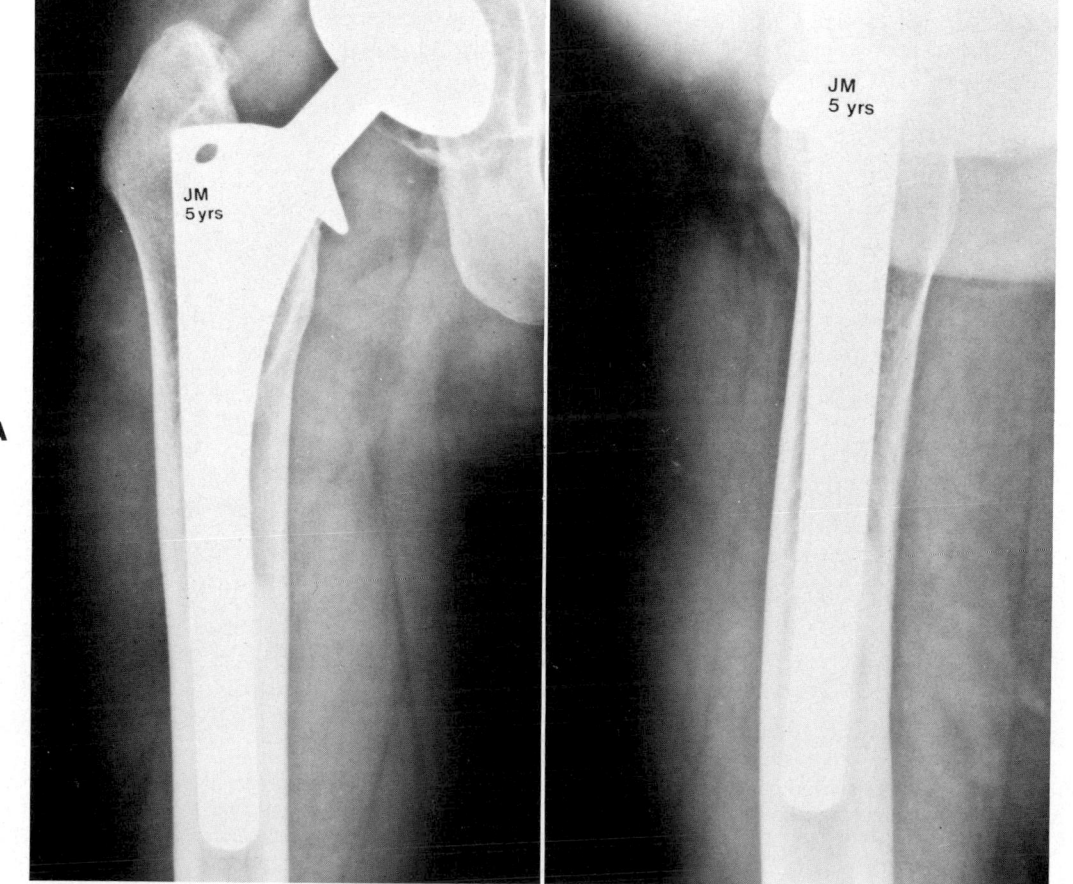

Fig. 4-15. 5 years postoperatively, AP **A,** and lateral, **B,** radiographs show the features of a porous-coated stem that failed to achieve bone ingrowth but achieved successful secondary stabilization by fibrous-tissue ingrowth and bone encapsulation. (Courtesy CA Engh, MD.)

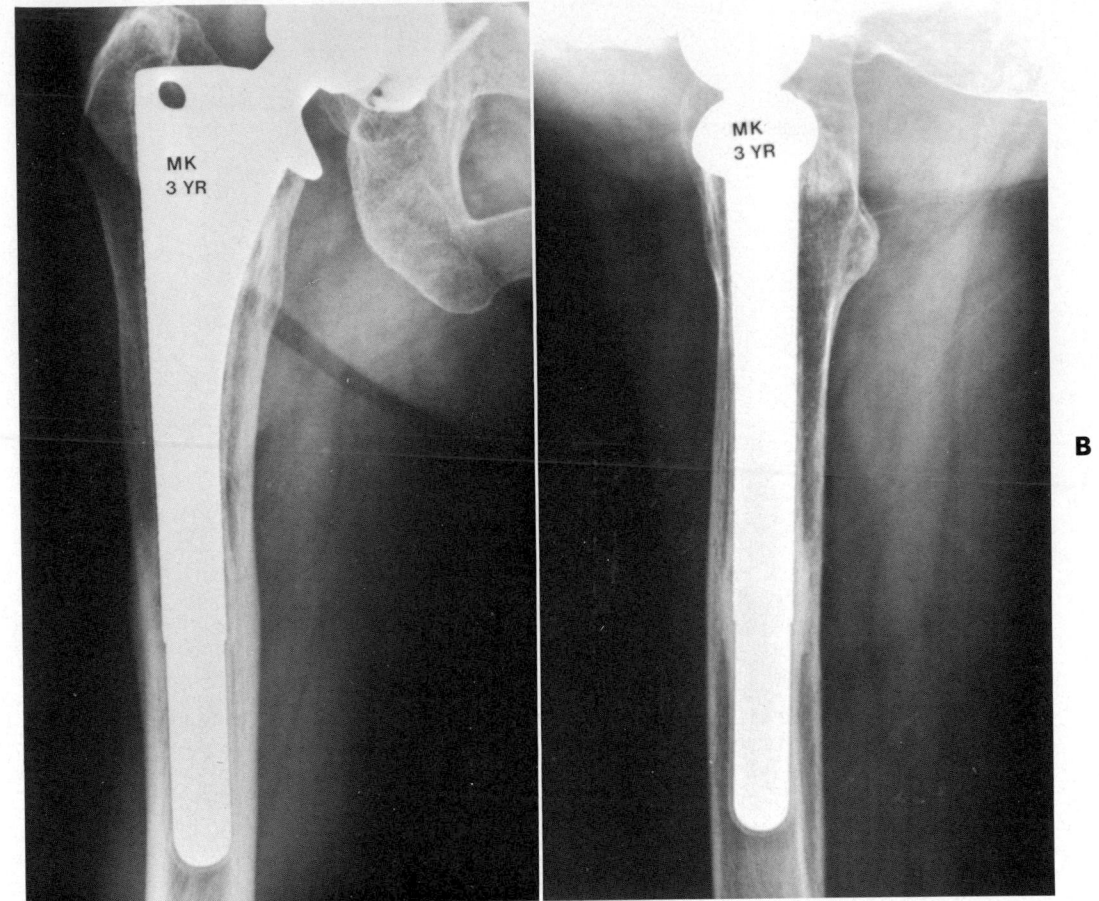

Fig. 4-16. Three years postoperatively AP, **A,** and lateral, **B,** radiographs show the features of a porous-coated stem that failed to achieve bone ingrowth but achieved successful secondary stabilization by fibrous-tissue ingrowth and bone encapsulation. (Courtesy CA Engh, MD.)

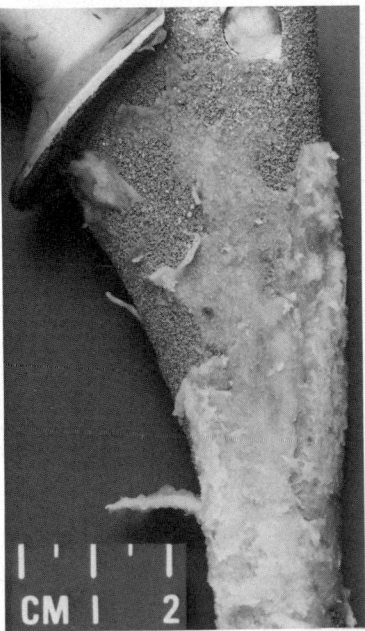

Fig. 4-17. Gross appearance of a retrieved porous-coated implant that was fixed by stable bone fibrous encapsulation. (Courtesy CA Engh, MD.)

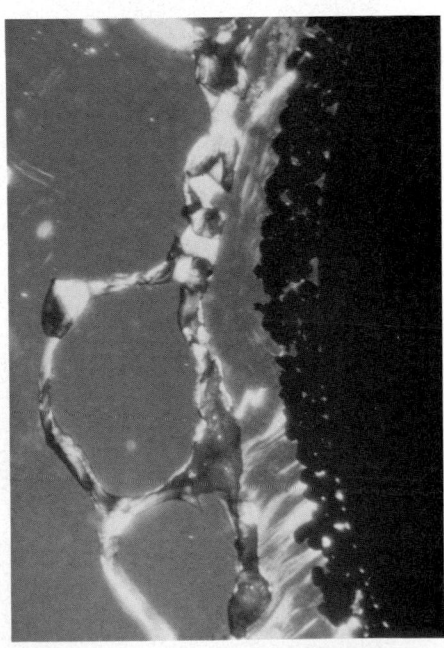

Fig. 4-18. Photomicrograph of a bone-implant interface retrieved after 6 years and viewed under polarized light. The radiographic appearance was of a radiopaque line. The surrounding shell of bone is separated from the implant by a space containing fibrous tissue. (Courtesy CA Engh, MD.)

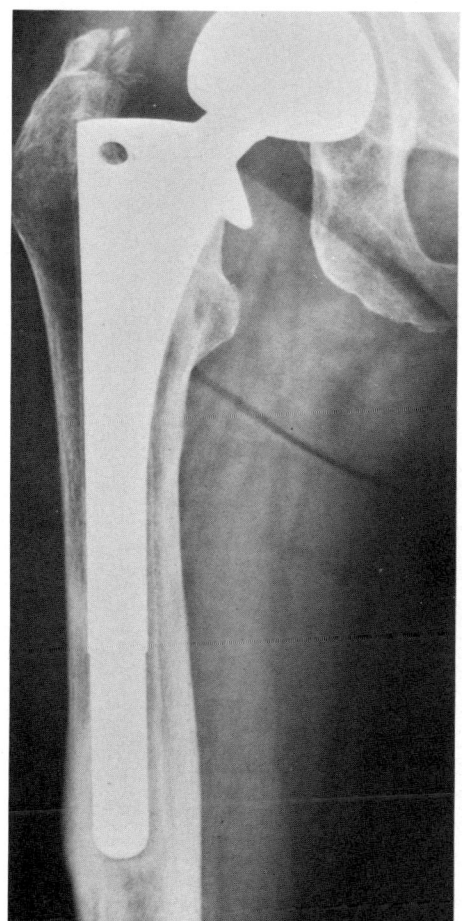

Fig. 4-19. AP radiograph depicts unstable AML prosthesis implanted in femur 2 years previously. (Courtesy CA Engh, MD.)

Fig. 4-20. A, A nearly fully porous coated AML stem was removed because of infection. The operation was extremely difficult since mostly "ingrown" section demonstrated strongly remodeled bone in the entire length of the porous-coated section. The metal fragments represent the sectioned collar pieces and diamond saw blades (used to section the collar for access by thin osteotomes). **B,** The rigidly fixed dense and cortical-like bone could not be separated from the stem by thin osteotome after explanation although the proximal bone *(metaphyseal region)* was more cancellous in nature and separated easily from the metal surface. **C,** Fibrous encapsulation of an AML prosthesis removed for thigh pain. Motion could be demonstrated at revision surgery. **D,** A threaded acetabular cup with its attached fibrous ingrowth removed for pain resulting in loosening. Nonporous surface of this type of implant frequently promotes fibrous ingrowth.

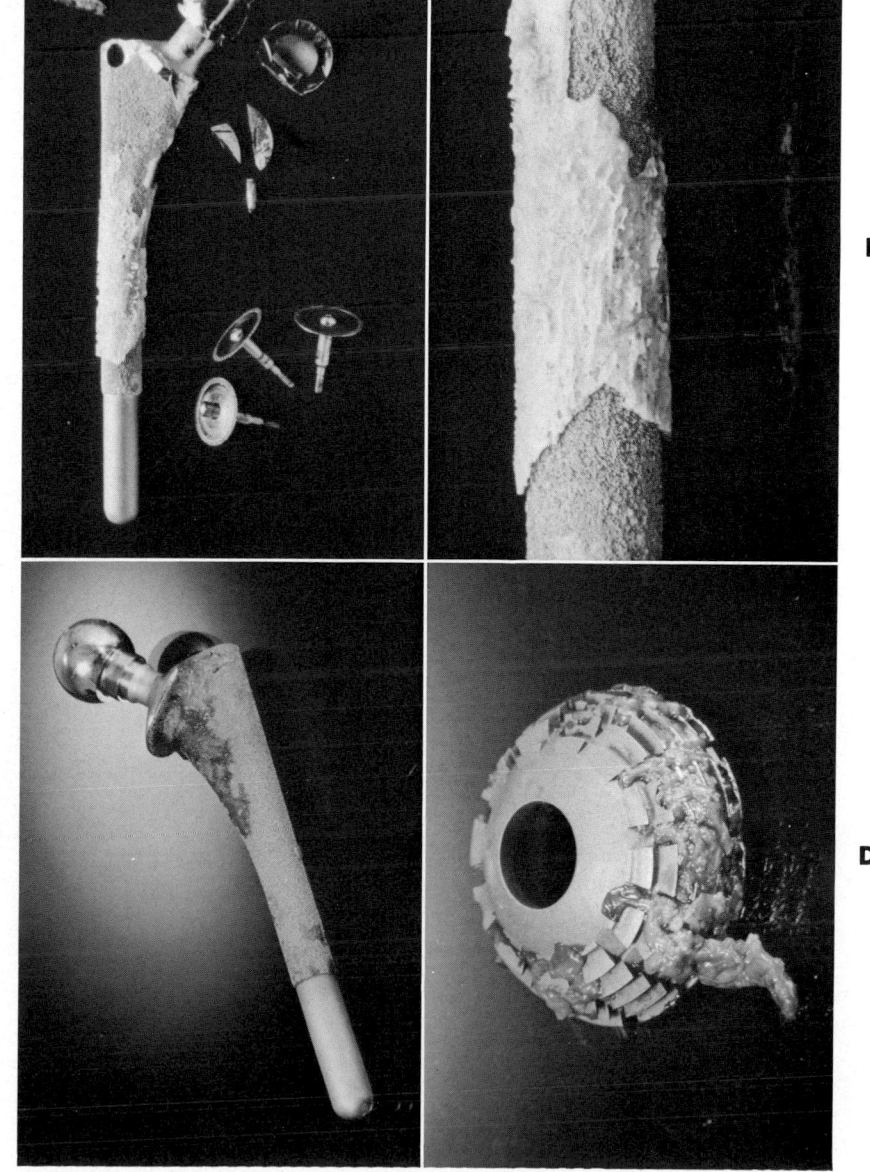

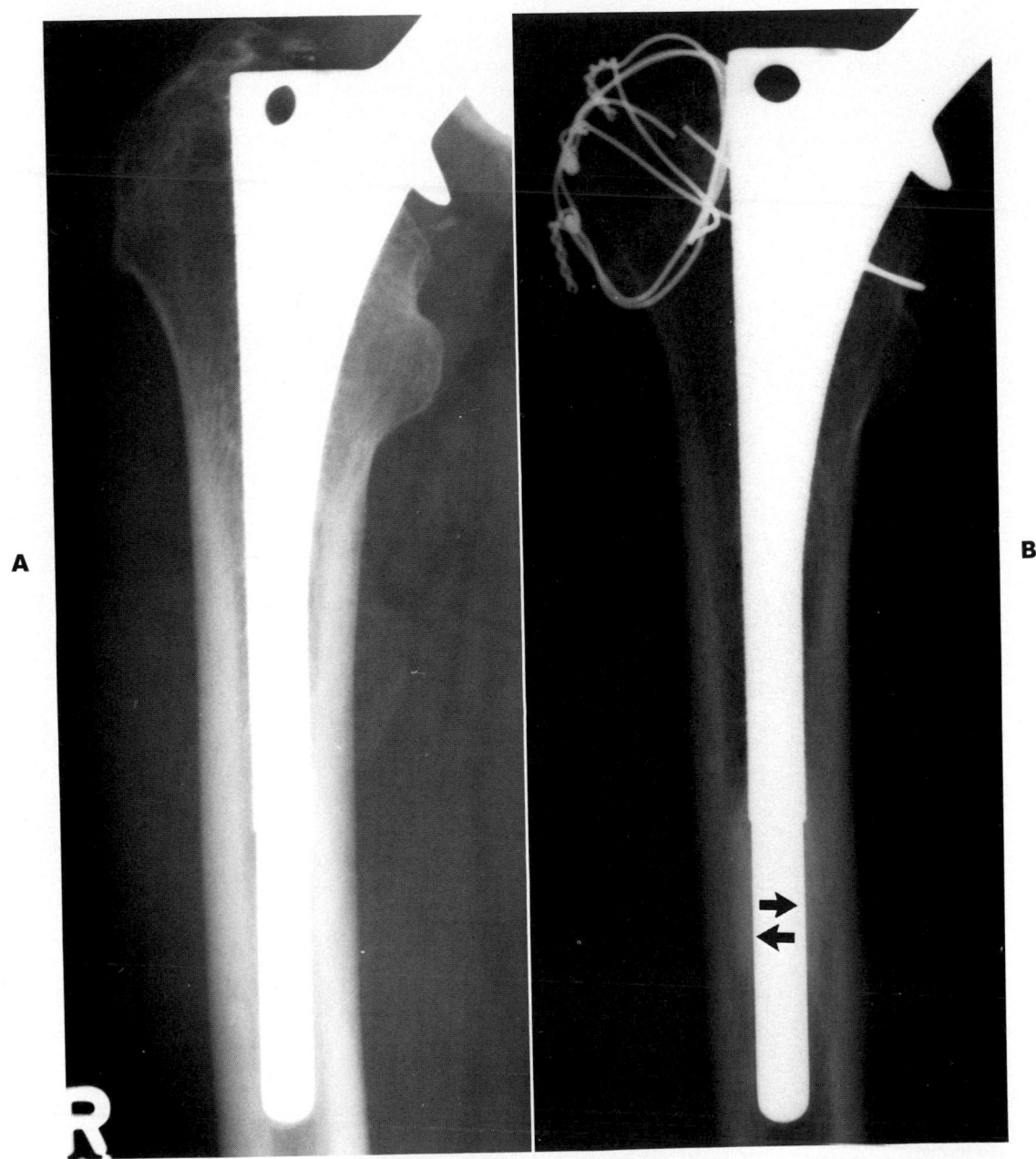

A

B

Fig. 4-21. A, AP radiograph of a 68-year-old female (D.P.) 1 year after AML arthroplasty with an 8 outer diameter stem. Note excellent adaptive remodeling of bone. **B,** 3 years after index operation, severe osteopenia has occurred. This suggests stress shielding phenomenon as the nonporous zone *(distal stem)* has hypertrophied since it has been load bearing *(arrows)*.

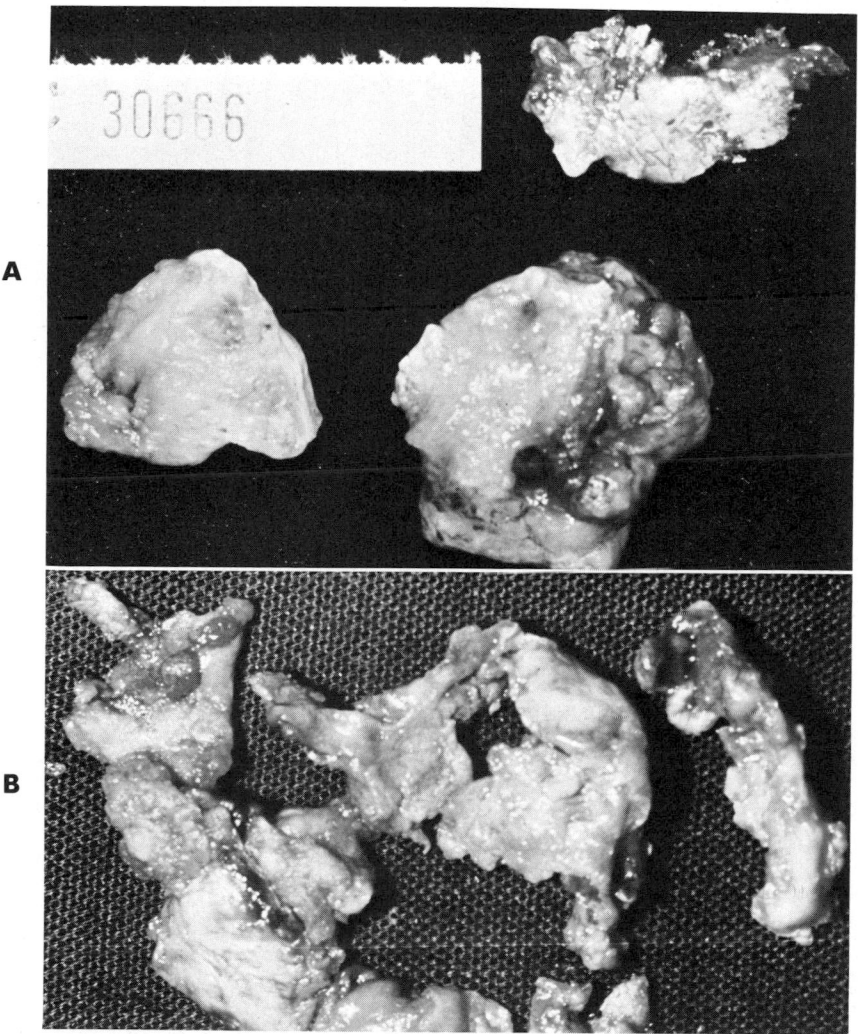

Fig. 4-22. A and **B,** Fibrous capsule formed around artificial joint usually contains plastic fragments, by-product of wear of HDP. This tissue is usually firm and gritty.

Continued.

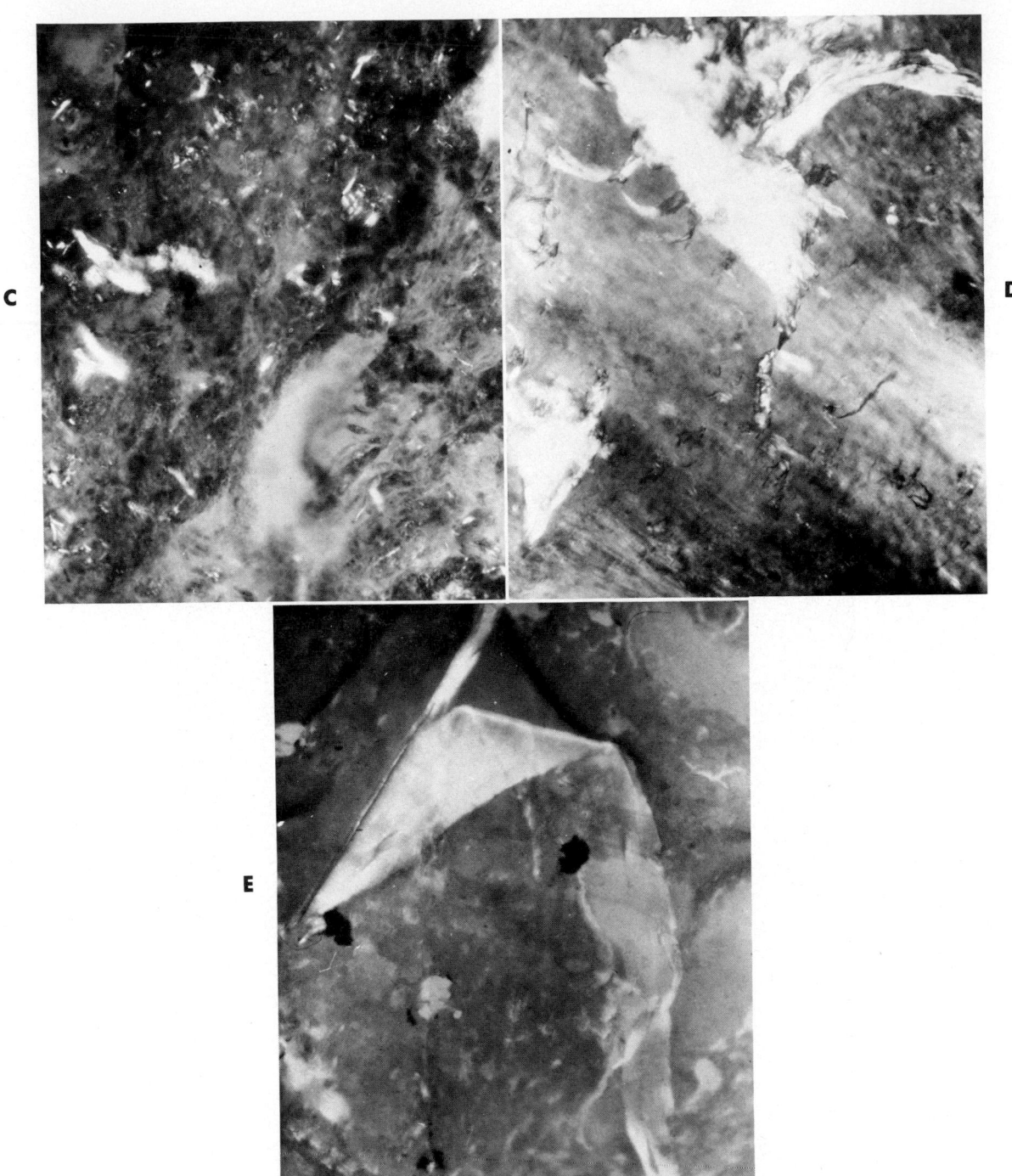

Fig. 4-22—cont'd. C to E, Large foreign body birefringent materials representing loose pieces of HDP within fibrous capsule are seen. This specimen is taken from a hip after recurrent dislocation. NOTE: adjacent tissue is also refractile but not vascular.

PROSTHETIC SYNOVITIS

For lack of a better term, I as well as my colleagues[126] have used the term *prosthetic synovitis* to describe the fibropseudosynovial lining of the prosthetic bed. Such material is often a natural response to the debris of PMMA, HDP, metal, bone, and other materials used in arthroplasty. The interface can also be the site of bacterial infection with or without bacteriological proof (see Chapter 32 for a discussion of infection).

Among other factors, the criteria for infected implants, the clinical history, an elevated sedimentation rate (more than 35 mm/hour), an elevated serum content of C-reactive protein (an electrophoretic plasma protein pattern compatible with an acute phase of reaction), and radiographic changes, including gallium bone scan, can be helpful to a pathologist in differentiating between an infected hip arthroplasty and aseptic loosening. Finally, and more importantly, four out of five positive bacterial cultures for the same microbe from the tissue adjacent to the cement (technique of Kamme and Lindburg) must be present to prove an infected implant.[142] Despite the criteria listed above, discord within these parameters casts doubt on whether the problem is a loose implant or an infected interface. The intraoperative decision whether to revise, stage, or excise the failed prosthesis depends on histological morphology at the time of surgery. This differentiation may be aided by light microscopy in three ways: (1) Gram stain for bacteria, (2) frozen sections of the interface membrane, and (3) touch imprints.

Mirra and others, using a semiquantitative method,[182] concluded that more than five polymorphonuclear cells per high-power field (2+ or greater polymorphonuclear cells) in tissues excluding those found in fibrin is the single most reliable indicator of infection at surgery. In 21 of 22 joints with 2+ or greater polymorphonuclear cells, the joint culture became positive. In the other one, because of a high clinical suspicion for infection, the prosthetic joint was excised despite a negative culture. Acute inflammatory cells are not seen in the pathology material with wear debris unless infection is also present. Wear debris generally provokes a chronic inflammatory response that is of no value in establishing the presence or absence of infection in pathology of joint implants. Based on 94 specimens examined by Mirra and co-workers, using a semiquantitative grading of the materials (0, 1+, 2+, 3+), chronic inflammation of 2+ to 3+ was not of any value in separating reaction to wear debris from infection.[181]

Johnston and colleagues at our institution reviewed the morphology and distribution patterns of the predominant cells, including giant cells, histiocytes, fibrinoid material, polyethylene, and cement from the material obtained at revision arthroplasty.[126] Fig. 4-23 demonstrates common cell types found in reactive prosthetic synovitis (noninfected) related to mechanically loose prostheses. The interpretations in the legends are by Johnston, Paresien, and Doty.

Quantitative estimates were based on a scale of 1 to 4+ of cells and foreign body materials using microscopic examination of tissue sectioning, stained with hematoxylin, phloxine, and saffron. Data summary relates to tissue samples obtained through debridement in 51 to 100 consecutive revision arthroplasties at our institution (Tables 4-1 to 4-3). The investigators concluded that the traditional Gram stain for bacteria has a limited value in determining the presence of low-grade infection and in verifying the presence or absence of infection at surgery. Of more than 200 consecutive revision operations, only on one occasion was the bacteriological report on Gram stain and cultures from the same specimen reported as positive. On three occasions, however, the reports were false positive. There was no growth of organisms from these specimens.

Histology of infection is well known to all pathologists. A frank bacterial infection evokes granulation tissue with proliferative capillaries and subsurface cellular exudates in which neutrophils are prominent or predominant. The use of a frozen section obtained during surgery for histological analysis is limited by the presence of fragments of bone or cement in the soft tissue. The amount of tissue to be examined in this way would require a small staff of pathologists familiar with and interested in this problem. The quality of sections may not be satisfactory to show adequate details for diagnosis. Sections limited to certain areas may not be representative and may not show the cellular details required to identify the state of the inflammatory cells (for example, neutrophils).

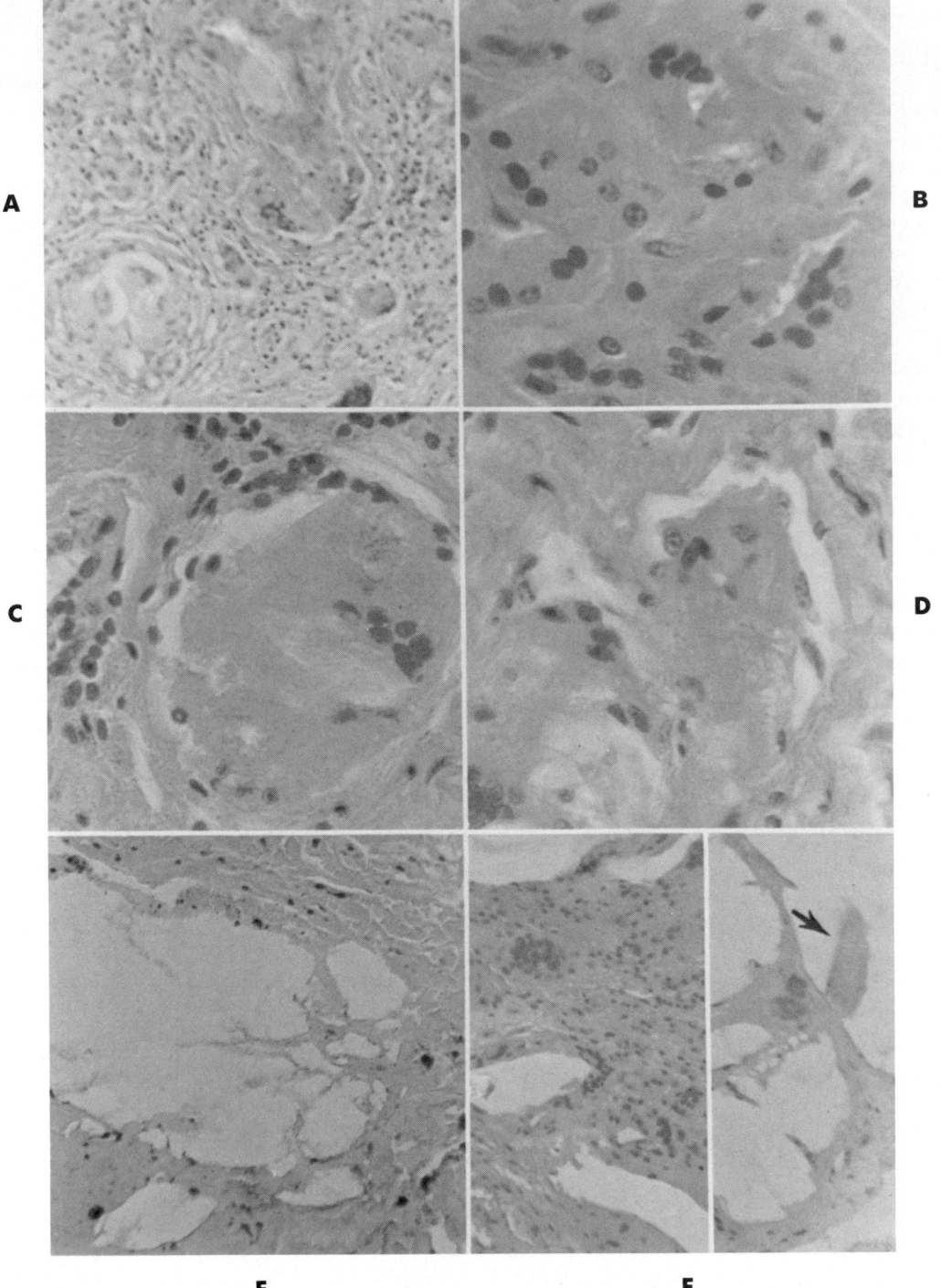

Fig. 4-23. A, Giant cells contain relatively large fragments of birefringent HDP, yellow in upper zone and pale blue in left part of center field (×160). **B,** Giant cells in upper and lower right field are apparently struggling with larger shards of birefringent HDP. Giant cell in upper center accommodates small particles of HDP, probably reflecting on its being formed amalgamation of mononuclear histiocytes (×500). **C,** Large distorted giant cell, having formed phagosome of nearly lethal proportions, has attracted halo of lymphocytes, evidently reflecting some immunological concern on part of host. Giant cell, undeterred, has generated a half-formed asteroid *(resembling as asterisk)* in right upper quadrant (×500). **D,** Especially large giant cell with even more voracious phagocytic appetites has formed two perfect asteroids in dead center and near lower left field. These bodies occur in sarcoidosis. Their pathogenesis is obscure (×500). **E,** Typical defect from which cement fragment has been dislodged. Incomplete septal patterns are most likely to be cytoplasmic extensions left behind by avulsed giant cells (×50). **F,** Large rounded defects with small loculations that undoubtedly housed fragments of acrylic cement. Small residual fragment composed of microspherules protrudes toward right upper corner of field *(arrow).* Oval, more sharply formed HDP fragments have also been avulsed, leaving one small residual shard left of center. Acidophilic histiocytes and giant cells form poorly vascularized background (×32). (From Johnston AD, Parisien MV: Pathology of reactive (prosthetic) versus septic (revisionary) synovitis. In Eftekhar NS, editor: *Infection in joint replacement surgery: prevention and management,* St Louis, 1984, Mosby–Year Book.)

Table 4-1 Quantitative Estimates of Cells and Foreign Body Material in Debridement Samples from Total Hip Arthroplasty Revisions

Case number	Fibrinoid	G. Histiocytes	Polyethylene	Cement
1	4+	3+	2+	1+
2	1+	2+	0.5	0
3	0	3+	1+	3+
4	0.5	3+	2+	3+
5 (infected)	3+	1+	2+	0.5+
6	1+	1+	0.5	0
7	0	2+	1+	3+
8	1+	3+	1+	1+
9 (infected)	2+	3+	1+	1+
10 (infected)	3+	4+	3+	2+
11	2+	3+	2+	2+
12	0	2+	3+	0.5+
13	2+	3+	3+	0
14	2+	3+	0.5+	0
15	2+	2+	3+	2+
16	2+	3+	2+	1+
17	3+	4+	2+	0
18	1+	4+	3+	0
19	0.5+	3+	3+	2+
20	3+	4+	3+	3+
21	0	2+	3+	1+
22	2+	3+	0	0
23	3+	3+	3+	0.5+
24	3+	1+	0	1.5+
25	1+	1+	1+	1+
26	1+	2+	3+	2+
27	1+	1+	0	1+
28	2+	4+	0.5+	1+
29	3+	3+	0	0
30	2+	3+	0	—
31 (infected)	3+	0	0	1+
32	0	4+	4+	0.5+
33	1+	2+	4+	0.5+
34	2+	1+	0	1+
35	2+	4+	0	1+
36	0	4+	3+	3+
37	3+	1+	0	4+
38	1+	3+	0	3+
39	3+	1+	1+	4+
40	0.5+	1+	0	0
41	2+	3+	3+	3+
42	0	3+	3+	4+
43	1+	1+	0	1+
44	4+	1+	1+	2+
45	0	0	0	1+
46	3+	4+	0	2+
47	1+	4+	2+	1+
48	3+	4+	3+	0.5+
49	0	2+	1+	2+
50	2+	2+	2+	1+
51	4+	2+	2+	3+

From Johnston AD, Parisien MV: Pathology of reactive (prosthetic) versus septic (revisionary) synovitis. In Eftekhar NS, editor: *Infection in joint replacement surgery: prevention and management,* St Louis, 1984, Mosby–Year Book.

Table 4-2 Prosthetic Synovitis Components: 50 Cases

Component	Percent of total
Acidophilic histiocytes	95+
Giant cells	80+
Cement	80+
HDP	75+
Metal	16
Fibrinoid	80+
Lymphocytes/plasma cells	26
Neutrophils	8

From Johnston AD, Parisien MV: Pathology of reactive (prosthetic) versus septic (revisionary) synovitis. In Eftekhar, NS, editor: *Infection in joint replacement surgery,* St Louis, 1984, Mosby–Year Book.

Table 4-3 Quantitative Concurrence of the Major Components of the Reactive System in Individual Cases

Components	HDP	Cement	G. Histiocyte
Fibrinoid	52%	60%	54%
G. histiocyte	74%	58%	—

From Johnston AD, Parisien MV: Pathology of reactive (prosthetic) versus septic (revisionary) synovitis. In Eftekhar, NS, editor: *Infection in joint replacement surgery,* St Louis, 1984, Mosby–Year Book.

Touch Imprint

Johnston and Parisien[126] developed a technique that has been applied since 1970 at our institution to circumvent the limitations of frozen sections mentioned above.[126] The specimen is cut at several levels into the subsurface to expose a wider cell population for examination by touch preparation. The preparation is made by touching the tissue fragments repeatedly to the surface of glass slides, producing imprints representative of the loose cellular population in the tissue. Neutrophils tend to cluster in a positive imprint. Actual neutrophils may be ruptured, and their nuclei may be extruded (and attenuated). Pus cells are neutrophils that have lost their cytoplasmic granules. They tend to cluster in almost pure colonies. We depend on the altered morphology and population density of neutrophils as our most reliable index for infection. The diagnostic value of this index is diluted by the tendency of neutrophils to appear in perivascular tissue within 1½ to 2 hours of surgery. However, in this case, neutrophils do not cluster nor do they show widespread

nuclear changes. If imprint does not include the exposed fibrous tissue and scar tissue, an error may arise because clusters of neutrophils may not be exposed during the touch preparation.[126] Sixty-six consecutive imprints correlated with final aerobic and anaerobic cultures showed a high index of diagnostic reliability for this technique. Tissue imprints were negative for infection in 44 operations (both aerobic and anaerobic cultures were negative) and positive for infection in 7 operations (all developed a positive culture). The remaining 13 imprints were judged to be borderline or suspicious for infection; of these, three developed a positive culture. Only one Gram stain indicated the presence of bacteria, which subsequently became positive in cultures obtained from the same specimen. Therefore we conclude that for distinguishing between infected and noninfected interface membrane, touch imprint is a superior intraoperative technique to Gram stain used for this purpose.

As shown in Table 4-2, acidophilic histiocytes were distinctive histological hallmarks of prosthetic synovitis (95%+); giant cells, fibrinoid materials, cement, and HDP fragments (75% to 80%) comprise the bulk of the most frequently encountered remaining components except scarred aponeurotic tissue from the articular capsule and fragments of bone.

Metallic deposits (16%) were rare. HDP fragments of widely varying sizes are derived from the acetabular components of most failed prostheses. The smaller fragments of HDP are difficult to detect even under polarized light; they probably occurred with greater than 7% frequency in our material.

The term *fibrinoid* was used to describe the amorphous proteinaceous debris that is interspersed with acellular collagen bundles and forms deposits on synovial-like folds of surfaces at the metal-cement interface of loose metallic components.

The more conventional inflammatory cellular exudate rarely was present in our material. Our ability to identify infected cases depended on the presence of neutrophils as previously described, which generally were not found in significant numbers in the classic pyogenic prosthetic synovitis. Lymphocytes and plasma cells seemed to contribute little to the recognition of infection. There was some tendency for these cells to gather in the vicinity of necrotic fibrinoid debris.

Table 4-3 presents the frequency with which various combinations of two out of the four major components of this reactive system are found concurrently in a given case. The concurrence is based on a reading within ±1 for each component on a scale of 1 to 4+.

Acidophilic Histiocytes

The relationship between granular acidophilic histiocytes and fragments of HDP established in our study[126] may be of significance. We noted 2 to 5 μm long birefringent shards of HDP in the cytoplasm of some cells. Characteristically, particles of this size could be incorporated by mononuclear histiocytes. This association is a dominant feature of the interaction between fine particles of HDP and tissue. Tissue morphology is dominated by small fragments of birefringent material associated with sheets of histiocytes. It is not possible to identify any small fragments of acrylic cement associated with these cells. Acrylic cement often consists of large fragments, which are associated with multinucleated giant cells or "walled off" by a connective tissue capsule. Small acrylic polymer spherules (30 to 80 μm) are too large to be phagocytized by histiocytes, although histiocytes could be associated with the surface of individual acrylic pearls.

Multinucleated Giant Cells

Evidently, giant cells are formed in response to large fragments of acrylic cement or high-density polyethylene. Fragments of cement are usually large and evidently require a syncytium of cells such as giant cells to encompass their bulk. As far as we have been able to determine, cement is not shed into the reactive tissue in the form of finely ground particles and does not appear to provoke increased numbers of mononuclear histiocytes. Whether it is only a spherule of the acrylic polymer or large fragments of acrylic, we are always able to identify giant cells in close relationship to the particles of PMMA, unlike that of a giant cell tumor. Fragments of cement, on the other hand, are larger and evidently require the cooperation of a modified syncytium of giant cells to encompass their bulk (Figs. 4-24 to 4-26). As far as we have been able to determine, cement is not shed into the reactive tissues in the form of finely ground particles and does not in all likelihood provoke an overgrowth of mononuclear histiocytes.

Text continued on p. 115.

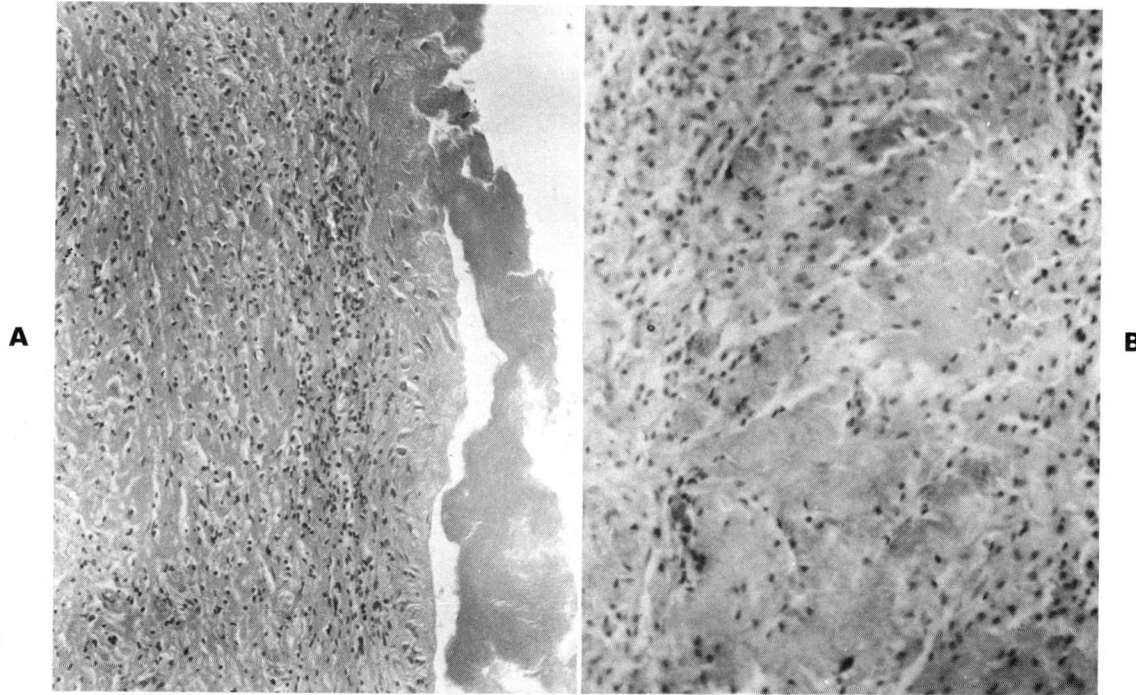

Fig. 4-24. A, Fibrinoid material found on surface of fibrous capsule is nonspecific to type of implant. It may be seen with loose prosthesis with or without cement. Severe fibrinoid material found in tissue may also suggest possibility of infection. This low-power photomicrograph is taken from loose Moore self-locking prosthesis. Specimen is from fibrous sleeve adjacent to stem of prosthesis. **B,** Intracellular amorphous material indicative of fibrinoid removed from tissue adjacent to loose cemented cup of total hip prosthesis.

Continued.

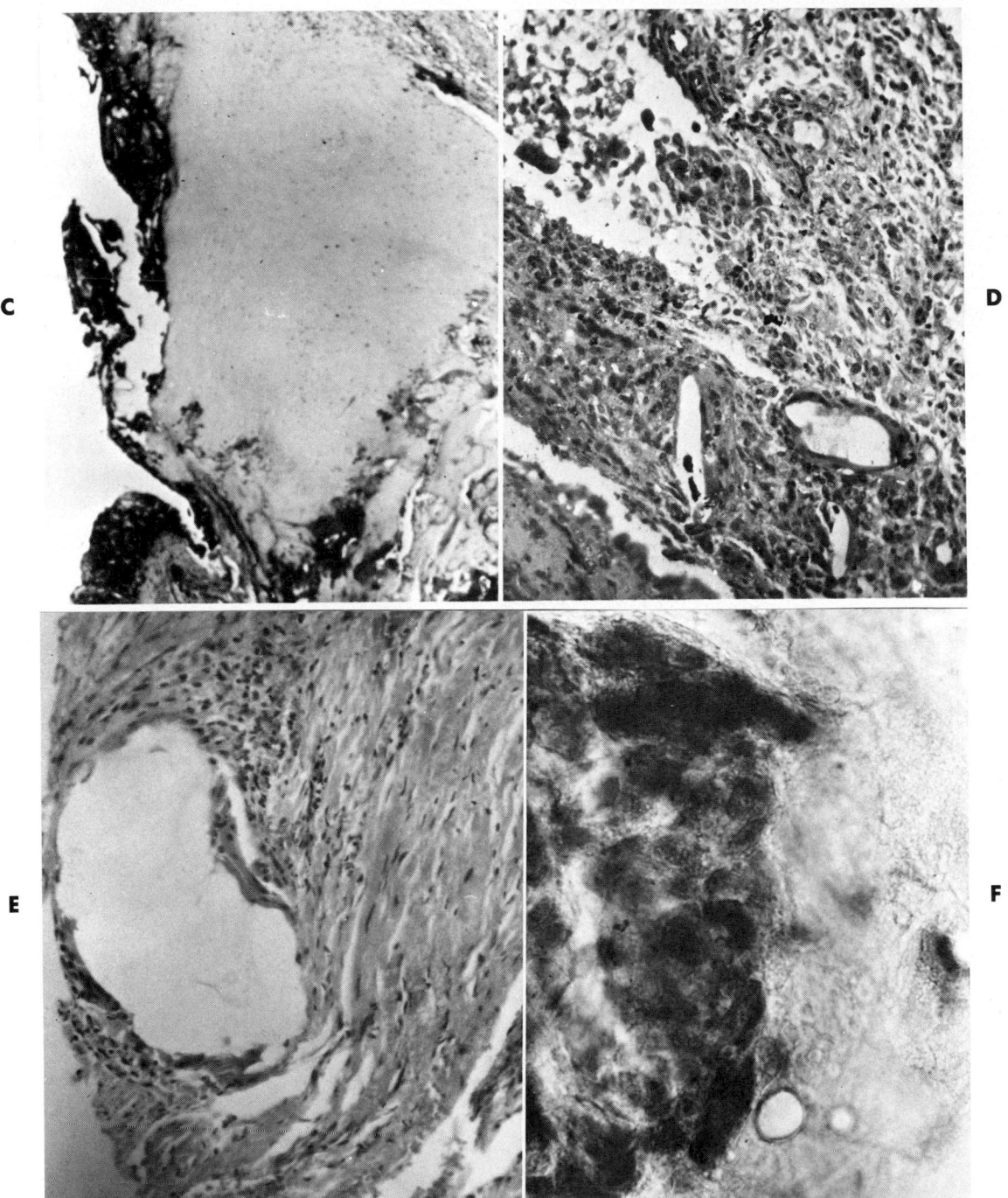

Fig. 4-24—cont'd. C, Caseation found in region of calcar. Severe caseous formation is evidence of motion between cement and bone, resulting in necrosis. No birefringent material was found. **D,** Considerable histiocytic reaction found in region of calcar. This histiocytic reaction is typical of loose cemented prosthesis. **E,** Foreign body granuloma reaction to loose cemented femoral prosthesis. Large void in field represents relatively large fragment of cement that has been removed from tissue during preparation. **F,** High-power magnification showing cluster of histiocytes. These cells usually contain acidophilic granular cytoplasm with tendency to cluster. If birefringent granules are seen within vicinity, most likely reaction relates to HDP; without their presence, reaction must be considered secondary to loose fragments of cement. Occasionally these cells may appear as large sheet within field resembling pseudocarcinoma-type appearance.

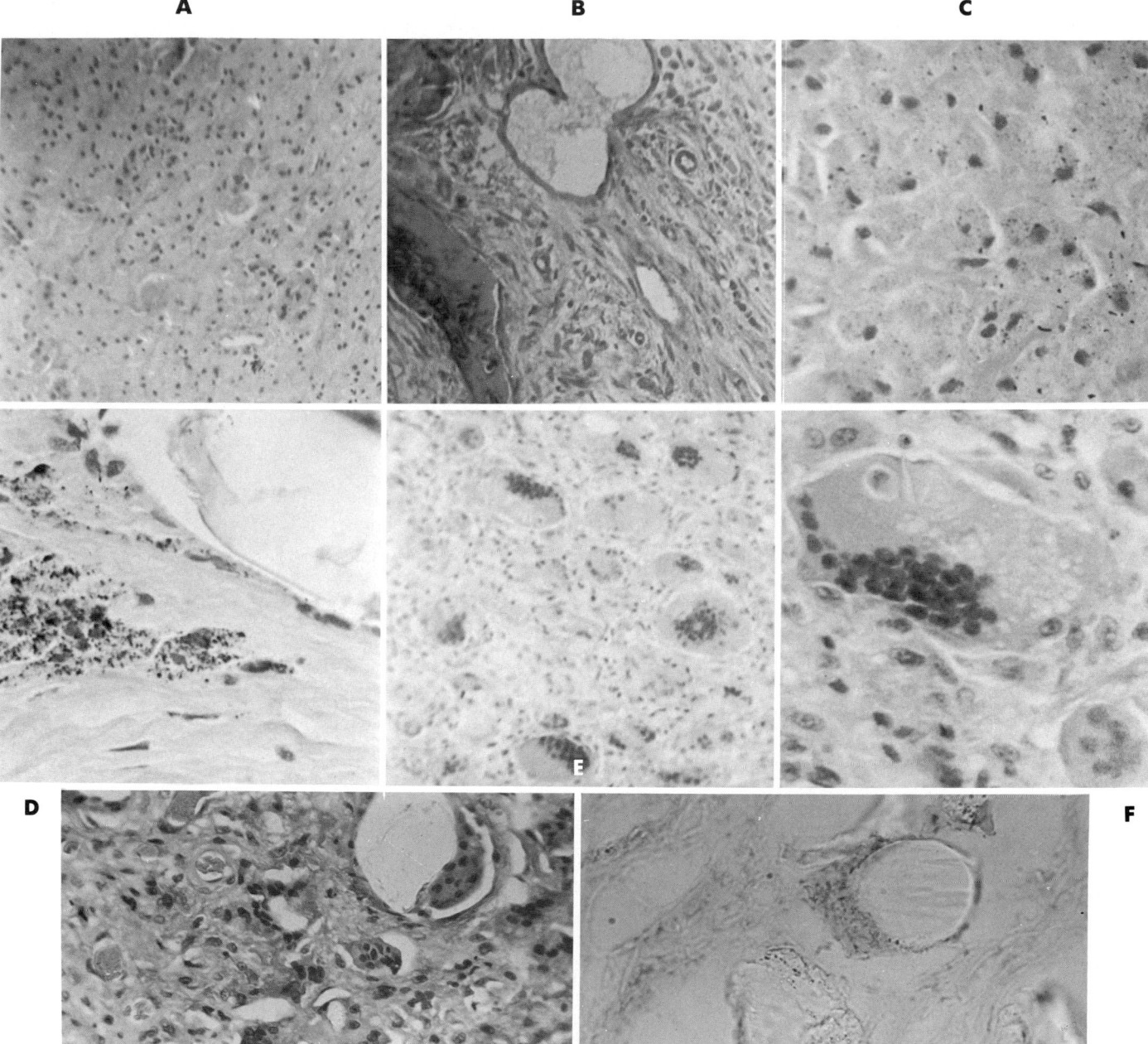

Fig. 4-25. A, Microscopic fragments of birefringent HDP highlight cytoplasm of acidophilic histiocytes with blue and yellow flecks. Larger fragments are trapped in multinucleated giant cells (×50). **B,** Histiocytic response to implant materials is shown occupying a defect in bone. Relatively large bilobed defect near left upper quadrant of this field almost certainly contained bone cement, which was dislodged during tissue processing (×160). **C,** Acidophilic histiocytes here contain small irregular black particles representing metallic deposits. These did not stain positively for iron (×500). **D,** Details of histiocytic cells are obscured by heavy metallic deposits (these also do not stain positively for iron). Relatively large fragment of HDP glows from tissue space in lower right, partially lined by giant cell (×500). **E,** Intermingled giant cells and mononuclear acidophilic histiocytes vaguely resemble giant cell tumor. Vascular supply is poor (×160). **F,** Giant cell in the center has evidently been inspired to insatiable phagocytic activity by unusually large number of nuclei. Vacuoles are phagosomes; recognizable remnants of a dead cell occupy one of these (×500). **G,** H and E stain of a giant cell wrapped around a spherule of PMMA polymer. Vascular supply is rich. **H,** Thin section of PMMA spherule surrounded by a large multinucleated giant cell. (**A** to **F** from Johnston AD, Parisien MV: Pathology of reactive (prosthetic) versus septic (revisionary) synovitis. In Eftekhar NS, editor: *Infection in joint replacement surgery: prevention and management,* St Louis, 1984, Mosby-Year Book.)

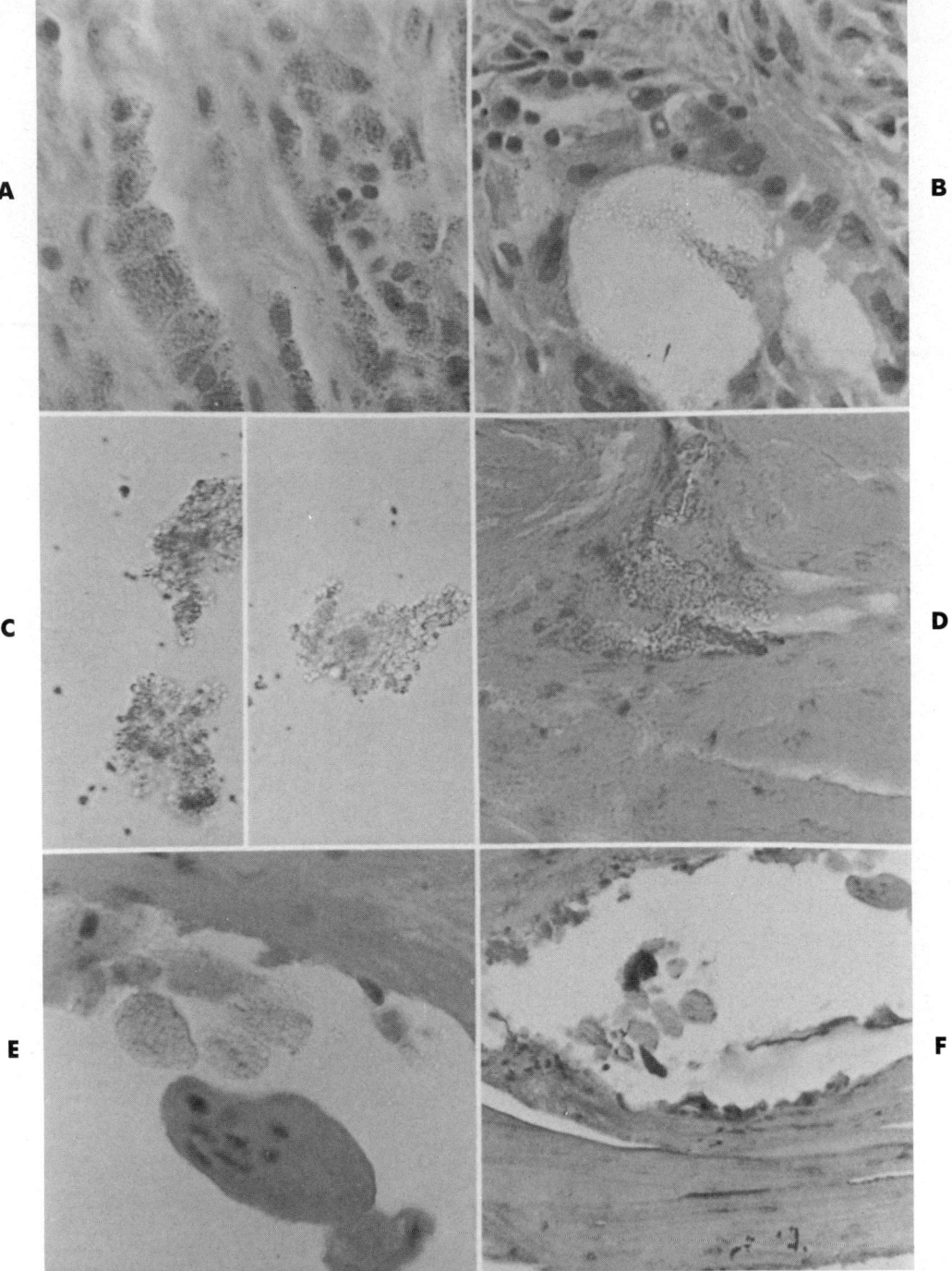

Fig. 4-26. A, Residual fragments of acrylic bone cement in cavity lined by giant cells and forming interface with bone (×50). **B,** Distorted giant cells from lower left of field in **A** simulate methacrylate egg laying. Bone cement in its reconstructed form would probably have occupied a phagosome around which foreign body giant cell would have formed intact enclosure (×500). **C,** Giant cells form a phagosome about indigestible small fragment of pale green microspherules representing bone cement. This is set in scar tissue. Light is not polarized (×500). **D,** Fragments of PMMA bone cement from surgical total hip arthroplasty revision scraped onto slide and photographed under polarized light (×500). **E,** Coalescent giant cells cradle defect from which PMMA cement has been displaced; almost colorless 0.5 to 1 µm spherules are rendered luminous by diffraction. This was not photographed under polarized light (×500). **F,** Ordinarily acidophilic histiocytes are discolored brown and accommodate fine, presumably vacuolar "bubbles" in their cytoplasm. Brown pigment does not stain like iron. These bubbles may represent PMMA, but we are not sure (×500). (From Johnston AD, Parisien MV: Pathology of reactive (prosthetic) versus septic (revisionary) synovitis. In Eftekhar NS, editor: *Infection in joint replacement surgery: prevention and management,* St Louis, 1984, Mosby–Year Book.)

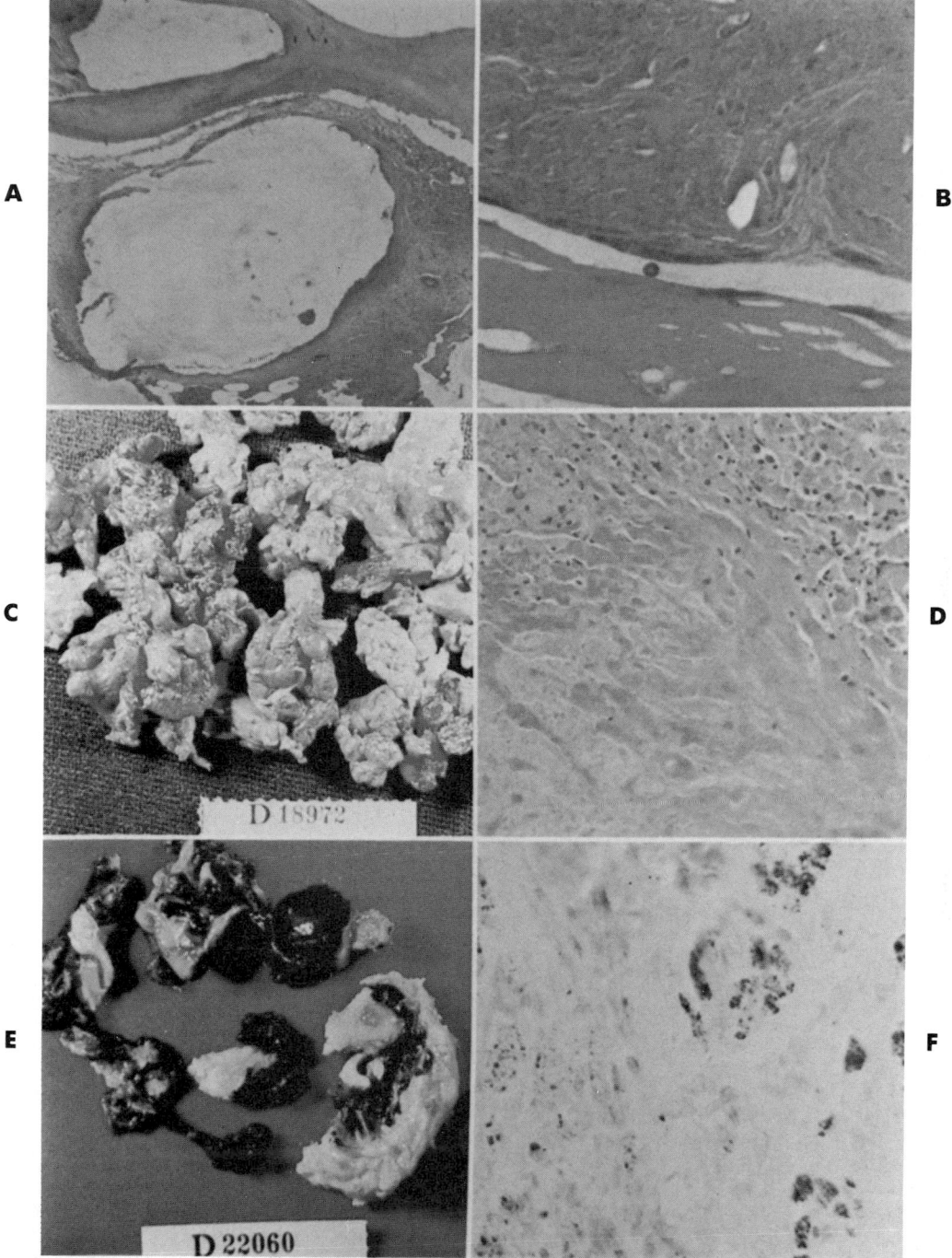

Fig. 4-27. Bone-cement interface. **A,** Cystlike defect originally contained cement and is housed in scar tissue. Bone shows no significant reactive change and is viable. In other fields some reactive bone appears at interface (×32). **B,** Interface between bone and histiocytic foreign body reaction we call *prosthetic synovitis* has been photographed under polarized light. Sizeable shards of birefringent HDP are trapped in giant cells and histiocytes. Margin of bone appears attenuated but is insulated from reactive histiocyte tissue by scar (×32). **C,** Prosthetic synovitis, though variable, is most frequently an irregularly villous, micronodular lesion that discolors parent tissue pale yellow or brown. It resembles underdeveloped or partially compromised pigmented villonodular synovitis (×1.5). **D,** Acidophilic histiocytic cells, some clustered in right upper corner, have destroyed most of aponeurotic fiber structure of articular capsule, leaving irregular acellular framework. Amorphous interfibrillary protein debris in places resembles fibrinoid (×160). **E,** Fragments of thickened and scarred synovium have been blackened rather dramatically by metallic deposits (×1.5). **F,** Black metallic deposits obscure histiocytic cells. Deposits do not stain positively for iron. This has been photographed under compensated polarized light, and birefringent fragment of HDP is clearly shown in upper margin of midfield (×160). (From Johnston AD, Parisien MV: Pathology of reactive (prosthetic) versus septic (revisionary) synovitis. In Eftekhar NS, editor: *Infection in joint replacement surgery: prevention and management,* St Louis, 1984, Mosby–Year Book.)

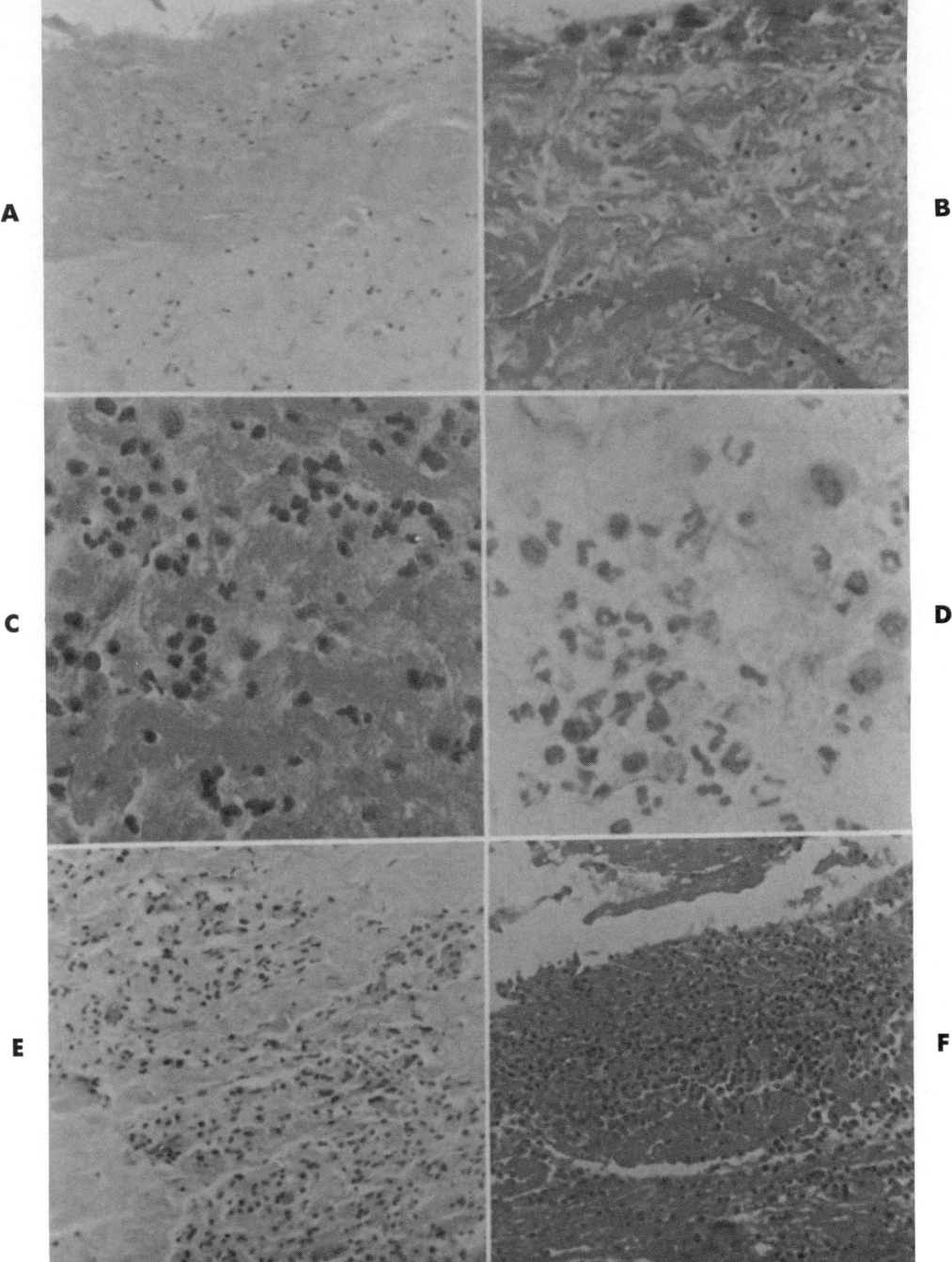

Fig. 4-28. A, The fibrinoid layer on this synovial surface was generated at metallic interface. Fibrinoid material is proteinaceous coagulum. Sublining tissue is scarred and shows no current evidence of inflammatory activity. Cells are viable, but tissue is virtually avascular (×50). **B,** Dark clusters represent bacterial colonies living on rich medium generated at fibrinoid interface with loose metallic prosthesis. This is not a common occurrence, although it offers good explanation for predisposition to infection in this circumstance (×50). **C,** Irregular cluster of neutrophils battens on fibrinoid debris, documenting evidence of infection (as opposed to saprophytic infestation, for example). Mononuclear cells are disintegrating histiocytes (×500). **D,** Cell cluster from cellular imprint of inflamed tissue from femoral canal has been photographed at high magnification. Polymorphic nuclei of neutrophils are extended. This distortion is frequently agonal; cell is often ruptured at this point, discharging lysosomal granules with activated proteolytic enzymes, etc. Larger cells are histiocytes, corresponding to acidophilic granular histiocytes previously described and shown in **E** (×500). **E,** Margins of these clusters of acidophilic granular histiocytes are sharply irregular; this suggests collagenase activity with little respect for fields of force. These cells are most prominently deployed as a rule in sublining or aponeurotic tissues (×160). **F,** Layer of pus cells on infected membranous surface; underlying zone is occupied by granulation tissue (×160). (From Johnston AD, Parisien MV: Pathology of reactive (prosthetic) versus septic (revisionary) synovitis. In Eftekhar NS, editor: *Infection in joint replacement surgery: prevention and management,* St Louis, 1984, Mosby–Year Book.)

Metallic Debris

Metallic deposits were prominent in our material. These particles were admixed in several instances with fine spherules of particulate colorless intracytoplasmic material that histologically resemble finely divided particles of cement but are less conclusively identifiable (Figs. 4-27 and 4-28).

Interfaces of Bone, Soft Tissue, and Prosthesis

The by-products of wear and tissue damage caused by loosened prostheses are visible at the interfaces of the bone, the soft tissue, and the prosthesis. Metallic debris is generated more prominently by the effects of wear on metal-to-metal prostheses than by metal on polyethylene. Considerable metallic debris can be generated after failure of metallic implants by corrosion and fretting. The multiple piece implants (modular systems or devices incorporating screw fixation design) are particularly prone to generate debris which in fact may cause accelerated wear of HDP as well (Fig. 4-29). The latter tends to produce fine shards and larger fragments of HDP, generating a histiocytic and giant-cell response that resembles a tumor (Figs. 4-30 to 4-33).

The histological patterns just reviewed have one characteristic in common that might enhance the vulnerability of the endoprosthetic host to infection. It is noteworthy that, in spite of very striking local hypercellularity, there were few blood vessels. This weakness of vascular support may be an important factor in the susceptibility to infection of patients with loosened prostheses, since mechanical injury helps to provide necrotic tissue as a culture medium for ambitious bacterial contaminants.

More sensitive methods might be tried for the detection of low-grade bacterial infection.

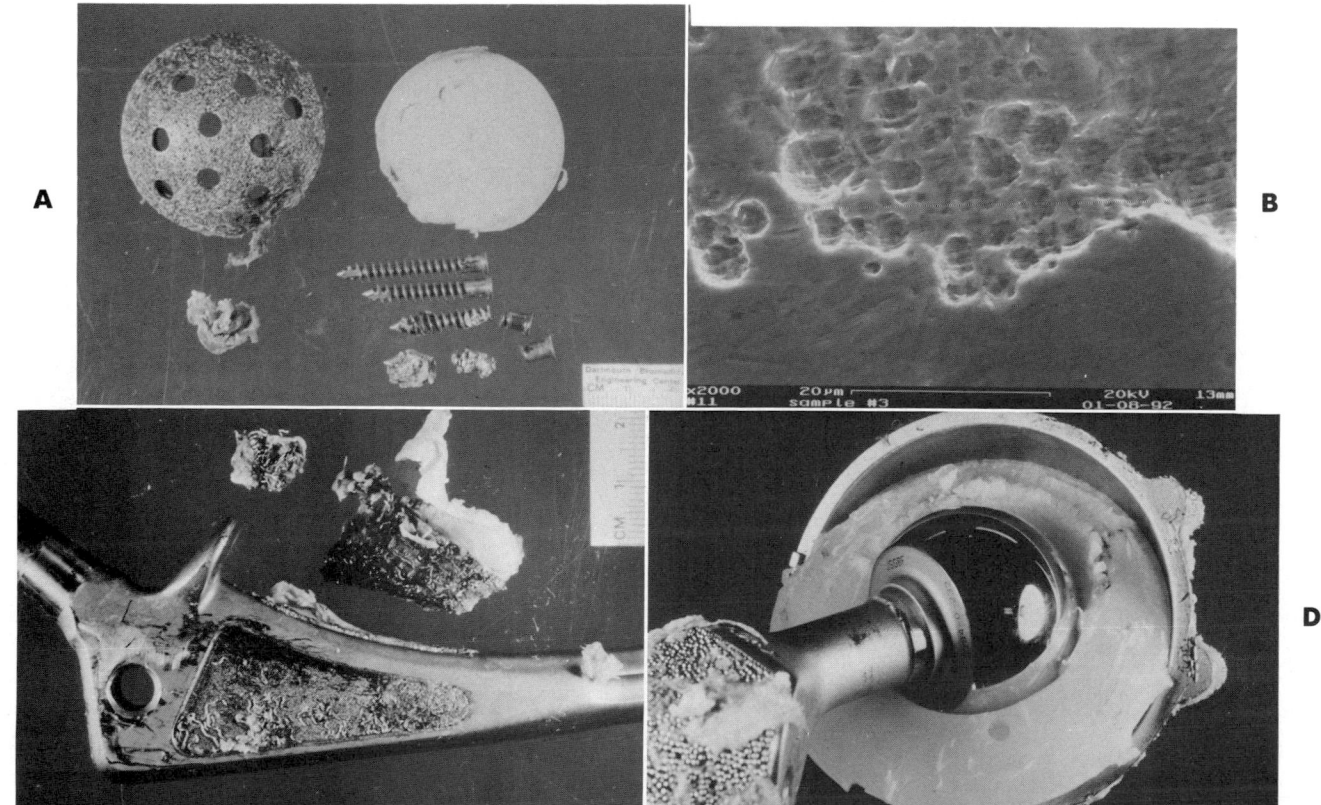

Fig. 4-29. A, Explanted Harris-Galante cup showing broken screw head with impingement on HDP. Darkened tissue is caused by titanium debris resulting from fretting between screw heads and the metal shell. **B,** Scanning electron microscopy (×2000) head showing pitting corrosion. The prosthesis was an Orthomet Perfecta cobalt-chromium alloy. This prosthesis was a retrieved postmortem specimen with a smooth, press-fit titanium stem. **C,** A Harris-Galante femoral stem showing loss of titanium ingrowth pad *(wire mesh)* and stem burnishing *(surgically explanted prosthesis).* **D,** Failure of HDP linear fixation to the metal backing *(surgically explanted specimen).*

Continued.

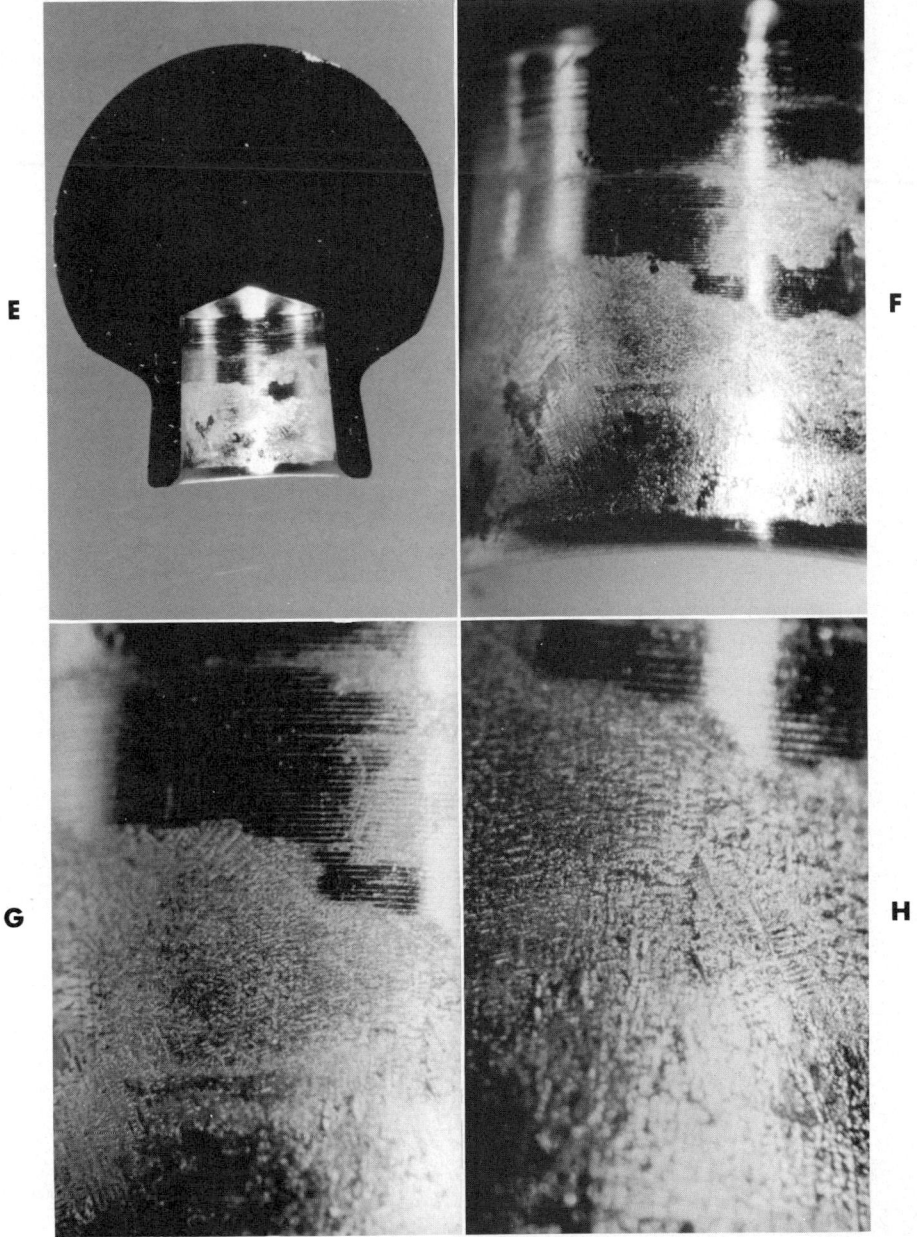

Fig. 4-29—cont'd. E, Corrosion attack phenomenon is revealed by sectioned femoral head in a chromium and cobalt alloy *(ball)* on the Harris-Galante stem. Explantation was at revision surgery only 17.9 months after surgery. **F to H,** Magnification of **E** at 10×, 20×, and 40×, respectively. (Courtesy John P. Collier D.E.)

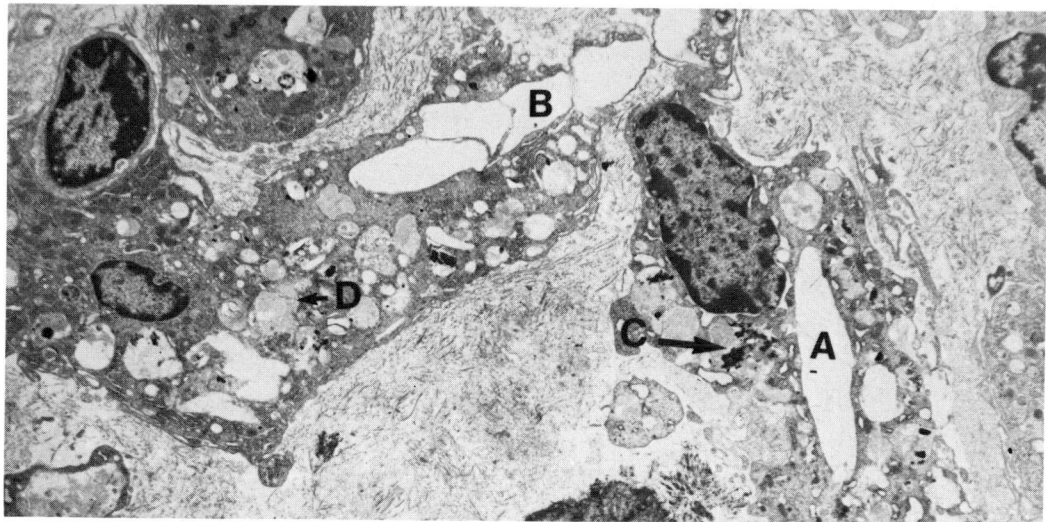

Fig. 4-30. Histiocytic cell in right midzone contains fusiform inclusion *(A)* resembling shape of polyethylene shards as visualized under polarized light microscopy. It should be noted that rounded electron-lucent defects (Fig. 4-31, *B*) do not appear in inclusion presumed to be HDP *(A)* but are visible in those presumed to contain cement *(B)*. A variety of inclusions is apparent in both cells; this corresponds to granular texture of cells under light microscopy. Some of the inclusions are slightly more electron-opaque than others. If this slightly opaque material were protein, acidophilic granular appearance of these cells under light microscopy would be explained. Irregular particulate fragments of electron-dense *(black)* material *(C)* represent intracellular metallic deposits. Such a variety of ingested debris identifies these cells as omnivorous phagocytes (×5850). (From Johnston AD, Parisien MV: Pathology of reactive (prosthetic) versus septic (revisionary) synovitis. In Eftekhar NS, editor: *Infection in joint replacement surgery: prevention and management,* St Louis, 1984, Mosby–Year Book.)

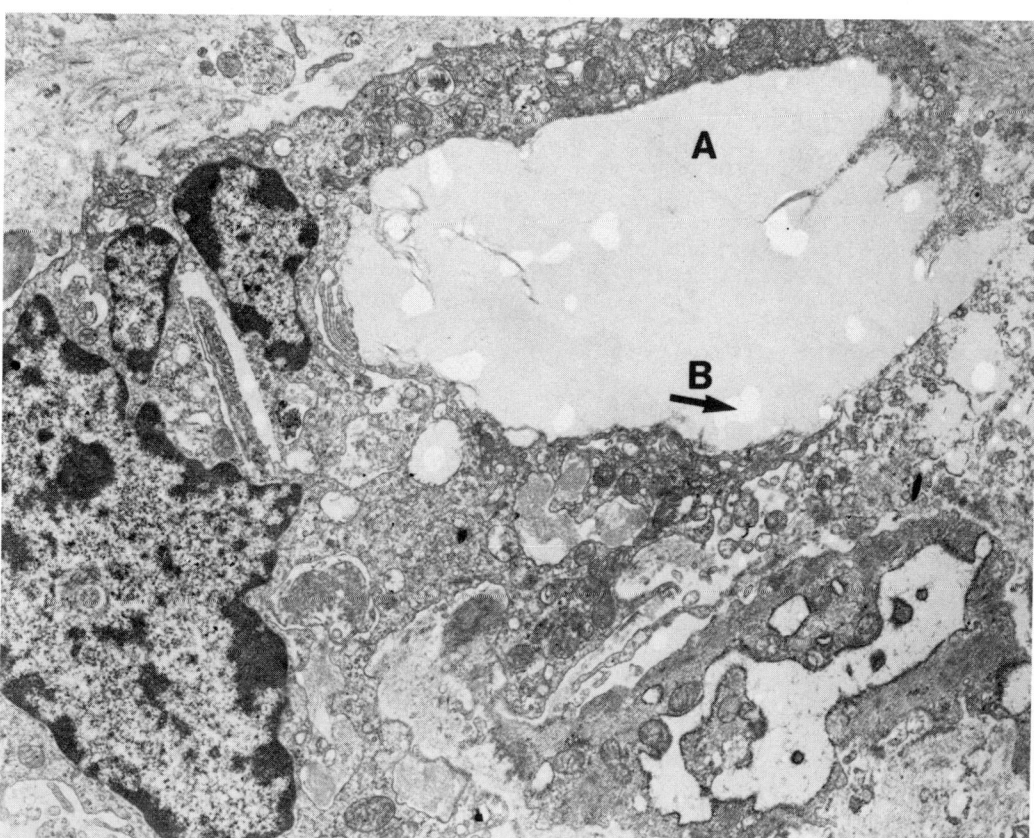

Fig. 4-31. Macrophagic histiocyte accommodates ovoid, incompletely loculated inclusions *(A),* which probably contained bone cement (MMA). Ordinarily particulate cement was lost in the course of processing these sections, possibly by solvents such as propylene oxide. Strange electron-lucent defects appear in this inclusion *(B)* and in cisternae lined by rough endoplasmic reticulum (×14,500). (From Johnston AD, Parisien MV: Pathology of reactive (prosthetic) versus septic (revisionary) synovitis. In Eftekhar NS, editor: *Infection in joint replacement surgery: prevention and management,* St Louis, 1984, Mosby–Year Book.)

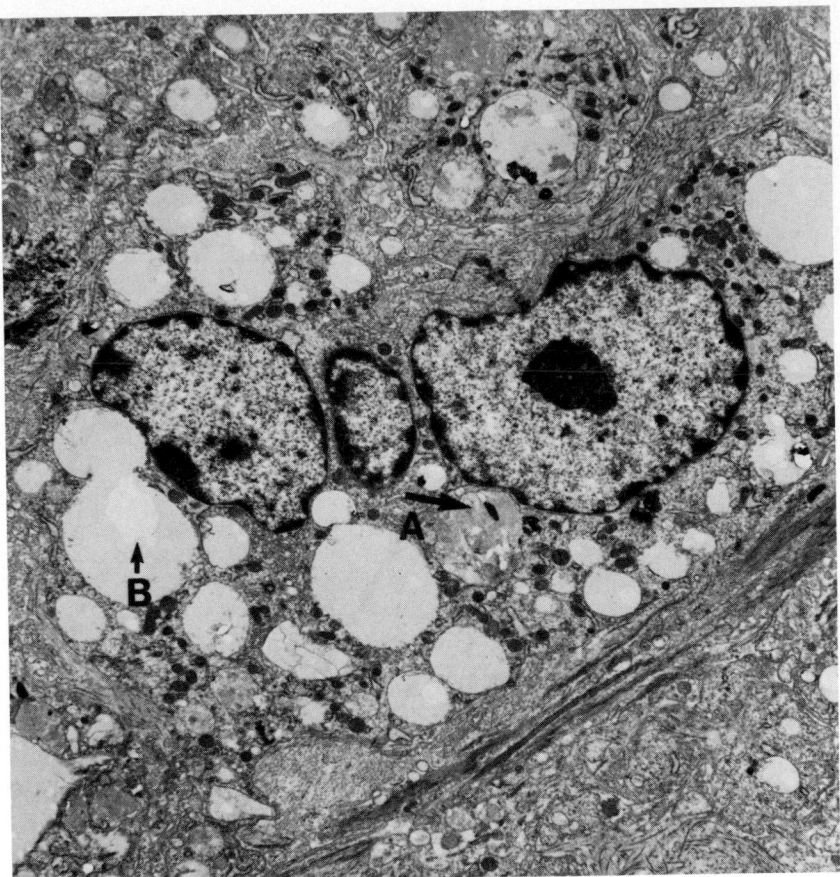

Fig. 4-32. Rounded cytoplasmic inclusions and their electron-lucent defects *(B)* are abundantly shown in this multinucleated giant cell. These defects also appear in slightly electron-opaque inclusions in which metallic particles appear *(A)*. We infer that this juxtanuclear inclusion contains protein and thus contributes to acidophilic granular cytoplasm in reactive histiocytes and giant cells under light microscopy (×7500). (From Johnston AD, Parisien MV: Pathology of reactive (prosthetic) versus septic (revisionary) synovitis. In Eftekhar NS, editor: *Infection in joint replacement surgery: prevention and management,* St Louis, 1984, Mosby–Year Book.)

RADIOLOGY OF PROSTHETIC INTERFACE

A radiological line of demarcation between bone and cement is often interpreted to be fibrous cartilage or fibrocartilage. Histologies corresponding to the interface may also contain particles of high-density polyethylene and small amounts of spherical acrylic cement. While the line of lucency may be a hallmark of future clinical failure, it has generally been appreciated that the incidence of loosening, that is, clinical failure, is much lower than that suggested by the radiographic lucency. Furthermore, radiolucency is especially important and regarded as evidence of loosening if (1) the lucency line is progressive in length, (2) the lucency line is expanding in width more than 2 mm, and (3) the lucency line borders a line of sclerosis, which is indicative of reaction to movement.[269] The bone lysis caused by widening of the radiolucency line appears to be erratic and expeditious, as if an associated "lytic process" may play a part in producing extensive bone loss.[105] As stated, the radiological sign alone is of no concern as long as it is not progressive and is associated with a line of sclerosis, the latter being an indication of stress causing a reactive process involving movement of the prosthesis.

HISTOCHEMISTRY OF THE INTERFACE MEMBRANE

Goldring and associates described the histochemical characteristics of the interface membrane of loose cemented prostheses, thus defining a pathomechanism of bone absorption and coining the term *synovial-like membrane.*[105] They recognized three distinct zones in the membrane: (1) the synovial-like lining forming papillary folds supported by fibrovascular tissue at the cement-bone interface, (2) a layer containing histiocytes and giant cells, including particles of high-density polyethylene and PMMA, and (3) a fibrocartilaginous layer blending into the adjacent bone.

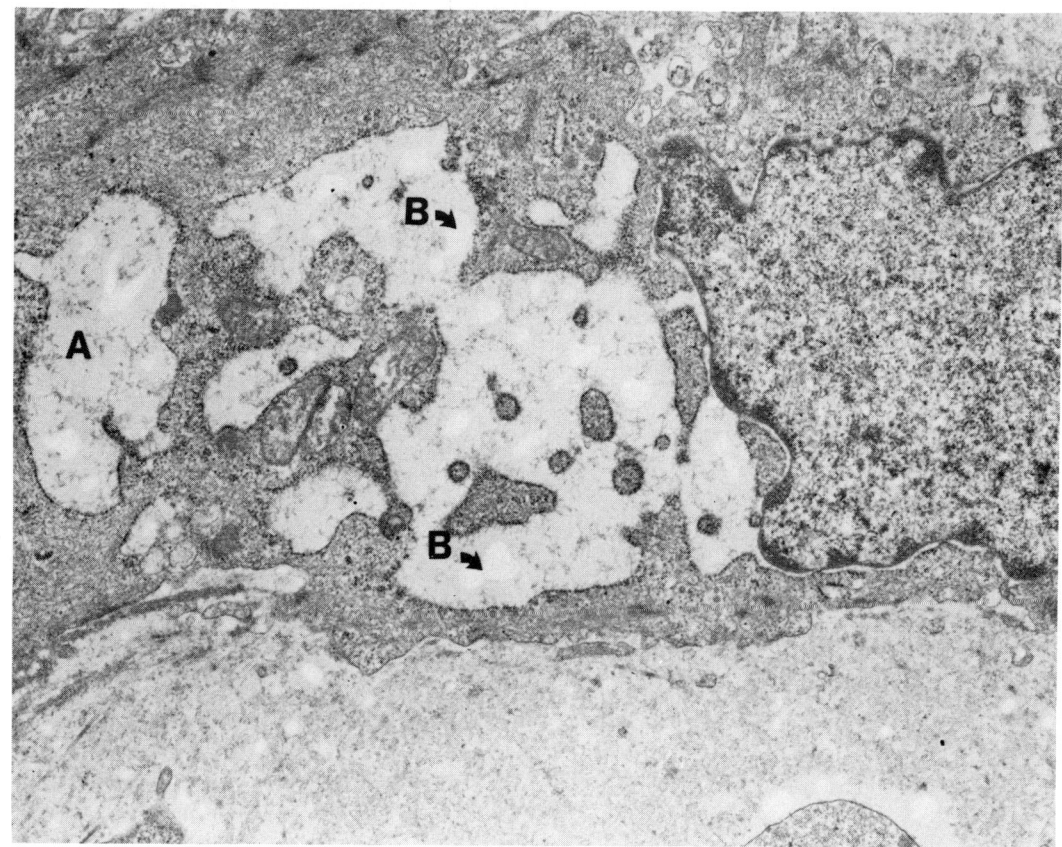

Fig. 4-33. Convoluted cisterna *(A)* almost certainly contains protein synthesized by rough endoplasmic reticulum lining cavity. This further contributes to acidophilic granular cytoplasm of histiocytic cells that dominate reactive response to HDP. We wish further to draw attention to rounded, electron-lucent *(B) (white)* defects in proteinaceous material filling cavity (×22,000). (From Johnston AD, Parisien MV: Pathology of reactive (prosthetic) versus septic (revisionary) synovitis. In Eftekhar NS, editor: *Infection in joint replacement surgery: prevention and management,* St Louis, 1984, Mosby–Year Book.)

The first layer is lined with large polygonal cells with an eccentric nuclei. The cells (one to two cell thickness) lacked a basement membrane. Occasional multinucleated giant cells were present with deeper lining of a loose fibrovascular stroma containing histiocytes and mononuclear infiltrates with occasional formation of papillary folds and features similar to a synovial membrane.

The second (midzone) layer was predominantly made of fibrovascular structures, containing sheets of granular histiocytes, mononuclear cells, and foreign body giant cells. The giant cells are often surrounded by large spaces, the site of dissolved PMMA containing the barium sulfate.

The third layer, being most adjacent to the bone and marrow, did not show evidence of acute or chronic inflammatory cells, but some areas of dissolved PMMA, residual granules of barium sulfate, and occasional giant cells were seen.

In general, enzymatically active cells, such as histiocytes and monocytes, were predominantly located in the middle zone and on the cement surface of the membrane that stained positively for nonspecific esterase, lysozome, and acid esterase, but were consistently positive for acid phosphatase.[105]

The synovial-like lining was positive only for acid phosphatase.

Based on the histochemical and cell cultures of membranes of failed total hip arthroplasty interfaces, Goldring and co-workers deduced that the stellate cells were similar to those found in cultures of normal tissue and rheumatoid synovial tissue. The membrane had the capacity to produce large amounts of prostaglandin E_2 and collagenase,[105] which can mediate resorption of bone and other connective tissues. It has been suggested that synovial tissue fails to develop in the absence of motion. Therefore traction or motion produces a biological signal that causes differentiation and organization of cells into the form of synovial tissue. In an independent in-vivo test, Edwards and associates showed that repeated injection of air into subcutaneous tissue after a period of 5 to 30 days created a lining indistinguishable from a synovial membrane.[80]

Doty, at our institution, reviewed several reactive membranes removed from loose cemented total hip prostheses,[81] confirming other investigators' conclusions[105] regarding the enzyme activities of the membrane formed between the loose prosthesis and bone (Tables 4-4 and 4-5).

Membranes removed during arthroplasty revisions were chemically preserved in glutaraldehyde-paraformaldehyde solutions and studied by light and electronmicroscopy. Methods were used for demonstrating acid phosphatase, alkaline phosphatase, beta-galactosidase, endogenous peroxidase, and glucose oxidase.[72]

Lysosomal enzyme activities, as indicated by acid phosphatase or naphthol esterase, were especially strong in the macrophage and giant cell populations of these membranes. The connective tissue cells within the membrane were also reactive for acid phosphatase but did not appear to change in activity regardless of their location within the membrane (Fig. 4-34).

The presence of methacrylate or HDP particles seemed to cause activation of the macrophage or giant cell, with resulting strong lysosomal response, especially in those cells with phagocytized wear particles. Beta-galactosidase, an enzyme specifically synthesized by macrophages during activation, was an especially good marker for cells that had phagocytized wear products. In most cases, the presence of these particles resulted in a cellular reaction for beta-galactosidase, whereas the other lysosomal enzymes did not always demonstrate this effect. Thus, lysosomal enzyme activity demonstrated focal areas of cellular response within an individual membrane. This result was further complicated by the presence of very large fragments of methacrylate, which appeared to be "walled off" by mononuclear connective tissue cells; these cells showed no significant increase in lysosomal enzyme activity.

Alkaline phosphatase was not demonstrable within the membrane. The enzyme would have been found in some of the leukocyte population, and endogenous peroxidase enzyme activity would have been abundant in activated leukocytes. However, these membrane samples indicated very little leukocyte activity. This also suggests that no infection was present. This conclusion was supported by our microscopic studies in which we were unable to find bacterial growth in these membrane samples.

Reactions for endogenous peroxidase and glucose oxidase were carried out as another indicator of macrophage activation. In general, these reactions were not uniform within our samples. Macrophages or giant cells that contained phagocytized wear particles did not always show high levels of these enzyme activities. Perhaps there is an original burst of enzyme activity when the particle is incorporated by the cell and, in time, these cells become quiescent. This would explain the "focal" localization of enzyme activities within these membranes. Goldring and colleagues found that different areas of a single membrane contained variable amounts of collagenase and prostaglandin activity and that different patient samples showed a large range of these same activities.[105] Our studies would confirm this sort of variability. It may be possible that large areas of a membrane may be undergoing continual active and quiescent phases during the lifetime of the prosthesis. Such a cyclic response by the membrane and the included cell populations might be mediated by the mechanical

Table 4-4 Hydrolytic Enzyme Content of Membranes—Removed from Interface of Loose Prostheses

Source	Number studied	Acid phosphatase activity/DNA (Pmol MUB/ min × μg DNA)
Cemented prosthesis	10	210–600
Noncemented prosthesis	3	85–240
Infected	3	1000–1200

Table 4-5 Hydrolytic Enzyme Content of Membranes—Source Loose Femoral and Acetabular Components

	Beta-galactosidase n = 6	Acid phosphatase n = 6	Tartrate res AP n = 4	B-Glucuronide n = 6
Femur	3.14 ± 0.95	358 ± 225	158 ± 76	14.1 ± 4.8
Acetabulum	2.55 ± 0.95	335 ± 229	131 ± 86	13.4 ± 6.2

Activity expressed as Pmol MUB/min × 4 gm DNA; ± 1 Standard Deviation.
Histochemical assays performed by Doty at Laboratory of Orthopaedic Department, NYOH, Columbia Presbyterian Medical Center.

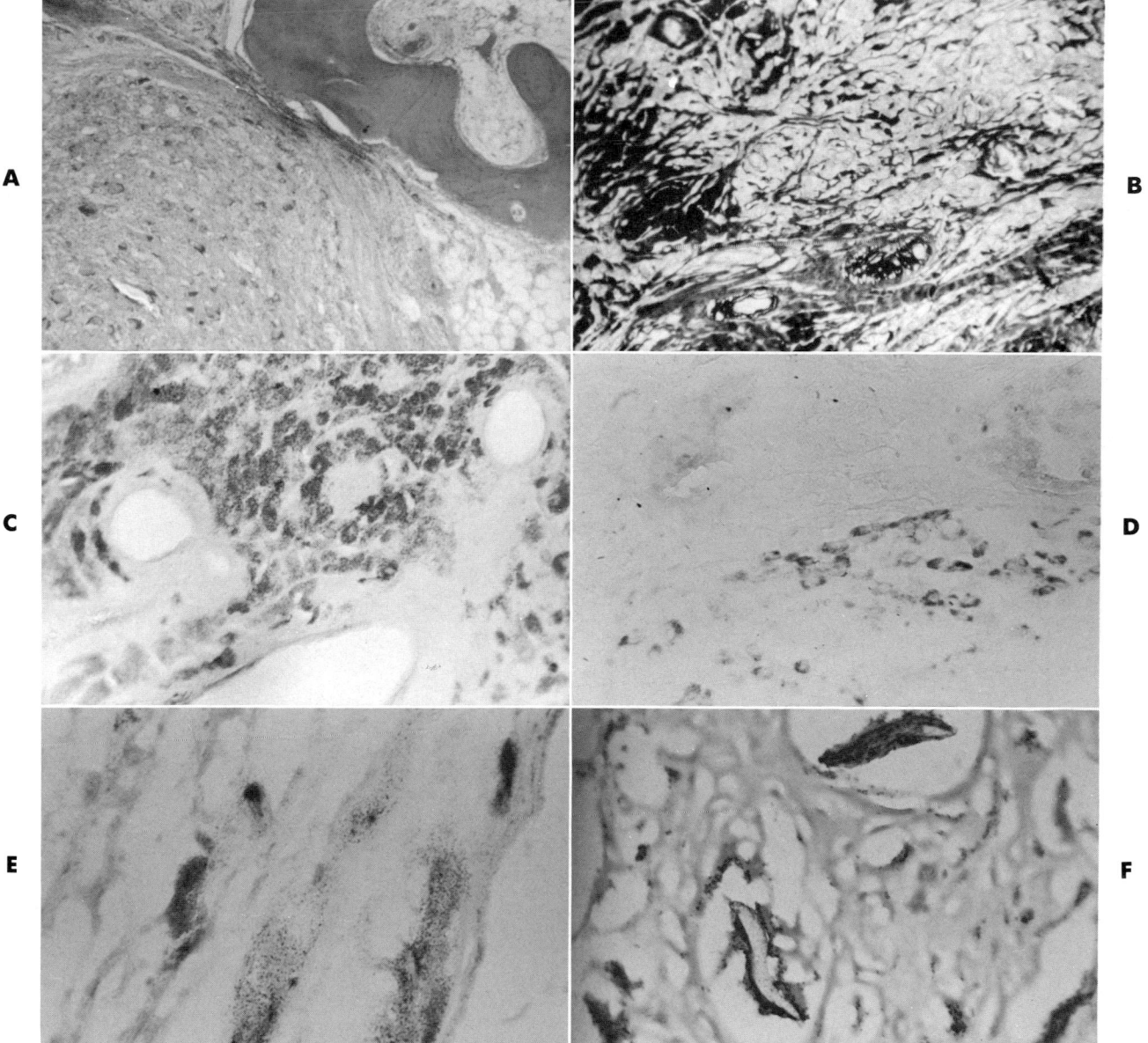

Fig. 4-34. A, Lower power magnification H and E stain of section through nonseptic prosthetic synovitis with an attached bone fragment showing evidence of bone necrosis. This highly cellular proliferative tissue is acting as a space occupying lesion at the interface (it contained many phagocytised particles of plastic material) and causing bone necrosis. **B,** Silver stain of the same specimen as shown in **A** illustrates the fibrotic and gritty nature of the gross tissue. **C,** Light microscopy of histological section stained for esterase activity. NOTE: high enzyme-related cellular activity about the vascular channels. The tissue is from a grossly loose cemented implant. **D,** Positive staining for beta galactosidase (note absence of acid phosphatase). Tissue is from same source as **A.** As in **A** and **B,** histochemical staining shows an increased endogenous peroxidase activity (beta-galactosidase, an enzyme specifically made by macrophages during activation) caused by the presence of PMMA or HDP and during active phase of membrane. **E,** Concurrent enzyme activities of acid phosphatase *(red)* and beta galactosidase *(blue)* within the same specimen (see text). **F,** Lysosomes are adsorbed to the surface of two shards of plastic (presumably HDP), indicating lysosomal activities in the tissue.

stimulation existing between the prosthesis and the supporting bone. The relationship of premacrophage stem cells to formation of giant cells, histiocytes, and osteoclasts is shown with an indication of their relative size and histochemical characteristics (Fig. 4-35).

MICROMOTION THEORY

Based on clinical, radiological, and histological observations, we believe that micromotion between cement and bone is the cause of failure of cement fixation. The amplitude of such motion need not exceed 30 μm of displacement since this is the smallest acrylic "spherule" displaced from its bed and incorporated into the shape of modified bone (bone caps).[47] These spherules

are the small particles recognizable from a mass of acrylic. In this theory the structure of the acetabulum is the cause of initiation of micromotion. The weight-bearing portion of the bone of the acetabulum after exposure of bony trabeculae by removal of the subchondral plate is responsible for the deformation of bone and micromotion at the interface. If the stiffness of the acetabulum is reduced by removal of the subchondral bone, plastic deformation of the bone may occur[82] (Figs. 4-36 to 4-37). Stress may then be concentrated at the exposed trabeculae which, in turn, results in bone necrosis. Necrotic bone, in time, is replaced by a fibrous membrane that may or may not turn into a strong fibrocartilaginous metaplastic

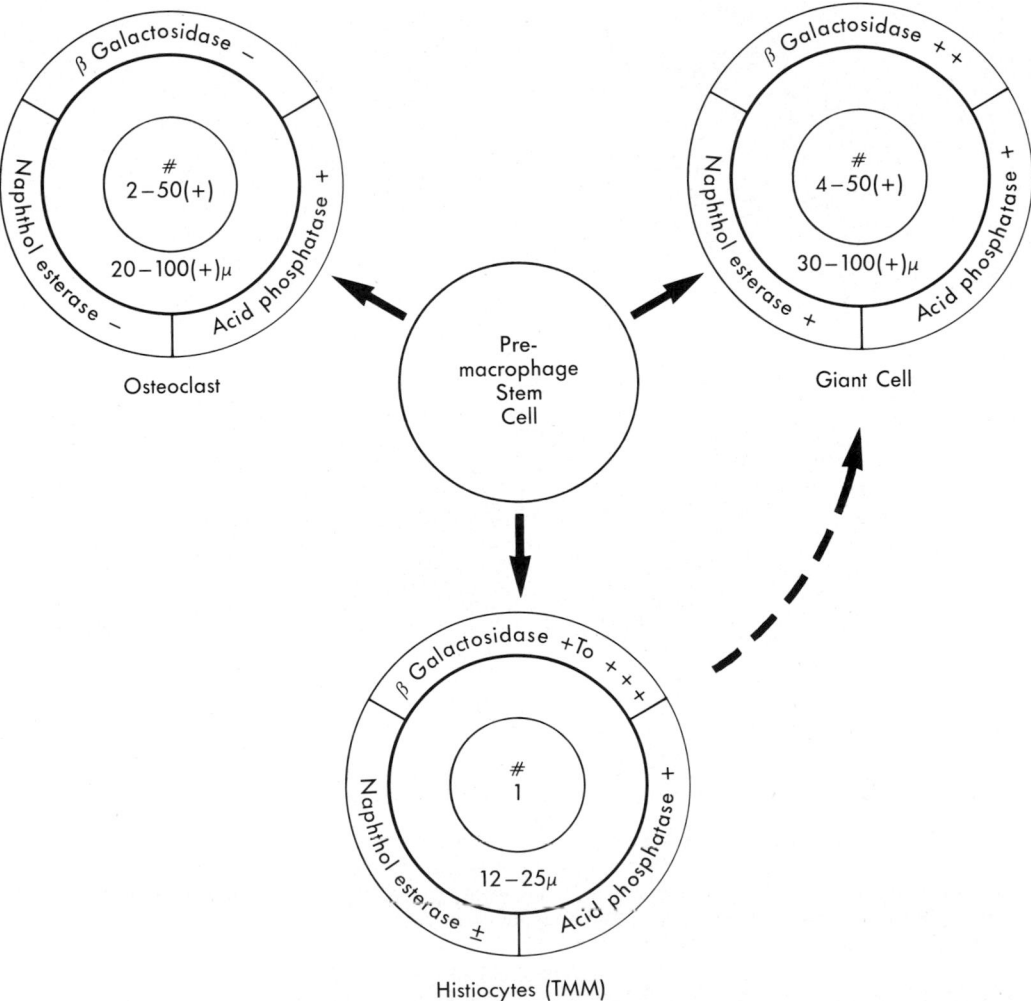

Fig. 4-35. Premacrophage stem cell and its relationship to cells frequently found at the interface: multinucleated giant cells, osteoclasts, and histiocytes. The inner circle illustrates the number of cell nuclei. Numbers at the space between the inner and middle circles indicate the average size of corresponding cells. The space between the second and third circles indicates the common enzymes specifically found within each cell type. The dotted arrow suggests the possibility of a relationship between histiocytes and formation of multinucleated giant cells. (From Eftekhar NS, Doty SB, Johnston AD, et al: Prosthetic synovitis. In The Hip Society: *The hip: proceedings of the thirteenth open scientific meeting of The Hip Society,* St Louis, 1985, Mosby–Year Book.)

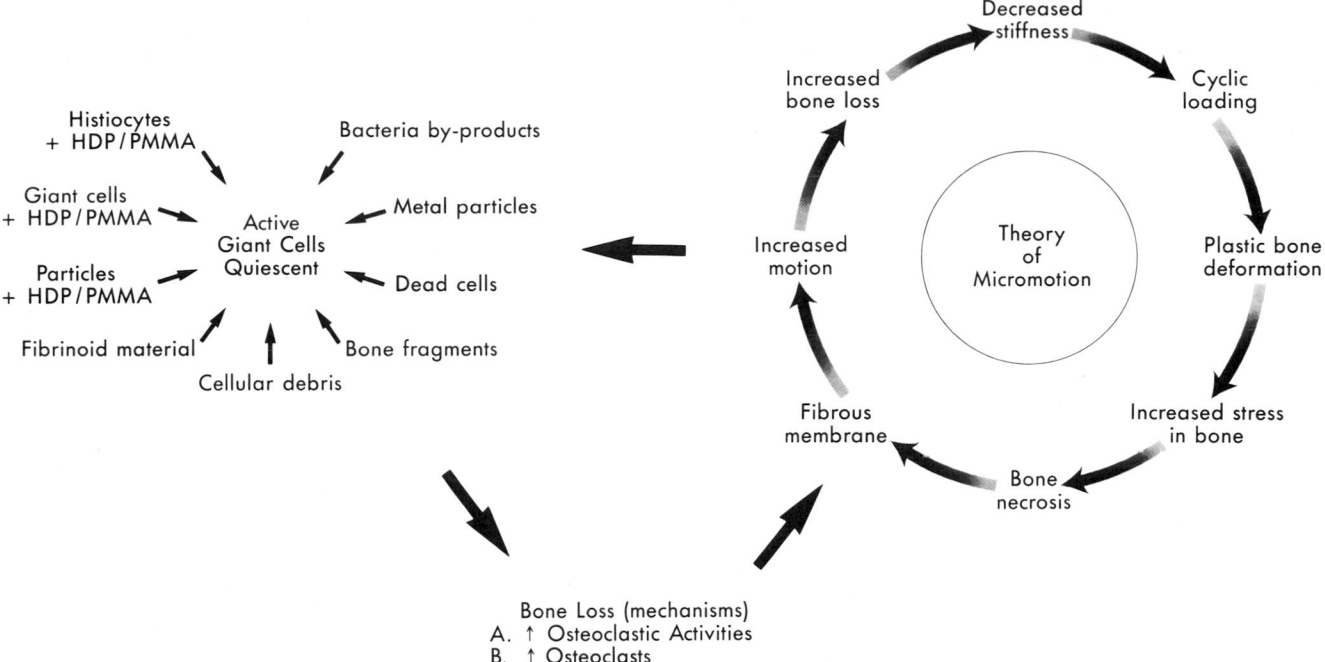

Fig. 4-36. The theory of micromotion and its contribution to giant cell formation and other causes of activation of giant cells. The mechanism of bone loss leading to further loss of stiffness is responsible for a vicious circle leading to ultimate failure of the implant. (From Eftekhar NS, Doty SB, Johnston AD, et al: Prosthetic synovitis. In The Hip Society: *The hip: proceedings of the thirteenth open scientific meeting of The Hip Society,* St Louis, 1985, Mosby–Year Book.)

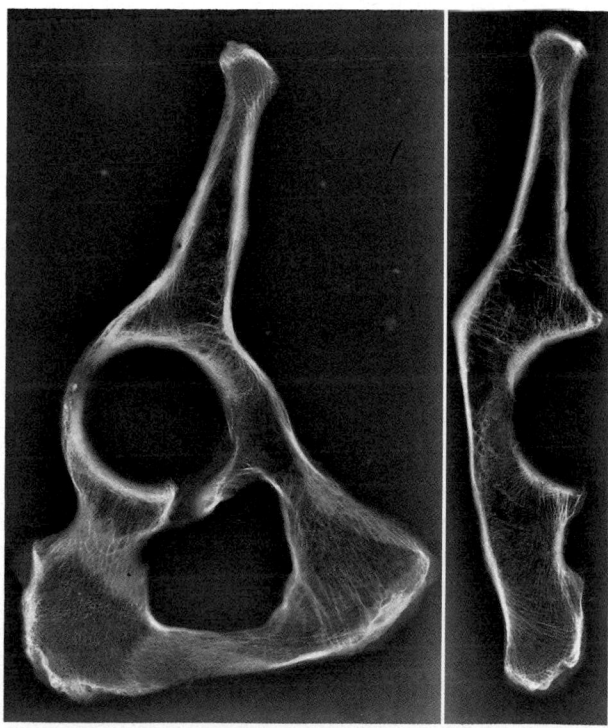

Fig. 4-37. A 5-mm cross section of iliac bone in a 68-year-old woman. This slab radiograph dramatically illustrates the paucity of cancellous bone and fine trabecula sparsely present beyond the subchondral bone of the acetabulum. (From Eftekhar NS, Doty SB, Johnston AD, et al: Prosthetic synovitis. In The Hip Society: *The hip: proceedings of the thirteenth open scientific meeting of The Hip Society,* St Louis, 1985, Mosby–Year Book.)

weight-bearing structure. If this fibrous interface results in significantly decreased stiffness, further motion will break down the acrylic and cause more looseness (micromotion).

We attribute histological changes observed at the proximal and medial aspects of the neck of the femur (proximal to the lesser trochanter) to the same phenomenon of micromotion. The histology differs from that found at the shaft of the femur where a close coaptation between cement and bone is possible.

During their attempt to degrade particles of PMMA and HDP, macrophages (histiocytes and multinucleated giant cells) continue to increase in number and enzyme activity level. Osteoclastic activity at the bone interface may also result from an increase in number of activities at the site. We believe that micromotion at the cement-bone interface in the acetabulum in patients with late loosening, as evidenced by progressive radiolucency, results from provocation of quiescent histiocytes and macrophages at the site and the attraction and proliferation of premacrophagic stem cells. Histologically and clinically, a stable interface may be provoked by the presence of these cells and eventually result in severe osteoclasis and bone loss (Figs. 4-36 to 4-38).

Clinically we have been able to identify four patient categories in which a stable interface has been altered,

undoubtedly related to micromotion between cement and bone: young and active patients with excess elasticity of bone, overweight individuals, patients with rheumatoid disease with disuse atrophy, and aged patients with progressive osteoporosis. In all of these patients the common pathway is increased motion as a result of loss of stiffness in the bone or relative motion accompanied by excess load (Fig. 4-38).

MASSIVE OSTEOLYSIS IN PRESENCE OF FIXED CEMENT

Bone resorption around the cemented total hip prosthesis, resulting from fragmentation of cement caused by the loss of fixation, is well documented (Fig. 4-39).* Extensive osteolysis resulting from particles of cement or high-density polyethylene was also documented originally by Charnley and Crawford (Fig. 4-40). Aggressive granulomatosis was first described by Harris and others in 1976. They defined this lesion based on the histology of four specimens removed from patients with loose prostheses as a "benign, noninflammatory tissue reaction" that caused extensive, localized tumorlike bone resorption around the cemented femoral component.[113]

---

* References 16, 44, 47, 183a, 195.

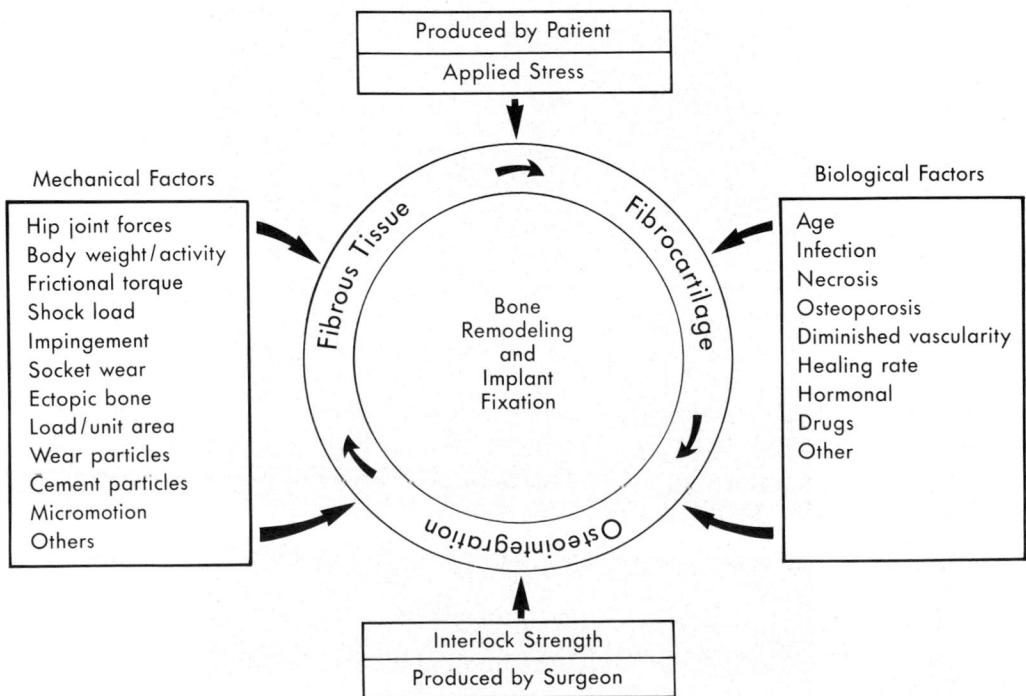

Fig. 4-38. The nature of the interface tissue (bone-cement junction) and its subsequent remodeling is affected by applied stress by patient (activity level, weight, etc.) and the quality of the initial fixation produced by the surgeon. Other factors such as mechanical properties of the prosthetic device and a series of biological factors may also be equally important in maintaining the strength and function of interface tissue.

Localized osteolysis has also been observed at the interface of a well-fixed prosthesis, between cement and bone (Fig. 4-41). A large number of particles of acrylic cement are present at the site of localized bone lysis without evidence of infection, neoplasm, or HDP. The histological response fails to demonstrate the synovial-like membrane similar to the one described by Goldring and co-workers.[105] Justy and others recently reported on four such rare lesions and offered a mechanism for their production.[128] The phenomenon is extremely rare; they were able to identify only 4 cases in more than 3000 total hip arthroplasties performed at the Massachusetts General Hospital between 1972 and 1986. Most recently, Maloney analyzed 25 cases of severe bone lysis from the same institution, including the 4 previously cited cases. In three hips, postmortem specimens were also available. Data related to the histology, back scatter scanning electronmicroscopy, and biochemical testing of the focal lesions confirmed a local cement fracture around an otherwise rigidly fixed implant. Maloney believed histiocytic reaction to the particulate PMMA to be the stimulus for local osteolysis.[157] This study and other reports on localized endosteal lysis[8a] in relation to fixed cemented femoral components suggest that a focal defect in the cement mantle must exist via which the contents of the joint cavity may reach the bone.

In a similar review of 16 such cases that required revision by a cementless prosthesis and that were followed from 2 to 6 years after surgery (mean follow up of 3½ years), Eskola has reported no recurrence of the lesion after revision.[84] Several other reports have pointed to the aggressive nature of the lesion, describing the histopathology of such lesions.[16,203,224a]

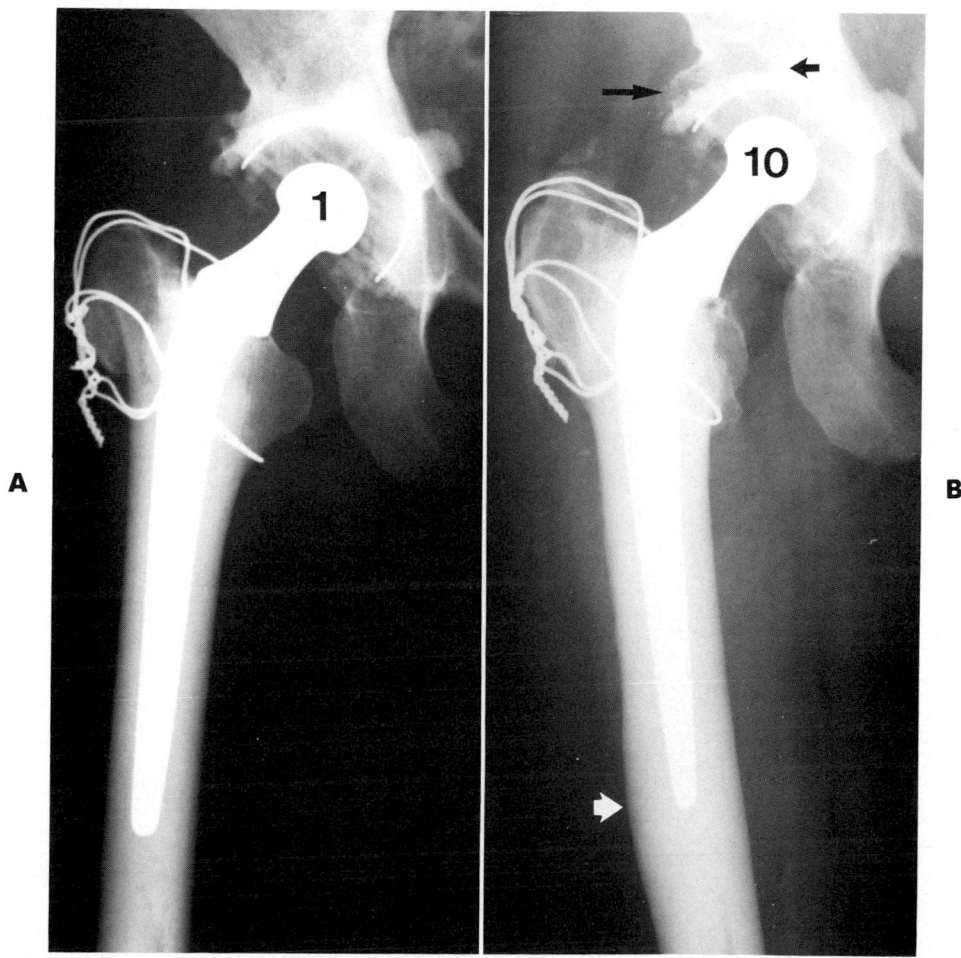

Fig. 4-39. A, 1 year after low-friction arthroplasty in a 41-year-old female patient (V.P.). NOTE: absence of demarcation or any radiolucency about either component (evidence of osteointegration of cemented stem). **B,** 10 years after surgery. NOTE: 3 mm wear of HDP with appearance of radiolucent line *(arrows)* and adaptive bone remodeling at level of stem tip (unicortical hypertrophy) *(arrows).*

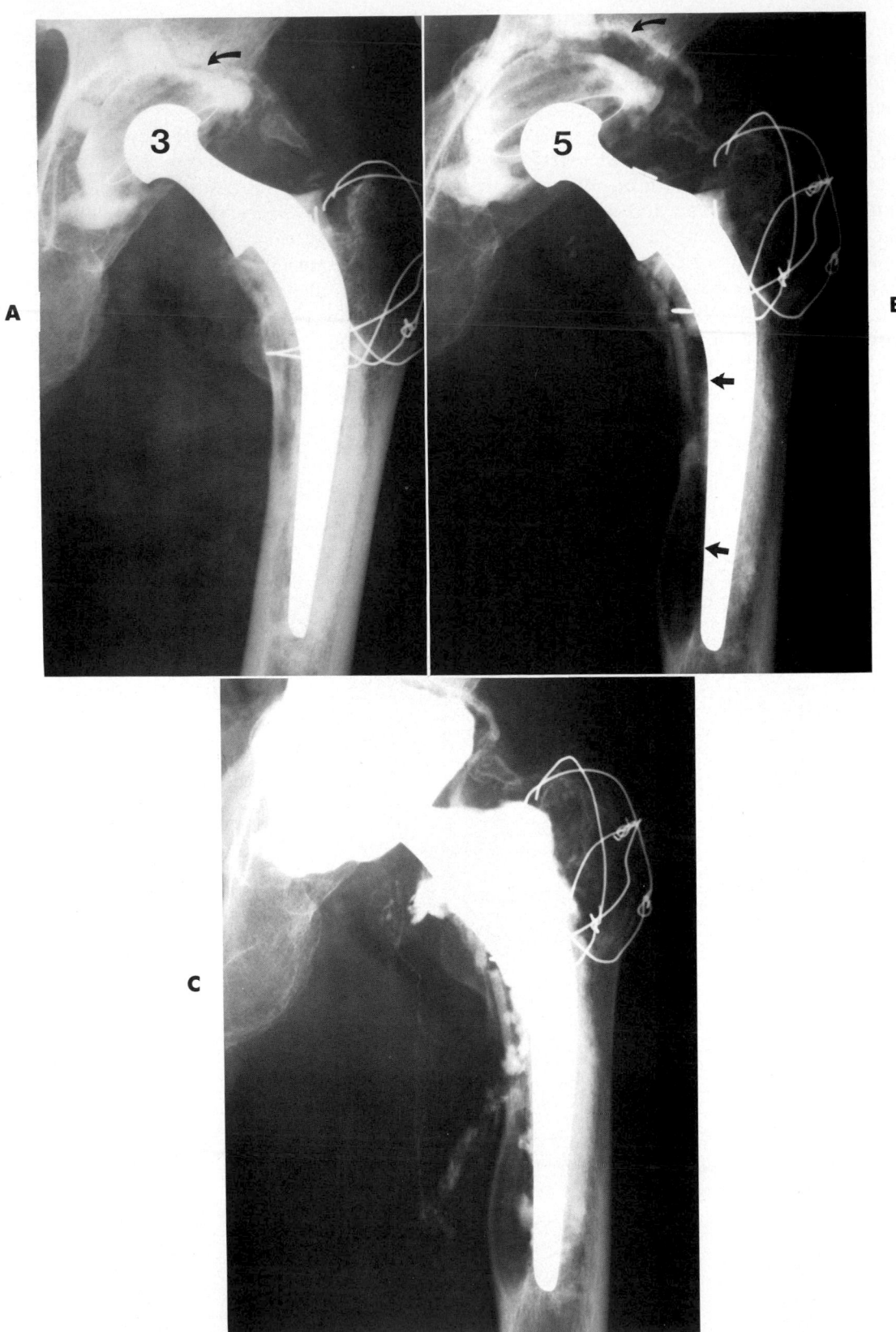

Fig. 4-40. A, Three years after insertion of Bechtol prosthesis in 63-year-old male (S.Z.) (performed at another institution). NOTE: plastic deformation of stem and radiolucent line at the cement bone interface about the cup has appeared. **B,** Extensive osteolysis along medial shaft of femur and acetabulum component *(arrows)* 2 years later (5 years after surgery.) **C,** Arthrogram shows extravasation, indicating spontaneous fracture of femoral cortex 5 years after index operation.

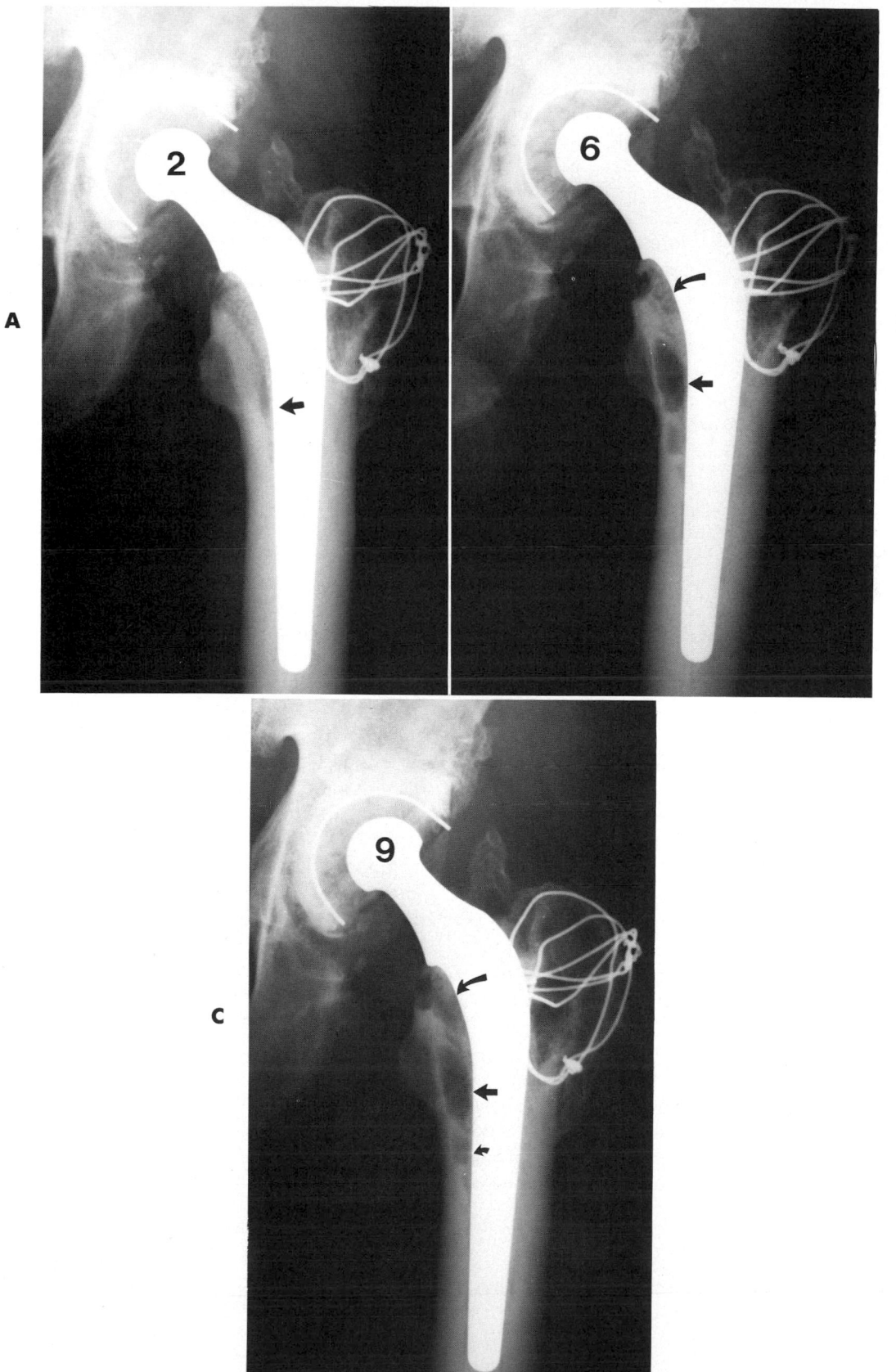

Fig. 4-41. A, Radiograph 2 years after low-friction arthroplasty in 68-year-old man (F.Z.) who weighs 84 kg and is extremely active. Arrow indicates very slight radiolucent zone appearing just at level of the junction of lesser trochanter. **B** and **C,** Progressive cystic erosions on medial side of femur at 6 years, **B,** and 9 years, **C.** Excellent distal stem fixation. Patient is asymptomatic despite radiological changes.

A report by Tallroth and others indicates that loosening of the implant is not an absolute prerequisite to bone lysis, which commonly occurs around a loose prosthesis.[250] Tallroth's observation is significant, however, because while it is believed that acrylic cement produces little or no reaction response while it remains fixed to the bone,[47] he indicates that occasionally a macrophage-mediated foreign body reaction can occur in the absence of cement loosening. The possible mechanism is either a localized fatigue of PMMA, leading to shedding of the particles, or, as suggested by Willert and associates, a portion of unpolymerized acrylic may be responsible for this phenomenon. Willert and co-workers observed unpolymerized acrylic polymer spherules in the cement bed of histological specimens implanted between 14 days and 5 years after surgery.[267] They thought these spherules were incompletely polymerized polymer.

In a recent study of the nature of the "aggressive granulomatous lesions" associated with total hip arthroplasty, Santavirta and others suggested that such lesions are a distinct entity, not only clinically, but also histopathologically and immunohistologically.[224] In their evaluation of 12 such lesions they found most cells were multinucleated giant cells, C^3 bireceptors, and nonspecific esterase-positive monocyte-macrophages, suggesting a rapidly progressive lytic nature of these lesions. In their view, the process is caused by uncoupling of the normal sequence of monocyte-macrophage-mediated clearance of foreign body and dead cells and normally followed by fibroblast-mediated synthesis.

Regarding bone resorption caused by HDP particles, Howie has shown that injection of particles measuring 20 to 200 μm produced osteolysis in an experimental animal model. In this model a plug of PMMA was first inserted in the distal femur and found to be encapsulated in a bony shell in control animals. However, after repeated injection of particles of HDP into the knee joint, bone resorption occurred at the stable interface. This experimental model was the first evidence to show a direct relationship between the presence and accumulation of polyethylene wear debris resulting from repeated injections and subsequent bone resorption.[121]

OSTEOLYSIS CAUSED BY HDP

Ultrahigh molecular weight polyethylene is generally accepted as an inert material when used in bulk, as in joint replacement; however, debris generated from the articulating surfaces is an accumulation process that relates to the size of the femoral component, the accuracy of surface finish (polish), and whether or not wear is accumulated by either an entrapped fragment of cement or batch variation of HDP blocks used in the manufacturing process. Wroblewski has documented a positive correlation between the wear of HDP and loosening and clinical failure.[276] Others also have implicated that wear of the socket and not cement will ultimately be responsible for osteolysis in the acetabulum.

Although the problem of wear has not been well studied, the wear of HDP has been radiographically measured to range from 0.0007 to 0.15 mm/year, including extreme wear of some sockets to as much as 0.3 mm/year.[50,52,108] Histologically the smallest wear particles (most common) appear as tiny splinters. Although the particles are not apparent in bright fields of microscopy, they show up clearly under polarized light, demonstrating their large distribution and large number in a relatively large portion of histological sections. These small, birefringent particles are usually phagocytized by or are associated with histiocytes while larger fragments are usually phagocytized by multinucleated giant cells. The largest pieces of HDP are encapsulated in a fibrous membrane.

Although most histological specimens related to failed total joint arthroplasty have been in patients whose arthroplasty included the use of HDP with PMMA, the collective reactive process was often thought to be caused by PMMA. Even today it is not generally realized that ultrahigh molecular weight polyethylene particles can induce massive osteolysis. Recently, I have observed patients in whom the ultrahigh molecular weight polyethylene wear was the sole contributor to the genesis of the erosions. Severe osteolysis at times includes severe loss of the cortex, which may be at a site distant to the site of articulation. There may be no evidence of metal or cement particles demonstrating that the wear of ultrahigh molecular weight HDP is the sole source of massive osteolysis by initiation of foreign body granuloma formation at the bone-cement interface.

The pathological material obtained often shows evidence of a thick membrane up to 1 to 2 cm eroding the bone of the femur and the bone of the acetabulum, appearing tumorlike and containing a large amount of HDP particles that had evidently caused the massive osteolysis by initiating foreign body granuloma formation at the bone-cement interface. The bone-cement interface remains intact beyond the osteolytic area.

The cellular morphology of foreign body granuloma is distinct under polarized light. The monocyte-macrophage system was stimulated by the presence of a large amount of ultrahigh molecular weight polyethylene particles shed from the ball heads of a "soft top" femoral head prosthesis.[268] The situation in this particular histological material was especially striking since the material was derived from soft top femoral head prostheses in which a high rate of wear is known to occur because of the convex rubbing surface of the polymer against cartilage and bone.[260]

Santavirta and others attributed an aggressive granulomatous lesion to HDP in six cases (only one had previously had a cemented total hip arthroplasty). They had performed revision at 4.8 years after five cementless Lord prostheses. At revision, a large granulomatous lesion showed uniform evidence of histiocytosis, which they attributed to plastic debris originating from the acetabular component.[223] Lord previously had described the cystic erosions associated with bone absorption related to HDP wear.[150] This study and others suggest that bone destructive lesions and absorptions, known as *cement disease*, are not unique to cemented devices but indeed may also be largely caused by HDP and other particles.

CARCINOGENICITY AND ONCOGENICITY OF IMPLANTS
Carcinogenicity of Polymers

PMMA has been found to be a bacterial mutagen (see Chapter 5). Polymers, including PMMA, in particulate form not only are capable of producing granulomatous reactions but also sarcomas under experimental conditions.[40,176] HDP generally is believed to be chemically inert and well tolerated in tissue. However, the carcinogenicity of HDP and other polymers is related to their physical properties, such as electrostatic charges, and their surface characteristics (hardness, roughness, nonwettability, etc.), which deteriorate their local tissue reactivity, and thus cause tumor formation.[28]

Most of the plastics implanted in the body have provoked sarcomas when implanted in rats and mice. Hueper advanced the idea that the chemical nature of the implant, and not its shape, is what offends,[123] but the authoritative work of Oppenheimer and Oppenheimer,[190] and Oppenheimer, Oppenheimer, and Stout[191] demonstrated that sarcomas are caused primarily by the size and shape of the implant. Concerning implantation of carcinogenic material in animals, however, a direct correlation between animal experimentation and human experiences has never been established. In spite of extensive implantation of plastics in the human body, only a very few authoritative cases of sarcomas have been reported to arise from the site of the joint prosthesis. Of special interest is the study of Hoopes and others in 1967, reporting a survey covering some 40,000 cases of breast augmentation with a variety of materials[120]; they found only 6 cases of cancer in these augmentations which, on detailed study, revealed no relationship between the implanted materials and cancer. Others have also attempted research to document the carcinogenicity of implanted materials in higher animals with notable failure.

Oncogenicity by implanted material has always been a concern of the orthopaedic surgeon. Although rarely do malignant tumors arise at the site of an implant, their occurrence, although regarded as unusual, causes speculation regarding implant application in young patients and centers on the materials and the time required to produce tumors. Whether the association is coincidental or there is a direct cause and effect relationship between the implanted material and tumors remains to be seen.

Carcinogenicity of Metals

Actually, very few examples exist in the literature concerning tumors in relation to implanted material in any animal phylogenetically above mice or rats. Clinical reports of tumors, presumably the result of inserted metals in the human body, are scarce[120,166,228] considering the large number of these implants currently being used, and all reports have failed to demonstrate a direct relationship between the implanted metals and cancer in humans.

Metallic orthopaedic implants have long been tested in laboratories for their potential for carcinogenicity, and a sporadic appearance of sarcomas at the site of insertion of various devices has been of special interest to orthopaedists.*

Metal implants for total hip arthroplasty also have been tested in the laboratory for potential carcinogenicity (Table 4-6, *A* and *B*).† Swanson, using wear particles generated by a wear apparatus made of chromium-cobalt and molybdenum, as well as other elements of chromium-cobalt-molybdenum prostheses, produced sarcoma in rats.[117,249] Elevated concentrations of chromium-cobalt in blood and urine[60] and significantly elevated levels of ionic metals in skeletal muscles[86] have been of concern for their systemic effects (Tables 4-6, *A* and *B* and 4-7). Because of widespread use of prostheses with expanded surfaces (porous coated), the issue of potential carcinogenicity related to release of ions by trace metals has surfaced.[160] Doll has shown a significant increase in carcinoma of lung and nasopharynx in workers exposed to nickel.[71] Arden and Bywaters[9] and Swann[247] have reported sarcoma arising from the site of a McKee-Farrar prosthesis (chromium-cobalt material). Additionally, a total knee replacement was associated with an epithelioid sarcoma also made of chromium and cobalt (Vitallium).[259]

Although implants made of chromium and cobalt have been used over the past 50 years, it is possible that the initiating factor in the increase of carcinogenicity may be related to the particles of the metal wear debris generated, thus causing a tumor at the site of the total hip implant. Evans and associates proposed a possible association between cobalt sensitivity in causing loosening of the implants, which might also cause carcinogenicity in certain individuals sensitive to these

---

* References 65, 69, 75, 137, 165, 251.

† References 11, 114, 155, 166, 229.

Table 4-6, A Cobalt-Based Alloy Composition

Cast Co–Cr–Co alloy (ASTM designation: F 75)	Wrought Co–Cr–W–Ni (ASTM designation: F 90)
Major alloy additions	
Cr: 27-30 (wt %)	Cr: 19-21 (wt %)
Ni: 1 (max)	Ni: 9-11
Mo: 5-7	W: 14-16
Trace components	
Fe: 0.75 (max)	Fe: 3 (max)
Si: 1 (max)	Si: 0.4 (max)
Mn: 1 (max)	Mn: 1-2
Co: 0.35 (max)	C: 0.05-0.15
	P: 0.04 (max)
	S: 0.03 (max)
Alloy base:	
Co: bal ($\cong$ 65 wt %)	Co: bal ($\cong$ 50 wt %)

From Black J: Metallic ion release and its relationship to oncogenesis. In The Hip Society: *The hip: proceedings of the 13th open scientific meeting of The Hip Society,* St Louis, 1985, Mosby–Year Book.

Table 4-6, B Elemental Content and Absorption

	Chromium	Cobalt	Nickel
Serum concentration[60b,256a] (μg/l)	0.2	0.3	5
Total body burden[152a] (μg)	6000	1200	10,000
Dietary intake[152a] (μg/day)			
In food	100	50	300-600
Absorbed (%)	?	?	9-18[3]
Implant release			
(μg/day)	9	18	0.3
(μg/year)	3285	6570	110

From Black J: Metallic ion release and its relationship to oncogenesis. In The Hip Society: *The hip: proceedings of the 13th open scientific meeting of The Hip Society,* St Louis, 1985, Mosby–Year Book.

metals.[85] According to one estimate,[21] in 1985, more than 90% of devices placed in patients were fabricated from chromium and cobalt. Therefore within the subsequent 20 years at least, these materials should be carefully watched for their potential side effects, since they have frequently been used. The various trace elements in the chromium-cobalt alloys may contribute to oncogenesis (see Table 4-6, A and B). Table 4-6, A shows two examples of chromium-based alloy compositions that are within the limits of two compositional standards of the American Society for Testing and Materials.[241,242]

For an agent to be considered carcinogenic in animal experiments, according to Furst, "tumors must appear at a site distant from the point of application; more

than one route must be affected; more than one species must respond; the growth must be transportable; and, if malignant, invasion and/or metastasis must be noted."[94]

Recent reviews of carcinogenicity related to chromium-cobalt alloys and nickel and its compounds considered them potentially carcinogenic in animals.[21,138,139] Of special interest, the U.S. Public Health Service lists chromium and some of its compounds among 22 known carcinogens in humans and lists nickel and some nickel compounds among 95 substances that may be carcinogenic.[22,23]

Malignancy at the Site of Total Hip Arthroplasty

Despite total hip arthroplasty now being one of the most common orthopaedic operations performed in the Western world, only a few neoplastic lesions have been reported as having arisen from the site of arthroplasty. Of interest, the neoplastic lesions reported are limited to a few case reports and almost all surfaced in the 1980s. Most are morphologically of rather uncommon types of malignancies, such as malignant fibrohistiocytoma (see Table 4-7). It is, however, worth noting that the emergence of late-appearing tumors might be the first such reports of malignancies related to thousands and even millions of total hip arthroplasties performed during the past three decades.

Most cases reported were in women in their sixties or seventies and most had a cemented prosthesis made of chromium-cobalt alloy. The length of time from surgery to discovery of the malignancy was from 2 to 11 years, with four cases being greater than 10 years after their index operation. The site of implant or adjacent bone was thought to be the origin of the tumor, which occurred mostly in the femur. Different brands of acrylic cement (with various compositions) had been used in most cases. The histological diagnosis was predominantly sarcoma, and most patients succumbed to their disease soon after the tumor was diagnosed or were lost to follow up (see Table 4-7).

Cancer at Remote Sites After Total Hip Arthroplasty

Because of the presence of metallic ions and wear products of total hip arthroplasty materials in tissues at the site of the total joint and remote areas of the body,* a fundamental and still plausible question is whether an increased incidence of cancer can be found in patients who undergo total hip arthroplasty using currently used combinations of metal and plastic. This is particularly significant since in-vitro studies and several animal models showed that cell mutagenesis, chromosomal damage, mammalian cell

---

* References 60, 67, 154, 257, 274.

Table 4-7 Malignancy Associated with Total Hip Arthroplasty

Author	Reference	Year published	Number of cases	Age	Sex	Histology	Implant type	Material implanted	Time since operation	Follow up after prescription	Comments
Haag and Adler	115	1990	1	69	F	Malignant fibrous histiocytoma	Webber-Huggler	HDP Protasul 10 Cr/Ni/Co PMMA	9 years	?	
Swann	247	1984	1	63	M	Malignant fibrous histiocytoma	McKee-Ferrar	Cr/Co PMMA	3 years	Died early	
Bagò-Grannell et al	10	1984	1	77	F	Malignant fibrous histiocytoma	Charnley-Müller	Cr/Co PMMA	2 years	?	Lost to follow up
Weber	259	1986	1	76	F	Epithelioid sarcoma	Variable axis	Cr/Co PMMA	5 years	Died early	At site of total knee replacement
Penmann and Ring	196	1984	1	75	F	Osteosarcoma	Ring	Co/Cr No cement	3 years	Died early	Died soon after diagnosis
Lamovec et al	135	1988	1	62	F	Synovial sarcoma	Charnley-Müller	HDP, S.S. PMMA	12 years	?	
Lamovec et al	135	1988	1	65	F	Spindle cell sarcoma (high-grade osteosarcoma)	Charnley-Müller	? Composit. PMMA	10 years	Died early	Died from ischemic heart disease
Martin et al	163	1988	1	66	F	Telengiectatic osteosarcoma	Charnley-Müller	Co/Cr/ Molybdenum, PMMA	10 years		Postoperative infection Hip disarticulation
Ryu et al	222	1987	1	53	M	Undifferentiated sarcoma	?	No cement Alum-oxide ceramic	15 months	11 months	
Arden and Bywaters	9	1978	1	58	?	Fibrosarcoma	McKee-Ferrar	?	2½ years	?	
Van der List et al	254	1988	1	72	F	Malignant epithelioid Hemangioendothelioma	Charnley-Müller	Co/Cr/Mo (Prutasal) PMMA	11 years	?	Three revisions of cemented hip before diagnosis of tumor

transformation, and disturbance of DNA replication can occur in the presence of chromium, cobalt, and nickel.[116,245,246,249]

Among others, Black has expressed concern regarding the lack of data and the use of chromium-cobalt alloys and their potential carcinogenicity at the site of implants and in remote areas.[20]

Gillepsie and co-workers reported on the incidence of tumors at remote sites in patients after total hip arthroplasty in 1358 patients who were followed up to 14,286 person-years after surgery.[102] They found that in the decade after total hip arthroplasty, the incidence of tumor of the lymphatic and hemopoietic systems was significantly higher, but breast, colon, and rectal cancers were less than expected. The association of other factors, such as the use of drug therapy and other factors that might also have affected the findings, could not be evaluated in this study. These authors concluded that "from the viewpoint of both the surgeon and the prospective recipient of the joint replacement, the evidence brought forward from this study should not detract from the potential benefit of joint replacement." It is this author's opinion, based on the data presented, that the prolonged biological effect of total hip arthroplasty cannot be determined based on the currently available data.

From the foregoing, this author has arrived at a conclusion similar to that related by Hamblen and Carter,[111] whose editorial annotation remains accurate in 1991:

> In conclusion we would emphasize that the number of reported cases of sarcoma is so minute, compared with the vast number of replaced hips, that no surgeon or patient should feel undue concern on this account; especially as the short latent period of the three cases described suggests that the malignancy could be coincidental.

TISSUE REACTION TO METALLIC IMPLANTS

Tissue reactions to metallic implants may be classified into four general types: injury, repair, corrosion, and metal particle reactions.

Injury Reaction

Injury reaction occurs at the time of the implantation of metal and includes damage to the bone and soft tissue as the result of drilling, reaming, and so on. This type of reaction naturally involves a local tissue repair reaction, accompanied by phagocytosis in the form of acute and, subsequently, subacute inflammatory cells, as well as osteoclastic activities to remove the necrotic bone.[62]

Repair Reaction

Repair reaction takes place as manifested by the healing of soft tissue and the formation of new bone and the replacement or removal of dead bone. Usually plump, active fibroblasts and macrophages are concentrated in the implant area, which is also rich in capillaries. This phenomenon is characteristically caused by the specialization of immature perivascular mesenchymal cells and monocytes for the removal of dead bone and the formation of new bone. In the initial phase, young fiber bone is formed, and this tissue is gradually converted to mechanically sound lamellar bone. Whether bone or fibrous tissue will be formed in any given situation during the multiphases of repair depends largely on the local properties (physical and chemical) at the site of repair.

Corrosion Reaction

The third type of reaction is corrosion reaction, which is characterized by redux reaction occurring at the interface between the metal (electrode) and the tissue fluids. For example, metals such as cobalt and nickel are mutagenic in cell cultures, while others are inert. The tissue response to metallic corrosion has been described by many authors. There is an electrochemical reaction adjacent to the metals that causes an inflammatory response to corrosion, leading to cell infiltration and fibrous tissue formation about the implant.[134] Bone reaction to this type of corrosion consists of osteolysis and osteoclasis, leading to loosening of the implant and formation of reactive bone in an attempt to encapsulate the implant. This reaction is very similar to that seen in osteomyelitis.

Metal Particle Reaction

Metal particle reaction is the fourth type of reaction. Vitallium (cobalt-chromium-molybdenum alloy) has been recommended because of its electrochemical inertness and its minimal tendency to self-welding.[84] This alloy has been used for internal fixation devices for over 40 years. Although Ferguson has demonstrated an increased concentration of metal ions around the implants,[86] it did not occur with chromium and cobalt in a static situation. When the alloy was used as a bearing joint component, the elements were released, found in the blood stream, and excreted in the urine.[89] It was also demonstrated that these alloy particles would partially dissolve when incubated in horse serum. Although hypersensitivity to cobalt, chrome, and nickel is well documented,[37] Evans and his associates were the first to draw attention to metal toxicity after total hip arthroplasty.[85] McKee and others have reported the cause of early failures of the McKee prosthesis to be a nonspecific inflammatory response in the absence of infection.[168] In analyzing seven patients with failed McKee-Farrar total hip arthroplasties, Jones and associates found that six of these patients were cobalt positive but nickel and chrome negative on skin patch testing.[127] Freeman and others found microscopic histological necrosis of bone, muscle,[92] and joint

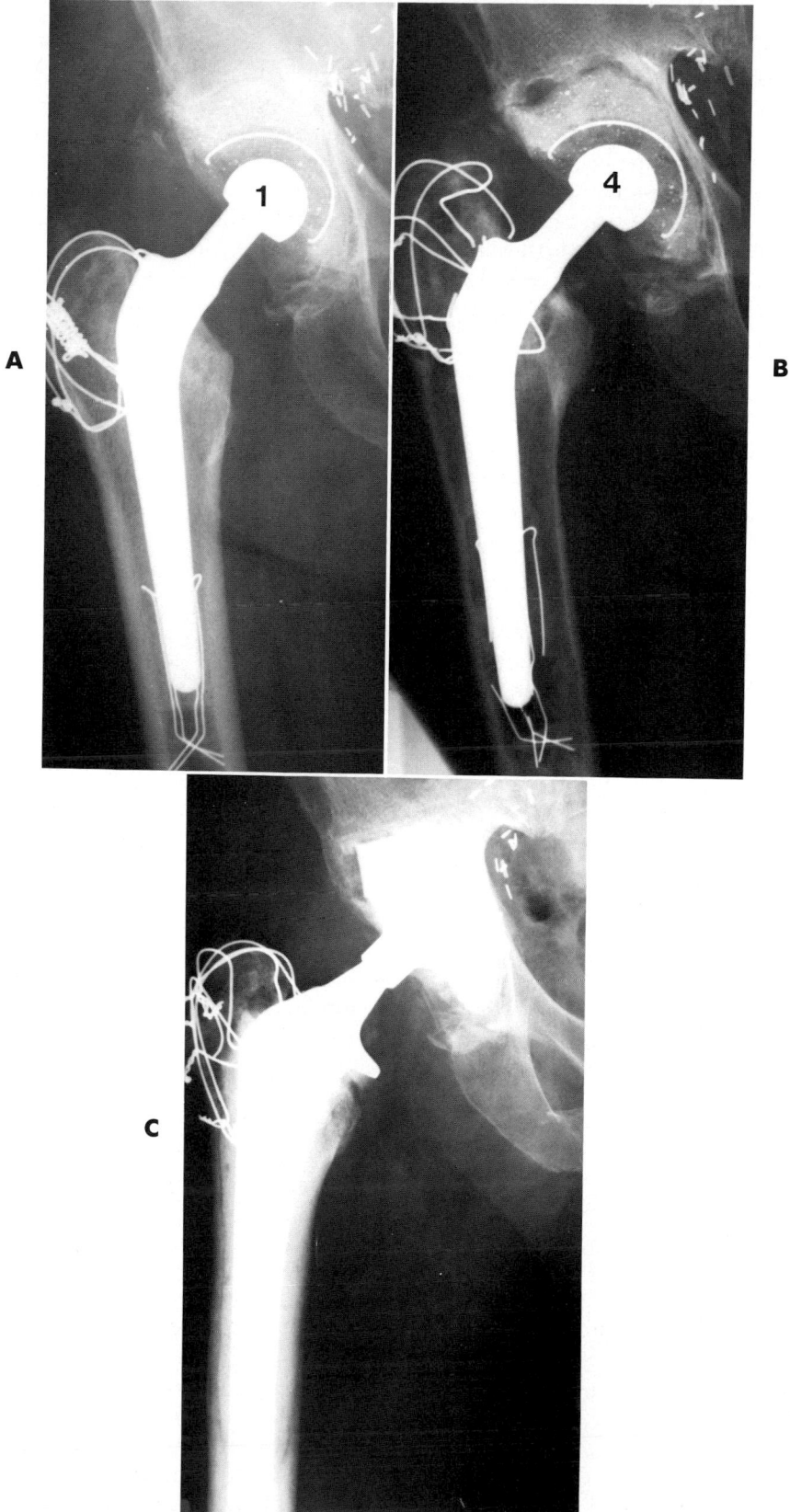

Fig. 4-42. A and **B,** Postoperative radiographs of a 68-year-old man whose all titanium femoral component was adequately fixed as judged by radiographs, **A.** Severe osteolysis and migration of both components are seen. NOTE: large particles of poorly mixed barium sulfate in cement might have initiated wear of the femoral head leading to failure. Severe metallosis was observed at revision surgery. **C,** Postrevision using a long-stem cemented component.

capsule around the prosthesis while exploring five patients' hips.[92] They observed severe bone resorption, pathological fracture of the acetabulum, and loosening or dislocations. They also reported increased cobalt concentrations in the urine and in a variety of tissues.

Reports indicate that Vitallium-alloy prosthetic components (metal against metal) provide excellent wear resistance under operating conditions, with a volumetric wear less than that of metal-to-plastic bearings.[258] But because of high "frictional torque" and the problems of loosening, tissue reaction, and remote accumulation of debris, it is probable that metal-to-metal prostheses will entirely be phased out and replaced by metal against HDP. The most accepted materials, coupled with HDP, are ceramics, chromium-cobalt, and high nitrogen content steel. Galante and Rostoker found that the wear of ultrahigh molecular weight polyethylene in sliding contact with titanium alloy was far greater than that generated by Vitallium alloy.[97-99] At a contact stress of only 238 to 277 psi, the wear rate of titanium was 15×10^{-9} mm/mm as compared with 1×10^{9} mm/mm with Vitallium; at higher contact stresses, wear rate was even greater. Also, the titanium specimens were severely scored after those tests (although contact was only with polyethylene, which became filled with a black powder); it appears that the passive oxide film covering the titanium surface was weakened by the sliding motion of the two materials. Although the conditions of wear testing may have influenced the results, recent work by Galante and Rostoker has shown that the wear resistance of titanium can be considerably improved by appropriately manipulating the passivation layer by either chemical or thermal techniques. However, despite in-vivo experiments concluding that titanium is at least as good as Vitallium (chromium-cobalt alloy) as tested in the laboratory,[100] titanium has not been favored as a bearing material because of abnormal wear in clinical practice (Figs. 4-42 to 4-44).

METALS FOR JOINT REPLACEMENT

Metals used in the body may fail from breakage or corrosion. Attempts to identify problems related to new metals used in orthopaedic surgery have led to a body of knowledge and standards that will continuously be revised on the basis of new studies and findings.* Metals commonly used for manufacturing of load-bearing joints include stainless steel, chromium-cobalt-molybdenum, and titanium alloy.

Stainless Steel

Impurities in stainless steel prostheses may initiate corrosion leading to failure of the implant; they can act as stress concentrators and, along with corrosion, may

cause fatigue fracture.[133] Two often found inclusions are magnesium sulfide and chromium oxide. A standard composition for stainless steel used in surgical implants taken from ASTM standard specifications X138 and F139 is shown in Table 4-8.[73,248] In the United States these standards are set by the F4 Committee on Surgical Implants. The steel used in the United States by manufacturers of implants is known as *AISI-316L*. A similar steel, known as *EN58J*, is used in England; this steel is susceptible to galvanic corrosions, especially in environments such as salt solutions (see Tables 4-8 and 4-9). The experimental (in-vitro) tests using atomic absorption analysis of Ringer's solution in two types of steel, F138 grade 2 (similar to 316L stainless steel) and F562 (MP35N), showed that the release rate of nickel was virtually the same for both types. This is a significant observation since F562 (MP35N) has three times greater nickel content than F138 grade 2 materials.[161]

Chromium Alloys

Just as iron can be made into alloys of steel, cobalt can be made into alloys that will resist corrosion and improve its physical properties (see Tables 3-1 to 3-3).[76,248] This alloy is commonly used as cast material (Austenal Laboratories).* Tissue reaction to long-term implantation of chromium-cobalt-molybdenum (Co-Cr-Mo) is minimal, although it does occur.[58,59,133] Microscopically, the tissue around the implants is generally free of excessive fibrous tissue, and the cellular reaction is usually slightly less than that seen around stainless steel implants. Small black particles have been observed in the phagocytes near Co-Cr-Mo implants, and spectral chemical analysis of adjacent tissue on both animals and plants has revealed ions of all three metals.

Titanium Alloys

Titanium ($Ti^{-6}Al^{-4}Va$) alloys have been used in orthopaedic surgery for cup arthroplasty prosthesis, plate and screws, and other hardware. Table 4-8 shows a standard composition for titanium.[76,248] It has been suggested that the tissue reaction to titanium is minimal in the absence of wear; when wear occurs, rapid oxidation of the particles may be expected with the formation of highly stable titanium salts. Spectral chemical analyses of tissue adjacent to implants have always demonstrated the presence of titanium in the tissues, even without severe tissue reaction. Previous studies have all documented that local biocompatibility of titanium is excellent because its corrosion resistance. A good compatibility is observed in the absence of wear and prosthetic instability.† Several attributes of

---

* References 58, 59, 122, 133, 200, 216, 255, 282.

* Vitallium is a trademark of Howmedica, Inc., Rutherford, NJ.
† References 27, 68, 90, 133, 134, 140.

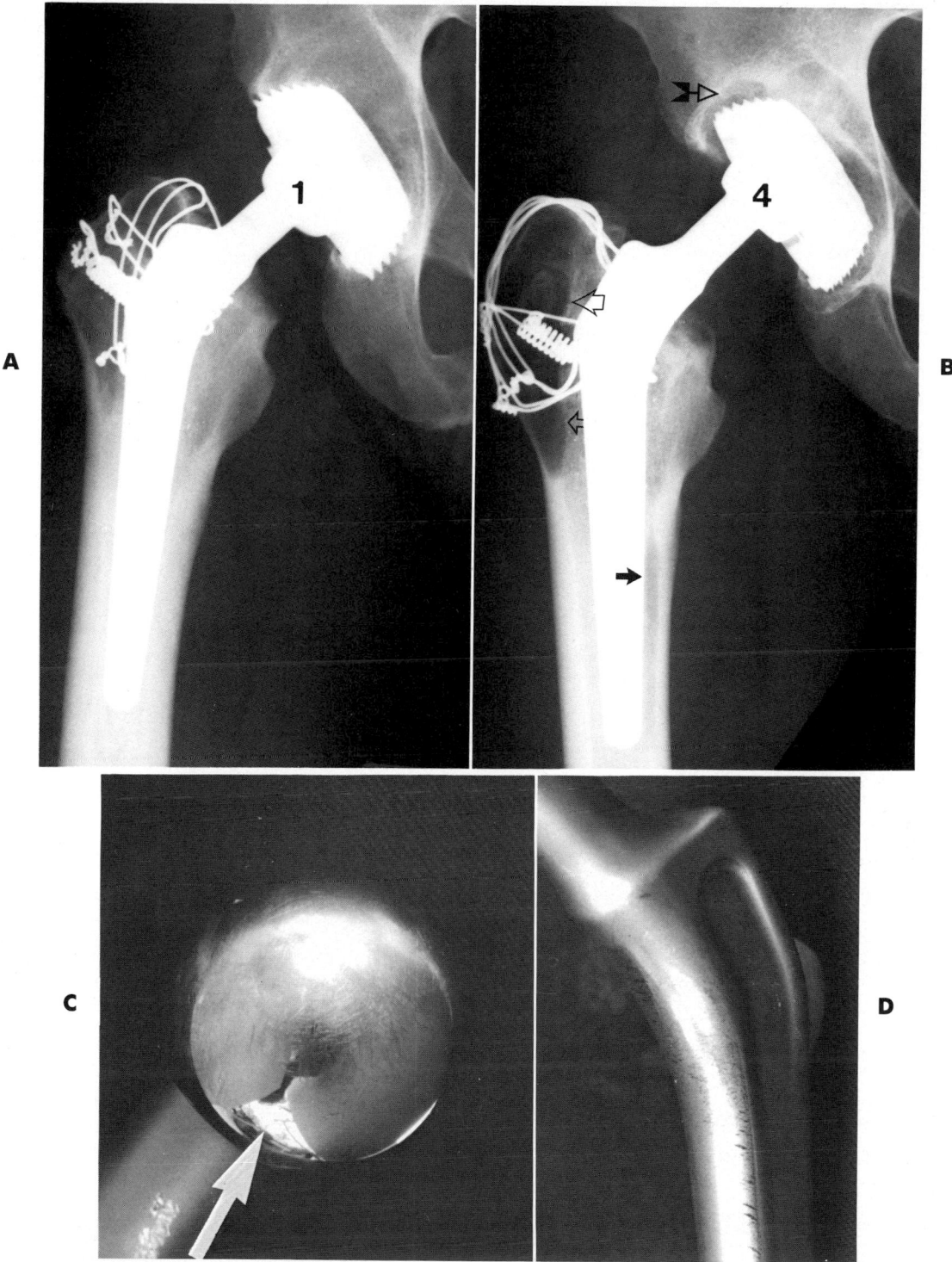

Fig. 4-43. A, One year postoperative radiograph of a 32-year-old athletic male. **B,** Evidence of severe osteolysis about the uncemented mecring cup *(top arrow)* and the cement-bone interface in the femur. At revision surgery, the acetabular component was grossly loose, and osteolysis of the trochanteric region *(hollow arrows)* was striking. Metallosis related to wear of titanium stem and moderate rim wear in the cup were present. **C** and **D,** Explanted stem shows burnishing of the head and many areas of wear along the heavily loaded region of the stem.

Continued.

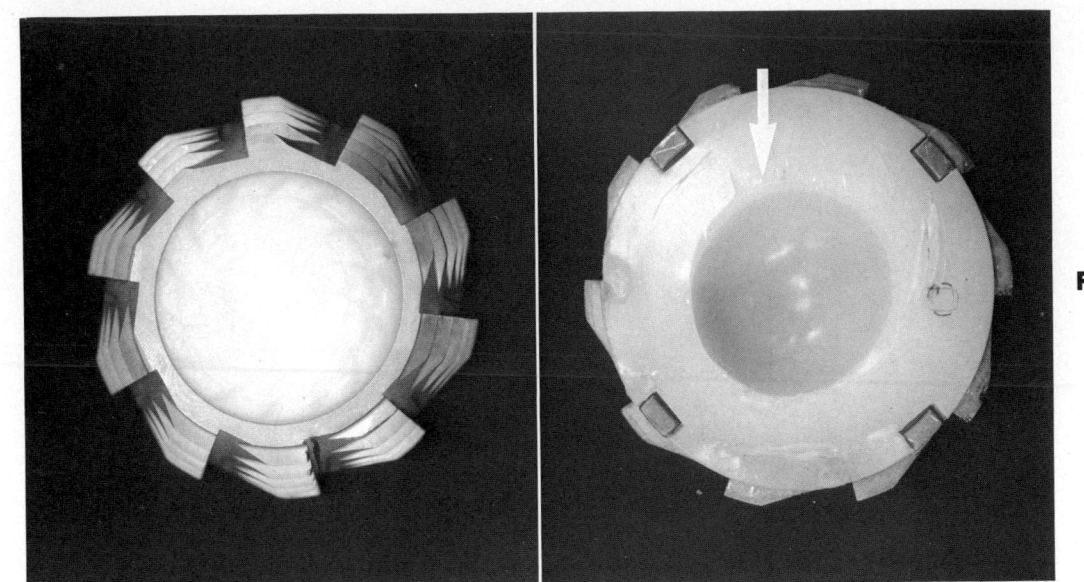

Fig. 4-43—cont'd. E, No evidence of wear can be seen on the convex side of the mecring cup. **F,** Moderate rim wear *(arrow)* and 2 mm linear wear were present.

Table 4-8 Chemical Composition of Commonly Used Metallic Alloys in Total Hip Arthroplasty

Material	Reference	ASTM standard	Trade names or common name	Chemical composition								
				C	Mn	P	S	Si	Cr	Ni	Mo	N
Stainless steel AISI 316	3	F55-grade 1		0.08 m	2 m	0.03 m	0.03 m	0.75 m	17-19 m	12-14 m	2-3 m	0.10 m
Stainless steel AISI 316L	263	F55-grade 2		0.03 m	2 m	0.03 m	0.03 m	0.75 m	17-19 m	12-14 m	2-3 m	0.10 m
Stainless steel	234		Ortron	0.054 m	3.74 m	0.017 m	0.003 m	0.19 m	21.41 m	9.32 m	2.72 m	0.39 m
Co-Cr alloy HS-21	8	F-75	Vitallium Zimalloy Micro-grain alloy	0.35 m	1 m			1 m	27-30 m	1 m	5-7 m	
Co-Cr alloy, wrought	8	F-563	Syntacoben	0.05 m	1 m		0.01 m	0.5 m	18-22 m	15-25 m	3-4 m	
Co-Cr-Ni alloy	8	F-562	MP-35 m	0.025 m	0.15 m	0.015 m	0.01 m	0.15 m	19-21 m	33-37 m	9-10.5 m	
Co-Cr-Fe alloy	183		Elgiloy	0.15 m	2 m				20 m	15 m	7 m	
Ti c.p. commercial purity	8	F-67, grade 1		0.10 m							0.03 m	
Ti-6Al-4V	8	F136,ELI	Tivanium	0.08 m							0.05 m	
Ti-5Al-2.5Fe	8,26			0.08 m							0.05 m	
Ti-6Al-7Nb	225											

From Ducheyne P, Cohen CS: In Steinberg ME, editor: *Reconstructive surgery of the adult hip*, Philadelphia, 1991, WB Saunders.

titanium make it useful in orthopaedic implants, including high resistance to fatigue and high tensile strength, low modulus of elasticity, low density, anticorrosion properties, and especially excellent ductility and biocompatibility.[5,61,131,146] Lintner and associates described the histology of four cementless prostheses made of titanium alloy, noting a direct bone-to-metal contact without interposed connective tissue, which was interpreted as osteointegration.[146] The design of the prosthesis was mainly a press-fit device with ungrooved, nonmesh, nonbeaded surfaces. However, titanium is a highly notch-sensitive metal that also is highly susceptible to wear and thus formation of metal debris leading to osteolysis.[1] McKellop et al showed in in-vitro studies that in contrast to stainless steel and chromium-cobalt alloy, titanium was highly susceptible to abrasive wear by acrylic cement particles in the joint, resulting in scoring of 80% of the prosthetic femoral head and formation of black residue.[169,171] The titanium alloy femoral heads were originally passivated to produce a protective layer by forming an oxide film to resist corrosion. Recently, as a result of new technologies borrowed from the aerospace industry, corrosion and fatigue properties of titanium alloys have improved.[148] In this process, the nitrogen ions are implanted into the surface of the component at a depth of 0.02 to 0.2 μm, which results in a substantial increase in the surface hardness, resulting in improved wear resistance.*

Aseptic Loosening of Titanium Prostheses

Several reports in recent years have documented osteolysis, which was caused by wear debris from titanium alloy. Of special reference in this regard was the wear of femoral heads made of titanium alloys that articulated with high-density polyethylene[1,148] or loose cemented titanium with obvious metal wear.

As stated before, Rostoker and Galante compared titanium alloy with chromium-cobalt alloy with regard to wear against high-density polyethylene. They found titanium alloy produced approximately ten times more wear than chromium-cobalt alloy.[218] Titanium alloy is especially susceptible to abrasive wear caused by particles of PMMA and possibly barium sulfate.[172,248]

The long-term side effects from titanium particles, as well as other metals implanted in the body, are not known, although allergic and hypersensitivity reactions, tissue toxicity, and carcinogenicity are theoretical possibilities. In a study of nine specimens recovered

---

* References 31, 32, 164, 170, 218, 230, 264.

Cu	Fe	Nb	Co	W	Ti	H	O	Al	V	Other each	Other total	BE
0.50 m	B											
0.50m	B											
	B	0.28										
	0.75m		B									
	4-6		B	3-4	0.5 -3.5							
	1m		B		1m							
	B		40									0.40
	0.2m				B	0.0125m	0.18m					
	0.25m				B	0.0125m	0.13m	5.5	3.5			
	2-3				B	0.0125m	0.2m	4.5		0.10	0.40	
		7			B		6					

B, balance; m, maximum.

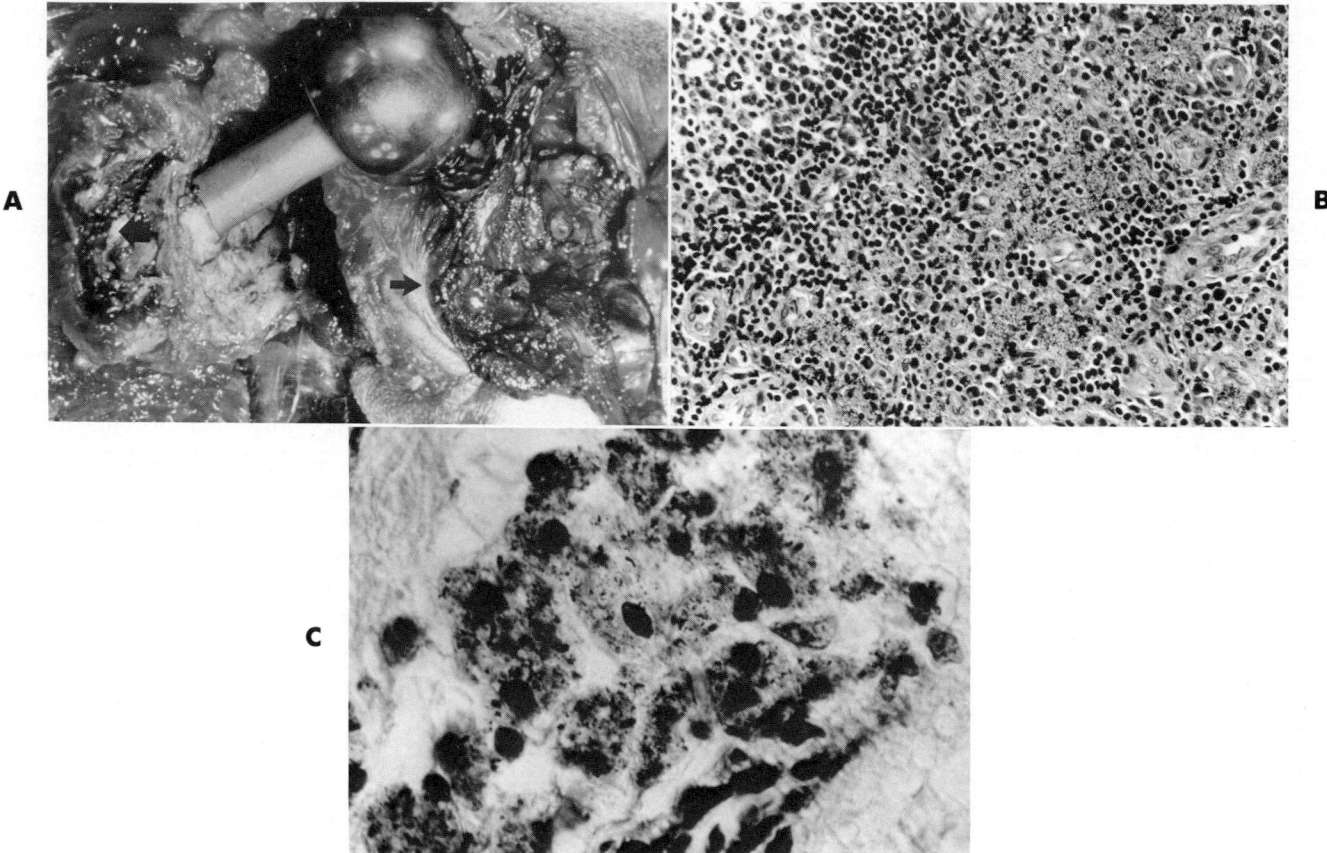

Fig. 4-44. A, Intraoperative photograph obtained at the time of revision surgery of a grossly loose all titanium (head and stem) femoral component. Severe black staining of the tissues is observed around the markedly burnished prosthetic head, under the osteotomized greater trochanter *(right small arrow)* and within the proximal intramedullary canal *(left large arrow).* (Courtesy EA Salvati, MD.) **B,** Photomicrograph showing extensive titanium metallic debris (approximately 1 to 3 μm in size) within the histiocytes. (Hematoxylin-eosin, ×800.) (Courtesy M. Bansal, MD.) **C,** High-power photomicrograph showing particulate titanium metal debris within macrophages in the parafollicular zones of a slightly hyperplastic lymph node. (H & E, ×350.) *G,* Germinal center. (Courtesy EF DiCarlo MD.)

from total hip devices with titanium heads, Agins and associates recovered high volumes of titanium, aluminum, and vanadium from tissue as a result of wear related to the heads or the stem made of titanium alloy.[1] Atomic absorption spectrophotometry revealed titanium values of 56 to 3700 μg/gm of dry tissue (average 1047 μg/gm). The value for normal tissue is 0 μg/gm. The value for aluminum ranged from 2.1 to 396 μg/gm of dry tissue (average 115 μg/gm of dry tissue). The value for aluminum in normal tissue is 0 μg/gm of tissue. For vanadium the values ranged from 2.9 to 220 μg/gm (average 67 μg/gm). The value for normal tissue for vanadium is 1.2 μg/gm.

Histological findings in the Agins study included synovial linings with moderate hypertrophy and histiocytes laden with black, opaque, metallic debris in addition to giant cells containing fragments of high-density polyethylene and diffuse lymphocytic reaction.[1]

The investigators concluded that when a titanium implant fails, copious metallic debris can be generated, which can be noxious to tissue and cause osteolysis and loosening. Black and co-workers have reported metallosis associated with stable (fixed) titanium alloy femoral component.[23] In this case no loosening occurred, and the entire source of metallosis was related to wear of the titanium head.

Metal Levels in Synovial Fluids and Tissue

Well-fixed cemented implants have relatively similar low metal levels. However, when an implant becomes loose, a large amount of metal particles are released that increase the level of metals in the synovial fluid and surrounding tissues.

In a prospective study, comparing a well-fixed chromium-cobalt implant with a loose implant, Brien et al[29] found that there was a seven-fold increase in

Table 4-9 Mechanical Properties of Biomaterials Used in Total Hip Arthroplasty

	Reference	Material	Yield strength (MPa)	Ultimate tensile strength (MPa)	Elongation (%)	Fatigue strength (MPa) ($R = -1$)	Source	Isotropy	Modulus of elasticity (MPa)
Stainless steel	8, 235	AISI 316 or 316L						Isotropic	200,000
	8, 235	Annealed	≥170	≥480	40	190-230	1,67		
		Cold-worked	310-690	655-860	28	530-700	1,67		
	234	Ortron	333 (torsional)	1150	15	583	65		
Cobalt-chromium	8, 183	Vitallium (cast)	≥450	≥655	≥8	245-280	1,48	Isotropic	220,000
		Syntacoben (wrought)							
	8	Annealed	≥276	≥600	≥50	—	1		
		Cold-worked	827-1310	1000-1590	12-18	—	1		
	8, 151	MP35N Annealed	241-448	793-1000	≥50	340	1,41		
	8, 151	Cold-worked	≥1586	≥1793	≥8	405	1,41		
	183	Elgiloy	1900	2500	17	617	48		
	95	PM processed	840	1270	14	725	26		
Titanium alloys	8	Ti cp, grade 1	≥170	≥240	≥24	—	1	Isotropic	107,000
	263	Ti-6Al-4V (a-B worked, annealed)	1000	1100	≥10	670	76	Isotropic	110,000
	263	Ti-6Al-4V (acicular structure)	838	948	12.5	440	76		
	177	Ti-5Al-2.5Fe	820	920	14	580	47		
	225	Ti-6Al-7Nb	900-1000	1000-1100	10-15	500-600	64		
Alumina,	104	Alumina, (single crystal)						Isotropic	362,700
		Alumina, polycrystal						Isotropic	408,900
HDP	192		See Table 4-13					Isotropic	410-1240
PMMA	192		See Chapter 5					Isotropic	3000-10,000

From Ducheyne P, Cohen CS: In Steinberg ME, editor: *Reconstructive surgery of the adult hip,* Philadelphia, 1991, WB Saunders.

metal levels with the loose implant. The difference was even more striking with titanium alloy prostheses. There was a 21-fold increase in metal levels in the loose prosthesis. Significantly, the metal levels as measured in dry tissues (removed at revision surgery) also showed a marked difference between a loose chromium-cobalt and titanium alloy prosthesis. The tissue-metal levels from revised cobalt-chromium implants averaged 45 μg/gm dry tissue weight compared with 4.470 μg dry tissue weight of titanium alloy prosthesis, representing a 100-fold difference. Severe burnishing and scratching of an all titanium alloy femoral head contributed to release of a large amount of metals that are not found in either stainless steel or chromium-cobalt prostheses. Tables 4-10 to 4-12 show

Table 4-10 Synovial Fluid Metal Levels

Metal	Well fixed (n = 11) (μg/L)	Loose (n = 13) (μg/L)
Stainless steel implants		
Cr	6 (1–16)*	17 (1–137)
Ni	7 (0.1–35)	20 (2–162)

Metal	Well fixed (n = 19) (μg/L)	Loose (n = 23) (μg/L)
Cobalt-Chromium Implants		
Co	2 (0.4–6)	21 (0.2–152)
Cr	6 (0.2–16)	19 (0.8–238)
Ni	9 (0.2–34)	12 (0.2–52)

Metal	Well fixed (n = 7) (μg/L)	Loose (n = 8) (μg/L)
Titanium Implants		
Ti	5 (0.1–13)	109 (13–194)
V	ND	0.4 (0.0–2)

From Brien NW et al: Metal levels in cemented total hip arthroplasty. A comparison of well-fixed and bone implants. *Clin Orthop* 275:66, 1992.
*Values are the means. The range is indicated in parentheses.

Table 4-11 Synovial Fluid Mean Total Metal Levels and Ratios

Metal	Well fixed (μg/L)	Loose (μg/L)	Ratio
SS	8*	42	1:5
CoCr	9	65	1:7
Ti-6Al-4V	6	119	1:21

From Brien NW et al: Metal levels in cemented total hip arthroplasty. A comparison of well-fixed and bone implants. *Clin Orthop* 275:66, 1992.
*Values are means.

Table 4-12 Tissue Metal Levels from Revised Hips

	Cobalt-chromium	Titanium
	(μg/g of dry tissue weight)	
Mean value	45	4470
Range	6–248	110–25,000

From Brien NW et al: Metal levels in cemented total hip arthroplasty. A comparison of well-fixed and bone implants. *Clin Orthop* 275:66, 1992.

values related to 37 well-fixed and 44 loose hip arthroplasties.[29] Concentrations of metallic elements in synovial fluid from well-fixed and loose prostheses made of stainless steel, cobalt-chromium, and titanium alloys are shown in Table 4-10. The ratio of levels of various metals in synovial fluid from well-fixed and loose prostheses is shown in Table 4-11. Table 4-12 shows that the total tissue-metal levels were 100 times greater in revised titanium alloy than chromium implants. Betts et al[17a] and Brien et al[29] concluded that the amount of cobalt-alloy metal debris in periarticular tissues from total hip revisions did not show any correlation with histological findings or other demographic variables or with duration of implantation. Also the ratios of individual constituent elements generally reflected the cobalt-chromium alloy composition suggesting that metal debris were present predominantly as wear particles and that low metal content in tissue appeared less important than loose particles of HDP or PMMA in producing response.

Endosteal Erosion in Stable Titanium Prostheses

In a recent study by Maloney and co-workers,[158] 12 of 16 stable cementless total hip arthroplasties were manufactured with titanium alloy (Harris-Galante design) using a porous-coated element for fixation. The authors observed osteolysis despite an excellent fixation of the implant. Two hip arthroplasties required revision, and in a third patient the lesion was biopsied. None of the patients had infection, hypersensitivity, or motion of the implant against bone, and the investigators could not explain localized lysis of the bone. This series of patients with localized bone loss is significant because of a relatively short time since the in-growth prostheses were first used and since their use is advocated for young and active individuals. The nature and implication of this complication need careful observation because of the ever-increasing popularity of the use of cementless devices, especially those made of titanium.

CORROSION OF METALS

As stated before, when two dissimilar metals are electrically coupled, they undergo galvanic corrosion owing to the flow of current stimulated by their differing electrical potentials. This corrosion may also occur when two identical electrodes are in contact with the solutions of different electrolytic composition. The types of metal corrosion occurring in the body include:

1. Uniform corrosion, in which the attack affects the entire surface (which undergoes corrosion).
2. Pitting corrosion, which is indicative of a local attack resulting in the formation of deep and shallow cavities (pits).
3. Intergranular corrosion, which occurs at the metal's grain boundaries and which may be deep and rapid.
4. Cracking, which is usually caused by tensile stresses causing fatigue fracture and exposing the interior of the metal to a corrosive environment; this is common in implants involving fracture fixation.

In general, reactions to metals relate not only to the ionic behavior in a biological situation (the body environment) but also to the size, shape, movement, and other physical parameters of the implant itself.[123]

Corrosion resistance of implants manufactured after 1950 has progressively improved. Historically, many instances of severe corrosion were related to steel components, as documented by removed hardware used for fracture fixation. Often severe corrosion was related to electrolytic reactions resulting from the use of different metals in the older devices, leading to localized metallosis and inflammatory process in the local tissues. This, among other factors, has presumably led to the removal of most orthopaedic devices used for fracture fixation.[60,63] Frank corrosion of three metal-based alloys used for implants—oron-based stainless steel (Ortron 90), cobalt-based alloys, and titanium-based alloys—is extremely rare because the metallurgical process used in the manufacturing of these devices, including surface treatment to resist corrosion, wear, and fatigue. Nevertheless, in animal studies using metals for joint arthroplasty or segmental bone arthroplasty, an elevated chromium and aluminum content in serum, urine, and other tissues, including hair, has been found.*

In a recent editorial, Black enumerated a list of biological effects that may result from the long-term release of metallic element into the recipient tissue.[22] He classified the effects under the main headings of metabolic, bacteriological, immunological, and onco-genic.[236] Black believes that since all metallic implants corrode with time and their active by-products are capable of causing tissue damage, their ultimate human side effects after implantation are not known; he thus urges caution, suggesting steps be taken to

limit risks by minimizing the patient's exposure to corrosive products.[22]

Steps taken to reduce corrosion related to the use of dissimilar metal combination have been controversial because of the lack of adequate basic scientific data. Until recently, the use of dissimilar metals was strongly discouraged. According to Mears, however, with the passive alloys and using the available electrochemical tests, accurate prediction of safe and unsafe combinations of metals is possible.[174] This offers the possibility of combining different metals by selecting an alloy with appropriate mechanical properties while transferring improved corrosion-resistant characteristics of another metal with which it is in contact. For example, by using a titanium-alloy stem and a chromium-cobalt head, a surgeon can achieve a satisfactory combination for a femoral component prosthesis. Various in-vitro laboratory tests, including electrochemical tests, have shown evidence that titanium in combination with dissimilar alloys appears to be compatible with chromium-cobalt alloys.[152,220,227] Long-term in-vitro tests and examination of retrieved specimens of prostheses made of titanium and chromium-cobalt heads have not shown any evidence of corrosion effect resulting from this combination. However, in clinical practice and from retrieved human specimens, corrosion at the site of dissimilar metals has been observed.

It is essential to recognize, however, that indiscriminate use of combined metals may lead to catastrophic corrosion. In an in-vitro compatibility test to determine the possibility of galvanic corrosion effect, Kummer and Rose tested cobalt-chromium alloy with either titanium alloy or stainless steel.[131] Results demonstrated that the chromium-cobalt alloy should not be used in combination with steel but can be used with titanium alloy.

METAL TOXICITY AND SENSITIVITY

Cellular toxicity from various metals is well established. In-vitro studies by Rae using culture of human synovial fibroblasts and three metals commonly used for total joint arthroplasty (chromium-cobalt, titanium, and stainless steel) demonstrated the cytotoxic level of each metal. The most potentially harmful components were those of cobalt-chromium alloy, nickel from stainless steel, and vanadium from titanium alloy. Rae suggested that under clinical conditions, chromium-cobalt alloy articulating against itself could produce an unacceptably high level of cobalt in the tissue. In-vivo, long-term effects of intraarticular cobalt-chromium alloy wear particles in rats demonstrated the cobalt-chromium particles and their associated macrophages persisted in the tissues for up to 2 years.[202] This is relevant in view of the use of chromium-cobalt alloy in cementless hips, since large numbers of macrophages and particles of this metal are present around the loose cementless hips[33] or where metallic wear acceleration is caused by abnormal operational conditions[213] such as entrapped wire within the total hip articulation with severe wear of the prosthetic femoral head.

The issue of metal sensitivity related to total hip arthroplasty surfaced after reports that metal-to-metal (McKee-Farrar) prostheses were capable of producing wear particles of chromium and cobalt in solution[249] and further discovery of metal traces of chromium and cobalt in the blood and urine[60] along with high local tissue concentration around these prostheses.[85] Evans and colleagues noted a high level of skin sensitivity in patients whose prostheses became loose, suggesting that metal sensitivity might be responsible for bone necrosis leading to loosening and failure of the implant.[85] Others have reported skin eruptions and eczema associated with metal sensitivity that were cured after removal of the implant.[173] The true incidence of metal sensitivity in patients after total hip arthroplasty remains unknown.

Several aspects of metal sensitivity must be considered:

1. Chromium, cobalt, and nickel are considered haptens and are capable of binding with proteins to form immunogenic complexes; 10% of nonimplant patients are sensitive to these metals.[93] A higher level of sensitivity has been detected in patients with orthopaedic implants using sensitive in-vitro cell inhibition migration tests.[178] The clinical relevance to the prosthetic joint of these observations remains unclear because of the lack of controlled prospective studies regarding acquisition of sensitivity after total joint arthroplasty.

2. With metal-to-metal chromium-cobalt alloy prostheses, there seems to be a unique correlation between wear by-products and loosening, both of which seem to increase the incidence of allergic reaction as manifested by skin sensitivity. For example, in those patients metal sensitivity has been reported as high as 74%[85] and 46%.[184]

3. Patients with repeated metal insertions (revision surgery) and loosening of metal to bone carry a higher incidence of metal sensitivity than the normal population or those with well-fixed metal-to-plastic devices.[66,159]

4. Patients appear to experience no increased sensitivity after metal-to-polyethylene replacements, and there appears to be no direct causal relationship between metal sensitivity and subsequent loosening in such patients after the use of such implants over three decades.

   It is possible that sensitivity occurs after loosening rather than before it. I agree with Rooker and Wilkinson that routine patch testing is not indicated in patients undergoing a metal-on-plastic total hip joint arthroplasty.[214] In a study of 54 (of 69) patients, total hip arthroplasty sensitivity tests were done before and after surgery. Six patients were metal-sensitive before surgery; only one remained so after surgery. Because of a history of metal sensitivity, this patient had a titanium prosthesis. All the other cases with a positive sensitivity test had good operative results without loosening. The preoperative patch test results, conducted by Benson and co-workers, were also similar to those of the normal population.[17]

5. A patch test (under the care of a dermatologist) is a good policy for patients who worry about metal sensitivity; this can be reassuring and yet might not relieve anxiety. The surgeon should not deny the patient a total hip arthroplasty because of a history of metal sensitivity because 10% of all female patients have a history of nickel sensitivity.

6. The interpretation of patch tests is not always easy, but a false positive reaction is rare. Erythema alone should not be taken as a sign of sensitivity. Significant sensitivity and any reaction occurring as part of an "angry back" can be misleading. The site and timing of the patch must also be considered.[87,88] Reactions are commonly graded as negative; minus (negative); erythema only; ± doubtful reaction; erythema and induration (positive); erythema, induration, and vesiculation (strongly positive reaction); severe induration with vesiculation or bullae formation ($+++$ very strong reaction).[87,88]

Patients undergoing total hip arthroplasty are commonly tested for the allergens listed in the following box as suggested and used by Rooker and Wilkinson.[214]

WEAR IN ARTIFICIAL JOINTS
Wear of Metals and Plastics

UHMWPE (ultrahigh molecular weight polyethylene) may be considered a serious obstacle in longevity of total hip arthroplasty. Although more wear-resistant plastics are currently being tested, ceramic balls against UHMWPE, based on the laboratory studies, are superior to other metal-to-plastic combinations (Fig. 4-45). By analyzing metal release, rates, and other results of metal-to-UHMWPE wear tests, it is now clear that in addition to the plastic, metals also wear with time. It has been demonstrated that cobalt-chromium-molybdenum alloy is more resistant to wear than stainless steel or titanium alloy. Davidson[6] demonstrated that the wear of chromium-cobalt-molybdenum alloy was 0.1 μm per year (10[6] cycles), while stainless steel (316L) was on the order of 0.2 μm per year, and tita-

---

Commonly Tested Allergens

Standard Patch Test Series
Allergens with special relevance to hip arthroplasty
   Potassium dichromate 0.5% pet*
   Cobalt chloride 1% pet
   Nickel sulfate 5% pet
   Dimethylparatoluidine 2% pet
   Hydroquinone 1% pet
   Benzoyl peroxide 5% pet
   MMA 5% pet

Intradermal Tests
   Nickel sulfate 0.025% and 0.01%
   Cobalt chloride 0.01%
   Potassium dichromate 0.05%
   Sterile saline (control)

---

*From Rooker GD, Wilkinson JD: Metal sensitivity in patients undergoing hip replacement. A prospective study. *J Bone Joint Surg* 62[Br]:502, 1980.

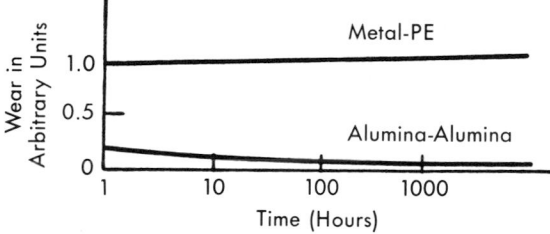

Fig. 4-45. Wear rates for alumina sliding against alumina and polyethylene. (From Dörre E, Beutler H, Geduldig D: *Arch Orthop Unfall-Chir* 82:269, 1975.)

nium is on the order of 1.0 μm per year. Significantly, surface hardening by nitrogen ion implantation was expected to give only a temporary resistance to the surface wear process as ceramic surfaces (AL203, aluminum 203 or ZRO02, zirconium 02) maintained their surface finish and thus minimized the wear of UHM-WPE wear significantly.[6] The long-term clinical results of ceramics are awaited as the improved ceramics have been in limited use during the past 5 or 6 years.

Teflon

Extensive surgical experience with Teflon has shown that this material is chemically inert; it was greatly surprising to find, however, that severe bone absorption and destruction resulted when it was used for sockets in total hip arthroplasty. Most of 344 Teflon sockets inserted from 1958 to 1962 had to be revised 2 to 3 years after surgery, not because of excessive wear but because of severe bone damage (acetabulum, calcar of femur, and trochanteric region).[46] On examining failed Teflon total hips, a porridge-like material was often observed. Cavities were often created at the interface between bone and cement, as if the wear products had been pumped into the osseous tissue, thus producing mechanical erosion. Charnley observed that, once the source of granulating Teflon particles was eliminated, the destructive process stopped (as evidenced by the presence of inspissated calcific Teflon granuloma). The mechanical erosion in the acetabulum (caused by Teflon) was also frequently observed in the upper femur when the stem had become loose, allowing entry of debris into clefts formed between the cement and bone. Teflon reactions were usually typified by multinucleated giant cells (often more than 100 nuclei), often within the vicinity of relatively large birefringent particles. Iliac and aortic lymph nodes, as one might anticipate, contained giant cells and plastic material, but it is of special interest that, strangely enough, particles of Teflon within the lymph nodes were not birefringent.[46]

High-Density Polyethylene
Wear vs Molecular Weight

It is essential to recognize that *polyethylene* is a generic term referring to a large group of materials that may have similar nominal chemical compositions with different properties because of different structural makeups. Furthermore, the resin used to mold the polyethylene may have varied mechanical and structural properties that may influence the mechanical properties of HDP polyethylene used for bearing. Notwithstanding, the molding process may produce variables because of changes in its density, oxidation, and mechanical deformation. For example, formation of voids resulting from incomplete fusion of the resin granules may influence its mechanical deformability. Among other variables that influence the structural and mechanical properties of polyethylene, the method of sterilization, such as radiation, may lead to degra-

Table 4-13 Mechanical Properties of UHMWPE

Property	Number of samples	Mean value (MPa) ± standard deviation*	Test method
Tensile yield	27	20.0 ± 0.49	ASTM D638
Tensile modulus	27	602 ± 36	Type IV bar 50.8 mm minutes^{-1}
Compressive yield (1.0% offset)	5	14.7 ± 0.76	ASTM D695
Compressive modulus	5	590 ± 50	1.27 mm minutes^{-1}
Flexural stress at 2% strain	11	13.3 ± 0.30	Method II, procedure B, 25.4 mm minutes^{-1}
Flexural modulus	11	656 ± 15	
Endurance limit	10	15.8	5×10^6 cycles R = 0.2 notched specimens (median value of maximum likelihood linear regression fit of the data, assuming a normal distribution)

Data from Fahrling GM, Greer K: In Hastings GW, William DF, editors: *Mechanical properties of biomaterials,* New York, 1980, John Wiley & Sons.

Table 4-14 Wear of Conventional Polyethylene Against Various Alloys

Counterface material	Maximum test duration (10^6 cycles)	Load and cycling rate	Coefficient of friction	Wear mm³/10⁶ cycles, average and range	μm/year
316 stainless steel	3.7	445 N 100/min	0.03–0.09	0.20 ± 15%	0.7
MP 35 N	3.0		0.04–0.10	0.13 ± 13%	0.4
Titanium 6–4	4.1		0.05–0.121	0.08 ± 50%	0.03
Nitrided titanium 6–4	3.3		0.07–0.11	0.27 ± 4%	0.9
316 stainless steel	3.7	223 N 60/min	0.03–0.15	0.12 ± 17%	0.4
Forged cobalt-chrome	2.1		0.03–0.16	0.18 ± 28%	0.6
Hot-pressed cobalt-chrome	3.3		0.05–0.15	0.14 ± 37%	0.5

From McKellop H et al: Friction and wear properties of polymer, metal and ceramic prosthetic joint materials evaluated on a multichannel screening device, *J Biomed Mater Res* 15:619, 1981.

Table 4-15 Wear of Alternate Polymers

Polymer	Counterface material	Coefficient of friction	Wear mm³/10⁶ cycles, average and range	μm/year	Ratio to extruded UHMWPE
Tested at 223-N axial load, 60 cycles/min					
Compression-molded UHMWPE	Stainless steel 316	0.05–0.12	0.11 ± 27%	0.4	1.0
Carbon fiber-polyethylene	Stainless steel 316	0.05–0.18		0.9–3.7	2.6–10.3
Composite	Cobalt-chromium			2.8	7.8
	Nitrided titanium 6–4			1.0	2.7
Polyacetal homopolymer (Delrin 150)	Stainless steel 316	0.15–0.23	3.7 ± 10%	12.1	34
Tested at 445-N axial load, 100 cycles/min, maximum duration, 3.2 million cycles					
Carbon-filter–polyethylene composite	Stainless steel 316	0.05–0.13	0.35 ± 9%	1.1	1.8

From McKellop H, Clarke I, Markolf K, et al: Friction and wear properties of polymer, metal and ceramic prosthetic joint materials evaluated on a multichannel screening device, *J Biomed Mater Res* 15:619, 1981.

Table 4-16 Ultimate Strength of Different Porous Materials and Ratio of Ultimate Strength to Strength of Fully Dense Parent Material

Material	Density (%)	Ultimate strength (MN m^{-2})	Ratio of ultimate strength (%)
Annealed stainless steel	50	100	18
AISI 316L, 50 μm fibers	65–70	200–230	35–40
Titanium, 250 μm fibers	50	30	8
Cast cobalt-chromium alloy powder	70	120	17
Alumina	50	42	12
	70	70	21
Titanium, VMC	50	172	15.6

From Rostoker W et al: Some mechanical properties of sintered fiber metal composites, *J Test Evaluation* 2:107, 1974.

Table 4-17 Some Typical Mechanical Properties of Porous Materials

Material	Density (%)	Pore size (μm)	Test method	UTS (MPa)	E (MPa)	References
Alumina, 96% pure	40	100–750	Compression	56	Not reported	42
HDP	Not reported	120	Tension	3.5–4.7	Not reported	62
Polysulfone	54–66	56–386	Tension	2.8–5.9	220–406	70
Co-Cr-Mo beads	65–70	~50	Tension	Not determined	101,000	54
Titanium, 250 μm fibers	50	200–400	Tension	25	Not reported	59

From Ducheyne P, Cohen CS: In Steinberg ME, editor: *Reconstructive surgery of the adult hip,* Philadelphia, 1991, WB Saunders.

dation and cross-linking.[189] Therefore polyethylene, which has proven to be an excellent industrial wear-resistant material, is structurally extremely sensitive to physical changes that may influence its wear characteristics.[64] The mechanical properties of UHMWPE are listed in Tables 4-13 to 4-17.

Dimensional Changes in Molecular Weight and Wear

In-vitro tests of HDP concluded that the true wear rate of HDP ranged from 0.3 to 10.2 mg of debris per year, which accounted for only small fractions from 1% to 30% of the dimensional changes that occurred in specimens.[217] Rose and associates concluded that most of the changes previously attributed to wear were, in fact, caused by creep or plastic flow. As a corollary, the clinical roentgenographic changes in patients are mostly dimensional changes observed by x-ray film.[217] This indicates that regarding the great discrepancy between the actual wear and dimensional changes of the socket, the former is far more significant because of tissue reaction resulting from polyethylene debris. The fact that some prostheses in the Rose study[217] were more than 30 times faster than the others was caused by the low molecular weights of polymer at the articulating face of the prosthesis. The prosthesis with the highest molecular weight had a negligible wear rate. Laboratory wear studies show considerable variation in wear of HDP based on the type of metal used or conditions of testing (see Fig. 4-9 and Tables 4-18 and 4-19). Direct in-vivo measurements by x-ray film of HDP wear in total hip arthroplasty and those of in-vitro studies suggest that the wear of polyethylene depends on structural variability of the HDP and especially on its molecular weight distribution.[215] Indeed, a relatively high rate of wear can occur (based on early experience with total hip arthroplasty using low molecular weight polyethylene) in the absence of acrylic

Table 4-18 Wear of Conventional Polyethylene Against Stainless Steel AISI 316L

Maximum test duration (10^6 cycles)	Polymer irradiation (Mrad)	Load (N)	Cycling rate (cycles/min)	Coefficient of friction	Wear mm^3/10^6 cycles, average and range	μm/yr
2.8	2.5	223	100	0.06–0.16	0.10 ± 20%	0.3
3.6	2.5	445	100	0.03–0.09	0.20 ± 15%	0.7
3.7	2.5	223	60	0.06–0.10	0.12 ± 17%	0.4
3.7	2.5	445	60	0.03–0.09	0.13 ± 38%	0.4
2.1	None	223	60	0.04–0.06	0.01 ± 82%	0.03
1.8	None	445	60	0.06–0.09	0.06 ± 27%	0.2

From McKellop H et al: Friction and wear properties of polymer, metal and ceramic prosthetic joint materials evaluated on a multichannel screening device, *J Biomed Mater Res* 15:619, 1981.

Table 4-19 Wear Rate of UHMWPE Acetabular Cup in Combination with Various Metal Hip Stems, as Measured in a Hip Simulator Test

Prosthesis type	Wear rate (mm/yr)	Friction coefficient
Charnley	0.15	0.05
McKee-Farrar	0.013	0.14
Charnley-Müller	0.08	0.07

From Weightman BO, et al: A comparative study of total hip replacement prostheses, *J Biomech* 6:299, 1973.

debris, since the latter has been frequently cited to cause rapid wear. It is hoped that with proper control of the molecular weight of the HDP a point may be reached where realistically, the wear approximates a negligible level.

Characteristics of HDP Wear In-Vivo

Wear of HDP in the body appears to be more rapid than in the laboratory.[47,50,73] Using optical and electronmicroscopy of Charnley low-friction cups removed post-mortem showed that sockets were worn on the superior portion in the direction of load and according to the orientation of the cup. Similar to Charnley and Kamangar's observation of the wear of Teflon cups, the socket had worn by a "boring-in effect" that could easily be recognized by direct examination of specimens. Electronmicroscopy studies showed that cups were worn predominantly by the mechanism of "adhesion"; however after 8 years the appearance of cracks suggested a surface fatigue as well. Such appearance did not explain the high clinical rate of wear. Based on specimens tested by Dowling and associates it was recognized that UHMWPE appeared to undergo several processes in the body up to 14 years as follows:[73]

1. The first period is the "bed-in" or running period;

the period at which machine marking and surface irregularities are removed by an abrasive process.
2. After use in the body, the high-wear area (superior half of the cup) becomes smooth and polished, presumably from adhesive wear.
3. The inferior (unloaded) portion of the cup often retains its original machine marks resulting from abrasive features of machining.
4. After 7 to 8 years of use in the body, the high-wear area (superiorly) shows creation of a new socket "worn out area" that is separated by a ridge from the low-wear area.
5. With further use (at 8 to 9 years), evidence of fine cracks and spall marks and adhesive wear appears at the site of the high-wear area, suggesting fatigue of the surface of the UHMWPE. Also with advanced states of wear, creeping takes place, which results in "cold flow" of plastic material in a direction away from the high-stress area to a low-stress zone of the cup. This explanation also seems to be in agreement with Rose and others that most postoperative findings of previously published wear studies were caused in part by creep and plastic flow and were not true wear.[215]

In summary, there appear to be several and perhaps combined mechanisms for wear of high-density polyethylene in human hip joints. These include abrasive wear, fatigue wear, possibility of a corrosion factor,[252] "third body" abrasive wear, and fretting fatigue.[119]

With longer follow up, the wear of HDP has increasingly become a concern, since a direct relationship exists between the wear of HDP and loosening of the acetabular component[280] (Table 4-20).

Charnley reported an increasing rate of migration of the socket after 12 to 15 years. Although similar to other observations, neither radiolucency nor migration necessarily caused clinical failure.

Several investigators have suggested that granulomatous tissue (giant cell foreign body reactions), not

Table 4-20 Correlation between Depth of Socket Wear and the Incidence of Socket Migration*

Wear (mm)	0	1	2	3	4	5	6
Cases (No.)	13	37	20	16	11	6	1
Sockets migrating (No.)	0	0	1	2	4	3	1
Cases of socket migration (%)	0	0	5	12.5	36	50	100

From Wroblewski BM: *Revision surgery in total hip arthroplasty,* New York, 1990, Springer-Verlag.

*Patients were under the age of 40 years at the time of surgery with average follow up 9.3 years.

the dimensional changes of the socket, causes socket loosening. Wear of HDP in the biological environment and in joint replacement surgery is complex. However, ingress of acrylic cement, causing a third body wear, has been implemented as the cause of excess wear. In this case, the highly polished femoral prosthetic head is damaged, leading to acceleration of wear. A good correlation between the wear measured by good-quality postoperative radiographs and the wear measured from actually retrieved specimens has been established. It has not been established that dimensional changes of the socket as a result of wear also cause neck-socket impingement, which in turn, causes loosening of the acetabular component. However, if a socket has bottomed in and there is direct contact between the outer diameter of the cup and bone, the external wear can cause a large amount of debris, resulting in severe bone lysis.

The possibility of the effects of high molecular weight polyethylene (HMWP) wear debris and their transport to the lymph nodes (iliac and aortic) remains unknown. However, along with other concerns the long-term effect of these changes in young patients cannot be completely dismissed.

Clinical Wear Studies

CHARNLEY (WRIGHTINGTON HOSPITAL) Charnley's interest regarding wear of high-density polyethylene was intensified based on his observations of the failure of Teflon because of wear. Three reports from Wrightington by Charnley and collaborators included the following:

1. Wear studies related to the 9 to 10 years after operation.[50]
2. Repeat of the same studies as in 1, but with improved techniques of measurement and average follow up of 10 years.[52]
3. Study of a separate group of 491 low-friction arthroplasties with a follow-up period of 8.3 years. Based on this research, Charnley arrived at the following conclusions:

a. A lack of correlation was found between weight and physical activity.
b. Considerable variation in wear was observed in young patients and was also associated with socket demarcation.
c. Male patients were more at risk for wear than female patients, except for Category A patients, (those with unilateral hip disease and no other disability) averaging 43 years of age.
d. A variation of wear by 50% was documented by Charnley and associates comparing two studies of the same unit of the same patients, which was attributed to possible difference in technique of wear measurements.
e. By plotting the average wear for a whole series year by year, the rate of wear after 5 years diminished, falling by 44.4%.
f. Prediction of the pattern of wear rate in a "high-wear group" was not possible; many hips showed rapid wear of 0.5 to 1 mm during the first 3 years, which slowed to stay within the medial range for rate of wear of no more than 2.5 mm after 9 to 10 years.
g. Because of the lack of data, it was not possible to determine the rate of wear in active and very young patients under 30 or even under 50 years of age. Nonetheless, a cautious attitude in selection of patients seemed advisable in this regard.[47]

WROBLEWSKI (WRIGHTINGTON HOSPITAL) As stated previously, in a study of 22 high-density polyethylene hip sockets of Charnley low-friction arthroplasty measured for wear (by acrylic case and shadow graph techniques), direct measurement showed a significant correlation with wear measurement by x-ray film. From this observation, similar to Charnley's, one can deduce that radiographic methods of wear measurement are reliable providing that each reading is corrected for x-ray magnification and that the femoral head size is known. The average rate of wear was 0.19 mm/year with a range of 0.52 mm/year to 0.017 mm/year for the 22.5 mm Charnley femoral head made of steel.

WEAR IN PATIENTS WITH 10- TO 20-YEAR FOLLOW UP Isaac and others[279] in a tribological study of 78 retrieved Charnley cemented cups found loosening the most common cause of failure. The examination of these cups showed six categories of damage: (1) socket erosion, (2) rim wear, (3) cement ingress, (4) cratering, (5) discoloration, and (6) articular surface scoring (Fig. 4-46). Frequent damage to the femoral stem was either caused by stem fracture of early stem design or roughening of the femoral head caused by Ba 504 used in the cement for radiographic contrast (Fig. 4-47). Fig.

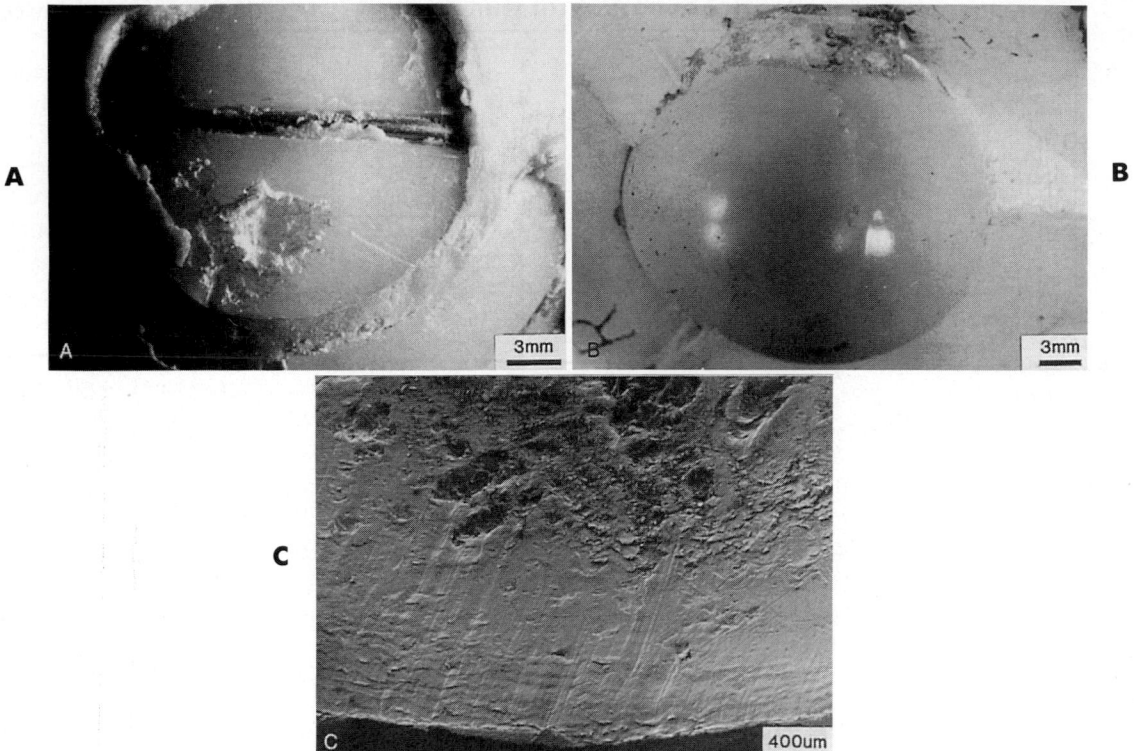

Fig. 4-46. Acetabular damage. **A,** Socket erosion showing the area of damage and the interrupted cement layer caused by bottoming out. **B,** Rim wear showing the damage to the rim of the acetabular cup. Cement ingress showing particles of acrylic cement on the articulating surface. **C,** Cratering showing a typical area of damage *(top)*. Scoring showing debris tracks running verticaly from the rim of the socket *(bottom)*. (From Isaacs GH et al: *Clin Orthop* 276:115, 1992

4-47 shows a graphic representation of the surface profile of the measured femoral heads causing an abnormally high wear rate. The amount of wear (the mean penetration) was 1.69 mm, and the mean penetration rate was 0.21 per year (range from less than 0.0005 mm to 0.6 mm per year) (Fig. 4-48). Similar to Wroblewski and Charnley's studies from Wrightington, a high penetration rate of the femoral head may be a major factor in limiting the life of the total hip arthroplasty. Fig. 4-49 demonstrates a positive correlation between penetration of the femoral head and the incidence of rim wear. Fig. 4-50 illustrates an inverse ratio between the penetration and the "service life" of the socket. Table 4-21 represents the longest series of wear studies in implants in hip joints in man (to date) from Wrightington Hospital Centre for Hip Surgery.[125] Fig. 4-46 shows typical socket wear related to socket erosion by cement, rim wear, and scoring caused by debris in the socket.

Unusual Wear of High-Density Polyethylene

Unusual and often catastrophic wear of HDP can cause severe tissue reaction after production of a large amount of debris requiring reoperation (Figs. 4-51 to 4-53). Histologically, Teflon cups (double cup) used by Charnley[42] produced such a large amount of caseating material that they had to be abandoned; the material was unsuitable for the design of the joint. Plastic surfaces that come in contact with osseous tissue may also generate a large amount of debris. A similar in-vivo study in dogs of HDP fixed by PMMA produced a similar tissue reaction with severe destruction caused by abraded HDP fragments.[176a] The large volume of HDP particles in total knee arthroplasty and wear from certain femoral endoprosthetic devices and total hip arthroplasties, in addition to patellar wear, are all from an unusual type of wear related to the mechanical failure of the devices, making revisionary surgery extremely difficult. Surgeons must consider direct wear of HDP against bone as a potential hazard that can be extremely and progressively destructive.

Effects of Radiation on High-Density Polyethylene

Dumbleton and Shen[77] and Dumbleton, Shen, and Miller[78] have suggested that a transfer film formed in nonradiated HDP favorably protected the surface of the material from continuous wear. However, the protec-

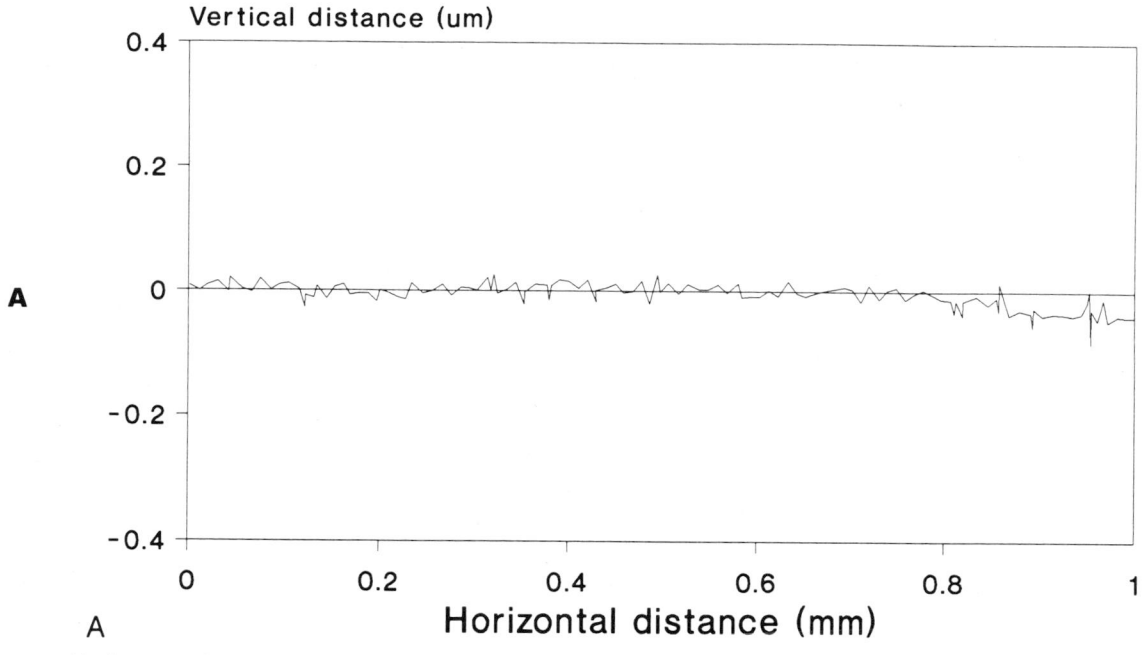

A

Undamaged, unused femoral head

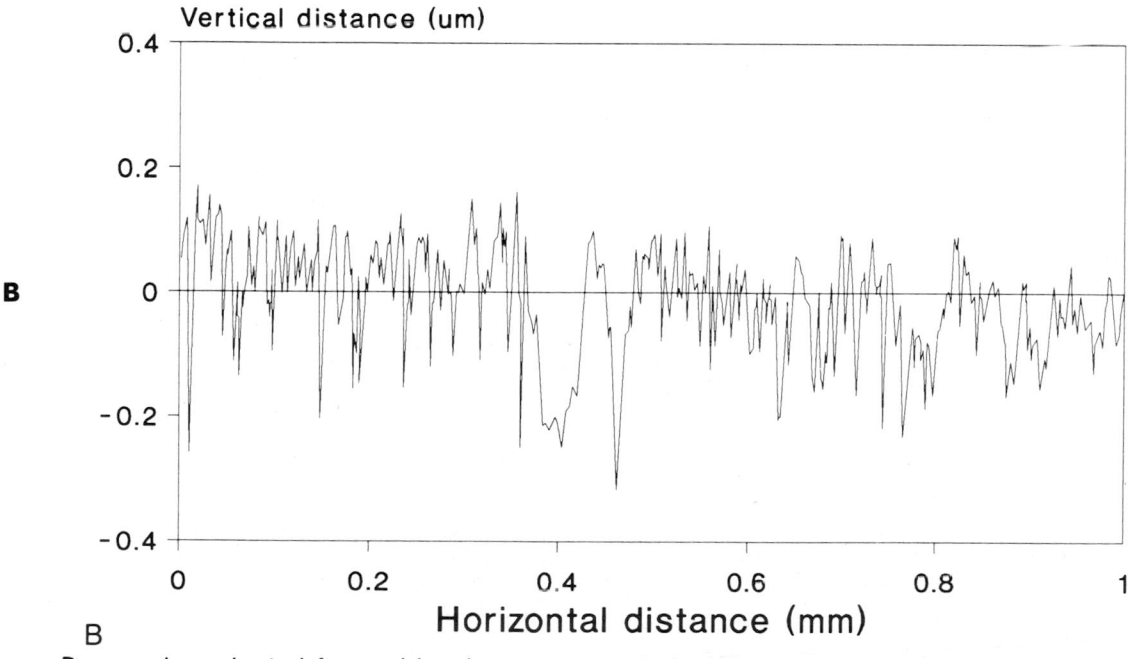

B

Damaged, explanted femoral head

Fig. 4-47. Graphic representation of surface profile of femoral heads as measured by Rotary Talysurf. **A,** Unused and thus undamaged specimen. **B,** In contrast, an explanted specimen showing an obvious increase in surface roughness. (From Isaacs GH et al: *Clin Orthop* 276:115, 1992.)

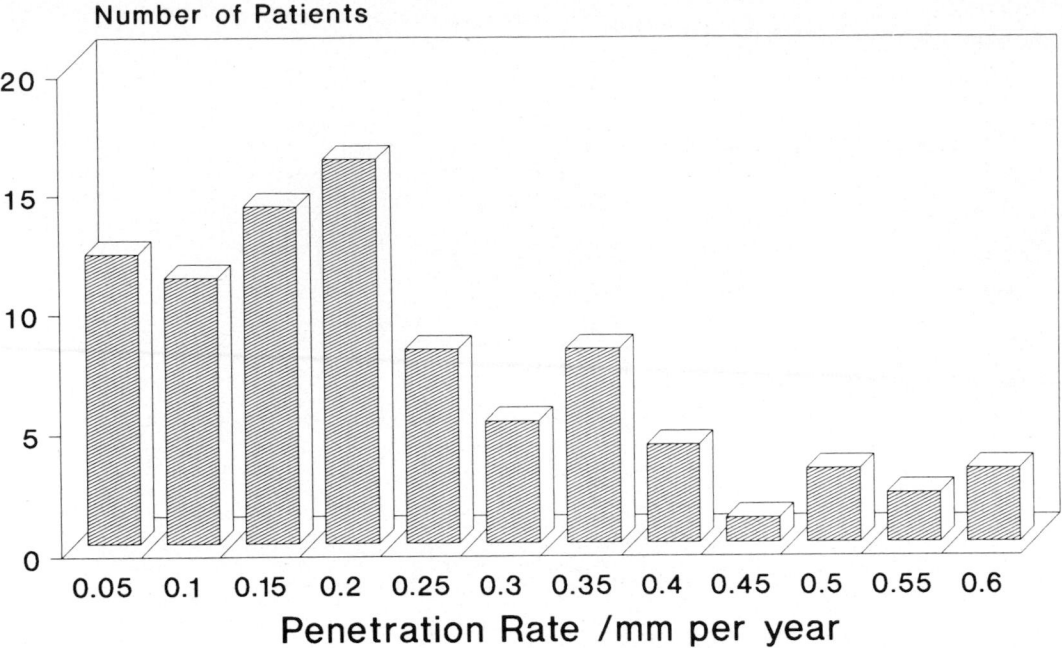

Fig. 4-48. Histogram of penetration rates demonstrating skewed distribution, with some cups exhibiting extremely high penetration rates. (From Isaacs GH et al: A tribiological study of retrieved hip prostheses, *Clin Orthop* 276:115, 1992.)

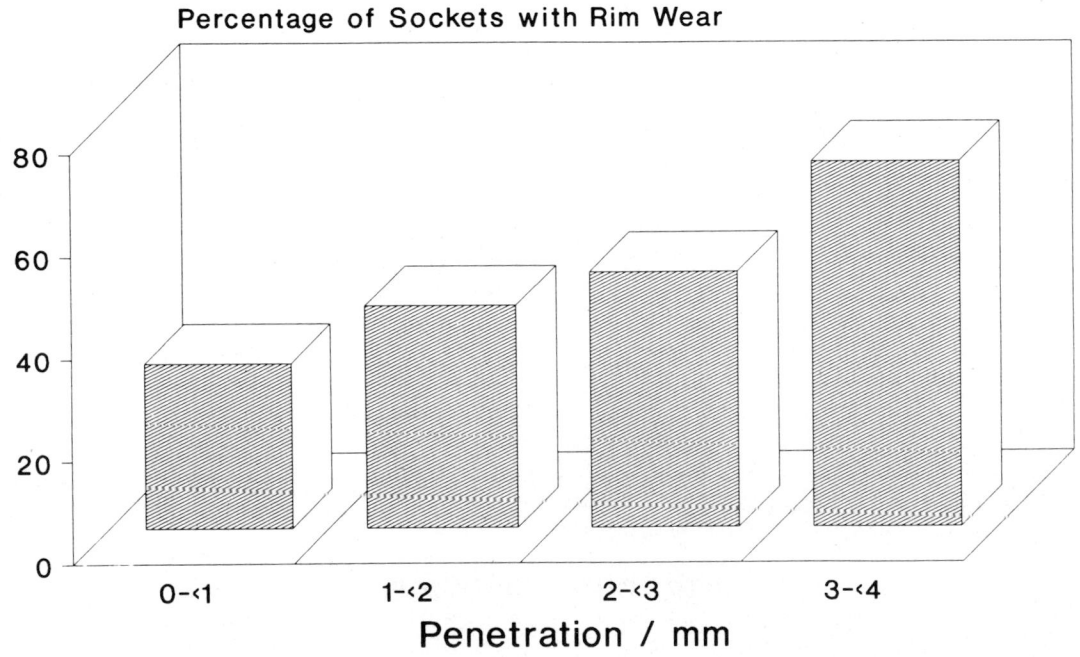

Fig. 4-49. Graph showing good correlation between penetration and incidence of rim wear. (From Isaacs GH et al: A tribiological study of retrieved hip prostheses, *Clin Orthop* 276:115, 1992.)

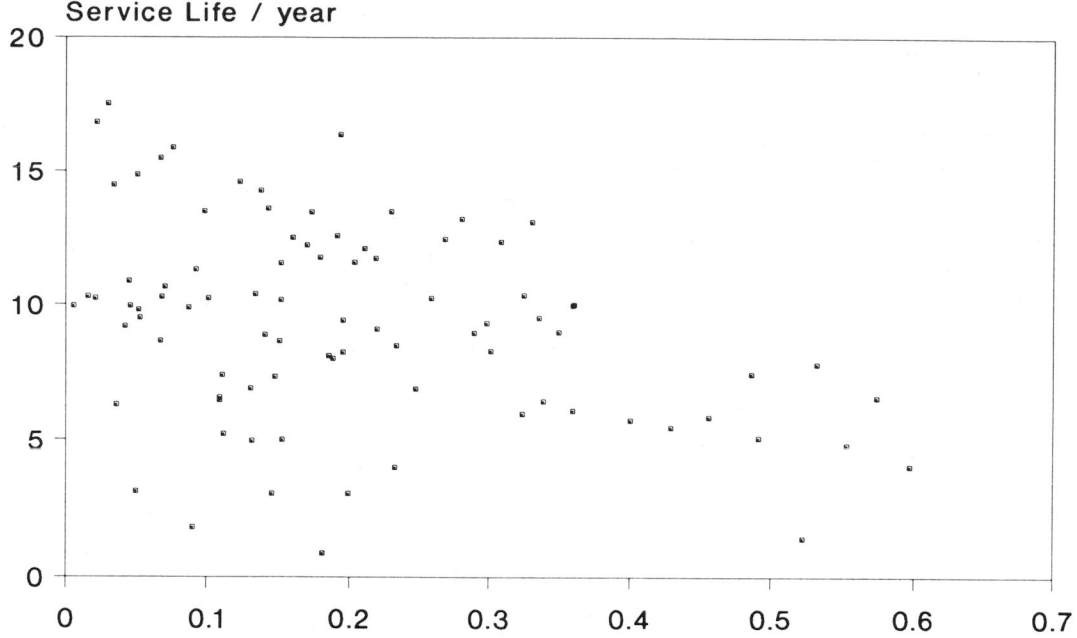

Fig. 4-50. Graph of service life versus penetration rate showing that there are no patients who have a high penetration rate and a long service life. (From Isaacs GH et al: A tribiological study of retrieved hip prostheses, *Clin Orthop* 276:115, 1992.)

Table 4-21 Summary of Wear Measurements

Study	Method	Number	Service life (years)	Age* (years)	Penetration rate (mm/year)	Penetration (mm)
Present	Shadowgraph	87	9	55	0.21	1.69
Wroblewski[301]	Shadowgraph	22	7.15	56	0.19	1.38
	Roentgenograph				0.21	1.51
Griffith[120]	Roentgenograph	491	8.3†	62‡	0.07	0.59

From Isaacs GH: A tribiological study of retrieved hip prostheses, *Clin Orthop* 276:115, 1992.
*Age at arthoplasty.
†Mean follow-up time.
‡Estimated.

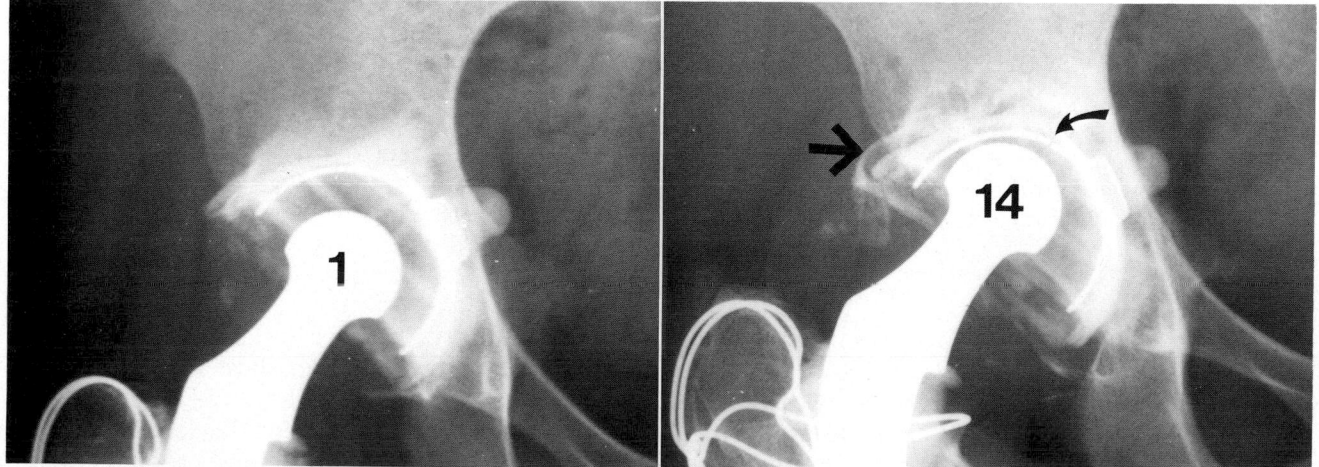

Fig. 4-51. A, 1-year postoperative radiograph of 20-year-old woman (F.B.) with juvenile rheumatoid arthritis. Patient was homebound before surgery because of severe hip pain, stiffness, and loss of function. **B,** 14 years after bilateral low-friction arthroplasty, note severe and rapid wear of both sockets associated with severe demarcation and socket migration.

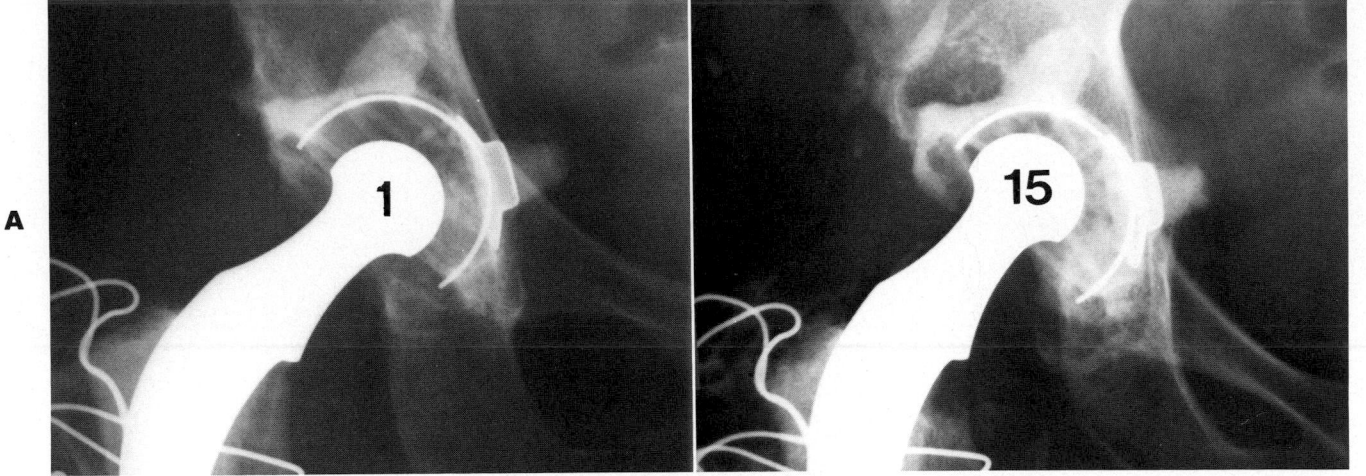

Fig. 4-52. A and **B,** 1 and 15 years postoperative radiographs of 35-year-old female social worker (D.W.) whose steroid-induced avascular necrosis was treated by low-friction arthroplasty. NOTE: Severe wear of the socket and associated osteolysis requiring revision. At revision surgery, the cup was not loose but almost being excavated by severe loss of bone because of worn out particles of HDP. At the time of revision, the patient was not symptomatic. Hip grades: B - R,6,6,6 and L,6,6,6. The operation was carried out to restore bone stock and arrest the rapid osteolysis.

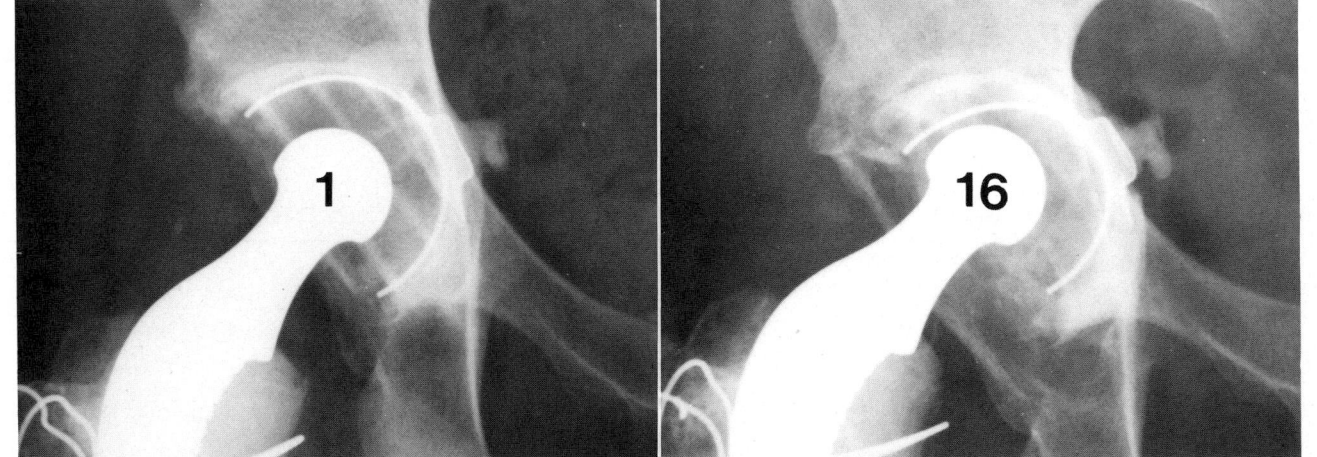

Fig. 4-53. A triad of "wear, loosening, and dislocation" was observed for which a revision arthroplasty became necessary at 16 years after low-friction arthroplasty. **A,** Radiograph of right hip is shown 1 year after low-friction arthroplasty performed for ankylosing spondylitis in a 29-year-old female (M.D.) whose hip began dislocating at 15 years after surgery and subsequently became painful because of loosening. **B,** Radiograph of same hip as shown in **A.** NOTE: wear and migration of the socket at 16 years after surgery and before revision.

tive layer formed (caused by cross-linking) may be prevented by irradiation of HDP, thus causing an increasing wear rate. In laboratory experiments, Grobbelaar and associates[110] and duPlessis and others[79] have shown that radiation cross-linking greatly improved its tensile strength, hardness, and softening point but only with a radiation dose of more than 400 kilogray. However, this level of radiation causes HDP to become brittle, markedly reduces its impact resistance, and de-

creases its wear resistance. In the presence of oxygen caused by radiolytic oxidation, these mechanical properties further deteriorate. However, by using cross-linking agents such as acetylene, the demands for high doses of radiation are reduced and cross-linking can occur at lower doses of radiation of 100 kilograys, thus increasing its tensile strength, hardness, and resistance against cold flow without changing its wear-resistance properties. Clinical application of these methods in total hip prostheses awaits control studies. Nussbaum and Rose, however, have concluded that low-dose radiation of typical radiation-sterilization might actually improve the mechanical properties of HDP against wear.[189]

Effects of Cup Thickness on Structural Stiffness

The structural stiffness imparted by the cup thickness is an important parameter that determines the amount of stress on the material and the displacement between HDP cup and bone. The stiffness of the total hip arthroplasty cup, made of a given homogenous block of HDP, depends on the ratio of the outer diameter to the inner diameter of the cup, which determines its thickness. For example, a given 50 mm outer diameter with a 32 mm inner diameter will result in 9 mm of plastic thickness as opposed to the same outer diameter with a 22 mm inner diameter, thus increasing the thickness to 14 mm and resulting in a considerable increase in its structural stiffness. Obviously, this increase can be achieved by either increasing the outer diameter or decreasing the inner diameter of the prosthesis. The common range of structural stiffness values in commonly used acetabular cups on the market is reported to be 10.1 mm.[36]

Reinforcement of HDP by carbon fibers can also produce a structurally stiffer acetabular component than plain HDP. However, adversity resulting from particulate matter (including carbon fibers) makes this material prohibitive for use in total joint arthroplasty materials. The relation of the structural thickness and wear of HDP awaits careful in-vitro and in-vivo studies.

Direction of Wear

Because of the frequency of wear noted in the vertical, upward, and lateral directions,[83] Charnley suggested that the hip socket must be implanted medially and be totally enclosed in bone. Although not proven in clinical studies, it is possible that with sockets oriented at surgery in an anteverted position there will be a greater amount of wear because of the lack of available plastic support, which can lead to an acceleration in wear of the anteverted socket.[47]

Failed Teflon used by Charnley produced a unique opportunity for the study of the pattern of wear of plastic in human hip joints. Several conclusions were derived from two studies by Charnley and co-workers,[47,83] including the following:

1. Socket wear did not occur randomly, but the head bored into the socket, creating a cylindrical path.
2. The volume of plastic generated by wear was proportional to the size of the worn cylinder (new cavity).
3. The wear was related to the functional activity of the patient and not to the patient's weight.

4. The smallest possible femoral head was considered to be 22 mm, which produced the smallest amount of debris (worn out material) without risking a rapid penetration or instability.

In Charnley and Halley's study, in 57 of 59 radiographs, the direction of wear was in a medial direction in 3.4% of sockets, in a lateral direction in 64.4%, and in a vertical line direction in 32.2%.

Wroblewski noted that of 22 HDP sockets in Charnley low-friction arthroplasty, the sockets wore lateral to a line drawn vertically from the center of the curvature of the socket in nine patients, medial to the same line in twelve patients, and in one patient, exactly in the same line. In the frontal plane, nine sockets wore in front of a similar line, two behind, and eleven wore exactly along the line.

Filler to Increase Wear Resistance

Enhancement of Teflon with glass fiber or with a synthetic material (Fluorosint-Polypenco) in laboratory conditions improved the wear resistance. However, results were discouraging when used in humans and exposed to body fluids after implantation.[47] Both Fluorosint and glass wore badly, resulting in a matte surface that did not become glazed as it did in the laboratory.

Socket Wear vs. Loosening

Wroblewski, in a study of two groups of patients after low-friction arthroplasty, found a positive correlation between the depth of socket penetration by the femoral head and the incidence of socket migration (see Table 4-20). One study included 103 sockets with an average follow up of 16.6 years (range from 15 to 21 years), and another included 104 sockets in patients 40 years of age or younger with an average of 9.3 years follow up (range from 4 to 17 years). Wroblewski concluded that progressive penetration of the head causes restriction of movement from the neck-socket impingement that may cause "shock load" and thus loosening of the cup. Impingement occurred in the same path as the direction of wear, that is, the coronal plane (Figs. 4-52 and 4-54 to 4-58).[278] The various wear characteristics of HDP based on explanted specimens are demonstrated in Figs. 4-59 to 4-62.

Wear and Neck-Socket Impingement

Increased penetration of the head as it bores through the socket thickness coincides with a reduction in the neck-socket angle and thus impingement (see Chapter 32) and increased rate of instability, dislocation, and deformity (erosion) of the acetabular rim. Wroblewski concluded that over half of the sockets (14 of 22) showed some degree of erosion of the rim; in this group the lowest depth of wear causing rim erosion was 0.56

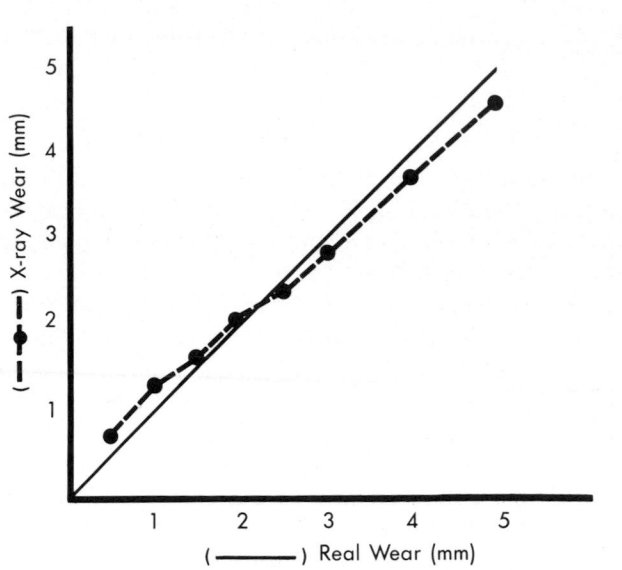

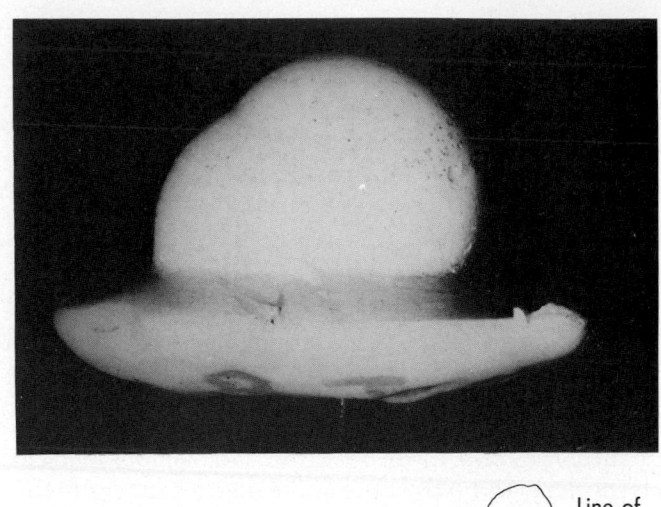

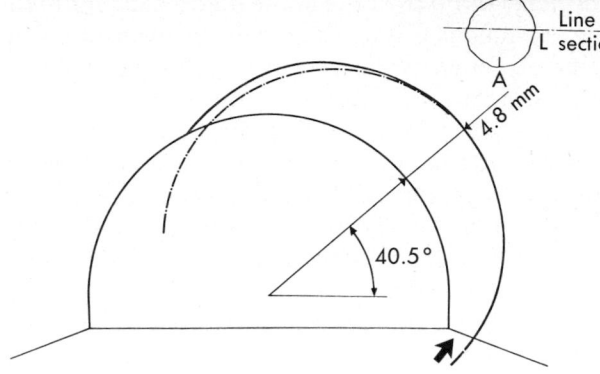

Fig. 4-54. Correlation between real and radiographic measurement of depth of socket wear. (From Wroblewski BM: *Revision surgery in total hip arthroplasty,* New York, 1990, Springer-Verlag.)

Fig. 4-55. A, Acrylic cast of worn socket at 9 ½ years. **B,** Shadowgraph showing depth of wear (4.8 mm) and direction of penetration (coronal plane). Note erosion of socket bore rim. (From Wroblewski BM: *Revision surgery in total hip arthroplasty,* New York, 1990, Springer-Verlag.)

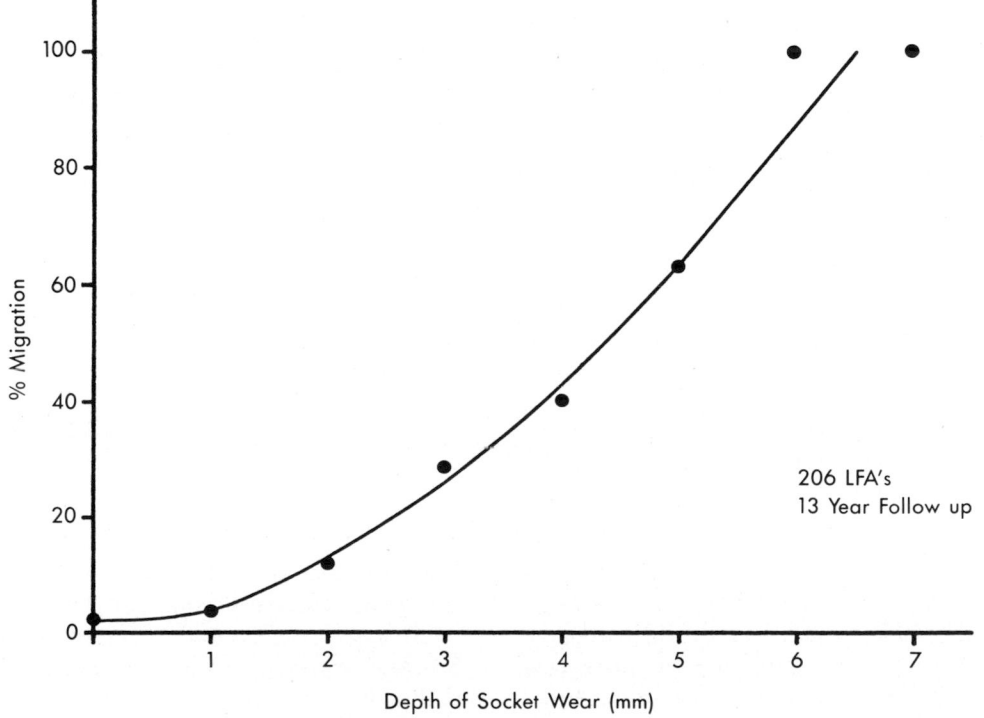

Fig. 4-56. Correlation between depth of socket wear and incidence of socket migration. (From Wroblewski BM: *Revision surgery in total hip arthroplasty,* New York, 1990, Springer-Verlag.)

Wear of Socket

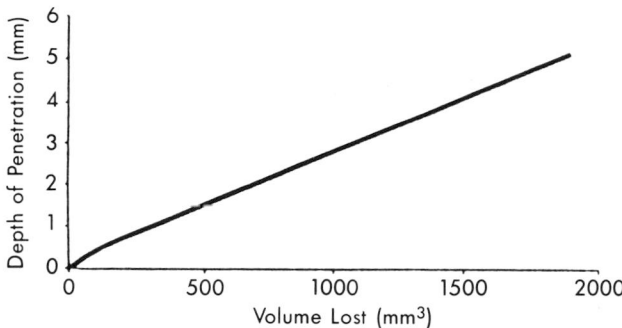

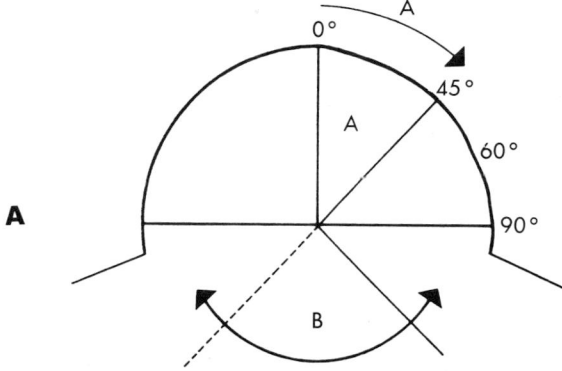

A- Direction of wear
B- Angular movement

Fig. 4-57. Volume of plastic lost in relation to depth of socket penetration with 22.25 mm diameter head. After 1 mm penetration, there is a straight-line relationship between the depth of penetration (mm) and the volume (mm³) of HDP lost. (From Wroblewski BM: *Revision surgery in total hip arthroplasty,* New York, 1990, Springer-Verlag.)

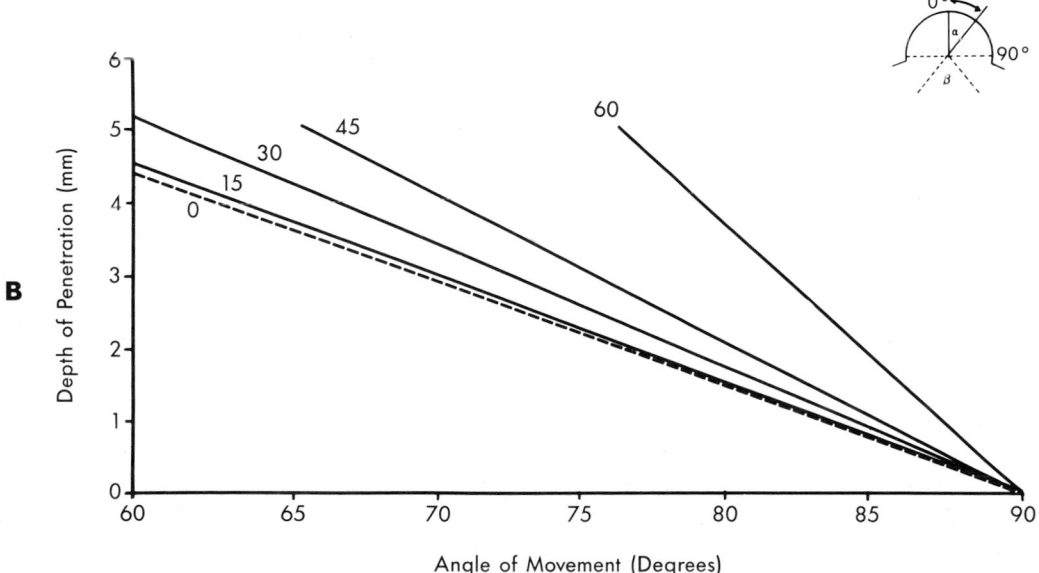

Fig. 4-58. Angular movements in relation to depth of socket wear. **A,** Schematic diagram of socket: *A,* direction of wear 0 to 90 degrees; *B,* angular movements. **B,** Restriction of angular movements (from the available 90 degrees) according to direction of socket wear (12.5 mm diameter neck); from 0 degrees central wear to 60 degrees peripheral wear. **C,** Improvement in angular range of movement with reduced (10 mm) diameter neck. The range of movements increased from 90 to 108 degrees. To restrict the movement to 90 degrees (as with the standard 12.5 mm diameter neck) at 45 degrees wear path, the depth of penetration must be 3 mm. (From Wroblewski BM: *Revision surgery in total hip arthroplasty,* New York, 1990, Springer-Verlag.)

Continued.

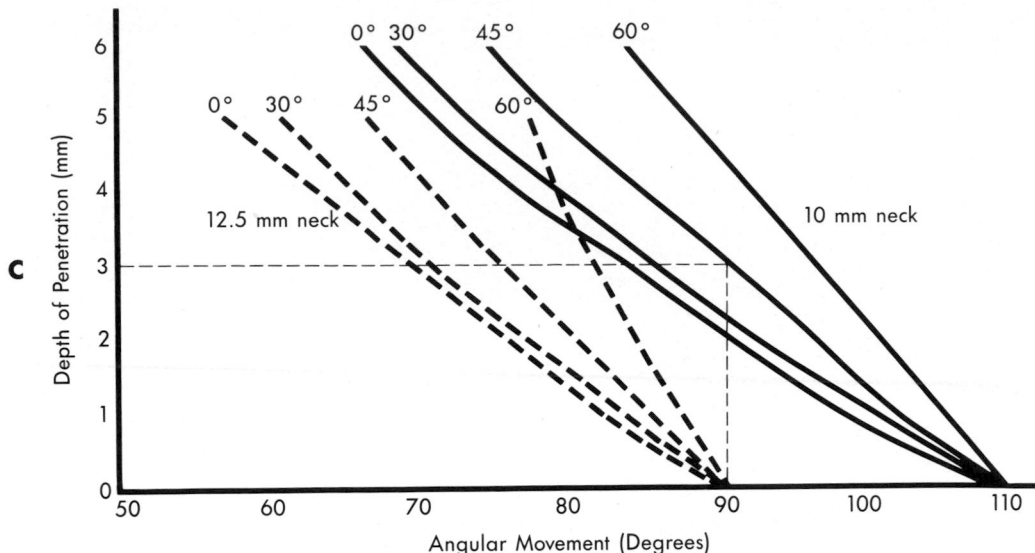

Fig. 4-58—cont'd. See legend on previous page.

mm. Of six sockets without rim wear, the greatest amount of socket wear was 0.4 mm, thus indicating that between 0.4 and 0.56 mm neck-socket impingement might be expected.[277] However, this observation was made on Charnley's prosthesis using the original neck design of 12.5 mm. As suggested by Wroblewski, the cross-sectional diameter of the neck can be reduced from 12.5 to 10 mm, which would allow an increase of 18 degrees of angular movement before impingement.[277] Increasing angular movement from 90 to 108 degrees can result in delaying the moment of impingement of the femoral neck on the rim of the cup, permitting an extra 3 mm wear of the cup. As a consequence, the life of the system is extended by an average of 15.8 years.

External Wear of the Socket

After loosening, it is not uncommon for the external surface of the cup to be subjected to wear. Such a wear mode can produce a large amount of HDP particles, leading to bone destruction. The incidence of socket wear at the external face of a Charnley low-friction arthroplasty prosthesis was documented to be frequent. Some 19 of 59 sockets (32%) examined after revision arthroplasty for loosening showed external wear. This observation is in contrast to earlier views that severe tissue reaction of the cemented socket was caused by wear debris, presumably entering into the space between bone and cement and causing loosening.[269a] To the contrary, Wroblewski has shown that most tissue reaction in some cases may be caused by the large number of wear particles generated from the external surface of the cup after loosening.[281]

Accuracy of Wear Measurements by Radiograph

Wroblewski has reported a high positive correlation between radiographic and real wear in 22 paired observations (P value = 0.001),[278] see Fig. 4-54. However, with less than 2 mm of real wear (measured directly from the specimens), x-ray measurements overestimated the linear wear, and with more than 2 mm of real wear, x-ray measurements underestimated the linear wear.

To make accurate measurements of wear by radiograph: (1) the cement used in arthroplasty must be radiopaque, (2) a radiographic marker must be incorporated on the cup, (3) anteversion of the cup (implanted at surgery) must be known, (4) the relationship of the x-ray tube to the hip must be correct, and (5) metal backing must not be present on the acetabular component.

Radiopaque Cement

It is possible to measure the distance between the femoral head prosthesis and the outer diameter of the cup using radiopaque cement. This measurement must be made at the site of maximum wear, that is, the thinnest portion of the cup in the direction of wear.

Radiographic Marker

Errors in measurement can occur if the original semicircular wire marker was not inserted in the coronal plane or was subsequently tilted after loosening. When the socket has been implanted more than 10 degrees from the coronal plane, a radiolucent crescent appears between the wire marker and cement. With

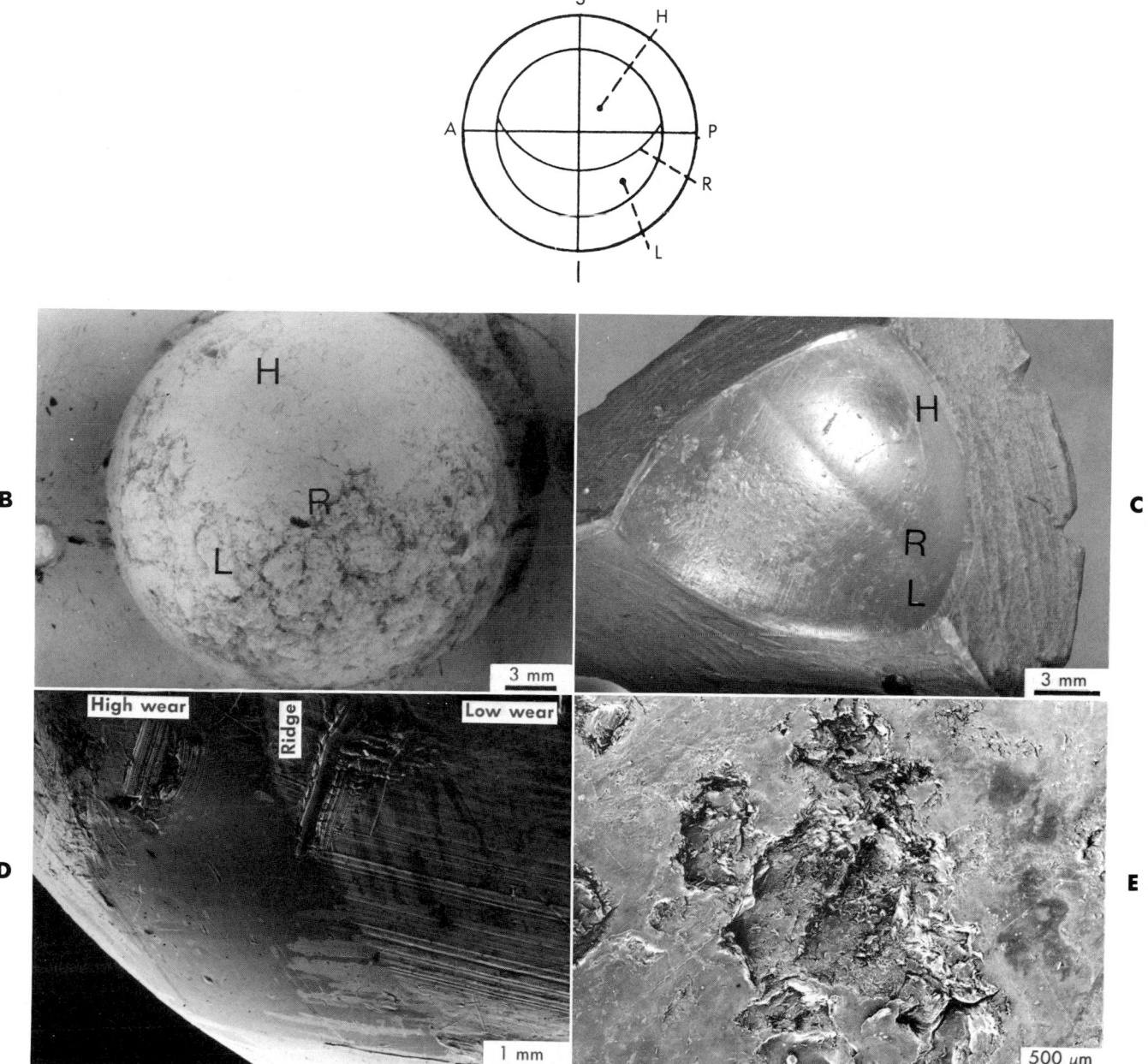

Fig. 4-59. Wear of HDP socket: characteristic areas. **A,** Diagrammatic representation of typical appearance of worn socket. *A,* Anterior; *P,* posterior; *S,* superior; *I,* inferior (parts of socket in relation to their position within the hip). *H,* High-wear area; *L,* low-wear area; *R,* ridge separating the low- and high-wear areas. **B,** Low-power view of the inside of the socket. *H,* High-wear area; *L,* low-wear area; *R,* ridge. **C,** Photograph of sectioned socket to show the characteristic appearance. **D,** High-power magnification. Note the smooth high-wear area with pits caused by cement ingress and the machining marks visible in the low-wear area. **E,** Damage caused by cement ingress. (From Wroblewski BM: *Revision surgery in total hip arthroplasty,* New York, 1990, Springer-Verlag.)

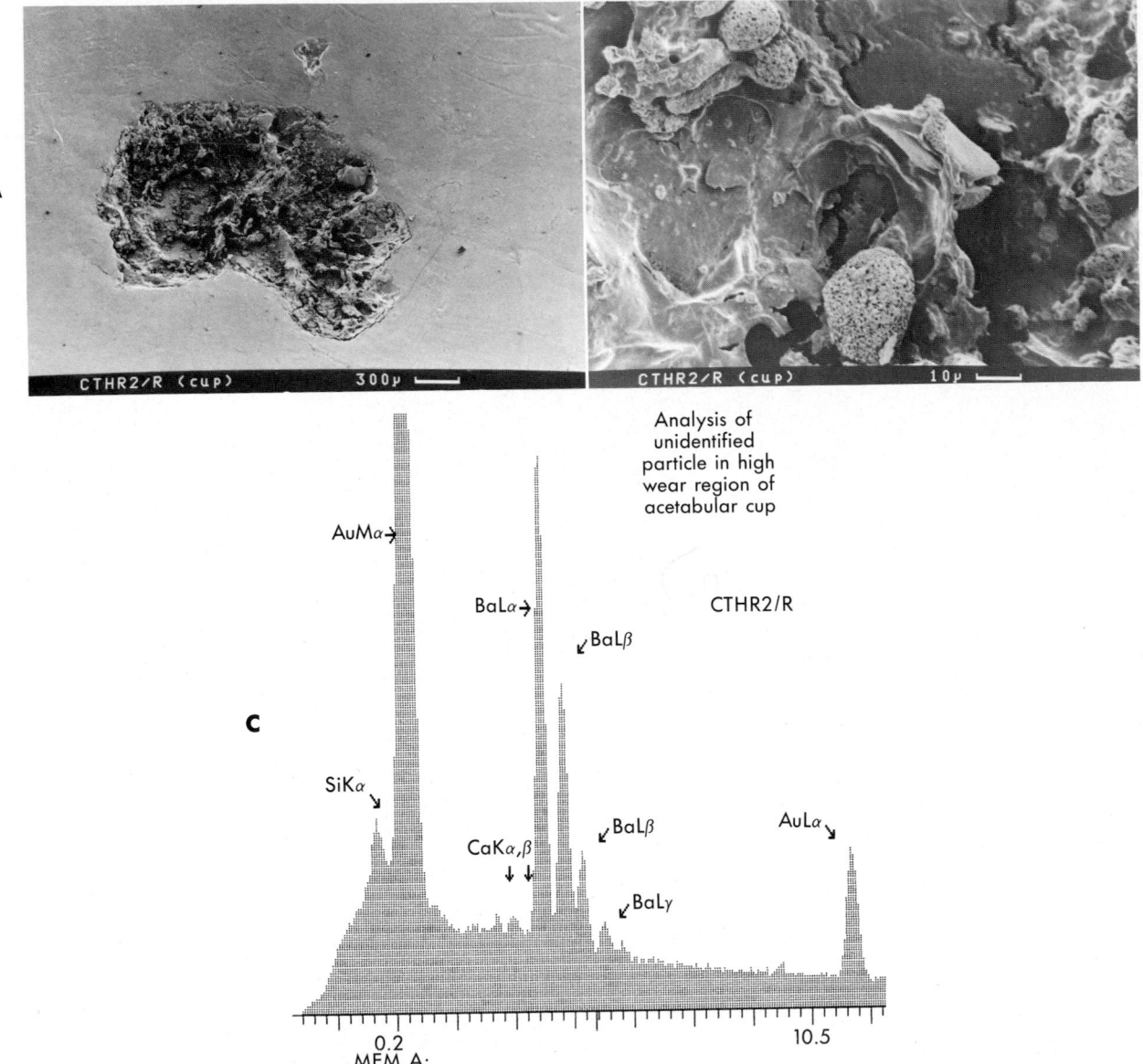

Fig. 4-60. Cement ingress into the articulation. **A,** Crater In HDP caused by acrylic cement. **B,** Pumicelike clumps of barium sulfate. **C,** Analysis of the clumps identifies them as barium. (The high peak for gold [Au] is caused by the preparation of the specimen to avoid damage when analyzed with the SEM; Si probably indicates presence of glove powder.) (**A** and **B** Courtesy Departments of Tribology and Mechanical Engineering, The University of Leeds; **C** from Wroblewski BM: *Revision surgery in total hip arthroplasty,* New York, 1990, Springer-Verlag.)

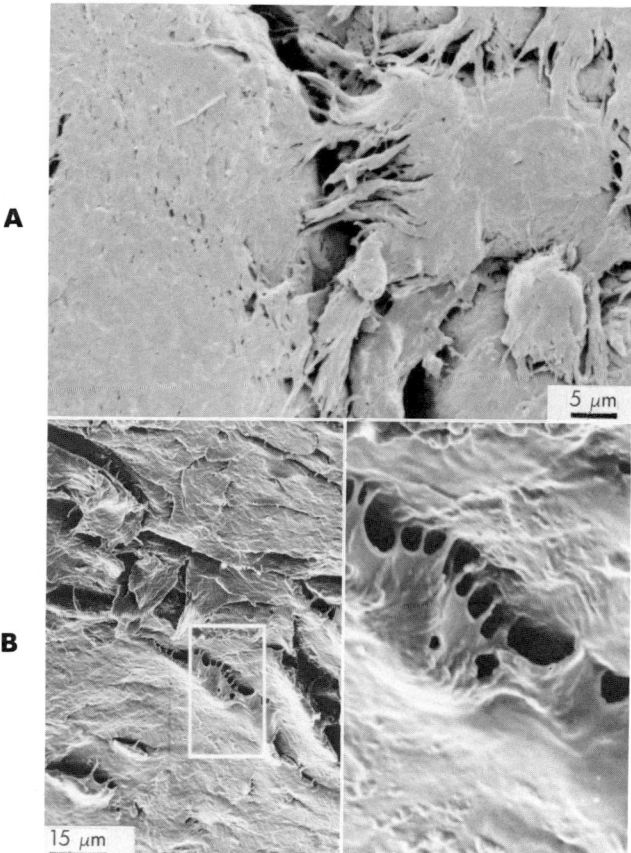

Fig. 4-61. Cracks within the HDP. **A,** Could this be caused by sintering? **B,** Does this picture show cold flow of the HDP? (From Wroblewski BM: *Revision surgery in total hip arthroplasty,* New York, 1990, Springer-Verlag.)

the presence of radiopaque cement it is possible to estimate the amount of wear by measuring the distance between the head and outer border of the radiolucent crescent rather than the radiolucent wire marker. Fig. 4-53, *A* illustrates the correct site of measurement for wear (between the head and radiographic wire marker). Fig. 4-54, *B* shows a radiographic marker in place, but the cup had not been implanted in the coronal plane; note the crescent between the wire marker and the radiopaque cement.

Anteversion of the Cup

When the cup is inserted with some degree of anteversion, it presents the radiographic wire more asymmetrically. In this case, the crescent portion appearing between the marker and cement should be included in the distance between the head and the cement.

Tube/Plate Orientation

Charnley pointed out that by using a 17 by 14 inch film and with the x-ray tube centered over the symphysis pubis, providing that the radiographic wire marker is in the coronal plane, variations in the placement of the x-ray tube cause differences of only approximately 0.2 mm in the thickness of the cup.[47]

Metal-Backed Acetabular Component

Metal-backed acetabular component renders radiographic measurements difficult if not impossible because of superimposed metal shell and femoral head on radiographs.

Interobserver Variability

The most significant variation in studies of wear may result from errors of different observers who may choose different radii for measurement. This interob-

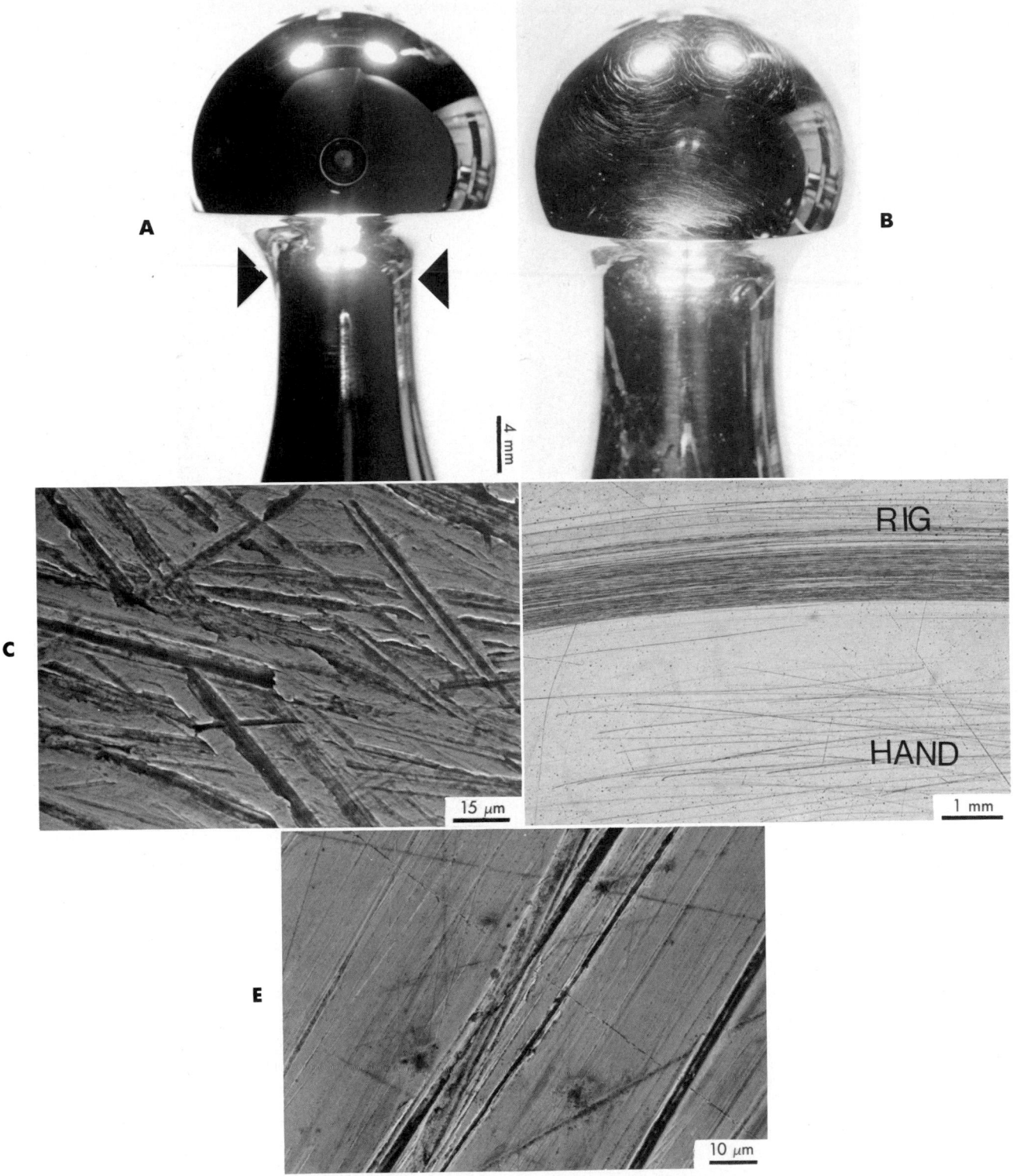

Fig. 4-62. Damage to head of femoral component. **A,** Appearance as delivered by manufacturer. Note the reduced diameter neck. **B,** Appearance at revision some 8 years later. **C,** SEM; damaged surface magnified. The grooves and the heaped-up ridges cause the damage to HDP socket. **D,** Damage reproduced using acrylic cement in test rig and by hand-held specimen. **E,** Magnified view of part of **D.** Note uniformity of direction as compared with **C.** (From Wroblewski BM: *Revision surgery in total hip arthroplasty,* New York, 1990, Springer-Verlag.)

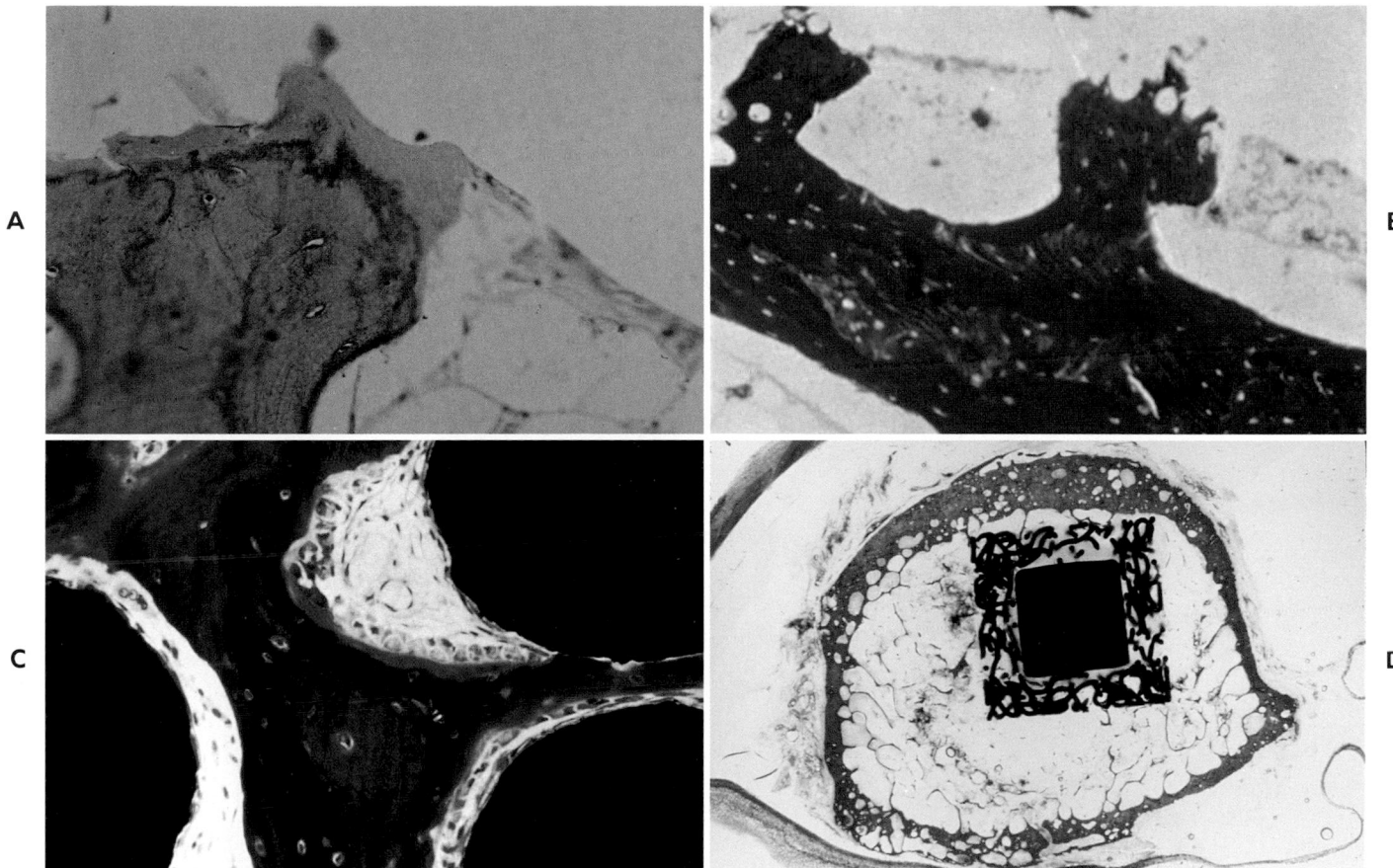

Plate 1. A, The load-bearing in a cemented femur is demonstrated histologically to occur through newly formed caps of fibrocartilage or modified bone matrix without any other interposing tissue. These caps in turn transmit load through selected points of the endosteal surface of the femur through its trabecular system to the cortex. Light microscopy H & E stain shows healthy marrow adjacent to caps after cement has been dissolved. **B,** Low-magnification areas of direct cement contact with bone. **C,** 6 weeks after implantation in canine model, lamellar bone with haversian systems is seen. Osteoid seams, multinucleated giant cells, and rimming osteoblasts are present. In many areas, a cellular layer remains interposed between bone and the fiber metal (×450). **D,** Matched canine femora explanted 6 months after bilateral total hip implantation with fully coated femoral stems. In the weight-bearing limb note the robust trabeculae extending from the cortex to implant and the dense ingrowth in the porous layer extending to the underlying prosthetic substrate. (**A** and **B** from Charnley J: *Low-friction arthroplasty of the hip: theory and practice,* Berlin, 1979, Springer-Verlag; **C** and **D** courtesy AG Rosenberg.)

Continued

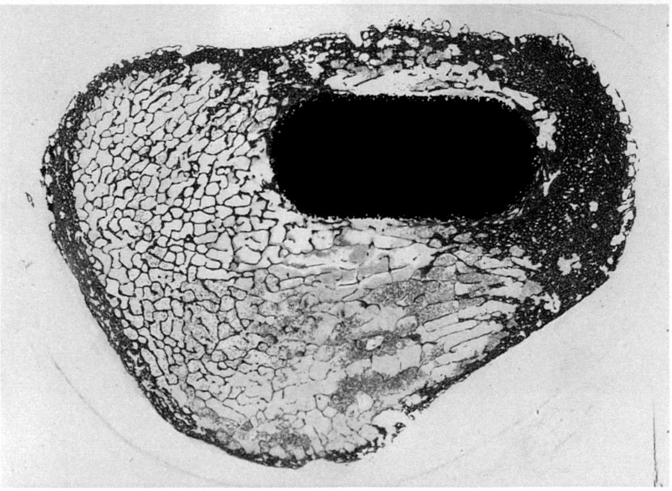

Plate 1–cont'd. E, Histological photograph of a transverse section taken at the isthmus through a 13.5 mm diameter 4/5 porous coated AML stem implanted for 2 years in a 77-year-old male (diagnosis: osteoarthritis). Note the generalized osteopenia of the cortex and the encapsulation of the implant by a thick, dense shell of bone. The bone has grown extensively into the porous coating, particularly on the lateral side *(right field).* **F,** Histological photomicrograph of a region of bone ingrowth on the posterior side just under the collar ($\times 20$). Note the lacunae and nutrient vessels deep within the porous coating. **G,** Histological photograph of a transverse section prepared about 1.5 cm distal to the collar. Note the bone ingrowth medially *(left field)* and laterally *(right field).* (**E** to **G** from Engh CA, Bobyn JD: *Biological fixation in total hip arthroplasty,* Thorofare, NJ, 1985, Slack, Inc.)

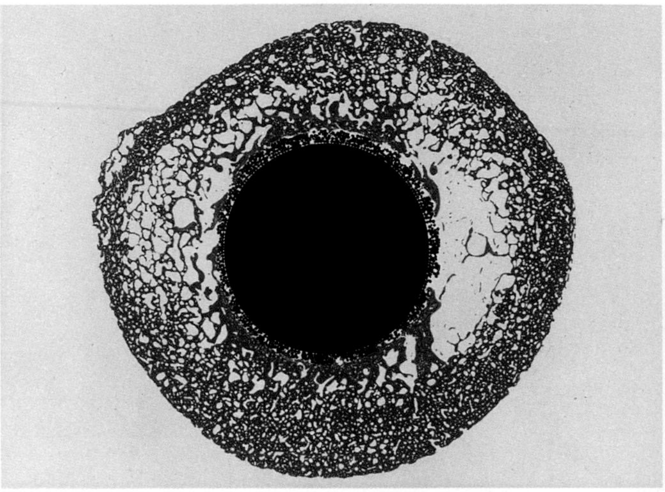

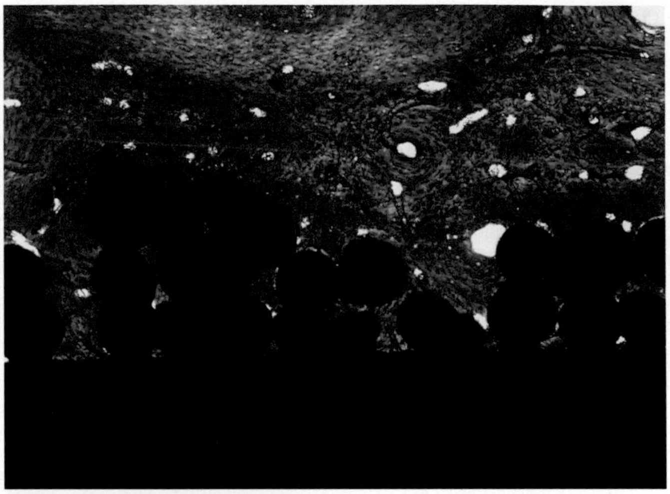

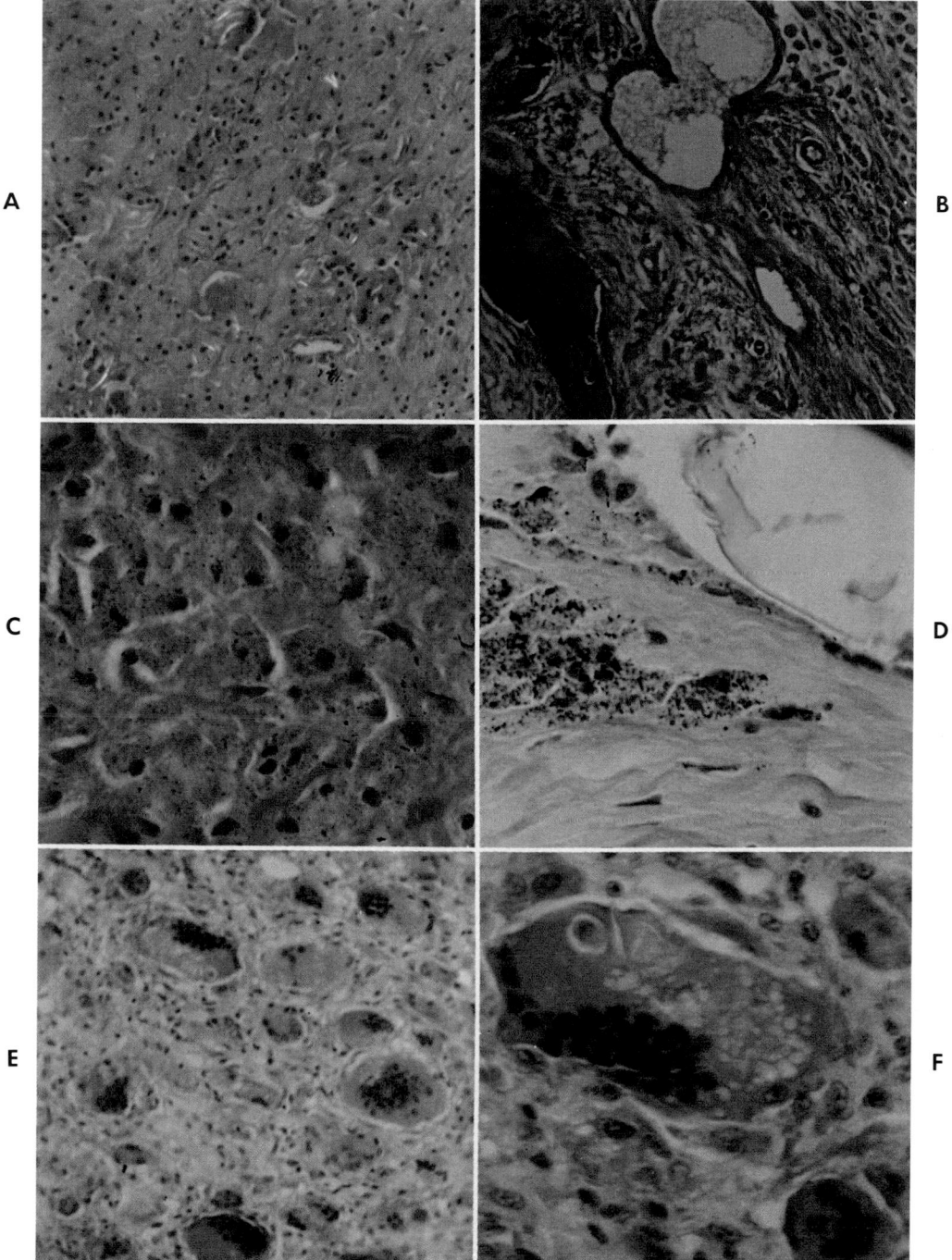

Plate 2. A, Microscopic fragments of birefringent HDP highlight cytoplasm of acidophilic histiocytes with blue and yellow flecks. Larger fragments are trapped in multinucleated giant cells (×50). **B,** Histiocytic response to implant materials is shown occupying a defect in bone. Relatively large bilobed defect near left upper quadrant of this field almost certainly contained bone cement, which was dislodged during tissue processing (×160). **C,** Acidophilic histiocytes here contain small irregular black particles representing metallic deposits. These did not stain positively for iron (×500). **D,** Details of histiocytic cells are obscured by heavy metallic deposits. These also do not stain positively for iron. Relatively large fragment of HDP glows from tissue space in lower right, partially lined by giant cell (×500). **E,** Intermingled giant cells and mononuclear acidophilic histiocytes vaguely resemble giant cell tumor. Vascular supply is poor (×160). **F,** Giant cell in the center has evidently been inspired to insatiable phagocytic activity by unusually large number of nuclei. Vacuoles are phagosomes, recognizable remnants of a dead cell occupy one of these (×500). (From Eftekhar NS, Doty SB, Johnston AD, et al: Prosthetic synovitis. In The Hip Society: *The hip: proceedings of the thirteenth open scientific meeting of The Hip Society,* St Louis, 1985, Mosby–Year Book.)

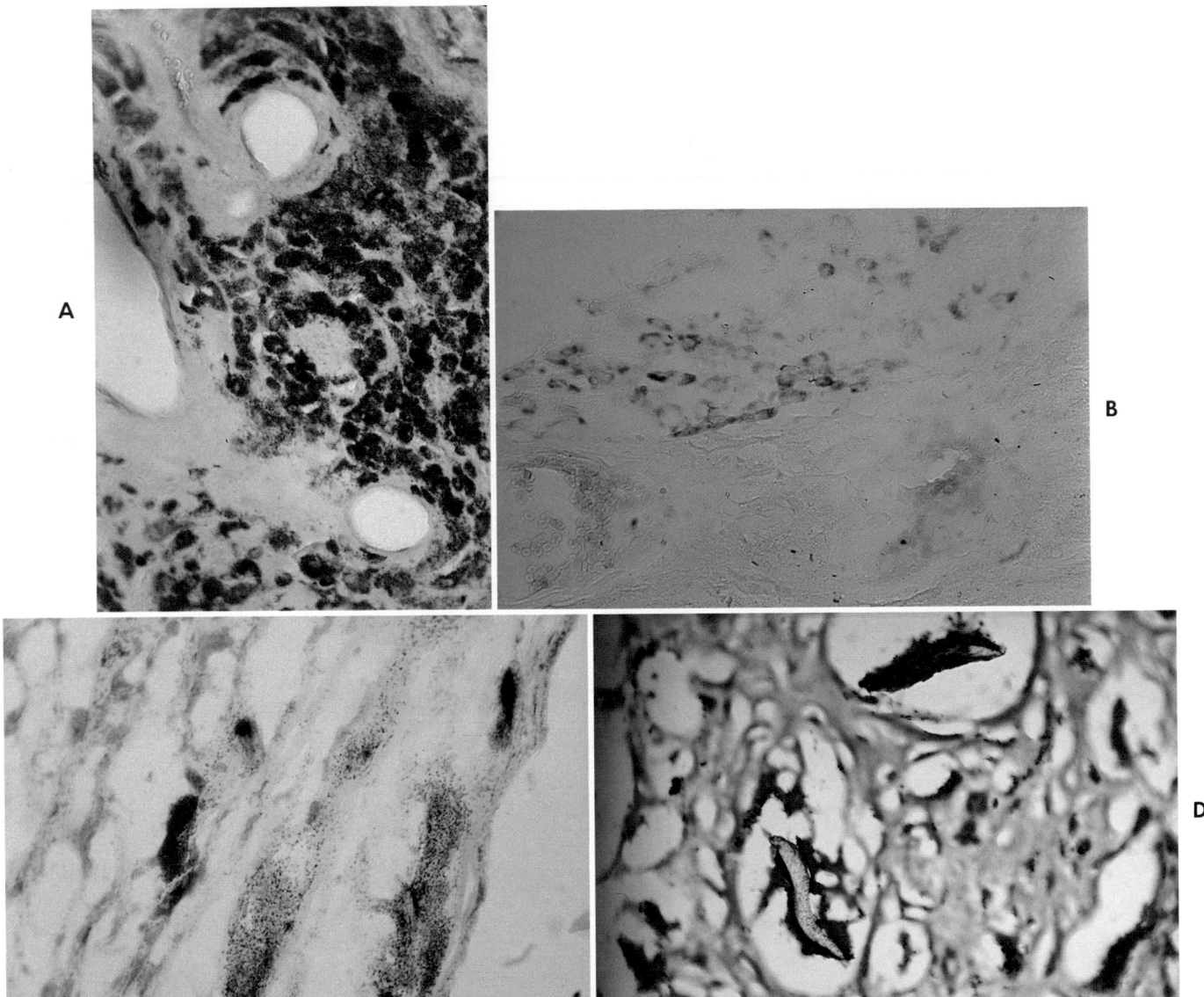

Plate 3. A, Light microscopy of histological section stained for esterase activity, note high enzyme-related cellular activity about the vascular channels. The tissue is from a grossly loose cemented implant. **B,** Positive staining for beta galactosidase (note absence of acid phosphatase). Tissue is section through nonseptic prosthetic synovitis with attached bone fragment. Histochemical staining shows an increased endogenous peroxidase activity (beta galactasidase, an enzyme specifically made by macrophages during activation) caused by the presence of PMMA or HDP and during active phase of membrane. **C,** Concurrent enzyme activities acid phosphatase *(red)* and beta galactosidase *(blue)* within the same specimen (see text). **D,** Lysosomes are adsorbed to the surface of two shards of plastic (presumably HDP) indicating lysosomal activities in the tissue.

servation error can be diminished by recognizing the correct direction of the radius, that is, the path of the femoral head penetration. Sequential (annual) radiographs of the same patient are helpful in determining the correct path of the head in the socket.

METAL BACK REINFORCEMENT OF HDP

At the time of this writing, some concern has been expressed regarding a possible detrimental effect imparted by metal backing of the acetabular component resulting in an increased HDP wear rate. Since the clinical use of metal-backed acetabular components has not been shown to be beneficial in prevention of loosening, this author anticipates that this design will be soon removed from the market.

CERAMICS

Although known for being brittle and fracturing under sufficient mechanical stress, ceramics have the advantage of being hard. Unlike ductile material such as metals they do not fail under "cyclic-load." The mechanical failure of ceramics is caused by the propagation of preexisting flaws or cracks. As a general rule a deformable (ductile) metal under stress undergoes plastic deformation and thus absorbs energy. On the other hand the brittle material such as ceramics under sufficient stress initiates a crack propagation through imperfections, leading to a sudden fracture and usually with associated increased impact resulting in many fracture pieces. Several ceramics used in orthopaedic implants include alumina, zirconia, calcium phosphate, such as tricalcium phosphate and hydroxyapatite, and carbon and other composites.

Aluminum oxide (A1203) is especially attractive for its wear characteristics against HDP and against aluminum oxide.[70] Alumina has very high elastic modulus and compressive strength, 380 GPa and 4500 MPa respectively. The tensile strength of surgical grade alumina is low and typically is 350 MPa. This marked difference between compressive strengths and tensile strength is because of the defects such as microscopic porosities and surface imperfections leading to failure of material in tension and relatively unaffected by compression. The effects of defects leading to a high degrees of variability in ceramics require that a "low variability" biomedical grade of ceramics be used in orthopaedic implants.

Characteristically alumina can be produced with a highly polished surface, a desirable feature in reducing wear in total hip arthroplasty. The alumina against alumina prosthesis has shown a superior wear characteristic to metal against metal, metal against HDP, and alumina against HDP. Dörre[5] and others demonstrated an order of magnitude reduction of wear of alumina versus alumina as compared with alumina

against HDP. It should be recognized that unlike HDP, alumina is not deformable. Therefore alumina against alumina requires a very precise sphericity of the mating surfaces to avoid high local stresses. A mismatch between the two nondeformable materials such as ceramics may lead to a localized wear and an accelerated wear caused by particles within the articular surfaces.[198,199] In addition to fracture of ceramics the other problem is the manufacturing control that demands exact and careful matching between the tapered metallic stem and the ceramic balls for articulation with either ceramic or HDP sockets. Improvement in manufacturing of ceramic joints has resulted in improved materials and manufacturing capabilities of the implants. For example the high wear rate of ceramics caused by "grain excavation" has now been addressed by keeping the particle size below 3 μm and by manufacturing the components of alumina-alumina bearings in matched pairs with a very high accuracy to within 1 μm. These efforts have now resulted in a low wear rate in ceramic total hip arthroplasty prostheses.[55]

Alumina is inert and biocompatible.[155] However, as a metal oxide in a biological environment, it degrades very slowly, which in time can cause tissue response.[109,129,197,212]

Zirconia (zirconium oxide) is another ceramic with a low surface roughness because of finer grain structure. It is stronger than alumina in tension and has a lower modulus of elasticity than alumina. Less is known about its biocompatibility, which is currently under investigation.[54,55,101] Aluminum oxide (alumina) has been investigated extensively for its potential use in joint replacement surgery for its excellent wear resistance against alumina and against high-density polyethylene. Reports of early clinical failure have been attributed to impurities and manufacturing defects. Mechanical grade of this material has now been recently improved because its strength and high-quality surface finish with an excellent report on in-vitro wear behavior. However, brittleness and catastrophic failure of this material combined with demand for its manufacturing quality require follow-up clinical studies on the recent vintage of this material.

Davidson recently examined (1) surface wettability and relative tendencies to form UHMWPE transfer film via adhesive wear, (2) oxidative wear of metal surfaces, (3) microabrasions from hard passive oxide film and metallic debris, and (4) generation of 3-body wear resulting from PMMA and bone debris.* By analyzing metal release rates, it was found that Co-Cr-Mo alloy wear was 0.1 μm per year. Ceramic surfaces can be arrested to maintain their initial surface finish, thus minimizing the wear of UHMWPE.

---

* Davidson JA, Personal communication, 1992, Washington, DC.

SUMMARY OF ESSENTIALS

- Because the development of implantable polymers (plastics) is relatively recent, their long-term compatibility and tolerance by the tissue are not fully documented. However, experience over the past three decades indicates that commonly used polymers such as HDP and acrylic cement, in addition to metals familiar to orthopaedic surgeons, have a good compatibility and are considered safe when they are used in bulk form for repair and replacement surgery.

- In-vivo research should be directed toward the selection of biocompatible materials for the bearing joints. Using new materials based on animal or laboratory testing cannot be transposed to expected results in human experience. Most, if not all, materials used for total hip arthroplasty can cause tissue reaction in particulate form.

- With the emergence of sarcomas reported at the site of metal or plastic joint materials, questions related to carcinogenicity of these materials when applied to very young patients must be answered only by very careful and prolonged documentation and follow up.

- When new materials are introduced or old materials are reintroduced in a different form, the surgeon should be particularly concerned about the potential harm of ionic release from metal trace elements of various alloys, as well as generation of particles from metals or plastics.

- A simple ball-and-socket bearing exposed to tissue fluid is most effective, provided that the plastic is wear resistant and the particulate matter released will not cause tissue reaction in the body because of wear. As such, the design and choice of materials should be aimed toward inertness of the wear by-product and tissue tolerance.

- A histologically stable interface between the implant and skeleton is of fundamental importance. Achieving stability of the total joint prosthesis is complex and challenging; it must be problem-free to perform a lifetime of service without failure.

- Materials selected for joint arthroplasties should be adequately fatigue resistant to withstand weight-bearing stresses. Wear must be minimal and the level of friction resistance reduced to a minimum to protect the fixation from excessive stress. These materials should also withstand corrosion and degradation in the hostile environment of the body.

- Although a stable cellular interface may be achieved between acrylic and bone, there is no agreement as to whether this stability can be maintained permanently and, if it cannot, what set of circumstances alters a histologically stable interface leading to bone destruction and mechanical loosening.

- The metals commonly used for bearings in human artificial joints include stainless steel, chromium-cobalt-molybdenum, and titanium alloys. The impurities or the elements of these alloys may lead to long-term failure of the implants, but their reactions in the short term may be minimal. Tissue reactions to long-term implantation of all of these metals do occur as analysis of the tissue adjacent to these metals reveals the ions of all elements of the metal alloys.

- Corrosion may be uniform, pitting, intragranular, and cracking type. In general, reactions to metals relate not only to the ionic behavior in a biological situation but also to the size, shape, movement, and other physical parameters of the implant itself.

- As a rule, most foreign bodies, regardless of their chemical constituency or physical makeup, will cause a local inflammatory process after implantation and finally become encapsulated by a fibrous membrane.

- It is generally agreed that foreign material influences the type of reaction at a cellular level depending on its size and shape, as well as its chemical composition.

- The influence of surface energy and roughness of implants on bone resorption has been documented to be related to microphage release mediators, which stimulate bone resorption.

- Tissue reaction to PMMA begins with injury and repair after implantation, followed by a sequence of events similar to fracture repair and finally by osteointegration if the state of stability is achieved. However, if motion persists between the implanted cement and bone, a condition known as prosthetic synovitis will develop, which typically leads to osteolysis and ultimate failure of the bond between PMMA and the host bone.

- Bone cement osteointegration occurs in the absence of mechanical stress, which includes filling of the existing gap between bone and implant with newly formed woven bone. Secondary remodeling process occurs resulting from revascularization of the cortex including replacement of necrotic bone as forces are being transmitted to bone via cement.

- In the femur, intimate contact between bone and cement occurs without interruption by fibrous or molecular connection. Without any tissue reaction, osteoblasts are conveniently deposited directly onto the bone cement interface as documented by histological specimens of long-term follow-up studies.

- Histological studies of bone in experimental models

indicate that the most significant changes occurred after reaming of bone leading to devascularization and apparent necrosis of large areas of trochanteric region of the femur. This necrotic region fully recovered within 6 months of surgery. However, necrosis produced in the inner layer of the diaphysis persisted beyond 1 year.

- After devascularization as a result of insertion of PMMA, the cortex vascularized without osteoclasia and the remodeling process was dramatically reduced.

- Tissue injury resulting from leaching of monomer from polymerizing bone cement indicated that the immediate effects from monomer were vascular flow interference including flow stasis and intravascular hemolysis; there was no indication that the polymerized cement exerted a toxic effect on the tissue.

- Quantitative measurements of bone mineral content have been established after injury and fractures. After total hip arthroplasty, an initial increase and a subsequent decrease occurred in the bone mineral content during the first postoperative year with a return to the initial value in men and a 10% net loss in women. The loss of bone mineral content was remarkably low compared with the results obtained after injuries of similar or even lesser magnitude.

- Histology related to tissue reaction to cement in absence of infection must be considered independently for the state of stability and the state of loosening. In the state of stability, the tissue reaction is minimal, and osteointegration is common. On the other hand, severe tissue reaction including severe bone lysis occurs resulting from physical movement or the presence of particulate matters of PMMA in the tissue.

- Specimens from well-fixed femoral components show fibrous interface as an extremely thin and never complete line in the whole endosteal surface of the femur. The load bearing appears to take place through caps of fibrocartilage or modified bone matrix; thus no tissue of any kind is interposed between the cement and bone. These points of contact indicate that a perfect fixation to skeleton is possible through these caps and that load is transmitted only through selected points of endosteal surface.

- Absence of radiolucencies after total hip arthroplasty in the femur and often lack of demarcation are the rule rather than the exception and can be interpreted as a positive and favorable response.

- Unlike the histology of the interface in the femur, repair of the acetabulum after 10 years may not reach an end point. The presence of histiocytes and a few giant cells may suggest an unstable state of repair, which is considered a "suspended animation" with neither positive repair nor positive destruction even after 10 to 15 years of successful clinical results.

- An extensive tissue reaction with giant cell formation and caseation suggests the presence of loosening of cement fragments in the bone for some time before surgical intervention. Similarly, cystic erosions encountered in the calcar region should be attributed to loosening of cement at this heavily loaded zone.

- Acrylic cement is not birefringent, and histologically birefringent material is indicative of wear debris from HDP.

- After loosening of a cemented component, histological characteristics of the interface membrane between cement and bone can be characterized as three zones: (1) the synovial-like lining forming papillary folds supported by fibril vascular tissue at the cement-bone interface; (2) a layer containing histiocytes and giant cells, including particles of high-density polyethylene and PMMA; and (3) fibrocartilaginous layer blending into adjacent bone.

- The synovial-like lining of the interface between a loose cemented prosthesis and bone is enzymatically very active, and tissue culture reveals stellate cells are similar to rheumatoid synovial tissue. The membrane has the capacity to produce large amounts of prostaglandin E2 and collagenase, which can mediate resorption of bone and other connective tissues. It has been suggested the traction or motion produces a biological signal that causes differentiation and organization of cells into synovial tissue. Lysosomal activities as indicated by acid phosphatase or naphtholesterase were especially strong in microphage and giant cell populations of these membranes. The connective tissue cells within the membrane were also reactive for acid phosphatase but did not appear to change in activity regardless of their location within the membrane.

- The presence of PMMA or HDP particles seemed to cause activation of microphage or giant cells with resulting strong lysosomal response especially in those cells with phagocytized wear particles. Beta galactosidase, an enzyme specifically synthesized by microphages during activation, was a special marker for cells that had phagocytized wear products. Therefore, lysosomal enzyme activity demonstrated focal areas of cellular response within an individual membrane.

- Massive osteolysis, also known as *aggressive granu-*

lomatosis, is a benign noninflammatory tissue reaction that has been observed in loose or, at times, in well-fixed prostheses. This phenomenon, when it occurs without detectable loosening of the prosthesis, is extremely rare and is caused by egress of the particulates HDP and PMMA in an area distant from the source of their origin because of hydrostatic pressure from the joint space.

■ Osteolysis caused by HDP wear particles is the ultimate cause of the failure of total hip arthroplasty in the long term, especially in young and active individuals.

■ Although most plastics implanted in the body have provoked sarcomas in rats and mice, in large studies involving humans, only a few cases of associated malignancy have been documented. Although total hip arthroplasty is one of the most commonly performed orthopaedic procedures in the Western world, only a few neoplastic lesions have been reported as having initiated from the site of arthroplasty.

■ A higher reaction to the particles released from titanium alloy than other metals has been reported. Titanium is particularly prone to release of a large amount of particles into the tissue because of wear of the articulating surface, poor design of the component, or mishandling at surgery.

■ Well-fixed cemented implants have relatively low metal levels in the synovial fluid and the surrounding tissues. However, when the implants become loose, a large amount of metal particles is released that increases the level of metals in the synovial fluid and the surrounding tissues. Studies comparing well-fixed and loose chromium-cobalt implants have shown a 20-fold increase in metal levels with the loose component.

■ Cellular toxicity from various metals has been demonstrated by culture of human synovial fibroblasts. The most potentially harmful components were those of cobalt-chromium alloys, nickel from stainless steel, and vanadium from titanium alloy.

■ Metal sensitivity related to joint arthroplasty has been especially pronounced in metal-to-metal prostheses that were capable of producing wear particles of chromium and cobalt in solution. Also, traces of chromium and cobalt have been found in the blood and urine, along with high tissue concentration around these prostheses.

■ It has been suggested that skin sensitivity in patients whose prostheses became loose was responsible for bone necrosis leading to loosening and failure of the implant. Others have reported skin eruptions and eczema associated with metal sensitivity which were

cured after removal of the implant.

■ HDP remains the material of choice for bearing, although an increasing number of failed total hips have been caused by excess wear of HDP.

■ *Polyethylene* is a generic term referring to a large group of materials that may have similar nominal chemical compositions but with different properties because of different structural make-up. Therefore a considerable variability in the wear of this material should be expected. Another variable that influences the structural and mechanical properties of polyethylene is the method of sterilization. For example, radiation may lead to degradation and cross-linking.

■ There appear to be several mechanisms for wear of HDP in human hip joints. These include abrasive wear, fatigue wear, and possibly corrosive wear. Fretting fatigue is also commonly present.

■ A high penetration rate of femoral head may be a major factor in limiting the life of the total hip arthroplasty. A positive correlation between the depth of socket penetration and socket loosening has been established. It may be caused by a biological response to the particles of HDP in addition to a progressive penetration of the head, which causes restriction of movement from the neck-socket impingement and may cause a "shock load" and thus loosening of the cup.

■ Wear of the external surface of the cup against the bone can produce a large amount of HDP particles. Incidence of the socket wear at the external surface of Charnley low-friction arthroplasty was documented in one third of sockets revised at surgery. This observation is in contrast to earlier views that loosening was caused by severe tissue reaction of the cemented socket, that was caused by wear debris presumably entering into the space between the bone and cement.

■ A positive correlation between radiographic and real wear of HDP sockets has been established. To make accurate measurements of wear by radiopaque, the cement used in arthroplasty must be radiopaque, a radiographic marker must be incorporated on the cup, anteversion of the cup as implanted at surgery must be known, the relationship of the x-ray tube to the hip must be correct, and metal backing must not be present under acetabular component.

■ Several clinical studies on the wear based on the postoperative radiographs reveal a lack of correlation between weight and physical activity and a considerable variation in wear in young patients associated with socket demarcation. Male patients were more at risk for wear than females except for category A (those with unilateral hip disease and no other disability).

- There was a suggestion that rate of wear after 5 years diminishes, but a prediction of the pattern of wear rate in a "high-wear group" was not possible. The average rate of wear of Charnley total hip with a 22.5 mm diameter femoral head was 0.19 per year with a range of 0.52 ml per year to 0.017 ml per year. The amount of wear (the mean penetration based on the measurements of explanted cups at the time of revision) was 1.69 ml and the mean penetration rate was 0.21 per year (range from less than 0.005 ml to 0.6 ml per year).

- Explanted cups have shown several types of damage: socket erosion, rim wear, cement ingress, cratering, dislocation, and articular surface scoring. Frequently found damage to the femoral head of the prosthesis and presence of barium sulfate used in cement for radiographic contrast may explain in part marked variability of the wear in explanted sockets.

- At the time of this writing, reinforcement of the cup by a metal shell seems to affect the fixation of the cemented cups and also appears to detrimentally affect the wear of the HDP. More research is needed to verify the role of metal backing of the acetabular cup as related to the wear of HDP.

REFERENCES

1. **Agins HJ, Alcock NW, Bansal M, et al:** Metallic wear in failed titanium-alloy total hip replacements. A histological and quantitative analysis, *J Bone Joint Surg* 70:347, 1988.
2. **Albrektsson T, Linder L:** A method for short- and long-term *in vivo* study of the bone-implant interface, *Clin Orthop* 159:269, 1981.
3. **Albrektsson T, Linder L:** A method for *in vivo* observations of cement-bone interface, *Adv Biomat* 3:309, 1982.
4. **Albrektsson T, Linder L:** Bone injury caused by curing bone cement. A vital microscopic study in the rabbit tibia, *Clin Orthop* 183:280, 1984.
5. **Albrektsson T, Branemark PI, Hansson HA, et al:** Osseointegrated titanium implants, Requirements for ensuring a long-lasting, direct bone-to-implant anchorage in man, *Acta Orthop Scand* 52:155, 1981.
6. **Andersson SM, Nilsson BE:** Changes in bone mineral content following ligamentous knee injuries, *Med Sci Sports* 11:351, 1979.
7. **Andersson SM, Nilsson BE:** Changes in bone mineral content following tibia shaft fractures, *Clin Orthop* 144:226, 1979.
8. **Annual Book of ASTM Standards:** *Medical devices,* vol 13.01, Philadelphia, 1984, American Society for Testing and Materials.
8a. **Anthony PP, Gie GA, Howie CR, et al:** Localized endosteal bone lysis in relation to the femoral components of cemented total hip arthroplasties, *J Bone Joint Surg* 72[Br]:971, 1990.
9. **Arden GP, Bywaters EGL:** Tissue reaction. In Arden GP, Ansell BM, editors: *Surgical management of juvenile chronic polyarthritis,* London, 1978, Academic Press.
10. **Bagò-Gramell J, Aquirre-Canyadell M, Nardi J, et al:** Malignant fibrous histiocytoma of bone at the site of a total hip arthroplasty. A case report, *J Bone Joint Surg* 66[Br]:38, 1984.
11. **Banks WC, Morris ERL, Herron MR, et al:** Osteogenic sarcoma associated with internal fracture fixation in two dogs, *J Am Veter Med Assoc* 167:166, 1975.
12. **Barclay AE:** *Micro-arteriography and other radiological techniques employed in biological research,* Oxford, 1951, Blackwell Scientific Publications.
13. **Barranco VP, Solomon H:** Eczematosis dermatitis from nickel, *JAMA* 220:1244, 1972.
14. **Bartalozzi A, Black J:** Chromium concentrations in serum, blood clot and urine from patients following total hip arthroplasty, *Biomateriuls* 6:2, 1985.
15. **Bechtel A, Willert HA, Freech HA:** Bestimmung des Monomergehalts von Metachrylsäuremetylester in Knochenmark. Fett und Blut nach dem Aushärten verschiedener "Knochenzemente," *Chromatographia* 5:226, 1973.
16. **Bell RS, Ha'eri GB, Goodman SB, et al:** Case Report 246: osteolysis of the ilium associated with a loose acetabular cup following total hip arthroplasty, secondary to foreign body reaction to polyethylene and methyl methacrylate, *Skeletal Radiol* 18:201, 1983.
17. **Benson MKD, Goodwin PG, Brostoff J:** Metal sensitivity in patients with joint replacement arthroplasties, *Br Med J* 4:374, 1975.
17a. **Betts F, et al:** Cobalt-alloy metal debris in periarticular tissues from total hip revision arthroplasties: metal contents and associated histological findings, *Clin Orthop* 276:75, 1992.
18. **Biozzini G, Halpern BN, Benacerraf B, et al:** Phagocytic activity of the recticulo-endothelial system in experimental infections. In Halpern BN, Benacerraf B, Delafresnaye JF, editors: *Physiopathology of the reticulo-endothelial system.* Symposium on the physiopathology of the reticulo-endothelial system, Oxford, 1957, Blackwell Scientific Publications.
19. **Björk L, Lemperg R:** Radiographic determination of the bone mineral content in amputation stumps, *Acta Radiol* 6:575, 1967.
20. **Black J:** Systemic effects of biomaterials, *Biomaterials* 5:11, 1984.
21. **Black J:** Metallic ion release and its relationship to oncogenesis. In The Hip Society: *The hip: proceedings of the thirteenth open scientific meeting of The Hip Society,* St Louis, 1985, Mosby–Year Book.
22. **Black J:** Does corrosion matter? *J Bone Joint Surg* 70[Br]:517, 1988.
23. **Black J, et al:** Metallosis associated with a stable titanium-alloy femoral component in total hip replacement, *J Bone Joint Surg* 72:126, 1990.
23a. **Bloch B, Hastings GW:** *Plastics in surgery,* Springfield, Ill, 1967, Charles C Thomas.
24. **Bobyn JD, Pilliar RM, Cameron HU, et al:** The optimum pore size for the fixation of porous-surfaced metal implants by the ingrowth of bone, *Clin Orthop* 150:263, 1980.
25. **Bobyn JD, Pilliar RM, Cameron HU, et al:** Osteogenic phenomena across bone-implant spaces with porous surfaced intramedullary implants, *Acta Orthop Scand* 52:145, 1981.
26. **Borowy KH, Kramer H-H:** On the properties of a new titanium alloy (TiA15Fe2.5) as implant material. In Lutjering G, Zwicker U, Bunk W, editors: *Titanium*

science and technology, vol II, Munich, 1985, Deutsche Gesellschaft für Metallkunde, EV.

27. **Bothe RT, Beaton LE, Davenport HA:** Reaction of bone to multiple metallic implants, *Surg Gynecol Obstet* 71:598, 1940.

28. **Brand KG:** Foreign body-induced sarcomas. In Becker FF, editor: *Cancer, a comprehensive treatise,* New York, 1975, Plenum Press.

29. **Brien NW, et al:** Metal levels in cemented total hip arthroplasty: a comparison of well-fixed and bone implants, *Clin Orthop* 275:66, 1992.

30. **Brookes M:** *The blood supply of bone: an approach to blood biology,* London, 1971, Butterworth & Co, Ltd.

31. **Buchanan RA, Rigney ED Jr, Williams JM:** Ion implantation of surgical Ti-6A1-4V for improved resistance to wear-accelerated corrosion, *J Biomed Mater Res* 21:355, 1987.

32. **Buchanan RA, Rigney ED Jr, Williams JM:** Wear-accelerated corrosion of Ti-6A1-4V and nitrogen-ion-implanted Ti-6A1-4V: mechanisms and influence of fixed-stress magnitude, *J Biomed Mater Res* 21:367, 1987.

33. **Buchert PK, Vaughn BK, Mallory TH, et al:** Excessive metal release due to loosening and fretting of sintered particles on porous-coated hip prostheses. Report of two cases, *J Bone Joint Surg* 68:606, 1986.

34. **Bullough PG:** Principles of cell injury, inflammation and repair. In Cruess RL, Rennie WRJ, editors: *Adult orthopaedics,* New York, 1984, Churchill Livingstone.

35. **Bullough PG, DiCarlo EF, Hansraj KK, et al:** Pathologic studies of total joint replacement, *Orthop Clin North Am* 19:611, 1988.

36. **Burstein AH:** Structural mechanical properties of polyethylene acetabular cups. In The Hip Society: *The hip: proceedings of the ninth open scientific meeting of The Hip Society,* St Louis, 1981, Mosby–Year Book.

37. **Cahoon JR, Paxton HW:** Metallurgical analyses of failed orthopedic implants, *J Biomed Mater Res* 2:1, 1968.

38. **Calnan J:** The use of inert plastic material in reconstructive surgery. I. A biological test for tissue acceptance. II. Tissue reactions to commonly used materials, *Br J Plast Surg* 16:1, 1963.

39. **Cameron HU, Pilliar RM, McNab L:** The effect of movement on the bonding of porous metal to bone, *J Biomed Mater Res* 7:301, 1973.

40. **Carter RL, Roe FJC:** Induction of sarcomas in rats by solid and fragmented polyethylene: experimental observations and clinical implications, *Br J Cancer* 23:401, 1969.

41. **Chambers TJ:** The cellular basis of bone resorption, *Clin Orthop* 151:283, 1980.

42. **Charnley J:** Tissue reactions to polytetrafluorethylene. Letters to the editors. *Lancet* 2:1379, 1963.

43. **Charnley J:** *Acrylic cement in orthopedic surgery,* Baltimore, 1970, Williams & Wilkins.

44. **Charnley J:** Fracture of femoral prostheses in total hip replacement: a clinical study, *Clin Orthop* 111:105, 1975.

45. **Charnley J:** Proceedings: the histology of loosening between acrylic cement and bone, *J Bone Joint Surg* 57[Br]:245, 1975.

46. **Charnley J:** In *Robert Jones lecture, combined meeting,* London, 1976.

47. **Charnley J:** *Low friction arthroplasty of the hip: theory and practice,* Berlin, 1979, Springer-Verlag.

48. **Charnley J:** The future of total hip replacement. In The Hip Society: *The hip: proceedings of the tenth open scientific meeting of The Hip Society,* St Louis 1982, Mosby–Year Book.

49. **Charnley J, Crawford WJ:** Histology of bone in contact with self-curing acrylic cement. In Proceedings and Reports of Universities, Colleges, Councils and Associations: British Orthopaedic Association, *J Bone Joint Surg* 50[Br]:228, 1968.

50. **Charnley J, Cupic Z:** The nine and ten year results of the low-friction arthroplasty of the hip, *Clin Orthop* 95:1, 1973.

51. **Charnley J, Follacci FM, Hammond BT:** The long-term reaction of bone to self-curing acrylic cement, *J Bone Joint Surg* 50[Br]:822, 1968.

52. **Charnley J, Halley DK:** Rate of wear in total hip replacement, *Clin Orthop* 112:170, 1975.

53. **Charosky CB, Bullough PG, Wilson PD Jr:** Total hip replacement failures: a histological evaluation, *J Bone Joint Surg* 55:49, 1973.

54. **Christel P, Meunier A, Heller M, et al:** Mechanical properties and short-term in vivo evaluation of yttrium-oxide partially stabilized zirconia, *J Biomed Mater Res* 23:45, 1989.

55. **Christel P, Meunier A, Dorlot J-M, et al:** Biomechanical compatibility and design of ceramic implants for orthopaedic surgery. In Ducheyne P, Lemons JE, editors: Biceramics: material characteristics versus *in vivo* behavior. *Ann NY Acad Sci* 523:234, 1988.

56. **Clarke EGC, Hickman J, Collins DH, et al:** Discussion on metals and synthetic materials in relation to tissues, *Proc R Soc Med* 46:641, 1953.

57. **Cohen J:** Assay of foreign-body reaction, *J Bone Joint Surg* 41:152, 1959.

58. **Cohen J, Hammond G:** Corrosion in a device for fracture fixation, *J Bone Joint Surg* 41:524, 1959.

59. **Cohen J, Wulff J:** Clinical failure caused by corrosion of a vitallium plate. Case report, new testing methods for crevice corrosion and new techniques for fashioning cobalt chromium alloys to be used in surgical implants, *J Bone Joint Surg* 54:617, 1972.

60. **Coleman RF, Herrington J, Scales JT:** Concentration of wear products in hair, blood, and urine after total hip replacement, *Br Med J* 1:527, 1973.

60a. **Cook SD, Rena EA, Barrack RL, et al:** Clinical and metallurgical analysis of retrieved internal fixation devices, *Clin Orthop* 194:236, 1985.

60b. **Cornelis R:** Chromium revisited. In Bratten P, Schramel P, editors: Proceedings: international workshop. *Trace element analytical chemistry in medicine and biology,* Berlin, 1985, DeGruyter.

61. **Crowninshield RD:** Mechanical properties of porous metal total hip prostheses. In The American Academy of Orthopaedic Surgeons: *Instructional course lectures,* vol 35, St Louis, 1986, Mosby–Year Book.

62. **Danckwardt-Lillieström G, Lorenzi GL, Olcrud S:** Intramedullary nailing after reaming. An investigation on the healing process in osteotomized rabbit tibias, *Acta Orthop Scand (Suppl)* 134:Suppl 1 + , 1970.

63. **Danzig LA, Woo SL-Y, Akeson WH, et al:** Internal fixation plates after fifty-six years of implantation: report of a case, *Clin Orthop* 149:201, 1980.

64. **Deanin RD, Patel LB:** Structure, properties, and wear resistance of polyethylene, *Adv Polymer Friction Wear* 5[Br]:569, 1975.

65. **Delgado ER:** Sarcoma following a surgically treated fractured tibia. A case report. *Clin Orthop* 12:315, 1958.

66. **Deutman R, Mulder TK, Brian R, et al:** Metal sensitivity before and after total hip arthroplasty, *J Bone Joint Surg* 59:862, 1977.

67. **Dobbs HS, Minski MJ:** Metal ion release after total hip replacement, *Biomaterials* 1:193, 1980.

68. **Dobbs HS, Scales JT:** Behavior of commercially pure titanium and Ti-318 (Ti-6A1-4V) in orthopaedic implants. In Luckey HA, Kubli F Jr, editors: *Titanium alloys in surgical implants,* Philadelphia, 1983, American Society for Testing and Materials.

69. **Dodion P, Putz P, Amiri-Lamraski MH, et al:** Immunoblastic lymphoma at the site of an infected vitallium bone plate, *Histopathology* 6:807, 1982.

70. **Dörre E, Beutler H, Geduldig D:** Anforderungen an oxidkeramische Werkstoffe as Biomaterial für künstliche Gelenke, *Arch Orthop Unfall-Chir* 83:269, 1975.

71. **Doll R:** Cancer of the lung and nose in nickel workers, *Br J Industr Med* 15:217, 1958.

72. **Doty SB, Schofield BH:** Ultrahistochemistry of calcified tissues. In Dickson GR, editor: *Methods of calcified tissue preparation,* Amsterdam, 1984, Elsevier.

73. **Dowling JM, et al:** The characteristics of acetabular cups worn in the human body, *J Bone Joint Surg* 60[Br]:375, 1978.

74. **Draenert K:** Histomorphology of the bone-to-cement interface: remodeling of the cortex and revascularization of the medullary canal in animal experiments. In The Hip Society: *The hip: proceedings of the ninth open scientific meeting of The Hip Society,* St Louis, 1981, Mosby–Year Book.

75. **Dube VE, Fisher DE:** Hemangioendothelioma of the leg following metallic fixation of the tibia, *Cancer* 30:1260, 1972.

76. **Dumbleton JH, Black J:** *An introduction of orthopaedic materials,* Springfield, Ill, 1975, Charles C Thomas.

77. **Dumbleton JH, Shen C:** The friction and wear of very high molecular weight polyethylene, *J Applied Polymer Science* 18:3493, 1974.

78. **Dumbleton JH, Shen C, Miller EH:** A study of the wear of some materials in connection with total hip replacement, *Wear* 29:163, 1974.

79. **du Plessis TA, Grobbelaar CJ, Marais F:** The improvement of polyethylene prostheses through radiation crosslinking, *Radiat Phys Chem* 9:647, 1977.

80. **Edwards JCW, Sedgwick AD, Willoughby DA:** The formation of a structure with the features of synovial lining by subcutaneous injection of air: an *in vivo* tissue culture system, *J Pathol* 134:147, 1981.

81. **Eftekhar NS, Pawluk RJ:** The role of surgical preparation in acetabular cup fixation. In The Hip Society: *The hip: proceedings of the eighth open scientific meeting of The Hip Society,* St Louis, 1980, Mosby–Year Book.

82. **Eftekhar NS, Doty SB, Johnston AD, et al:** Prosthetic synovitis. In The Hip Society: *The hip: Proceedings of the thirteenth open scientific meeting of The Hip Society,* St Louis, 1985, Mosby–Year Book.

83. **Elson RA, Charnley J:** The direction of the resultant force in total prosthetic replacement of the hip joint, *Med Biol Engineering* 6:19, 1968.

84. **Eskola A, Santavirta S, Konttinen YT, et al:** Cementless revision of aggressive granulomatous lesions in hip replacements, *J Bone Joint Surg* 72[Br]:212, 1990.

85. **Evans EM:** Metal sensitivity as a cause of bone necrosis and loosening of the prostheses in total joint replacement, *J Bone Joint Surg* 56[Br]:626, 1974.

85a. **Fahrling GM, Greer K:** An improved bearing material for joint replacement prosthesics: carbon fiber reinforced ultrahigh-molecular weight polyethylene. In Hastings GW, Williams DF, editors: *Mechanical properties of biomaterials,* New York, 1980, John Wiley & Sons.

86. **Ferguson AB Jr, Laing PG, Hodge ES:** The ionization of metal implants in living tissues, *J Bone Joint Surg* 42:77, 1960.

87. **Fisher AA:** *Contact dermatitis,* ed 2, Philadelphia, 1973, Lea & Febiger.

88. **Fisher AA, Chargin L, Fleischmajer A, et al:** Pustular patch test reactions; with particular reference to those produced by ammonium fluoride, *AMA Arch Dermatol* 80:742, 1959.

89. **Fornasier VL, Cameron HU:** The femoral stem/cement interface in total hip replacement, *Clin Orthop* 116:248, 1976.

90. **Fraker AC, Ruff AW, Sung P, et al:** Surface preparation and corrosion behavior of titanium alloys for surgical implant. In Luckey HA, Kubli F Jr, editors: *Titanium alloys in surgical implants,* Philadelphia, 1983, American Society for Testing and Materials.

91. **Freeman MAR, Bradley GW, Revell PA:** Observations upon the interface between bone and polymethylmethacrylate cement, *J Bone Joint Surg* 64[Br]:489, 1982.

92. **Freeman MAR, Swanson SAV, Heath JC:** Study of the wear particles produced from cobalt-chromium-molybdenum-manganese total joint replacement prostheses, *Ann Rheum Dis* 28:Suppl:29, 1969.

93. **Fregert S, Hjorth N, Magnusson D, et al:** Epidemiology of contact dermatitis, *Trans St Johns Hosp Dermatol Soc* 55:17, 1969.

94. **Furst A:** An overview of metal carcinogenesis, *Adv Exp Med Biol* 91:1, 1977.

95. **Fuson RI, Bardos DL:** Improved properties of HIP Co-Cr-Me powder alloy, *Metal Powder Rep* 34:306, 1979.

96. **Gaschter A, Alroy J, Andersson GBJ, et al:** Metal carcinogenesis: a study of the carcinogenic activity of solid metal alloys in rats, *J Bone Joint Surg* 59:622, 1977.

97. **Galante JO, Rostoker W:** Wear in total hip prostheses. An experimental evaluation of candidate materials, *Acta Orthop Scand* (Suppl) 1:1, 1973.

98. **Galante JO, Rostoker W:** Wear rates of candidate materials for total hip arthroplasty. In The Hip Society: *The hip: proceedings of the first open scientific meeting of The Hip Society,* St Louis, 1973, Mosby–Year Book.

99. **Galante J, Rostoker W:** Materials, wear, and potential late complications. In American Academy of Orthopaedic Surgeons: *Instructional course lectures,* vol 23, St Louis, 1974, Mosby–Year Book.

100. **Galante JO:** Personal communications.

101. **Garvie RC, Urbani C, Kennedy DR, et al:** Biocompatibility of magnesia partially stabilized zirconia, *J Mater Sci* 19:3224, 1984.

102. **Gillespie WJ, Frampton CMA, Henderson RJ, et al:** The incidence of cancer following total hip replacement, *J Bone Joint Surg* 70[Br]:539, 1988.

103. **Gitelis S, Anderson GEJ, Galante JO, et al:** The effect of weight bearing on the bone-cement interface after total hip arthroplasty: an experimental study in dogs. In The Hip Society: *The hip: proceedings of the seventh scientific meeting of The Hip Society,* St Louis, 1979, Mosby–Year Book.

104. **Gitzen WH,** editor: *Alumina as a ceramic material,* Columbus, Ohio, 1970, American Ceramic Society.

105. **Goldring SR, Schiller AL, Roetke M, et al:** The synovial-like membrane at the bone-cement interface in loose total hip replacements and its proposed role in bone lysis, *J Bone Joint Surg* 65:575, 1983.

106. **Goodman SB, Fornasier VL, Kei J:** The effects of bulk versus particulate polymethylmethacrylate on bone, *Clin Orthop* 232:255, 1988.

107. **Goodman SB, Fornasier VL, Kei J:** The effects of bulk versus particulate ultra-high-molecular-weight polyethylene on bone, *J Arthroplasty* 3(Suppl),S41, 1988.

108. **Griffith MJ, Seidenstein MK, Williams D, et al:** Socket wear in Charnley low-friction arthroplasty of the hip, *Clin Orthop* 137:37, 1978.

109. **Griss P, Heimke G:** Biocompatibility of high density alumina and its applications in orthopaedic surgery. In Williams DF, editor, *Biocompatibility of clinical implant materials*, vol I, Boca Raton, 1981, CRC Press.

110. **Grobbelaar CJ, du Plessis TA, Marais F:** The radiation improvement of polyethylene prostheses. A preliminary study, *J Bone Joint Surg* 60[Br]:370, 1978.

111. **Hamblen DL, Carter RL:** Sarcoma and joint replacement, *J Bone Joint Surg* 66[Br]:625, 1984.

112. **Harris WH, Jasty M:** *Bone ingrowth into porous coated canine acetabular replacements: the effect of pore size, apposition, and dislocation.* The Hip Society: The Hip, St Louis, 1985, Mosby–Year Book.

113. **Harris WH, Schiller AL, Scholler JM, et al:** Extensive localized bone resorption in the femur following total hip replacement, *J Bone Joint Surg* 58:612, 1976.

114. **Harrison JW, McLain DL, Hohn RB, et al:** Osteosarcoma associated with metallic implants. Report of two cases in dogs. *Clin Orthop* 116:253, 1976.

115. **Haag M, Adler CP:** Malignant fibrous histiocytoma in association with hip replacement, *J Bone Joint Surg* 71[Br]:701, 1989.

116. **Heath JC:** The histogenesis of malignant tumours induced by cobalt in the rat, *Br J Cancer* 14:478, 1960.

117. **Heath JC, Freeman MAR, Swanson SAV:** Carcinogenic properties of wear particles from prostheses made in cobalt-chromium alloy, *Lancet* 1:564, 1971.

118. **Henrichsen E, Jansen K, Krogh-Poulsen W:** Experimental investigation of the tissue reaction to acrylic plastics, *Acta Orthop Scand* 22:141, 1952.

119. **Hoeppner DW, Goss GL:** Metallographic analysis of fretting fatigue damage in Ti-6A1-4V MA and 7075-T6 aluminum, *Wear* 27:175, 1974.

120. **Hoopes JE, Edgerton MT Jr, Shelley W:** Organic synthetics for augmentation mammaplasty: their relation to breast cancer, *Plast Reconstr Surg* 39:263, 1967.

121. **Howie DW, Vernon-Roberts B, Oakeshott R, et al:** A rat model of resorption of bone at the cement-bone interface in the presence of polyethylene particles, *J Bone Joint Surg* 70:257, 1988.

122. **Hudack S:** High chromium, low nickel steel in the operative fixation of fractures, *Arch Surg* 40:867, 1940.

123. **Hueper WC, Conway WD:** *Chemical carcinogenesis and cancers*, Springfield, Ill, 1965, Charles C Thomas.

124. **Hughes AW, Sherlock DA, Hamblen DL, et al:** Sarcoma at the site of a single hip screw. A case report, *J Bone Joint Surg* 69[Br](3):470, 1987.

125. **Isaacs GH, et al:** A tribiological study of reviewed hip prostheses, *Clin Orthop* 276:115, 1992.

126. **Johnston AD, Parisien MV:** Pathology of reactive (prosthetic) versus septic (revisionary) synovitis. In Eftekhar NS, editor: *Infection in joint replacement surgery: prevention and management*, St Louis, 1984, Mosby–Year Book.

127. **Jones DA, Lucas HK, O'Driscoll M, et al:** Cobalt toxicity after McKee hip arthroplasty, *J Bone Joint Surg* 57[Br]:289, 1975.

128. **Justy MJ, Floyd WE, Schiller AL, et al:** Localized osteolysis in stable, non-septic total hip replacement, *J Bone Joint Surg* 68:912, 1986.

129. **Krainess FE, Knapp WJ:** Strength of a dense alumina ceramic after aging, *J Biomed Mater Res* 12:241, 1978.

130. **Krause WR, Krug W, Miller J:** Strength of the cement-bone interface, *Clin Orthop* 163:290, 1982.

131. **Kummer FJ, Rose RM:** Corrosion of titanium/cobalt-chromium alloy couples, *J Bone Joint Surg* 65:1125, 1983.

132. **Kurokawa KM, Pawluk RJ, Eftekhar NS:** The response of canine bone to self-curing methyl methacrylate (unpublished data).

133. **Laing PG:** Compatibility of biomaterials, *Orthop Clin North Am* 4:249, 1973.

134. **Laing PG, Ferguson AB Jr, Hodge ES:** Tissue reaction in rabbit muscle exposed to metallic implants, *J Biomed Mater Res* 1:135, 1987.

135. **Lamovec J, Zidar A, Cuček-Pleničar M:** Synovial sarcoma associated with total hip replacement. A case report, *J Bone Joint Surg* 70:1558, 1988.

136. **Leake ES, Wright MJ, Gristima AG:** Comparative study of the adherence of alveolar and peritoneal macrophages, and of blood monocytes to methyl methacrylate, polyethylene, stainless steel, and Vitallium, *J Reticuloendothel Soc* 30:403, 1981.

137. **Lee YS, Pho RW, Nather A:** Malignant fibrous histiocytoma at site of metal implant, *Cancer* 54:2286, 1984.

138. **Leonard A, Gerber GB, Jaquet P:** Carcinogenicity, mutagenicity and teratogenicity of nickel, *Mutat Res* 87:1, 1981.

139. **Leonard A, Lauwerys RR:** Carcinogenicity and mutagenicity of chromium, *Mutat Res* 76:227, 1980.

140. **Leventhal GS:** Titanium, a metal for surgery, *J Bone Joint Surg* 33:473, 1951.

141. **Lindberg H, Nilsson B:** Changes in bone mineral content in the femur following total hip arthroplasty, *Clin Orthop* 183:276, 1984.

142. **Lindberg LT:** Replacement operation for infected total hip arthroplasty. In Eftekhar NS, editor: *Infection in joint replacement surgery: prevention and management*, St Louis, 1984, Mosby–Year Book.

143. **Linder L, Hansson HA:** Ultrastructural aspects of the interface between bone and cement in man: report of three cases, *J Bone Joint Surg* 65[Br]:646, 1983.

144. **Linder L, Romanus M:** Acute local tissue effects of polymerizing acrylic bone cement. An intravital microscopic study in the hamster's cheek pouch on the chemically induced microvascular changes, *Clin Orthop* 115:303, 1976.

145. **Lindwer J, Van Den Hooff A:** The influence of acrylic cement on the femur of the dog, *Acta Orthop Scand* 46:657, 1975.

146. **Lintner F, Zwetmuller K, Brand G:** Tissue reactions to titanium endoprostheses. Autopsy studies in four cases, *J Arthroplasty* 1:183, 1986.

147. **Ling RSM:** Observations on the fixation of implants to the bony skeleton, *Clin Orthop* 210:80, 1986.

148. **Lombardi AV Jr, et al:** Aseptic loosening in total hip arthroplasty secondary to osteolysis induced by wear debris from titanium-alloy modular femoral heads, *J Bone Joint Surg* 71:1337, 1989.

149. **Lord G, Bancel P:** The madreporic cementless total hip

arthroplasty: new experimental data and a seven-year clinical follow-up study, *Clin Orthop* 176:67, 1983.

150. **Lord G, Marotte JH, Blanchard JP, et al:** Cementless madreporic and polarised total hip prostheses: a ten-year review of 2688 cases, *French J Orthop Surg* 2(1)·82, 1988.

151. **Lorenz M, Semliesch M, Panis B, et al:** Fatigue strength of cobalt-base alloys with high corrosion resistance for artificial hip joints, *Eng Med* 7(4):241, 1978.

152. **Lucas LC, Buchanan RA, Lemons JE:** Investigations on the galvanic corrosion of multialloy total hip prostheses, *J Biomed Mater Res* 15:731, 1981.

152a. **Luckey TD, Venugopal B:** *Metal toxicity in mammals.* I: *Physiological and chemical basis for metal toxicity,* vol 1, New York, 1977, Plenum Press.

152b. **Ludinghausen M, von Meister P, Probst J:** Metallosis after osteosynthesis, *Pathol Eur* 5:307, 1970.

153. **Lundberg BJ, Nilsson BE:** Osteopenia in the frozen shoulder, *Clin Orthop* 60:187, 1968.

154. **Lux F, Zeisler R:** Investigations of the corrosive deposition of components of metal implants and of the behaviour of biological trace elements in metallosis tissue by means of instrumental multielement activation analysis, *J Radioanal Chem* 19:289, 1974.

155. **Madewell BK, Poot RR, Leighton RL:** Osteogenic sarcoma at the site of a chronic nonunion fracture and internal fixation device in a dog, *J Am Vet Med Assoc* 181:187, 1977.

156. **Maier HR, Stark N, Krauth A:** Reliability of ceramic-metallic hip joints based on strength analysis, proof, and structural testing. In Hastings GW, Williams DF, editors: *Mechanical properties of biomaterials,* Chichester, 1980, Wiley.

157. **Maloney WJ, Justy MJ, Rosenberg A, et al:** Bone lysis in well-fixed cemented femoral components, *J Bone Joint Surg* 72[Br]:966, 1990.

158. **Maloney WJ, Justy M, Harris WH, et al:** Endosteal erosion in association with stable uncemented femoral components, *J Bone Joint Surg* 72:1025, 1990.

159. **Malton KE, Nater JP, van Ketel WG:** *Patch testing guidelines,* Nijmegen, the Netherlands, 1976, Dekker and van da Vegt.

160. **Manley MT:** Biological accommodation of bone to hip implants. In Stillwell WT: *The art of total hip arthroplasty,* Orlando, 1987, Grune and Stratton.

161. **Marek M, Treharne RW:** An *in vitro* study of the release of nickel from two surgical implant alloys, *Clin Orthop* 167:291, 1982.

162. **Markolf KL, Amstutz HC:** Penetration and flow of acrylic bone cement, *Clin Orthop* 121:99, 1976.

163. **Martin A, Bauer TW, Manley MT, et al:** Osteosarcoma at the site of total hip replacement. A case report, *J Bone Joint Surg* 70:1561, 1988.

164. **Matthews FD, Greer KW, Armstrong DL:** The effect of nitrogen ion implantation on the abrasive wear resistance of the Ti-6A1-4V/UHMWPE couple, *Mater Res Soc Sympos Proc* 55:243, 1986.

165. **McDonald I:** Malignant lymphoma associated with internal fixation of a fractured tibia, *Cancer* 48:1009, 1981.

166. **McDougall A:** Malignant tumour at site of bone plating, *J Bone Joint Surg* 38[Br]:709, 1956.

167. **Maguire JK Jr, Coscia MF, Lynch MH:** Foreign body reaction to polymeric debris following total hip arthroplasty, *Clin Orthop* 216:213, 1987.

168. **McKee GK:** McKee Farrar total prosthetic replacement of the hip. In Jayson M, editor: *Total hip replacement,* London, 1971, Sector Publishing, Ltd.

169. **McKellop H, Clarke I, Markolf K, et al:** Friction and wear properties of polymer, metal and ceramic prosthetic joint materials evaluated on a multichannel screening device, *J Biomed Mater Res* 15:619, 1981.

170. **McKellop H, Clarke I:** Wear of artificial joint materials in laboratory tests, *Acta Orthop Scand* 59:349, 1988.

171. **McKellop H, Kirkpatrick J, Markolf K, et al:** Abrasive wear of Ti-6A1-4V prostheses by acrylic cement particles, *Trans Orthop Res Soc* 5:96, 1980.

172. **McKellop H, Clarke I, Markolf K, et al:** Friction and wear properties of polymer, metal and ceramic joint materials evaluated on a multichannel screening device, *J Biomed Mater Res* 15:619, 1981.

173. **McKenzie AW, Aitken CVE, Ridadill-Smith R:** Urticaria after insertion of Smith-Petersen Vitallium nail, *Br Med J* 4:36, 1967.

174. **Mears DC:** The use of dissimilar metals in surgery, *J Biomed Mater Res* 9:133, 1975.

175. **Meachim G:** Histological interpretation of tissue changes adjacent to orthopaedic implants. In Williams D, editor: *Biocompatibility of implant materials,* London, 1976, Sector Publishing.

176. **Memoli VA, Urban R, Alroy J, et al:** Malignant neoplasms associated with orthopedic implant materials in rats, *J Orthop Res* 4:346, 1986.

176a. **Mendes DG, Walker PS, Figarola F, et al:** Total surface hip replacement in the dog: a clinical and pathological study. In Proceedings of the Orthopaedic Research Society, *J Bone Joint Surg* 54:1124, 1972.

177. **Merger M, Adinger F:** Influence of technological parameters on the fatigue strength of Ti5A12.5 Fe — a new material for endoprostheses. In Lutjering G, Zwicker U, Bunk W, editors: *Titanium science and technology,* vol 2, Munich, 1985, Deutsche Gesselschaft für Metallkunde.

178. **Merritt K, Brown SA:** Biological effects of corrosion products from metals. In Fraker AC, Griffin CD, editors: *Corrosion and degradation of implant materials: second symposium,* Philadelphia, 1985, American Society for Testing and Materials.

179. **Miller EH, Heidt RS, Fox BE, et al:** Endosteal surface temperature during total hip replacement, *Orthop Rev* 12(4):87, 1983.

180. **Miller JE, Heidt RS, Fox DE, et al:** A study of the interface between polymethylmethacrylate and living cortical bone under conditions of load bearing, *Trans Orthop Res Soc* 1:191, 1976.

181. **Mirra JM, Marder RA, Amstutz HC:** The pathology of failed total joint arthroplasty, *Clin Orthop* 170:175, 1982.

182. **Mirra J, Amstutz HC, Mates M, et al:** The pathology of the joint tissues and its clinical relevance in prosthesis failure, *Clin Orthop* 117:221, 1976.

183. **Morrall FR:** Cobalt alloys as implants in humans, *Materials* 384, 1966.

183a. **Mundy CR, Altman AJ, Gondck MD, et al:** On direct resorption of bone by human monocytes, *Science* 196:1107, 1977.

184. **Munro-Ashman AD, Miller AJ:** Rejection of metal to metal prosthesis and skin sensitivity to cobalt, *Contact Dermatitis* 2:65, 1976.

185. **Murray DW, Rae T, Rushton N:** The influence of the surface energy and roughness of implants on bone resorption, *J Bone Joint Surg* 71[Br]:632, 1989.

186. **Nilsson BE:** Post-traumatic osteopenia. A quantitative study of the bone mineral mass in the femur following fracture of the tibia in man using americium-241 as a

photon source, *Acta Orthop Scand* 37(Suppl) 91:1, 1966.

187. **Nilsson BE, Westlin NE:** Osteoporosis following injury to the semilunar cartilage, *Calcif Tissue Res* 4:185, 1969.

188. **Nilsson BE, Westlin NE:** Bone mineral content in the forearm after fracture of the upper limb, *Calcif Tissue Res* 22:329, 1977.

189. **Nussbaum HJ, Rose RM:** The effects of radiation sterilization on the properties of ultrahigh molecular weight polyethylene, *J Biomed Mater Res* 13:557, 1979.

190. **Oppenheimer BS, Oppenheimer ET, Danishefsky, et al:** Further studies of polymers as carcinogenic agents in animals, *Cancer Res* 15:333, 1955.

191. **Oppenheimer BS, Oppenheimer ET, Stout AP, et al:** Studies of the mechanism of carcinogenesis by plastic films, *Acta Un Int Cancer* 15:659, 1959.

192. **Park JB:** *Biomaterials science and engineering*, New York, 1984, Plenum Press.

193. **Paul HA, Bargar WL:** Histologic changes in the dog femur following total hip replacement with current cementing techniques, *J Arthroplasty* 1:5, 1986.

194. **Paul HA, Bargar WL:** Histological changes in the dog acetabulum following total hip replacement with current cementing techniques, *J Arthroplasty* 2:71, 1987.

195. **Pazzaglia U, Byers PD:** Fractured femoral shaft through an osteolytic lesion resulting from the reaction to a prosthesis. A case report, *J Bone Joint Surg* 66[Br]:337, 1984.

196. **Penman HG, Ring PA:** Osteosarcoma in association with total hip replacement, *J Bone Joint Surg* 66[Br]:632, 1984.

197. **Plenk H Jr:** Biocompatibility of ceramics in joint prostheses. In Williams DF, editor, *Biocompatibility of orthopaedic implants,* vol I, Boca Raton, 1982, CRC Press.

198. **Plitz W, Griss P:** Clinical, histomorphological and material related observations on removed alumina-ceramic hip joint components. In Weinstein A, Gibbons D, Brown S, et al, editors: *Implant retrieval: material and biological analysis,* Washington DC, 1981, Nat Bureau of Stds.

199. **Plitz W, Hoss HU:** Wear of alumina-ceramic hip joints: some clinical and tribiological aspects. In Winter G, Gibbons D, Plenk H Jr, editors: *Biomaterials,* Chichester, 1982, Wiley.

200. **Poss R, Thilly WG, Kaden DA:** Methylmethacrylate is a mutagen for *Salmonella typhimurium, J Bone Joint Surg* 61:1203, 1979.

201. **Radin EL, Rubin CT, Thrasher EL, et al:** Changes in the bone-cement interface after total hip replacement. An in vitro animal study, *J Bone Joint Surg* 64:1188, 1982.

202. **Rae T:** The toxicity of metals used in orthopaedic prostheses. An experimental study using culture human synovial fibroblasts, *J Bone Joint Surg* 63[Br]:435, 1981.

203. **Reinus WR, Gilula LA, Kyriakos M, et al:** Histiocytic reaction to hip arthroplasty, *Radiology* 155:315, 1985.

204. **Rhinelander FW:** Circulation in bone. In Bourne GH: *The biochemistry and physiology of bone,* ed 2, vol II, New York, 1972, Academic Press.

205. **Rhinelander FW:** Effects of medullary nailing on the normal blood supply of diaphyseal cortex. In American Academy of Orthopaedic Surgeons: *Instructional course lectures,* vol 22, St Louis, 1973, Mosby–Year Book.

206. **Rhinelander FW:** Tibial blood supply in relation to fracture healing, *Clin Orthop* 105:34, 1974.

207. **Rhinelander FW, Nelson CL:** Experimental implantation of porous materials into bones—proplast for low modulus fixation of prostheses, *Acta Orthop Belg* 40:771, 1974.

208. **Rhinelander FW, Rouweyha M, Milner JC:** Microvascular and histogenic responses to implantation of a porous ceramic into bone, *J Biomed Mater Res* 5:81, 1971.

209. **Rhinelander FW, Nelson CL, Stewart CL, et al:** Experimental reaming of the proximal femur and acrylic cement implantation: vascular and histologic effects, *Clin Orthop* 141:74, 1979.

210. **Rich A, Harris AK:** Anomalous preferences of cultured macrophages for hydrophobic and roughened substrata, *J Cell Sci* 50:1, 1981.

211. **Rietz KA:** Polymer osteosynthesis. III. Segmental resection of femur and fixation of endoprosthesis with methylmethacrylate in dogs, *Acta Chir Scand Suppl* 388:4, 1968.

212. **Ritter JE, Greenspan DC, Palmer RA, et al:** Use of fracture mechanics theory in lifetime predictions for alumina and bioglass-coated alumina, *J Biomed Mater Res* 13:251, 1979.

213. **Ritter MA, Meding JB:** Intraarticular trochanteric wire migration following bilateral total hip arthroplasty. A case report, *Orthopedics* 11:1295, 1988.

214. **Rooker GD, Wilkinson JD:** Metal sensitivity in patients undergoing hip replacement. A prospective study, *J Bone Joint Surg* 62[Br]:502, 1980.

215. **Rose RM, Radin EL:** Wear of polyethylene in the total hip prosthesis, *Clin Orthop* 170:107, 1982.

216. **Rose RM, Schiller AL, Radin EL:** Corrosion-accelerated mechanical failure of a Vitallium nail-plate, *J Bone Joint Surg* 54:854, 1972.

217. **Rose RM, Nussbaum HJ, Schneider H, et al:** On the true wear rate of ultra high-molecular-weight polyethylene in the total hip prosthesis, *J Bone Joint Surg* 62:534, 1980.

218. **Rostoker W, Galante JO:** Some new studies of the wear behavior of ultrahigh molecular weight polyethylene, *J Biomed Mater Res* 10:303, 1976.

219. **Rostoker W, Galante JO, Shen G:** Some mechanical properties of sintered fiber metal composites, *J Test Evaluation* 2:107, 1974.

220. **Rostoker W, Pretzel CW, Galante JO:** Couple corrosion among alloys for skeletal prostheses, *J Biomed Mater Res* 8:407, 1974.

221. **Rotblat J, editor:** *Aspects of medical physics: review of papers presented at the First International Conference on Medical Physics,* London, 1966, Taylor & Francis.

222. **Ryu RK, Bovill EG Jr, Skinner HB, et al:** Soft tissue sarcoma associated with aluminum oxide ceramic total hip arthroplasty. A case report, *Clin Orthop* 216:207, 1987.

223. **Santavirta S, Hoikka V, Eskola A, et al:** Aggressive granulomatous lesions in cementless total hip arthroplasty, *J Bone Joint Surg* 72[Br]:980, 1990.

224. **Santavirta S, Konttinen YT, Bergroth V, et al:** Aggressive granulomatous lesions associated with hip arthroplasty. Immunopathological studies, *J Bone Joint Surg* 72:252, 1990.

224a. **Scott WW Jr, Riley LH Jr, Derfman HD, et al:** Focal lytic lesions associated with femoral stem loosening in total hip prosthesis, *AJR* 144:977, 1985.

225. **Semlitsch M, Staub F, Weber H:** Development of a vital, high-strength wrought Ti-6A1-7Nb alloy for surgical implants. In Chrissel P, Meunier A, Lee AJC, editors: *Biological performance of biomaterials,* Amsterdam, 1985, Elsevier.

226. **Sew Hoy AL, Hedley AK, Clarke IC, et al:** The acetabular cement-bone interface in experimental arthroplasties in

dogs, *Clin Orthop* 155:231, 1981.

227. **Shaw BJ, Pessall N, Zervins A:** A crevice corrosion study of HS21 alloy in contact with Ti and Ti-6A1-4V. Scientific Paper 72-509-CRCOR-P1, Pittsburgh, 1972, Westinghouse Research Laboratories.

228. **Siddons AHM, MacArthur AM:** Carcinomata developing at the site of foreign bodies in the lung, *Br J Surg* 39:542, 1952.

229. **Sinibaldi K, Rosen H, Liu S-K, et al:** Tumors associated with metallic implants in animals, *Clin Orthop* 118:257, 1976.

230. **Sioshansi P:** Medical applications of ion beam processes, *Nucl Instr Meth Physics Res* B19/20:204, 1987.

231. **Slooff TJ:** *The influence of the acrylic cement on the fixation of the hip endoprosthesis,* doctoral dissertation, 1970, The Catholic University of Nigmegen.

232. **Slooff TJ:** The influence of acrylic cement, *Acta Orthop Scand* 42:465, 1971.

233. **Slooff TJ:** Experiments with acrylic cements. In *Orthopedic surgery and traumatology. Proceedings of the twelfth congress of SICOT,* Amsterdam, 1972, Excerpta Medics.

234. **Smethurst E:** A new stainless steel alloy for surgical implants compared to 316 S12, *Biomaterials* 2:116, 1981.

235. **Smith DJE, Hughes AN:** *The influence of frequency and cold work on the fatigue strength of 316 stainless steel in air and 0.17 M saline,* AWRE Rep 44/83/189. Aldermaston, Berkshire, 1977, Atomic Weapons Research Establishment.

236. **Smith GK, Black J:** Models for systemic effects for metallic implants. In Weinstein A, Horowitz E, Ruff AW, editors: *Retrieval and analysis of orthopaedic implants.* Proceedings of Symposium in March 1976. NBS special publication. Washington, DC, 1977, US Government Printing Office.

237. **Smith GK, Black J:** Estimation of in vivo type 316L stainless steel corrosion rate from blood transport and organ accumulation data. In Fraker AC, Griffith CD, editors: *Corrosion and degradation of implant materials.* 2nd Symposium, Philadelphia, 1985, American Society for Testing and Materials.

238. **Sorensen WG, Bloom JD, Kelly PJ:** The effects of intramedullary methylmethacrylate and reaming on the circulation of the tibia after osteotomy and plate fixation in dogs, *J Bone Joint Surg* 61:417, 1979.

239. **Spector M, Harmon SL, Kreutner A:** Characteristics of tissue growth into proplast and porous polyethylene implants in bone, *J Biomed Mater Res* 13:667, 1979.

240. **Spinelli R:** *A study of the interface between bone and acrylic cement by scanning electron microscopy,* Rome, 1975, Institute of Clinical Orthopaedics and Traumatology, University of Rome.

241. **Standard specification for thermomechanically processed cobalt-chromium-molybdenum alloy for surgical implant applications.** Designation: F 799-82. In *1984 annual book of ASTM standards,* vol 13.01. Medical devices, Philadelphia, 1984, American Society for Testing and Materials.

242. **Standard specification for wrought cobalt-chromium-tungsten-nickel alloy for surgical implant applications.** Designation: F 90-82. In *1984 annual book of ASTM standards,* vol 13.01. Medical devices, Philadelphia, 1984, American Society for Testing and Materials.

243. **Stinson NE:** The tissue reaction induced in rats and guinea-pigs by polymethylmethacrylate (acrylic) and stainless steel (18/8/Mo), *Br J Exp Pathol* 45:21, 1964.

244. **Stinson NE:** Tissue reaction induced in guinea-pigs by particulate polymethylmethacrylate, polythene and nylon of the same size range, *Br J Exp Pathol* 46:135, 1965.

245. **Sunderman FW Jr:** Carcinogenic effects of metals, *Fed Proc* 37:40, 1978.

246. **Sunderman FW Jr:** Recent advances in metal carcinogenesis, *Ann Clin Lab Sci* 14:93, 1984.

247. **Swann M:** Malignant soft-tissue tumour at the site of a total hip replacement, *J Bone Joint Surg* 66[Br]:629, 1984.

248. **Swanson SAV, Freeman MAR:** *The scientific basis of joint replacement,* New York, 1977, John Wiley & Sons.

249. **Swanson SAV, Freeman MAR, Heath JC:** *Laboratory tests on total joint replacement prostheses,* J Bone Joint Surg 55[Br].759, 1973.

250. **Tallroth K, Eskola A, Santavirta S, et al:** Aggressive granulomatous lesions after hip arthroplasty, *J Bone Joint Surg* 71[Br]:571, 1989.

251. **Tayton KJ:** Ewing's sarcoma at the site of a metal plate, *Cancer* 45:413, 1980.

252. **Traveniou SZM:** Irregularities in the wear of plastics materials in the hip joint, *Plastics Rubber* 1:194, 1976.

253. **Trueta J, et al:** *Studies of the renal circulation,* Oxford, 1947, Blackwell Scientific Publications.

254. **van der List JJJ, van Horn JR, Slooff TJJ, et al:** Malignant epithelioid hemangioendothelioma at the site of a hip prosthesis, *Acta Orthop Scand* 59:328, 1988.

255. **Venable CS, Stuck WG:** Three years' experience with Vitallium in bone surgery, *Ann Surg* 114:309, 1941.

256. **Vernon-Roberts D, Freeman MAR:** The tissue response to total joint replacement prostheses. In Swanson SAV, Freeman MAR, editors: *The scientific basis of joint replacement,* Wells UK, 1977, Pitman Medical.

256a. **Versieck J, Cornelis R:** Normal levels of trace elements in human blood plasma or serum, *Anal Chim Acta* 116:217, 1980.

257. **Walker PS, Bullough PG:** The effects of friction and wear in artificial joints, *Orthop Clin North Am* 4:275, 1973.

258. **Walker PS, Salvati E, Hotzler RK:** The wear on removed McKee-Farrar total hip prostheses, *J Bone Joint Surg* 56:92, 1974.

259. **Weber PC:** Epithelioid sarcoma in association with total knee replacement. A case report, *J Bone Joint Surg* 68[Br]:824, 1986.

260. **Weightman B:** Friction, lubrication and wear. In Swanson SAV, Freeman MAR, editors: *The scientific basis of joint replacement,* Tunbridge Wells, United Kingdom, 1977, Pitman Medical.

261. **Weightman BO, Paul H, Rose RM, et al:** A comparative study of total hip replacement prostheses, *J Biomech* 6:299, 1973.

262. **Westlin NE:** Loss of bone mineral after Colles' fracture, *Clin Orthop* 0(102):194, 1974.

263. **Williams DF:** Titanium as a metal for implantation. I. Physical properties. *J Med Eng Technol* 1:195, 1977.

264. **Williams JM, Buchanan RA:** Ion implantation of surgical Ti-6A1-4V alloy, *Mater Sci Eng* 69:237, 1985.

265. **Willert HG:** Reactions of the articular capsule to wear products of artificial joint prostheses, *J Biomed Mater Res* 11:157, 1977.

266. **Willert HG, Frech HA, Bechtel A:** *Measurements of the quantity of monomer leaching out of acrylic bone cement into the surrounding tissues during the process of polymerization,* Chicago, 1973, 166th National Meeting of the American Chemical Society.

267. **Willert HG, Ludwig J, Semlitsch M:** Reaction of bone to

methacrylate after hip arthroplasty: a long-term gross, light microscopic and scanning electron microscopic study, *J Bone Joint Surg* 56:1368, 1974.

268. **Willert HG, Bertram H, Buchhorn GH:** Osteolysis in alloarthroplasty of the hip. The role of ultra high molecular weight polyethylene wear particles, *Clin Orthop* 258:95, 1990.

269. **Willert HG, Semlitsch M:** Problems associated with the anchorage of artificial joints. In Schldach M, Hohmann D, editors: *Advances in artificial hip and knee joint technology*, New York, 1976, Springer-Verlag.

269a. **Willert HG, Semlitsch M:** Reaction of the articular capsule to artificial joint prostheses. In Williams D, editor: *Biocompatibility of implant materials*, Tunbridge Wells, United Kingdom, 1977, Pitman Medical.

270. **Wiltse LL, Hall RH, Stenehjem JC:** Experimental studies regarding possible use of self-curing acrylic in orthopaedic surgery, *J Bone Joint Surg* 39:961, 1957.

271. **Winter GD:** Wear and corrosion products in tissues and the reactions they provoke. In Williams D, editor: *Biocompatibility of implant materials*, London, 1976, Sector Publishing.

272. **Woodman JL, Black J, Jiminez SA:** Isolation of serum protein organometallic corrosion products from 316LSS and HS-21 in vitro and in vivo, *J Biomed Mater Res* 18:99, 1984.

273. **Woodman JL, Black J, Nunamaker DM:** Release of cobalt and nickel from a new total finger joint prosthesis made of Vitallium, *J Biomed Mater Res* 17:655, 1983.

274. **Woodman JL, Jacobs JJ, Galante JO, et al:** Titanium release from fiber metal composites in baboons: a long term study, *Trans Orthop Res Soc* 7:166, 1982.

275. **Woodman JL, Jacobs JJ, Galante JO, et al:** Metal ion release from titanium-based prosthetic segmental replacements of long bones in baboons: a long-term study, *J Orthop Res* 1:421, 1984.

276. **Wroblewski BM:** Wear of high-density polyethylene on bone and cartilage, *J Bone Joint Surg* 61[Br]:498, 1979.

277. **Wroblewski BM:** Charnley low-friction arthroplasty. Review of the past, present, status and prospects for the future, *Clin Orthop* 210:37, 1986.

278. **Wroblewski BM:** Direction and rate of socket wear in Charnley low-friction arthroplasty, *J Bone Joint Surg* 67[Br]:757, 1985.

279. **Wroblewski BM:** 15-21-year results of the Charnley low-friction arthroplasty, *Clin Orthop* 211:30, 1986.

280. **Wroblewski BM:** Wear and loosening of the socket in the Charnley low-friction arthroplasty, *Orthop Clin North Am* 19:627, 1988.

281. **Wroblewski BM, Lynch M, Atkinson JR, et al:** External wear of the polyethylene socket in cemented total hip arthroplasty, *J Bone Joint Surg* 69[Br]:61, 1987.

282. **Zierold AA:** Reaction of bone to various metals, *Arch Surg* 9:365, 1924.

ADDITIONAL READINGS

Atkinson JR, Dowson D, Isaac GH, et al: Laboratory wear tests and clinical observations of the penetration of femoral heads into acetabular cups in total replacement hip joints. II. A microscopical study of the surfaces of Charnley polyethylene acetabular sockets, *Wear* 104:217, 1985.

Atkinson JR, Dowson D, Isaac GH, et al: Laboratory wear tests and clinical observations of the penetration of femoral heads into acetabular cups in total replacement hip joints. III. The measurement of internal volume changes in explanted Charnley sockets after 2-16 years in vivo and the determination of wear factors, *Wear* 104:225, 1985.

Black J, Maltin EC, Coleman H, et al: Serum concentrations of chromium, cobalt and nickel after total hip replacement: a six month study, *Biomaterials* 4:160, 1983.

Black J, Oppenheimer P, Morris DM, et al: Release of corrosion products by F-75 cobalt base alloy in the rat. III. Effects of a carbon surface coating, *J Biomed Mater Res* 21:1213, 1987.

Bullough PG: Tissue reaction to wear debris generated from total hip replacements. In The Hip Society: *The hip: proceedings of the first open scientific meeting of The Hip Society*, St Louis, 1973, Mosby–Year Book.

Charnley J: A biomechanical analysis of the use of cement to anchor the femoral head prosthesis, *J Bone Joint Surg* 47[Br]:354, 1965.

Charnley J: An artificial bearing in the hip joint: implications in biological lubrication, *Fed Proc* 25:1079, 1966.

Charnley J, Kamangar A, Longfield MD: The optimum size of prosthetic heads in relation to the wear of plastic sockets in total replacement of the hip, *Med Biol Engin* 7:31, 1969.

Clarke JC, Black K, Rennie C, et al: Can wear in total hip arthroplasties be assessed from radiographs? *Clin Orthop* 121:126, 1976.

Crock HV, Crock C: *The blood supply of the lower limb bones in man*, Edinburgh, 1967, E & S Livingstone Ltd.

Danckwardt-Lilliestrom G: Reaming of the medullary cavity and its effect on diaphyseal bone. A fluorochromic, microangiographic and histologic study on the rabbit tibia and dog femur, *Acta Orthop Scand* (Suppl) 128:Suppl − 1 +, 1969.

DeLee JG, Charnley J: Radiological demarcation of cemented sockets in total hip replacement, *Clin Orthop* 121:20, 1976.

Follacci FM, Hammond BT, Charnley J: The long-term reaction of bone to self-curing acrylic cement, *J Bone Joint Surg* 50[Br]:822, 1968.

Gitelis S: The effects of weight bearing on the bone-cement interface after total hip arthroplasty, *Proc Inst Med Chi* 32:95, 1979.

Hodgkinson JP, Shelley P, Wroblewski BM: The correlation between the roentgenographic appearance and operative findings at the bone-cement junction of the socket in Charnley low friction arthroplasty, *Clin Orthop* 228:105, 1988.

Howie DW, Vernon-Roberts B: Long-term effects of intraarticular cobalt-chrome alloy wear particles in rats, *Arthroplasty* 8:327, 1988.

Isaac GH, Atkinson JR, Dowson D, et al: The role of cement in the long term performance and premature failure of Charnley low friction arthroplasties, *Eng Med* 15:19, 1986.

Issac GH, Atkinson JR, Dowson D, et al: The causes of femoral head roughening in explanted Charnley hip prostheses, *Eng Med* 16:167, 1987.

Jones LC, Hungerford DS: Cement disease, *Clin Orthop* 225:192, 1987.

Lipsky PE, Jasin HE: Monocytes and macrophages. In McCarty DJ, editor: *Arthritis and allied conditions*, Philadelphia, 1979, Lea & Febiger.

Livermore J, Ilstrup D, Morrey B: Effect of femoral head size on wear of the polyethylene acetabular component, *J Bone Joint Surg* 72:518, 1990.

McKellop HA: Metallic wear in total knee replacements. In Goldberg VM, editor: *Controversies of total knee arthroplasty*, New York, 1991, Raven.

McKellop HA, Röstlund TV: The wear behavior of ion-implanted Ti-6Al-4V against UHMW polyethylene, *J Biomed Mater Res* 24:1413, 1990.

McKellop HA, Sarmiento A, Schwinn, CP, et al: In vivo wear of titanium-alloy hip prostheses, *J Bone Joint Surg* 72:512, 1990.

Nusbaum HJ, Rose RM, Paul IC, et al: Wear mechanisms for ultrahigh molecular weight polyethylene in the total hip prosthesis, *J Appl Polymer Sci* 23:777, 1979.

Rhinelander FW, Baragry RA: Microangiography in bone healing. I. Undisplaced closed fractures, *J Bone Joint Surg* 44:1273, 1962.

Rook AJ, Wilkinson DS, Ebling FJG: *Textbook of dermatology*, vol 1, ed 2, Oxford, 1972, Blackwell Scientific Publications.

Rose RM, Nussbaum HJ, Crugnula A, et al: The effect of ionizing radiation on ultrahigh molecular weight polyethylene. In *Transactions of the Third Annual Meeting of the Society for Biomaterials*, 1977.

Rose RM, Schneider H, Ries M, et al: A method for the quantitative recovery of polyethylene wear debris from the simulated service of total joint prostheses, *Wear* 51:77, 1978.

Rostoker W, Galante JO, Lercim P: Evaluation of couple/crevice corrosion by prosthetic alloys under in vivo conditions, *J Biomed Mater Res* 12:823, 1978.

Scales JT, Winter GD, Shirley HT: Corrosion of orthopaedic implants: screws, plates and femoral nail-plates, *J Bone Joint Surg* 41[Br]:810, 1959.

Spealman CR, Main RJ, Haag HB, et al: Monometric methyl methacrylate: studies on toxicity, *Ind Med* 14:292, 1945.

Trueta J: *Studies of the development and decay of the human frame*, London, 1968, William Heinemann Ltd.

Trueta J, Cavadias AX: Vascular changes caused by the Kuntscher type of nailing: an experimental study in rabbits, *J Bone Joint Surg* 37[Br]:492, 1955.

Venable CS, Stuck WG, Beach A: The effects on bone of presence of metals: based on electrolysis; experimental study, *Ann Surg* 105:917, 1937.

Willert HG, Bertram H, Buckhorn GH: Osteolysis in alloarthroplasty of the hip. The role of bone cement fragmentation, *Clin Orthop* 258:108, 1990.

Wroblewski BM: Charnley low-friction arthroplasty in patients under the age of 40 years. In Sevastik J, Goldie I, editors: *The young patient with degenerative hip disease*, Stockholm, 1985, Almqvist & Wilsell International.

Wroblewski BM: *Revision surgery in THA*, Berlin, 1990, Springer-Verlag.

See Chapters 5, Acrylic Cement: Properties and Application; and 32, Dislocation and Instability for additional information.

CHAPTER FIVE

Acrylic Cement: Properties and Application

- There is no doubt that in orthopaedic surgery acrylic cement is going to be widely used in many different parts of the world; there is equally no doubt that its use by uninformed operators will produce complications which might seriously threaten its reputation and might hold back the progress of science.
  Sir John Charnley

Acrylic cement has been used in orthopaedics since its introduction by Sir John Charnley 30 years ago, and it has remained an important tool for fixation of bone implants.

The surgeon must thoroughly understand the background and properties of self-curing acrylic cement to appreciate the mechanism of fixation and the biological interaction between bone and cement and to deal with problems arising from defective fixation of a total hip prosthesis related to methods of fastening. Space limits a complete account of self-curing cement; the reader is strongly urged to review Charnley's original report of its use in orthopaedic surgery[30] and the appropriate references at the end of this chapter. Some aspects of acrylic cement are also discussed in Chapters 4 and 6.

HISTORICAL BACKGROUND

Acrylic cement was first synthesized in 1843.[119] Ester-saturated ethyl methacrylate was prepared in 1865 and 1877, at which time investigators observed its tendency to polymerize. Industrial techniques for polymerization of cement were developed by Rohm and Haas in Germany at the turn of the century, and by 1927, the first commercially produced acrylic ester polymer was available. Polymethyl methacrylate (PMMA) was developed in Britain principally by Hill and Crawford.[106] PMMA can spontaneously polymerize, but the reaction is very slow. However, heat, ultraviolet light, or chemical activating agents accelerate polymerization. Heat

is used for commercial polymerization of MMA to form Plexiglas (Rohm & Haas), Perspex (ICI, Ltd.), and Lucite (Dupont).

Heat-cured MMA was first used in the human body as a denture base material in 1937.[155] Acrylic resin was first used in Germany during World War II and became available commercially as Rapid Paladon and subsequently as Simplex Pentrocryl. Since then, acrylic cement has been used in medicine, dentistry, neurosurgery, thoracic surgery, plastic surgery, ophthalmology, otology, and other areas.[28,35] In 1946, the Judet brothers introduced the heat-cured material for replacement of the femoral head, the first clinical application of such a large-sized acrylic prosthesis in hip surgery.[91]

In 1940, Zander[172] performed the first acrylic cranioplasty in humans; since that time many reports have been published on its use in such surgery.*

Cabanela and associates[22] have reported a long-term follow-up of patients with MMA cranioplasties. Dutton[55] has also used PMMA as intracranial investment, and in 1959 Knight[97] reported using self-curing MMA for more than 10 years to stabilize the spine, especially the cervical spine, with considerable success.

Among the first surgeons to use self-curing acrylic cement in hip surgery were Kiaer and Jansen of

---

* References 17, 54, 57, 95, 145, 189, 152, 153, 169, 170.

Copenhagen, before 1951. Kiaer[96] used PMMA to fix the hip prosthesis into the upper femur. Subsequently, Haboush[72] at the Hospital for Joint Diseases in New York used self-curing PMMA as a setting compound to distribute the load to the calcar of the prosthesis during extensive biomechanical analysis of the prosthetic femoral head replacement. However, he did not use the cement for transmitting the load through the intramedullary canal of the femur. Charnley's experience with acrylic cement started in 1958 after discussion with Dr. DC Smith, who was in charge of the Materials Laboratory of the Turner Dental School, Manchester University, England. He is responsible for the present popularity of the cement and for clarifying the principles and technique by which prosthetic arthroplasty fixation can be successfully achieved.[30–33,36,38] McKee and Watson-Farrar[114] and Müller[122] have attributed their successes to Charnley's advocacy of self-curing acrylic cement during the early development of total hip surgery. The Food and Drug Administration in the United States considers acrylic cement a "drug," and at the present time only one brand, Simplex cement, is approved for clinical use.†

CONSTITUENTS AND CHEMISTRY OF PMMA

The basic MMA polymer formula is $R \cdot CH_2 \cdot C(CH_3) \cdot COO(CH_3)$. The box at the right details the chemical formula. For orthopaedic surgery several acrylic products are available, which usually consist of separately packaged liquid monomer and sterile polymer powder. The different brands vary in their chemical composition, powder:liquid ratio, and consistency of powder. CMW* is used in Europe, and Charnley's work is based solely on the use of CMW cement. The bone cement presently available in the United States is Simplex P radiopaque.† The powder of Simplex P consists of fine granules of prepolymerized PMMA (15% W/W), copolymerized MMA styrene (75% W/W), and barium sulfate (10%). PMMA is produced by an aqueous redox system and is free from initiator residues. MMA styrene copolymer is produced by dispersion using benzoyl peroxide as the polymerization initiator and tertiary dodecyl mercaptan as the chain regulator.[4] A cellulose derivative is used as a dispersing agent. This copolymer contains small quantities of initiator and modifier residues but is free from dispersing agent residues. The total weight of the radiopaque bone cement powder is 40 gm per package; the powder without barium sulfate is also 40 gm. The latter, therefore, has relatively more prepolymerized

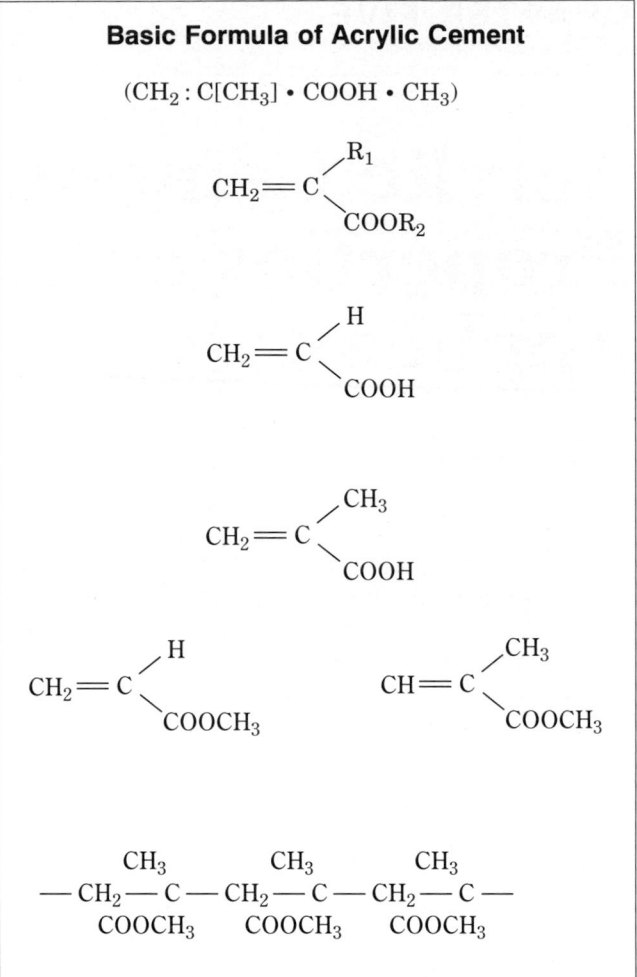

Basic Formula of Acrylic Cement

$(CH_2 : C[CH_3] \cdot COOH \cdot CH_3)$

---

* CMW Laboratories, Ltd., Blackpool, England.

† Northill Plastics, Inc., London, England.

PMMA (16.7% W/W) and MMA styrene copolymer (83.3% W/W).

The liquid monomer contains 97.4% V/V and has N,N-dimethyl-para-toluidine (DMPT) (2.6% V/V) and traces of hydroquinone (75 ± 15 ppm.). DMPT is the amine accelerator that permits the cold curing of acrylic cement; hydroquinone is added to prevent premature spontaneous polymerization of the monomer. The volume per vial is 20 ± 1 ml. The Simplex P is supplied already sterilized by gamma radiation. The liquid is sterilized by passing it through a Seitz bacterial filter.[3–5]

A suitable formulation for self-curing acrylic cement (according to Charnley and Smith[38]) consists of a liquid component of 97.9% MMA, 2% DMPT as initiator, and 0.1% hydroquinone as inhibitor.

The powder typically consists of 97% PMMA and 2% benzoyl peroxide as activator. Pigment and fillers constitute 1%.[38]

In collaboration with a dental manufacturing company (EMC), Charnley formulated the CMW cement used today in orthopaedic surgery. The powder is of low

Table 5-1 Chemical Composition of Two Acrylic Cements

Chemical composition	Simplex P radiopaque*	Zimmer low-viscosity cement†
Powder	75.0% wt/wt MMA styrene copolymer	89.25% wt/wt PMMA
	15.0% wt/wt PMMA	10.00% wt/wt barium sulfate
	10.0% wt/wt barium sulfate	0.75% wt/wt benzoyl peroxide
Liquid	97.4% vol/vol MMA	97.25% vol/vol MMA
	2.6% vol/vol *N,N*-DMPT	2.75% vol/vol *N,N*-DMPT
	75 ± 15 ppm hydroquinone	75 ± 10 ppm hydroquinone

Modified from Gates IE, Carter DR, Harris WH: Comparative fatigue behavior of different bone cements, *Clin Orthop* 189:294, 1984.

molecular weight in granular form (PMMA) with no other additives. The granules are formed in a dispersion medium by the "pearl polymerization" process. The liquid is first distilled to remove the hydroquinone inhibitor, which is then replaced by 0.02% ascorbic acid as an inhibitor; 1.2% DMPT is added as accelerator. Charnley felt that the use of ascorbic acid instead of hydroquinone was advantageous in its medical application.[30,38]

Table 5-1 shows the chemical composition of two cements, Simplex P and Zimmer low-viscosity cement. Several different commercially available bone cements possess different chemical and physical characteristics.[100] For example, LVC and CMW cement contain powdered PMMA polymer, and Palacos K powder is an MMA–methacrylate copolymer. The Simplex P is a mixture of PMMA and MMA–styrene copolymer. Most commonly used cements, including Zimmer Regular, LVC, CMW, and Simplex P, use barium sulfate for radioopacification; zirconium oxide is used in Palacos R. Chlorphyll also is added to Palacos R to provide a green color for identification during surgery.

The viscosity of different cements largely accounts for variations in the bead sizes in polymer as determined by each manufacturer.[103] Lowest viscosity is found in LVC cement followed by Zimmer Regular and Simplex P cement. Palacos R and CMW have the highest viscosity.

STERILIZATION OF SELF-CURING ACRYLIC CEMENT

Sterilization of the cement poses certain technical problems. The liquid monomer possesses some self-sterilization power as verified by Charnley.[30] With exposure to monomer, cultures of *Staphylococcus aureus* were sterilized in 1 minute, but spore bearers required 4 days. Towers[158] found that *Staphylococcus aerogenes* survived exposure for up to 20 minutes, while the spore-forming *Bacillus cereus* was viable up to exposure for 14 days. Because of self-polymerization, sterilization of monomer by autoclaving or gamma radiation is not possible. Seitz filtration is used for purification.

Based on laboratory tests, it was concluded that over a period of weeks, common organisms tend to die out spontaneously in acrylic cement powder.[30] This is consistent with observations made in 1962 by Hullinger, who did not encounter any growth of organisms in tissue cultures to which unsterilized Palacos powder had been added.[82,86,151] Charnley felt that formaldehyde vapor was quite safe for sterilization of powder. He recommended double-wrapped polyethylene packaging and placing a porous packet containing formaldehyde vapor within each pack, to be thrown away when the pack is opened. The powder may also be sterilized by gamma rays, which also prolong the setting time by approximately 2 minutes. Irradiation of the mixed barium sulfate and cement powder must be avoided, however, since this prolongs the setting time by 20 minutes or more.[30,38] Simplex P powder as supplied for surgical use is sterilized with 2.5 megarads from a cobalt 60 source.

RADIOPACITY OF CEMENT

Radiopacity is an extremely important feature that should be preserved in all formulas for cement used in total hip surgery. Without this property the presence and amount of cement cannot be determined (Fig. 5-1). The best radiographic density for the acetabulum was produced by the addition of 2.5 gm barium sulfate to 40 gm powder; the amount of barium sulfate is doubled (5 gm) for the shaft and femur. Initially, the barium sulfate was supplied in two separate 2.5-gm packets sterilized in the packet by gamma irradiation. Each was then added to the cement at the time of mixing. A premixed barium sulfate PMMA powder is preferred because mixing at surgery may be incomplete and resulting in severe weakening of the cement. Currently in most brands of cement, barium sulfate is added to the powder at the time of manufacture and constitutes a 10% W/W of the total polymer powder. Barium sulfate particles may be a major factor in producing osteolysis following loosening of the cemented total hip arthroplasty components (see Chapter 4).

MECHANICAL AND PHYSICAL PROPERTIES

Several investigators have determined the mechanical properties of self-curing cements (see Table 5-2).[38,56,80,109] Charnley and Smith[38] evaluated self-curing acrylic cement as used in orthopaedic surgery and found a positive relationship between the mechan-

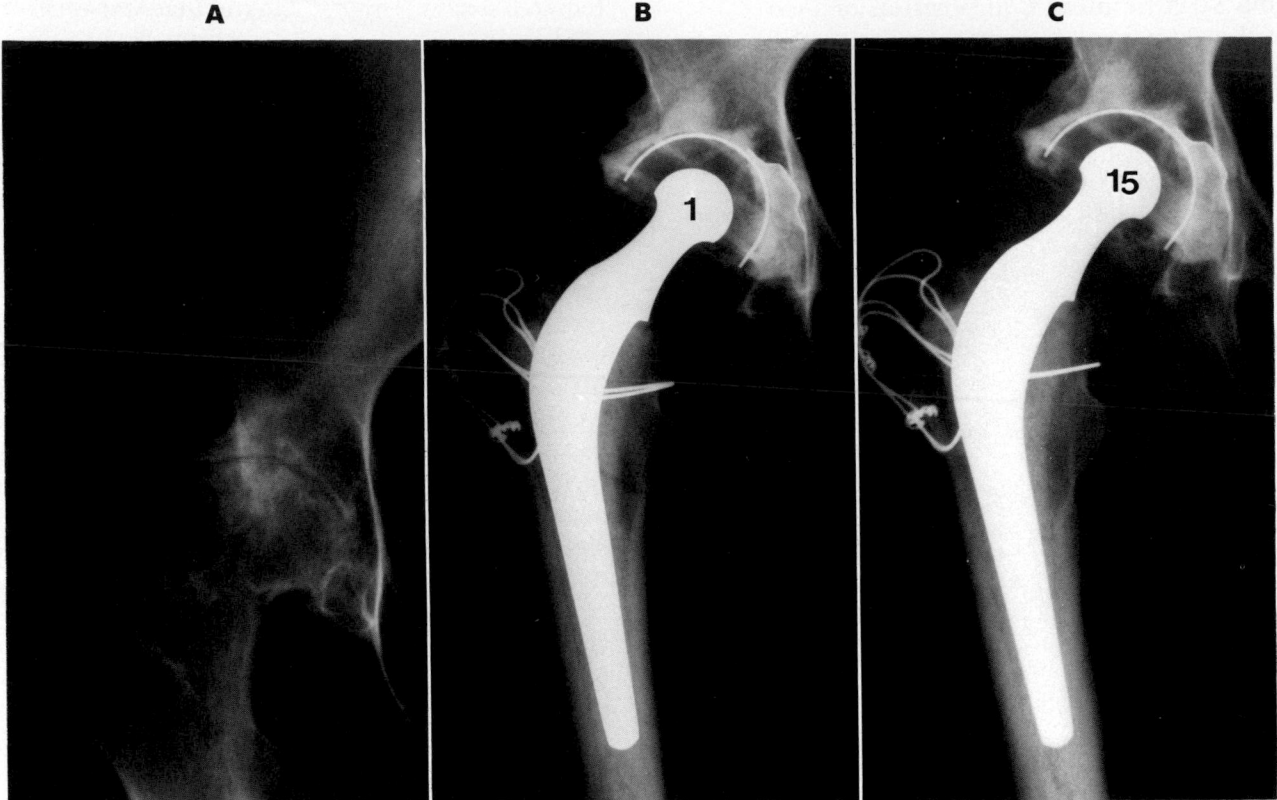

Fig. 5-1. Radiopacity of cement permits visualization of the cement-bone interface because of differences in their radiopacity. **A,** Preoperative radiograph of a 38-year-old woman (M.W.) with degenerative osteoarthritis who weighed 83 kg. **B,** 1 year after surgery, there is no demarcation or radiolucent zone between cement and bone of either component. **C,** 15 years after surgery, radiographs have remained unchanged except for mild degrees of bone adaptive remodeling including increased canalization of the superior acetabular bone in zone 1 and evidence of hypertrophy of the femoral cortex; osteointegration. Preoperative hip grade A: 3,3,2. Postoperative hip grade A: 6,6,6. This case represents perfect clinical and biological compatibility of cement and bone.

Table 5-2 Mechanical Properties of Two Cements

	Regular simplex*	Low-viscosity cement†
Tensile strength (MPa)*	36.12 ± 11.46	35.02 ± 8.20
Fracture strain (mm/mm)	.0148 ± .0042	.0147 ± .0034
Elastic modulus (GPa)†	2.93 ± 0.48	2.72 ± 0.28
Fatigue results		
Log N (N = cycles to failure)	3.38 ± .61	3.05 ± .37
Weilbull parameters (m)	4.77	8.45
β (MPa)	3.72	3.23

From Gates EI, Carter DR, Harris WH: Comparative fatigue behavior of different bone cements, *Clin Orthop* 189:294, 1984.
*Howmedica, Rutherford, N.J.
†Zimmer, Warsaw, Ind.

ical properties of pure polymer and that used in actual surgery. Compared with heat-cured material containing a minimum of residual monomer, the tensile strength was reduced by 10% and the stiffness by 5% because of 2% residual monomer.[151] However, Charnley maintains that more important alterations in mechanical behavior result from porosity induced by mixing air in the mass of cement, or as happens during surgery, by inclusion of blood in the mass of cement during insertion. Barring inclusion of air or blood, he presents the average following figures[38]:

Compressive strength	15,000 psi
Flexural strength	15,000 psi
Tensile strength	10,000 psi
Modulus of elasticity	0.3×10^6 psi

Commercially available bone cement polymer has an average molecular weight of 198,000. Its molecular weight increases by curing to 242,000. Approximately 90% of its tensile strength is reached by 4 hours and

100% by 24 hours after polymerization.

The mechanical properties of Simplex P acrylic cement mixed for orthopaedic use, as determined by Lee and co-workers,[107] are listed in Table 5-3.

Wilde and Greenwald found the average shearing strength of surgical Simplex P bone cement to be 5762 ± 180 psi,[165] whereas average shearing strength of compact bone is about 10,000 psi. They therefore concluded that surgical Simplex P does not resist shear

forces as well as compact bone and should not be used as a substitute for bone when avoidable. Approximate tensile and compressive strengths and modulus of elasticity (expressed in megapascal [MPa]) are 32, 100, and 2700 respectively. These values are considerably lower than those of cortical bone; by 25% in tensile strength, 50% in compressive strength, and 15% in modulus of elasticity.[26]

Because of the viscoelastic properties of PMMA, it becomes stiffer and stronger at a higher strain rate than at a low strain rate. Fig. 5-2 shows the relationship between the strain rate, modulus of elasticity, and ultimate compressive strength.[108]

The mechanical properties of radiopaque cement and nonradiopaque cement have been compared (Table 5-4) with those of commercial heat-cured acrylic resins. Note the reduction in the tensile and compressive strength of cement caused by added barium sulfate. Water solubility and sorption for both radiopaque and radiolucent cement are shown in Tables 5-5 and 5-6. In a later study by Lee and co-workers,[108] the inclusion of 10% barium sulfate for radiographical purposes did not adversely affect the shear strength. This amount of barium was the same percentage by weight as that found in radiopaque Simplex P in clinical use. The shear force at failure increased slightly with increased time of curing. The curing periods in their experiments varied from 2 to 168 hours. They estimated all strengths to be approximately 25% lower than the upper limits of normal bone and the stiffness five to ten times less.[38]

Table 5-3 Mechanical Properties of Acrylic Cement as Determined by Lee and Ling*

Parameters tested	Unit (newton/mm²)	Number of specimens tested
Compression		
Ultimate stress	−77	
0.1% proof stress	−60	324
	2270	
Tension		
Ultimate stress	25	24
Torsion		
Ultimate stress	37	
Modulus of rigidity	850	24
Shear		
Ultimate stress	41	42

*From Lee AJC, Ling RSM, Wrighton JD: *Clin Orthop* 95:281, 1973.

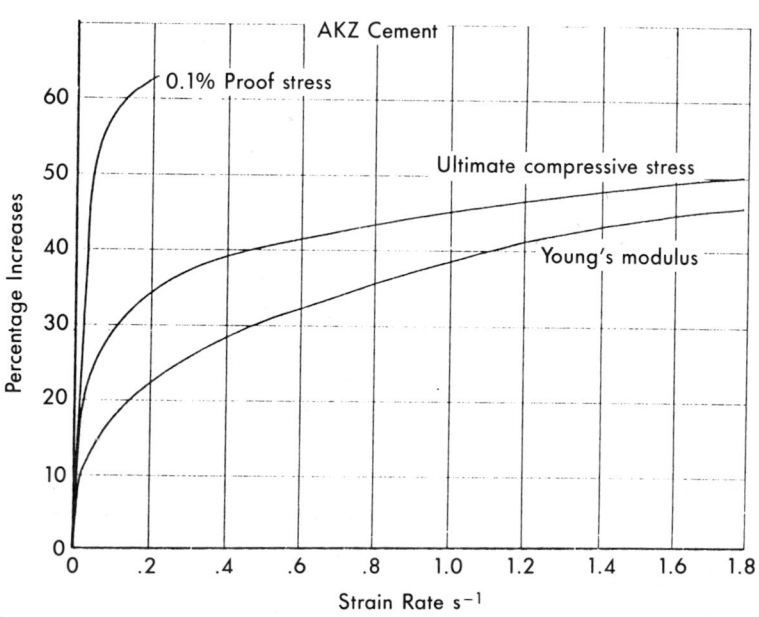

Fig. 5-2. Relationship of strain rate to mechanical properties of cement. (From Lee AJC, Ling RSM, Vangala SS: Some clinically relevant variables affecting the mechanical behavior of bone cement, *Arch Orthop Traumat Surg* 92:1, 1978.)

Table 5-4 Mechanical Properties of Bone Cement

	Radiopaque cement	Radiolucent cement	Commercial acrylic resins
Tensile strength, MPa*	28.9 (1.6)†	32.6 (1.2)	55–76
Compressive strength, MPa	91.7 (2.5)	93.1 (3.9)	76–131
Transverse breaking load, N‡	41.9 (3.1)	47.9 (1.3)	–
Modulus of rupture, MPa	51.5 (3.1)	56.9 (1.6)	83–117
Young's modulus			
From transverse loading data, MPa	2070 (90)	2200 (80)	2690–3280
From compressive loading data, MPa	2200 (60)	2300 (50)	2690–3280

From Haas SS, Brauer GM, Dickson G: A characterization of polymethylmethacrylate bone cement, *J Bone Joint Surg* 57:380, 1975.
*To convert MPa to psi multiply by 145.
†Standard deviations are shown in parentheses.
‡To convert N to lb force multiply by 0.225.

Table 5-5 Effect of Powder-to-Liquid Ratio on Compressive Strength and Modulus of Elasticity of Cement*

Powder-to-liquid ratio (gm/ml)	Number of specimens	Compressive strength (MPa)	Modulus of elasticity (MPa)
3/1	8	94.1 (0.7)†	2320 (40)
2/1	8	91.7 (2.5)	2250 (60)
3/2	8	93.5 (2.1)	2390 (60)

*Cement used for this comparison contained $BaSO_4$.
†Standard deviations are shown in parentheses.

Table 5-6 Water: Sorption and Solubility

	Radiopaque cement (mg/cm²)	Radiolucent cement (mg/cm²)	Requirements (mg/cm²)
Sorption	0.5	0.4	0.7 max.
Solubility	0.03	0.04	0.04 max.

From Haas SS, Brauer GM, Dickson G: A characterization of polymethylmethacrylate bone cement; *J Bone Joint Surg* 57:380, 1975.

Table 5-7 Effects of Variables Tested

	Variable	Possible % change in strength	
		UCS	UTS
A	Environmental temperature 37° C	−10%	
	Equilibrium moisture content	−3%	
	Strain rate—impact rates	+67%	
	Aging	−10%	
	Fatigue	Uncertain	Uncertain
B	Radiopaque fillers	−5%	
	Antibiotics (1 gm A.B./40 gm polymer)	−4%	
	Mixing technique	−21%	
	Insertion technique —delay	−40%	−54%
	—pressure	+20%	
C	Inclusion of blood and tissue debris	−16%	−70%
	Stress raisers	Profound	Profound
	Constraint	Profound	Profound
	Cement thickness	Uncertain	Uncertain

From Lee AJC, Ling RSM, Vangala SS: Some clinically relevant variables affecting the mechanical behavior of bone cement, *Arch Orthop Traumat Surg* 92:1, 1978.

Mechanical properties of cement were not significantly affected by a variation of mixing techniques studied by Lee and associates.[109] They suggested that in clinical practice the presence of blood in the cement may cause weakness, although the adverse effect was not significant. Lamination was minimized when the mixture of blood with cement was kept to a minimum and when the cement was under pressure (Table 5-7).

At our laboratories,[23] we studied the mechanical properties of a cemented stem when (1) the medullary canal is vented with a catheter during the insertion of cement, (2) blood is included in cement during insertion, and (3) a prosthesis is recemented. In addition, we evaluated the strength imparted by cement to a prosthesis. In this study, we minimized biological variables by using paired wet formalin-

preserved femurs, one acting as control. We applied a single static load until failure (Fig. 5-3). The results showed that the PMMA-bone-metal system consistently produced good results with reasonable, but not careless, variations in technique. Venting the canal, recementing the prosthesis, or admixing with blood under these conditions did not alter the mechanical properties of the cement fixation.[18]

Astleford and co-workers[8] evaluated the acetabular hole configuration of the prosthesis fixation in the pelvis as related to the strength of PMMA. They

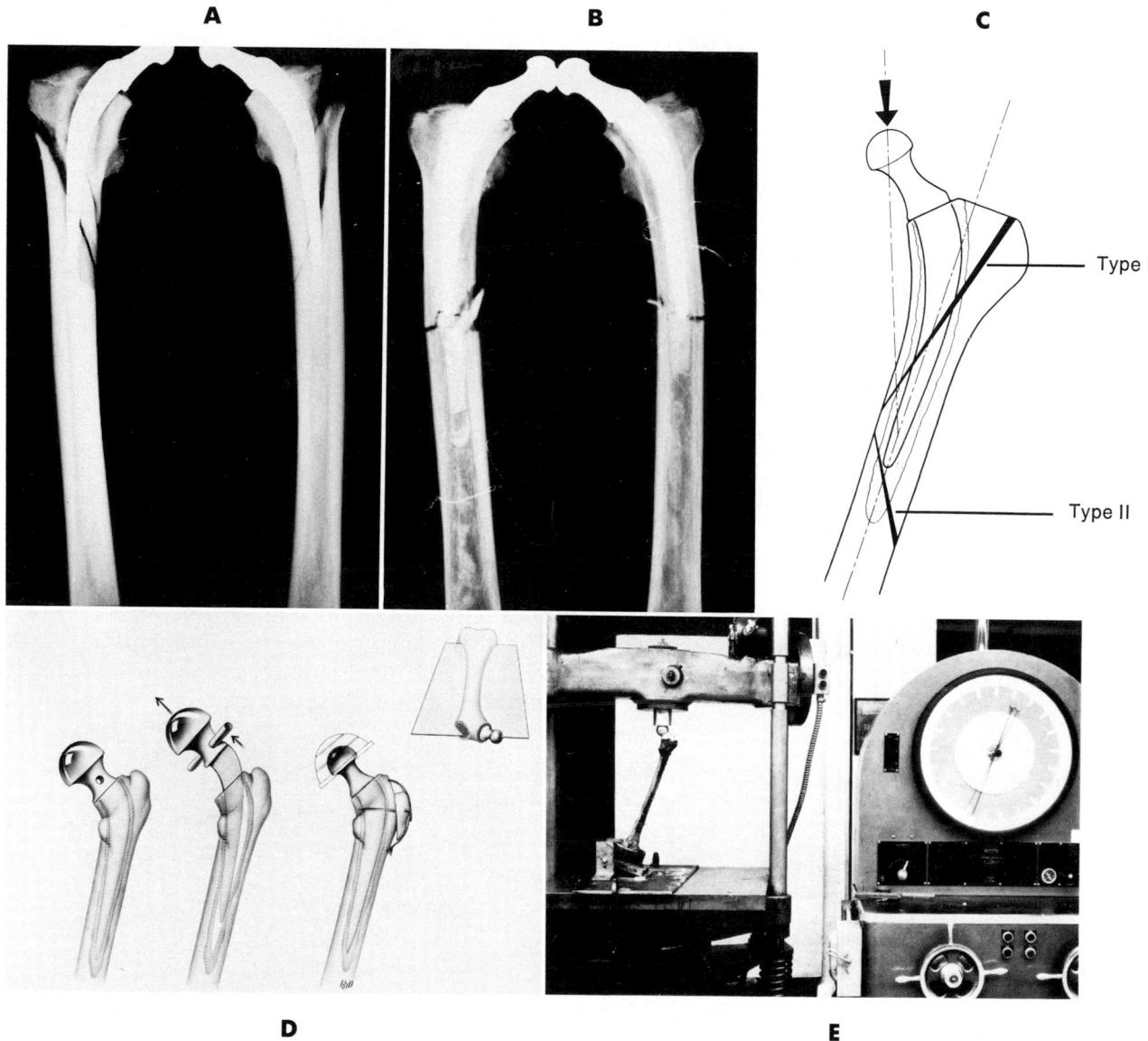

Fig. 5-3. A, Radiograph of paired specimens subjected to loading. X-ray films reveal oblique fracture extending from greater trochanter to medial cortex at level of tip of prosthesis. This mode of failure was far more common in specimens tested. **B,** Posttest radiographs of femur with fracture of cement at level of tip or prosthesis. NOTE: reverse obliquity of fracture, which extends from medial side outward and distalward. **C,** Diagrammatic drawing of line of application of load. Direction of lines of fracture has occurred in two patterns, Type I and Type II. *Type I.* Prosthesis settled into varus. There was failure of trochanteric cancellous bone parallel to trochanteric line. *Type II.* Diaphyseal fracture of cortical bone was produced with reversed obliquity of fracture line beginning at tip of prosthesis. All specimens showed cement fractures at tip of prosthesis, at junction of stiff column with more elastic column of shaft. Twenty tests showed type I fractures, and eight showed type II fractures, All showed cement fractures at tip of stem of prosthesis. **D,** Charnley's low-friction arthroplasty stem (standard) compared with author's stem. Latter design is similar to Charnley's standard stem but 10% proportionately larger in all dimensions. In recementing tests Eftekhar prosthesis was knocked out of channel, and Charnley stem cemented in place using only small amount of cement. *Inset,* Transcondylar plane (neutroversion) of preparation of femur. **E,** Testing setup using a Baldwin 10-ton press. NOTE: for testing, femoral condyles were placed in epoxy molds. Long axis of bone was placed at 20 degrees to vertical in press to produce resultant joint force of one-legged stance plus normal varus inclination of femur. Rate of loading was slow, 400 lb/min. At fatigue, or shatter, failure, the force noted on the scale would drop despite continued compression. End point was taken as peak force applied.

concluded that the geometric configuration did not significantly affect the maximum shear load-carrying capabilities of the PMMA.

Tests on stability of the mechanical properties of self-curing acrylic bone cement (both Simplex P and CMW) have revealed that storage of cement up to 2 years in bovine serum at 37° C caused no significant deterioration or change in the mechanical properties (neither static properties nor compression fatigue behavior). Data on compression fatigue suggested that working stresses in the cement should be limited to less than 1.4×10^{-8} dynes/cm^2 to ensure long-term viability of any design or implantation technique.[88]

This author and Thurston studied the effect of irradiation on acrylic cement, with special reference to fixation of pathological fractures.[56] We tested to determine the mechanical properties of the two commonly used bone cements, Simplex P radiopaque and CMW, and the effect of irradiation on each (Fig. 5-4). We concluded that there was no significant difference in mechanical properties of irradiated and nonirradiated cement and that postoperative irradiation may be safely performed after fixation of pathological fractures or pathology of the pelvis without adverse effects on the mechanical properties of the cement.

POROSITY OF CEMENT

It has been estimated that the method of cement preparation affects shrinkage, density, and porosity of cement[71] (Table 5-8). Cement porosity is caused by the presence of air spaces between polymer beads and formation of "bubbles" during cement mixing. In addition to air entrapment, voids may result from evaporation of monomer and thermal expansion of bubbles. Air bubbles, especially micropores, constitute 5% to 10% of hand-mixed cured cement mass because of the viscosity of cement. Evidently a low-viscosity cement contains fewer macropores since such cement allows large bubbles to escape, leaving the micropores. A large variation in porosity of cement occurs when cement is mixed per the manufacturer's instructions but in an uncontrolled environment.[59,111]

Eyrer demonstrated that kneading of Palacos cement for 20 to 30 seconds reduced air bubbles, thus decreasing porosity. Similarly, for hand-mixed cement the best results (approximately 5% porosity) can be obtained by allowing the mixed cement to sit undisturbed after initial mixing of the monomer with polymer. Without vigorous and continuous mixing the air bubbles rise to the surface, and the macropores are diminished for the most part.

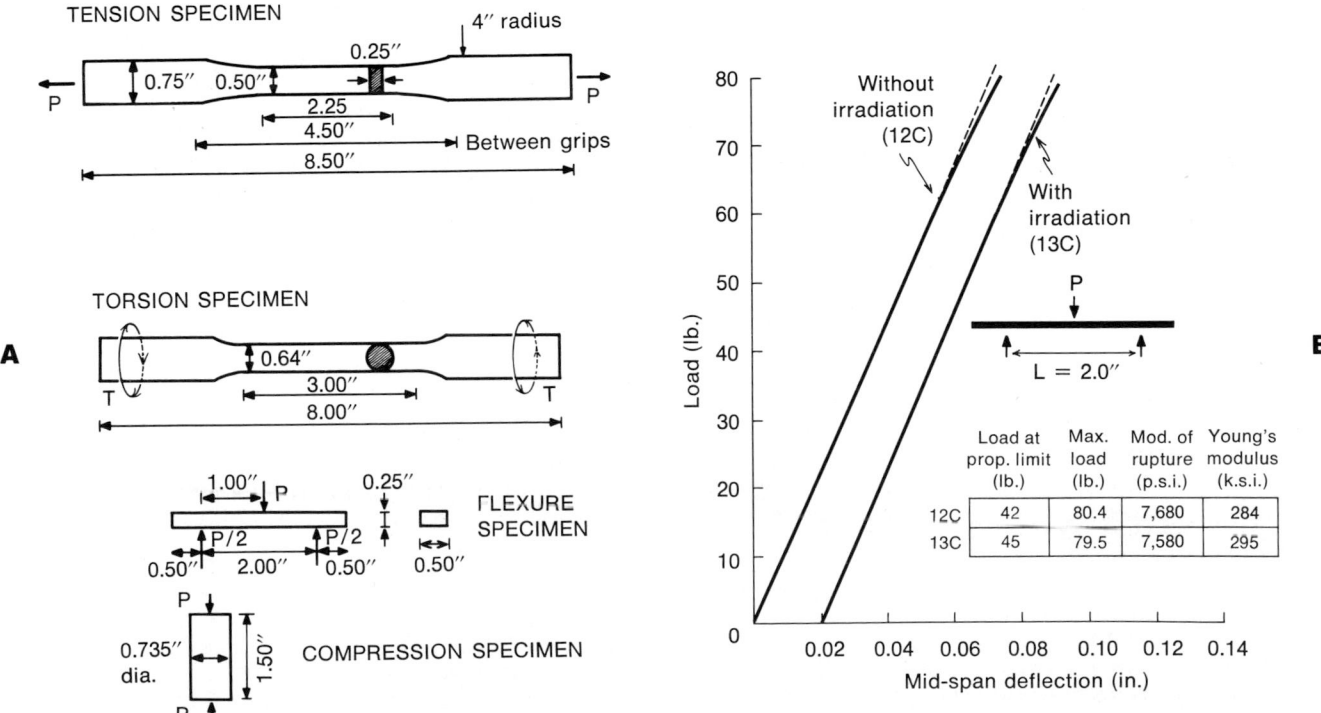

Fig. 5-4. **A,** Tests were conducted for both CMW and Simplex cements with and without barium sulfates and with and without irradiation. Specimens were molded by hand in molds machined from Teflon stock. Dimension and arrangement for tension, torsion, and compression specimens are shown. **B,** Typical load-deflection curve using irradiated and nonirradiated specimens.

Table 5-8 Effects of Preparation Variables on Shrinkage, Density, and Porosity of Bone Cement

Variable	Number of specimens	Shrinkage (percent)	Density (gm/cm³)	Porosity (percent)
BaSO₄ content				
Polymerized in water				
BaSO₄ present	8	2.7 (0.6)*	1.17 (0.02)	6.7 (1.8)
BaSO₄ absent	4	3.2 (0.6)	1.09 (0.02)	8.4 (1.5)
Polymerized in compression mold				
BaSO₄ present	15	–	1.19 (0.01)	4.5 (0.7)
BaSO₄ absent	13	–	1.13 (0.01)	4.7 (0.6)
Polymerized in constant-pressure mold				
BaSO₄ present	1	5.2	1.23	1.6
BaSO₄ absent	1	5.3	1.18	0.8
Rate of mixing				
Polymerized in water				
Vigorous mixing	2	2.3 (0.3)	–	9.0 (1.5)
Normal mixing	6	2.8 (0.7)	–	7.4 (1.3)
Minimum mixing	4	3.2 (0.5)	–	6.1 (1.6)
Polymerized in compression mold				
Vigorous mixing	1	–	1.127	9.8
Normal mixing	1	–	1.134	9.3
Minimum mixing	1	–	1.150	8.0
Powder-to-liquid ratio (gm/ml)				
3/1	8	–	1.22 (0.01)	3.5 (0.4)
2/1	10	–	1.20 (0.01)	4.3 (0.5)
3/2	9	–	1.19 (0.01)	4.2 (0.7)
Molding pressure				
Polymerized in water	6	2.8 (0.7)	–	7.4 (1.8)
Polymerized in compression mold	28	–	–	4.6 (0.7)
Polymerized in constant-pressure mold	2	5.2 (0.1)	–	1.2 (0.6)

From Haas SS, Brauer GM, Dickson G: A characterization of polymethylmethacrylate bone cement, *J Bone Joint Surg* 57:380, 1975.
*Numbers in parentheses are standard deviations.

Porosity of cement can be reduced by centrifugation or under partial vacuum (Figs. 5-5 and 5-6). Centrifugation is not as effective in highly viscous cements such as Palacos. It is most effective in less doughy cements such as Simplex P. Centrifugation can reduce the porosity of Simplex P from 10% to 5%.

Chilled cement is poured immediately after mixing into a syringe and spun at 3000 to 4000 rpm for 1 minute. A partial vacuum between 400 to 730 mm Hg below atmospheric pressure reduces the porosity to 1% in set specimens.[53,168] A partial vacuum at 500 to 550 mm Hg at slow speed (2 Hz) is most effective in eliminating most porosities in most cements tested, including Palacos.[167]

Porosity Vs. Shrinkage and Fracture Toughness

Changes in cement volume during polymerization are caused by polymerization shrinkage, thermal expansion, and thermal shrinkage (Figs. 5-7 and 5-8).

Volumetric changes as a function of the polymerization process have long been established. Charnley[30] and others[2,71,118] reported on volumetric changes in self-curing acrylic cement. Shrinkage in PMMA is caused by shrinkage of monomer molecules to form chains of PMMA. During the process, there is approximately 21% volumetric shrinkage by monomer. Monomer is one third of polymer in cements used in orthopaedics, which results in a 7% shrinkage of the entire mass.[51]

Thermal expansion of cement during the polymerization process depends largely on the size of the mass. For example, in Mayer's experiment, the peak temperature for a 3-mm specimen was 60° C, whereas the peak temperature for a 10-mm cement mass was 107° C.[118] In this context, measurements of expansion and shrinkage of large masses of cement resulting from exothermic reaction overestimate the condition that applies in practice. A significant amount of generated heat is dissipated through the prosthesis (a process known as *heat sink*) and ab-

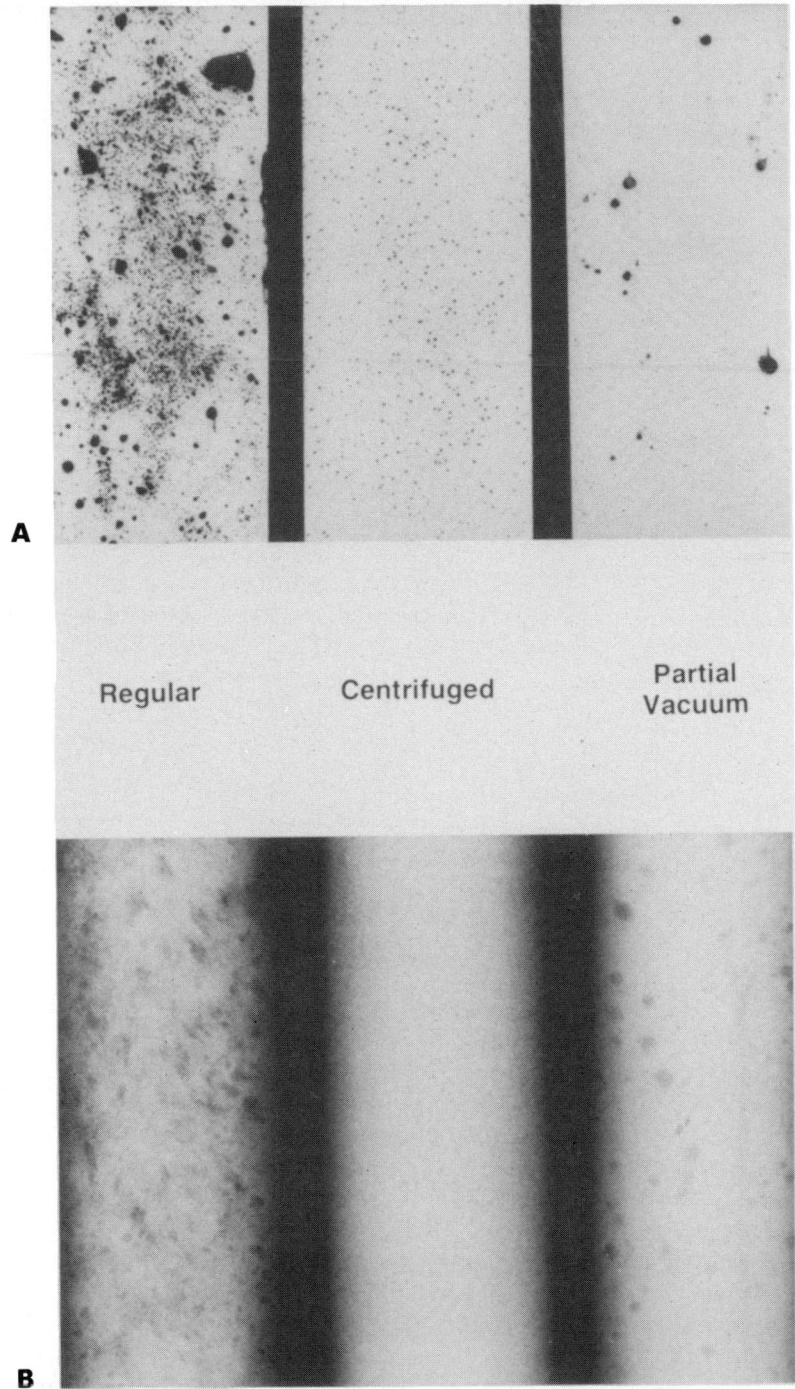

Fig. 5-5. Comparison of stained section **(A)** and radiograph **(B)** of bone cement. Cement polymerized in a Miller cartridge was sectioned longitudinally and then stained with black shoe polish to visualize the voids. The same specimen was also radiographed to learn the porosity of the solid mass. The porosity in these samples is exaggerated because of the high temperature resulting from the large mass of the polymerizing cement. *(Left)* Micropores and macropores are present in large numbers in hand-mixed cement prepared under atmospheric pressure. *(Center)* Centrifugation completely eliminates the macropores. Stained section shows the remaining micropores. These micropores are barely visible, even on special high-resolution radiographs. *(Right)* Partial vacuum mixing eliminates many of the micropores as well as the macropores. Residual voids are still present. The residual porosity is most evident on the high-resolution radiographs. (From Chan KH, Ahmed AM: Polymethyl methacrylate in joint replacement arthroplasty. In Morrey BF, editor: *Joint replacement arthroplasty,* New York, 1991, Churchill-Livingstone.)

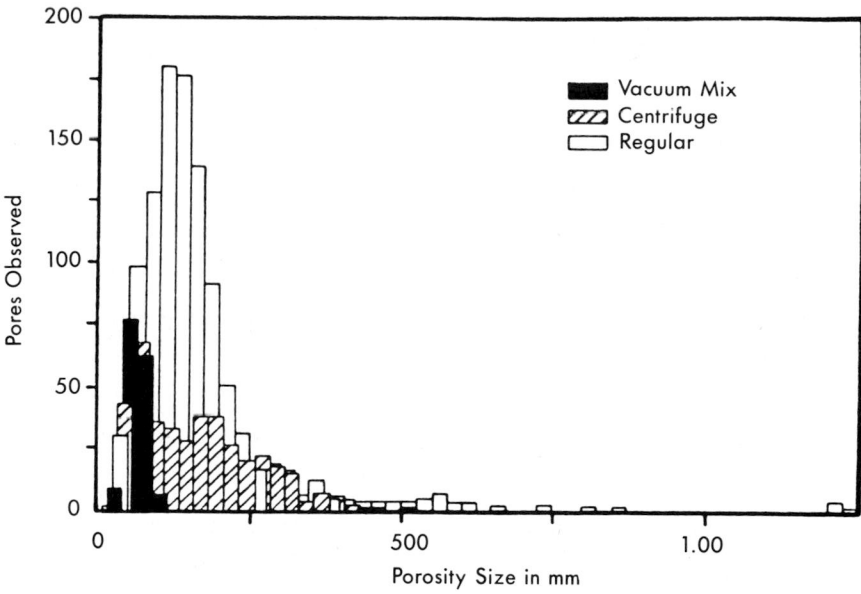

Fig. 5-6. Distribution of pores in 0.025-mm size intervals for Simplex P mixed by various techniques. (From Wixson RL, Lautenschlager EP, Novak MA: Vacuum mixing of acrylic bone cement, *J Arthroplasty* 2:141, 1987.)

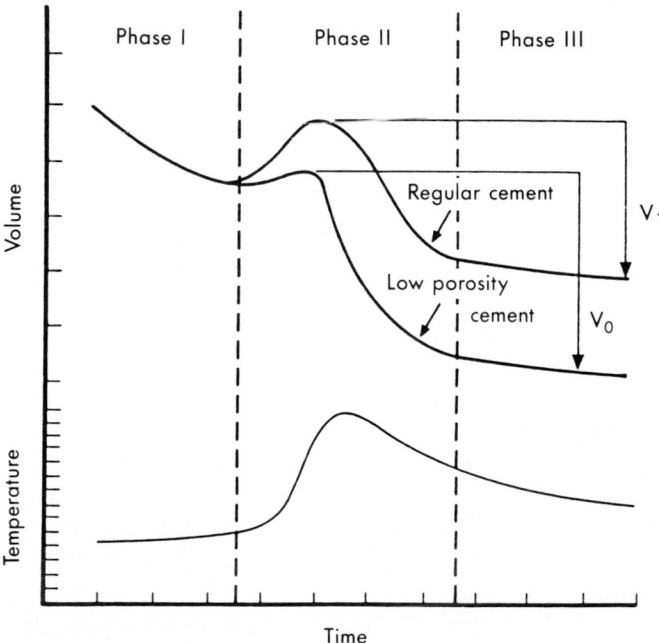

Fig. 5-7. Schematic representation of volume change during polymerization of bone cement. During phase I, the volume change is mainly caused by polymerization shrinkage. In phase II there is simultaneous volume expansion caused by thermal expansion of the gaseous bubbles and volume contraction caused by polymerization. The volume change in phase III after solidification of the cement is caused by thermal contraction as the cement cools. (From Chan KH, Ahmed AM: Polymethyl methacrylate in joint replacement arthroplasty. In Morrey BF, editor: *Joint replacement arthroplasty,* New York, 1991, Churchill-Livingstone.)

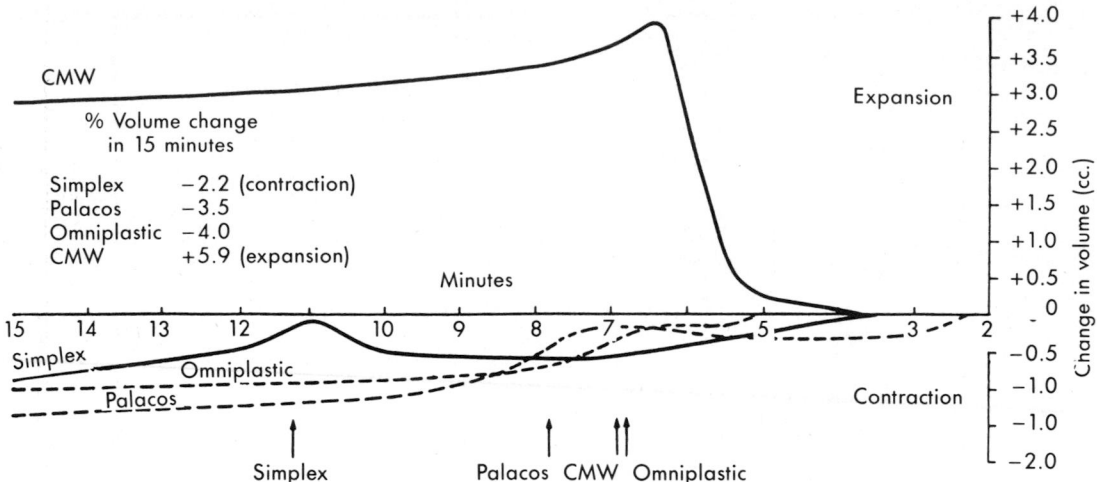

Fig. 5-8. Dimensional changes of four commonly used orthopaedic cements: Simplex, Palacos, CMW, and Omniplastic. (From Amstutz HC, Gruen T: In Ahstrom JP, editor: *Current practice in orthopaedic surgery,* St Louis, 1973, Mosby–Year Book.)

sorbed by the implant. The expansion of cement is caused by the heat of polymerization of cement resulting from the expansion of gaseous bubbles within the PMMA mass. The expansion phase coincides with acceleration of polymerization shrinkage[26] (see Fig. 5-6). If the gas bubbles (porosities) are removed, the net result would be greater net shrinkage of the mass from cooling of the solid cement, a process known as *thermal contraction*.[143]

While net shrinkage of cement mass is greater if cement porosity is reduced, this effect may be neutralized by increased static and fatigue strengths in cement without porosity. However, since porosity may act as a crack terminator, removal of pores from polymerized cement may possibly produce an adverse effect by reducing its fracture toughness.[143]

Rimnac and co-workers[143] have argued that irregularities of the surface of acrylic cement after implantation control the fracture toughness of the cement. Therefore fracture toughness cannot necessarily be enhanced by reducing porosity alone. Additional shrinkage resulting from centrifugation may further reduce fracture strength in in-vivo situations. Rimnac's observation that irregularities of the cement surface and not the internal void are the controlling factors in limiting the fatigue strength has subsequently been supported by Chin and associates.[39] In Chin's in-vitro model, the static failure test of the cement-stem composite (in centrifuged and hand-mixed models) showed a significantly greater static strength in centrifuged specimens than in hand-mixed specimens. However, when they tested similar specimens, under low-cycle fatigue tests, they found no significant difference.[39] The model used for the tests by

Chin and co-workers is thought to be more realistic concerning practical application of cement than other investigators' data, which were derived from fracture-mechanics models.

Centrifugation caused one of the cements tested (Simplex) to shrink significantly, which theoretically can adversely affect the quality of the microinterlock between bone and cement. It may be concluded from these observations that because the low-cycle fatigue strength of PMMA did not show significant improvement after centrifugation in in-vitro simulated models, centrifugation to rid the cement of porosity currently cannot be justified, since centrifugation increases the overall cost and operation time.[48,62] Further, centrifugation of cement to reduce porosity may substantially increase cement shrinkage, which can result in failure of fixation at the interface between bone and cement.[74] Based on experimental data Hamilton has suggested that pressurization of cement to 4 atmospheres may result in tensile strength increases to levels comparable with those produced by centrifugation.[74]

The strength of PMMA can also be increased by mixing it under vacuum (Figs. 5-9 to 5-12) in both low-viscosity and high-viscosity gentamicin-loaded cements. Using three different mixing procedures—hand, vibration, and vacuum stirring—Lidgren and co-workers[110] achieved an improvement of 15% to 30% in the flexural and compression strength and modulus of elasticity. Ferracane and associates[61] found an admixture of liquid fat with PMMA up to only 5% (by weight) caused a significant reduction (P value = 0.05) in tensile and compressive strength of both low-viscosity and conventional cement.[61] This adverse effect in lowering the strength of liquid low-viscosity

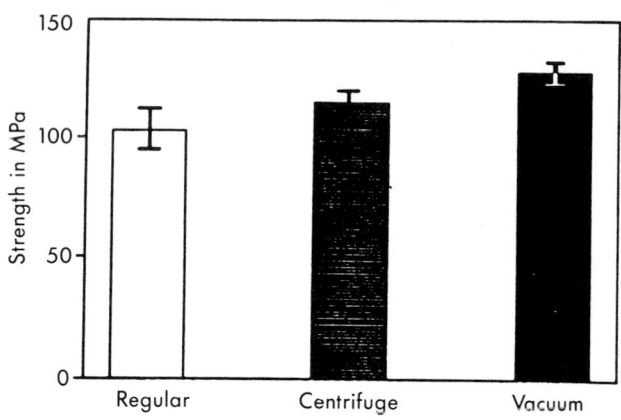

Fig. 5-9. Compression strength averages ± standard deviations for Simplex P mixed by various techniques. (From Wixson RL, Lautenschlager EP, Novak MA: Vacuum mixing of acrylic bone cement, *J Arthroplasty* 2:141, 1987.)

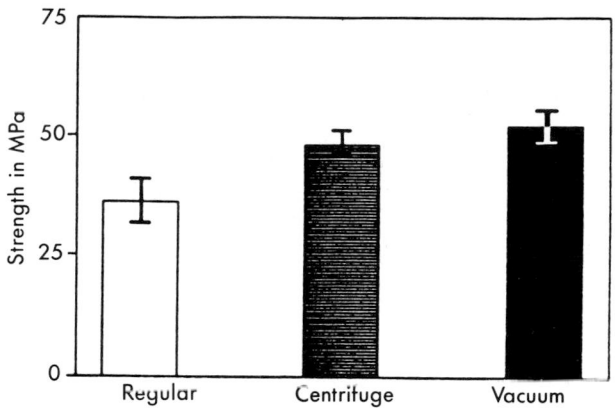

Fig. 5-10. Uniaxial tension averages ± standard deviations for Simplex P mixed by various techniques. (From Wixson RL, Lautenschlager EP, Novack MA: Vacuum mixing of acrylic bone cement, *J Arthroplasty* 2:141, 1987.)

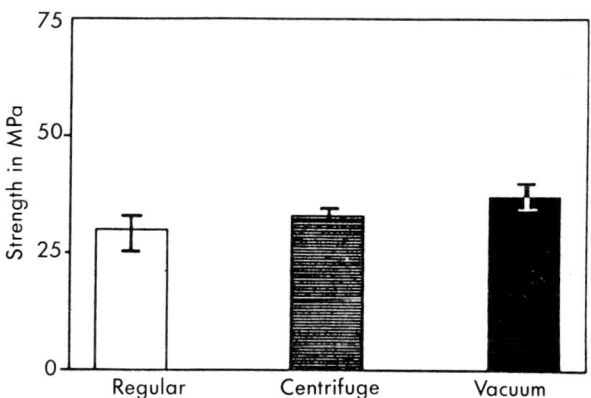

Fig. 5-11. Diametral tension averages ± standard deviations for Simplex P mixed by various techniques. (From Wixson RL, Lautenschlager EP, Novack MA: Vacuum mixing of acrylic bone cement, *J Arthroplasty* 2:141, 1987.)

cement was greater than for conventional cement.

Two other studies have reported on the subject. One showed an improved fracture toughness imparted by either centrifuged or undervacuum mixing of the cement by 10% to 20% respectively.[104] Lange and Pilliar[163] concluded that slowly hand-mixed specimens possess comparable fracture toughness to centrifuged specimens. From these observations it may be concluded that further investigation into the role of centrifugation or vacuum mixing of cement in the fracture toughness of acrylic cement is warranted.

Porosity vs. Static and Fatigue Strengths

In-vitro studies[25] on PMMA have shown that porosity distribution plays a major role in determining the tensile and fatigue strengths of PMMA. Investigators also have observed regional variations in the shear strength of the bone cement, which could be attributed

partially to the nonhomogeneity of the MMA related to porosity.[11]

Jasty and co-workers measured the total and mean pore sizes of various bone cement preparations. They found that in different commercial bone cements the porosity varied from 5% to 16% when these cements were mixed in the usual fashion. After 30 seconds of centrifugation a substantial reduction of the overall number of pores (mean pore size) occurred in Simplex P, Zimmer Regular, and CMW. However, porosity reduction after centrifugation in other types of cements including LVC, Palacos R, and Palacos R with gentamicin bone cement was not significant.[89]

Fatigue Properties

A modest but significant improvement (10% to 40%) in the tensile strengths of PMMA results from removal of porosity by either centrifuging or vacuum mixing of cement (Table 5-9).

The fatigue properties of cement have been of considerable interest, since they pertain to long-term results of cemented total joint arthroplasties and have been the subject of several biomechanical studies.[20,39,48,143] The fatigue porosity of cement as indicated by its fatigue strength is of special concern because of its expected long-term use and cyclic loading conditions. Typically the fatigue strength of materials used for tensile strength is demonstrated by plotting stress (expressed in MPa) against the number of cycles of failure. Increasing applied stress decreases the number of cycles to failure. Conversely, by decreasing the stress, the number of cycles to failure increases in a nonlinear manner until the curve flattens out (Fig. 5-13). At this point the stress is below the limit to cause failure of the material. Such a stress level is called the *endurance* or *fatigue limit,* which is approximately

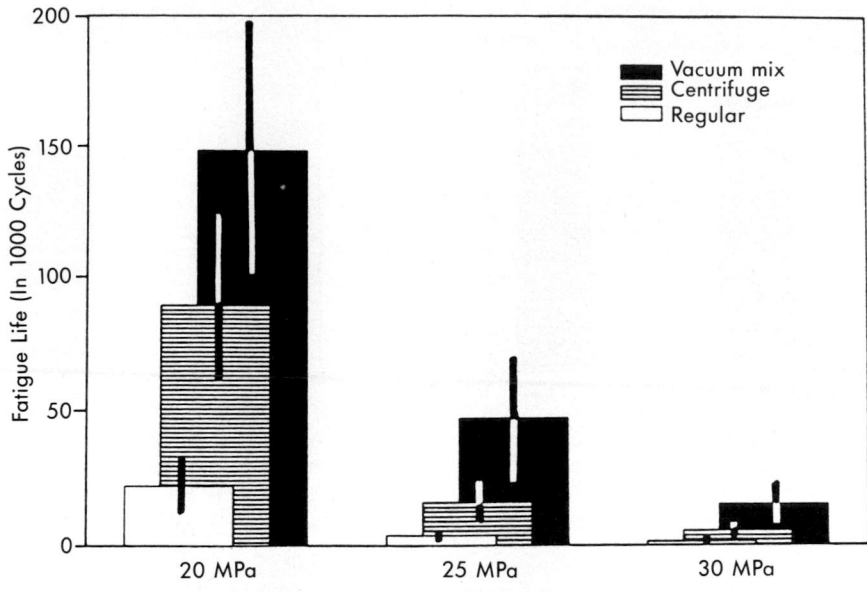

Fig. 5-12. Weibull average cyclic fatigue lives for Simplex P mixed by various techniques. The cited stressing levels (in MPa) represent the maximum in a sinusoidal cycling between 1 MPa and the maximum (20 MPa, 25 MPa, or 30 MPa). (From Wixson RL, Lautenschlager EP, Novack MA: Vacuum mixing of acrylic bone cement, *J Arthroplasty* 2:141, 1987.)

Table 5-9 Effect of Porosity Reduction on Tensile Strength (MPa) of Simplex P

Author/ Year*	Conventional	Centrifugation	%†	Partial vacuum	%‡
Davies et al[47]	36.2	44.7	23		
(1987)	(10.1)‡	(5.2)			
Burke et al[20]	32.5	42.0	29		
(1984)	(10.5)	(5.5)			
Noble et al[124]	37.4	43.5	16	40.7	8
(1984)	(7.0)	(5.4)		(7.2)	
Wixson et al[167]	36.0	48.0	33	52.0	44
(1987)	(5.0)	(3.0)		(4.0)	
Wixson et al[168]	44.8			58.5	31
(1985)	(5.0)			(2.6)	
Arroyo[6]	31.4			41.4	31
(1986)	(5.1)			(4.3)	

From Chan KH, Ahmed AM: Polymethylmethacrylate in joint replacement arthroplasty. In Morrey BF, editor: *Joint replacement arthoplasty,* New York, 1991, Churchill-Livingstone.

*Author/Year: The leading author of the referenced article and the year published.

†The percentage increase in tensile strength after porosity reduction.

‡Figures in parentheses are standard deviations.

20% to 30% of the static strength. The endurance limit of Simplex P has been estimated from less than 3 MPa to over 12 MPa.[26,47,98] Thus a modest decrease in stress or an increase in mechanical strength can be imparted by centrifugation of cement, resulting in increased tensile strength of PMMA.

As Davies and associates and others have shown, in-vitro tests indicate that a considerable reduction in the porosity of cement is achieved by centrifugation of the cement, which improves its mechanical properties (Fig. 5-14).[48–50] In addition, these investigators concluded that centrifugation might increase the long-term survival of total hip arthroplasty by improving the mechanical properties of cement. Davies and co-workers tested the porosity and fatigue life of centrifuged and noncentrifuged specimens of Simplex P, Zimmer low-viscosity cement, Zimmer Regular, CMW, and Palacos R. The fatigue life varied for different cements by a factor of 100; it was influenced more by the composition of the cement than by porosity alone (Fig. 5-15). Simplex P, under the conditions tested, had the highest fatigue life (Tables 5-10 and 5-11).[48] Low-viscosity cement has the lowest porosity, so centrifugation resulted in an insignificant reduction of porosity. Simplex P mixed with chilled monomer had one of the lowest porosities among cements tested when centrifuged for 120 seconds.[89] Centrifuging also resulted in a significant improvement in fatigue life.[48] The investigators thought failure of centrifugation to improve the fatigue life of Palacos R and CMW bone cement was related to their high viscosity.[48]

LOSS OF MONOMER BY EVAPORATION AND LEACHING

Loss of monomer during mixing has been studied by Charnley and Smith[38] and Lee and associates.[107,109]

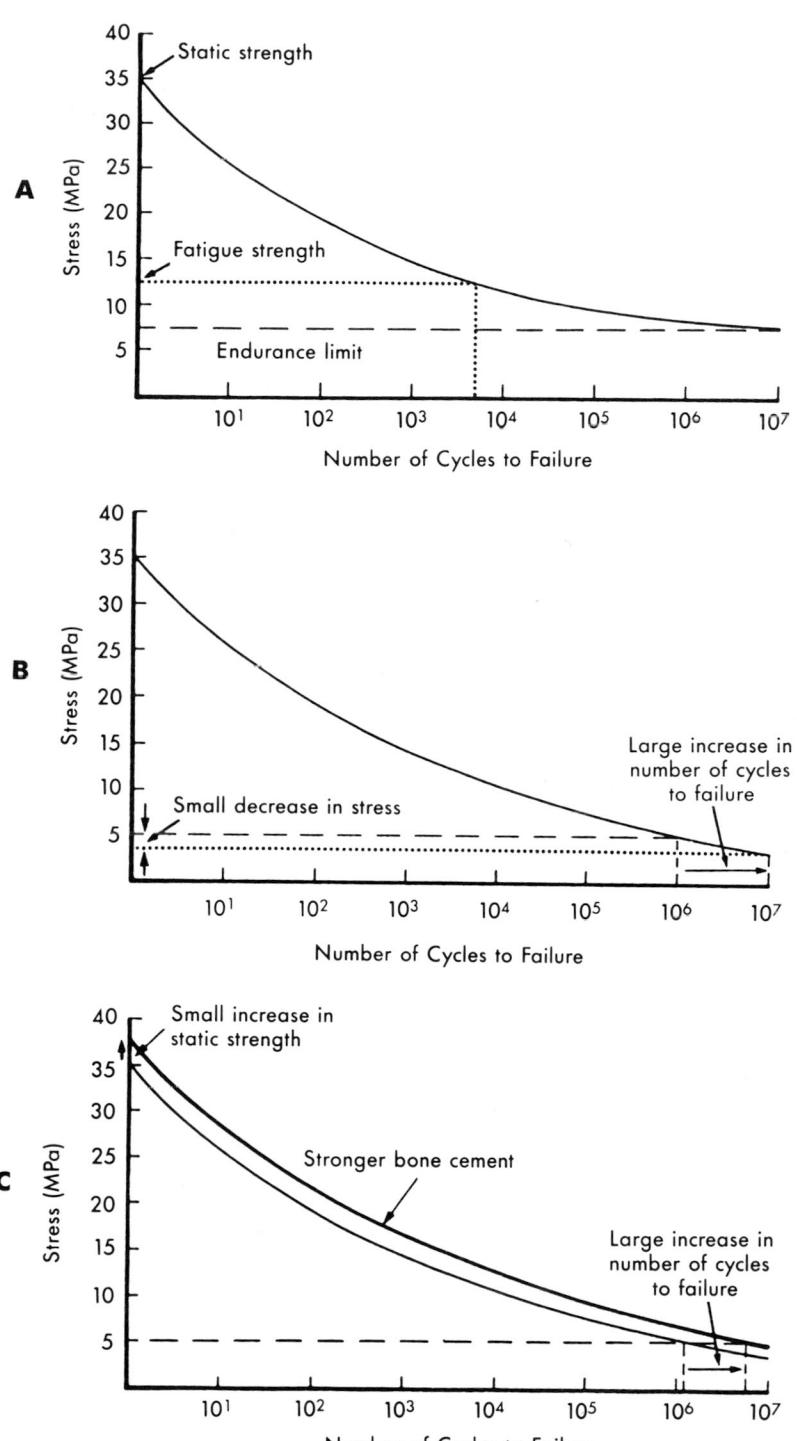

Fig. 5-13. A, Schematic representation of a theoretical S-N curve for bone cement. **B,** Large increase in fatigue life with small decrease in the applied stress. **C,** Large increase in fatigue life with small increase in the strength of the bone cement. (From Chan KH, Ahmed AM: Polymethyl methacrylate in joint replacement arthroplasty. In Morrey BF: *Joint replacement arthroplasty,* New York, 1991, Churchill-Livingstone.

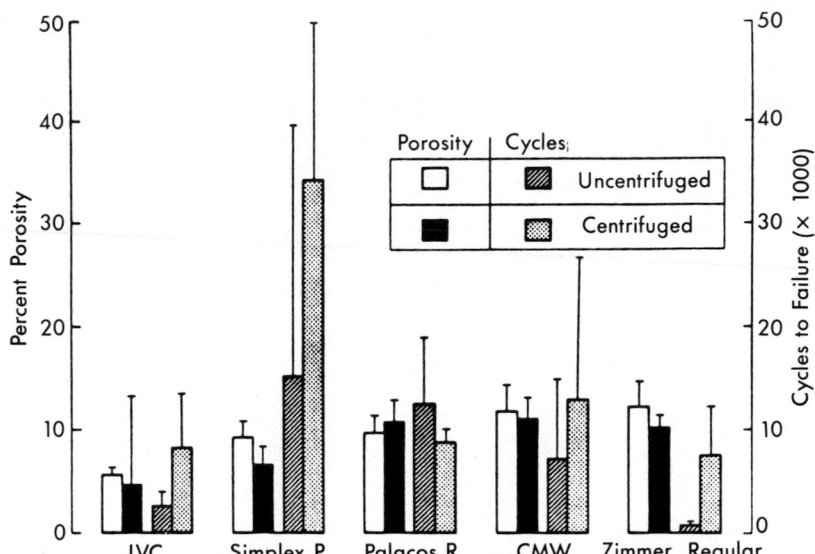

Fig. 5-14. The porosity *(black and white)* and cycles to failure *(shaded)* for commercial bone cements. The uncentrifuged cements were mixed with monomer at room temperature. The centrifuged cements were mixed with chilled monomer (except LVC) and spun for 30 seconds (except Palacos R, which was spun for 60 seconds). (From Davies JP, Jasty M, O'Connor DO, et al: The effect of centrifuging bone cement, *J Bone Joint Surg* 71[Br]:39, 1989.)

Table 5-10 Porosity of Fatigue Life of Common Bone Cements

Cements*		Porosity (percent) mean†				Cycles to failure mean†			
LVC		5.06 (0.52)				2575 (1,375)			
Simplex P	S	9.39 (1.53)	S		S	15,147 (24,690)	S		
		S				NS			
Palacos R	S	9.70 (1.83)	S		S	11,504 (6,387)	S		
		S				S			
CMW		11.99 (2.18)		S	S	S	7043 (7,806)		S	NS
		NS							
Zimmer Regular		12.38 (2.51)		S		879 (493)		S	

From Davies JP, Jasty M, O'Connor DO, et al: The effect of centrifuging bone cement, *J Bone Joint Surg* 71[Br]:40, 1989.
*Listed in order of increasing porosity.
†Figures in parentheses are standard deviations.
S—significant difference ($p < 0.05$).
NS—no significant difference.

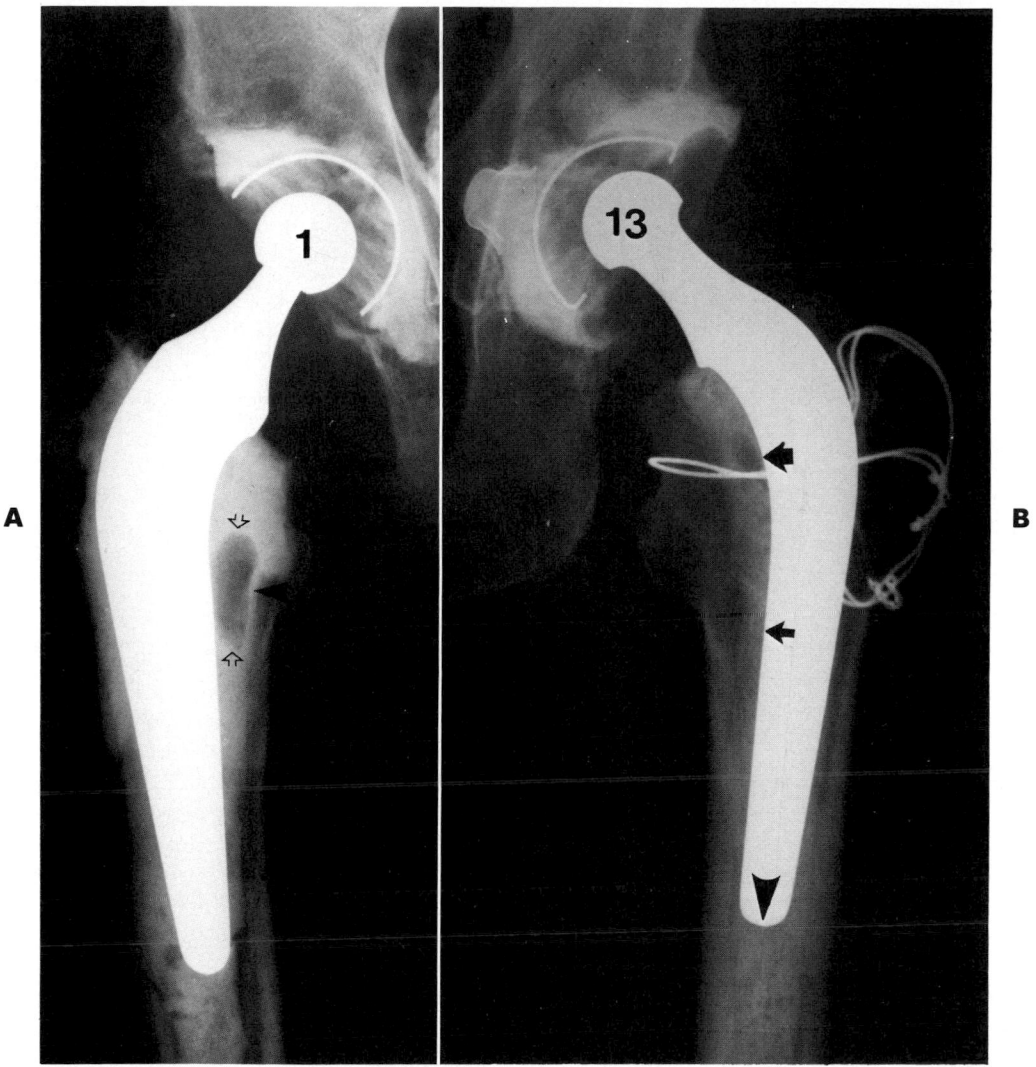

Fig. 5-15. A, 1 year postoperative radiograph of a revision total hip arthroplasty (E.F.) using noncentrifuged Palacos R cement. Arrows show a large void representing an air bubble measuring 3.1 cm. No failure has occurred. **B,** Radiograph 13 years postoperatively of a 61-year-old woman (L.K.) whose hip grade is A:6,6,6. Note many large, intermediate, and small porosities *(arrows)*. In practice, porosities did not cause failure as cement mantle is thick and thus unaffected by porosities.

The major monomer loss from evaporation of acrylic cement dough appears to take place during periods of mixing of the dough rather than at the final stage of mixing (from surface of the bolus before insertion) (Tables 5-12 to 5-14). It is of special interest that, irrespective of the amount of beating in preparation, cement became stronger with the passage of time up to 1 week after polymerization. Lee and co-workers observed a very satisfactory mechanical strength of PMMA in a specimen examined 7½ years after implantation.[109]

PMMA monomer is a very volatile substance. Its solubility in water is about 1.5% at 30° C, and it is rapidly eliminated from the body. The total concentration of leached-out monomer must therefore be low.[30]

The residual monomer in self-curing acrylic cement is measured by a calorimetric test using potassium permanganate. With this test, Smith and Bains[150] showed that two specimens of acrylic cement demonstrated no further loss of monomer after immersion for 36 hours in distilled water at 37° C. With heat-cured cement, the leaching of the monomer was completed experimentally at 17 hours in large volumes of water at 37° C and also after a similar period in a large group of volunteer patients. Smith examined four types of self-curing acrylic cement from different manufacturers for residual monomer from 1 hour to 58 weeks after curing. The four products demonstrated that fall in residual monomer was related to the "after-cure" process of further polymerization of the cement. The

Table 5-11 Effects of Centrifugation on Porosity and Fatigue Life

Cements*	Centrifugation time (seconds)		Porosity (percent) mean†			Cycles to failure mean†		
LVC	30		4.47 (0.85)			8233 (5185)		
Simplex P	30	S	6.62 (1.88)	S	S	34,239 (15,889)	S	
			|			|		
			S			S		
Zimmer Regular	30	NS	10.35 (1.34)	S	NS	7941 (4662)		NS
			|			|		
			NS			NS		
Palacos R	60	NS	10.76 (1.27)	S	S	NS	8687 (1258)	NS	S
CMW	30		11.11 (2.01)		S		12,127 (14,051)		NS

From Davies JP, Jasty M, O'Connor DO, et al: The effect of centrifuging bone cement, *J Bone Joint Surg* 71[Br]:40, 1989.
*Listed in order of increasing porosity.
†Figures in parentheses are standard deviations.
S—significant difference (p < 0.05).
NS—no significant difference.

Table 5-12 Mean Monomer Loss in gm/½ min During Mixing at Different Mixing Frequencies

Number of cements	Beat frequency/min	Mean monomer loss in gm/½ min during mixing
22	60	0.133
12	120	0.213
7	184	0.355
29	260	0.436

Table 5-13 Monomer Loss at Polymerization Testing Three Different Commercially Available Acrylics

Type of cement	Total loss over 1½ min	Loss/min
Simplex	0.165 gm	0.055 gm
Simplex opaque	0.192 gm	0.064 gm
CMW opaque	0.273 gm	0.091 gm

From Lee AJC, Wrighton JD: Some properties of polymethyl-methacrylate with reference to its use in orthopaedic surgery, *Clin Orthop* 95:281, 1973.

Table 5-14 Total Monomer Loss in gm/15 min at Different Mixing Frequencies

Beat frequency/min	Monomer loss in gm
60	0.85–1.28
120	1.01–1.96
184	1.67–2.24
260	2.4–3.4

From LEE AJC, Wrighton JD: Some properties of polymethyl-methacrylate with reference to its use in orthopaedic surgery, *Clin Orthop* 95:281, 1973.

four specimens started the test with retained monomer ranging from 3.5% to 1.9%. The residual monomer contents fell slightly over the period of the test, and for all specimens the drop averaged 0.3% over 58 weeks.[30] Monomer loss by evaporation from acrylic cement dough takes place to a significant degree only during periods in which the dough is being mixed and cannot be significantly altered after the mixing period. If the cement mass is left undisturbed until implantation, the concentration of monomer at the surface becomes low, but manipulation of the mass (during insertion into the medullary cavity of the femur, for example) will expose the deeper layer of the dough, and thus the monomer, to the bone surface.[107] It is, therefore, logical to suggest a vigorous mixing during doughing time to rid the cement of monomer. It should continue until cement is pasty and thick and starts giving "fine hairs" from the surface. However, this increases the air trapped in the cement as it is being polymerized, which in turn causes an increased porosity that may affect the fatigue life of the cement. The amount of monomer that reaches systemic circulation during in-vivo polymerization does not seem to cause any significant toxicity.

Smith and Schoonover[151] also determined residual activator (benzoyl peroxide) in the powder. Two of four specimens started with peroxide contents of approximately 0.35%, which fell in the first 58 weeks to a value of about 0.05%, which further fell to a final level of 0.02%.[91]

WORKING TIME AND SETTING TIME CHARACTERISTICS

During surgery, the full amount of liquid monomer is added to the preweighed polymer and thoroughly mixed with a spoon. For about 30 seconds there appears to be insufficient liquid for the powder, but the

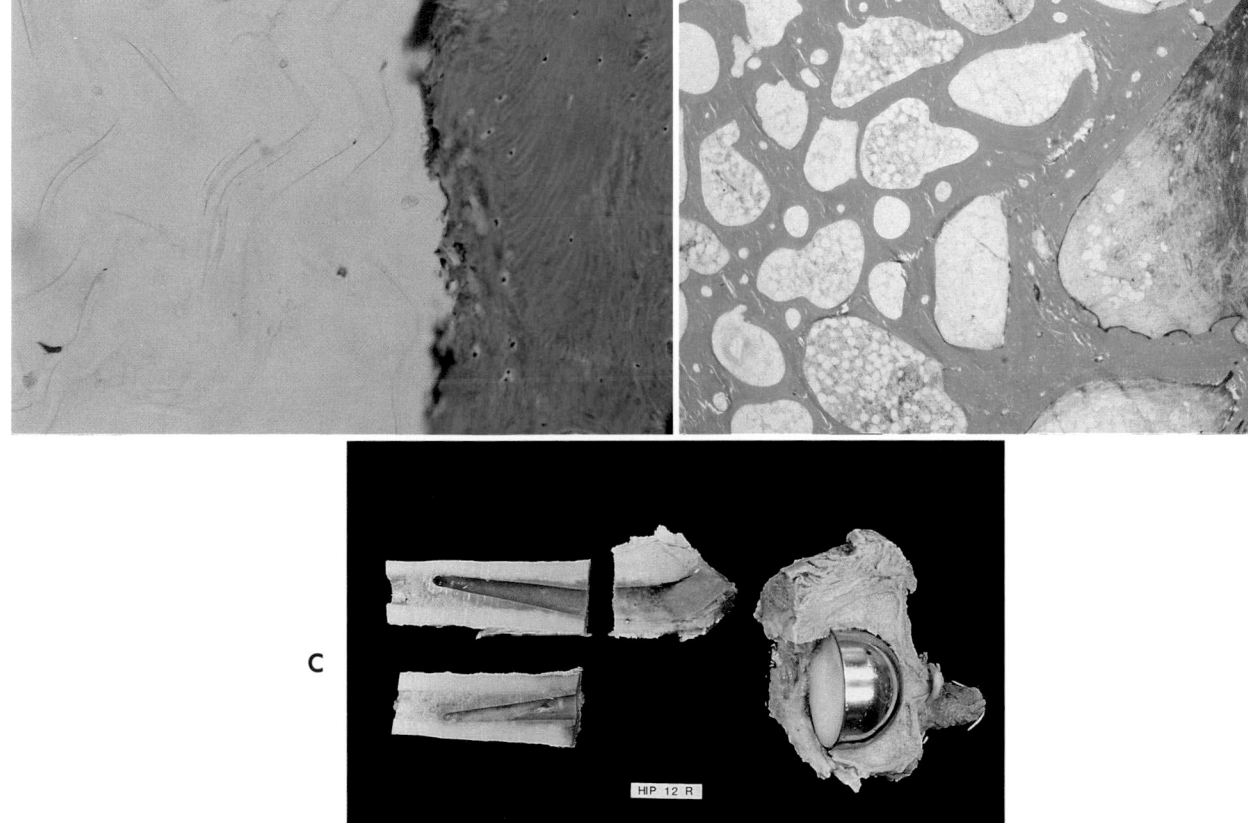

Plate 4. A, A higher magnification (x6) of wrinkled cement with mineralized bone showing that the osteocytes are still viable. **B,** A thick fibrous tissue was regular finding at the interface between the cemented cup and bone of the acetabulum. It was uncommon between the cemented femoral component and bone of the femur. The thick fibrous membrane contained wear particles of high density polyethylene. **C,** A longitudinal section of a cemented femur (pink dental cement was used by Sir John Charnley) and acetabulum. Horizontal cut confirmed evidence of osteointegration. Severe fibrosis was present around the press-fit metal-backed acetabular component (H.D.P.). (Reproduced from Sir John Charnley's Histological Collections, courtesy of Dr. AJ Malcolm).

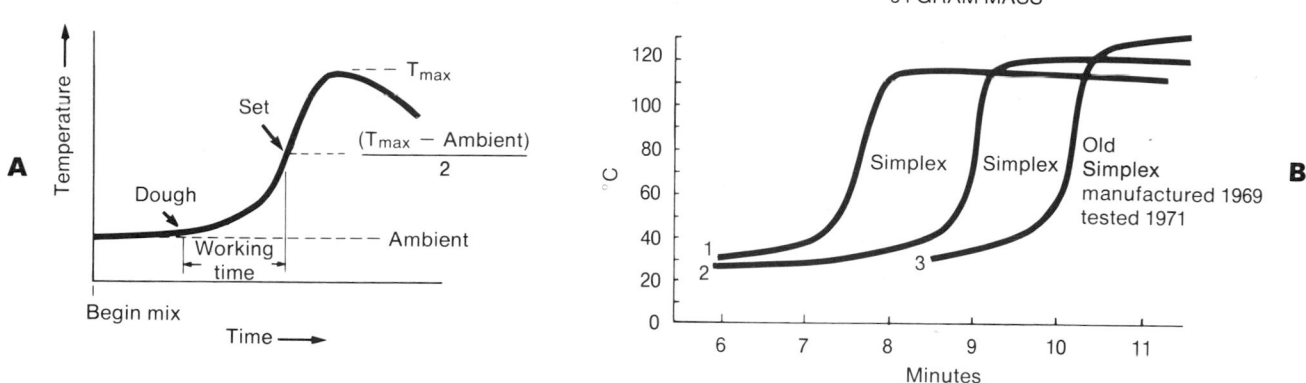

Fig. 5-16. A, Setting and working time characteristics of cement and its relationship to exothermic reaction. **B,** Effect of storage on setting characteristics of acrylic cement. Examples presented here: 1, Simplex fresh, 1969; 2, Simplex fresh, 1971; 3, old Simplex manufactured in 1969 and tested in 1971 using a 54-gm mass. (From Amstutz HC, Gruen T: In Ahstrom JP, editor: *Current practice in orthopaedic surgery,* St Louis, 1973, Mosby–Year Book.)

mass soon liquifies further and becomes rubbery. With mixing and aeration, tenacious "hairs" form, indicating readiness for removal from the bowl. When hairs no longer form, the glistening liquidlike appearance disappears, and a soft doughlike consistency allows removal from the bowl by scraping. The working time of the cement is approximately 2 to 4 minutes. During this period the surgeon inserts it into the bone (see Chapter 12). The setting characteristics (Fig. 5-16, *A*) of commercially available cements vary from brand to brand, batch to batch, and with the age of the liquid monomer (Fig. 5-16, *B*). An increase in ambient temperature decreases the working time of the dough; setting time (usually 12 to 13 minutes) depends on humidity, molecular weight of the polymer, texture of the powder, proportion of activator and initiator, and proportion of liquid to powder. Meyer and associates[118] concluded that in one batch of PMMA tested, the surface temperature of the setting cement never exceeded 70° C; the setting time was prolonged by lowering the ambient temperature, decreasing the powder:liquid ratio, and increasing the mass of cement. Although working time is not altered materially by changing the powder:liquid ratio, rise in maximum temperature occurs when excess monomer is used (Fig. 5-16, *A*). As a rule, CMW cement sets in about two thirds the time of Simplex P. The most significant and practically important factor is a decreased working time with rises in ambient temperature. Most investigators have concluded that batch-to-batch variations in cement composition should be expected.[27,109,113,118] Setting characteristics of cement as related to exothermic temperature and working time are shown in Figs. 5-16 to 5-19 and Tables 5-15 and 5-16.

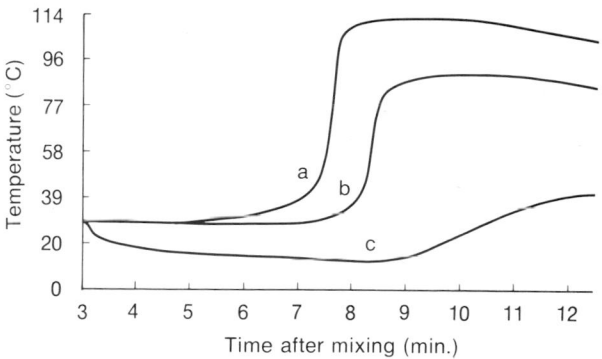

Fig. 5-17. Effect of ambient temperature on setting characteristics of PMMA. **A,** Thermal profile of mass center polymerizing at room temperature. **B,** Thermal profile of center. **C,** Periphery of mass setting with plastic bag immersed in ice water. (From Amstutz HC, Gruen T: PMMA cement. In Ahstrom JP, editor: *Current practice in orthopaedic surgery,* St Louis, 1973, Mosby–Year Book.)

RISE OF TEMPERATURE AND DENATURING OF PROTEIN

The degree of temperature elevation in the polymerizing cement mass is directly proportional to the size of the mass and to the ambient temperature. For example, a mass 1 inch in diameter may become too hot to hold in the hand. The temperature in the center of such a mass may rise to the boiling point, whereas the exterior temperature may be somewhat lower. When cement is used in conjunction with the prosthesis, considerable heat may be absorbed by metal and plastic, thus diminishing the surface temperature. Occasionally, however, one may see darkening of the blood adjacent to a thick layer of cement, suggesting heat denaturation of hemoglobin. When the rise in

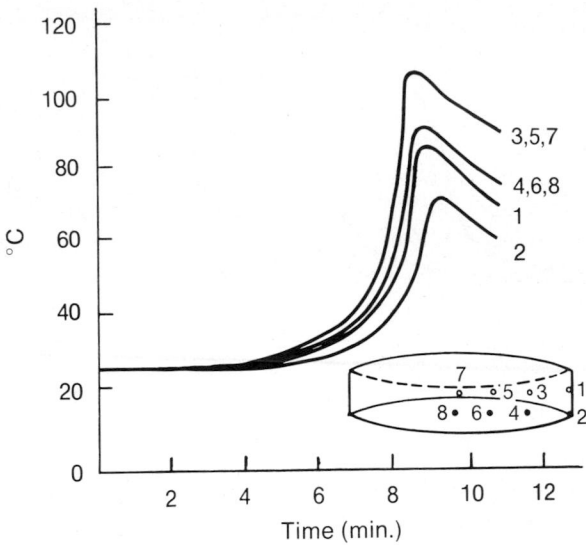

Fig. 5-18. Differences in temperature rise with respect to location in setting cement. Cement is insulating material capable of withstanding a large temperature gradient. At the surface, considerable heat can be conducted away by prosthesis or bone; in the interior mass of cement, temperature rise is considerably greater. (From Meyer PR, Lautenschlager EP, Moore BK: On the setting properties of acrylic bone cement, *J Bone Joint Surg* 55:149, 1973.)

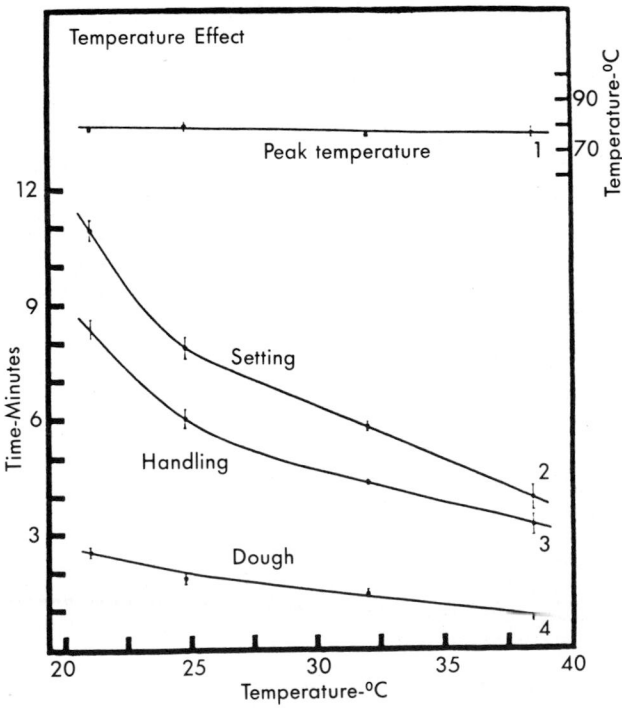

Fig. 5-19. Effects of mixing temperature (temperature of cement, mixing bowl, and atmosphere) on dough time, handling time, setting time, and peak temperature. Points for dough time are averages of two to seven determinations; other points are averages of four to fourteen determinations. Brackets on points show standard deviations. All specimens were made from material with the same manufacturer's batch number. (From Haas SS, Brauer GM, Dickson G: A characterisation of polymethylmethacrylate bone cement, *J Bone Joint Surg* 57:380, 1975.)

Table 5-15 Effect of Ambient Temperature of Setting Properties of Acrylic Cement

Ambient temperature (°C)	Dough time (min)	Set time (min)	Working time (min)	T_{max}* (°C)
4	34.0	60.0	26.0	53
15	10.5	21.5	11.0	89
20	4.5	13.0	8.5	101
25	3.0	8.0	5.0	107
30	2.0	5.0	3.0	111
37	1.0	3.0	2.0	125

From Meyer PR Jr, Lautenschlager EP, Moore BK: On the setting properties of acrylic bone cement, *J Bone Joint Surg* 55:149, 1973. *Measured in center of 36-gm specimen, 10 mm thick, mixed at P/L = 2.0, and placed in a 60-mm diameter Teflon mold.

Table 5-16 Effect of Thickness and Weight in Setting Properties*

Thickness (mm)	Weight (gm)	Set time (min)	T_{max} (°C)
10	36	8.0	107
6	22	7.0	86
3	11	6.2	60

From Meyer PR Jr, Lautenschlager EP, Moore BK: On the setting properties of acrylic bone cement, *J Bone Joint Surg* 55:149, 1973. *Ambient temperature = 25° C. All specimens set in 60-mm Teflon mold. T_{max} measured in center of disk at a depth of 5, 3, and 1.5 mm respectively.

temperature can be palpated, the working time is cut; thus cement becomes too hard to allow insertion of cement or prosthesis, and the surgeon is well advised to discard it (Figs. 5-17 and 5-18).

DIMENSIONAL CHANGES DURING POLYMERIZATION OF ACRYLIC CEMENT

Shrinkage of the acrylic cement mass after polymerization is expected. This shrinkage of pure monomer is approximately 20% with an increase in density from 0.94 gm/cm^3 to 1.19 gm/cm^3 after polymerization.[4,15] Since acrylic (combined liquid and powder) as used in orthopaedics comprises only one third of the total mass, the shrinkage of the mass should be approximately 7%. Smith and Schoonover[151] observed that polymerization shrinkage with dental cement was concentrated in localized areas and was not uniform throughout the mass.

When the bulk of cement is polymerized, shrinkage

of the final mass is attributed to volumetric shrinkage of the liquid component. Volumetric changes of CMW cement were determined by Charnley.[30] Several other investigators conducted similar studies and concluded that Simplex P, Omniplastic, and Palacos initially contracted, then expanded minimally, and finally contracted 2.2%, 4%, and 3.5% respectively (see Fig. 5-8).[30,80,162] The expansion of CMW was considerably greater; the net dimensional change after 15 minutes was 5.9%. Ideally, the cement would expand at the final stages of polymerization for better penetration into the bony interstices. In 1957, Wiltse and associates[166] reported a shrinkage of about 6% by volume. Charnley[38] concluded that the air bubbles trapped in the mix during preparation were responsible for expansion of the volume of cement and compensated for shrinkage of the total mass. This is the basis for his recommendation of vigorous beating for aeration.[30] However, as stated, increased porosity of cement reduces the fatigue life of cement, which may affect its long-term clinical behavior.

MICROSTRUCTURE OF PMMA CEMENT

The powder of PMMA is composed of two forms of PMMA, one consisting of tiny spherical beads formed by suspension polymerization methods and the other of finely ground amorphous PMMA. In surgical Simplex P, 83.8% of the polymer is MMA styrene copolymer, whereas in CMW the polymer is pure PMMA.

Polymerized cement has a biphasic structure consisting of aggregates of small spheres or granules of the previously described polymer (powder) cemented together by recently polymerized monomer (liquid)[24,30] (Fig. 5-20). The balls of polymer are from 10 to 80 μm in diameter and are said to be responsible for the semicircular impression on the surface of endosteal bone in histological specimens. Charosky and Walker,[44] using scanning electron microscopy, concluded that the cast surfaces and polished sections of two different types of cement (Simplex P and CMW) demonstrate spherical domes 5 to 30 μm in diameter. The domes are bubbles in the material seen in polished sections, and therefore the cement probably is a monophasic material.

The presence of bubbles and voids in the texture of the cement is clearly seen under the microscope. In studying the porosity of self-curing acrylic cement, Smith and co-workers[151] observed two types of porosities: (1) large irregular voids, which were attributed to polymerization contraction, and (2) fine spherical bubbles similar to those of gaseous porosity in heat-cured materials. They cited work showing that acrylic monomer can contain up to 10% dissolved air by volume and suggested that these bubbles are caused by the separation of dissolved air as the monomer solidifies.

MECHANICAL FIXATION BY INTERLOCK

Some of the principles involved in mechanical fixation have been detailed in Chapters 4 and 6.

Uninitiated surgeons often use the term *glue* for the cement used in replacement surgery. The distinction between a glue and a "filler" is not merely semantic but is based on real differences in the mechanisms by which the two operate. Understanding how acrylic cement can transfer the load from the stem of a prosthesis to the shaft of the femur and diffuse the load onto the endosteal surface of the bone is the sine qua non of correct application of the cement. When used as a stiff paste or dough, it has space-filling properties not possessed by thin liquid glue. If a prosthesis were glued to the bone, it would be advantageous to have a tight mechanical fit using the thinnest possible layer of glue. The stem would be wet with the glue and then be driven firmly into a tight bed. In this situation, obviously the surfaces must be shaped to make an accurate fit, which is not possible in this surgery. Also, glue depends on a chemical reaction for adhesion, and a thin adhesive could not withstand the incumbent stresses. On the other hand, a filler, or cement, does not require any chemical interaction between the two surfaces; the cement serves as an interface. Thus an accurate fit between bone surface and prosthesis is not required, since the cement fills in bulk inaccuracies and gaps between the two structures. In this context, therefore, the cement is used thickly and has the mechanical advantage of withstanding a considerable amount of stress. Indeed, a thin layer may weaken and become brittle, inevitably fragmenting.

Because most forces in the hip are compressive, cement is most suitable for bonding, since its best mechanical property is compressive strength. By interdigitation of the cement into the bone during cyclic loading and unloading of the transmission of body weight, the whole surface of the interior of the bone is subjected to the load, thus preventing concentration of stress at any given area of contact. Therefore shearing forces between prosthesis and bone are reduced by the absence of friction between the two surfaces. Lack of motion prevents fretting movements that cause bone necrosis. The most common cause of failure of fixation is principally related to the stress concentration often produced by "mechanical-interference-fit" (also known as Press-fit) of bone implants.

Inability to understand the mechanism by which cement functions led to early surgeons' failure to achieve successful results.[72,96] Apparently they used a small amount of cement only to improve the seating of the collar of the prosthesis against the cut surface of the femoral neck. This also explains the failure of fixation when cement was delicately applied to the

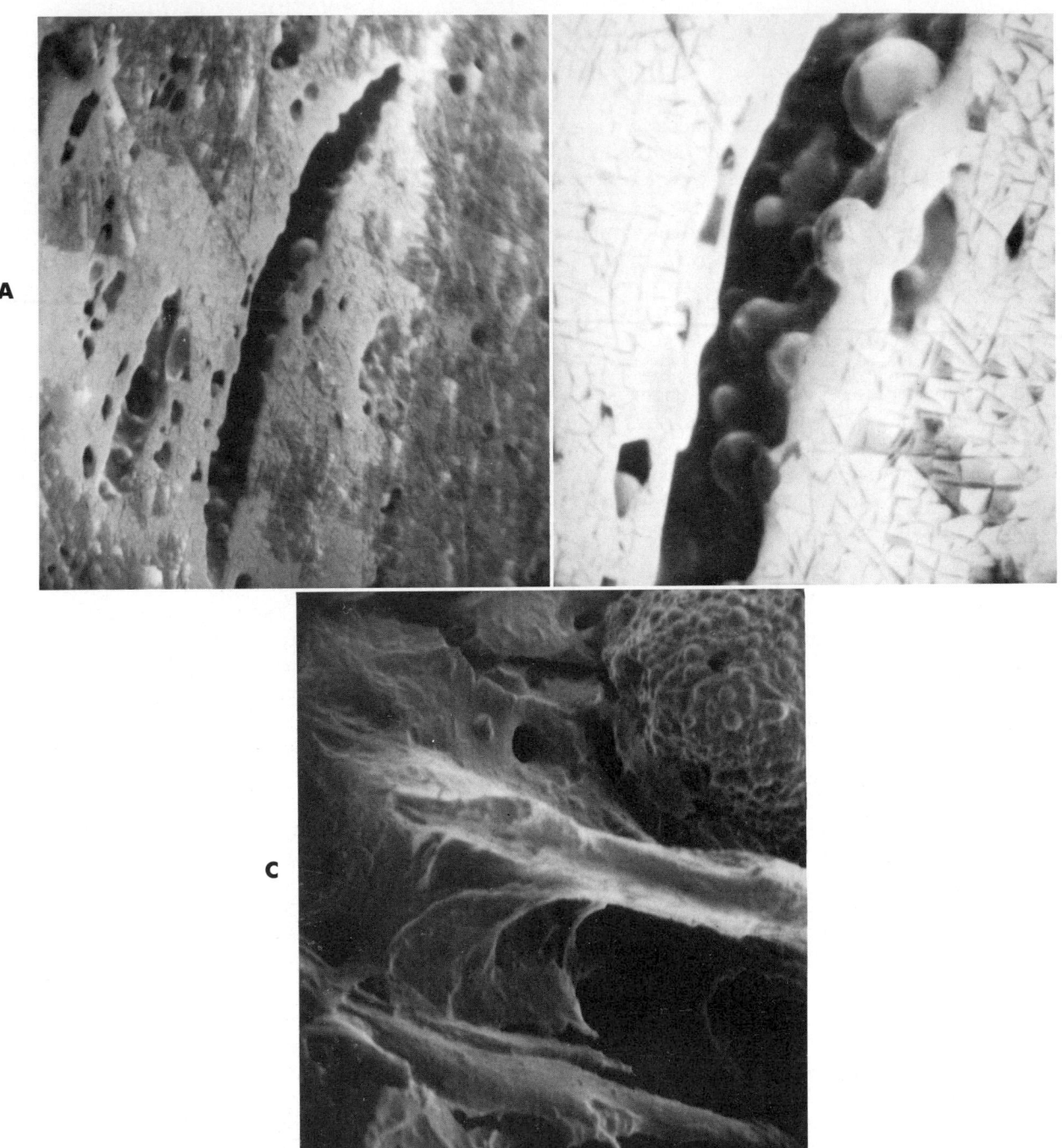

Fig. 5-20. A, At low magnification of the cut surface of acrylic cement (prepared during surgery), an elongated void in the internal mass of bolus can be seen (scanning electron microscopy). **B,** Higher magnification of **A** shows features of the surface of the void, revealing small spheres of polymer on internal surface (scanning electron microscopy). **C,** Moderate magnification of the cement-bone interface, showing blob of cement at upper right corner of field. NOTE: characteristic feature of cement surface—spheres of polymer (scanning electron microscopy).

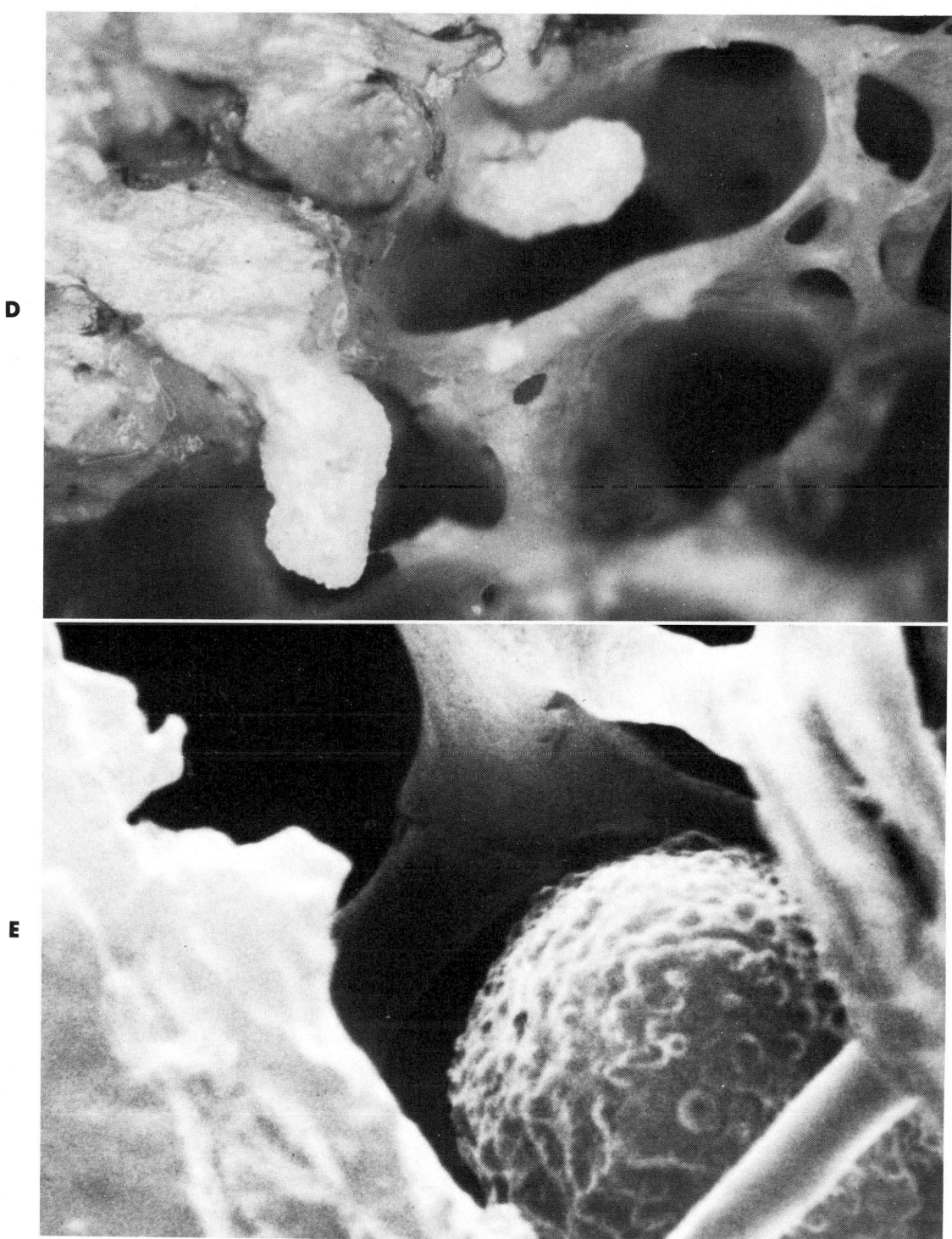

Fig. 5-20—cont'd. D, High-power magnification of cement in contact with polymethyl methacrylate cement. NOTE: intimacy of cement with trabeculae. Note also healed fractured trabeculae *(center of field)* presumably from trauma at surgery. **E,** Scanning electron microscopy of PMMA cement-bone interface. Close coaptation of cement with bone in specimen is observed. Polymeric spheres again are seen here. (Courtesy James Pugh, Ph.D.)

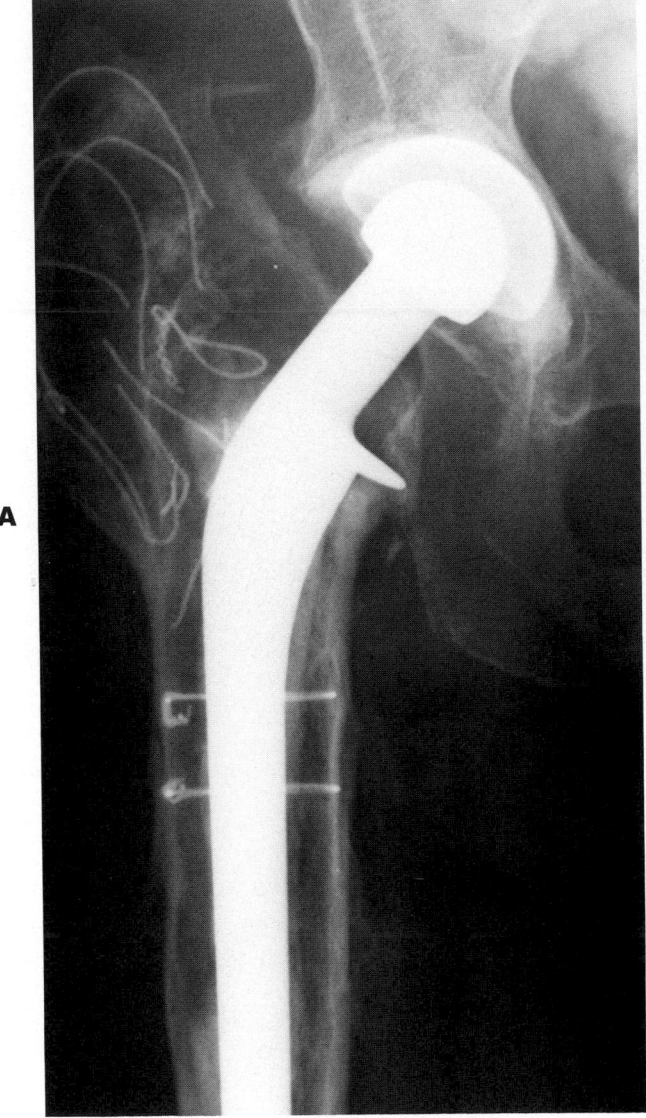

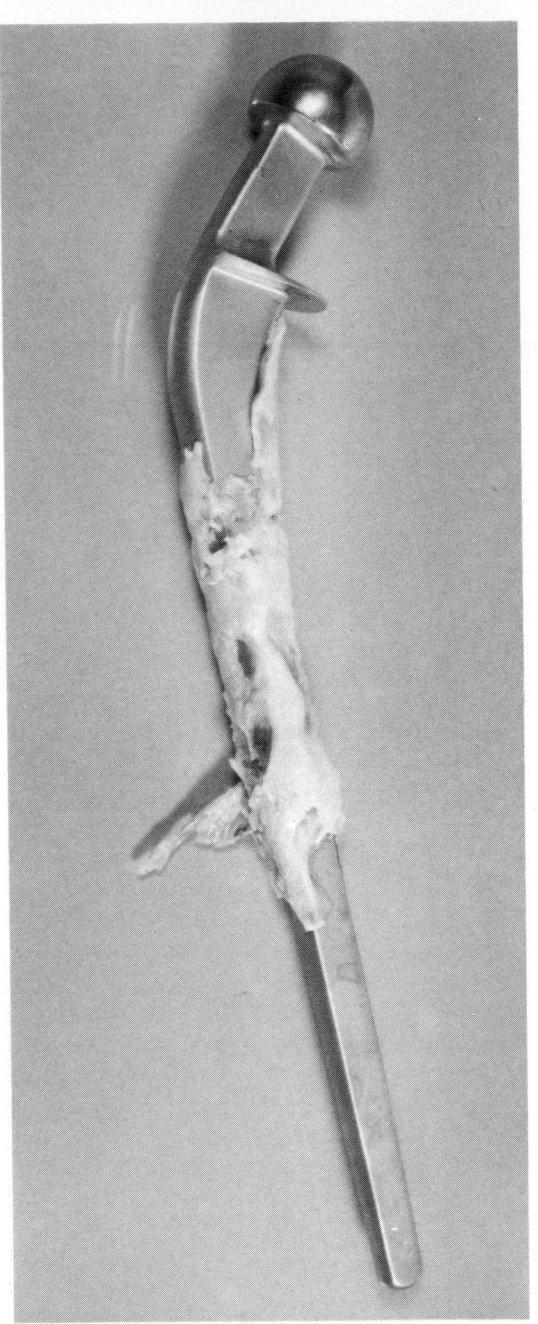

Fig. 5-21. An example of inadequate bonding of cement with bone caused by inadequate amount of cement and bleeding pressure caused at surgery. **A,** Postoperative radiograph of 67-year-old woman (B.A.) with revision arthroplasty for a fractured femur after total hip arthroplasty (performed at another institution) with immediate failure. **B,** The long stem prosthesis removed at surgery was found to be grossly loose.

upper femur. Failure will occur if the surgeon does not appreciate that interosseous injection of cement provides adequate thickness and bonding over a relatively large surface area. Fixation of a prosthesis into the medullary canal is analogous to a flagpole being pushed into a hole filled with wet concrete. The larger the volume of concrete and the greater the interdigitation of its surface with the ground, the more stability against compressive and shearing stresses is provided for the flagpole (Fig. 5-21).

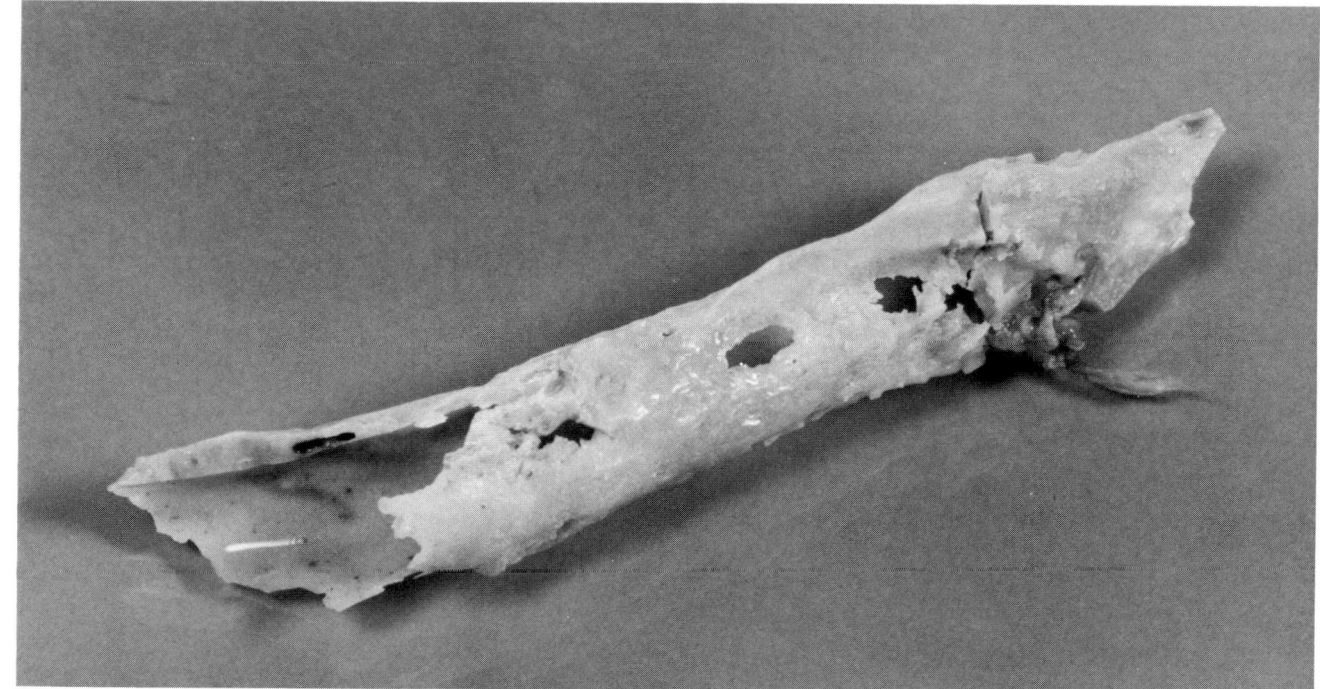

Fig. 5-21 – cont'd. C, Note inadequate (incomplete) cement mantle without any evidence of interdigitation of cement into bone.

Charnley is credited with the use of cement in orthopaedic surgery as a filler rather than an adhesive. He contended that it forms an accurate filling for cavities of the interior surface of the bone. Thus it transmits the load evenly over a fairly large area between the outer surface of the metal and the inner surface of the bone.[29,32,33]

BONDING OF PMMA TO METAL SURFACES

Without adhesive properties, PMMA has the capability of bonding to irregular surfaces by an interlocking mechanism. Cook and associates[43] increased shear strength properties by treating the surface of metal with a porous-coating process. They tested the shear properties of TI6-AL4-V alloy of smooth satin finish and comparably sized, porous-coated cylindrical specimens. The sintered surfaces, with beads ranging from 294 to 1400 μm and porosities of 165 to 550 μm, created a surface porosity between 40% and 44%.[43] They found a significantly increased shear strength in the coated specimens, as the pore size increased from 285 μm to 345 μm; shear strength increased from 18.1 MPa to 23.6 MPa.[43]

Other techniques to improve bonding of PMMA to metal surfaces have included precoating of the metal surface by PMMA before using it during surgery.[128,140,141] The PMMA precoating involves depositing a thin film of PMMA comprising high-quality acrylic, normally used in the manufacturing of bone cement, which does not contain impurities such as antioxidants, inhibitors, initiators, plasticisors, or radiographic markers such as barium sulfate. The thickness of the film may vary from 0.0001 to 0.0250 inches (2.5 μm to 635 μm) depending on the method of application, but a typical thickness is 12.7 to 76.2 μm. The film is applied after a fine microfinish, cleaning, and normal passivation of the metal surface. The process of precoating the metal surface is a relatively simple but effective way to improve bonding between the prosthesis and the cement by optimizing the "adhesive bond" between the metal surface and the PMMA. Crowninshield and Tolbert[44] have shown the effectiveness of a firm bonding between the precoated PMMA and PMMA. In testing the pullout strength of PMMA precoated and standard implant finish using cobalt-chromium-molybdenum alloy test pins, they found a significant improvement after precoating: 335 (±224.9) versus 527 (±79.1) pounds for the precoated and standard implant finish, respectively. Park and co-workers[127a] have demonstrated that the shear strength of a rod/interface also can be enhanced substantially (585%) by precoating. Sandblasting increases the shear strength between the implant and cement by 337% (from 1.17 to 3.84 MPa).[127,127a] The value of precoated stems of total hip prostheses awaits testing in controlled clinical studies.

VARIABLES CAUSING ALTERATIONS IN MECHANICAL PROPERTIES OF PMMA

Several variables can affect the basic mechanical properties of acrylic cement. These variables may directly or indirectly influence the strength of the cement and thus the strength of fixation by microinterlock or macrointerlock, influencing the ultimate stability of the prosthesis and the clinical outcome. Some of these variables are interrelated and coexist. They can be deleterious in the effort to achieve a perfect bond between the prosthesis and bone or can influence the long-term results as a result of general fatigue and failure of the material. Some of these variables are controlled by the surgeon; others are inherent in the mechanical properties and can be influenced only by the surgeon's choice of the type of cement or by manipulation and application of the material. These variables include (1) cement thickness, (2) contamination by blood, fat, and debris, (3) mixing techniques, (4) layering of cement, (5) environmental effects, (6) additives, (7) physical constraint of cement, (8) implants, (9) viscosity, (10) aging of PMMA, (11) loading rate, (12) bone strength, and (13) cement-bone interface.

Cement Thickness

Because of the relative weakness of cement in shear and tension, it is suitable for application in joint replacement only if it is used in bulk and in a thickness sufficient to withstand applied forces. A crack can be initiated and propagated with much less energy in a thin layer of cement than in a thick layer. Any defect resulting from impurities or the polymerization process, such as shrinkage or porosity, will affect a thin layer of cement more. However, the flow of a very thick layer of cement may be more difficult to control during insertion of the prosthesis. A thick layer also generates a greater exothermic reaction and surface monomer release to tissue, and thus in theory, greater cytotoxicity and dimensional changes by surface shrinkage.

Contamination by Blood, Fat, and Debris

In practice, during manipulation of the cement by hand, blood, fat, and bone debris can contaminate the cement and alter its mechanical properties to a lesser or greater degree. Contaminants can also increase stress after polymerization of the cement, the extent of which is often unpredictable. In one study,[108] blood contamination of cement reduced the ultimate compression stress of acrylic cement between 8% and 16% with a significantly high standard deviation. Gruen and associates[70] have shown that admixture of blood reduces the tensile strength and shear strength by as much as 77% and 69%, respectively. Homsey and co-workers[80] have made similar observations, demonstrating reductions of more than 50% in the tensile strength of their specimens. While a decrease in mechanical strength can be shown dramatically in test specimens, as evidenced by these studies, the composite of prosthesis-bone, cement-bone in a simulated implanted prosthesis may not be as sensitive to inclusion of blood using static loads.[18] Continuous bleeding remains a major problem and challenge to the surgeon while cement is being applied to the bone during surgery. Bleeding pressure occurs at the bone surface (unless a tourniquet is applied) and may compromise the integrity of bone-cement and cement fixation. Such undesirable effects were demonstrated by Benjamin et al in a simple laboratory experiment using a low-viscosity cement; by maintaining adequate pressure on the cement until it increases its viscosity, the surgeon can resist displacement of cement caused by bleeding pressure.[12a,16] However, this beneficial effect may be upset by a decrease in its fracture toughness caused by centrifugation.

Mixing Techniques

Rapid beating of the cement before polymerization increases porosity, thus lowering its strength.[10,71,109]

Layering of Cement

In addition to avoiding contaminants such as fat, blood, and debris, the surgeon must protect the cement from lamination, which can occur during the late stages of polymerization, that is, after 5 to 7 minutes.[70] Gruen demonstrated that up to a 54% reduction in tensile strength can occur after lamination. Lamination of cement tends to occur late in polymerization. During the early phase of polymerization cement is less viscous, but toward the end (exothermic phase) any residual folds in the cement tend to persist. Another factor that may influence layering of cement is lack of pressure on the cement, which allows introduction of fat and blood. Although the old and new cement will bond chemically and mechanically,[18,66,87] layering of cement can seriously weaken the mechanical properties of cement as a result of large voids and impurities trapped between the layers.[14,18] This may also occur if a new batch of cement is added to a polymerizing batch of cement. In an experiment by Greenwald and associates, the shear strength of the added cement was decreased by between 63% and 78%. This dramatic effect was thought to be the result of exothermic reaction of the initial cement, which in turn decreases the density of the new cement by initiating numerous voids and porosities.[67]

Environmental Effects (Temperature and Moisture)

During mixing under laboratory conditions at temperatures between 20° and 21° C, Lee and associates[109] showed a subsequent temperature increase to the level of body temperature, that is, 37° C, can reduce the mechanical properties of cement by 10% (Fig. 5-22). Lee also has reported that a 3% reduction in ultimate compressive strength can occur from moisture content in the cement, which reaches equilibrium after insertion in the body.[108]

Haas et al characterized PMMA by its physical properties such as dough time, handling time, setting time, and temperature rise as these parameters were affected by relative humidity (Table 5-17).[71]

Additives

The addition of radiopaque materials (barium sulfate) decreases ultimate compressive strength by 5%. It can be as great as 8% if mixed as recommended by the manufacturers. If barium sulfate is added during surgery, it must be thoroughly mixed with polymer to avoid scattered stress risers, which can weaken cement. Like barium sulfate, antibiotics in powder form can weaken the cement; their effect is based on the ratio of antibiotic to the quantity of cement used (Table 5-18).

Bargar and associates[9] have tested the effects of adding 1 ml of aqueous methylene blue dye to give visual contrast for Simplex P radiopaque bone cement, Zimmer bone cement, and low-viscosity Zimmer ce-

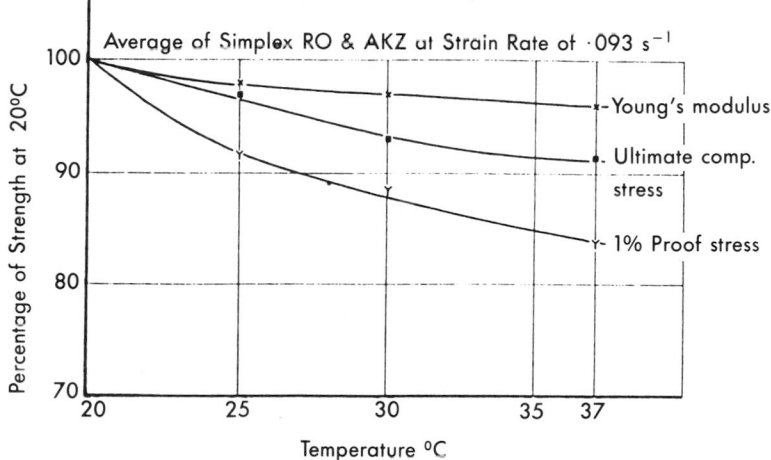

Fig. 5-22. Relationship of environmental temperature to mechanical properties of cement. (From Lee AJC, Ling RSM, Vangala SS: Some clinically relevant variables affecting the mechanical behavior of bone cement, *Arch Orthop Traumat Surg* 92:1, 1978.)

Table 5-17 Effect of Relative Humidity (RH), Combinations of Variables, and Aging on Setting Behavior

	Dough time (sec)	Handling time (sec)	Setting time (sec)	Peak temperature (°C)
Effects of relative humidity				
Powder desiccated (mixed at 45% RH)	142	519	661	77
Mixed at 20% RH	147	410	556	82
Mixed at 74% RH	120	369	489	82
Powder stored over water (mixed at 48% RH)	114	298	412	85
Water added to mix	106	302	408	87
Effects of combinations of variables				
Radiolucent, 32° C, kneaded, 3/1	88	224	312	72
Radiopaque, 24° C, not kneaded, 2/1	222	404	626	76
Effect of age of material				
Initial trial	170	322	492	75
After 5 months	161	325	486	77

From Haas SS, Brauer GM, Dickson G: A characterization of polymethylmethacrylate bone cement, *J Bone Joint Surg* 57:380, 1975.

Table 5-18 Effect of Antibiotic Additions

Cement	Antibiotic added (gm)	Number of samples	Ultimate compressive stress (Nmm^{-2})*
Simplex P	0	9	87.7 (2.0)
Simplex P	1	5	82.0 (2.3)
Simplex P	2	5	73.0 (1.9)
Simplex P	5	4	70.9 (4.6)
CMW	0	9	87.25 (2.45)
CMW	1	5	80.17 (2.03)
CMW	2	6	71.98 (3.74)
CMW	5	5	64.32 (8.47)

From Lee AJC, Ling RSM, Vangala SS: Some clinically relevant variables affecting the mechanical behavior of bone cement, *Arch Orthop Traumat Surg* 92:1, 1978.
All samples 2 days old. Strain rate = 0.003 s^{-1}.
Antibiotic = Nebacetin.
*Standard deviations are shown in parentheses.

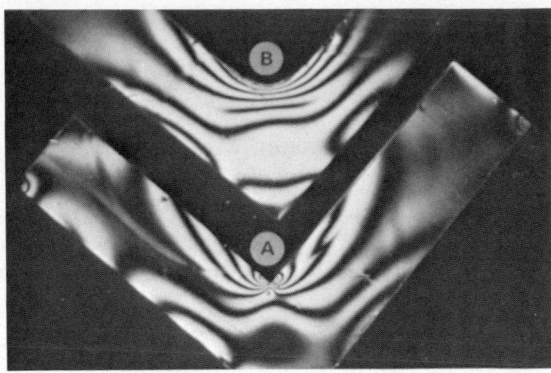

Fig. 5-23. Comparison of stress concentration at sharp corner *(A)* with more even distribution of stress at the radiused corner *(B)* demonstrated by photoelastic fringes. (From Lee AJC, Ling RSM, Vangala SS: Some clinically relevant variables affecting the mechanical behavior of bone cement, *Arch Orthop Traumat Surg* 92:1, 1978.)

ment. Their study indicated that the mechanical properties of these cements, tested for torsion, compression, and three- or four-point bending strength under laboratory conditions, were not changed and appeared safe and effective for use in primary and revision surgery. However, the working time, including dough and set, was decreased by 30 to 150 seconds. Also, tests showed that adding 1.2 gm of tobramycin weakened the cement to 87% of the control (100%), but no further weakening occurred as a result of adding methylene blue dye to the composite.

Antibiotics in powder form (never in liquid form) may be mixed with cement in a ratio of 1 to 2 gm per 20-gm packet of cement without any serious deleterious effect. Large amounts of antibiotics (4 to 6 gm) should not be used because this significantly alters the mechanical properties of the cement. Antibiotics should be mixed well with the polymer before adding the monomer. Centrifugation does not affect the distribution of antibiotics in the cement. The percentage of weakening of cement by varying amounts of antibiotics (Nebacetin) is shown in Table 5-18.

Other additives, such as carbon, polyethylene, and stainless steel fibers, cause alterations in the mechanical properties of cement and changes in the working time and handling of the material.[42]

Load-Bearing Capacity of PMMA

Because of the relatively inferior mechanical properties of cement in comparison with bone, overstressing of cement by the prosthesis must be avoided. The following conditions, which may lead to abnormal strain and thus failure of cement from excess stress, are related to poor prosthesis design or to the lack of constraint and support for cement by the bone.

High stresses resulting from design of the implant observed in clinical practice and by finite element stress analysis[44] have been shown to cause cement failure. Early prostheses with a diamond cross-sectional design often failed because of high compression stress at the sharp corners (wedge effect). In laboratory conditions, cement failure resulting from a loaded triangular pin and a circular tapered pin were compared. The load at cement failure with the triangular taper was below the limit of the resolution of the machine, whereas in the circular taper (control) the average was 11 kN. A comparison of stress concentration resulting from sharp corners can also be made between a triangular taper and a round taper using photoelastic methods (Fig. 5-23). These data clearly imply that high stress is generated by sharp corners, which must be avoided in stems designed to be used with cement (see Chapter 6).

Hoop stresses generated in the cement mantle resulting from vertical load of the tapered stem have been recognized as a cause of cement failure. The hoop stress can exceed the ultimate tensile stress of acrylic cement that is partly caused by polymerization shrinkage of acrylic cement.[154]

It is believed that high degrees of creep resulting from high stress occur within cement. An unconstrained cement column may undergo an increasingly significant creep as time passes under load. The cement's capacity to carry considerable load when it is constrained was demonstrated by Lee by a simple experiment (Fig. 5-24) that entailed loading tapered pins in constrained and nonconstrained conditions. A great load-bearing capacity was imparted by constraining the acrylic cement in a metal tube. The constrained specimens failed at 11 kN, but the load was transmitted to a very high level, 45 kN and 91 kN (despite cement cracking within constraint).[108]

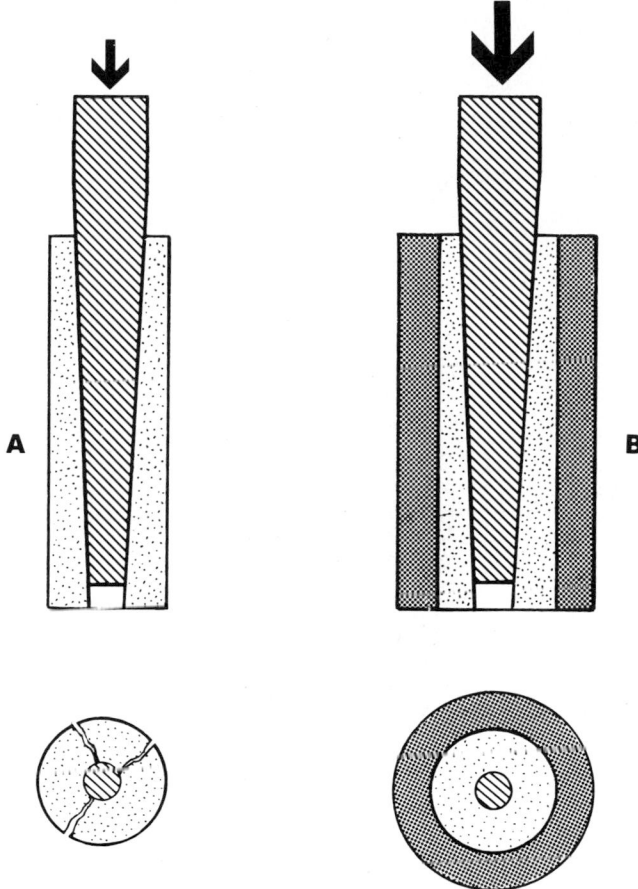

Fig. 5-24. **A,** Circular sections *(bottom)* and tapers *(top)* in acrylic cement without variable constraint. **B,** Circular sections *(bottom)* and tapers *(top)* in acrylic cement with constraint. (Redrawn from Lee AJC, Ling RSM, Vangala SS: Some clinically relevant variables affecting the mechanical behavior of bone cement, *Arch Orthop Traumat Surg* 92:1, 1978.)

When the surgeon fails to produce support for cement by bone, the hoop stresses may exceed the strength of the cement, causing the cement to fail. The case illustrated in Fig. 5-25 shows that a surgeon's failure to produce a good cement mantle by using too little cement in a large medullary canal caused a sudden failure of the cement mantle under unusually heavy load.

Aging and Fatigue

Wagner and associates[161] found a reduction in tensile strength and Young's modulus of elasticity but an increase in compressive strength as a result of aging. In their study they stored specimens at 37° C for 6 months. In a similar study using Simplex and CMW bone cement, Jaffe and co-workers[88] stored specimens in bovine serum at 37° C for up to 2 years and found no deleterious effect in the mechanical properties of these cements. Lee and associates[108] tested samples at 2 hours, 2 days, and 7 days after mixing with some

samples tested up to 2 years. They estimated that the reduction in the ultimate compressive strength over 10 years was approximately 10%; however, during the first weeks of aging the ultimate compressive strength of cement always increased (Fig. 5-26). In specimens obtained from a hip at 7½ years after surgery, they found evidence of a significant reduction in ultimate compressive strength and Young's modulus of elasticity. The results of fatigue tests performed in the laboratory may be biased by whether an implanted prosthesis (simulated conditions) is tested or not.[88] Although a reduction in the mechanical properties of cement caused by aging has been well documented, the long-term clinical failure after 10 or 15 years has not been fully determined.

Bone Strength and Fixation Strength

The strength of fixation cannot be considered independent of the mechanical properties of bone. While bone strength cannot be controlled by the surgeon, the significance of the surgeon's operative technique cannot be overestimated. Laboratory tests have shown that loosely attached and fragile trabeculae cannot withstand the stresses that affect a heavily loaded femur. Proper cleansing and removal of the soft cancellous bone enhance fixation. PMMA also has been used extensively as an adjunct to conventional fixation of pathological bone (after metastatic lesions) for prevention and management of fractures. Studies have shown that augmentation of fixation by PMMA is effective for this purpose. A properly designed and cement-augmented fluted intramedullary rod and low-viscosity cement have produced strength approaching that of an intact femur, which can make immediate mobilization of the patient possible.[120]

Cement-Bone Interface

In-vitro studies suggest that strong bone support is a prerequisite for good fixation by cement. Lee[108] has concluded that, in general, the strongest trabecular bone is located near the cortex. However, the strength of fixation also depends on the relationship of the trabeculae to the plane of shear. As might be expected, Lee found that in-vitro preparation affected the strength of the interface between the cement and bone; maximal cement/bone interface shear strength was obtained by exposing the strong trabecular bone and applying low-viscosity cement under pressure. Since shear forces must be resisted in the bone of the femur and since failure of the prosthesis is probably a result of shear force, good-quality bone is necessary to resist the incumbent shear forces.

The strength of bone and cement increases with increased pressure introduced when inserting low-viscosity cement. The cement penetration is a decreas-

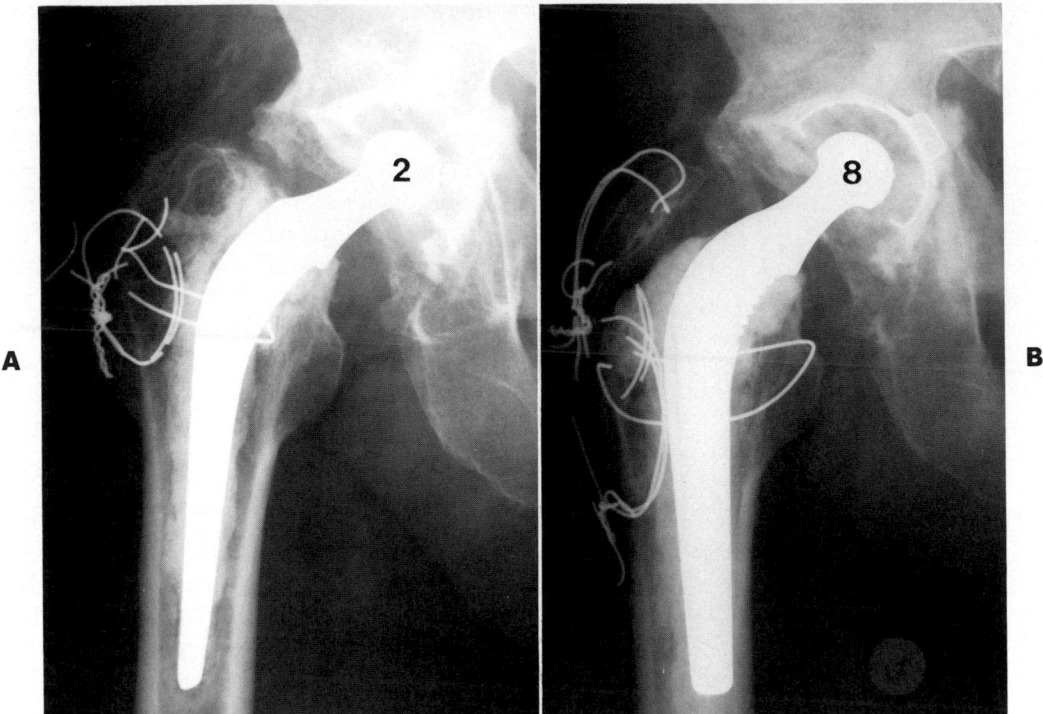

Fig. 5-25. Total hip arthroplasty was performed in a 63-year-old man (J.L.) with osteoarthritis. The original Charnley flat-back stem was used. **A,** Two years postoperatively, note inadequate medullary canal filling. The stem failed early when patient lifted a large piece of furniture, experiencing a sudden sensation of "cracking" in the upper thigh. **B,** Radiograph 8 years after revision surgery demonstrates excellent fixation of stem by PMMA. This demonstrates failure because of technique rather than cement.

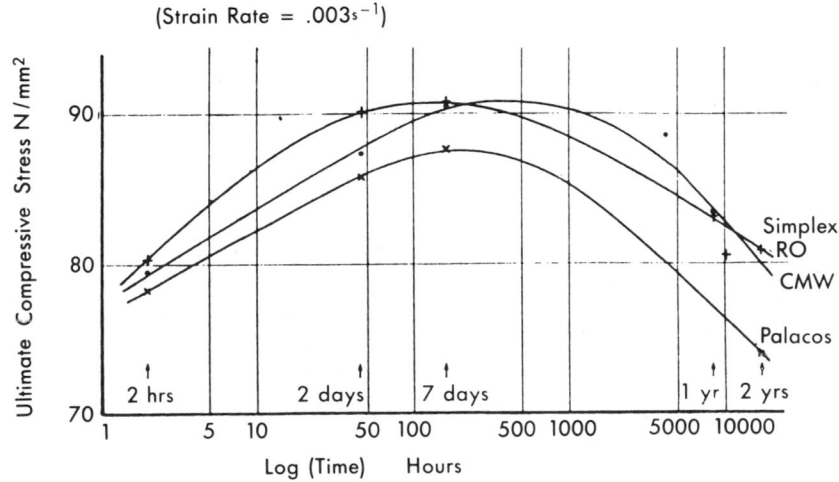

Fig. 5-26. Relationship of ultimate compressive strength of cement to time after curing. (From Lee AJC, Ling RSM, Vangala SS: Some clinically relevant variables affecting the mechanical behavior of bone cement, *Arch Orthop Traumat Surg* 92:1, 1978.)

ing function of bone strength and porosity. The strength of the bone/cement composite achieved is limited by the intrinsic mechanical properties of the bone. A weak bone cannot produce strong fixation in vitro despite good penetration of cement.[7]

In attempting to define the mechanical properties of soft tissue interface after implantation in canines, Hori and Lewis[83] found that the interface fibrous tissue is very compliant and deformable and can withstand large strains from a load with a nonlinear stress/strain curve. However, with increasing load the material became stiffer and with high loads, linear. The mechanical properties of the interface tissue are substantially different from the mechanical characteristics of other related materials, that is, HDP, metal, bone, and cement. This tissue may influence the behavior of the entire system once it develops between the implant and bone.[85]

Conventional mechanical testing, that is, push-out tests, commonly used to measure the interface strength between PMMA and bone, have produced inconsistent results because of the variability of strength in bony trabeculae (by quantity and quality) and the depth of penetration of the cement, among other factors. In this regard, Bean and associates[11] have proposed a more reliable model for testing shear failure of the interface using rectangular specimens of bone/cement interface. This method may shed light on some of the discrepancies of the results related to the bone properties and accuracy of bonding by cement that have been reported in the literature.

SYSTEMIC AND LOCAL SIDE EFFECTS
Toxicity Studies

Wiltse and co-workers[166] observed no harmful effects when an amount of PMMA cement equivalent to a dose in humans of 2 pounds was implanted in animals. Thus they concluded that the toxicity of MMA was not very high. When dogs were given large doses in an intravenous drop over a period of 19 seconds, the fatal dose calculated from the blood volume was 125 mg/L.[81,82] Injection of pure monomer into the veins of experimental animals such as guinea pigs, rabbits, and rats produced vascular irregularities and eventual cardiac arrest and death, showing that monomer is cytotoxic.[57,80,115] When injected intravenously in rabbits, a monomeric dose of 0.03 ml/kg body weight produced a sudden and transient fall in arterial blood pressure.[91] Although Homsey was able to produce localized pulmonary hemorrhage in dogs after intravenous administration of 5 mg/100 ml, morbidity did not occur in the animals even when a dose of 50 mg/100 ml was given for up to a year. However, when the dose was increased to 125 mg/100 ml, the blood pressure dropped severely, and the animal died of respiratory failure.[80] Homsey

further investigated the PMMA in clinical use and found that its monomer level in the central venous system reached a maximum of 1.26 mg/100 ml, preceding by 1 to 3 minutes the heat generation of hand-held acrylic. The monomer was also detected in expired anesthetic air.[79,81] The effect of pulmonary changes reported by Homsey has not been found in routine radiological examination of the human chest.[41,46]

Charnley explicitly discussed the concerns expressed in the papers presented by Henrichsen and co-workers,[76] Wiltse and co-workers,[166] Scales,[146] Reitz,[142] and Homsey and co-workers[80,81] in his monograph on acrylic cement.[30] He suggested that the widespread bone and animal death related to intramedullary filling in experimental animals should be carefully considered and compared when small doses are introduced in human bone at the time of total hip arthroplasty. Fortunately, because cement is fully polymerized in 15 minutes and there is only minimal residual monomer at the time of full polymerization, tissue is exposed to a negligible amount of monomer.

Histological and hemodynamically toxic effects of MMA monomer were also studied by Holland and associates.[78] From their animal experimentation, they concluded that the toxic effects were dose related. When they injected MMA monomer into dogs in the range of 59 mg/100 ml by three different routes (portal vein, carotid artery, and thoracic aorta), they observed histological changes of congestion, edema, hemorrhage, degeneration, or necrosis in the lungs, liver, and kidneys, depending on the route of injection. These authors were unable, however, to demonstrate histological changes in the brain, heart, gastrointestinal tract, or spleen.

Investigators have studied blood clearance of monomer and acute pulmonary toxicity in dogs after simulated arthroplasty and intravenous injections. McLaughlin and associates[142] determined clearance of ^{14}C-labeled monomer from the blood in beagles during simulated hip arthroplasties and after intravenous injection of the monomer. They found blood clearance to be rapid, with the lungs apparently functioning as a major clearing organ for MMA. Decreased pulmonary function (documented by decreased P_{O_2}, elevated P_{CO_2}, and metabolic acidosis) occurred only when the dose of monomer was more than 35 times the amount liberated in humans during total hip arthroplasty procedures.

Teratogenicity, Fetal Toxicity, and Carcinogenicity

McLaughlin and associates[116] have studied the teratogenicity of PMMA in vivo in mice by exposing pregnant mice to 1330 parts per million vapor of PMMA during days 6 to 15 of pregnancy. Except for a slight increase in the weight of the fetuses of exposed pregnant animals, no evidence of fetal toxicity or teratological effects existed. The average vapor concentration used in this study is far in excess of human exposure during total hip arthroplasty. The concentration of PMMA vapor in the operating room during total hip arthroplasty never rose above 280 parts per million during testing of three total hip arthroplasties. The Occupational Safety and Health Administration (OSHA) of the Department of Labor has restricted the exposure of PMMA during any 8-hour work shift of a 40-hour work week to not more than the 8-hour weighted limit of 100 parts per million or 410 mgm.[160]

In an independent study, Poss and co-workers[138] measured the mutagenicity of PMMA for *Salmonella typhimurium*. At levels of 34 millimolar, PMMA monomer showed 28% of mutogenic activity of an equimolar dose of dimethylnitrosamin, which is a known mutagen and carcinogen of similar chemical structure.

As with all mutagens, the high-risk individuals theoretically are those who are frequently exposed to the agent, such as operating room personnel, the patient, and the surgeon handling the PMMA. However, monomer is not the agent to be implanted, and only a very small residue of PMMA monomer is retained in the solid form, that is, 0.2% to 0.5%, which is leached out and excreted from the body. To what extent the vapor of PMMA in the operating room or residual monomer in the patient is harmful cannot be scientifically determined at this time. After 50 years of use of PMMA in many forms (dentures, implants, etc.), there is no evidence that this material has been carcinogenic in humans. This impression is not intended to be optimistically complacent, but further work might be needed to elucidate this matter.[73,102]

Intraoperative Hypotension and Cardiac Arrest
Early Observations

Charnley showed the effect of monomer on blood pressure in the human after implantation of acrylic cement. He considered this lowering effect to be transient and recovery uneventful when it appeared during anesthesia; he suggested no special precautions during surgery at the time of cement insertion based on his extensive experience. However, he recommended aeration of the mix during cement preparation to rid it of excess monomer and leaving the bolus of cement undisturbed at the time of insertion to prevent bringing interior monomer to the surface of the bolus just before its insertion.[23]

In subsequent literature, several isolated cardiac arrests and sudden deaths were attributed to the monomer lowering the blood pressure and causing circulatory collapse. However, controversy still exists as to the cause of death in these cases.*

Fearn and co-workers[60] and Phillips and co-workers[135] reported their experiences with changes in systolic blood pressure during total hip arthroplasty operations. Fearn cited systolic blood pressure changes in 45 patients during total hip arthroplasty with cement. At the acetabular stage of the operation, blood pressure rose in 16 (35%), fell in 24 (53%), and remained unchanged in 5 patients (12%). He found that when the femur was packed with cement, the systolic blood pressure rose in 24 (54%), fell in 20 (44%), and remained steady in one patient (2%). Phillips and associates[135] also measured arterial blood pressure, central venous pressure, ECGs, blood gases, and intrafemoral pressure in patients undergoing total hip arthroplasty. They measured monomer level in blood samples taken during the operation and demonstrated that there was usually a substantial fall in arterial blood pressure after the introduction of cement into the upper end of the femur but rarely after introducing the cement into the acetabulum. Packing cement into the femoral canal resulted in intramedullary pressure rising as much as 1900 mm Hg. They concluded that the rise in medullary canal pressure did not appear to cause the fall in blood pressure. They felt that the time relationship between the two phenomena was inconsistent with a reflex effect via baroreceptors in the bone. The measurement of monomer level in the blood was small only after acetabular implantation but relatively large after introducing the cement into the femoral canal. They concluded that the fall in blood pressure had always been transient and should not be considered a cause for alarm during total hip arthroplasty.

The cardiovascular effect of monomer was studied by Ellis and associates,[58] who compared the effects of the liquid components of commercial acrylic cement and pure MMA monomer on mean arterial blood pressure, central venous pressure, heart rate, and cardiac output. They concluded that the cardiovascular disturbance is caused by monomeric PMMA alone, rather than by any other constituents in the liquid monomer. Berman and associates[13] evaluated the blood pressure lowering effect of monomer in 12 normovolemic and hypovolemic dogs and concluded that the monomer influenced arterial blood pressure and cardiac output, as well as peripheral resistance. Furthermore, they concluded that the monomer produced vasodilation of the small blood vessels and that peripheral resistance and blood pressure were decreased in both normovolemic and hypovolemic dogs. There was, however, a significant increase in the cardiac output of normovolemic dogs and a decrease in hypovolemic dogs (Fig. 5-27).

---

* References 19, 40, 65, 68, 69, 75, 93, 117, 123, 129, 139.

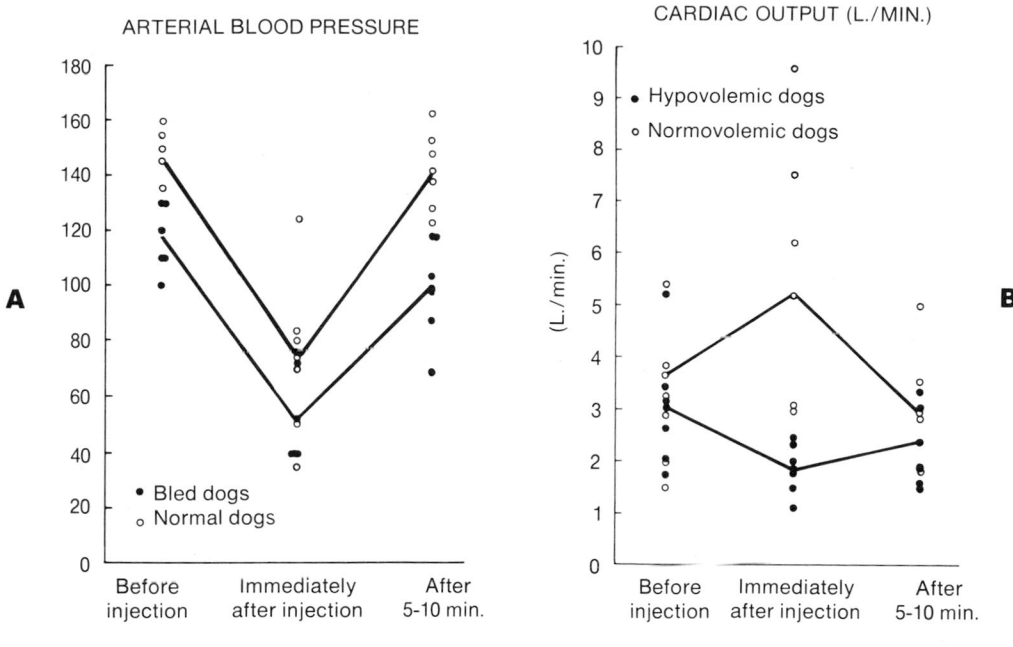

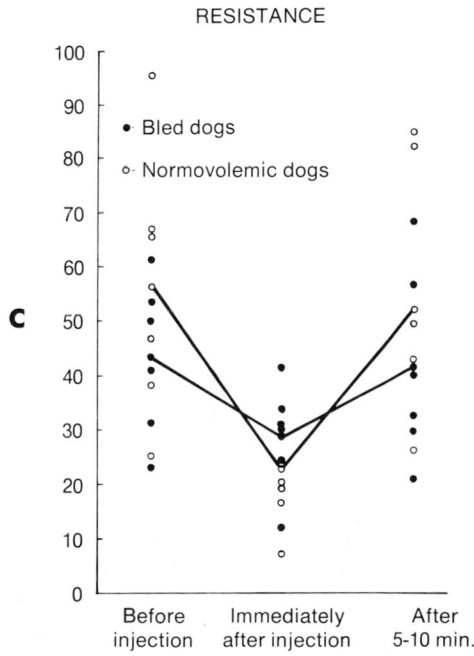

Fig. 5-27. A, Arterial blood pressure in normovolemic and hypovolemic dogs showing lower initial blood pressure in hypovolemic dogs but equal decrease in blood pressure after administration of monomer. **B,** Cardiac output in normovolemic and hypovolemic dogs showing rise in cardiac output in normovolemic dogs and decrease in hypovolemic dogs. **C,** Peripheral resistance in normovolemic and hypovolemic dogs showing greater decrease in resistance in normovolemic dogs. (From Berman AT, Price HL, Hahn JF: The cardiovascular effects of methylmethacrylate in dogs, *Clin Orthop* 100:265, 1974.)

McMaster and associates,[117] in their study of the blood pressure–lowering effect of monomer, concluded that with intravenously injected monomer the depletion of blood volume potentiates the lowering of blood pressure. Therefore these authors felt that peripheral vasodilation with myocardial depression is the main mechanism by which peripheral arterial blood pressure is lowered, thus confirming the findings of Charnley and Smith[38] and Homsey.[80,82]

It is clear from presently available literature that the pathophysiology of blood pressure lowering by monomer is not fully understood, and the cause of cardiac arrest attributed to implantation of monomer is not being fully investigated.[157] It is agreed, however, that hemorrhagic shock and inadequate blood replacement might have been a predisposing factor in the severe blood pressure–lowering effect of circulating monomer in many cases of operative death.

Because embolization of monomer as a cause of death in humans has not been documented, it is logical to presume a mechanical migration of air or fat or both as the etiological factor for a drop in blood pressure. This view is augmented since the fall in pressure is not often seen when the cement is inserted into the acetabulum but usually is present when it is inserted into the femur. Furthermore, this does not occur in all patients. In addition, during bilateral operations on the same patient, only one hip surgery may cause blood pressure lowering. It must also be recognized that blood pressure lowering occurs in humans even with a smaller dose of monomer as compared with animal experimentation such as Homsey's. This theory of the erratic occurrence of fall in blood pressure owing to air and fat embolization would also explain the rapid onset of drop in blood pressure after insertion of cement into the bone causes extrusion of the fat and air into the circulation.[112]

McLaughlin and co-workers[115] established that lung parenchyma functions as the major clearing tissue for monomer after intramedullary cement insertion. A decreased pulmonary function (as measured by decreased Po_2) occurred only when the monomer was more than 35 times the equivalent of the amount liberated in humans during total hip arthroplasty. However, fat particles in the lung have been histologically demonstrated in several autopsies.[40] In some cases, air and fat were noted in pelvic veins and coronary vessels.[87] Fat embolization has been experimentally produced in animals after reaming of the medullary canal, and marrow tissue has been observed in blood samples from the femoral vein during reaming in animals. The elevation of pressure within the medullary canal has been blamed for massive mobilization of fat and marrow, especially the pressure created by the impact of the acrylic cement into the canal of the femur. Based on these observations, venting has been suggested by some investigators to reduce the pressure in the femur. Ohnsorge[125] experimentally recorded a pressure rise of 4.2 atm (61.7 psi) during insertion of the prosthesis into acrylic cement. The pressure could be reduced to 1.4 atm (20.6 psi) if a drill hole was made in the femoral cortex. Tronzo and co-workers[159] measured the intramedullary pressure of the femoral canal during total hip arthroplasty in 12 patients and found transitory pressure changes. Pressure was high when the femoral prosthesis was inserted without cement, higher when the PMMA was forced into the cavity, and highest when the femoral prosthesis was finally positioned into the cement. He concluded that although venting of the femur proximally was ineffective, a distal vent prevented the rise in pressure and suggested that distal venting is a good prophylactic procedure against embolization or cardiac arrest.

After a comprehensive review of the literature and a clinical prospective study on physiological emboli changes observed during total hip arthroplasty, Jones[90] concluded that fat embolization occurs with introduction of the femoral component and can be prevented by distal venting of the femur at the time of insertion of the cement. Alternatively, a plastic suction tube may be inserted as a method of venting the femoral canal during packing of the cement to eliminate the problem of fat embolization. Because of animal experimental work and the personal preferences of those teaching in educational centers, venting has become a popular procedure.

Herndon and associates[77] reviewed the literature in 1974 and did an in-depth study. They noted 28 deaths, 20 of which had a postoperative autopsy; in 16 of these, fat emboli were found, some of which were massive. Three of the 16 also had documented bone marrow emboli, some of which were associated with both pulmonary and systemic fat emboli; others were associated with acute myocardial infarction, pulmonary emboli, and suggestion of air emboli.

The true incidence of fat embolization in patients who died of sudden circulatory collapse is not known. Similarly, the incidence of pulmonary fat embolism in patients who survived cardiac arrest by resuscitation during the operation cannot be defined. Herndon and associates[77] studied 34 unselected patients in an attempt to quantify the incidence of fat embolism. They demonstrated the phenomena associated with fat embolization in most patients during the procedure, although none of these patients exhibited clinical or laboratory evidence of the fat embolism syndrome. They used an ultrasound probe over the femoral vein and performed serial analysis of venous blood fat. Computer energy–density spectrum analysis of the sounds was recorded by the ultrasound probe. "Chirps" were heard during insertion of the femoral component in all patients. Individual chirps lasting 2 to 5 milliseconds occurred every 10 to 15 milliseconds. Mean duration of activity was 4.2 minutes. Chirps were rarely heard during seating of the acetabular component, reaming, or insertion of cement into the femur. Blood samples* taken during peak ultrasound activity showed 79 globules per high-power field by cryostat test (contrasted with a control of 1.7), or 360 globules per high-power field by the Millipore filter test (control, 6.8), and a mean drop in triglycerides of 27.8 mg/100 ml (control, + 1.2) after filtration. They concluded that although no clinical evidence of fat embolism was observed, venting of the femoral medullary canal at insertion of the femoral stem reduced the amount of fat emboli.

Kallos and associates[92] demonstrated that femoral medullary pressures and pulmonary embolization of medullary contents during insertion of cement and medullary rods in greyhounds were considerable. In three animals they found that insertion of cement into the femoral shaft resulted in medullary pressures between 290 and 900 torr, with the appearance of medullary contents in the lungs within 10 to 120 seconds. They also could prevent this phenomenon by drilling the shaft to release the pressure at the time of insertion.

Our own and Charnley's larger experience indicates that venting of the femur is unnecessary. We prefer to have the anesthetic agents discontinued 2 to 3 minutes before inserting cement into the acetabulum and femur, with the patient maintained on pure oxygen at the time of cement insertion. We make every effort to keep the patient normotensive and normovolemic before inserting cement. For the past 20 years, approximately 12,000 low-friction arthroplasties have been performed at the New York Orthopaedic Hospital without venting the femur at the time of stem insertion, which maximizes pressurization and presumably causes fat mobilization into the system. No significant hypotensive episodes have been observed, and there have not been any cardiac arrests as the result of cement insertion into the femur. However, this author is aware of two intraoperative deaths at our institution that were attributed to insertion of cement used for fracture fixation during insertion of an endoprosthesis. In one case, the patient had metastatic carcinoma and in the other case, the patient was a 70-year-old debilitated individual with known heart disease. An autopsy was not done in either case, and the cause of death was unknown.

* The fat emboli were counted in the blood samples by two histological techniques, and the plasma was analyzed for triglycerides before and after filtration.

Clinical Picture

Although many intraoperative deaths are reported related to the insertion of acrylic cement, a number must remain unrecorded. Of 33 cases recorded and reviewed by Keret and Reis,[94] only three followed total knee arthroplasty. Interestingly, 21 of the 30 remaining followed insertion of a Thompson prosthesis. Some 14 cases of intraoperative cardiac arrest reviewed by Keret were successfully resuscitated. Autopsy findings were available in 21 of the cases. Fat emboli (some massive) were found in 16 of 21 patients.* Marrow emboli were also seen in 3 of the 16 with emboli.[93,94,147] In some instances evidence of pulmonary and systemic fat emboli existed,† while in the others there was also evidence of myocardial infarction,[37,94,139] pulmonary embolism,[46,134] or air embolism.[87]

Although in most reports the exact onset of the hypotensive episode is not recorded, it usually immediately follows application of the cement into the medullary cavity of the femur.[87,129] It is not clear why neither significant hypotension nor cardiac arrest occurs after insertion of the cement into the acetabulum. The classic pattern of cardiovascular collapse begins in a sudden and significant fall in arterial blood pressure immediately after insertion of cement into the medullary cavity of the femur. Cardiac arrest follows the cardiovascular collapse and hypoxia. In general, as recorded by several investigators, only one third of the patients show any hypotensive episode. These episodes were transient, beginning between 19 and 90 seconds after insertion of the cement into the medullary cavity of the femur and lasting from 20 seconds to 20 minutes. A severe hypotensive episode after insertion of the cement is unique in that (1) it occurs after introduction of cement into the femur and not into the acetabulum, and (2) it rarely occurs during elective total hip arthroplasty procedures, occurring most often in patients with fractured hips who have had a femoral head replacement. The latter group may constitute somewhat older and debilitated patients with prior compromised cardiopulmonary status who have suffered from a pulmonary embolic episode before their operation.

Based on biochemical disturbance associated with total hip arthroplasty, Alexander and Barron[2a] have suggested that pulmonary microembolism occurs consistently when acrylic cement and the prosthesis are placed in the femur. This coincides with a fall in arterial oxygen tension and hypoxemia that extends to the postoperative period. Based on their prospective study of 227 patients undergoing total hip arthroplasty with elevation of serum lipase and concomitant fall in

* References 19, 40, 45, 75, 93, 94, 134.

† References 1, 68, 69, 87, 94, 147.

triglycerides, they suggested that a fat marrow embolization occurs. Venting of the femur did not influence the biomechanical disturbances described.

Anaphylaxin Release and PMMA

Because anaphylaxins are potent mediators and can influence vascular permeability and significant cardiopulmonary disturbances, they have been suggested as a possible mechanism in producing cardiopulmonary embarrassment during total hip arthroplasty.[84]

Anaphylaxins (C3A and C5A) have been reported to appear in the plasma of patients undergoing total hip arthroplasty in which acrylic cement is used. Because anaphylaxins can induce hypotension and hypoxia by disturbing oxygen uptake, they have been implicated as one cause of hemodynamic instability when the cement is used.[12] In addition to PMMA, which is released into the blood circulation, surgical trauma, release of fat, bone particles, and even air into the circulation can possibly cause anaphylaxins to be activated during total hip arthroplasty. However, in a prospective study of 30 patients who had total hip arthroplasty by the Charnley low-friction arthroplasty technique using acrylic cement and 15 patients who underwent a cementless total hip arthroplasty, Bengtson and associates[12] found activation of complements when PMMA was used. When a prosthesis was used without cement, they observed no formation of anaphylaxins and only slightly reduced whole complement activity and concentrations of C3, C4, and C5 in the plasma.

Fat Embolization Theory

Fat embolization occurs during reaming of the medullary canal or the acetabulum. Fat embolization (without surgical intervention) has been documented in patients with femoral shaft fractures and in multiple trauma victims. The introduction of the prosthesis into the cement, leading to a great rise in medullary pressure, can lead to mobilization of fat into the circulation.[92,121,123,147]

Three recent independent studies have clearly pointed to mobilization of fat and its embolization as giving rise to cardiopulmonary dysfunction observed after cemented total hip arthroplasty. In the first study, an experimental model using dogs, Sherman and co-workers[148] demonstrated that during cemented arthroplasty a thorough irrigation and plugging of the medullary canal before insertion of cement and prosthesis was capable of eliminating the hypoxemia and increased intrapulmonary shunt fraction that characterize the fat pulmonary embolism.

In a second study, Byrick and associates[21] demonstrated that a high-volume, high-pressure pulsatized lavage during cemented total hip arthroplasty reduced pulmonary embolization of fat to 25.7% of the control

(nonlavaged) group, thus significantly reducing the changes in pulmonary artery pressure, pulmonary vascular resistance, arterial oxygen tension, and intrapulmonary shunt fraction (QS/QT).

In the third study, a laboratory study of the cardiopulmonary function and embolization phenomenon during total hip arthroplasty, Orisini et al[126] isolated the pathological changes caused by fat embolization from those caused by PMMA. In a randomized selection of 24 mongrel dogs into three groups, one group received a noncemented implant, the second group received a cemented implant, and the third group received an implant fixed with bone wax. In the first group (implant without cement or wax), low intramedullary pressure was generated and caused few microemboli; no significant cardiopulmonary changes were observed. In the second and third groups (those with implant and cement or bone wax), a high intramedullary pressure was generated that coincided with significant cardiopulmonary changes, including decreased arterial pressure and increased intrapulmonary shunt fraction. This study clearly demonstrated that increased intramedullary pressure and fat embolization, not the PMMA monomer, were responsible for cardiopulmonary changes. Thus the procedures that do not require high pressurization of the medullary canal, such as the use of prostheses without cement, are less likely to cause massive fat embolization. It might also be concluded indirectly that patients with a predisposition for cardiopulmonary dysfunction are prone to cardiopulmonary dysfunction resulting from increased fat/marrow embolization during insertion of the stem and cement.

Allergic Reactions

Obscure complications at times have been attributed to allergic reactions to MMA, including radiological changes of bone simulating those of osteitis, wounds from which no organisms can be grown, mechanical loosening of the prosthesis, and unexplained pain after total hip arthroplasty. Occupational asthma related to PMMA exposure in an operating room nurse and in patients has been reported.[48,136] After a detailed study of the literature and my personal experience with nearly 3000 total joint arthroplasties using acrylic cement, I conclude (similar to Charnley)[30] that allergic reactions are exceedingly rare. An occasional isolated allergic reaction, however, cannot be denied.

Numerous sensitivity studies are available in dental literature,* mostly relating to heat-cured acrylic. Sensitivity to acrylic resins has been studied by skin testing to demonstrate a true sensitivity in patients who had symptomatic reactions to their acrylic dentures. A

---

* References 16, 62, 63, 64, 105.

single exposure for a sensitized individual working with the dental material may produce dermatitis that may last for several weeks or months. Fries and associates[64] collected 13 cases of contact dermatitis attributed to handling MMA; Fries himself was a victim. They tested a variety of commercially available gloves for penetration of monomeric PMMA and suggested that most of these gloves were inadequate in protecting a sensitive individual's skin and that improved surgical gloves were needed to prevent penetration of PMMA monomer. They recommended that sensitive individuals add an extra pair of gloves, to be removed at once after handling cement. It has been suggested that the monomer may permeate rubber surgical gloves to produce contact dermatitis,[130] and the possibility of reactions to additives of PMMA has also been argued. It is suggested that benzoyl peroxide can occasionally cause sensitivity.[62] Charnley[30] proposed avoiding hydroquinone stabilizer (used in Simplex P) and replacing it with ascorbic acid (as in CMW). In addition to hydroquinone and benzoyl peroxide, DMPT may also be allergenic.[23]

Intraarticular Lodgement

PMMA can lodge between the articular surfaces in a total hip arthroplasty. This can occur inadvertently during the arthroplasty, or it may result from loosening of the total hip arthroplasty, or even from trauma occurring after arthroplasty. This condition occurs more often than has been discussed in the literature. It is frequently seen in revision surgery for loose components or when revision is performed for severe wear of the socket. Because of the abrasive nature of PMMA, socket wear and failure can be seen as a late complication of total hip arthroplasty. Despite lodgement, the patient may remain asymptomatic during the early postoperative course.[156]

Wroblewski,[171] in a study of socket wear in total hip arthroplasty, observed great variation in the wear of ultramolecular HDP. He postulated that the variations might be caused by entrapment of cement between the metal head and HDP of the socket, resulting in an accelerated wear rate. This untoward effect of PMMA may prove to be a significant drawback to its use in total joint arthroplasty.

Effects of Chemotaxis on Polymorphonuclear Leukocytes

Charnley recognized that total hip arthroplasty using PMMA made patients more susceptible to infection than other operations.[30] He considered the presence of a foreign body, the use of plastics, and mobility of the joint in total hip arthroplasty to be predisposing factors to infection.

Petty and co-workers[132,133] reported on the adverse

effect of PMMA on the antibacterial activities of normal human serum against *Staphylococcus epidermidis* and on complement activity. They found that adding PMMA to polymorphonuclear suspensions during the growth of *Staphylococcus aureus, S. epidermidis,* and *Escherichia coli* produced a significant depression of cells. This occurred at 0.312% of PMMA. At concentrations of 0.625% and 1.25%, no leukocyte migration occurred.[131] The implication of the depression of chemotaxis by PMMA (either by formation of chemotaxic factors or depression of mobility of polymorphonuclear leukocytes) is that it allows the bacteria with its known pathogenicity to multiply by incompetence of the immune system (see Chapters 4 and 8).

Intravenous PMMA

One of the uncommon findings on postoperative x-ray films after total hip arthroplasty is the presence of acrylic cement in the soft tissue unrelated to violation of bone. The findings are often incidental and appear to be unique to the soft tissue adjacent to the femoral prosthesis. Configuration of the radiopaque cement in the soft tissue suggests that the PMMA may be present in a vein adjacent to the cement in the femur. Weissman and associates[162] reported eight such cases; two of which developed cardiac problems (one myocardial infarction and the other congestive heart failure). The significance of PMMA found in the vein cannot be determined at this time.

Liver Dysfunction

Convery and associates[42] studied in detail the relative safety of PMMA, comparing two groups of patients, one group undergoing Charnley low-friction arthroplasty and the second undergoing other methods of total hip arthroplasty, the former with the use of PMMA and the latter without. They concluded that the postoperative alterations, erythrocyte sedimentation rate, serum glutamic-oxaloacetic transaminase (SGOT), and lactic acid dehydrogenase (LDH) were related to the surgical intervention and not to the use of cement. Postoperative serum alkaline phosphatase was increased over the preoperative level and remained elevated for up to 12 months in all patients. This elevation was attributed to the formation of ectopic bone rather than hepatic toxicity of the cement. Intraoperative alterations in cardiovascular function were attributed to the use of cement. In one patient in the cemented group there was evidence of myocardial depression.

Until recently there has been very little concern about the possible effect of PMMA monomer on patients with cemented total joint arthroplasty other than cardiac dysfunction during insertion of cement. Ritter and co-workers[144] noted that a small percentage of patients had changes in their liver function tests

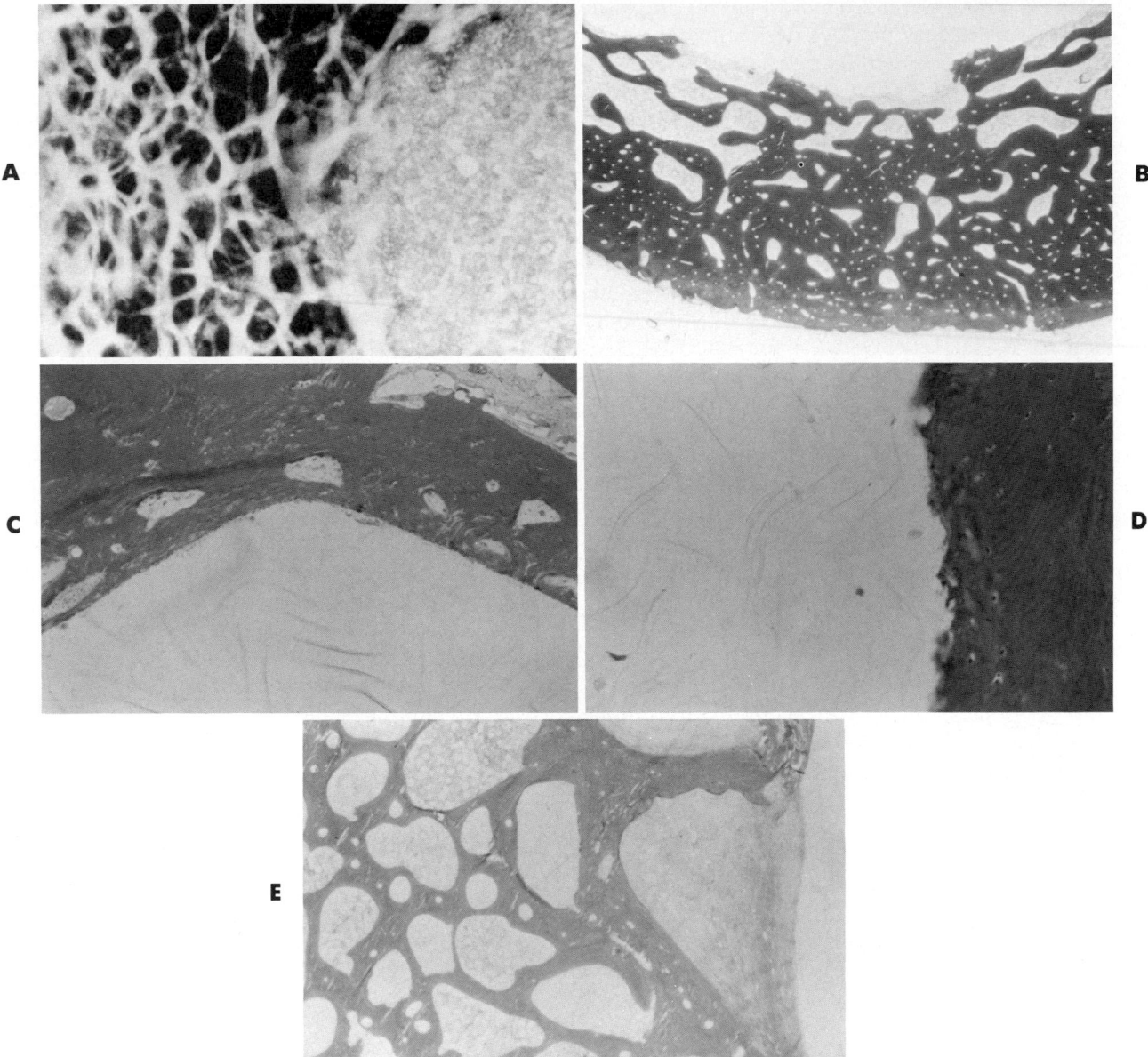

Fig. 5-28. A, A specimen radiograph showing intimate osteointegration of bone with cement (containing barium sulfate). **B,** A ×40 photograph of the bone-cement interface in an LFA performed 14 years before death. Note that Masson Goldner stain is used—mineralized bone stains green and unmineralized bone or fibrous tissue is red. Note absence of fibrous tissue between the bone and the homopoietic marrow is viable. **C,** Stained as in **B**; wrinkled material is the bone cement. The bone is in contact with cement. **D,** A higher magnification (×6) of wrinkled cement with mineralized bone showing that the osteocytes are still viable. **E,** A thick fibrous tissue was regularly found at the interface between the cemented cup and bone of the acetabulum. It was uncommon between the cemented femoral component and bone of the femur. The thick fibrous membrane contained wear particles of high-density polyethylene. **F,** A longitudinal section of the femur and the acetabular specimen, was implanted before 1962. Note severe wear of Teflon socket but excellent fixation of stem by acrylic cement (Charnley used pink dental cement). Severe osteolysis over the medial neck and calcar region (because of invasive Teflon granuloma) did not cause loosening of the stem. **G,** A longitudinal section of a cemented femur (Charnley used pink dental cement) and acetabulum. Horizontal cut confirmed evidence of osteointegration. Severe fibrosis was present around the press-fit metal-backed acetabular component (HDP). (From Sir John Charnley's histological collections, courtesy Dr. AJ Malcolm.)

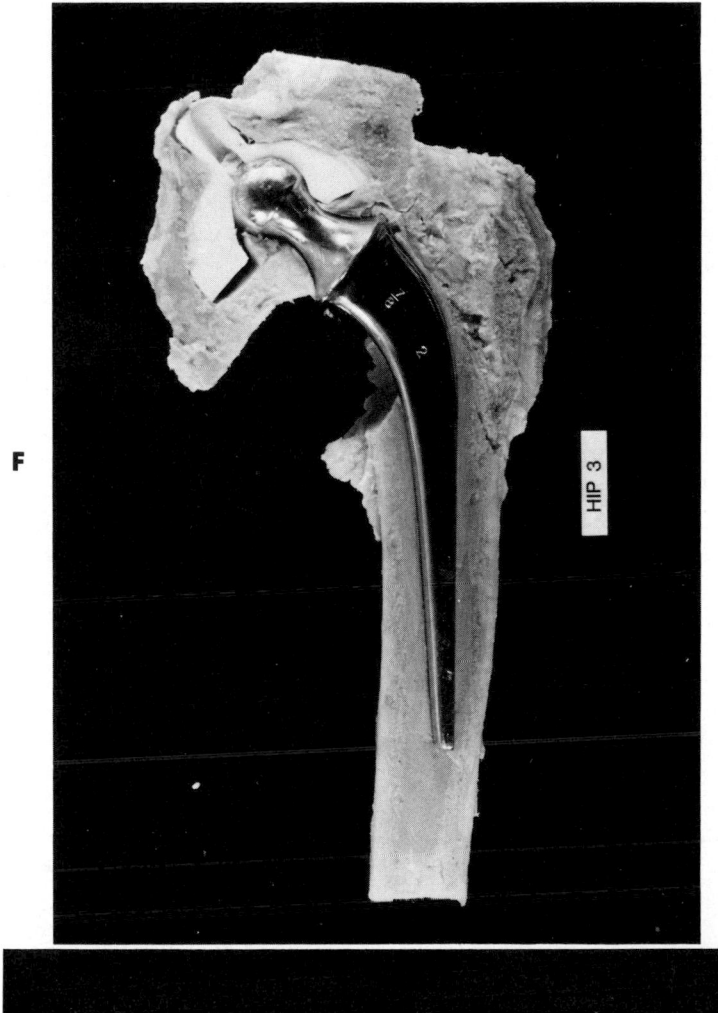

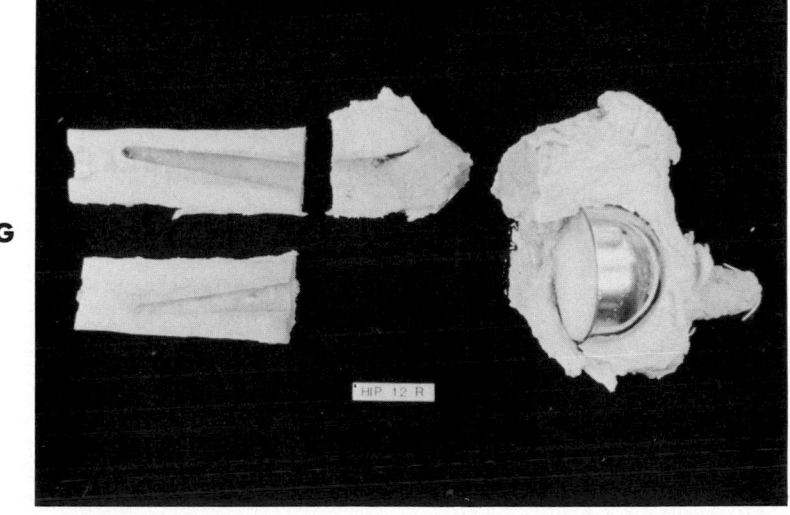

after cemented total hip arthroplasty, as evidenced by increased serum levels of gammaglutamyltranspeptidase. However, this was thought to be insignificant. In a comparative study of liver function after total hip arthroplasty using acrylic cement in 40 consecutive patients, Pople and Phillips[137] compared preoperative and postoperative patients with cemented total hip arthroplasty with a control group (total knee arthroplasty and Thompson prosthesis) in whom no cement had been used. In 12 of 40 patients (32%) who had had cemented arthroplasty, serum gammaglutamyltransferase (SGGT) was abnormally elevated for more than 4 days. This contrasted with only one patient in the control group. Interestingly, the changes in the SGGT levels correlated with the amount of cement used. This was statistically significant (P value less than 0.001). However, this elevated SGGT returned to normal in all patients, indicating a transient dose-related effect of PMMA on liver function. Although none of the patients in the study developed jaundice as a result of cement use, symptoms such as nausea and pyrexia, which occurred in 28% of patients in the group receiving cement, could have been attributed to hepatic malfunction. Duration of anesthesia and blood transfusion were greater in the cemented group than in the noncemented patients. However, these differences were not statistically significant. Evidently, careful double-blind, randomized studies are needed to elucidate the issue of liver toxicity and systemic effects of PMMA in humans.

BIOLOGICAL COMPATIBILITY

To study the safety and compatibility of acrylic cement, Charnley postulated that retrieved specimens for histological studies must be from clinically successful cases after total hip arthroplasty.[26a,30] He obtained 78 specimens from patients of his who had bequeathed their hip joints to him for scientific studies. Charnley had performed all of the surgery using a low-friction arthroplasty technique 8 to 22 years previously. Although Charnley carried out fairly extensive histological studies on those specimens and interpreted the results with utmost authority[26a,30] Charnley's trust funded further histological study of the long-term outcome. Dr. Archie J. Malcolm of the University of Newcastle-on-Tyne was selected to carry out this work. Following is a summary of Dr. Malcolm's findings (Fig. 5-28)[101]:

Femur

1. Of 78 femoral specimens, 60 showed osteointegration throughout the length of cement fixation and 18 specimens showed various amounts of fibrous tissue.
2. Viable tissue consisting of mineralized pegs of viable lamellar bone and a thin layer of osteoid was found in 60 specimens.
3. Scanning electron microscopy of some cases also showed evidence of osteointegration.
4. Fibrous tissue was present (up to 2.6 mm in thickness) between the cement and living bone; it was more prominent proximally and often disappeared distally in the femur.
5. When a membrane was present, there also was a histological reaction and associated wear particles of HDP and metals.

Acetabular Component

1. In contrast to evidence of osteointegration in the femur, a fibrous membrane was found in every acetabular specimen between cement and bone.
2. In all cases, the fibrous membrane contained wear particles of HDP and metal particles with evidence of macrophagic reaction.
3. In contrast to the femoral specimens, in the acetabulum between the bone and cement the surface was often smooth.

SUMMARY OF ESSENTIALS

- Acrylic cement was first synthesized in 1843. In 1937, its heat-cured form was first used in humans as denture base material. Zander first performed an acrylic cranioplasty in 1940. Judet introduced the heat-cured femoral head replacement in 1946. Its early use in hip surgery by Kiaer in 1952 and Haboush is of special interest.

- Charnley is credited with formulating and elucidating the principles of using acrylic cement in orthopaedic surgery. His analysis of the mechanism for achieving fixation is one of the greatest milestones in the history of orthopaedic surgery of this century.

- The use of acrylic cement has not changed and is still based on the original observations Charnley made in his 1970 monograph on acrylic cement.

- The cement must have the proper chemistry and constituents to be effective. Its liquid component is methylmethacrylate (MMA), a tertiary amine that acts as an initiator and inhibitor. The powder typically consists of polymethyl methacrylate (PMMA) as an activator. The monomer is added to polymer, initiating the polymerization process that produces the solid polymerized acrylic intraoperatively.

- Radiopacity is an essential feature of acrylic cement used in orthopaedic surgery, without which the presence and amount of cement cannot be determined. It is this author's opinion that a nonradiopaque cement must not be used in surgery. Barium sulfate is the radiographic marker in most cements used in surgery and does not significantly weaken the cement's mechanical properties.

- Commercially available bone cement polymer has an average molecular weight of 198,000, which curing increases to 242,000; approximately 90% of its tensile strength is reached by 4 hours after polymerization. Approximate tensile and compressive strengths and modular self-elasticity expressed in megapascal (MPa) are 32, 100, and 2700. These values are considerably lower than those of cortical bone — by 25% in tensile strengths, 50% in compressive strengths, and 15% in modular self-elasticity. Additives such as barium sulfate reduce the compressive strength and tensile strength of the cement to a small degree.

- The mechanical properties of acrylic cement are somewhat affected by variations in mixing techniques and can be significantly altered by lamination or mixture of blood and fat during surgery, especially when the cement is not kept under pressure at surgery.

- Neither irradiation, ambient temperature, nor added antibiotics alter the mechanical properties of cement to a significant degree as used in clinical practice. However, unsupported cement, lack of constraint, or use of cement in a thin layer may be inadequate to provide support and function. Aging of cement does not seem to be a significant problem except for a modest reduction in its fatigue properties. Of all variables affecting the mechanical properties of cement, the technical aspects of its application seem to have the greatest influence.

- The porosity of cement can be reduced to increase its fatigue life by either centrifugation or partial vacuum mixing. In practice the value of reduced porosity has not been documented, although laboratory tests have verified that it increases the life of the cement.

- The working and setting times of acrylic cement vary in different brands of cement and circumstances of its use. These variables include ambient temperature, ratio of monomer to polymer, humidity, molecular weight of the polymer, texture of the polymer, proportions of activator and initiator, and degree of aeration. Mixing and insertion instructions must be accurately followed to achieve optimum results.

- The major monomer loss from acrylic mass occurs during its mixing. Only a very small amount of acrylic cement monomer enters the circulatory blood, and it is rapidly eliminated.

- Temperature elevation during polymerization (exothermic reaction) of the cement mass is directly proportional to the size of the mass. Under normal circumstances, the heat of polymerization and dimensional changes (expansion and shrinkage) during polymerization do not appear to interfere with clinical fixation.

- While the ambient temperature significantly influences the setting and working times of PMMA, the polymerization process can also be influenced by the temperature of the equipment used to mix the cement and the temperature of the prosthesis used with it.

- The aeration of cement that occurs during mixing by rapid beating is partly responsible for volumetric expansion, which compensates for shrinkage of the total mass. However, increased porosity reduces the fatigue life of cement and possibly its fracture toughness, which may affect its long-term clinical behavior.

- PMMA has a biphasic structure consisting of aggregates of small spheres or granules of the polymer cemented together by recently polymerized monomer (liquid). The balls of polymer, which range from 10 to 80 μm in diameter, are responsible for the semicircular impression on the endosteal bone in histological specimens after the cement is dissolved.

- Acrylic cement should not be considered a glue because it possesses no adhesive properties. It acts as a filler when it is used in conjunction with the prosthetic component. When used as a filler it occupies the space between prosthesis and bone, creating an accurate fit between the two. Because most forces in the hip are compressive and acrylic is most suitable for bonding, it makes an ideal grout for fixation of the prosthesis. Cement fills the cavities of the interior bone surfaces and allows transmission of the load over a fairly large area between the prosthesis and the inner surface of the bone.

- Bonding of PMMA to metal surfaces has been developed as a thin film of industrial PMMA applied by manufacturers to a portion of the prosthesis to improve its fixation to the freshly applied cement at surgery. As tested in the laboratory, a precoated prosthesis is superior from a mechanical standpoint. However, the long-term clinical significance of this method requires further documentation.

- Several variables can affect the basic mechanical properties of cement, which can directly or indirectly influence the cement strength and long-term performance. These include thickness of cement, contamination by blood, fat, and debris, mixing techniques, layering of cement, environmental effects, additives, physical constraint and support by bone, design of implants, viscosity and aging of cement, rate of loading, bone strength, and cement/bone interface. Surgeons should familiarize themselves with the mechanical and physical properties of cement before attempting to use it.

- Of all the factors that affect mechanical properties during the application of cement, the single most important is proper application at surgery.
- Toxicity studies related to acrylic cement focus primarily on cell toxicity and toxicity resulting from monomer and its effect on the cardiovascular system.
- Many cumulative data related to intraoperative hypotension and cardiac arrest focus on allergic reaction, the vasodilatory effect of the monomer, and air and fat embolism during insertion of the cement. The most significant hypotensive changes related to cement occur during its insertion into the medullary cavity of the femur. Postmortem studies of patients who died in surgery from cardiac arrest are inconclusive. However, release of anaphylaxin, and most significantly, fat embolism have become accepted as pathological mechanisms for cardiovascular collapse after the use of acrylic cement. Other factors predisposing the patient to cardiovascular collapse in addition to intramedullary pressure and fat embolism are prior hypotension and preexisting fat or pulmonary embolism. Anaphylactic shock resulting from insertion of cement has less acceptance as a cause for intraoperative cardiovascular collapse.
- Although acrylic cement has been shown to be a mutagen for certain bacteria, its carcinogenicity has been of little concern. Based on clinical experience over 30 years in thousands of patients, cement may be considered an acceptable and biologically compatible material as used in total hip arthroplasty. Most effects from intravenous release of monomer, transient intraoperative dip in blood pressure, and reported liver dysfunction after its use are of limited consequence, and these risks can be minimized by protective measures.

REFERENCES

1. **Adams JH, Graham DI, Mills E, et al:** Fat embolism and cerebral infarction after use of methylmethacrylate cement, *Br Med J* 3:740, 1972.
2. **Ahmed AM, Pak W, Burke DL, et al:** Transient and residual stresses and displacements in self-curing bone cement. Part I: Characterization of relevant volumetric behavior of bone cement, *J Biomech Eng* 104:21, 1982.
2a. **Alexander JP, Barron DW:** Biochemical disturbances associated with total hip replacement, *J Bone Joint Surg* 61[Br]:101, 1979.
3. **Amstutz HC, Gruen T:** Clinical application of polymethyl methacrylate for total joint replacement, *Curr Pract Orthop Surg* 5:158, 1973.
4. **Amstutz HC, Gruen T:** Prosthetic fixation with polymethyl methacrylate. In *Proceedings of National Academy of Science Symposium on Internal Structural Prosthetics*, 1973.
5. **Amstutz HC, Lurie L, Bullough P:** Skeletal fixation with self-curing polymethyl methacrylate. A report of 23 canine total hip replacements, *Clin Orthop* 84:163, 1972.
6. **Arroyo NA:** Physical and mechanical properties of vacuum mixed cement. In *Transactions of the 12th Annual Meeting of the Society for Biomaterials*, Minneapolis–St Paul, 1986.
7. **Askew MJ, Steege JW, Lewis JL, et al:** Effect of cement pressure and bone strength on polymethyl methacrylate fixation, *J Orthop Res* 1:412, 1984.
8. **Astleford WJ, Asher MA, Lindholm US, et al:** Some physical and mechanical factors affecting the simple shear strength of methylmethacrylate, *Clin Orthop* 108:145, 1975.
9. **Bargar WL, Martin RB, deJesus R, et al:** The addition of tobramycin to contrast bone cement. Effect on flexural strength, *J Arthroplasty* 1:165, 1986.
10. **Bayne SC, Lautenschlager EP, Compere CL, et al:** Degree of polymerization of acrylic bone cement, *J Biomed Mater Res* 9:27, 1975.
11. **Bean DJ, Convery FR, Woo SL, et al:** Regional variation in shear strength of the bone–polymethyl methacrylate interface, *J Arthroplasty* 2:293, 1987.
12. **Bengtson A, Larsson M, Gammer W, et al:** Anaphylatoxin release in association with methylmethacrylate fixation of hip prostheses, *J Bone Joint Surg* 69:46, 1987.
12a. **Benjamin JB, Gie GA, Lee AJ, et al:** Cementing technique and the effects of bleeding, *J Bone Joint Surg* 69[Br]:620, 1987.
13. **Berman AT, Price HL, Hahn JF:** The cardiovascular effects of methylmethacrylate in dogs, *Clin Orthop* 100:265, 1974.
14. **Black JD, Greenwald AS:** Structural weakening of layered acrylic bone cement, *Clin Orthop* 171:94, 1982.
15. **Blumenthal LM:** Recent German developments in the field of dental resins, F.I.A.T. Report No. 1185, May, 1947.
16. **Borzelleca JF, Larson PS, Henningar GR Jr, et al:** Studies on the chronic oral toxicity of monomeric ethyl acrylate and methyl methacrylate, *Toxicol Appl Pharmacol* 6:29, 1964.
17. **Bricolo A, Benati A, Bazzan A:** Cranioplastiche con ressiva acrilica, con rete di acciaio inossidokile pesante e con framenti di teca, *Renerva Neurochir* 11:208, 1967.
18. **Buerkle AR Jr, Eftekhar NS:** Fixation of the femoral head prosthesis with methylmethacrylate, *Clin Orthop* 111:134, 1975.
19. **Burgess DM:** Cardiac arrest and bone cement, *Br Med J* 3:588, 1970.
20. **Burke DW, Gates EI, Harris WH:** Centrifugation as a method of improving tensile and fatigue properties of acrylic bone cement, *J Bone Joint Surg* 66:1265, 1984.
21. **Byrick RJ, Bell RS, Kay JC, et al:** High-volume, high-pressure pulsatile lavage during cemented arthroplasty, *J Bone Joint Surg* 71:1331, 1989.
22. **Cabanela ME, Coventry MB, MacCarty CS, et al:** The fate of patients with methyl methacrylate cranioplasty, *J Bone Joint Surg* 54:278, 1972.
23. **Calnan CD, Stevenson CJ:** Studies in contact dermatitis. XV. Dental materials, *Trans St. John Hosp Derm Soc* 49:9, 1963.

24. **Cameron HU, Mills RH, Jackson RW, et al:** The structure of polymethyl methacrylate cement, *Clin Orthop* 100:287, 1974.

25. **Carter DR, Gates EI, Harris WH:** Strain-controlled fatigue of acrylic bone cement, *J Biomed Mater Res* 16(5):647, 1982.

26. **Chan KH, Ahmed AM:** Polymethylmethacrylate. In Morrey BF, editor: *Joint replacement arthroplasty.* New York, 1991, Churchill-Livingstone.

26a. **Charnley J:** *Low-friction arthroplasty of the hip: theory and practice,* Berlin, 1989, Springer-Verlag.

27. **Charnley J:** Long-term results of low-friction arthroplasty of the hip performed as a primary intervention, *J Bone Joint Surg* 54[Br]:61, 1972.

28. **Charnley J:** The reaction of bone to self-curing acrylic cement. A long-term histological study in man, *J Bone Joint Surg* 52[Br]:340, 1970.

29. **Charnley J:** The fixation of prostheses in living bone. In Simpson DC, editor: *Modern trends in biomechanics,* New York, 1970, Appleton-Century-Crofts.

30. **Charnley J:** *Acrylic cement in orthopaedic surgery,* Baltimore, 1970, Williams & Wilkins.

31. **Charnley J:** A biomechanical analysis of the use of cement to anchor the femoral head prosthesis, *J Bone Joint Surg* 47[Br]:354, 1965.

32. **Charnley J:** The bonding of prostheses to bone by cement, *J Bone Joint Surg* 46[Br]:518, 1964.

33. **Charnley J:** Anchorage of the femoral head prosthesis to the shaft of the femur, *J Bone Joint Surg* 42[Br]:28, 1960.

34. **Charnley J, Crawford WJ:** Histology of bone in contact with self-curing acrylic cement, *J Bone Joint Surg* 50[Br]:228, 1968.

35. **Charnley J, Follacci FM, Hammond BT:** The long-term reaction of bone to self-curing acrylic cement, *J Bone Joint Surg* 50[Br]:822, 1968.

36. **Charnley J, Kettlewell J:** The elimination of slip between prosthesis and femur, *J Bone Joint Surg* 47[Br]:56, 1965.

37. **Charnley J, Murphy JCM, Pitkeathly DA, et al:** Fractured femur and fat embolism, *Br Med J* 3:474, 1971.

38. **Charnley J, Smith DC:** The physical and chemical properties of self-curing acrylic cement, Internal Publication No. 16, 1968, Center for Hip Surgery, Wrightington Hospital, England.

39. **Chin H-C, Stauffer RN, Chao EYS:** The effect of centrifugation on the mechanical properties of cement. An in vitro total hip-arthroplasty model, *J Bone Joint Surg* 72:363, 1990.

40. **Cohen CA, Smith TC: The intraoperative hazard of acrylic bone cement: report of a case,** *Anesthesiology* 35:547, 1971.

41. **Convery FR, Gunn DR, Hughes JD, Martin WE:** The relative safety of polymethyl methacrylate. A controlled clinical study of randomly selected patients treated with Charnley and Ring total hip replacements. *J Bone Joint Surg* 57:57, 1975.

42. **Convery FR, Devine SD, Hollis JM, et al:** Cement composite delivery system, *Orthop Rev* 15:581, 1986.

43. **Cook SD, Thongpreda N, Anderson RC, et al:** Optimum pore size for bone cement fixation, *Clin Orthop* 223:296, 1987.

44. **Crowninshield RD, Tolbert JR:** Cement strain measurement surrounding loose and well-fixed femoral component stems, *J Biomed Mater Res* 17(5):819, 1983.

45. **Dandy DJ:** Fat embolism following prosthetic replacement of the femoral head, *Injury* 3:85, 1971.

46. **Daniel WW, Coventry MB, Miller WE:** Pulmonary complications after total hip arthroplasty with Charnley prosthesis as revealed by chest roentgenograms, *J Bone Joint Surg* 54:282, 1972.

47. **Davies JP, Burke DW, O'Connor DO, et al:** Comparison of the fatigue characteristics of centrifuged and uncentrifuged Simplex P bone cement, *J Orthop Res* 5:366, 1987.

48. **Davies JP, Jasty M, O'Connor DO, et al:** The effect of centrifuging bone cement, *J Bone Joint Surg* 71[Br]:39, 1989.

49. **Davies JP, O'Connor DO, Burke DW, et al:** Comparison and optimization of three centrifugation systems for reducing porosity of Simplex P bone cement, *J Arthroplasty* 4:15, 1989.

50. **Davies JP, O'Connor DO, Burke DW, et al:** The effect of centrifugation on the fatigue life of bone cement in the presence of surface irregularities, *Clin Orthop* 156, 1988.

51. **Debrunner HU, Wettstein A, Hofer P:** The polymerization of self-curing acrylic cements and problems due to the cement anchorage of joint prostheses. In Schaldach M, Holmann D, editors: *Advances in artificial hip and knee joint technology,* Berlin, 1976, Springer-Verlag.

52. **Deichmann W:** Toxicity of methyl, ethyl, and n-butyl methacrylate, *J Indust Hyg Toxicol* 23:343, 1941.

53. **Demarest VA, Lautenschlager EP, Wixson RL:** Vacuum mixing of acrylic cement. In *Transactions of the 9th Annual Meeting of the Society for Biomaterials,* Birmingham, Alabama, 1983.

54. **Dodge HW Jr, Craig WM:** Acrylic cranioplasty: a newer rapid method for repair of cranial defects; preliminary report, *Proc Staff Meet Mayo Clin* 28:256, 1953.

55. **Dutton J:** Acrylic investment of intracranial aneurysms. A report of 12 years' experience, *J Neurosurg* 31:652, 1969.

56. **Eftekhar NS, Thurston CW:** Effect of irradiation on acrylic cement with special reference to fixation of pathological fractures, *J Biomech* 8:53, 1975.

57. **Elkins CW, Cameron JE:** Cranioplasty with acrylic plates, *J Neurosurg* 3:199, 1946.

58. **Ellis RH, Mulvein J:** The cardiovascular effects of methyl methacrylate, *J Bone Joint Surg* 56[Br]:59, 1974.

59. **Eyerer P, Jin R:** Influence of mixing technique on some properties of PMMA bone cement, *J Biomed Mater Res* 20:1057, 1986.

60. **Fearn CBD'A, Burgidge HC, Bentley G:** Effect of methyl methacrylate cement on systolic blood pressure in operations for total hip replacement, *J Bone Joint Surg* 55[Br]:210, 1973.

61. **Ferracane JL, Wixson RL, Lautenschlager EP:** Effects of fat admixture on the strengths of conventional and low-viscosity bone cements, *J Orthop Res* 1:450, 1984.

62. **Fisher AA:** *Contact dermatitis,* Philadelphia, 1967, Lea & Febiger.

63. **Fisher AA:** Allergic sensitization of the skin and oral mucosa to acrylic denture materials, *JAMA* 156:238, 1954.

64. **Fries IB, Fisher AA, Salvati EA:** Contact dermatitis in surgeons from methyl-methacrylate bone cement, *J Bone Joint Surg* 57:547, 1975.

65. **Frost PM:** Cardiac arrest and bone cement, *Br Med J* 3:524, 1970.

66. **Greenwald AS, Combs SP, Wilde AH, et al:** Comparative studies of the bonding strength of new and old acrylic bone cements, *Surg Forum* 26:505, 1975.

67. **Greenwald AS, Narten NC, Wilde AH:** Points in the

technique of recementing in the revision of an implant arthroplasty, *J Bone Joint Surg* 60[Br]:107, 1978.

68. **Gresham GA, Kuczynski A:** Cardiac arrest and bone cement (correspondence), *Br Med J* 3:465, 1970.

69. **Gresham GA, Kuczynski A, Rosborough D:** Fatal fat embolism following replacement arthroplasty for transcervical fractures of femur, *Br Med J* 2:617, 1971.

70. **Gruen TA, Markolf KL, Amstutz HC:** Effects of laminations and blood entrapment on the strength of acrylic bone cement, *Clin Orthop* 119:250, 1976.

71. **Haas SS, Brauer GM, Dickson G:** A characterisation of polymethylmethacrylate bone cement, *J Bone Joint Surg* 57:380, 1975.

72. **Haboush FJ:** A new operation for arthroplasty of the hip based on biomechanics, photoelasticity, fast-setting dental acrylic, and other considerations, *Bull Hosp Joint Dis* 14:242, 1953.

73. **Hamblen DL, Carter RL:** Sarcoma and joint replacement, *J Bone Joint Surg* 66[Br]:625, 1984.

74. **Hamilton HS, Cooper DF, Fels M:** Shrinkage of centrifuged cement, *Orthop Rev* 17:48, 1988.

75. **Harris NH:** Cardiac arrest and bone cement (correspondence), *Br Med J* 3:523, 1970.

76. **Henrichsen E, Jansen K, Krogh-Poulsen W:** Experimental investigation of tissue reaction to acrylic plastics, *Acta Orthop Scand* 22:141, 1952.

77. **Herndon JH, Bechtol CO, Crickenberger DP:** Fat embolism during total hip replacement. A prospective study, *J Bone Joint Surg* 56:350, 1974.

78. **Holland CJ, Kim KC, Malik MI, et al:** A histologic and hemodynamic study of the toxic effects of monomeric methyl methacrylate, *Clin Orthop* 90:262, 1973.

79. **Homsy CA:** *Prosthesis seating compounds of rapid cure acrylic polymer.* Paper presented at the National Academy of Science–American Academy of Orthopaedic Surgeons Joint Workshop on Total Hip Replacement and Skeletal Attachment, Washington, DC, November 1969.

80. **Homsy CA, Tullos HS, Anderson MS, et al:** Some physiological aspects of prosthesis stabilization with acrylic polymer, *Clin Orthop* 83:317, 1972.

81. **Homsy CA, Tullos HS, King JW:** Evaluation of rapid-cure acrylic compound for prosthesis stabilization, *Clin Orthop* 67:169, 1969.

82. **Homsy CA, Tullos HS, King JW:** Physiological sequel from implantation of rapid-cure acrylic compounds, *J Bone Joint Surg* 51:805, 1969.

83. **Hori RY, Lewis JL:** Mechanical properties of the fibrous tissue found at the bone-cement interface following total joint replacement, *J Biomed Mater Res* 16:911, 1982.

84. **Hugli TE, Muller-Ebergard HJ:** Anaphylatoxins: C3a and C5a, *Adv Immunol* 26:1, 1978.

85. **Huiskes R:** Some fundamental aspects of human joint replacement. Analyses of stresses and heat conduction in bone-prosthesis structures, *Acta Orthop Scand* 185(suppl):1, 1980.

86. **Hullinger L:** Unterschungen uber die Wirkung von Kunstharzen (Palacos und Ostamer) in Gewbekulturen, *Arch Orthop Unfallchair* 54:581, 1962.

87. **Hyland J, Robbins RH:** Cardiac arrest and bone cement, *Br Med J* 4:176, 1970.

88. **Jaffe WL, Rose RM, Radin EL:** On the stability of the mechanical properties of self-curing acrylic bone cement, *J Bone Joint Surg* 56:1711, 1974.

89. **Jasty M, Davies JP, O'Connor DO:** Porosity of various preparation of acrylic bone cements, *Clin Orthop* 259:122, 1990.

90. **Jones RH:** Physiologic emboli changes observed during total hip replacement arthroplasty, *Clin Orthop* 112:192, 1975.

91. **Judet J, Judet R:** The use of an artificial femoral head for arthroplasty of the hip joint, *J Bone Joint Surg* 32[Br]:166, 1950.

92. **Kallos T, Enis JE, Gollan F, et al:** Intramedullary pressure and pulmonary embolism of femoral medullary contents in dogs during insertion of bone cement and a prosthesis, *J Bone Joint Surg* 56:1363, 1974.

93. **Kepes ER, Undersood PS, Becsey L:** Intraoperative death associated with acrylic bone cement, *JAMA* 222:576, 1972.

94. **Keret D, Reis DR:** Intraoperative cardiac arrest and mortality in hip surgery. Possible relationship to acrylic bone cement, *Orthop Rev* 9:51, 1980.

95. **Kerr AS:** The use of acrylic resin plates for the repair of skull defects, *J Neurol Neurosurg Psychiatry* 6:158, 1943.

96. **Kiaer S:** Hip arthroplasty with acrylic prosthesis, *Acta Orthop Scand* 22:126, 1952.

97. **Knight G:** Paraspinal acrylic inlays in the treatment of cervical and lumbar spondylosis and other conditions, *Lancet* 2:147, 1959.

98. **Krause WR, Krug W, Miller J:** Strength of the cement-bone interface, *Clin Orthop* 163:290, 1982.

99. **Krause WR, Mathis RS, Grimes LW:** Fatigue properties of acrylic bone cement: S-N, P-N, and P-S-N data, *J Biomed Mater Res* 22:221, 1988.

100. **Kusy RP:** Characterization of self-curing acrylic bone cements, *J Biomed Mater Res* 12:271, 1978.

101. **Langlais F, Tomeno B, editors:** *Limb salvage—major reconstruction in oncologic and nontumoral conditions,* Berlin-Heidelberg, 1991, Springer-Verlag.

102. **Laskin DM, Robinson IB, Weinmann JP:** Experimental production of sarcomas by methyl methacrylate implants, *Proc Soc Exp Biol Med* 87:329, 1954.

103. **Lautenschlager EP, Stupps I, Keller JC:** Structure and properties of acrylic bone cement. In Duchaynep Hasting GW, editor: *Functional behavior of orthopedic biomaterials,* vol II, *Applications,* CRC Series in structure-property relationships of biomaterials, Fla, 1984, CRC Press.

104. **Lautenschlager EP, Wixson RL, Novak MA:** Fatigue and fracture toughness of Simplex P. In *Transactions of the 32nd Annual Meeting of the Orthopaedic Research Society* 11:118, 1986.

105. **Lawrence WH, Bass GE, Purcell WP, et al:** Use of mathematical models in the study of structure toxicity relationships of dental compounds. I. Esters of acrylic and methacrylic acids, *J Dent Res* 51:526, 1972.

106. **Lazansky MG:** Materials for total hip replacement, Part I: Methyl methacrylate: chemical properties and clinical uses. In American Academy of Orthopaedic Surgeons: *Instructional course lectures,* vol 23, St Louis, 1974, Mosby–Year Book.

107. **Lee AJC, Ling RSM:** Further studies of monomer loss by evaporation during the preparation of acrylic cement for use in orthopaedic surgery, *Clin Orthop* 106:122, 1975.

108. **Lee AJC, Ling RSM, Vangala SS:** Some clinically relevant variables affecting the mechanical behavior of bone cement, *Arch Orthop Traumat Surg* 92:1, 1978.

109. **Lee AJC, Wrighton JD:** Some properties of polymethyl methacrylate with reference to its use in orthopaedic surgery, *Clin Orthop* 95:281, 1973.

110. **Lidgren L, Drar H, Möller J:** Strength of polymethyl methacrylate increased by vacuum mixing, *Acta Orthop Scand* 55(5):536, 1984.

111. **Linden U:** Porosity in manually mixed bone cement, *Clin Orthop* 231:110, 1988.

112. **Ling RSM, James ML:** Blood pressure and bone cement, *Br Med J* 2:404, 1971.

113. **Luskin LS, Myers RJ:** Acrylic ester polymers. In Mark HF, editor: *Encyclopedia of polymer science and technology*, vol 1, New York, 1964, John Wiley & Sons.

114. **McKee GK, Watson-Farrar J:** Replacement of arthritic hips by the McKee-Farrar prosthesis, *J Bone Joint Surg* 48[Br]:245, 1966.

115. **McLaughlin RE, DiFazio CA, Hakala M, et al:** Blood clearance and acute pulmonary toxicity of methyl-methacrylate in dogs after simulated arthroplasty and intravenous injection, *J Bone Joint Surg* 55:1621, 1973.

116. **McLaughlin RE, Reger SI, Barkalow JA, et al:** Methylmethacrylate: a study of teratogenicity and fetal toxicity of the vapor in the mouse, *J Bone Joint Surg* 60:355, 1978.

117. **McMaster WC, Bradley G, Waugh TR:** Blood pressure lowering effect of methyl methacrylate monomer. Potentiation by blood volume deficit, *Clin Orthop* 98:254, 1974.

118. **Meyer PR Jr, Lautenschlager EP, Moore BK:** On the setting properties of acrylic bone cement, *J Bone Joint Surg* 55:149, 1973.

119. **Miles DC, Briston JH:** *Polymer technology*, New York, 1965, Chemical Publishing.

120. **Miller GJ, VanderGriend RA, Blake WP, et al:** Performance evaluation of a cement-augmented intramedullary fixation system for pathologic lesions of the femoral shaft, *Clin Orthop* 221:246, 1987.

121. **Modig J, Olerud S, Malmberg P, et al:** Medullary fat embolism during total hip replacement surgery: a preliminary report, *Injury* 5:161, 1973.

122. **Müller ME:** Total hip prostheses, *Clin Orthop* 72:46, 1970.

123. **Newens AF, Volz RG:** Severe hypotension during prosthetic hip surgery with acrylic bone cement, *Anesthesiology* 36:298, 1972.

124. **Noble PC, Jay JL, Lindahl LJ, et al:** Methods of enhancing acrylic bone cement. In *Transactions of the 13th Annual Meeting of the Society for Biomaterials*, New York, 1987.

125. **Ohnsorge J:** Some aspects of polymerizing bone cement, *J Bone Joint Surg* 53[Br]:758, 1971.

126. **Orsini EC, Byrick RJ, Mullen JB, et al:** Cardiopulmonary function and pulmonary microemboli during arthroplasty using cemented or non-cemented components. The role of intramedullary pressure, *J Bone Joint Surg* 69:822, 1987.

127. **Park JB, Malstrom CS, von Recum AF:** Intramedullary fixation of implants pre-coated with bone cement; a preliminary study, *Biomater Med Devices Artif Organs* 6:361, 1978.

128. **Park JB, von Recum AF, Gratzick GE:** Pre-coated orthopedic implants with bone cement, *Biomater Med Devices Artif Organs* 7:41, 1979.

129. **Peebles DJ, Ellis RH, Stride SD, et al:** Cardiovascular effects of methylmethacrylate cement, *Br Med J* 1:349, 1972.

130. **Pegum JS, Medhurst FA:** Contact dermatitis from penetration of rubber gloves by acrylic monomer, *Br Med J* 2:141, 1971.

131. **Petty W:** The effect of methylmethacrylate on chemotaxis

132. **Petty W:** The effect of methylmethacrylate on the bacterial inhibiting properties of normal human serum, *Clin Orthop* 132:266, 1978.

133. **Petty W, Caldwell JR:** The effect of methylmethacrylate on complement activity, *Clin Orthop* 128:354, 1977.

134. **Phillips H, Cole PV, Lettin AW:** Cardiovascular effects of implanted acrylic bone cement, *Br Med J* 3:460, 1971.

135. **Phillips H, Lettin AWF, Cole PV:** Cardiovascular effects of implanted acrylic cement, *J Bone Joint Surg* 55[Br]:210, 1973.

136. **Pickering CAC, Bainbridge D, Birtwistle IH, et al:** Occupational asthma due to methylmethacrylate in an orthopaedic theatre sister (correspondence), *Br Med J* 292:1362, 1986.

137. **Pople IK, Phillips H:** Bone cement and the liver. A dose-related effect, *J Bone Joint Surg* 70[Br]:364, 1988.

138. **Poss R, Thilly WG, Kaden DA:** Methylmethacrylate is a mutagen for *Salmonella typhimurium, J Bone Joint Surg* 61:1203, 1979.

139. **Powell JN, McGrath PJ, Lahiri SK, et al:** Cardiac arrest associated with bone cement, *Br Med J* 3:326, 1970.

140. **Raab S, Ahmed AM, Provan JW:** Thin film PMMA precoating for improved implant bone cement fixation, *J Biomed Mater Res* 16:679, 1982.

141. **Raab S, Ahmed AM, Provan JW:** The quasistatic and fatigue performance of the implant/bone-cement interface, *J Biomed Mater Res* 15:159, 1981.

142. **Reitz KA:** Polymer osteosynthesis, *Acta Chir Scand Supp* 3:388, 1968.

143. **Rimnac CM, Wright TM, McGill DL:** The effect of centrifugation on the fracture properties of acrylic bone cements, *J Bone Joint Surg* 68:281, 1986.

144. **Ritter MA, Gloe TJ, Sieber JM:** Systemic effects of polymethylmethacrylate. Increased serum levels of gamma-glutamyltranspeptidase following arthroplasty, *Acta Orthop Scand* 55:411, 1984.

145. **Roberts AC:** The surgical application of autopolymerizing acrylic resin, *Biomed Eng* 2:392, 1967.

146. **Scales JT:** In Kenedi RM, editor: *Symposium on biomechanics and related bioengineering topics*, Oxford, 1965, Pergamon Press.

147. **Sevitt S:** Fat embolism in patients with fractured hips, *Br Med J* 2:257, 1972.

148. **Sherman RMP, Byrick RJ, Kay JC, et al:** The role of lavage in preventing hemodynamic and blood-gas changes during cemented arthroplasty, *J Bone Joint Surg* 65:500, 1983.

149. **Small JM, Graham MP:** Acrylic resin for the closure of skull defects. Preliminary report, *Br J Surg* 33:106, 1945.

150. **Smith DC, Bains MED:** The detection and estimation of residual monomer in polymethyl methacrylate, *J Dent Res* 35:16, 1956.

151. **Smith DL, Schoonover IC:** Direct filling resins: dimensional changes resulting from polymerization shrinkage and water sorption, *J Am Dent Assoc* 46:540, 1953.

152. **Spence WT:** Form-fitting plastic cranioplasty, *J Neurosurg* 11:219, 1954.

153. **Spence WT:** Ten years' experience using form-fitting plastic for cranioplasty, *Bull Georgetown Univ Med Cent* 10:154, 1957.

154. **Stachiewicz JW, Miller J, Burke DL:** *Hoop stress generated by shrinkage of polymethyl methacrylate as a source of prosthetic loosening.* Paper read at the 11th

International Conference on Medical and Biological Engineering, Ottawa, 1976.

155. **Sweeney WT:** Acrylic resins in prosthetic dentistry, *Dent Clin North Am* 2:593, 1958.

156. **Tailor CC, Murphy WA, Smith EL:** Intraarticular methyl methacrylate: a complication of hip surgery, *Am J Roentgenol* 131:1055, 1978.

157. **Thomas TA, Sutherland IC, Waterhouse TD:** Cold curing acrylic bone cement. A clinical study of the cardiovascular side effects during hip joint replacement, *Anesthesiology* 26:298, 1971.

158. **Towers AG:** Viability of common pathogens in cold-curing acrylic resin used in orthopaedic surgery, *Br Med J* 2:1046, 1966.

159. **Tronzo RG, Kallos T, Wyche MQ:** Elevation of intramedullary pressure when methylmethacrylate is inserted in total hip arthroplasty, *J Bone Joint Surg* 56:714, 1974.

160. **U.S. Food and Drug Administration:** Guidelines for reproduction studies for safety evaluation of drugs for human use, 1, 1966.

161. **Wagner J, Hermans M, Bourgois R:** Etude en durimétrie sur du plastique acrylique retiré de hanches humaines, *Acta Orthop Belg* 38(Supp. 1):111, 1972.

162. **Walker PS, Bienenstock M:** Fixation properties of acrylic cement, *Rev Hosp Spec Surg* 1:27, 1971.

163. **Wang CT, Pilliar RM:** Fracture toughness of acrylic bone cement, *J Mater Sci* 24:3725, 1989.

164. **Weissman BN, Sosman JL, Braunstein EM, et al:** Intravenous methylmethacrylate after total hip replacement, *J Bone Joint Surg* 66:443, 1984.

165. **Wilde AH, Greenwald AS:** Shear strength of self-curing acrylic cement, *Clin Orthop* 106:126, 1975.

166. **Wiltse LL, Hall RH, Stenehjem JC:** Experimental studies regarding the possible use of self-curing acrylic in orthopaedic surgery, *J Bone Joint Surg* 39:961, 1957.

167. **Wixson RL, Lautenschlager EP, Novak MA:** Vacuum mixing of acrylic bone cement, *J Arthroplasty* 2:141, 1987.

168. **Wixson RL, Lautenschlager EP, Novak MA:** Vacuum mixing of methylmethacrylate bone cement. In *Transactions of the 31st Annual Meeting of the Orthopaedic Research Society* 10:327, 1985.

169. **Woolf JI, Walker AE:** Cranioplasty. Collective review, *Int Abstr Surg* 81:1, 1945.

170. **Woringer E, Schwieg B, Brogly G, et al:** Nouvelle technique ultra-rapide pour la réfection de brèches osseuses craniennes à la resine acrylique. Avantages de la résine acrylique sur le tantale, *Rev Neurol* 85:527, 1951.

171. **Wroblewski BM:** *Revision surgery in total hip arthroplasty,* London, 1990, Springer-Verlag.

172. **Zander, Cited by Kleinschmidt O:** Plexiglas zur Deckung von Schädellücken, *Chirurg* 13:273, 1941.

ADDITIONAL READINGS

American Society of Testing Materials: Standard specification for acrylic bone cement, *ASTM* F451:767, 1976.

Ayer M, Stone R, Eftekhar NS: Operating room asepsis and sterilization techniques. In Eftekhar NS, editor: *Infection in joint replacement surgery,* St Louis, 1984, Mosby–Year Book.

Breed AL: Experimental production of vascular hypotension, and bone marrow and fat embolism with methylmethacrylate cement, *Clin Orthop* 102:227, 1974.

Byrick RJ, Kay JC, Mullen JB: Pulmonary marrow embolism: a dog model simulating dual component cemented arthroplasty, *Can J Anaesth* 34:336, 1987.

Charnley J, guest editor: Total hip replacement (Symposium), *Clin Orthop* 72:1, 1970.

Charnley J: The fixation of prostheses in living bone. In Simpson DC, editor: *Modern trends in biomechanics,* New York, 1970, Appleton-Century-Crofts.

Charnley J, Cupic Z: The nine and ten year results of the low-friction arthroplasty of the hip, *Clin Orthop* 95:9, 1973.

Charnley J, Eftekhar N: Postoperative infection in total hip prosthetic replacement arthroplasty of hip joint. With special reference to the bacterial content of the air of the operating room, *Br J Surg* 56:641, 1969.

Charosky CB, Walker PS: The microstructure of polymethyl methacrylate cement, *Clin Orthop* 91:221, 1973.

Crout DHG, Corkill JA, James ML, et al: Methylmethacrylate metabolism in man. The hydrolysis of methylmethacrylate to methacrylic acid during total hip replacement, *Clin Orthop* 141:90, 1979.

Dall DM, Miles AW, Juby G: Accelerated polymerization of acrylic bone cement using preheated implants, *Clin Orthop* 211:148, 1986.

Daumas-Duport C, Hanau J, Abelanet R: Cerebral fat emboli. Apropos of a case of a perioperative complication associated with the use of a bone cement in orthopedic surgery, *Ann Anat Pathol* (Paris) 22:269, 1977.

Eftekhar NS: Charnley "low-friction torque" arthroplasty. A study of long-term results, *Clin Orthop* 81:93, 1971.

Engesaeter LB, Strand T, Raugstad TS, et al: Effects of a distal venting hole in the femur during total hip replacement, *Arch Orthop Traumat Surg* 103:328, 1984.

Fernandez-Fairen M, Vazquez JJ: The aging of polymethyl methacrylate bone cement, *Acta Orthop Belg* 49:512, 1983.

Fisher AA: Allergic sensitization of the skin and oral mucosa to acrylic resin denture materials, *J Prosthet Dent* 6:593, 1956.

Gates EI, Carter DR, Harris WH: Comparative fatigue behavior of different bone cements, *Clin Orthop* 189:294, 1984.

Giercksky KE, Bjørklid E, Prydz H, et al: Circulating tissue thromboplastin during hip surgery, *Eur Surg Res* 11:296, 1979.

Halawa M, Lee AJC, Ling RSM, et al: The shear strength of trabecular bone from the femur, and some factors affecting the shear strength of the cement-bone interface, *Arch Orthop Traumat Surg* 92:19, 1978.

Hallin G, Modig J, Nordgren L, et al: The intramedullary pressure during the bone marrow trauma of total hip replacement, *vol(issue): pages, year.*

Hamati FI, Wixson RL, Novak MA, et al: The effect of notching of Simplex-P bone cement on the fatigue lives of regular versus vacuum-mixed specimens. In *Transactions of the 33rd Annual Meeting of the Orthopaedic Research Society,* San Francisco 12:226, 1987.

Jefferiss CD, Lee AJC, Ling RSM: Thermal aspects of self-curing polymethylmethacrylate, *J Bone Joint Surg* 57[Br]:511, 1975.

Kallos T: Impaired arterial oxygenation associated with use of bone cement in the femoral shaft, *Anesthesiology* 42:210, 1975.

Krause WR, Mathis RS: Fatigue properties of acrylic bone cement: review of the literature, *J Biomed Mater Res* 22(A1 Suppl.):37, 1988.

Loshaek S, Fox TG: Cross-linked polymers. I. Factors influencing the efficiency of cross-linking in copolymers of methyl methacrylate and glycol dimethacrylates, *J Am Chem Soc* 75:3544, 1953.

Lozewicz S, Davison AG, Heckirk A, et al: Occupational asthma due to methyl methacrylate and cyanoacrylates, *Thorax* 40:836, 1985.

Memoli VA, et al: Malignant neoplasms associated with orthopaedic implant materials in rats, *J Orthop Res* 4.346, 1986.

Modig J, Busch C, Olerud S, et al: Arterial hypotension and hypoxaemia during total hip replacement. The importance of thromboplastic products, fat embolism and acrylic monomers, *Acta Anaesthesiol Scand* 19:28, 1975.

Modig J, Busch C, Olerud S, et al: Pulmonary microembolism during intramedullary orthopaedic trauma, *Acta Anaesthesiol Scand* 18:133, 1974.

Monteny E, Oleffe J, Donkerwolke M: Methylmethacrylate hypersensitivity in a patient with cemented endoprosthesis. A case report, *Acta Orthop Scand* 49:554, 1978.

Ngai SH, Stinchfield FE, Triner L: Air embolism during total hip arthroplasties, *Anesthesiology* 40:405, 1974.

Park WY, Balingit P, Kenmore PI, et al: Changes in arterial oxygen tension during total hip replacement surgery, *Anesthesiology* 39:642, 1974.

Parsons DW: Cardiac arrest and bone cement, *Br Med J* 3:710, 1970.

Rinecker H: New clinico-pathophysiological studies on the bone cement implantation syndrome, *Arch Orthop Trauma Surg* 97:263, 1980.

Saha S, Pal S: Mechanical properties of bone cement: a review, *J Biomed Mater Res* 18:435, 1984.

Schuh FT, Schuh SM, Viguera MG, et al: Circulatory changes following implantation of methylmethacrylate bone cement, *Anesthesiology* 39:455, 1973.

Sikorski JM, Millar AJ: Systemic disturbance from Thompson's arthroplasty: an age-matched and sex-matched controlled retrospective survey, *J Bone Joint Surg* 59[Br]:398, 1977.

Spealman CR, Main RJ, Haag HB, et al: Monomeric methylmethacrylate; studies on toxicity, *Indust Med* 14:292, 1945.

Spengler DM, Costenbader M, Bailey R: Fat embolism syndrome following total hip arthroplasty, *Clin Orthop* 121:105, 1976.

Stinchfield FE, guest editor: Statistics on total hip replacement, *Clin Orthop* 95:1, 1973.

Turnbull KW, Berezowsky JL, Pouisen JB, et al: General anaesthesia and total hip replacement, *Can Anaesth Soc J* 21:546, 1974.

Weightman B, Freeman MAR, Revell PA, et al: The mechanical properties of cement and loosening of the femoral component of hip replacements, *J Bone Joint Surg* 69[Br]:558, 1987.

Weinstein AM, Bingham DN, Barry BW, et al: The effect of high pressure insertion antibiotic inclusions upon the mechanical properties of polymethylmethacrylate, *Clin Orthop* 121:67, 1976.

Wong KC, Martin WE, Kennedy WF, et al: Cardiovascular effects of total hip placement in man. With observations on the effects of methylmethacrylate on the isolated rabbit heart, *Clin Pharmacol Ther* 21:709, 1977.

See Chapters 4, Biomaterials, Compatibility, and Wear; 6, Applied Biomechanics and Loosening; and 8, Prevention of Infection for additional information.

CHAPTER SIX

Biomechanics: Fixation and Loosening

■ Every change in the . . . function of a bone . . . is followed by certain definite changes in . . . internal architecture and external conformation in accordance with mathematical laws.
  Wolff's law

FORCES ABOUT THE HIP

It is established that the static force on the femoral head is greater than the weight of the body (Fig. 6-1) during stance, perhaps two or three times greater.[90,129] Assuming that "maximum wear" occurs at the maximum force location, Elson and Charnley, after examining worn-out Teflon acetabular cups, calculated the direction of the actual resultant force to be 10 to 15 degrees from the midaxis of the body. They determined this to be the most common direction of wear, although in a small percentage of their cases it was as much as ±20 degrees toward or away from the midline.[50]

Forces acting on the hip joint are influenced considerably by the pelvic angle and the position of the trunk and limbs.[105] Joint reaction force, determined by a simple two-dimensional free-body diagram, is calculated from the formula

$$J = W \times 1 + a/d$$

The force is calculated as the muscle positions alter (Fig. 6-2). During the walking cycle, the angle between the line of action of the joint force and the femoral axis changes, as determined by Paul.[128] Joint reaction force during walking has been determined by Seirig and Arkivar,[153] Crowninshield and associates,[42] Bergmann and colleagues,[11] Röhrle,[142] and Davy and co-workers.[46] With the pelvis in a normal walking attitude and the limbs symmetrically disposed, muscle forces range from 1.0 to 1.8 times the body weight, joint forces from 1.8 to 2.7 times the body weight; even small changes in the positions of the lever arms of the muscles involved will alter these forces considerably. With simple calculations the load on the hip joint,

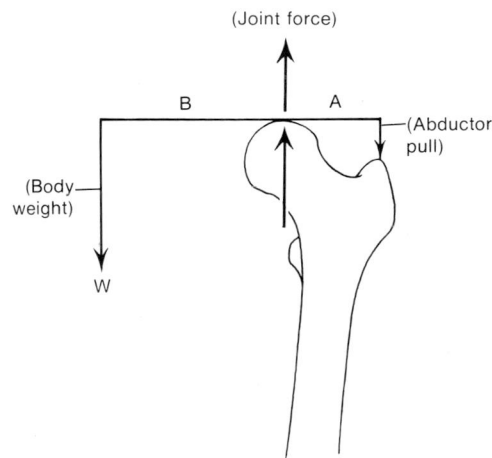

Fig. 6-1. Force on femoral head is equal to abductor pull (force) times *A* (distance) plus body weight times *B* (distance). Static force on femoral head is greater than weight of body, *W*, during stance, being two to three times greater in magnitude than body weight. NOTE: The vector of abductor pull is shown in same direction as body weight for clarity.

when the person lies supine and raises a leg 2 inches off the ground, is approximately twice that of the body weight; obviously, then, the forces generated in the hip by muscle action must be kept in mind when recommending exercises to a patient not yet ready for weight bearing.[63] The clinical implication is a paradox: keeping a patient nonweight bearing while emphasizing active straight-leg-raising exercises.

While static force is considerably greater than body weight, an even greater force is generated in dynamic

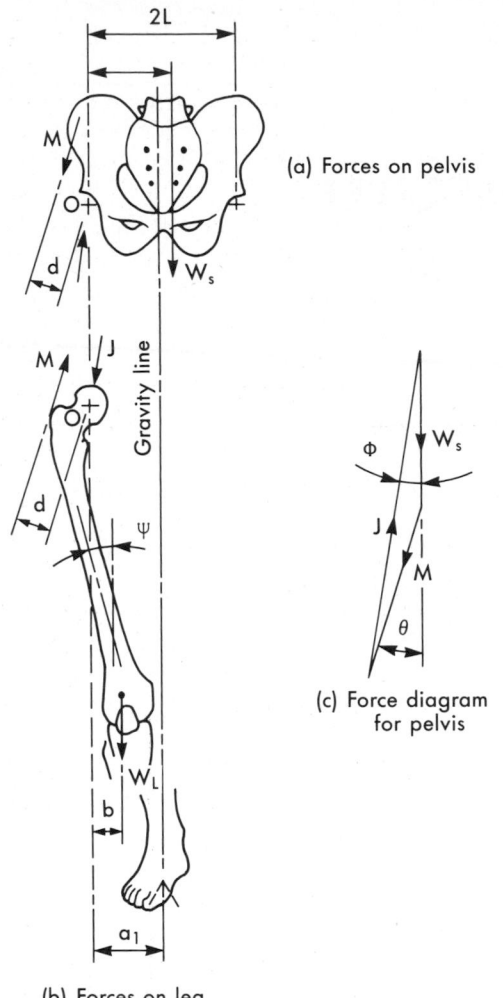

(a) Forces on pelvis

(b) Forces on leg

(c) Force diagram for pelvis

Fig. 6-2. Hip joint mechanics. (From McLeish RD, Charnley J: Abduction forces in the one legged stance, *J Biomechanics*, 3:192, 1970.)

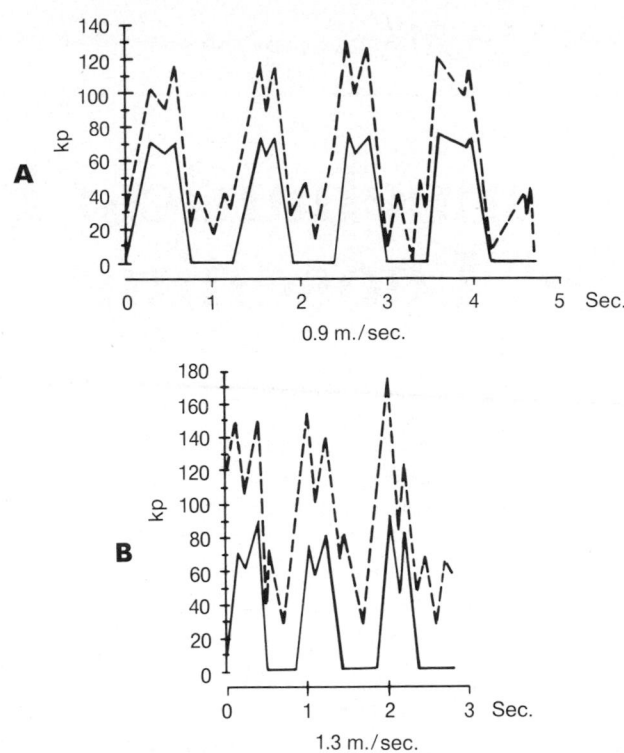

Fig. 6-3. While static force is considerably greater than body weight, even greater force is generated in dynamic situations, such as acceleration and deceleration. Instrumented prosthesis indicates that with walking speed of 1.3 m/sec maximum force of 3.8 times body weight is generated. **B,** Reduction of speed to 0.9 m/sec diminished force on hip joint to 1.8 times body weight, **A.** (Modified from Rydell MW: Forces acting on the femoral head prosthesis: a study on strain gauge supplied prostheses in living persons, *Acta Orthop Scand [Suppl]* 88:Suppl, 1966.)

situations such as acceleration and deceleration (Fig. 6-3).

Using an instrumented Moore self-locking prosthesis, studies measured the forces acting directly across the hip joint.[145,146] A walking speed of 1.3 m/second, they determined, generated a maximum force of 3.8 times the body weight; reducing this rate to 0.9 m/second reduced the force on the hip to 1.8 times the body weight. In other words, the forces on the hip joint were reduced by 50% simply by reducing the walking speed (see Fig. 6-3).

To measure in-vitro contact pressures in human hip joints opposing the natural acetabular cartilage, Hodge collected data telemetrically; he used an instrumented femoral head prosthesis, which measured the intraarticular pressure at 10 discrete locations 253 times per second.[80] At various periods after implantation, the

researchers made continuous records of data regarding the dynamic forces of the hip joint. They obtained significant data indicating that muscle contractions play an important role in creating those forces; with their data they calculated the net forces generated during walking, sitting, standing, and other normal daily activities, such as stair climbing and rising from a chair. The last-mentioned function generated much higher forces on the posterior acetabular wall than had previously been estimated.[80]

Using an instrumented hip arthroplasty 3 days postoperatively, Davy and co-workers[46] found that the joint reaction force increases to 2.1 times body weight with one-legged stance with the subject using contralateral hand support. Walking between parallel bars produced a maximum joint reaction force of 2.4 times body weight. Instrumented hip prostheses in experimental animals also showed that load-bearing force increases progressively with time elapsed from the operation (in contrast to the animal's walking speed).[11] The peak resultant (average) joint contact force increases linearly from about 3.5 times body weight at 0.7 m/second to seven times body weight at 1.75 m/second.[142] These figures are similar to those obtained by instrumented prostheses[46,59] and somewhat lower than estimates based on mathematical calculations.[42,74,128] The figures recorded via instrumented prostheses are lower because patients with artificial joints have uneven gaits and may also take smaller steps.[173] At 3 days after surgery, joint force equaled body weight only when the patient used a walker for support.[46]

It seems that active young patients can generate extraordinary forces in the hip that would exceed the reductions produced by any surgical or prosthetic modification designed to lower incumbent forces. Even so, it seems logical to reduce all excessive forces from the joint to increase the life and function of the prosthesis.

Dynamic data obtained by using a force plate to determine ground reaction indicate that the force generated may be even greater than that generated by the use of an instrumented prosthesis. During the stance phase of the gait, forces on the femoral head may be approximately five or six times the body weight; they at least equal body weight during the swing phase of the gait. The reason is that during the "swing phase," the mass of the limb with the muscular and ligamentous action produces the load on the joint; in the "stance phase," ground reaction adds to the forces generated.

As mentioned earlier, the pelvic angle and the position of the trunk and limbs affect forces considerably. Forces acting on the abductor muscles and femoral head have been determined experimentally in a range of "pelvic attitudes."[105] In these studies, the location of the body's center of gravity was determined by simultaneously recording force measurements with radiography to determine how the forces relate to the position of the skeleton. The forces were calculated using muscle positions, cadaveric dissections, and radiography of specimens. Calculations based on the recorded data revealed that, with the pelvis in the normal walking attitude and the limbs symmetrically disposed, muscle forces ranged from 1.0 to 1.8 times body weight and joint forces from 1.8 to 2.7 times body weight.

Joint reaction forces increase considerably during stair climbing. Kinematic studies of lower-extremity joints have indicated that ascending or descending stairs requires a larger range of hip and knee motion than walking. And although stair climbing creates moments of high joint stress, the highest moment occurs during descent.[3] According to Andriacchi, the hip's mean maximal sagittal plane motion was 42 degrees; its mean maximal net flexion-extension moment was 123.9 newton-meters while climbing and 112.5 newton-meters while descending stairs. The magnitude of flexion-extension moments required to climb stairs is greater than that used when walking on a level surface.[16a,110] The largest increase occurs at the knee joint. The difference in increased force results largely from the muscle activities required to move the body vertically. It is important to consider these greater forces both in establishing prosthetic design criteria and in planning the patient's postoperative activity level.

To measure pressure contact, Mizrahi and colleagues placed pressure transducers in experimental models; the transducers were placed in the subchondral bone in contact with the cartilage to measure force transmission patterns in the hip joint. The transducers were placed throughout the hip loaded in flexion-extension, abduction-adduction, and extension and internal rotation. Their data revealed that the highest pressures were in the anterior and posterior segments of the acetabulum; the lowest pressures occurred at the zenith of the acetabulum.[111]

With a force plate it is possible to measure and analyze the pattern of forces in the hip joint both qualitatively and quantitatively.[29,125–127] A force plate (also called a *gait recorder*) traces the quantitative measure of force versus time to analyze gait objectively.[31] This device is far more sensitive and objective than clinical observation or cinematography. It is so sensitive to gait measurements that, for example, it records an asymmetrical tracing in cases of bilateral hip disease that clinically show symmetrical involvement. These measurements provide a sensitive indicator of the patient's preoperative and postoperative gait pattern (Fig. 6-4).

Reduction of Hip Joint Forces

Imbalanced muscles or diseases such as congenital dysplasia of the hips or osteoarthritis can create abnormal forces on the hip joint, leading to excess load per unit area of the joint and causing wear of the cartilage and exposure of the bone, leading to pain. Logically, therefore, an alternative to joint arthroplasty is to reduce the load and the forces that generate pain in a malfunctioning hip joint.

A simple way to reduce forces in the hip is to have the patient lean over the affected hip. His or her center of gravity then moves laterally toward the center of the femoral head, thus shortening its lever arm. This simple action reduces the magnitude of forces needed in the abductor muscles for balance and thus reduces the net force across the hip joint.

Another way to reduce forces in the hip is to increase the weight-bearing surface in the joint by osteotomy; this procedure places a major portion of the head underneath the weight-bearing zone of the acetabulum;

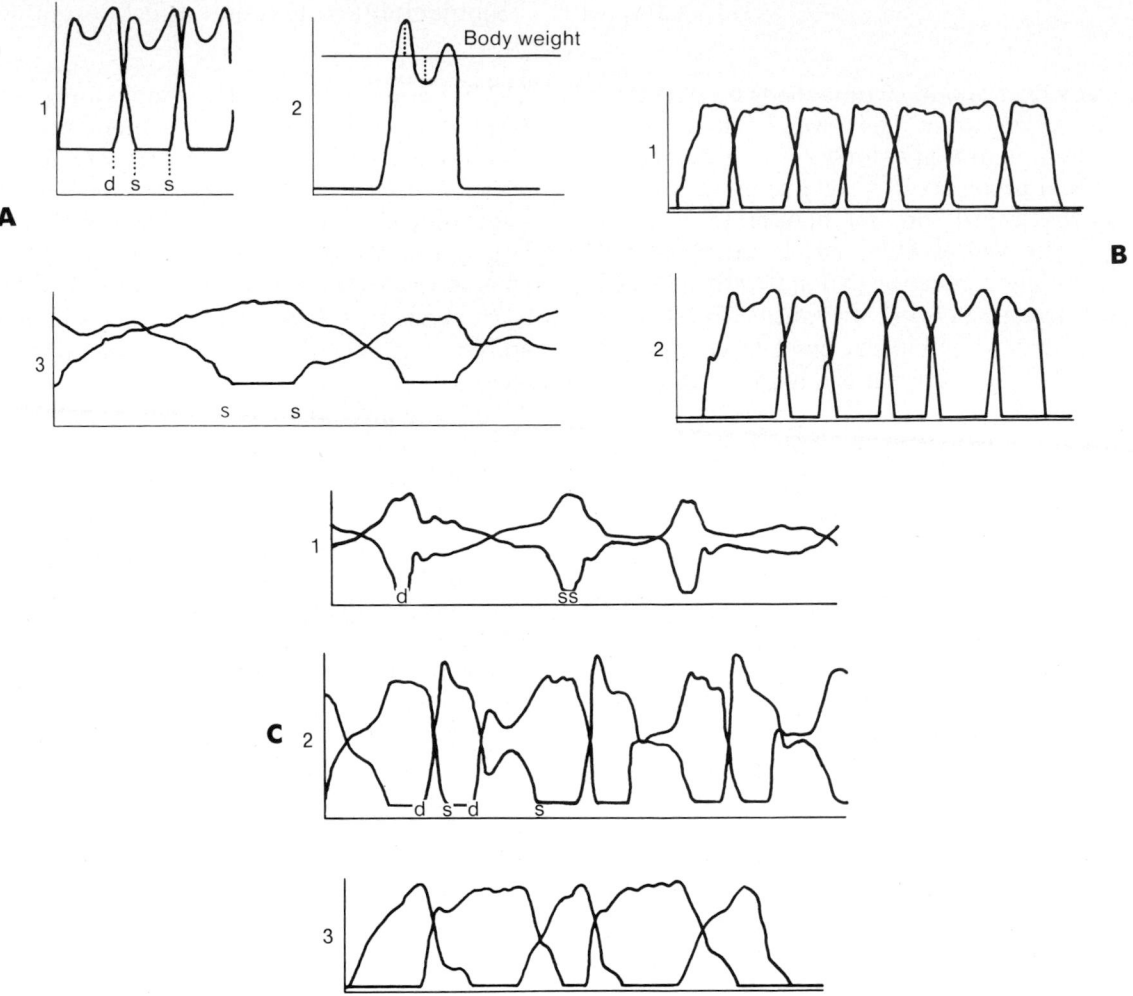

Fig. 6-4. A, Subject walking on recording platforms of gait recorder. *(1)* Characteristic trace in normal gait of young subject; *ds,* double support phase; *ss,* single support phase. *(2)* Level of body weight in relation to peaks caused by acceleration and deceleration of body mass. One mm vertical height equal to 5 pounds actual weight is recorded with both feet on one trace. *(3)* Short steps made very slowly. Part only of very long trace needing 20 steps to cover 11 feet. **B,** *(1)* Gait of elderly person (normal) or symmetrical arthritis of hips. *(2)* Notch on ascending limb of pulse probably indicating incoordination of knee extension. **C,** *(1)* Symmetrical slow progress of "alternate-standing" type. *(2)* Marked asymmetry of *ds* phase. Patient not stepping through with right foot, merely bringing one foot up to other and leading again with same foot. *(3)* Severe limp from unilateral hip disease. NOTE: for normal limb *ss* phase is too long to show "first and second peaks" of normal gait as seen in **A** *(1).* (Modified from Charnley J, Pusso R: The recording and the analysis of gait in relation to the surgery of the hip joint, *Clin Orthop* 58:153, 1968.)

the logic is congruent with that behind a varus osteotomy in congenital dysplasia of the hips. Weight reduction is the simplest principle for reducing the force on the femoral head and thus on the hip joint. For each pound of weight lost, the force is reduced by approximately 2.5 to 3 pounds; therefore a reduction of even a few pounds in weight is significant (Fig. 6-5). Another way to reduce the weight on the hip joint is to have the patient use a cane in the opposite hand; Blount and others have demonstrated the effectiveness of this method (Fig. 6-6).[13]

As noted previously, the force can also be reduced by slowing the speed of walking[125,126] and by reconstruct-

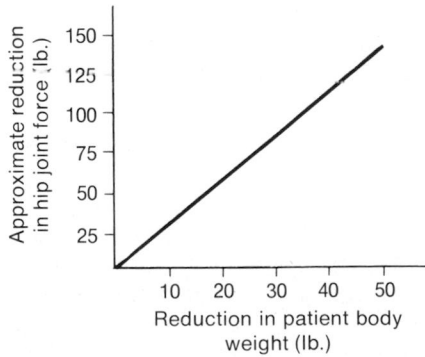

Fig. 6-5. Graph shows correlation between weight loss and hip joint force; reduction is by ratio of 1:3.

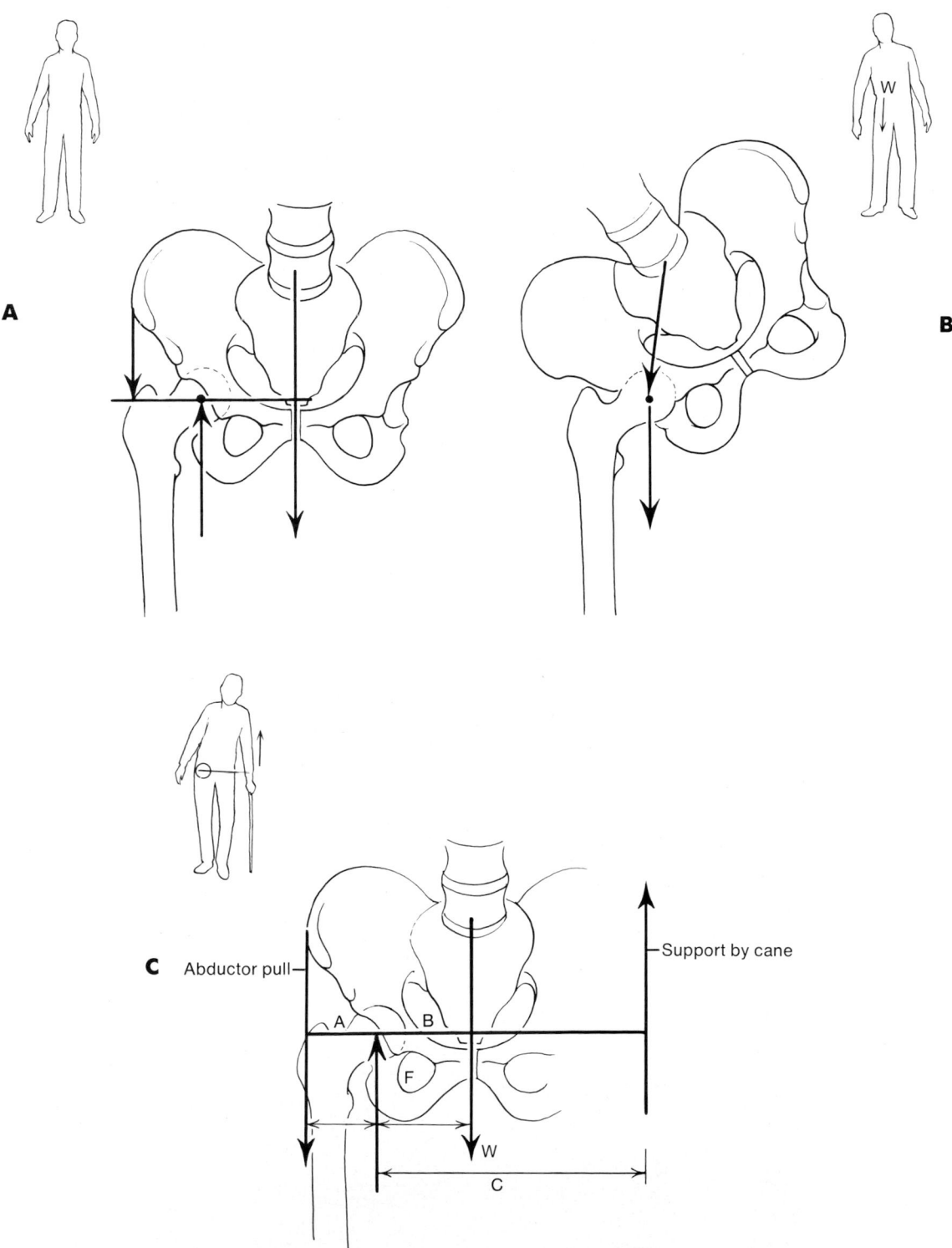

Fig. 6-6. A and **B,** Mechanics of painful hip may be changed by reduction of force generated by having patient lean over affected hip. In this situation center of gravity moves laterally toward center of femoral head, thus shortening its lever arm. **B,** This action simply reduces magnitude of forces needed in abductor muscles to produce "balance," thus reducing net force across hip joint. **C,** Another means of reducing force, *F,* on hip joint is use of cane. Supporting force is provided by cane applied through favorable lever arm and greatly reduces force that abductors must exert to produce balance. In this diagram *A* represents abductor lever arm; *B,* body weight lever arm; and *C,* hip support (cane) lever arm. *W* represents weight.

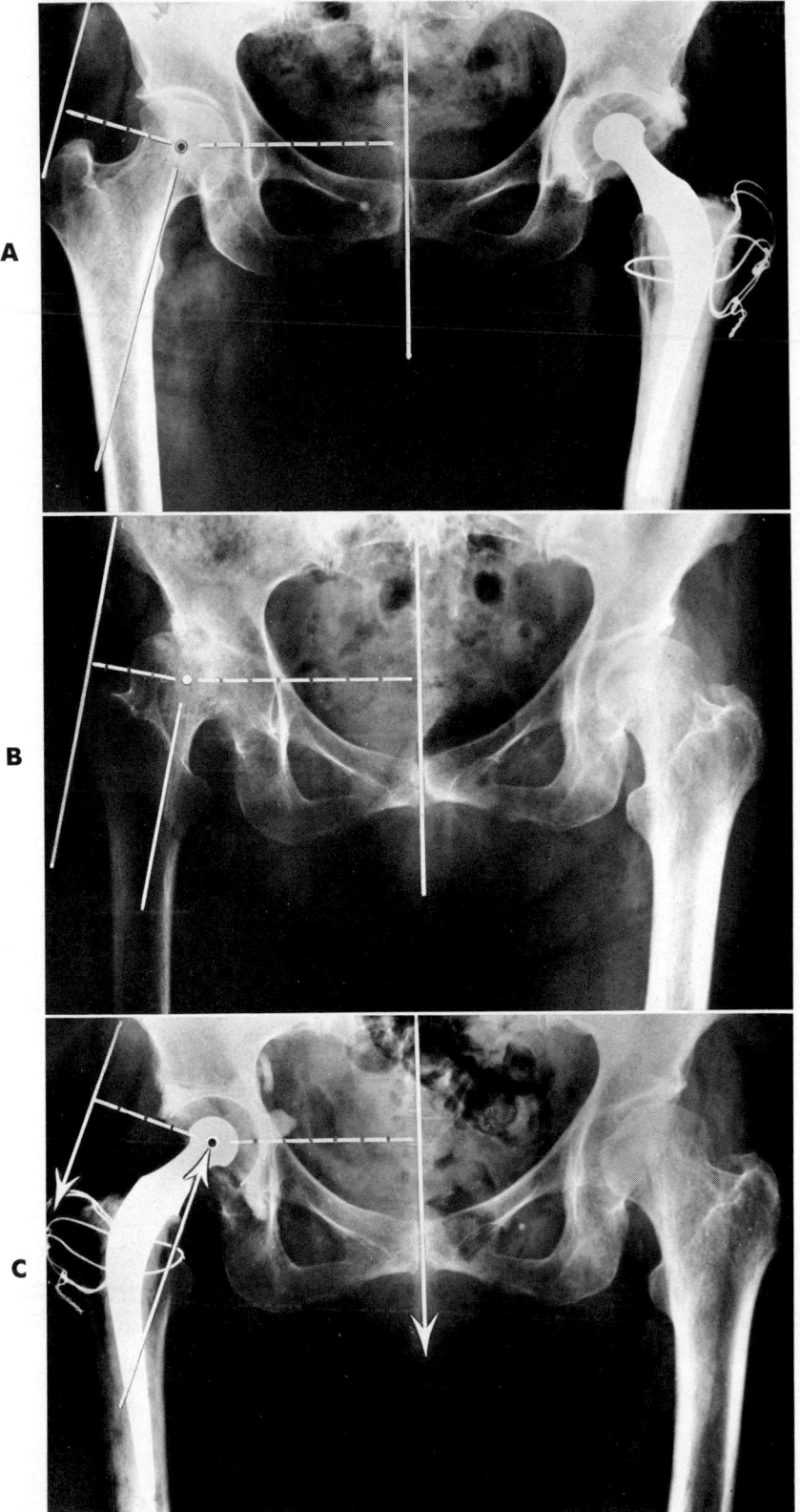

Fig. 6-7. Reduction of load after arthroplasty is achieved by reducing body weight moment arm through maximal deepening of acetabulum, thus moving center of rotation medially, and by increasing gluteal moment arm via lateral transfer of greater trochanter. **A,** Normal; **B,** osteoarthrosis; **C,** after arthroplasty.

ing the joint at arthroplasty.

Various investigators have documented how forces are affected by disease-related geometrical alterations,[60,136] surgical reconstruction,[23,94,95] and design-related effects.[4,7]

Charnley advocated restoring hip function via lateralizing the abductor forces and medializing the center of rotation of the hip.[26,27] He also advanced the theory of mechanical improvement by reconstruction, which may reduce the socket load, sparing the artificial joint from excessive stress, which could otherwise considerably affect wear, loosening, and failure of the stem (Fig. 6-7).[25,29] There are two ways to achieve this reconstruction: (1) reduce the body-weight moment arm by deepening the acetabulum maximally, thus moving the center of rotation medially, and (2) increase the gluteal moment arm by transferring the greater trochanter laterally.

The optimal geometrical relationships after total hip arthroplasty have been determined mathematically.[95] Johnston and associates demonstrated several ways in which total hip arthroplasty reduces the forces: (1) it minimizes the effort required to perform normal activities, (2) it produces minimal joint contact force, and (3) it minimizes the bending moment at the neck-stem junction of the stem. The model these researchers used considered the surgical effects of altering the site of acetabular placement in the pelvis, the femoral shaft–prosthesis neck angle, the neck length of the femoral prosthesis, and the role of transfer of the greater trochanter in reconstruction. They reached the following conclusions:

1. The loads on the hip joint were significantly reduced by placing the center of the acetabulum (hip joint) as far medially, inferiorly, and anteriorly as possible.
2. A prosthesis with a short offset (i.e., short neck) and reduced neck-shaft angle (i.e., 130 degrees) lowered the moment of force on the stem.
3. Lateral transfer of the trochanter (abductor moment arm), although desirable, had a less significant effect.

From the foregoing it can be noted that the shorter the body-weight-moment arm, the less the pull of the abductors required to balance the pelvis; conversely, by lengthening the abductor-moment arm, the gluteal tension required to balance the pelvis is reduced, also reducing the total load on the hip joint (Fig. 6-8).

To illustrate this mechanical situation, attempt to balance a beam on a fulcrum (for example, an 18-inch ruler on a fingertip) (Fig. 6-9). As shown in the diagram, balancing the ruler on the finger requires no extra force if the fulcrum is exactly at the midpoint of the ruler (marked 9 inches). The weight transferred to

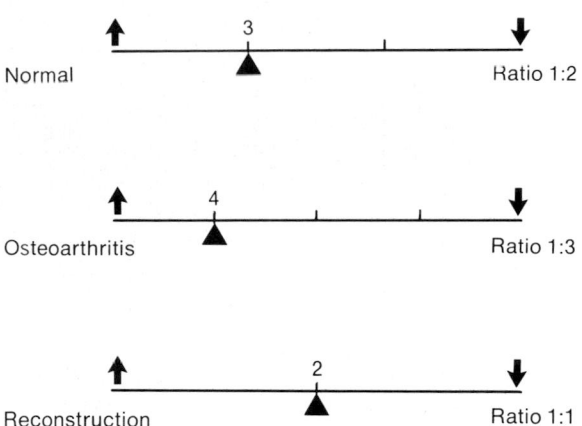

Fig. 6-8. Mechanical principles involved in arthroplasty. Normal hip has ratio of about 1:2, but in osteoarthritis this ratio can change to 1:3 or more. By low-friction arthroplasty (deep socket, small head, and transposition of greater trochanter) it is possible to bring lever ratio to 1:1, thus reducing socket load. (Solid triangles represent socket load in each situation.)

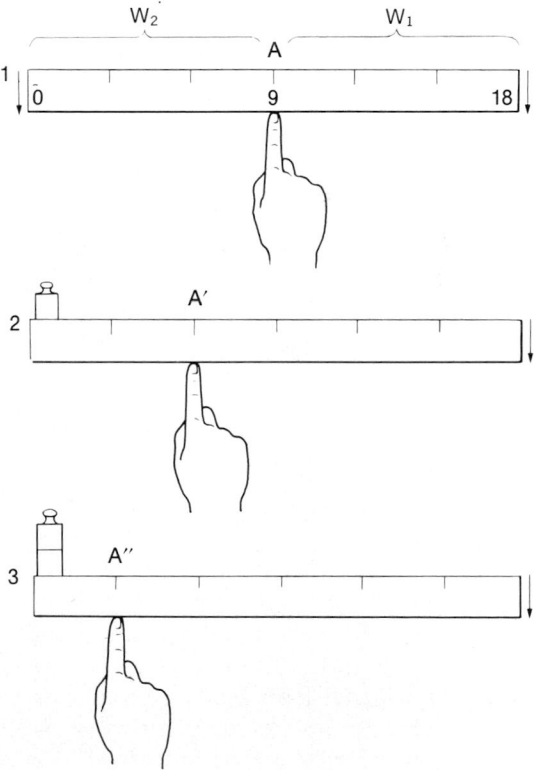

Fig. 6-9. Analogy of hip joint forces as related to changes in lever arm systems. *1,* Beam (18-inch ruler) is balanced on fingertip. Fulcrum point is exactly at midpoint of ruler. Weight transferred to tip of finger is equal to weight of ruler acting at that point ($W_1 + W_2$). *2,* By transferring finger (fulcrum) to point A′ added force is required to balance ruler. *3,* Even greater force is needed for balance if distance between weight and fulcrum on acting moment arm is further reduced (point A″). Consequently, forces on fulcrum are proportionately increased, that is, weight of ruler ($W_1 + W_2$) plus weight required to balance beam.

the tip of the finger is equal to the weight of the ruler acting at point A. By transferring the finger (fulcrum) to point A, we readily see that force must be added to balance the ruler. Balance requires even greater weight (force) if the distance between the weight and the fulcrum on the acting moment arm is further reduced (point A); consequently, the forces on the fulcrum also increase. This simple analogy demonstrates the importance of recognizing the moments of the forces about the hip in attempting to reduce the socket load (fingertip, in the experiment).

By applying these principles to hip arthroplasty, we see that laterally transposing the trochanter does not provide stability solely by stretching the elastic muscle fibers. The stability achieved by these means also increases the abductor-moment arm, placing less demand from the abductor on the joint and so less load. The marked external rotation of the hip reduces the distance between the abductor tendons and the hip's center of rotation (a fact not commonly appreciated); in other words, the muscle must act severely to compensate for the "effective" shortening of the abductor-moment arm. Therefore transposing the greater trochanter laterally after removing the external deforming force (short rotators) increases the effective neck length, thus reducing the demand on the abductors.

Another important advantage of arthroplasty is that a smaller-diameter head makes it possible to move the hip's center of rotation more medially. At surgery, it is possible to elongate the abductor-moment arm and reduce the "body-weight moment arm" conveniently without excessively deepening (and thus damaging) the acetabular floor.

Practical Application of Moment of Forces
Offset of the Femur and Prosthesis

Offset of the femur is designated by a perpendicular line drawn from the center of the femoral head to the axis of the femur. Charnley originally accepted a 45-mm offset for an average adult femur. In this case, after arthroplasty, the center of the head coincides with the anatomical center of the femur.

Clearly, for a given joint load, a prosthesis with a short offset provides greater strength while maintaining the neutral axis of the prosthesis in the same line as the femur and also maintaining the normal offset of the femur (Fig. 6-10). Fig. 6-10 shows a short offset prosthesis (35 mm) maintaining the normal offset without grossly exaggerated valgus in a short-statured patient. Clinical examples of arthroplasty-induced changes in hip biomechanics are shown by changes in offset in Figs. 6-11 to 6-14.

There are two main disadvantages to a short-offset prosthesis:

1. The length of the abductor lever arm is reduced, in turn requiring greater abductor power, thus negating the benefits of the short offset.
2. The joint force becomes more vertical by changing the abductor force to a more vertical angle (more parallel to the axis of the femur), thus increasing the demand on abductor pull. The main disadvantages of increased offset after arthroplasty include increased stress on the medial neck, medial femoral cement, and stem, with potential for loosening and stem failure. However, an increased abductor lever arm resulting from an increased offset may improve the abductor function, which may reduce joint reaction force and increase joint stability.

Lateralization of the Abductors

To facilitate the function of the abductors, it is essential to (1) maintain the abductor lever arm, and (2) maintain the angle of inclination of the abductor muscle pull. By using a short-offset prosthesis (to reduce the bending moment on the femur), it is essential to increase the length of the abductor lever arm by slight lateral displacement of the trochanter. Charnley emphasized that lateral displacement need not be extreme; only 1 cm or so lateral and distal displacement is sufficient to alter the angle of inclination of the abductors.

Deepening of the Socket

Severe deepening of the socket, once thought to be essential, is no longer practiced at surgery. McLeish[105] concluded that one-legged stance transposes the greater trochanter more laterally, making the abductor arm more sensitive to changes in length than the medialization of the socket and the body lever arm.[29] Therefore 0.5 cm of lateralization of the abductor lever arm is equivalent to 1.0 to 1.5 cm medialization of the body lever arm. To keep the angle of the abductors normal, be sure to maintain the lateral projection of the greater trochanter. Excessive deepening of the acetabulum eliminates the lateral projection, especially when using a short-offset prosthesis. Charnley[29] compared the combined effects of variables related to the offset of the prosthesis (45-mm offset, 40-mm offset, and 35-mm offset), deepening of the socket (normal socket deepening 1 cm), and lateralization of the trochanter (normal trochanter 0.5 cm lateral displacement). He reached the following conclusions:

• *Prosthesis with 45-mm offset:* 1 cm socket deepening reduced joint reactive force by 10% and increased the bending moment of the stem by 20%. The optimal use of a 45-mm offset prosthesis was 0.5 cm lateral displacement of the trochanter and no deepening of the socket.

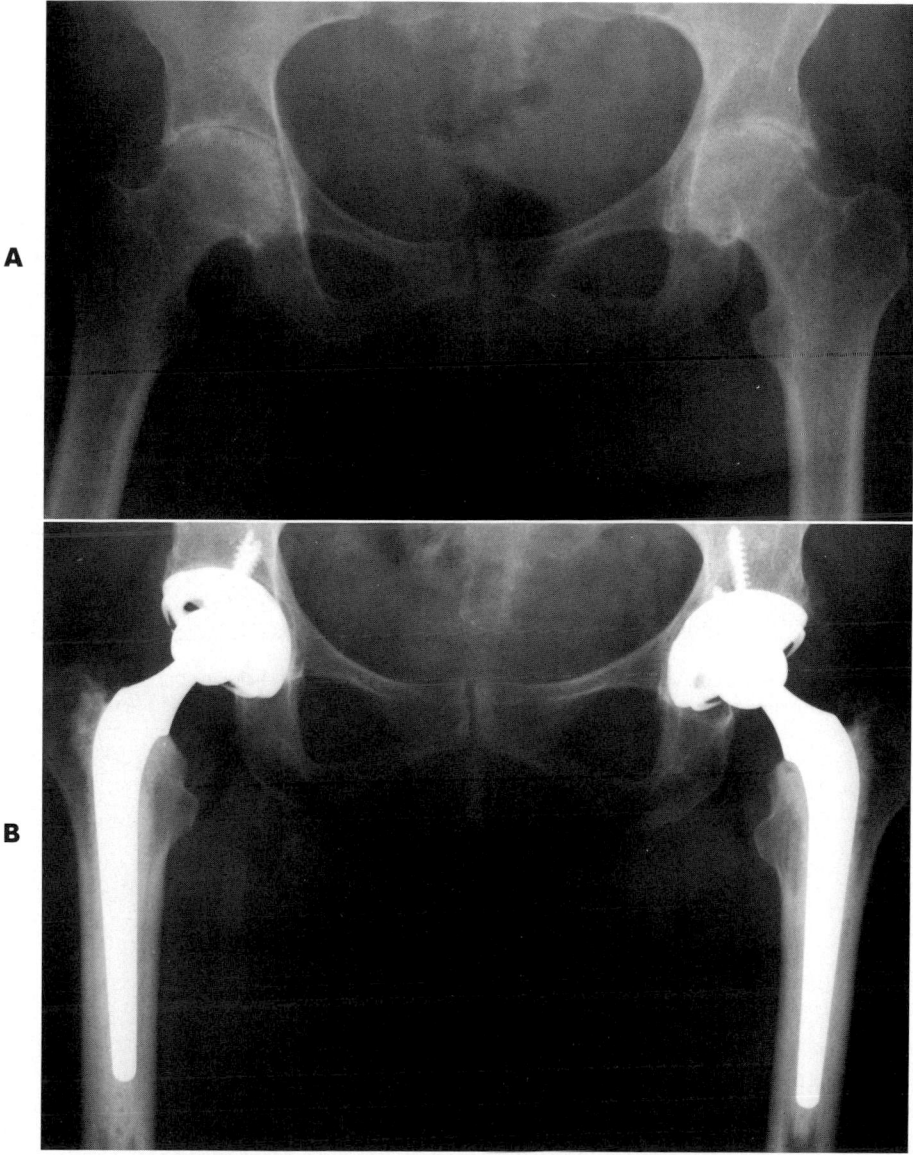

Fig. 6-10. Restoration of hip biomechanics by prosthesis and surgery is essential. **A,** Bilateral hip disease in 47-year-old woman (E.S.) with rheumatoid arthritis. **B,** Well-centered stems and use of modular Charnley prosthesis (Elite) and 26-mm femoral component with straight narrow stems and 35-mm offset reproduced the patient's own anatomical abductor and body lever arms. Reconstruction was carried out based on preoperative planning using radiographic templates (see Chapters 11 and 15).

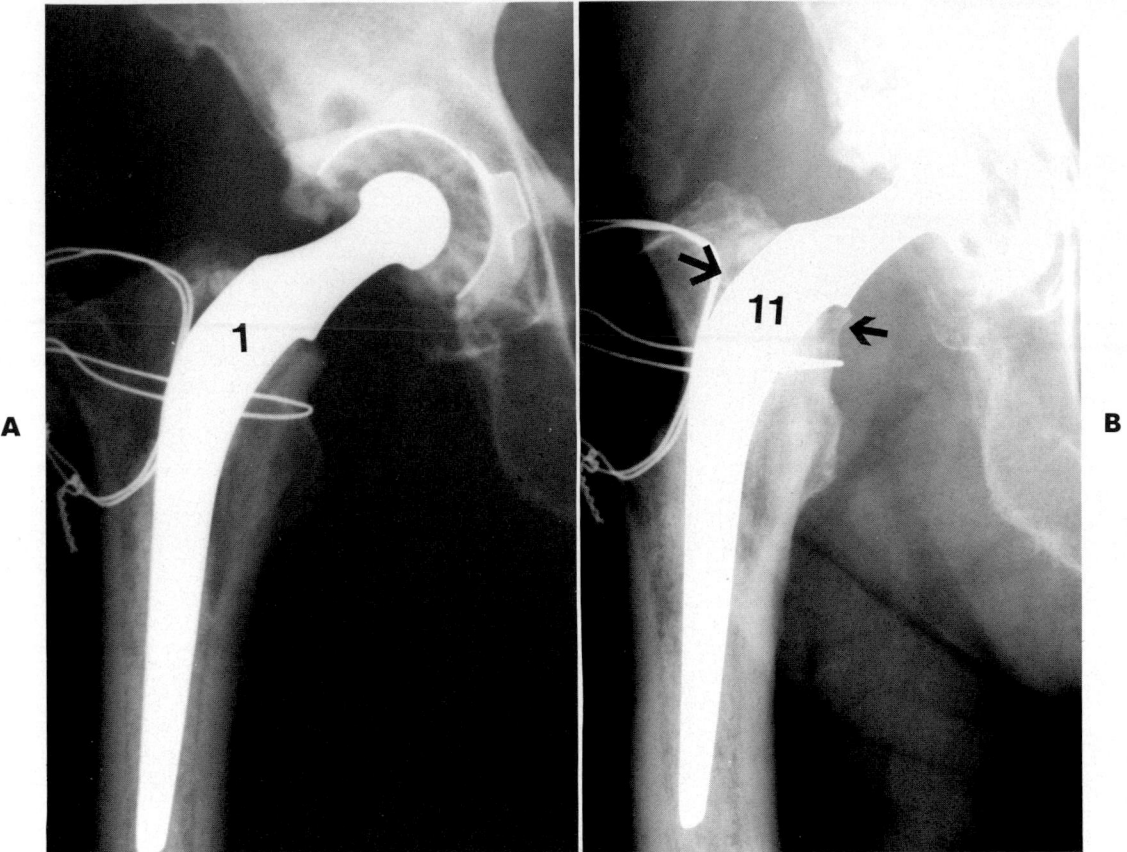

Fig. 6-11. Adverse effect by a varus stem orientation is shown. **A,** 1 year postoperative radiographs of 68-year-old army general (L.F.). NOTE: varus orientation of stem causing stress at the medial neck region, as evidenced by neck absorption and plastic deformation of stem and separation of stem from cement. Preoperative grades A-3,3,3. Patient's weight was 68 kg. **B,** 11 years postoperatively, the hip clinically remains successful. Hip grade A-6,6,6. Patient's weight is 65 kg.

- *Prosthesis with 40-mm offset:* Deepening the socket also produced an adverse effect of 5%, which was neutralized by displacing the trochanter laterally. The optimal result of using a 40-mm offset prosthesis was a lateral transfer of the trochanter without deepening the socket, resulting in a bending moment of 30% with a significant change in joint reaction force.
- *Prosthesis with 35-mm offset:* Without deepening the socket and 0.5 cm lateral trochanteric displacement, the bending moment on the 35-mm offset prosthesis is reduced by 47%; the joint reactive force increases by 3.8% with 0.5 cm lateral transfer of the trochanter; and with a 1.0 cm lateral transfer the bending moment is reduced by 23.7% and the joint reaction force is reduced by 6.6%.

Based on these observations, we can conclude that when using a prosthesis with 40- to 45-degree offset, it is imperative to guard against deepening the socket excessively, although it is essential to deepen enough to achieve acetabular coverage. For a short-offset prosthesis, it is necessary to medialize the center of the femur and to lateralize the abductor muscles.[29]

FRICTIONAL FORCE

The frictional forces acting on the acetabular component of total hip prostheses depend on several factors:

1. The magnitude of the resultant compressive force: 2½ times to 3 times the body weight.
2. The direction of the forces: 15 degrees inclined medially from the vertical.
3. The frictional moment and the axes around which they act.

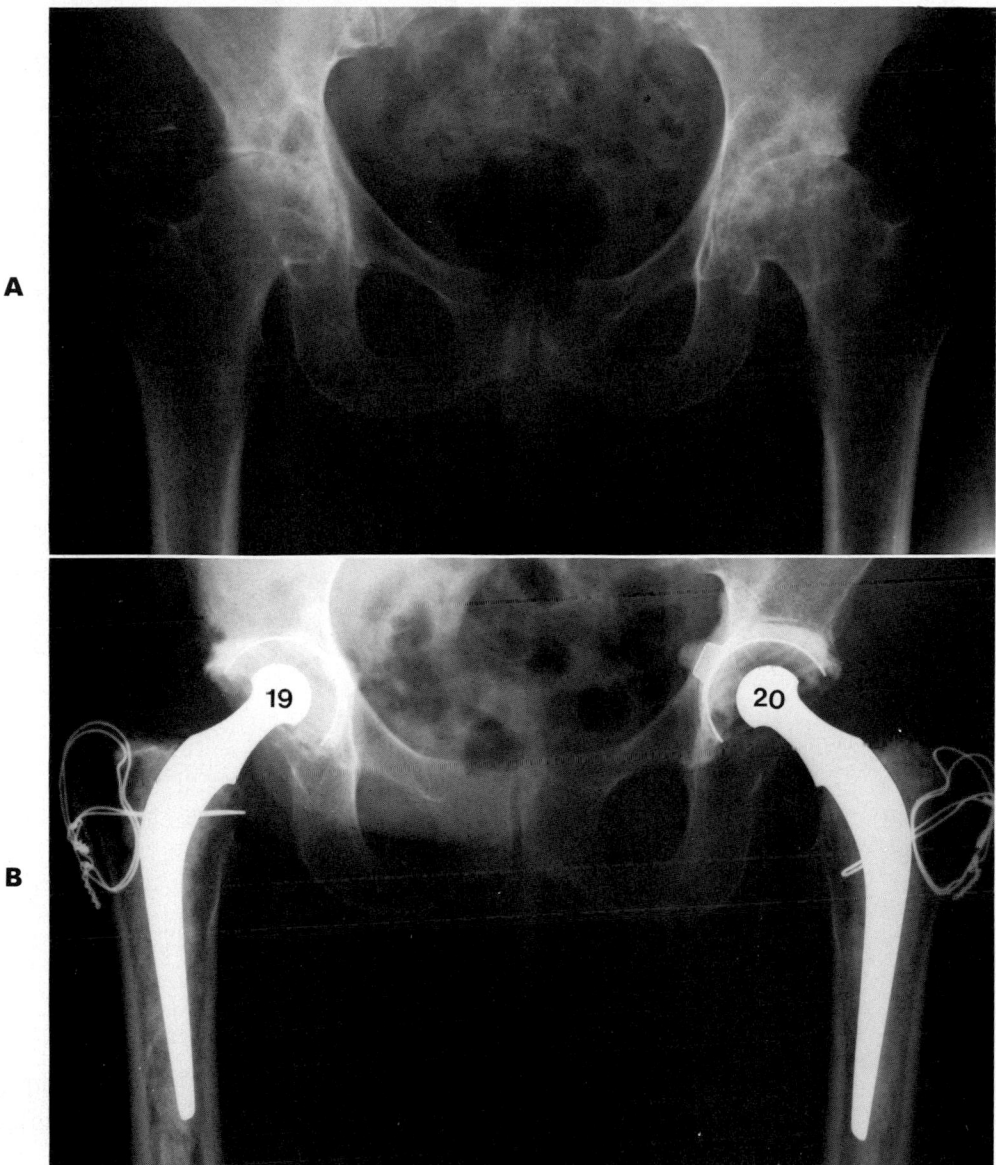

Fig. 6-12. Slight valgus orientation of cemented stem is well tolerated. **A,** Preoperative radiograph of 58-year-old woman (A.C.) with degenerative osteoarthritis of the hips. Grade B-R,3,2,2 and L,3,2,2. **B,** Postoperative radiograph at 19 and 20 years after low-friction arthroplasty. NOTE: absence of any radiolucency or demarcation in either femora or the right acetabulum. Demarcation measuring 1 mm is noted between bone and cement in zone 1 on the left side. Patient has been very active, walking 2 to 3 miles a day. Grades B-R,6,6,6 and L,6,6,6. Stems were in a slight valgus. NOTE: cortical atrophy on the medial neck and calcar region.

4. The geometry of the prostheses (that is, ball size). The frictional torque is calculated by multiplying the radius of the ball by the frictional force acting tangentially to the surface; consequently, the smaller the radius, the smaller the frictional torque (Fig. 6-15).
5. The coefficient of friction between the mating surfaces (for example, metal-on-plastic devices have a lower frictional coefficient than do metal-on-metal devices).

The frictional forces that act on the artificial hip joint have been measured by several investigators. They must be considered in both dynamic and static modes, which have different effects on human hip joint function.

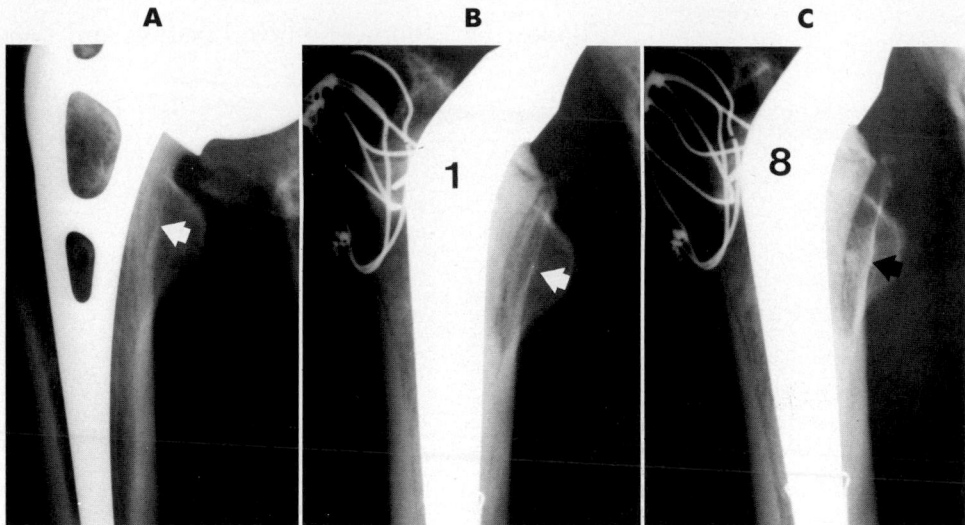

Fig. 6-13. **A,** 5 years after insertion of Austin-Moore prosthesis for fracture of femur in 55-year-old man (V.L.). NOTE: collar contact and presence of good-quality bone of the medial neck and calcar region *(arrow)*. Hip grade A: 3,3,2. Patient's weight was 70 kg. **B** and **C,** At 1 and 8 years after low-friction arthroplasty, stem of extra-heavy 1 cm long neck has been placed in valgus position. Note progressive stress shielding resulting from changes of stress distribution. Patient remains active. Hip grade A-6,6,6.

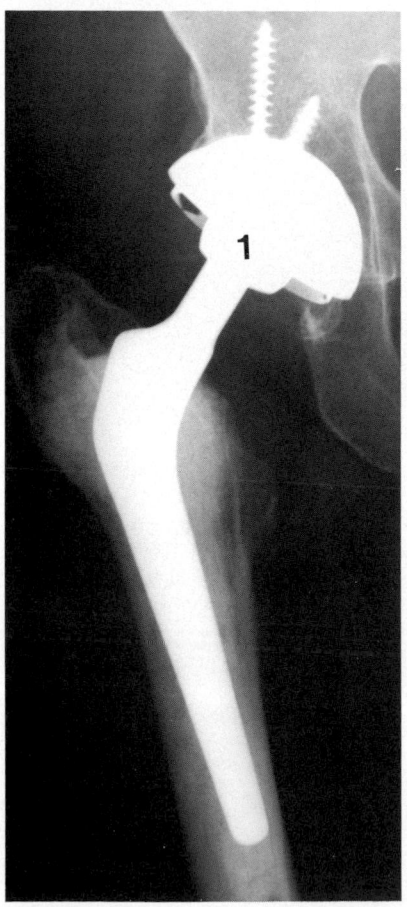

Fig. 6-14. Postoperative radiograph of a 65-year-old woman whose osteoarthritis (secondary to avascular necrosis) was treated with a total hip arthroplasty. Note excess valgus orientation of stem, which is undesirable, and has reduced stresses from the medial neck and upper femur leading to severe atrophy.

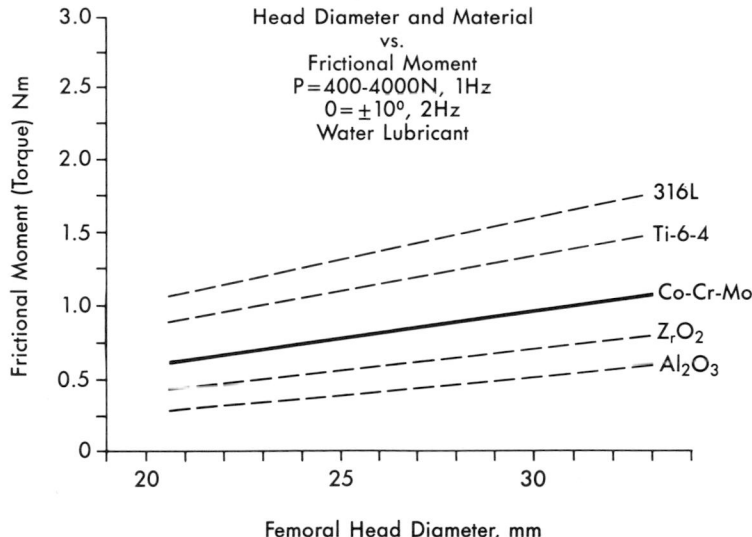

Fig. 6-15. The effects of femoral head diameter and material on the frictional moment or torque. (From Davidson JA, Brasher T: *Technical memo OR-90-13,* Memphis, 1990, Smith and Nephew Richards.)

Frictional Torque: Measurement and Significance

The literature reflects that the coefficient of friction between two sliding surfaces varies depending largely on the method used to measure it and the combinations of materials used to make the prosthesis. Simon and Radin[156] have given a coefficient of friction of between 0.05 and 0.01 for metal against HDP lubricated with synovial fluid; the coefficient of friction of normal animal joints is lower by one order of magnitude.

Using photoelastic methods, Charnley demonstrated that when the diameter of the head of the prosthesis was reduced from 50 mm to 22.5 mm, the frictional torque decreased by a factor of 1.5.[26,27] Ma and colleagues[103] measured the frictional torque of a total hip prosthesis with a 28-mm femoral head; they compared the result with that obtained when two-surface arthroplasty prostheses (with application) were loaded with up to 890 newtons, while the femoral component went through a 60-degree arc at 40 cycles/minute. They arrived at three conclusions: (1) the frictional torque of the prostheses tested was proportional to the diameter of femoral heads tested, but the relationship was not linear. (2) For a head of a given size, thick HDP effectively lowered the frictional torque. Metal backing reduced the rate of increase in frictional torque when the device had a thin acetabular component as compared to one of the same internal diameter but with a thicker-walled component. (3) Greater frictional torque was generated when contact was more peripheral than when it was polar.

Several factors may influence frictional torque and

the torque-diameter relationship: the degrees of surface finish, relative fit, thickness of the acetabular wall, deformation of plastic under load, and use of various lubricants. All of these factors can be tested in the laboratory using a multichannel joint simulator that incorporates a load cell and a pendulum.

Using the comparator pendulum method, Charnley demonstrated that frictional torque varies in different prostheses; the tests were performed under both dry and wet conditions using various lubricants. The lowest level of frictional torque occurred with a 22-mm stainless-steel head against HDP; the highest, with a metal-to-metal prosthesis of the McKee-Farrar type.[29]

As we see, in addition to head size, the material used to design the components affects frictional resistance and wear in total hip prostheses. Ceramics (aluminum oxide and zirconium oxide) produce lower frictional moments than most metal heads against HDP. Among metals, cobalt-chromium heads produced lower values than those made of stainless steel or titanium alloy. Extensive clinical trials are currently being initiated to test newer ceramics, which also exhibit a lower rate of wear and friction against ultramolecular-weight high-density polyethylene (UMWHDP).[44]

In most bearings it takes more force to initiate motion than to maintain it. At a low speed (that is, normal walking) poor lubrication gives rise to stick-slip motion (what is commonly known by engineers as *static friction* or *stiction friction*). Under physiological conditions, static friction differs very little from "dynamic friction" in metal-to-metal and metal-to-plastic prostheses, as long as there is a fluid film between the

Table 6-1 Frictional Moments Measured in Charnley and McKee-Farrar Prostheses

Type of prosthesis	Material of head	Material of cup	Diameter of head (millimeters)	Source of results	Lubricant	Frictional moment in newton-meters (pounds-force-inches) under	
						Constant load of 890 newtons (200 pounds force)	Load varying from 0–890 newtons (0–200 pounds force)
Charnley	Stainless steel	HDP	23	Freeman and Swanson	Ringer's solution	0.4–1.2 (4–11)	—
					Synovial fluid	0.47 (4.2)	—
				Wilson and Scales	Bovine serum	0.90 (8)	0 hours: 1.1 (10); 500 hours: 0.67 (6)
McKee-Farrar	Cobalt-chromium	Cobalt-chromium	41	Freeman and Swanson	Ringer's solution	17.4 (154)	8.5 (7.5)
					Bone fat	2.3 (20)	1.7 (15)
					Synovial fluid	8.9 (88)	7.9 (70)
				Wilson and Scales	Bovine serum	4.5 (40)	0 hours: 4.5 (40); 500 hours: 3.1 (27)
			35	Freeman and Swanson	Synovial fluid	2.7–4.4 (24–39)	—

From Andersson GBJ, Freeman MAR, Swanson SAV: Loosening of the cemented acetabular cup in total hip replacement, *J Bone Joint Surg* 54[Br]:590, 1972.

two components. However, static friction increases significantly after a relatively long period at high load. These frictional forces in prostheses are usually at least 40 times higher than those generated in normal joints.[155]

Charnley argued that although the patient might be unaware of increased frictional torque after total hip arthroplasty (even in the worst case, metal against metal), in the long term, increased frictional torque may help loosen the acetabular component of the total hip arthroplasty. Despite cadaveric studies indicating that loosening a cemented socket takes a frictional torque as much as 20 times greater than that generated between the femoral head and HDP, Charnley believed that high frictional torque by itself could prevent a cemented socket from functioning.[29]

In hip simulators, the frictional moments have been measured using Ringer's solution, synovial fluid, and bovine serum and under a variety of load conditions (Table 6-1).[2]

DEFORMATION OF ACETABULUM UNDER LOAD

In vitro, Markolf tested and compared for gross and relative compressive deformation of the acetabulum under loads of up to 2000 newtons.[107] When fresh-frozen acetabula were potted in PMMA and loaded, he conducted tests for hemiarthroplasty, cemented sockets with and without subchondral bone removal, and cemented surface replacement. As one might expect, the deformations were sensitive to the size of the hemiarthroplasty under load conditions. Additionally, the overall compressibility was increased with intact subchondral plates. After removal of the subchondral plate, relative deformation beneath the cup increased by an average of 0.035 mm for all 11 specimens tested. The average percentage increase was 91% in specimens with good bone quality and 18% in the three specimens with poor bone quality, indicating a relatively greater support function by the subchondral plate for the pelvis with good cancellous bone.

ACETABULAR CUP FIXATION

Our laboratory measured the strength of the fixation (bond) of the acetabular cup in pairs of cadaveric hemipelvises.[49,130] In the experimental situation, cadaveric bone was used and surgical conditions were simulated (Figs. 6-16 and 6-17). In a static situation, the lowest turning moment required to twist a prosthetic socket loose out of its bone in the tests was 44.5 newton-meters (394 in/lb)—more than four times the highest frictional moment (10.4 newton-meters or 92 inch/lb force). When the joint was lubricated with serum, it required more than twice the highest frictional moment as when lubricated with Ringer's solution. These observations suggest that the frictional moment exerted on the fixation of the cup is unlikely

to approach the failure strength of the fixation (cup-cement or cement-bone interface). These conditions may not, however, represent the surgical conditions, the development of necrosis after polymerization of the cement (exothermic reaction), or the role played by cyclically applied frictional forces.

Differences in the coefficient of friction between the all-metal and metal-plastic total hip designs of today are of such magnitude (see Table 6-1) that metal-to-metal components can be safely assumed to have a greater tendency to cause bone fatigue leading to loosening than metal-to-plastic designs. A low frictional moment in metal-to-metal prostheses depends far more on the presence of a "designed" lubricating fluid film than does the higher moment in metal-to-plastic designs (mechanism of elastohydrodynamic lubrication); therefore the occasional marked increases in frictional torque resulting from "squeezed out" fluid film in metal-to-metal joints may cause the metallic seizures that trigger the sudden onset of loosening.

Because the failures in clinical situations occur at the cement-bone interface, efforts are directed to (1) maximize the bond strength at surgery, and (2) preserve supporting bone at the site of fixation (providing the bone is healthy and in continuity). Pay special attention to preserving the bone close to the acetabular rim, because the periphery of the acetabulum provides the greatest resistance against the frictional force.

Stress distribution in a normal acetabulum has been characterized by the following parameters: (1) the resultant forces under loading conditions are superior and medial[162]; (2) the stresses are significantly higher in the acetabular region of the pelvis than in other areas[68]; and (3) more stress (by as much as seven times) is transferred to the cortical portion (i.e., medial and lateral plates) than to the cancellous portion of the ilium.[91]

These stress patterns are greatly affected by surgical technique and cup design after total hip arthroplasty. Success derives largely from achieving a stress pattern as normal as possible after cup insertion. Relevant factors include the following:

- Surgical technique vis-à-vis clinical results
- Subchondral plate
- Anchor holes
- Containment of the cup
- Pressurization and containment of cement
- Design features of the cup

Surgical Techniques Vis-à-Vis Clinical Results

Cemented sockets are currently disfavored because a substantial number of cement radiolucencies and

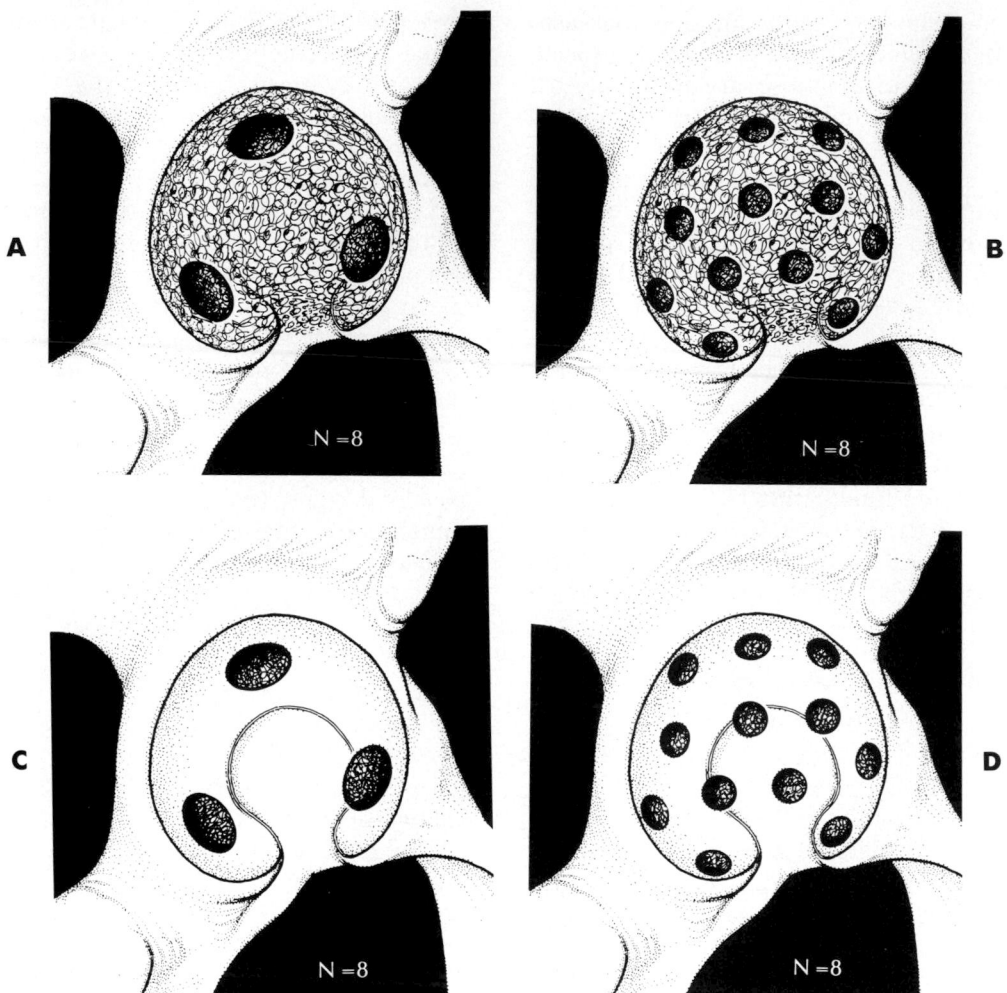

Fig. 6-16. Four types of acetabular preparation of paired cadaveric specimens. **A** and **B,** Removed subchondral bone; three large (12.5-mm) drill holes were made in **A;** 12 6.2-mm anchor holes were made in **B. C** and **D,** After removal of cartilage, the subchondral bone was retained using large and small holes similar to **A** and **B** respectively.

migrations have been encountered.[29,47] In studies by De Lee and Charnley, loosening and migration in cemented sockets occurred in approximately one quarter of patients followed from 10 to 15 years. Double-cup resurfacing operations failed in the past because this procedure required great expansion of the acetabulum by reaming at surgery, and the cup used in conventional total hip arthroplasty at that time was thinner.

Radiolucency and loosening of the cemented acetabular cup appear late, so they may also coincide with advanced degrees of wear in the HDP socket. Griffith and colleagues[70] observed that within the first 5 to 10 years of follow up, only six hips (or 4.5%) showed loosening. However, by between 11 and 15 years after surgery, 24% of the hips had loosened. It is of particular interest that demarcation (grade III) and socket migration (grade IV) were four times more common in patients with rheumatoid arthritis, who were less active than patients with osteoarthritis.[29]

Subchondral Plate and Anchor Holes

Several independent in-vitro studies on cemented acetabular cup fixation have applied torque to failure: Andersson and colleagues,[2] Chen and associates,[32] and Volz and Wilson.[165] They studied such variables as articular cartilage removal, acetabular reaming, cup intrusion, anchor-hole diameter, and numbers of anchor holes. The results of their collective work indicate that little additional benefit derives from securing good fixation of the cup after removing cartilage and soft tissue from the acetabular fossa. The

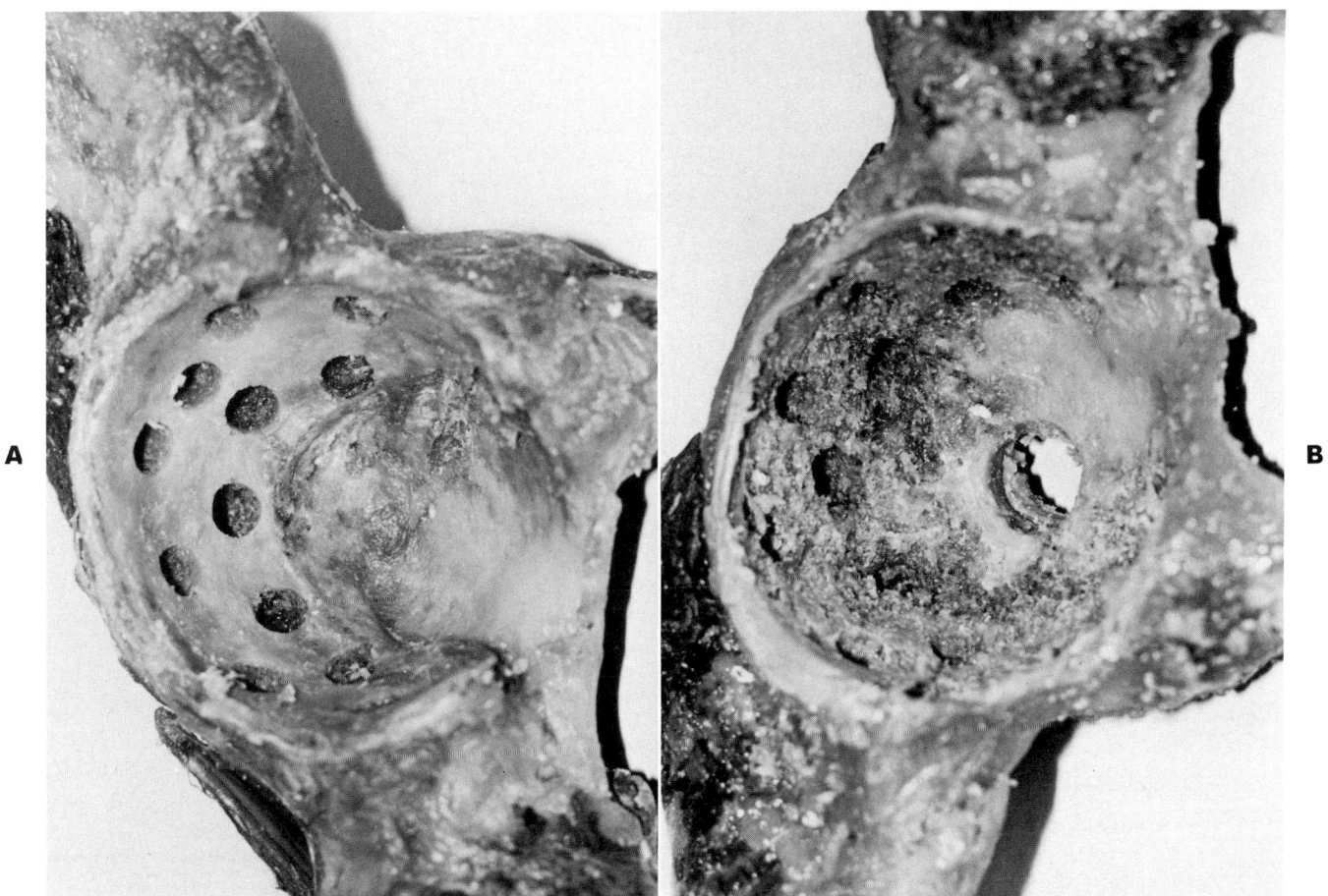

Fig. 6-17. Specimens used in testing the role of acetabular preparation in acetabular cup fixation. **A,** Subchondral bone has been preserved. Ten to twelve 6-mm (outer diameter) drill holes are made. **B,** Subchondral bone has been removed by Charnley deepening and expanding reamers (center spigot hole is seen at the level of Pulvinar), and multiple 6-mm (outer diameter) drill holes are drilled.

measured torsional moments to failure in another study[2] were 4 to 20 times higher than the frictional moments encountered for the present designs of metal-to-plastic prostheses. These in-vitro studies have primarily concentrated on torque to failure as it relates to the range of materials used for acetabular fixation, and not on the mechanical events preceding the failure. Volz and Wilson[165] tested six types of bony preparations in a static load and concluded that stability increased when the prosthetic cup was completely intruded into the acetabulum once all cartilage had been removed and when the socket rim and anchoring holes (three of 6.5 mm outer diameter) were used for cement fixation.

At our laboratories, tests for cup fixation revealed the critical importance of preserving subchondral bone during cemented total hip arthroplasty.[49] Several finite element analysis studies also have demonstrated the apparent value of retaining the subchondral bone and thus of the stiffness of the bone as a function of acetabular preparation. If subchondral bone is preserved, it creates a more normal and uniform load and thus a more normal strain pattern.[21,22] Also, use of a strain-gauge instrumented pelvis has demonstrated that when the socket is prepared with preserved subchondral bone, it maintains a normal pattern of stress distribution, but it becomes abnormal if the subchondral plate is removed. To reverse these abnormal stress patterns, insert a cup with a metal backing, which increases the stiffness of the acetabular component.[61]

We designed our study to analyze the mechanical factors associated with different acetabular preparations relating to their ranges of stiffness.[49] Torque was measured with respect to angular motion at the cement-bone interface. A 475-pound axial load was

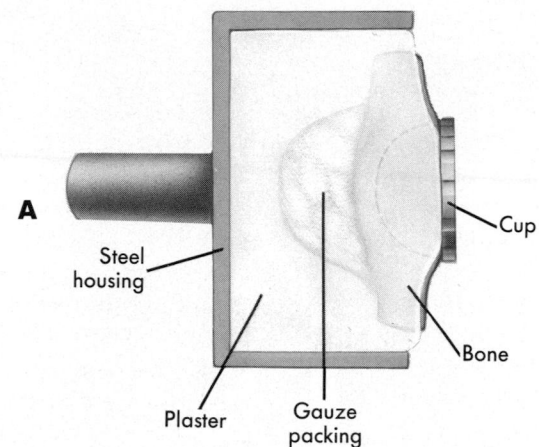

A

Steel
housing

Plaster   Gauze
packing

Cup

Bone

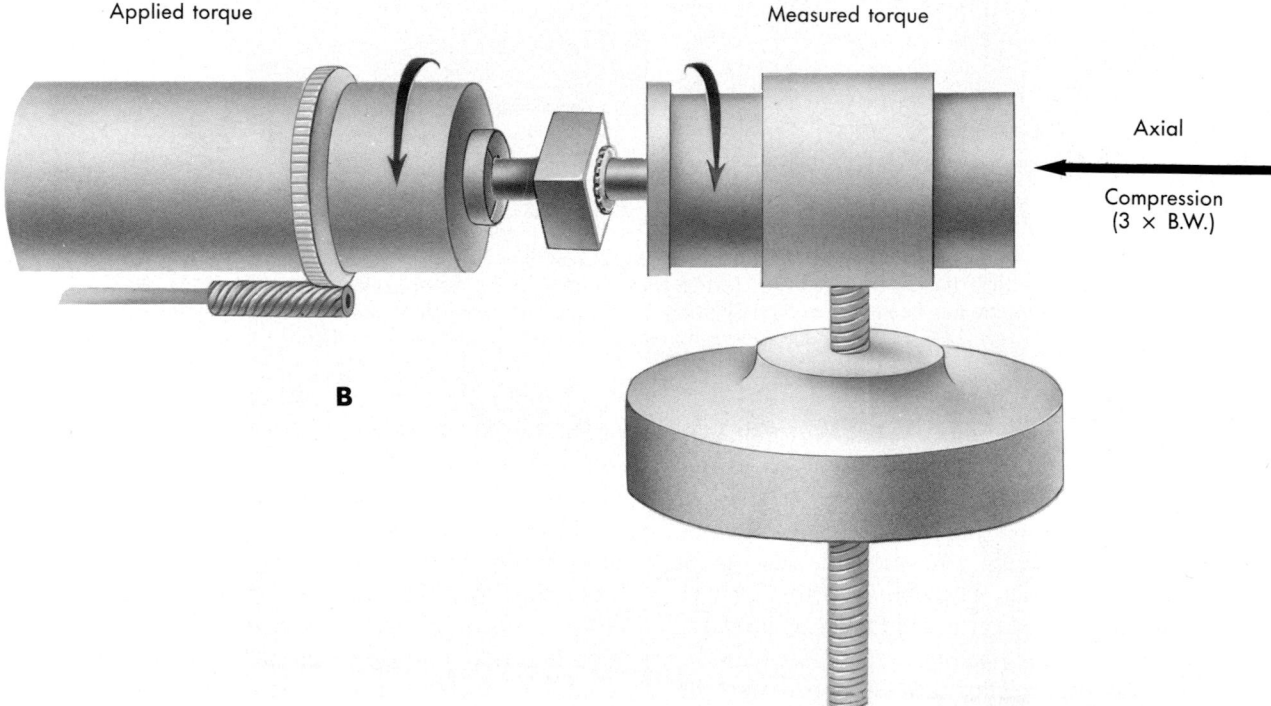

Applied torque

Measured torque

Axial

Compression
(3 × B.W.)

B

Fig. 6-18. A, Mounting of cups and bone. NOTE: gauze packing was interspersed between the bone and plaster to avoid modifying the mechanical characteristics of bone. **B,** Drawing of Amsler torque testing machine (capacity 0.2 to 2400 pounds) used in the study. (From Eftekhar NS, Pawluk RJ: Role of surgical preparation in acetabular cup fixation. In The Hip Society: *The hip: proceedings of the eighth open scientific meeting of The Hip Society,* St Louis, 1980, Mosby–Year Book.)

Table 6-2 Clinical Range Analysis

Surgical procedure (preparation)	Angular displacement (degree)	Torsional strength (ft/lb)	Stiffness (ft/lb/degree)
Retained subchondral bone Multiple holes	0.890 ± 0.037	76.38 ± 14.10	85.17 ± 4.58
Retained subchondral bone Three holes	0.955 ± 0.018	62.86 ± 17.89	61.31 ± 6.89
Reamed subchondral bone Multiple holes	0.915 ± 0.057	59.50 ± 14.84	67.02 ± 4.37
Reamed subchondral bone Three holes	0.935 ± 0.028	57.13 ± 15.04	59.30 ± 5.23

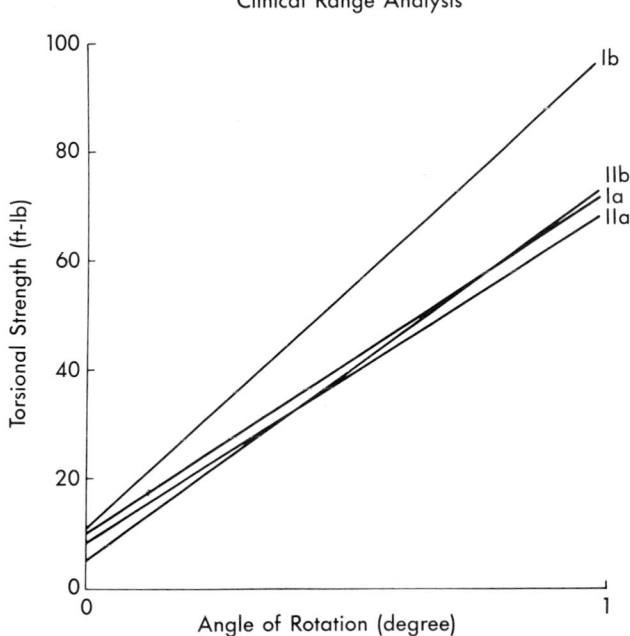

Fig. 6-19. Clinical range analysis of torque measured as a function of angular displacement. *I,* preservation of subchondral bone; *II,* removal of subchondral bone; *a,* three ½-inch anchor holes; *b,* multiple holes. (From Eftekhar NS, Pawluk RJ: Role of surgical preparation in acetabular cup fixation. In The Hip Society: *The hip: proceedings of the eighth open scientific meeting of The Hip Society,* St Louis, 1980, Mosby–Year Book.)

applied after the specimen was mounted in a steel casing (Fig. 6-18). Using stiffness as a function of acetabular preparation, cross-correlating the results of 48 specimens demonstrated that nonreamed multiple ¼-inch anchor-hole specimens are most resistant to applied torque at a 95% level of significance (Table 6-2). This outcome contrasted sharply to the results using three ½-inch holes in other specimens where the subchondral bone had been removed, exposing cancellous bone (Fig. 6-19).

Torque was measured as a function of angular displacement (0 to 1 degree) for each specimen, and data were compiled with respect to each type of surgical preparation (see Fig. 6-19). Linear regression analysis was performed for each group by the least-squares-fit methods. This analysis that defines the stiffness provided a slope for each of the groups tested (Fig. 6-20). The stiffness values were then compared for statistical significance at a 95% confidence level. Table 6-2 represents stiffness for four types of acetabular preparation. The nonreamed, multiple ¼-inch hole specimens provided a stiffness of 85.17 ft/lb/degree in contrast to 59.3 ft/lb/degree for reamed bone with three holes (Charnley's preparation). As in other studies, the values obtained were recorded to torque failure, failure being 5 degrees or more of angular displacement (Fig. 6-21). In this analysis, although specimens were tested to failure, we were primarily concerned with micromotion, that is, the first degree of rotation of the specimen.

The rationale for clinical range analysis (see Fig. 6-19) is (1) to emphasize mechanical events preceding clinical failure, and (2) to analyze "clinical loading" conditions rather than material failure properties as previous studies have done. Clinical range torque analysis accounts for low frictional torque present in clinical situations with a metal-to-HDP prosthesis and fatigue failure of bone. We suggest that local stress concentrations must be of much greater magnitude when a vertical load such as cyclic walking is applied to the interface.

MICROMOTION VS. SUBCHONDRAL BONE From a mechanical standpoint, preserved subchondral bone with multiple holes offers more resistance to torque for small angular displacement, increases distribution of load-bearing forces, reduces local stress concentration in bone, conserves bone by retaining maximal surface areas, and — as stiffness increases — may reduce the micromotion that leads to late acetabular loosening. We may conclude that after removing subchondral bone and bone of the acetabular roof, the drop in stiffness

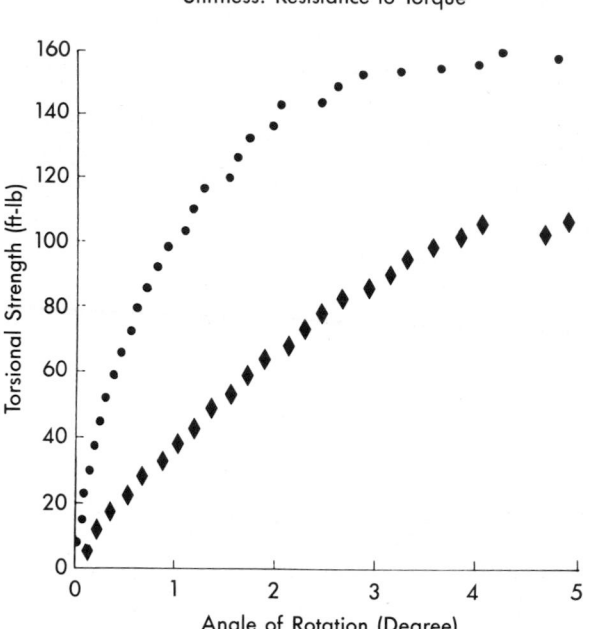

Stiffness: Resistance to Torque

Fig. 6-20. Stiffness and resistance to torque for two specimens. Circles represent torsional strength (ft/lb) plotted against angle of rotation (degree) for a specimen in which subchondral bone has been preserved and multiple holes have been used, contrasted with a curve *(diamonds)* in a specimen where subchondral bone has been removed and three ½-inch anchor holes have been used for fixation. (From Eftekhar NS, Pawluk RJ: Role of surgical preparation in acetabular cup fixation. In The Hip Society: *The hip: proceedings of the eighth open scientific meeting of The Hip Society,* St Louis, 1980, Mosby–Year Book.)

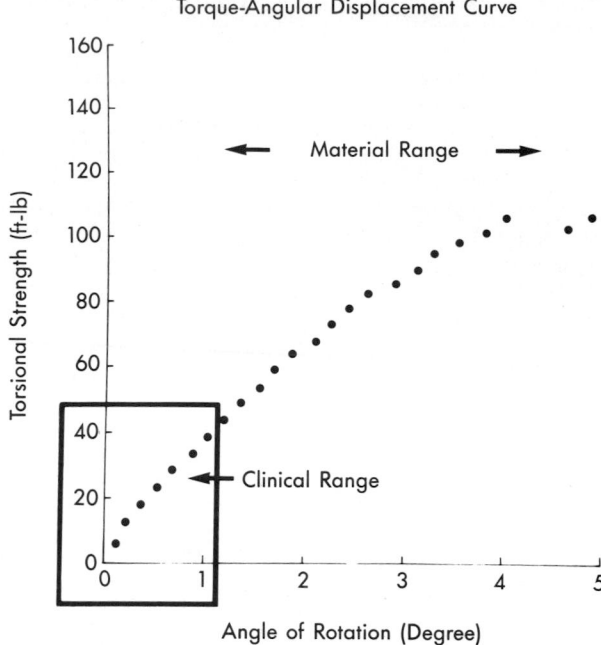

Torque-Angular Displacement Curve

Fig. 6-21. Torque angular displacement curve. All specimens were taken to failure, which occurred at 5 degrees or more of angular displacement (material range failure). The square indicates the clinical range analysis used in the study. (From Eftekhar NS, Pawluk RJ: Role of surgical preparation in acetabular cup fixation. In The Hip Society: *The Hip: proceedings of the eighth open scientific meeting of The Hip Society,* St Louis, 1980, Mosby–Year Book.)

leads to plastic deformation of cancellous bone under cyclic load. If individual unsupported bony trabeculae are subjected to stress concentration, they may develop necrosis and eventually be replaced by a fibrous membrane; the resulting increased motion leads to further bone resorption and decreased stiffness. Clinical failure is the end stage of such a vicious circle (Figs. 6-22 and 6-23). Several clinical facts support this theory:

1. Early demarcations are prevalent in young and active or heavy individuals.
2. Demarcation and loosening are time-dependent phenomena.
3. Demarcation and loosening appear with the aging process and with increased osteoporosis.
4. A higher incidence of loosening is observed in rheumatoid patients than in osteoarthritic patients.

From a biomechanical point of view, this theory of micromotion, as applied to clinical studies, may explain the role of these etiological factors in loosening the cemented acetabular cup.

Oh also studied the effect of the size and depth of anchor holes as a function of fixation of the cemented acetabular cup[119]; his results were consistent with our studies. In his experiments, the highest torque was required to loosen six 0.85-cm holes drilled 0.8 cm deep. In actual surgery, larger and deeper holes are unnecessary, especially in small acetabula, and they present the hazard of penetrating or fracturing the pelvis, causing flow and decompression of the cement during pressurization that will result in early loosening and migration.

The surgical technique practiced by the author is presented in Chapter 19. The biomechanical principles described in this chapter support the theory that preservation of subchondral roof helps prevent loosening of a cemented acetabular component (Figs. 6-24 and 6-25) (see Chapter 28).

Containment of the Cup

It has long been recognized that cups inserted out of the bony confinement of the acetabulum are likely to fail sooner than those supported by bone. Experimental work by Volz and associates[165] and clinical studies by Charnley and others support this view.

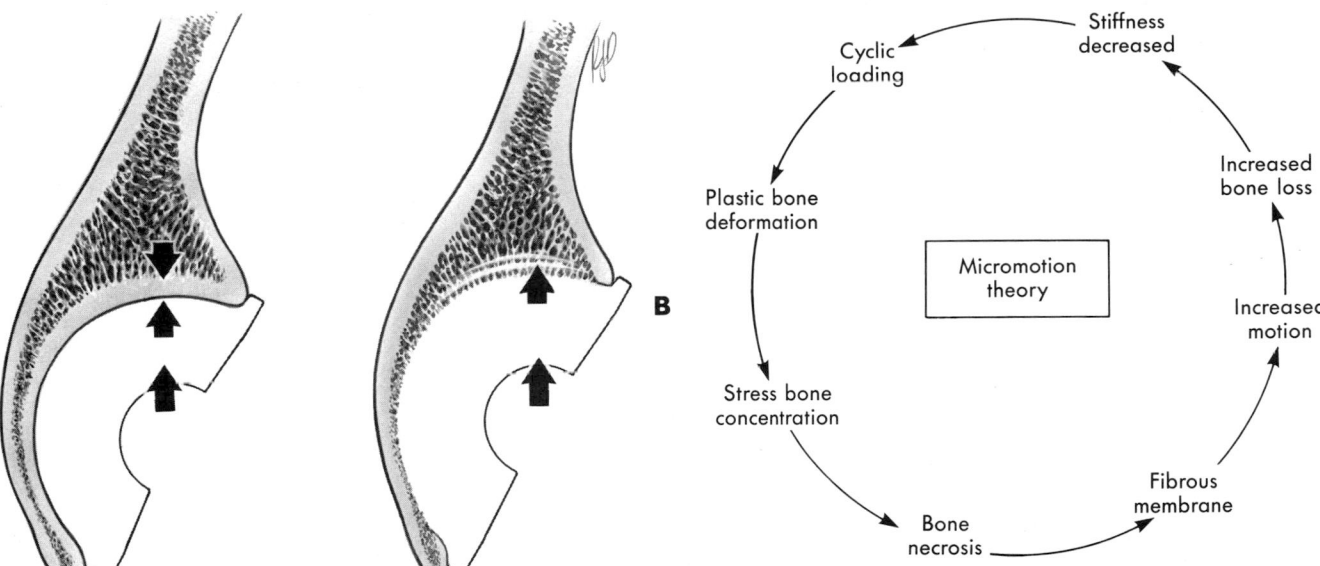

Fig. 6-22. Concept of micromotion after removal of subchondral bone and exposure of cancellous trabeculae. **A,** Subchondral bone is preserved (resistance against upward movement is indicated by top arrow) while load is applied from weight bearing and muscle tension *(bottom arrows)*. **B,** Unprotected roof of acetabulum after removal of subchondral bone indicates micromotion in weight-bearing zone of acetabulum. (From Eftekhar NS, Pawluk RJ: Role of surgical preparation in acetabular cup fixation. In The Hip Society: *The hip: proceedings of the eighth open scientific meeting of The Hip Society,* St Louis, 1980, Mosby–Year Book.)

Fig. 6-23. Vicious circle created by micromotion. Stiffness of roof is reduced by removal of subchondral bone, after which plastic deformation of bone leads to stress concentration in exposed trabeculae, in turn resulting in bone necrosis. Necrotic bone in time is replaced by fibrous membrane, leading to increased motion and further loss of stiffness. The end of the vicious circle is failure. (From Eftekhar NS, Pawluk RJ: Role of surgical preparation in acetabular cup fixation. In The Hip Society: *The hip: proceedings of the eighth open scientific meeting of The Hip Society,* St Louis, 1980, Mosby–Year Book.)

Cement Pressurization and Containment

For cement to work successfully, an intimate micro-interlock between cement and bone is essential (see Chapters 4 and 5). Cement can be pressurized either by applying pressure via a pressurization device[99] or via a cup with a flanged design, such as Charnley's pressure injection cup (Fig. 6-26).[121] A cup without a flange produces very low intrusion pressure, which is lost as the cup "bottoms out" in the acetabular cavity.[154] Although the cup designs with "spacers" prevent the bottoming of the cup and retain cement between the cup and the acetabulum, they cannot help pressurize the cement (see Fig. 6-26).

To sustain pressurization throughout polymerization, the flanged cup is essential; it consistently produces a higher injection pressure that can be maintained throughout the cement polymerization.[154] Maintaining cement pressure to resist bleeding pressure is essential to prevent blood from pooling between bone and cement (see Chapter 19).[9] Be sure to use a uniform mantle of cement to maintain an optimal level of stress in the cement and at the cement-bone interface. As stated, a flange or spacers introduced between the cup and bone centralize the cup and optimize cement thickness.[124,132,133]

In a study comparing the effectiveness of a pressurizer versus a flanged cup, the Exeter pressurizer produced only marginally better results than the OGEE flanged cup (Fig. 6-27).[154] These findings were consistent with Oh's experience using a flanged cup for his experiment.[123] He demonstrated that a cup with pods and a continuous flange positioned concentrically in the acetabular cavity surrounded by a uniform cement thickness was well contained in the cavity.[123]

ACETABULAR CUP DESIGN Charnley attributed several advantages to incorporating a thick (rather than thin) plastic cup into the design of the acetabular component. In most cases, using a small head (22 mm) allows space to accommodate a 10-mm acetabular component thickness in the standard size and an 8-mm thickness in the small version (Fig. 6-28). Using photoelastic models, Charnley demonstrated that plastic cups with a thick wall (against a small head) diffuse load better and more uniformly than thin plastic cups of the same outer diameter used with a larger head (Fig. 6-29). A thin cup is more likely to produce "high

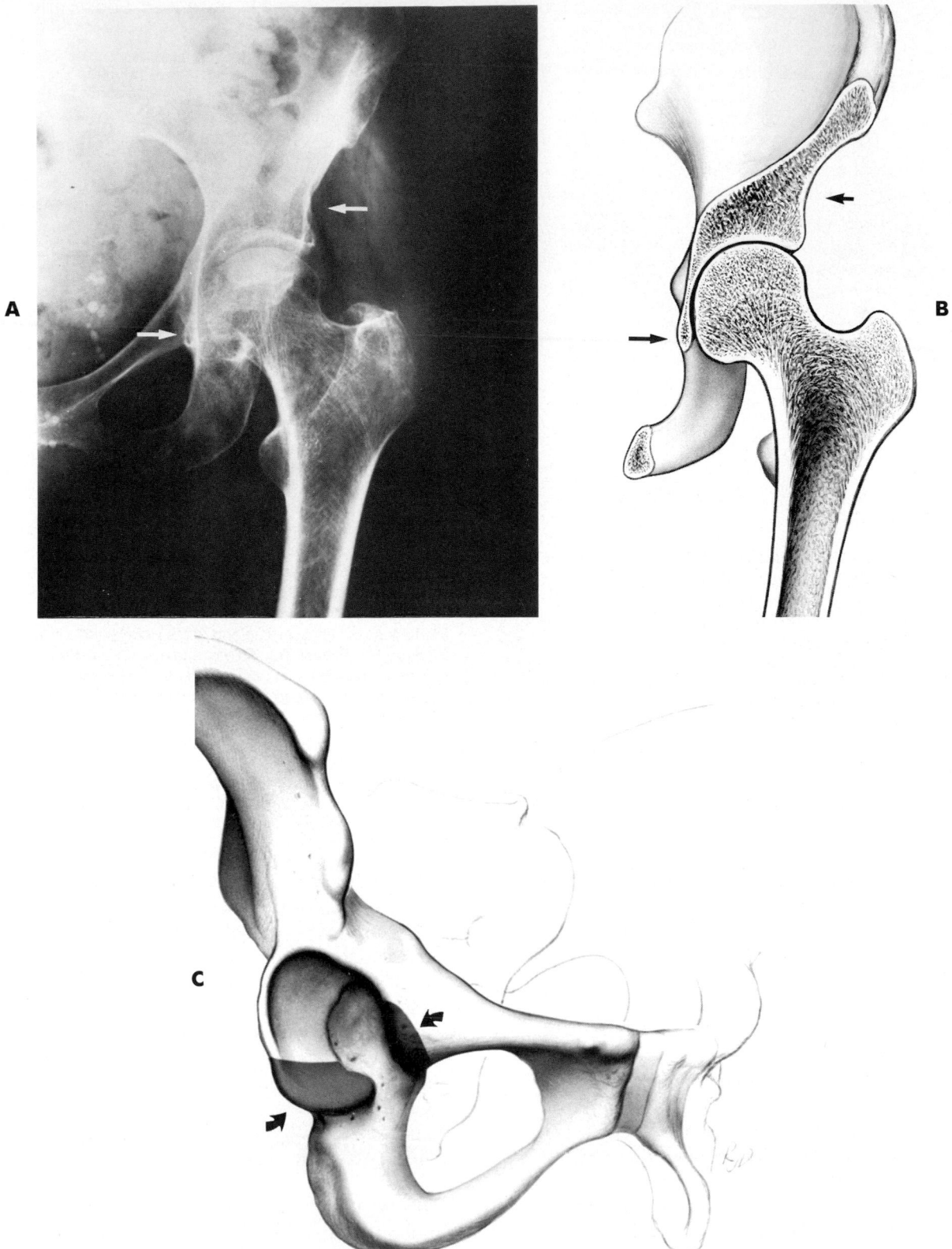

Fig. 6-24. A, Frontal view of hip joint, anteroposterior representation of normal hip joint. Arrows indicate teardrop and cancellous zones of weight-bearing portion of acetabulum. **B,** Cross-sectional view of hips in frontal plane illustrates the teardrop and thinnest segment of acetabular floor. Top arrow indicates superior weight-bearing cancellous zone of hip at level of the acetabular roof. **C,** Anterior and posterior edges of articulating portion of acetabulum *(arrows)* is the usual site of osteophytes. This area *(shaded)* should be excised to allow lowering of the socket and to protect the roof of the acetabulum. (From Eftekhar NS, Pawluk RJ: Role of surgical preparation in acetabular cup fixation. In The Hip Society: *The hip: proceedings of the eighth open scientific metting of The Hip Society,* St Louis, 1980, Mosby–Year Book.)

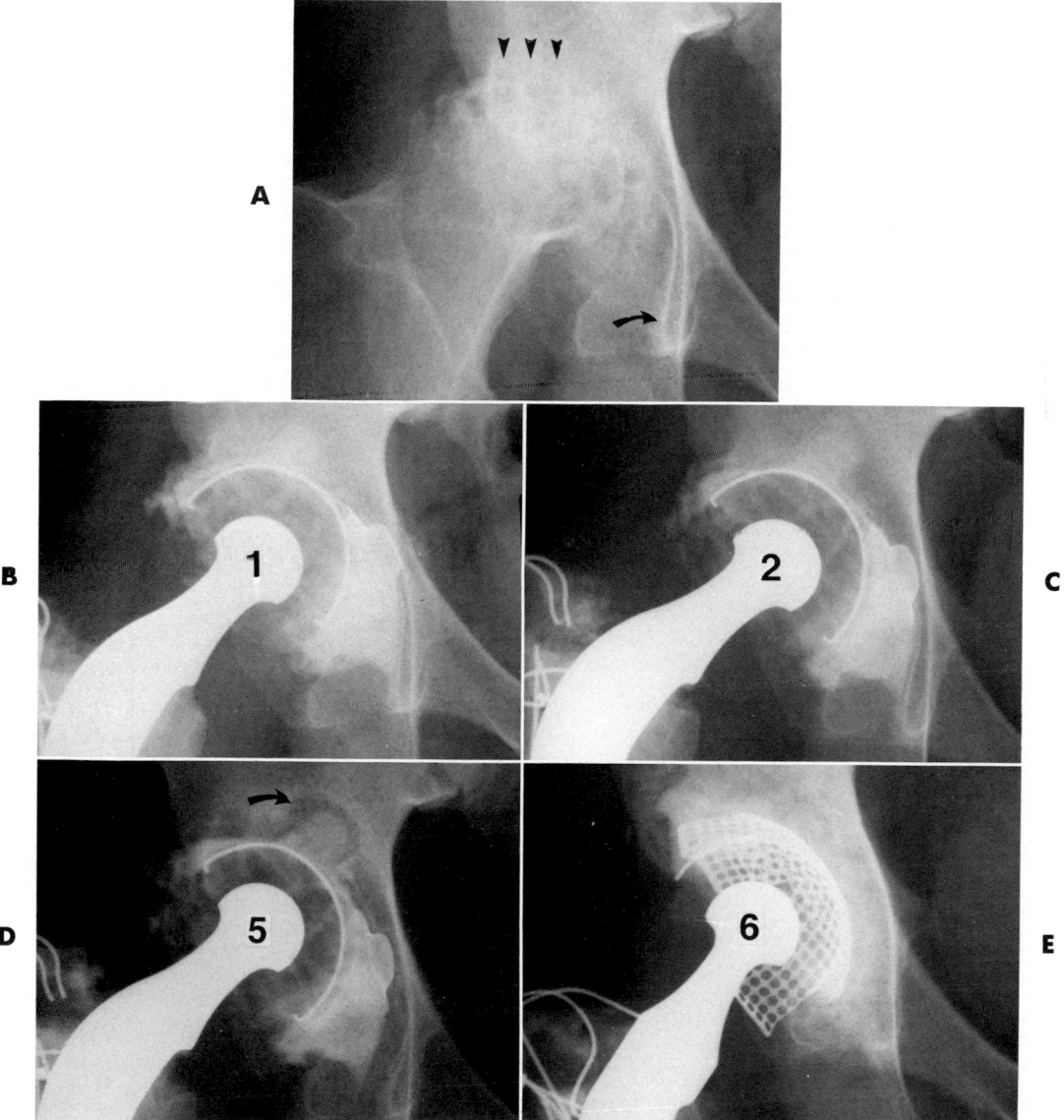

Fig. 6-25. A, Preoperative radiograph of 29-year-old male (P.L.) with monoarticular rheumatoid arthritis in the right hip. Patient's weight was 96 kg. NOTE: cystic erosions of acetabulum and migratory-type arthritis *(arrows)* with proximal migration of femoral head in relationship to teardrop sign. **B,** 1 year postoperatively, note a slightly high position of socket and a thin layer of cement superiorly. **C,** Evidence of demarcation 2 years postoperatively. **D,** Progressive demarcation to complete loosening *(arrow)* at 5 years. **E,** 6 years after revision arthroplasty. This case illustrates the absence of subchondral bone at the initial surgery accentuated by a thin layer of cement between the cup and bone in a heavy, active person.

ACETABULAR CUP DESIGN

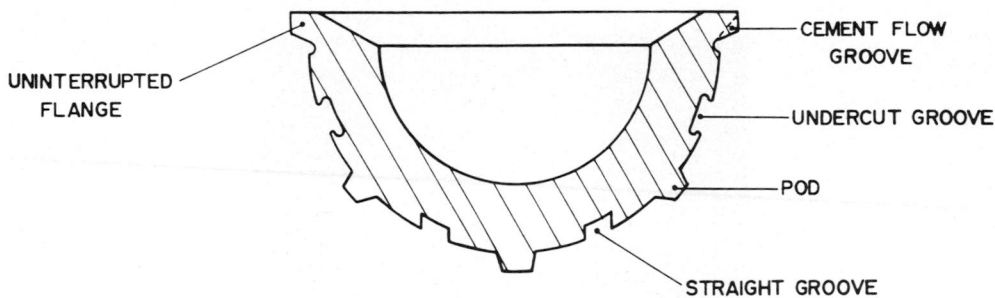

Fig. 6-26. Surface design features of HDP acetabular component. (From Oh I: A comprehensive analysis of factors affecting acetabular cup fixation and design in total hip replacement arthroplasty. A series of experimental and clinical studies. In *The Hip Society: The hip: proceedings of the eleventh open scientific meeting of The Hip Society,* St Louis, 1983, Mosby–Year Book.)

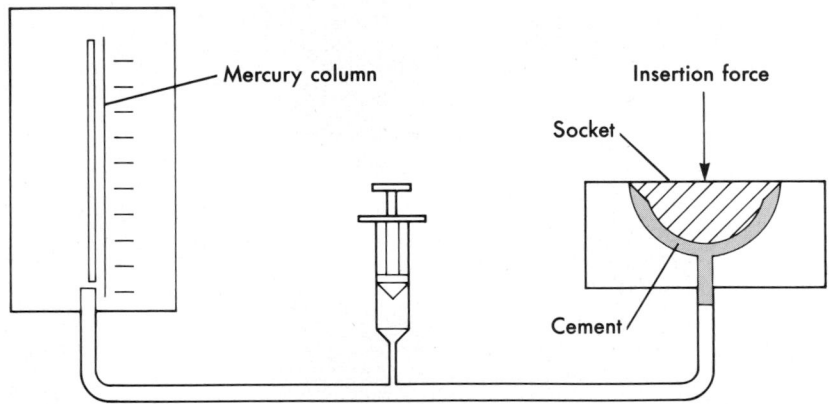

Fig. 6-27. The experimental apparatus. (From Shelley P, Wroblewski BM: Socket design and cement pressurization in the Charnley low-friction arthroplasty, *J Bone Joint Surg* 70[Br]:358, 1988.)

spots" at the cement-bone interface, which might precipitate minute, localized movement between cement and bone. This movement in turn might lead to a histiocytic reaction, bone cavitation, and loosening (Fig. 6-30).

Finite-element stress analysis has demonstrated that the stress distribution becomes more concentrated after socket implantation (Fig. 6-31).[162] Also, a thick component reduces stress, whereas a thin acetabular wall component increases stress in cement-polythylene and bone. Using a component with the same outer-diameter size and changing the femoral head diameter from the smallest (22 mm) to the largest (44 mm), thus reducing wall thickness, substantially increases stress within the cement. For example, changing the femoral head size from 22 mm to 44 mm increases the maximum stress by 400% and the maximum compressive stresses by 200%.[131] Acetabular cup strength can also be affected by changes in the design of the anchoring mechanism such as grooves, pods, and spacers.[119] As in Charnley's design, however, grooves are introduced in most cups to improve fixation of PMMA. Make sure the grooves are not too thick, however, because excessively deep grooves have several drawbacks: (1) fatigue and failure of the HDP, especially in thin polyethylene sockets, (2) reduced thickness of the polyethylene, causing the inherent problems mentioned above, and (3) grooves acting as a stress riser could lead to creep and failure of the implant.[122,148,161,168] Finite stress analysis has demonstrated that stress is greater when subchondral bone is removed or a thin layer of

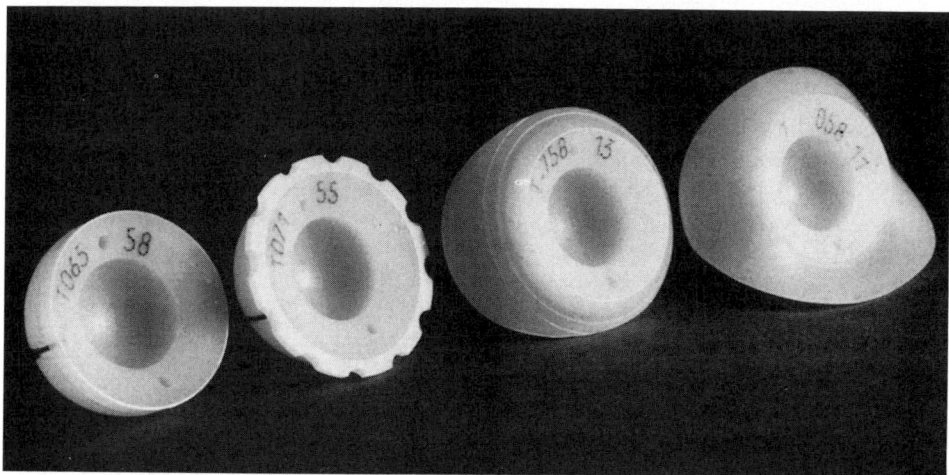

Fig. 6-28. Evolution of Charnley socket from rimless type to OGEE-flanged model. (From Shelley P, Wroblewski BM: Socket design and cement pressurization in the Charnley low-friction arthroplasty, *J Bone Joint Surg* 70[Br]:358, 1988.)

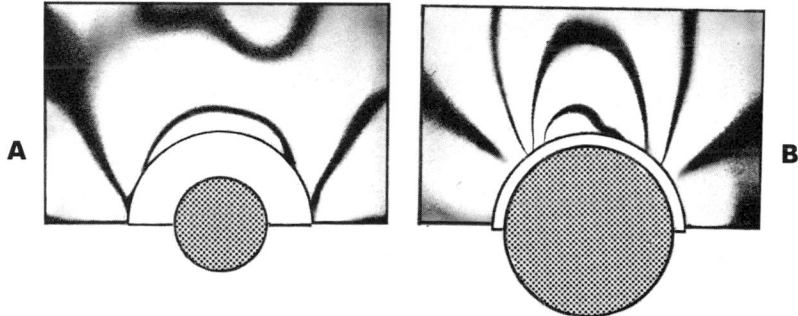

Fig. 6-29. Effect of thickness of socket wall. **A** shows the thick socket under load from small-diameter metal prosthetic head. Fringes are distributed evenly over whole surface of socket. **B** shows thin socket and large-diameter metal prosthetic head under same load as above. Stresses are now concentrated over only 90-degree quadrant of socket surface and are nearly 1.5 × higher than in **A**. (Modified from Charnley J: *Low-friction arthroplasty*, Berlin, 1979, Springer-Verlag.)

cement is applied, both of which can result from the use of a large femoral head prosthesis against an HDP socket (Figs. 6-32 to 6-34).

METAL-BACKED COMPONENT Harris was the first to use a metal-backed acetabular component with the idea of replacing the HDP liner as needed without disturbing the fixation.

A significant number of analytic (finite-element stress analysis) and strain gauge studies supporting the use of metal-backed acetabular components appeared in the literature in the 1980s* (Figs. 6-32 and 6-35).

Charnley believed that to produce a more normal pattern of stress, one should simply keep the size of the

femoral head as small as possible, permitting a thick acetabular wall; the small ball diffuses the load more evenly over the socket-cement bone than a large one (Fig. 6-36). Charnley found no need for a metal backing to stiffen the HDP.

To date, unfortunately, there is no evidence that metal-backed acetabular components have any long-term clinical success in preventing loosening, despite the obvious experimental advantages (as can be seen from Chapter 28). This lack of correlation may be explained by several factors: (1) additional metal thickness mandates use of a thinner HDP component, possibly increasing deformation and wear, (2) metal-backed acetabular components reduce available space, forcing the use of a thin layer of cement or excessive

*References 21, 41, 43, 76, 78, 79, 109, 131, 161, 162.

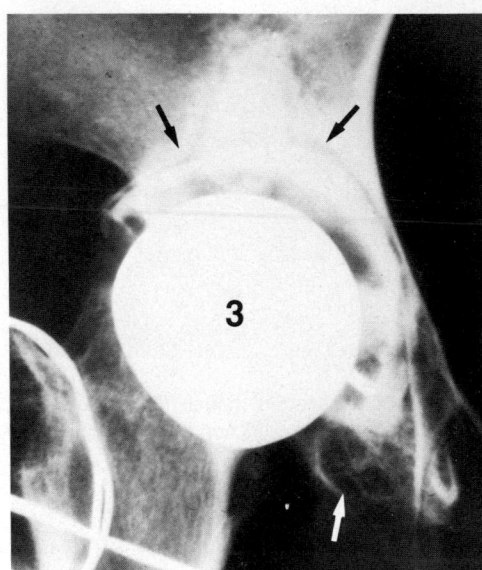

Fig. 6-30. Radiograph of 23-year-old woman 3 years after resurfacing procedure. Arrow indicates radiological demarcation of socket measuring 1.5 mm in three zones. NOTE: proximal migration of socket *(lower arrow)* 39 months after migration of the cup. The socket was revised.

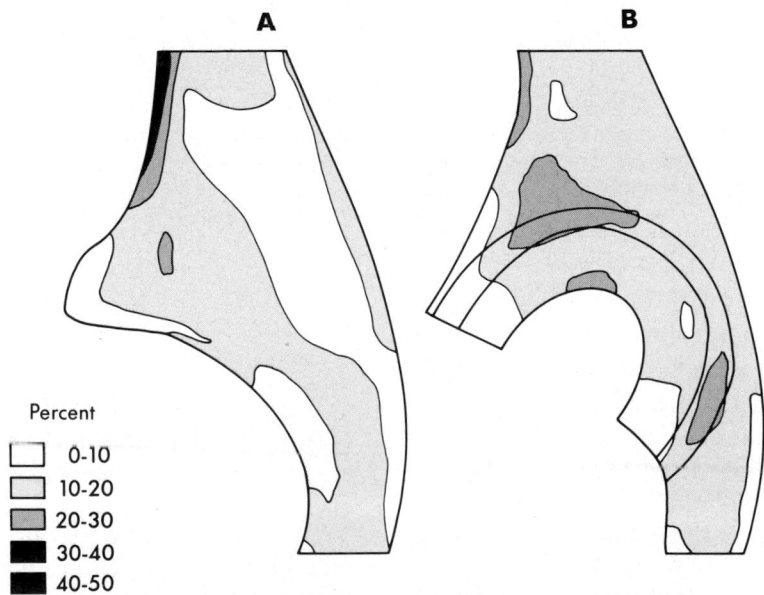

Percent

- ☐ 0-10
- ☐ 10-20
- ▨ 20-30
- ■ 30-40
- ■ 40-50

Fig. 6-31. Von Mises' stresses in the normal, **A,** and cemented, **B,** acetabular component. Notice the more concentrated stress distributions with the implant. (From Vasu R, Carter DR, Harris WH: Stress distributions in the acetabular region. I. Before and after total joint replacement, *J Biomechanics* 15:155, 1982.)

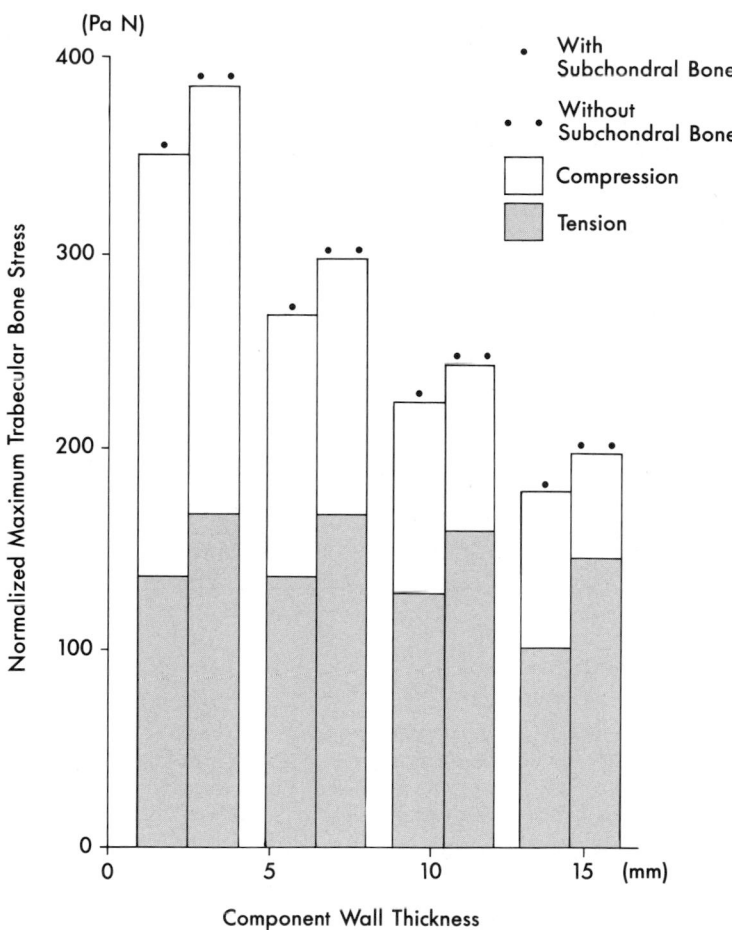

Fig. 6-32. Greater bone stress is present when the subchondral bone has been removed. (From Crowninshield RD, Brand RA, Pedersen DR: The effect of femoral stem cross-sectional geometry on cement stresses in total hip reconstruction, *J Bone Joint Surg* 65:495, 1983.)

removal of bone from the subchondral plate, (3) the excess stiffness produced by a thick metal shell can cause stress shielding, and (4) wear of the HDP over the convex surface in some acetabular cups has been reported. In conclusion, although a metal backing of the acetabular component may improve the mechanical stress distribution in analytic studies, the significant clinical disadvantages offset its advantages.

Methods of Acetabular Cup Fixation

The acetabular cup can be fixed in several ways, including use of (1) acrylic cement, (2) cups with a single screw for attachment, (3) press fit, (4) threaded cups, (5) porous-coated ingrowth, and (6) threaded cups with ingrowth.

Socket Fixation by Acrylic Cement

Two historical disadvantages of cemented socket fixation deserve comment: (1) to deepen the acetabulum maximally, surgeons removed excessive subchondral bone, and (2) the rudimentary cement techniques of the past did not include careful bone preparation or cement pressurization. These drawbacks have been overcome by new techniques, however, that preserve subchondral bone, pressurize the cement, and incorporate a modified cup design.

Acetabular Fixation by Press-Fit

In 1963, Charnley was the first to use a press-fit socket. A highly polished stainless steel Smith-Peterson cup with a 50-mm outer diameter was designed to provide adequate resistance against bone, allowing motion between the small 22-mm outer-diameter ball and the HDP. This design was introduced to compensate for a significant drawback of cemented sockets using HDP: radiolucencies invariably developed between the bone and the cemented cups. Because of the evidence that the cemented-cup radiolucencies related to this press-

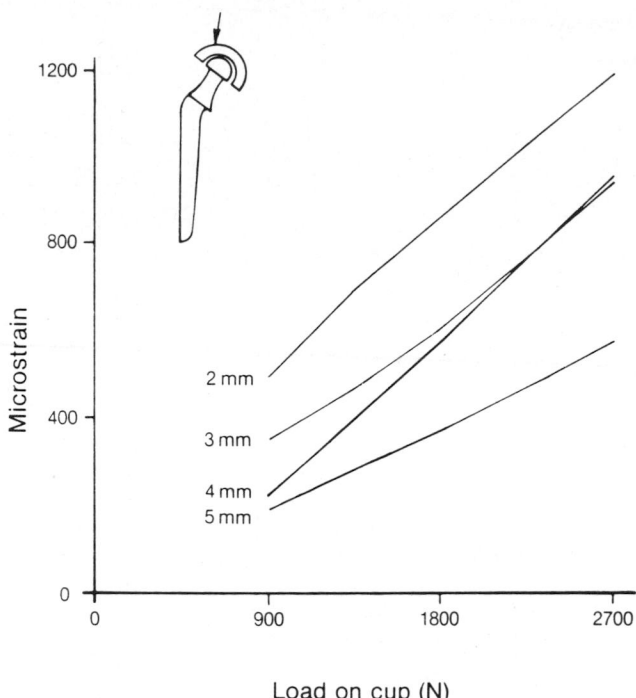

Fig. 6-33. Increased strain is observed in the PMMA for the thin 2-mm HDP component compared with the thicker 4- and 5-mm models. (From Oh I: A comprehensive analysis of factors affecting acetabular cup fixation and design in total hip replacement arthroplasty. A series of experimental and clinical studies. In The Hip Society: *The hip: proceedings of the eleventh open scientific meeting of The Hip Society,* St Louis, 1983, Mosby–Year Book.)

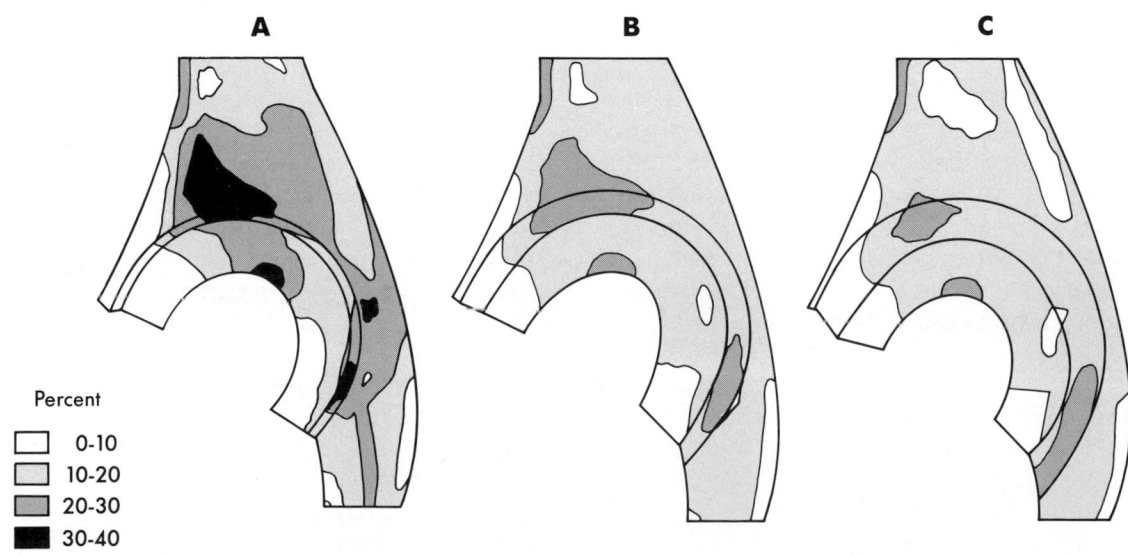

Fig. 6-34. Von Mises' yield contours for total hip arthroplasty with **A,** 1 mm PMMA; **B,** 3 mm PMMA; and **C,** 5 mm PMMA. Notice the lessening of the peak stresses with the thicker PMMA preparation. (From Carter DR, Vasu R, Harris WH: Stress distribution in the acetabular region. II. Effects of cement thickness and metal backing of the total hip acetabular component, *J Biomechanics* 15:165, 1982.)

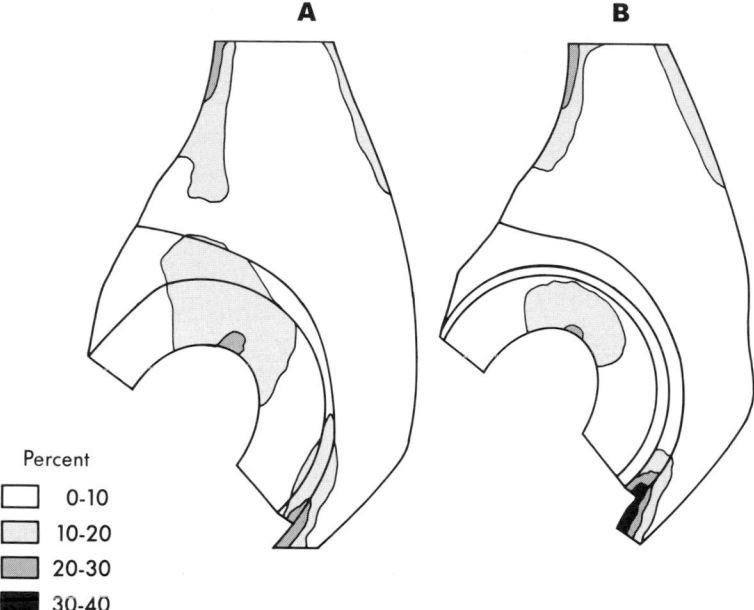

Fig. 6-35. Von Mises' yield contours for total hip arthroplasty and subchondral bone retention for **A,** conventional and **B,** metal-backed acetabular components. (From Carter DR, Vasu R, Harris WH: Stress distribution in the acetabular region. II. Effects of cement thickness and metal backing of the total hip acetabular component, *Acta Orthop Scand* 54:29, 1983.)

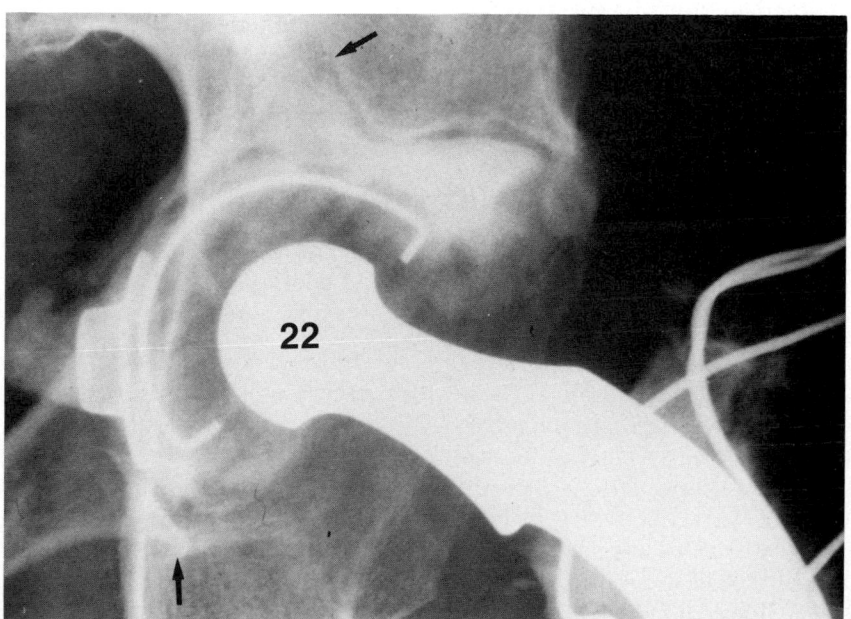

Fig. 6-36. Radiograph of left hip in woman with unilateral hip degenerative osteoarthrosis. Patient was 25 years of age at index operation and weighed 61 kg. NOTE: complete demarcation (wider than 2 mm) with migration 22 years after surgery. Hip has remained asymptomatic, but plans for revision of the acetabular component are being made.

fit modification were nonprogressive, it was used popularly in 1965. On the other hand, while most press-fit sockets did well and were mechanically sound, some 15% gradually migrated or tilted, requiring revision by a cemented version. And at 12 to 15 years, 20 of the press-fit sockets (35.5%) had tilted or migrated[29]—three times the migration rate of the cemented socket over the same period of time.

Rising interest in cementless fixation of the acetabular component seems to be related to the increasing reports of late cemented acetabular loosening (occurring after 10 to 15 years). However, it has not been established whether the long-term failures of the acetabular component should be attributed primarily to poor surgical technique in preparing the bone and inserting the cemented socket or to wear of the acetabular component, with subsequent osteolysis and loosening.

There are four basic designs for cementless sockets: (1) HDP sockets without metal backing, (2) threaded acetabular shells with an HDP insert, (3) porous-coated press-fit designs without screw fixation, and (4) porous-coated press-fit designs with screw fixation. A fifth combines threaded sockets with a porous-coated surface.

HDP sockets without metal backing may be used exclusively with PMMA. Theoretically, based simply on mechanics, direct contact between HDP and bone should be a very attractive choice, because the mechanical properties of polyethylene sockets more closely approximate those of bone than do those of a metal shell. In clinical practice, however, placing HDP in contact with bone has been shown to cause wear, granulomatous tissue formation, and osteolysis (see Chapter 4). Consequently, no design should use direct contact between the HDP and bone; all HDP cups are now supported by a metal shell made of chromium and cobalt or titanium alloy.

Threaded acetabular cups (Fig. 6-37, *A*) have several distinct advantages: they provide immediate mechanical fixation to the acetabular bone at surgery; the plastic liner is replaceable; and the cups can be applied even when the bony acetabula is defective (the latter two qualities are particularly attractive for revision surgery). However, these advantages are offset by reports of a high incidence of early clinical loosening.[5,58] In this author's own series of 32 Mecring acetabular cups, failures occurred between 3 and 6 years after insertion, so revision surgery became necessary in six patients.[48] Based on in-vivo finite element modeling, the mechanical failure of threaded acetabular components has been attributed to several factors: (1) the high rigidity of the implant and the overstressed acetabular bone, (2) stress shielding of the trabecular bone, (3) cortical load transference, (4)

limited areas of contact and load transfer pattern via individual threads (i.e., first and last threads), (5) significant peak stresses in subchondral bone with generally more stress than with cemented sockets, and (6) a high medial wall strain, as recorded at insertion.

Two versions of the porous-coated press fit design have gained great popularity despite their relatively short-term clinical use:

1. Without screws for fixation. The sockets were manufactured from chromium and cobalt alloys and incorporated porous surfaces, antirotational elements, and pegs (PCA) (Fig. 6-37, *B*) or spikes (AML) (Fig. 6-37, *C*). Several investigators have demonstrated through in-vivo studies that to obtain enough ingrowth for this approach to succeed, the design must allow maximum contact between the porous surface and bone. It has been suggested that ingrowth in these designs depends upon a precise fit with maximum contact.[55] Justy observed that 12.5% bone ingrowth occurred in specimens with intimate contact and only 7% in those without contact. For improved contact and a stable fit, some surgeons have advocated use of an oversized (by 1 to 2 mm) cup after the last reamer. However, an oversized component can theoretically cause an overstressed pelvis, another drawback to the use of threaded acetabular shells.

2. Concentric shells with additional screws. The design in these shells is similar to the design described above, but screws have been added to enhance initial fixation of the shell to the bone; once ingrowth through the porous coating has taken place, the screws become superfluous (Fig. 6-37, *D*). Two concerns have arisen regarding the screw fixation of these implants: (1) the potential that fretting will occur between the screws and the metal shell, leading to osteolysis or damage to the polished femoral head, and (2) bone incorporated around the screws will absorb some of the stress, affecting stress transfer through the cup.

At this time, because of the short clinical follow up of these designs, it is not yet possible to determine their design merits or disadvantages.

*Threaded shells with porous-coated sockets** are intended to take advantage of the initial fixation by a threaded cup as well as the subsequent long-term benefits of ingrowth of bone onto the shell. Although the idea is somewhat novel because of the complexity of bone remodeling, it is not possible to quantify the potential of this concept. Long-term, well-controlled

---

*Joint Medical Products Corp., Stamford, Ct.

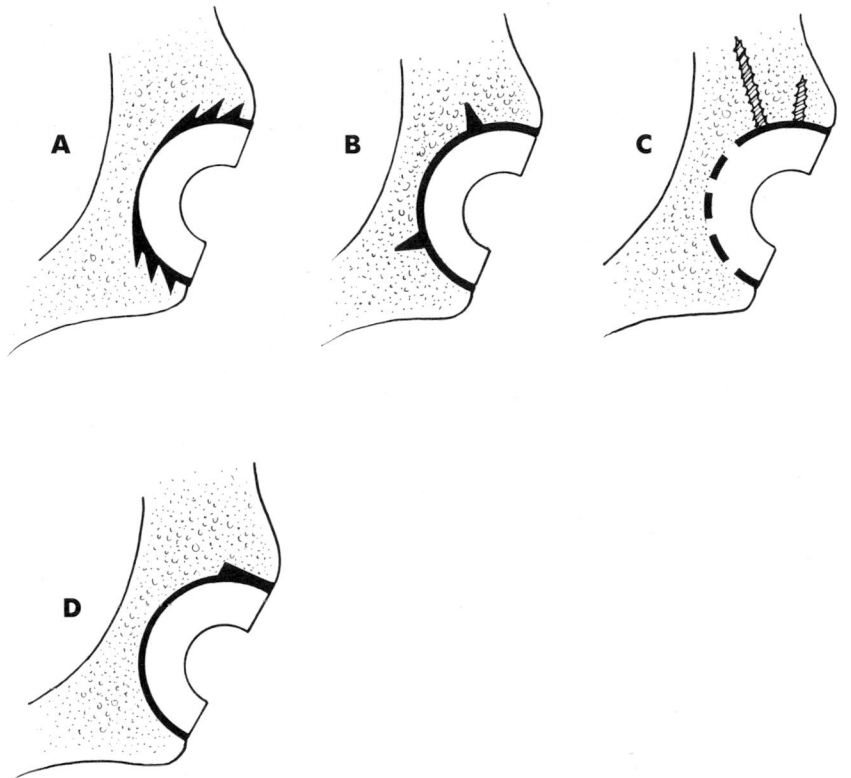

Fig. 6-37. Four modes of acetabular fixation by mechanical fit. **A,** Threaded cup (without dependence on biological bone ingrowth). **B** to **D,** Permanent fixation depends on biological ingrowth. In **C,** additional screws are used as a temporary means of fixation, until osteointegration occurs.

clinical studies related to the clinical application of this design will be needed to judge its effectiveness.

FEMORAL FIXATION AND ADAPTIVE BONE REMODELING

The biomechanical behavior of the stem and adaptive bone changes are significantly influenced by the geometrical design of the stem, its modulus of elasticity, and the method of fixation, which may determine its immediate and long-term durability (Figs. 6-38 to 6-40). Additionally, its permanent success depends not only on the immediate fixation but on the future maintenance of normal strain patterns to allow continuously favorable adaptive changes in bone. In this context, the theoretical and practical aspects of various methods of fixation can be grouped in nonbonded and bonded categories.

Nonbonded Fixation Methods
Plates and Screws

To avoid cancellous bone load transfer in uncemented total hip arthroplasty, prostheses have been designed with the object of preserving load transfer to the lateral proximal femur and in an attempt to reproduce the normal physiological stress transfer to the bone.[84] In

fact, Phillip Wiles used this concept in the first design of total hip arthroplasty.[172]

Prostheses may be attached to the bone by means of plate and screws; this method was used early and discussed in the early orthopaedic literature on total hip arthroplasty. This method has been criticized because of failures owing to varying stress concentrations of materials and different modula of elasticity at the fixation site. In fact, loss of fixation results from motion at the plate-screw-bone site and leads to a vicious cycle of bone absorption and necrosis, which in turn causes further absorption and necrosis and greater loss of fixation.

A "shear force" is generated at the site of fixation, which acts on the screws and ultimately causes failure at the screw-plate-bone junction. When the frictional resistance between a plate and the underlying bone disappears, the main part of the shearing force acting on the plate shifts onto one or more of the screws. The high concentration of stress and bone necrosis leads to failure as various forces shift onto the remaining screws via repeated patterns of stress concentration at each screw level. In surgical practice, when a screw is subjected to repeated loading and unloading after operation, the screws generally

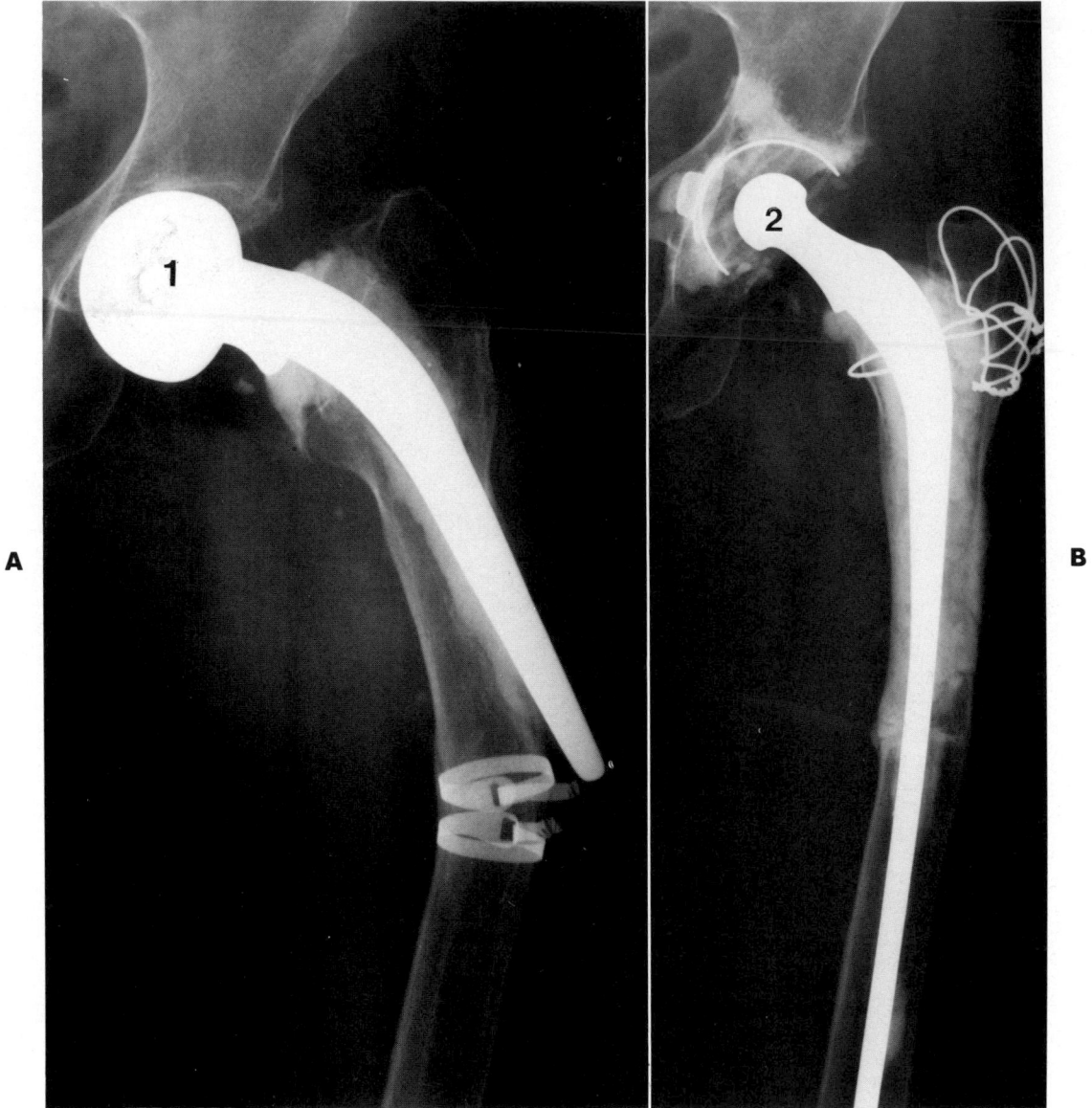

Fig. 6-38. Long-term bone remodelling based on varying stress transmission along the stem of a partially bonded and partially nonbonded prosthesis. **A,** Cemented endoprosthesis used to fix a fracture of femoral neck in 52-year-old woman (M.B.) at another institution. Surgery was complicated by intraoperative fracture of femur. **B,** 2 years after conversion to a Charnley long-stem low-friction arthroplasty. NOTE: good cement filling proximal to the fracture site.

become loose and easily extractable. Ease of extractability is presumably a result of bone absorption caused by abnormal stress. Conversely, in conditions of unloaded but fixed screws, osteointegration can occur. If it does it indicates that load transfer has not occurred; thus the screw becomes tighter than it was when originally inserted. Chromium-cobalt screws are characteristically difficult to extract at reoperation. This type of mechanical fixation is not predictable because its effectiveness depends on the magnitude

and direction of the forces; therefore a permanent fixation of the same magnitude cannot in all cases be reproduced. When osteointegration occurs, it can no longer be regarded as a mechanical fixation but must be characterized as bonded fixation.

Fixation by Interference Fit

Spike impaction of a tapered stem produces an engineering action known as *press fit* or *interference fit*. Morse taper is an example of a "perfect interference

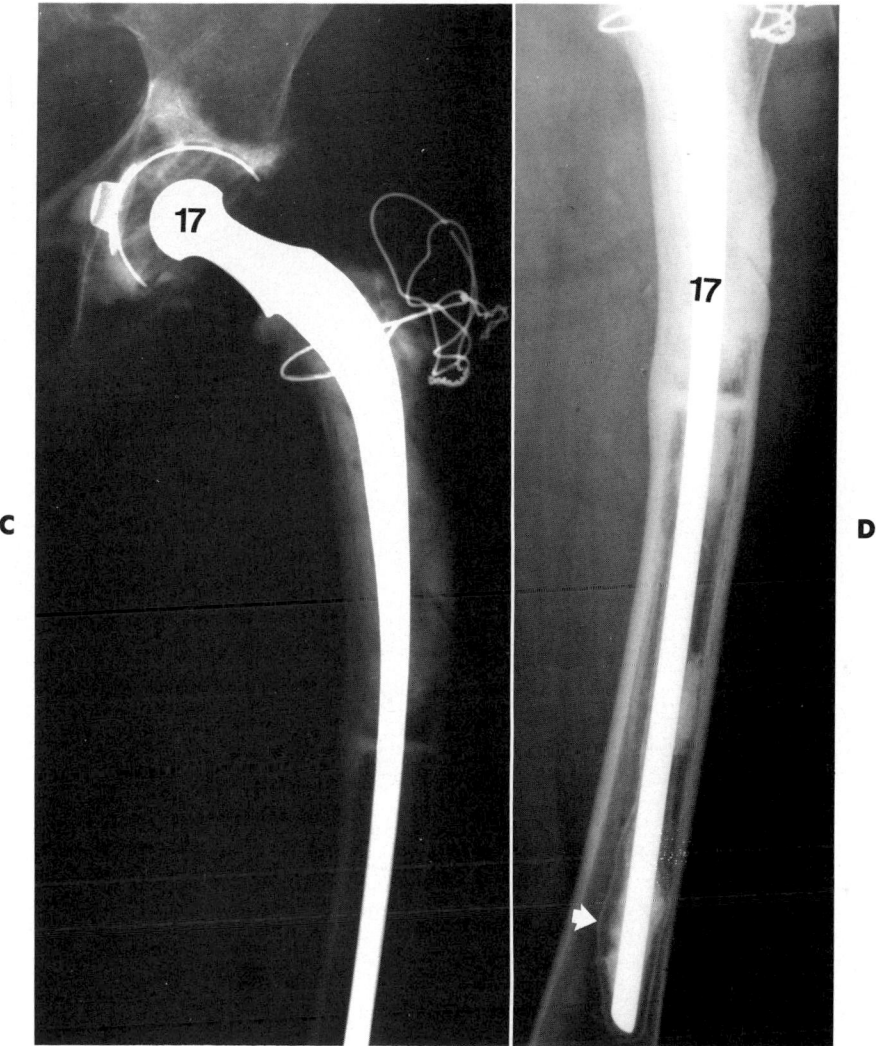

Fig. 6-38—cont'd. C and **D,** Stem has become bowed (not fractured) because of stress. The amplitude of the motion is significantly distal and has resulted in a "windshield wiper sign." Grade A-6,6,6 17 years after conversion surgery. Patient's weight was 65 kg.

fit." In a conventional, noncollared femoral prosthesis, weight bearing is transferred through the tapered segment of the stem to the bone (Fig. 6-41, *A* to *F*).

By definition, this type of fit calls for a line-to-line or surface-to-surface contact, which is stabilized under loading conditions. A perpetual self-locking system provides the stability resulting from ever-increasing friction between the prosthesis and bone caused by the load applied to the system (Fig. 6-41, *A* and *B*). Because of the difference in the modulus of elasticity of bone and of metals with a straight, smooth surface driven into the bone, the femoral cavity is expected to subside unless it becomes bonded to the bone. With the nonbonded interface, shear stress develops to equilibrate the compressive force of the load applied to it

(Fig. 6-41, *C* and *D*). On the other hand, when the tapered stem is smooth, a slight subsidence is needed to develop adequate stress values to resist further subsidence and produce a state of stability. The amount of subsidence for a given tapered angle of the pin largely depends on the rigidity of the bone and the tapered radius of the pin (Fig. 6-41, *C* and *D*). A loosely fitted pin, a nontapered pin and cone, or a deformable cone (Fig. 6-41, *A* and *B*) allows continuous subsidence until (1) adequate resistance (stress) is generated by the cone (Fig. 6-41, *E* and *F*) or (2) the system fails because the cone is inadequate to generate enough resistive stress to put the two forces in equilibrium (Fig. 6-41, *F*). Ideally, the tapered angle (radius) of the tapered pin must be infinitely large (Fig. 6-41, *G*) or the

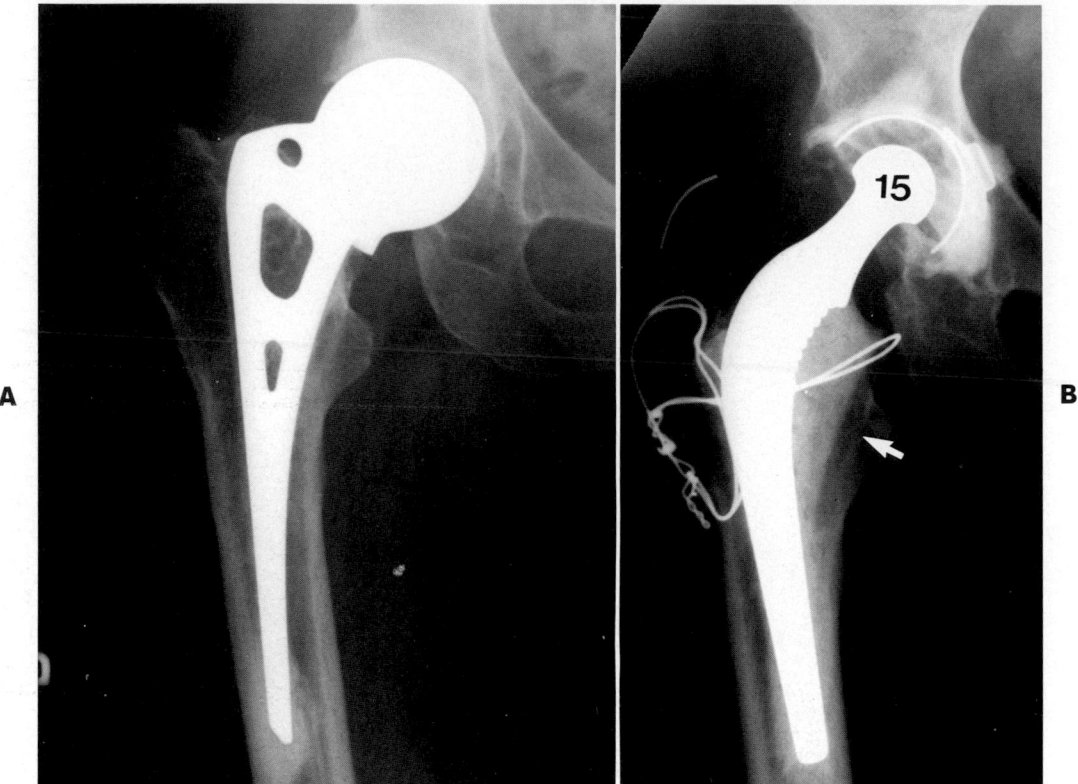

Fig. 6-39. A, Radiograph of right hip in 55-year-old woman (A.C.) with failed Austin-Moore prosthesis for hip fracture. Grade A-3,3,5. Patient's weight was 88 kg. **B,** 15 years after low-friction arthroplasty. NOTE: asymmetrical cement mantle caused by exaggerated valgus position of an undersized prosthesis. NOTE: cancellous transformation of cortical bone at the medial neck caused by altered stress pattern (stress shielding) and adaptive bone remodelling. Radiolucency of proximal medial is trabecular bone, which continues to support cement mantle *(solid arrow).* Grade A-6,6,6. Patient's weight was 85 kg.

largest possible (Fig. 6-41, *H*) to resist failure.

Using a two-dimensional finite element model (and assuming line-to-line contact), Huiskes estimated various stress patterns for a nonbonded stem[86]:

1. In the press-fit stem interface, stresses were more affected by the geometrical shape of the stem and less by stem rigidity. The patterns of load transfer of the nonbonded press-fit stem designs also depend very much on the geometrical shape of the prosthesis.[89]
2. Considering the mechanical properties of the stem, titanium was expected to produce more favorable results than the chromium-cobalt-molybdenum alloys.
3. A nonbonded press-fit stem provoked only calcar stress shielding. As in the midstem region, the stress in the cortex was even greater than in the natural case.
4. Lack of uniformity between the bone of the upper femur (metaphysis) and the lower femur (diaphy-

sis) generates a nonuniform progressive stress pattern (Figs. 6-42 and 6-43). While the distal portion of the femur and the stem act similarly to a tapered pin within a cone, because of the curvature of the stem, the proximal portion of the neck and shaft junction behaves differently. As the prosthesis subsides, the surrounding bone is forced under axial load to straighten out, thus developing a high compressive stress at the proximal and medial aspects of the femur. In this situation, a properly designed prosthesis is necessary to fill up the flare of the canal of the femur to reduce a high stress concentration at the medial-femoral neck.

Design Criteria for Nonbonded Stem (Press-Fit)

- Fit and fill vs. stability
- Fit and fill vs. stress distribution
- Fit and fill vs. micromotion
- Fit and fill and surgical technique

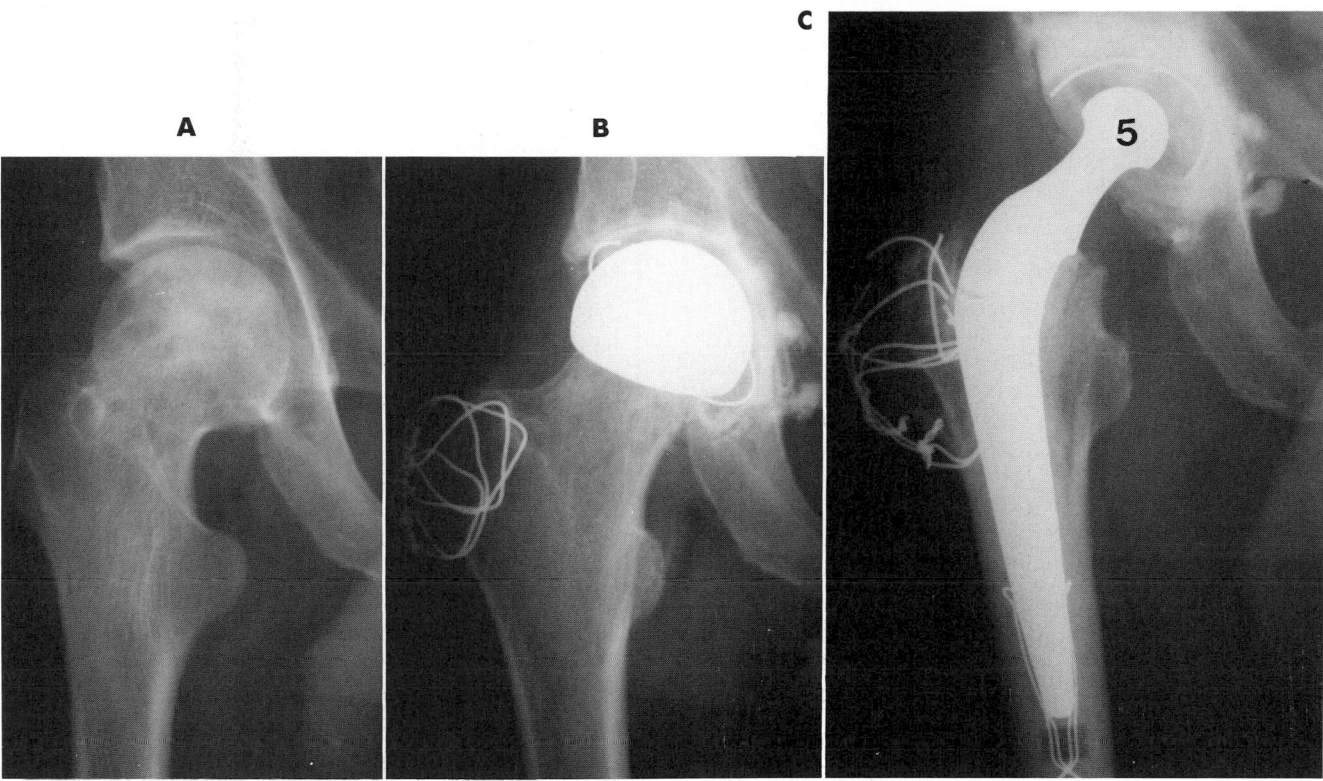

Fig. 6-40. A, Radiograph of 40-year-old man (G.G.) with unilateral avascular necrosis of femoral head. Patient has postpolio paralysis of the opposite hip and extremity and uses a brace and one crutch. **B,** 4 years after Wagner resurfacing procedure and progressive pain. NOTE: only modest atrophy of neck of femur has occurred. **C,** 5 years after low-friction arthroplasty, cement mantle is asymmetrical. Further atrophy (cancellous transformation) has occurred with the stemmed prosthesis. Grade C-6,4,6. Patient's weight was 95 kg.

• Fit and fill vs. materials

MAXIMUM FIT AND FILL VS. STABILITY That initial fit and stability are prerequisites common to all arthroplasties is undeniable.[16,53,114,137] A poor fit generates micromotion, which promotes fibrous tissue interface and bone stimulation, resulting in pain. Because adult femora vary so greatly in the size and shape of the internal and external architectural design, it is impossible to fit the medullary canal perfectly with an off-the-shelf prosthesis[116] (see Chapter 2).

A nonbonded, press-fit design must be fitted with maximum contact against the strong bone of the femoral cortex and the load-bearing trabeculae of the femur (Figs. 6-44 and 6-45).

Deformable or weak cancellous bone cannot withstand compressive and torsional forces transmitted via the femoral head. Because of the complex geometry and variability in the shape of the femur, prefabricated stems cannot produce perfect fit and fill.[116] The femur's complex geometry results from a number of variables: cervical-femoral angle, torsional angle, medial-lateral width, anteroposterior width, anterolateral diaphyseal bow, and posterior metaphyseal bow. The shape and size of the medullary canal are also disproportionate. Additionally, as a result of genetic and environmental influences, there seems to be no association between the size and shape of the femur in man. Consequently, there is no predictable relationship between the size and shape of the metaphysis and diaphysis. In addition, aging affects the femur disproportionately: the diaphysis expands at a rate of 1.3 mm per decade, but the metaphysis remains relatively unaffected by age.[6,137,144,160] As a result of diaphyseal expansion after age 40, the diameter ratio of the metaphysis to that of the diaphysis—known as the *flare index*—is typically reduced in older patients; the flare index is categorically larger in the younger population (see Chapter 2 and Fig. 6-46). Because the flare index varies so greatly, there is no "average" ratio that could be scaled to fit perfectly all skeletal sizes.[116]

Text continued on p. 263.

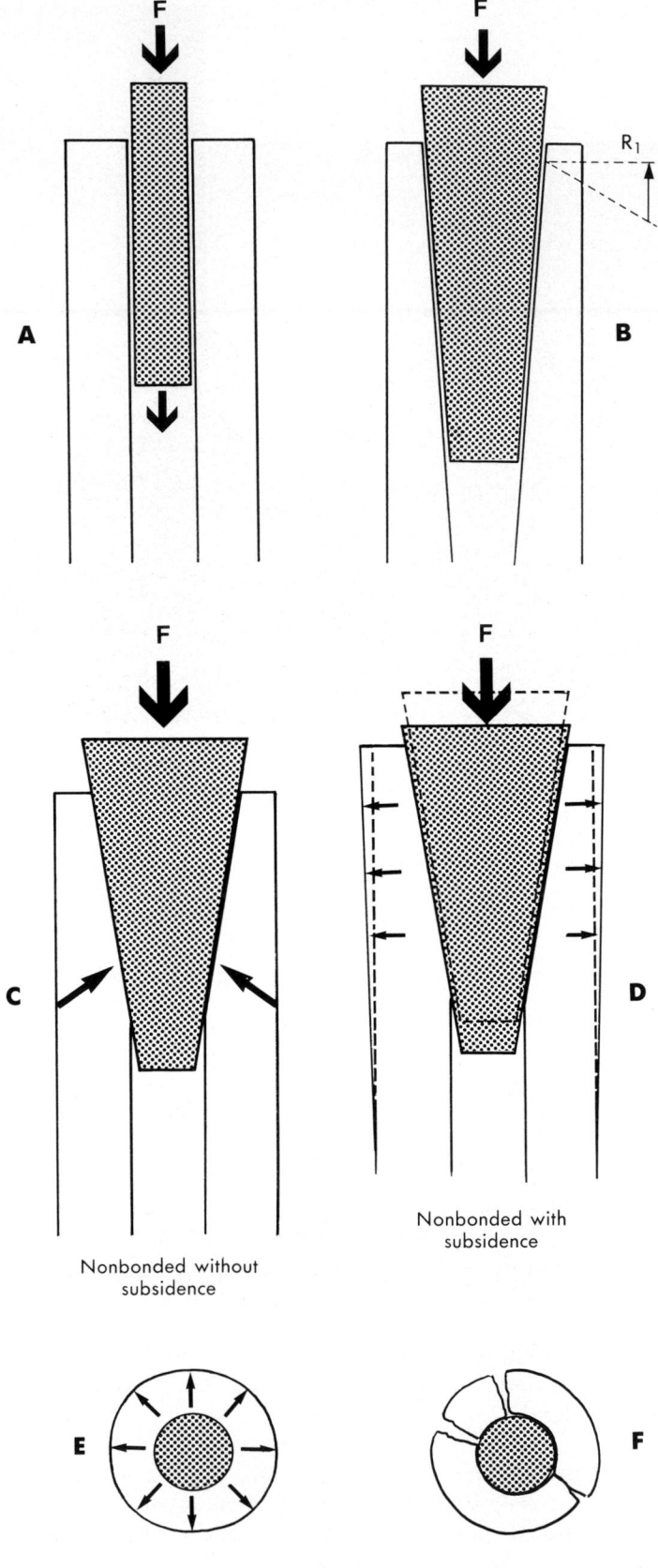

Nonbonded without
subsidence

Nonbonded with
subsidence

Hoop stress

See legend on opposite page.

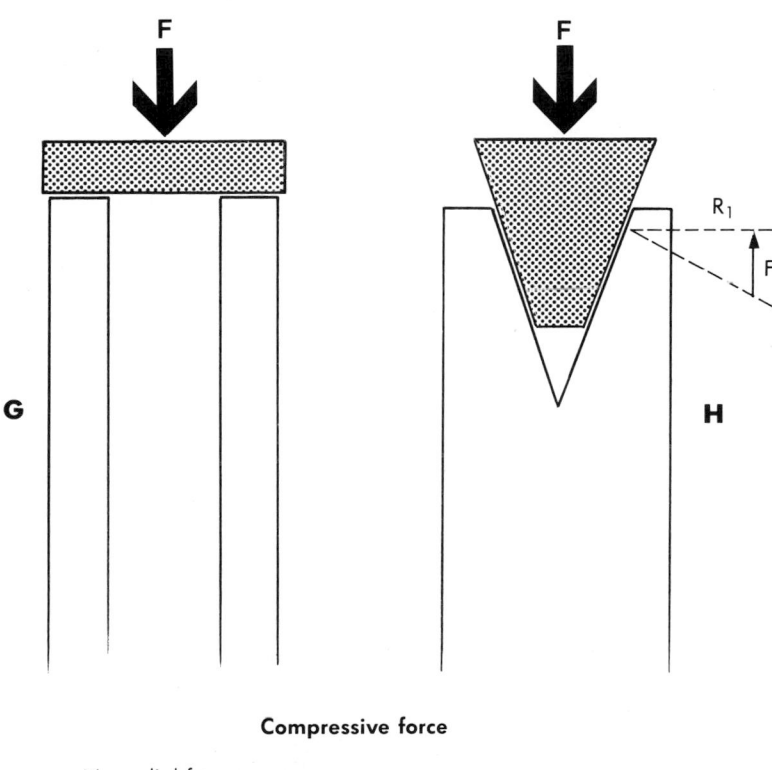

Compressive force

No radial force
No hoop stress

Low radial force

Fig. 6-41. A, Demonstration of nonbonded, noncollared, nontapered pin within a cylindrical tube. Load transfer via such a system is not possible because of lack of support by cylinder. **B,** Demonstration of perpetual self-locking by ever-increasing friction between tapered pin and cone. F = force, R = tapered radius. **C,** Shear stress generated at interface between the two elements is resisted by rigidity of cone *(arrows)*. **D,** Lack of rigidity (elasticity) of cone causes expansion of cone until sufficient resistance (frictional force) is created or system ends in failure. Amount of subsidence is governed by amount of applied force *(F)*. The frictional characteristics between the two elements and the taper radius *(R)*. **E,** Subsiding forces of tapered pin have resulted in hoop stress within the cone (cross section). Balanced forces results in equilibrium in the system. **F,** A greater subsiding force (than frictional force) has led to failure of system caused by excess hoop stress. **G,** A zero radial force results in a zero hoop stress irrespective of amount of applied force *(F)*. **H,** The lowest radial force is generated by the widest tapered angle (R_1).

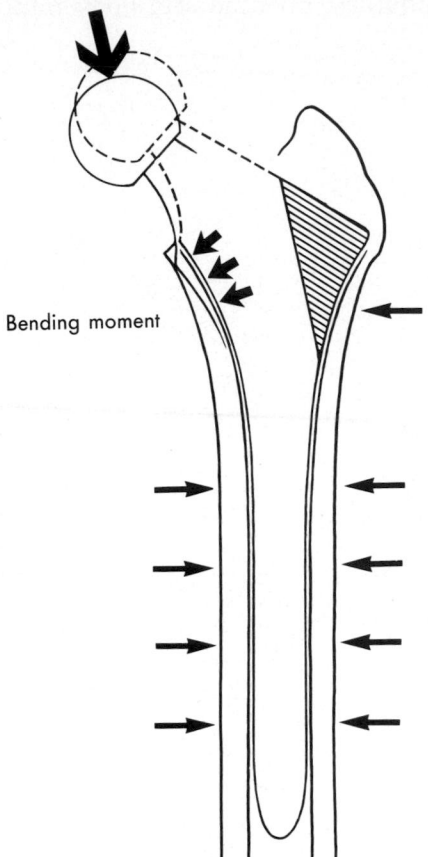

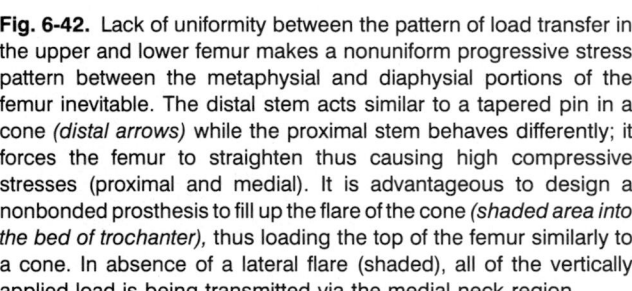

Fig. 6-42. Lack of uniformity between the pattern of load transfer in the upper and lower femur makes a nonuniform progressive stress pattern between the metaphysial and diaphysial portions of the femur inevitable. The distal stem acts similar to a tapered pin in a cone *(distal arrows)* while the proximal stem behaves differently; it forces the femur to straighten thus causing high compressive stresses (proximal and medial). It is advantageous to design a nonbonded prosthesis to fill up the flare of the cone *(shaded area into the bed of trochanter),* thus loading the top of the femur similarly to a cone. In absence of a lateral flare (shaded), all of the vertically applied load is being transmitted via the medial neck region.

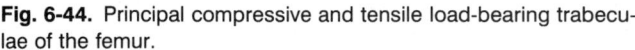

Fig. 6-43. Various forces transmitted to the femur via a prosthesis are shown: tensile (anteroposterior, *APT,* and mediolateral, *ML*) compressive (subsiding), *S,* and torsional (twisting), *T.*

Fig. 6-44. Principal compressive and tensile load-bearing trabeculae of the femur.

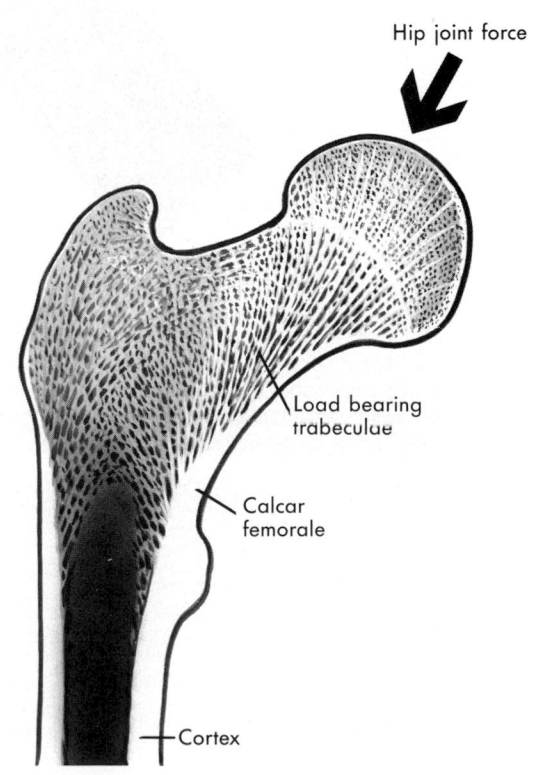

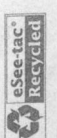

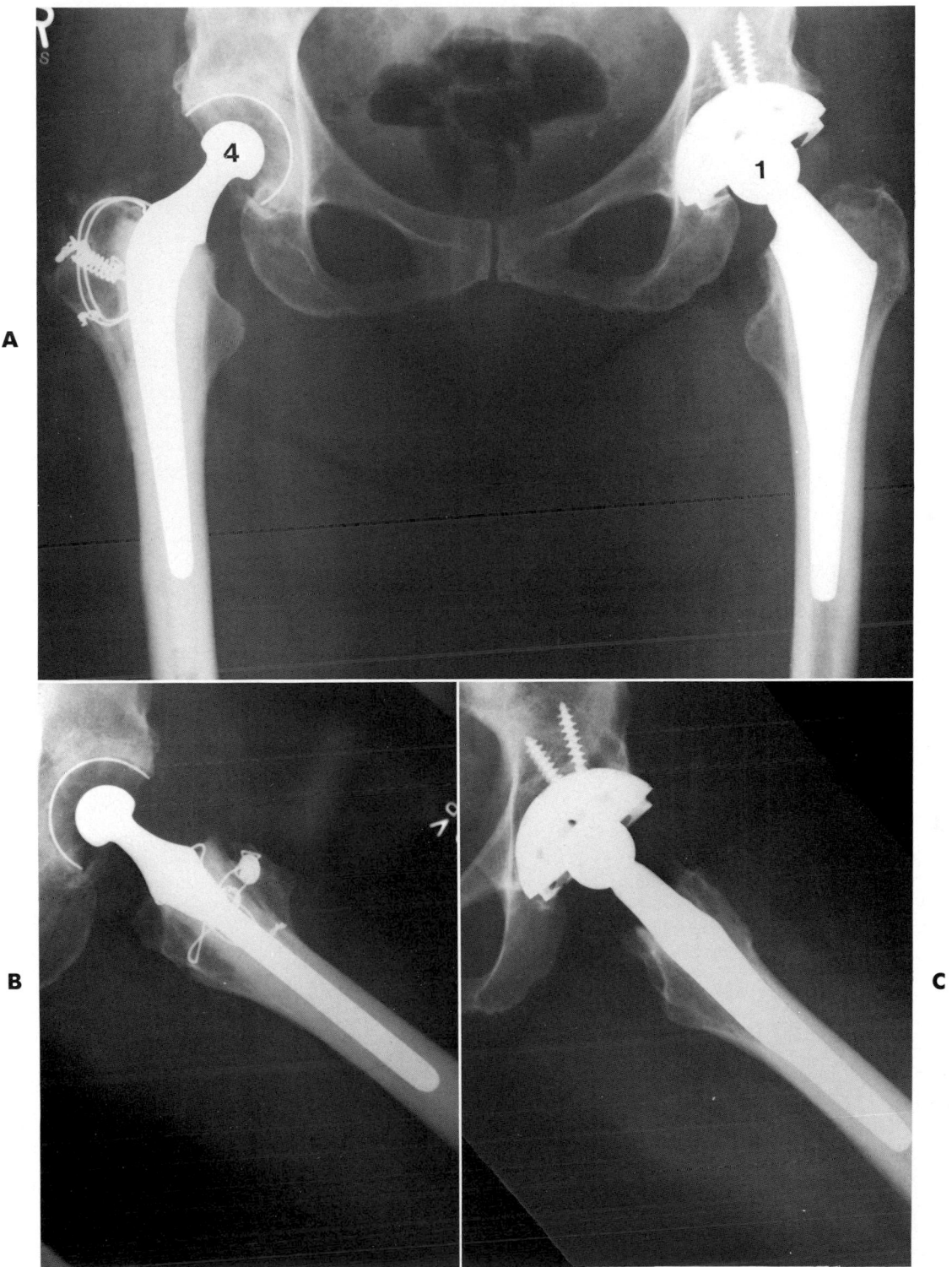

Fig. 6-45. One and 4 years after bilateral total hip arthroplasty in 61-year-old woman (E.M.) who demanded a cementless hip on the left hip despite the excellent clinical and radiographic results at 4 years on the right side. NOTE: space filling of the metaphysis and diaphysis by titanium on the left side versus stainless steel (Ortron 90 and cement on the right side). **B,** Fit and fill of both prostheses on lateral views are satisfactory. Bone remodelling cannot be determined because of short follow up.

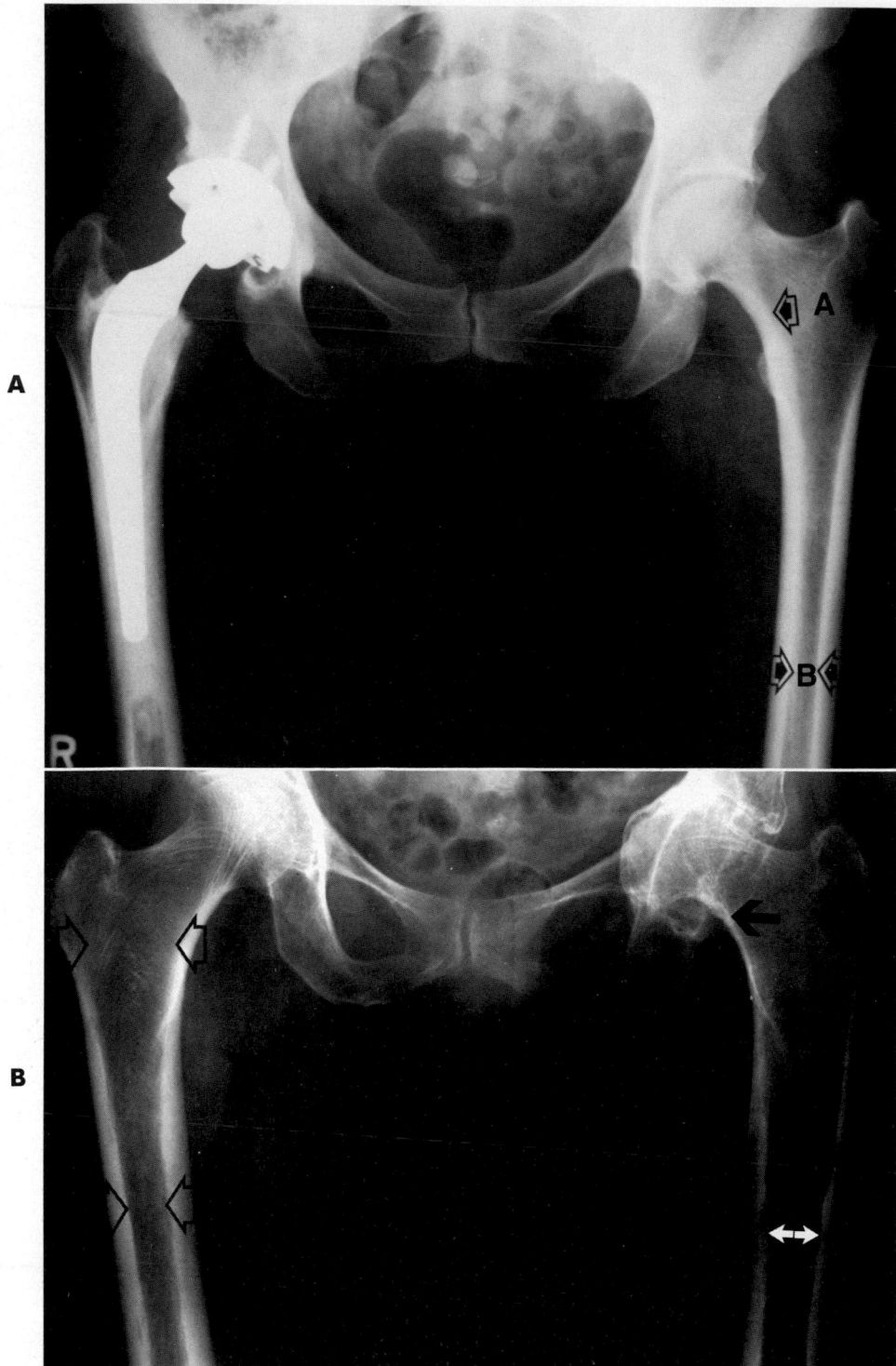

Fig. 6-46. A, Radiograph of 46-year-old woman (S.D.) after a right hip replacement. NOTE: a high flare index (ratio of metaphysial internal diameter at 20 mm proximal to the midsection of the lesser trochanter *A* to the inner diameter of the isthmus *B* measuring $\frac{A}{B} = 5.5$). This type of femur, known as *champagne flute*, is suitable for prosthetic load transfer. **B,** Example of a "normal" femur (flare index = 3.2) on the right and a "stove-pipe" femur (flare index = 2.0) on the left. A successful intramedullary fixation is more difficult to achieve in femurs with a stove-pipe configuration regardless of the method of fixation; that is, bonded or nonbonded prostheses (see text and Chapter 2).

FIT AND FILL VS. STRESS DISTRIBUTION Clinical studies have demonstrated that a close match between the implant and bone in a nonbonded stem is essential for success.* To meet the need for a better fit, cementless prostheses are now available in a larger range of stem sizes. In fact, the dramatically improved clinical results can be attributed to the variety of component sizes now available.† It has been well established that an undersized, nonbonded stem is likely to produce micromotion leading to thigh pain, subsidence, or loosening, eventually requiring revision surgery. Conversely, an oversized, mismatched bone prosthesis ultimately causes fracture of the trochanter (4% to 21%) or of the femoral shaft (1% to 17%).[16,138] Some surgeons have suggested that to achieve maximal canal fill, intraoperative fractures of the femur are unavoidable.[92,138]

Currently there are only a few studies on nonbonded anatomically shaped prostheses with ideal fit. Using strain-gauge study of an anatomically shaped stem with a vertical force of 1000 newtons, Walker and co-workers found the compressive strains of the proximal, medial-lateral femur to be between 45% and 56% of normal[167]; the hoop strains, on the other hand, were elevated to 125% of normal. In a similar study of loading conditions using a long-stem press-fit, the compressive strains were further reduced to 50% of normal with a collared prosthesis and to only 15% without a collar.[82] Others have demonstrated that the degree to which a fit approximates perfection significantly influences the amount of strain in the bone. For example, Jasty and associates found that a tight distal fit produced only 20% of normal strains proximally, but a distally loose fit and a collar produced a strain 130% of normal. In their studies, a close fit reduced the proximal strain optimally (70% to 90%).[93]

From the foregoing, it is apparent that a prosthetic fit designed to closely resemble the anatomical shape of the femur with priority loading produces a strain closer to normal than do bonded prostheses, such as those with ingrowth or cemented stems. In addition to excess hoop strain generated by wedge action, torsional forces—which can be significant—must be resisted.

Based on 200 anatomical specimens, Noble concluded that the anatomical shape of the femur may be represented as a "unique shape" called a *somtype*. By mathematical calculations, a set of somtypes could be recognized to include the anatomical range of canal geometry with the smallest error possible.[116] By describing the medial and lateral endosteal contour of the proximal femur to an accuracy of ± 1 mm, 45 somtypes were derived; only 17 of these occurred with an incidence of more than 1%. When the tolerance was reduced to 2 mm in the proximal implant-bone interface, the original 17 could be reduced to a set of eight unique geometries. If these data are taken at face value, a "press-fit" prosthesis is by definition a misnomer, because in a true press-fit, even ± 1 mm mismatch is unacceptable. Additionally, despite the large range of sizes, press fits are not adequate to all situations, and thus there is no justification for the high cost of maintaining a large inventory.

FIT AND FILL VS. MICROMOTION For the sake of discussion, we can argue that when two materials of dissimilar modulus of elasticity are put in conjunction, micromotion always occurs between them when they are placed under cyclic load—even if this motion is so minuscule that it cannot be seen or measured by ordinary devices.

The lock-wedge action, which also causes micromotion under cyclic load, can be minimized only by making the radius of the tapered angle of the wedge so large that it reduces the load transfer to a level that the bone can tolerate. An extreme example of force reduction is a zero angle; at zero degrees, the tapered stem is transformed to a horizontal plate (such as a collar), which can transfer the entire load to the top of the femur. Let us now assume that the load is shared proximally by an effective collar, such as a Thompson prosthesis, and the tapered stem.

When a Thompson prosthesis is inserted by simple interference fit (with no interposing material, such as cement), the collar of the prosthesis rests against the cut end of the femur. Motion takes place between the collar of the prosthesis and the cut end of the femur during the loading and unloading of "walking cycles," as has been demonstrated; the stem acts only as a stabilizing element to prevent the prosthesis from tilting. The motion between the prosthesis and the bone seems to relate to the difference in modulus of elasticity between the steel and the bone; the modulus of elasticity of steel is 2.8×10^7 lb/in^2 (1.93×10^8 KN/m^2); for bone, it is approximately 2×10^6 lb/in^2 (1.38×10^7 KN/m^2). Because the stem length remains constant while the load is applied and transmitted via the collar, the femur is shortened; the amount of shortening can be calculated from the load, the elastic modulus, and the size of the section of bone. Basing our calculations on the assumptions that the entire load is transmitted via the collar and that the 15-inch femur has an internal diameter of 1.25 inches and an external diameter of 1.5 inches, we can calculate that the femur under a load of 150 lb contracts 0.001 inch.

According to these calculations, when the femur is under load, every inch of it shortens by 0.000066 inch; keeping in mind that the 5-inch length of the stem of the prosthesis under load remains constant and that

*References 51, 52, 77, 147, 149.
†References 16, 139, 140, 166, 177, 178.

the corresponding segment of bone shortens, there must be a fretting movement of 0.00033 between the stem and the tip of the endosteal surface of the bone. Considering that the load of the hip joint for dynamic and static situations is three times that of the body weight, the actual displacement between the stem and the endosteal surface of the bone would be three times greater, that is, $\frac{1}{1000}$ inch or 25 μm. The cyclic loading and unloading, which cause relative motion between metal and bone, have been implicated in causing bone absorption. This phenomenon, well known by engineers as *fretting*, causes failure between dissimilar materials under loading conditions. Because of the persistent fretting motion between the prosthesis and the bone, this mode of failure can result even if the two materials (bone and steel) have the same modulus of elasticity.

Studies have demonstrated that when a prosthesis mismatch resulted from undersizing, a load of four times body weight produced a relative motion of more than 200 μm.[104,118,152a] When endosteal bone is in direct contact with the prosthesis by cortical bone, micromotion is remarkably reduced.[104,118,167]

In their micromotion studies, Walker and associates[167] found that in micromotion at the stem-bone interface the rotations were small (5 to 52 μm) and reversible (because of bone elasticity) using 1000 N vertical force. By adding rotational forces of 100 N about the vertical axis, a significant degree of stem-bone displacement occurred, from a mean of 18 to 47 μm. Added torsional forces in this study also significantly increased rotation about the vertical axis, from 0.017 to 0.050 degree.

Consider the following situation: a tapered 5-inch stem with a collarless prosthesis without fenestration or rough texture (i.e., a nonfenestrated Austin-Moore prosthesis made of polished stainless steel) is driven into the medullary cavity. If we calculate that the tapering of the stem is 1:7 (1 inch proximally to 0.14 inch at the tip) and a 120-pound patient loads such a prosthesis, the total transverse force available to dilate the femoral canal is $120 \times 3 \times 7 = 2520$ lb. Assuming plane surfaces and a wedge of $\frac{5}{16}$ inch (0.3126 inch) in thickness, with the entire length (both medial and lateral surfaces) in firm contact with bone, the area of contact would be approximately $5 \times 2 \times 0.313$, equal to 3.3 square inches, given a stress on the bone of $3.12/25201 = 800$ lb per square inch. Quite obviously, the fretting movements resulting from the "wedge action" of such a theoretical prosthesis would be considerable; "lock wedge" would inevitably cause failure from sinking unless further sinking is prevented by moving the prosthesis to a new position.

To achieve the best clinical and radiological results in fixation of a poorly fitted intramedullary stem (that

is, Austin-Moore), transmission must be shared by the collar, the tip of the stem (Fig. 6-47), and the bone of the fenestration. This optimal situation usually results when the prosthesis has fallen (tilted) into a varus or valgus orientation (Fig. 6-48). In these cases, a local strengthening of the cortex is a manifestation of weight-bearing phenomena (Wolff's law). This situation often occurs after a period of sinking, usually in strong, active patients with good functional capacity.

Another possibility, however, is that the growth of cancellous bone into the fenestration of the Moore self-locking prosthesis might withstand some vertical stress and some torsional force (see Fig. 6-48). Unfortunately, this outcome is seldom achieved: space/fibrous tissue between the prosthesis and the bone cannot be entirely eliminated, so the fretting movement and high-stress concentration continue. When the bone in the fenestration is visible by x-ray films—and even when the fenestration is completely obliterated by bone—it is doubtful that a true state of "locking" exists. Despite difficulties encountered in the removal of such a prosthesis, motion between the prosthesis and the bone can frequently be demonstrated at surgery (see Fig. 6-48).

To maximize fixation, one popular method uses a longer prosthetic stem; but, as stated before, because the collar is the main weight-bearing region, the stem offers no advantage except to prevent toggle. It can be argued that an extremely long stem, like that of the Matchet-Brown prosthesis, increases the amplitude of fretting movements. For example, the amplitude of fretting at the tip of a 15-inch (37.5-cm) stem is three times that of a 5-inch (12.5-cm) stem; thus, a greater range of motion is transferred to a further distal zone with resultant increased fretting movement and bone necrosis without preventing loosening.

EFFECTS OF COLLAR ON NONBONDED STEM

When examining the load on the upper femur via the collar of the prosthesis, it is important to consider the role played by the length of the neck. If the resultant forces (pull of the abductors and the body weight load) are in equilibrium—with the force directed to the neck of the femur—the length of the neck has no effect on the forces applied to the cut end of the femur (see Fig. 6-47). On the other hand, if the abductors are weak, the forces on the hip are more vertical, so the long neck increases the pressure on the calcar; conversely, a short neck would reduce the pressure caused by weight bearing.

It is also important to note that bone absorption occurs under vertical load and under the stress produced by any tangential movement; therefore, the collar of the prosthesis must be ideally inclined so that it distributes the load throughout the cut surface of the femur and prohibits tangential movement. As already

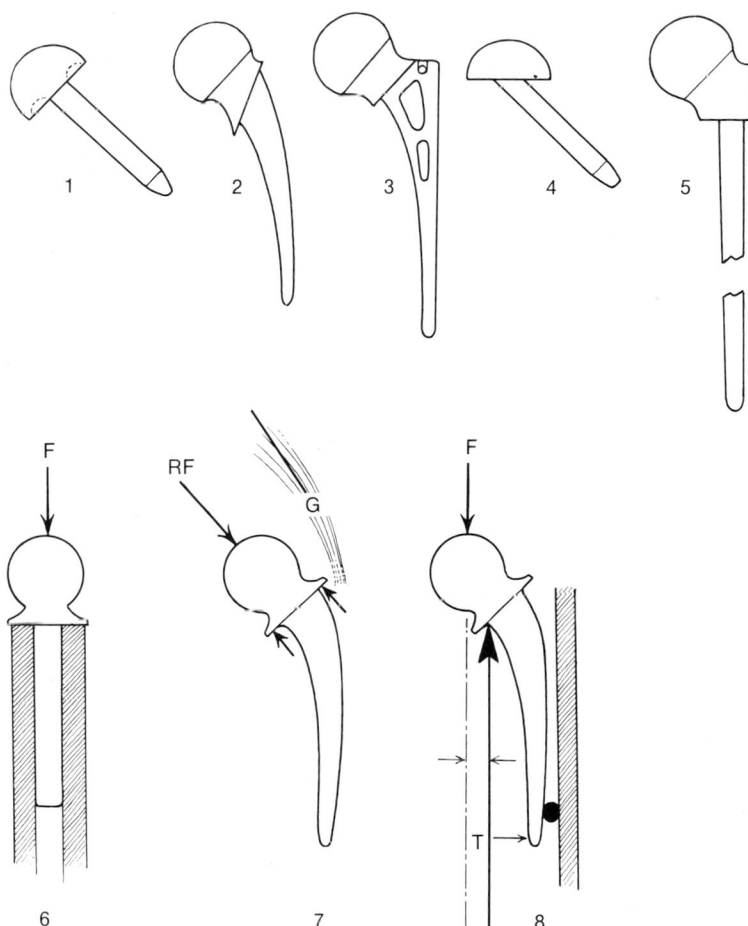

Fig. 6-47. Examples of different neck designs in several prostheses used in past by interference fit. *1,* Original Judet, *2,* Thompson, *3,* Moore self-locking, *4,* modified Judet, and *5,* Leinbach. Ideal inclination of neck depends entirely on efficiency of abductor mechanism. For example, *6* illustrates prosthesis with collar that is most efficient if abductor pull is not present; *7* illustrates that if abductor pull is normal, plane of collar should be at 90 degrees to resultant forces, *RF.* Compare direction of forces of *7* with *6. 8,* Illustrates resultant forces acting on intramedullary stem prosthesis. Vertical load, *F,* causes bending moment in absence of abductor muscle tending to turn prosthesis into varus direction. Force, *T,* neutralizes moment of force, *F,* tending to rotate prosthesis. Schematic drawing illustrates major compressive forces present at calcar and lateral side of prosthesis.

mentioned, the ideal inclination depends entirely on the efficiency of the abductor power. For example, if the abductor muscles and their force angle are normal, the plane of the collar should be at 90 degrees to the resultant forces (see Fig. 6-47),[25] but as the abductor system becomes more defective, the collar must be inclined at a more horizontal angle.

For this discussion, consider a tapered nonbonded stem with a smooth surface. Successful fixation of such a stem is limited by the significant hoop stress generated in the femur, which can cause fracture, bone lysis, or both (Figs. 6-49 and 6-50). It has been demonstrated that after the femoral component is inserted, the pattern of strain in the proximal femur

changes dramatically compared with that of the intact femur.[120] In cemented prostheses, the pattern of stress was reversed; stress decreased massively in the calcar region and maximum strain became focused around the tip of the prosthesis. Transferring the load via a collar restored the strain toward normal by shifting 30% to 40% of the normal strain to the calcar. This study demonstrated conclusively that use of a collar improves the load distribution pattern. In cemented fixation, it revealed the collar is ineffective if the cement mantle is bound to both the implant and the bone (i.e., with precoated stems) (Fig. 6-51). When a nonbonded, tapered stem is used, the collar may reduce pistoning of the femoral component inside the

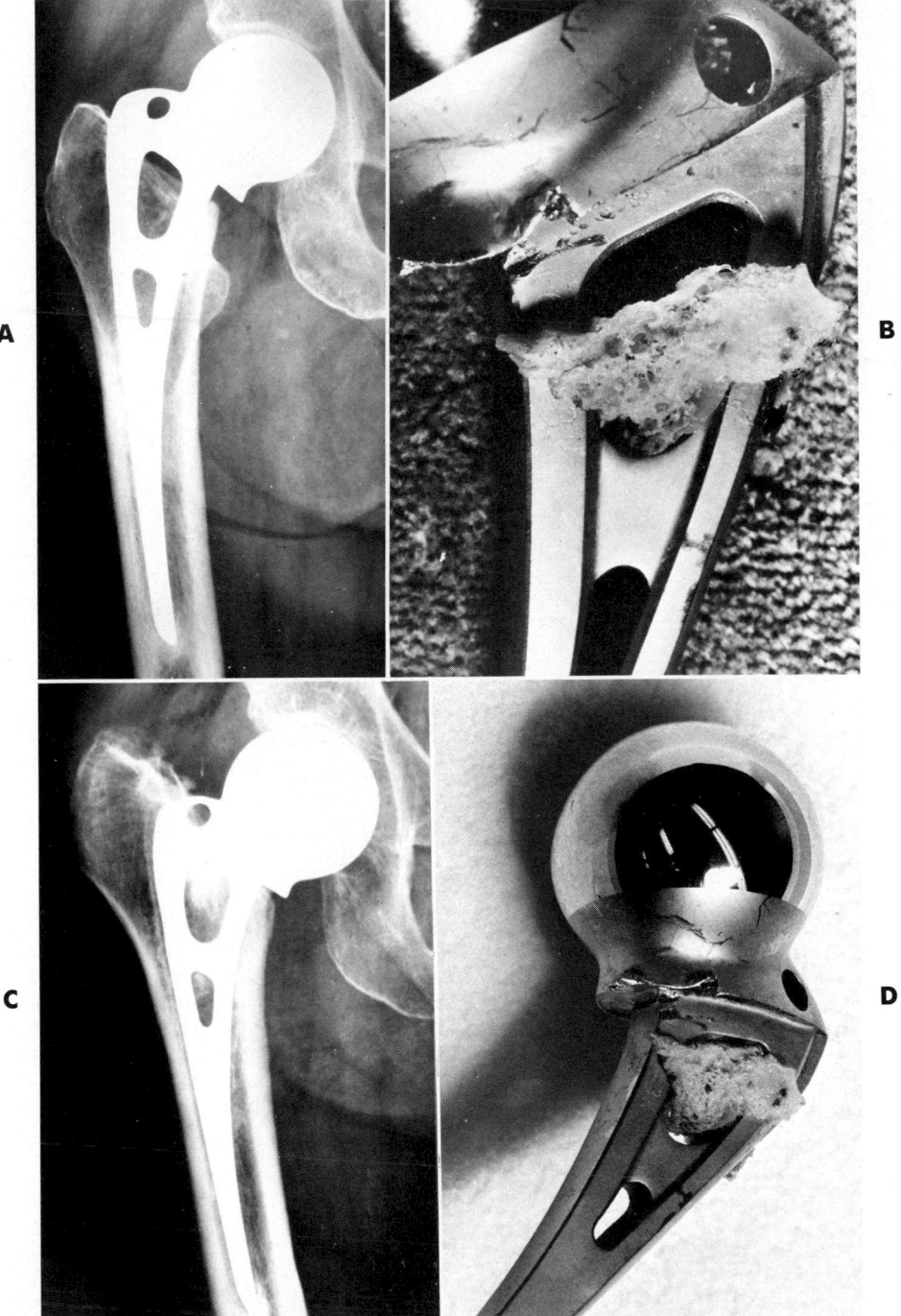

Fig. 6-48. A, 4 years after successful Moore self-locking prosthesis inserted for fracture of neck of femur. Weight-bearing film shows space between top end of femur and collar of prosthesis. NOTE: weight-bearing zone at tip of prosthesis indicating that although weight bearing is eliminated from collar, it is shared by tip of stem and tapered segment of stem. **B,** Considerable violent trauma was necessary to extract this prosthesis despite gross motion (wobble) noted at surgery. **C,** Example of "sunk-in" prosthesis that has eventually stabilized itself by same mechanism shown in **A.** Observe extreme neck absorption before stabilization of prosthesis. It is presumed that stabilization was achieved by three-point fixation of tapered segment and tip, as well as bone of fenestration. **D,** Considerable difficulty experienced while extracting this prosthesis. No detectable motion was observed at surgery.

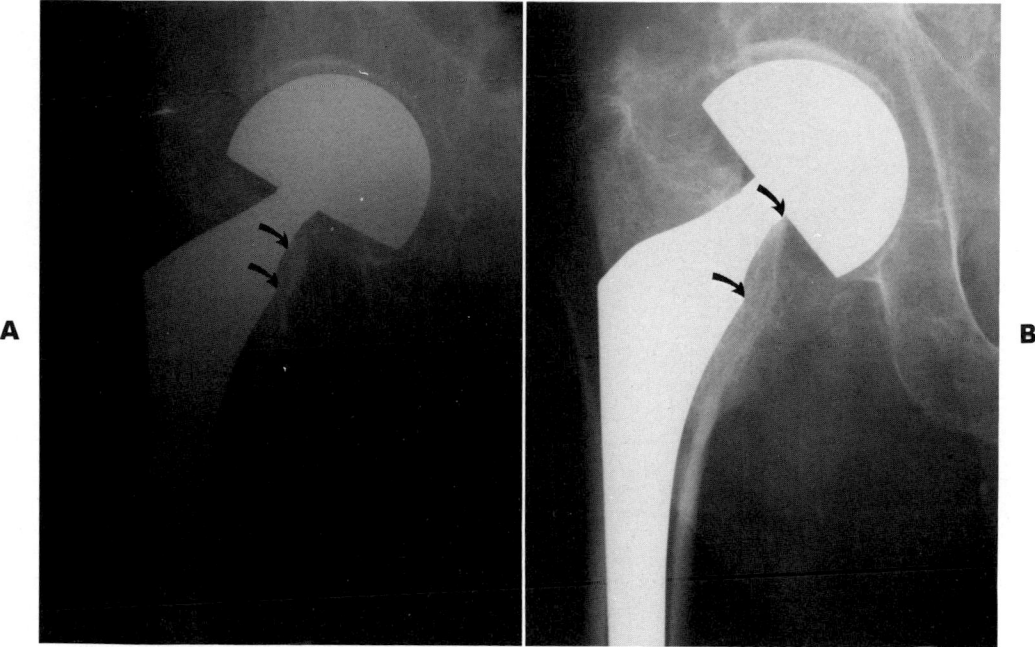

Fig. 6-49. A, Postoperative radiograph taken in the recovery room shows stem subsidence into medullary cavity *(distance between the two arrows).* The patient is an 80-year-old man (J.B.) who was treated by an Osteonics long-stem prosthesis, and the prosthesis was driven to the level of neck resection at surgery with a modest amount of hammering. A tight fit was achieved. **B,** Press-fit prosthesis further subsided (to the level of lesser trochanter) as patient noted a progressive shortening of his leg. A wide, stovepipe-shaped femur in the elderly makes a good fill and fit difficult.

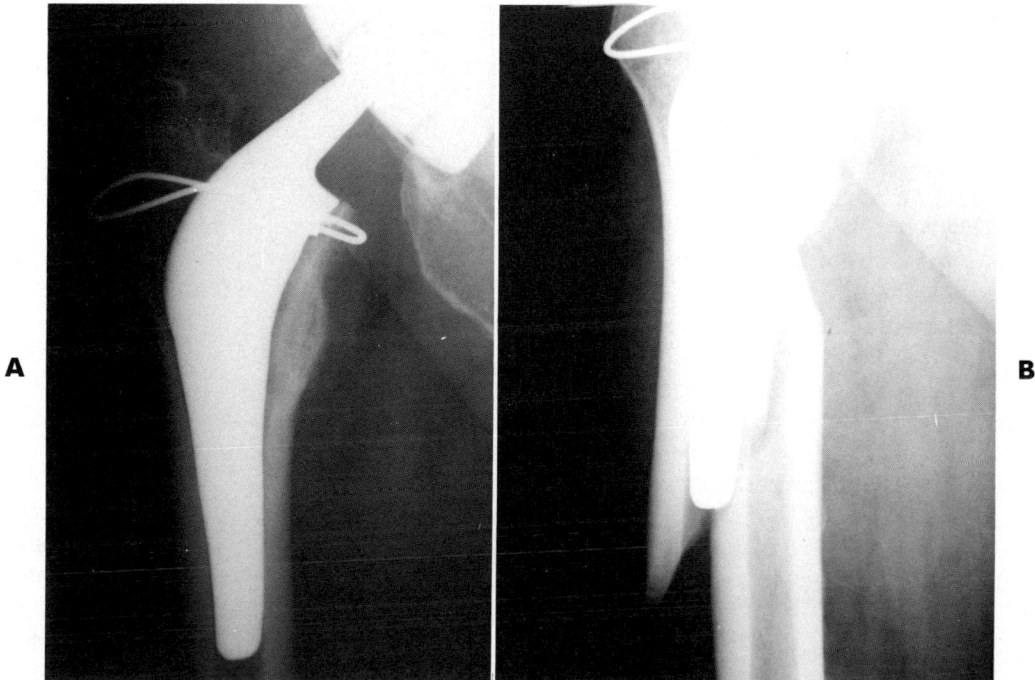

Fig. 6-50. A, Total hip arthroplasty using an Identifit prosthesis was performed at another institution on 61-year-old man (J.S.). NOTE: a prophylactic wire cerclaged the femur. Patient weighed 235 pounds and was 6'4" in height. **B,** Patient sustained a spiral femoral fracture in a forceful attempt to bring the leg up and rotate it to place his leg into his trousers. Excessive torsional stress generated by flexing the hip and hoop stress was thought to produce a fracture since surgery was completely uneventful and satisfactory (see Chapter 36).

Fig. 6-51. **A,** Radiograph of 58-year-old man (T.P.) 6 months after low-friction arthroplasty. He was a "steel bender" who weighed 100 kg at surgery. **B,** Same hip 1 year after surgery (excellent calcar collar contact with minimum cement interposition) shows femoral neck cortical atrophy *(arrows).* **C,** Complete loss of support by bone caused by absorption 13 years after surgery. NOTE: wear of socket. Grade A-6,6,6. Weight was 105 kg.

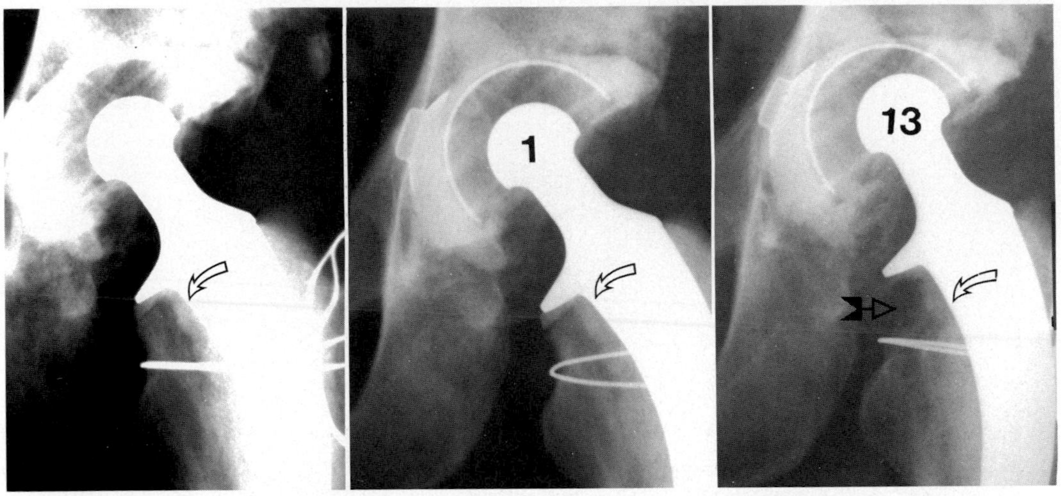

medullary canal.[3,108] The maximum tensile strains in the stem were inversely proportional to the stiffness of the collar support. Other studies using uncemented femoral components and a collar have shown abnormal stress distribution and thus abnormal strain in the bone after insertion of a nonbonded stem.[86-88,115] Others have demonstrated in the laboratory that collar contact with the upper femoral cortex and control of stem subsidence have beneficial effects[70]: collar seating substantially decreased subsidence and increased axial load to failure. In a recent study, Whiteside and Easley,[171] using collared and collarless prostheses in cadaveric femora, demonstrated the independent effects of collar and distal stem fixation in cementless prostheses. Their study concluded that achieving distal fixation minimized micromotion distally and proximally and that the collar primarily controlled the axial load transfer. A lateral toggle of the stem has been suggested as the cause of failure in most prostheses resulting from loss of proximal support by bone.[28,73,159a]

EFFECT OF DISTAL STEM FIT Distal stem fit is the most significant factor in achieving rigidity against toggle in cementless total hip prostheses.[171] It is also most effective in reducing and abolishing micromotion. Although a collar cannot prevent distal micromotion, a well-fixed distal stem can. In their study, Whiteside and Easley[171] demonstrated that the cylindrical distal portion of the stem allows a distal tight fit to control side-to-side and front-to-back motion and that it also allows distal slippage so the prosthesis

can subside and wedge to avoid proximal stress shielding. It can be argued that a tight distal fit is only temporary (see Chapter 4) because of femoral endosteal overstressing, which can lead to bone absorption, or because of the expansion that results from aging. However, changes in bone caused by an optimal strain about the distal stem (either a neocortex or thickening of the bone in that region of the femur) may cause the medullary canal to narrow and thus improve its fixation. Also, critics question a tight permanent distal fit because of the possibility of unloading of the proximal femur, causing stress shielding in that region (Fig. 6-52).[10]

SURGERY AND FILL AND FIT Surgical preparation of bone is aimed at sculpting the bone to the shape of the prosthesis to produce maximum contact. As noted previously, because of the nonlinear relationship of metaphyseal and diaphyseal sizes, a single design for a broach cannot accommodate all femurs. Because vertical and torsional forces can be significantly reduced by proximal intramedullary fill and fit and because stabilization of the stem depends upon a proximal and distal load transfer, proximal and distal fit are essential[86,166] (Figs. 6-45, 6-53, and 6-54). Engh recognized this need and the difficulties of achieving it: "Ideally the stem should fit tightly both proximally and distally with the tightest fit proximally; unfortunately, this seldom occurs."[54]

To improve fit and fill, a prefabricated anatomically curved stem (such as PCA) has been advocated by some surgeons for proximal and distal fit. Straight

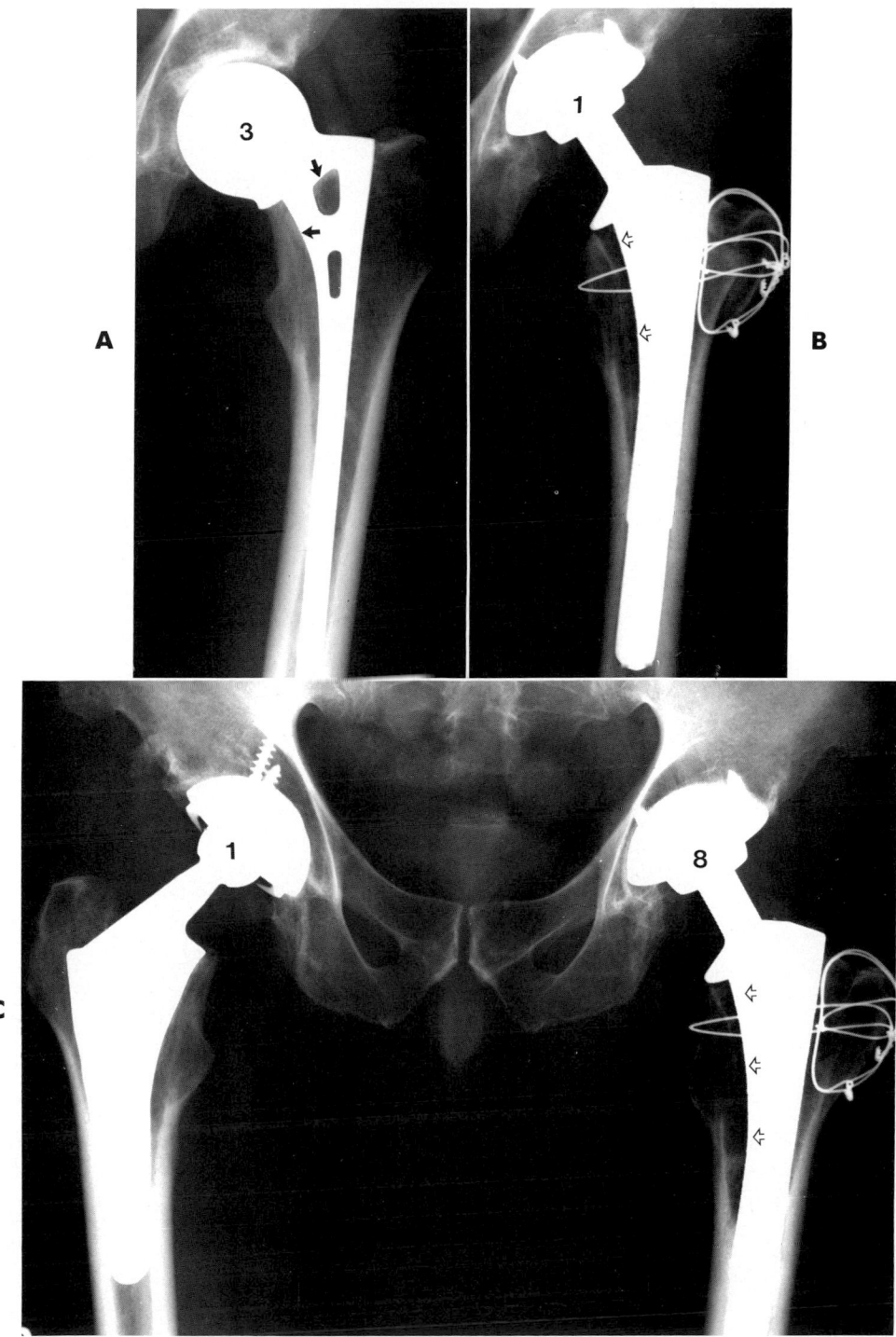

Fig. 6-52. **A,** Radiograph of 39-year-old man (F.H.) with bilateral avascular necrosis of femoral head 3 years after insertion of endoprosthesis. Grade R,3,3,3 and L,3,3,3. NOTE: only minor degrees of stress shielding caused by prosthesis. **B,** 1 year after surgery, severe bone loss *(arrows)* is caused by proximally two-third coated prosthesis (AML), and evidence of end-bearing by the noncoated segment exists. **C,** 8 years after surgery, progressive and severe osteopenia caused by abnormal load transmission is becoming a great concern to the surgeon and the patient. The hip remains without pain. The opposite hip was treated by a nonporous-coated prosthesis, customized intraoperatively by Mulier's technique (Identifit).

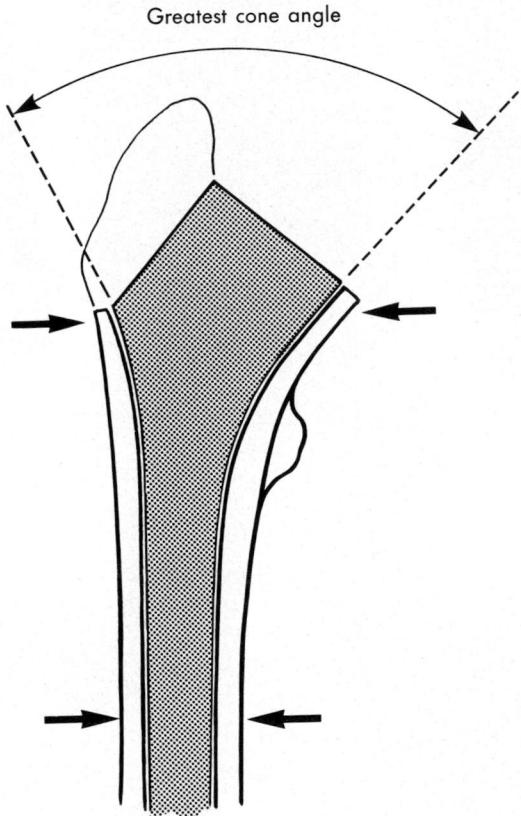

Fig. 6-53. The "greatest cone angle" idealizes the load-transfer pattern between the metaphysis and diaphysis. A nonbonded prosthesis must continuously and uniformly load the femur (proximally and distally) as a progressively converging tapered pin in a cone.

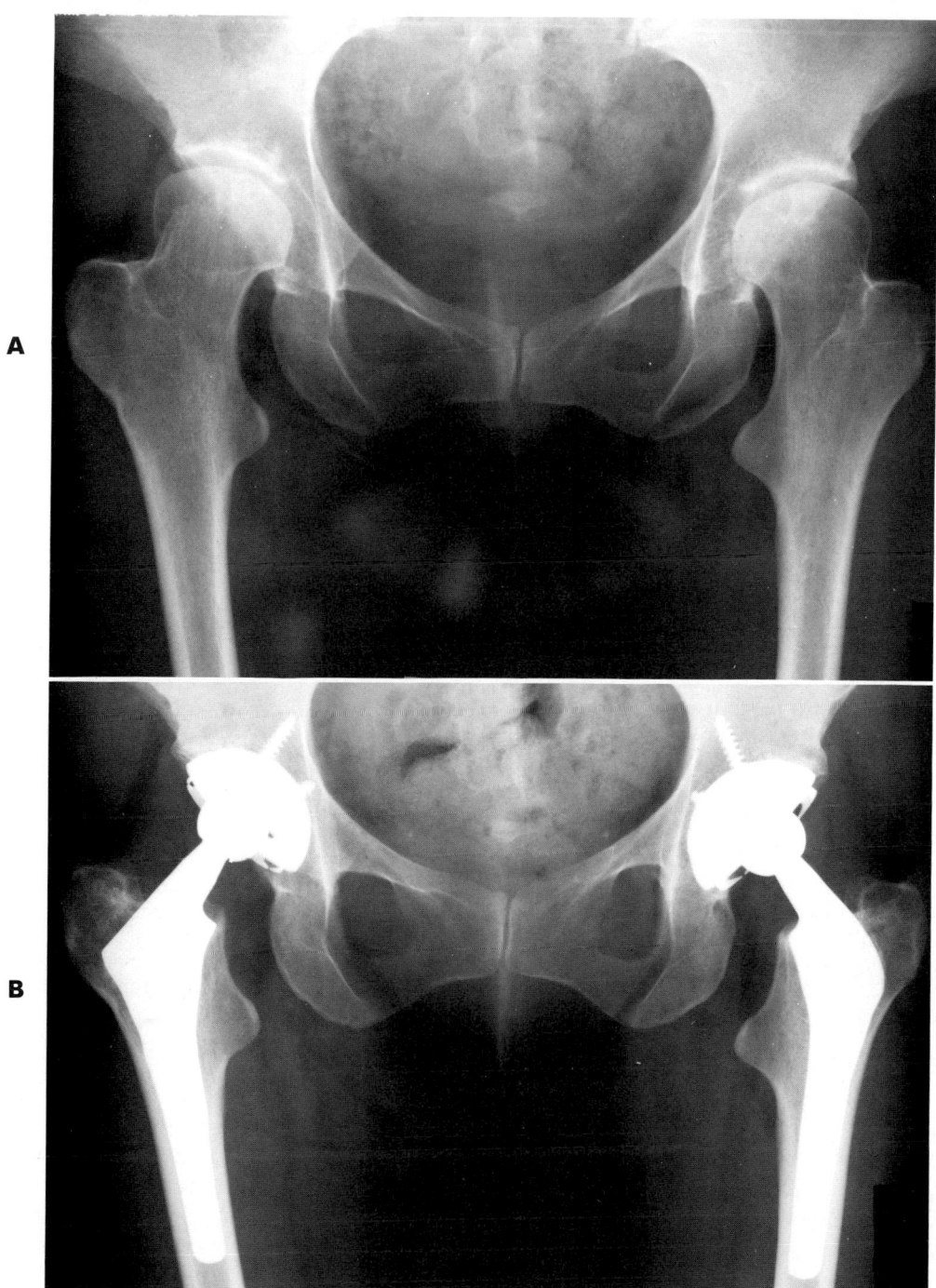

Fig. 6-54. A, Preoperative radiograph of 32-year-old female (M.T.) with bilateral congenital subluxation of the hips and status of postoperative bilateral core decompression for avascular necrosis of femoral head. **B,** 1 year after customized total hip arthroplasty. Stems were manufactured intraoperatively. NOTE: high flare index of both hips, also different shape and design of stems by intraoperative molds taken by the same surgeon on the same individual. The design of the prosthesis with a lateral flare is preferred.

Continued.

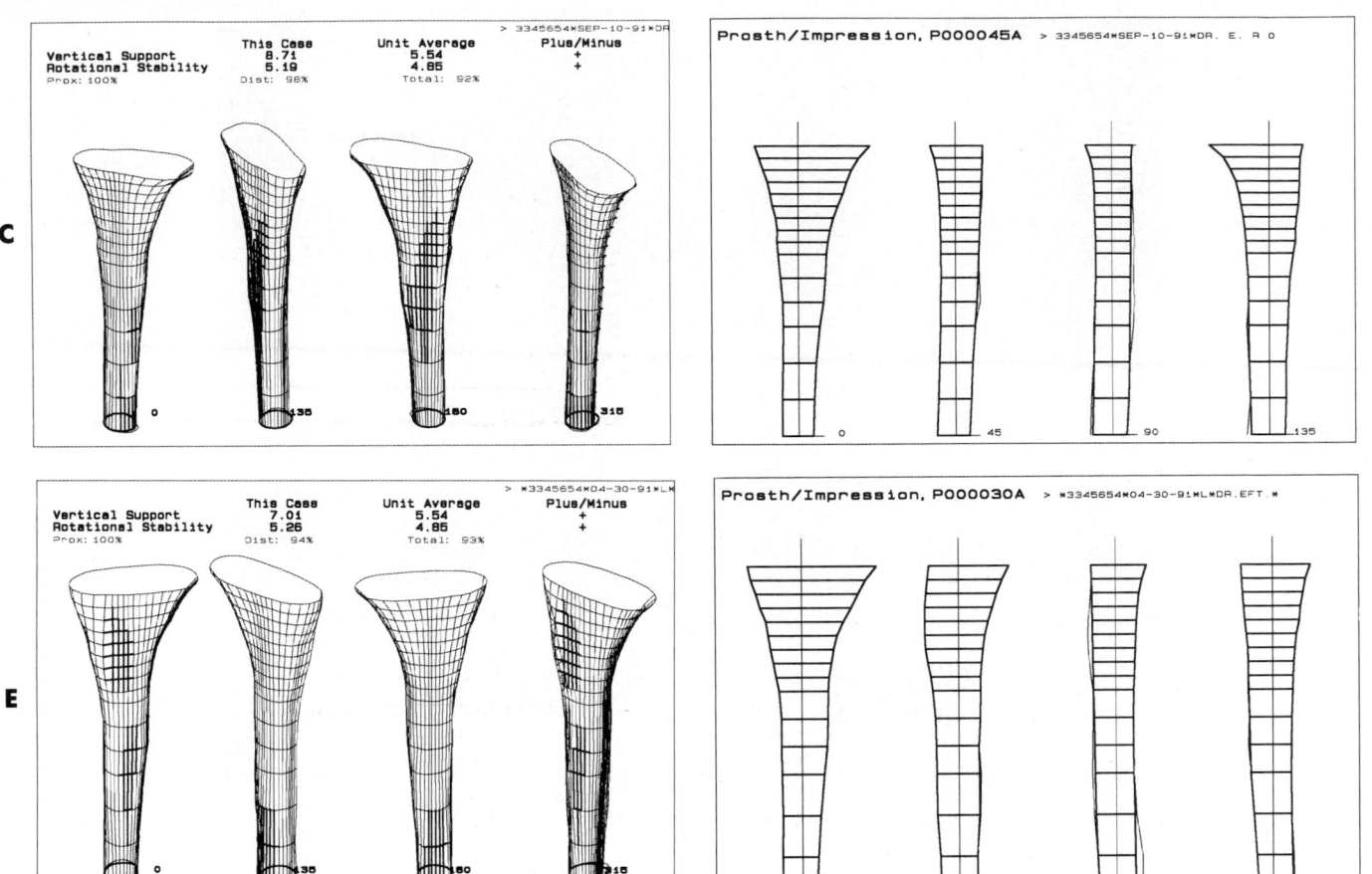

Fig. 6-54—cont'd. C, Computer printout shows design configurations and statistics related to contact, vertical support, and rotational stability of the design, comparing the latter values with the unit average at author's institution (right hip as in **A** and **B**). **D,** Prosthesis profile at 0, 45, 90, and 135 degrees of rotation (right hip as in **A** and **B**). **E** and **F,** The same as in **C** and **D**, except the left hip. NOTE: the shaded areas denote portions of the mold to be deleted because of reentrants, a procedure that is necessary to allow insertion and extraction of the prosthesis without risking a fracture.

reamers are used to prepare the diaphysis, and broaches are used to produce maximum contact between bone and stem in the metaphyseal region of bone. However, without some degree of mismatch between the tapered metaphysis and the more cylindrical diaphysis, insertion might be impossible without fracturing the bone.

Other surgeons advocate a nonanatomical straight stem to enhance initial fixation (AML prosthesis). Here again, the difficulty is to achieve a perfect fit proximally and distally. By using a straight stem in the curved femur, it certainly is possible to achieve the initial fixation via a three-point fixation (Fig. 6-55). However, the contact areas between the stem and bone seemingly are small, and overreaming provides only modest improvement. To improve fit and fill in straight stems, it is often necessary to alter the level of the neck resection by shortening the femur and removing the widest portion of the metaphysis (Fig. 6-56). A longer neck prosthesis adds length and stability for the hip. This practice contradicts principles of biomechanical fixation, since the uppermost portion of the femur produces the greatest resistance against rotation (Fig. 6-57). A near-perfect fill and fit only achievable by intraoperative customization proximally and distally is demonstrated in Fig. 6-58.

FIT AND FILL VS. MATERIALS The criteria for selecting the materials with which to manufacture the stem include strength, corrosion resistance, and biocompatibility. All three metals (stainless steel, chromium and cobalt, and titanium alloy) used in manufacturing total hip prostheses meet these criteria (see Chapter 4). The stiffer materials, such as chromium and cobalt alloy and stainless steel, are favored for use with cement; the stiffer metal increases stress within the stem but decreases stress in the cement mantle. On

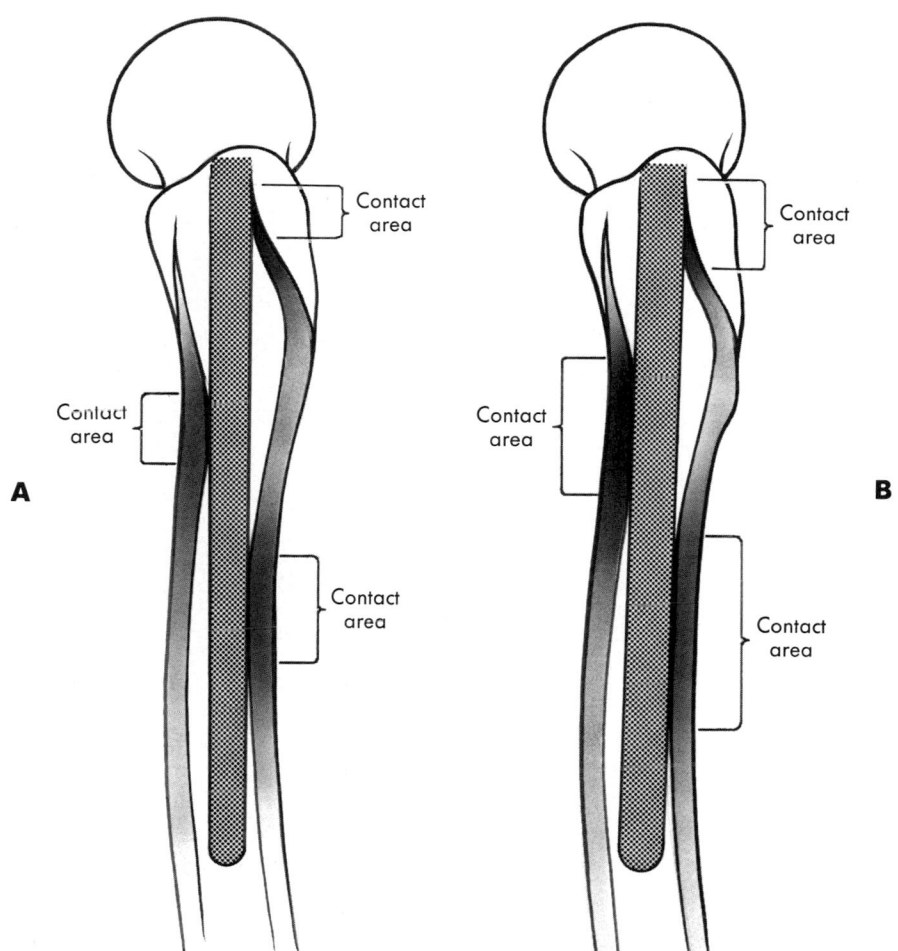

Fig. 6-55. Paradox of fill and fit. **A,** Nonanatomical straight stem can be fitted tightly in a curved femur by 3 points of fixation (contact). However, a fill is not possible. **B,** By expanding the three points of contact, the fill can be improved only by a modest amount, but a complete fill cannot be achieved without severe damage to the femur (modified from Engh CA: Instructional manual, 1989.)

the other hand, cementless devices require materials with a reduced modulus of elasticity to reduce stresses from surrounding bone. Reducing the modulus of elasticity (thus the stiffness of the prosthesis) is especially important in the large-caliber prostheses commonly used in large and heavy individuals, because the stiffness increases with the diameter of the femoral stem. Unfortunately, even a low-modulus metal, such as titanium, may not be of sufficiently low modulus of elasticity to protect the bone from stress during a normal remodeling process. Both chromium and cobalt and newer process stainless steel (high nitrogen content stainless steel [Ortron]) are acceptably corrosion resistant. Because of their structural density, titanium and its alloys depend significantly upon surface treatment, such as anodization processes (see Chapter 4). It remains unknown whether micromotion

occurs between bone and cement in a nonbonded stem; it could be damaging to the surface of a titanium alloy. Transmission electronmicroscopy of pure titanium has revealed mineralized osteoid directly on the surface of titanium.[1,177,178] A high tensile and shear strength at the junctional tissue between the bone and the titanium surface has been observed as an indication of mechanical bonding.[157] The relative geometrical shape and size and the role played by the surface reattachment of the bone to the prosthetic surface remain to be verified. Similarly, alternative methods and composite materials to manufacture the stem deserve investigation.

Fixation by Adhesives

Prosthetic fixation with adhesives appears to have several drawbacks: the "glue" must be partially water-

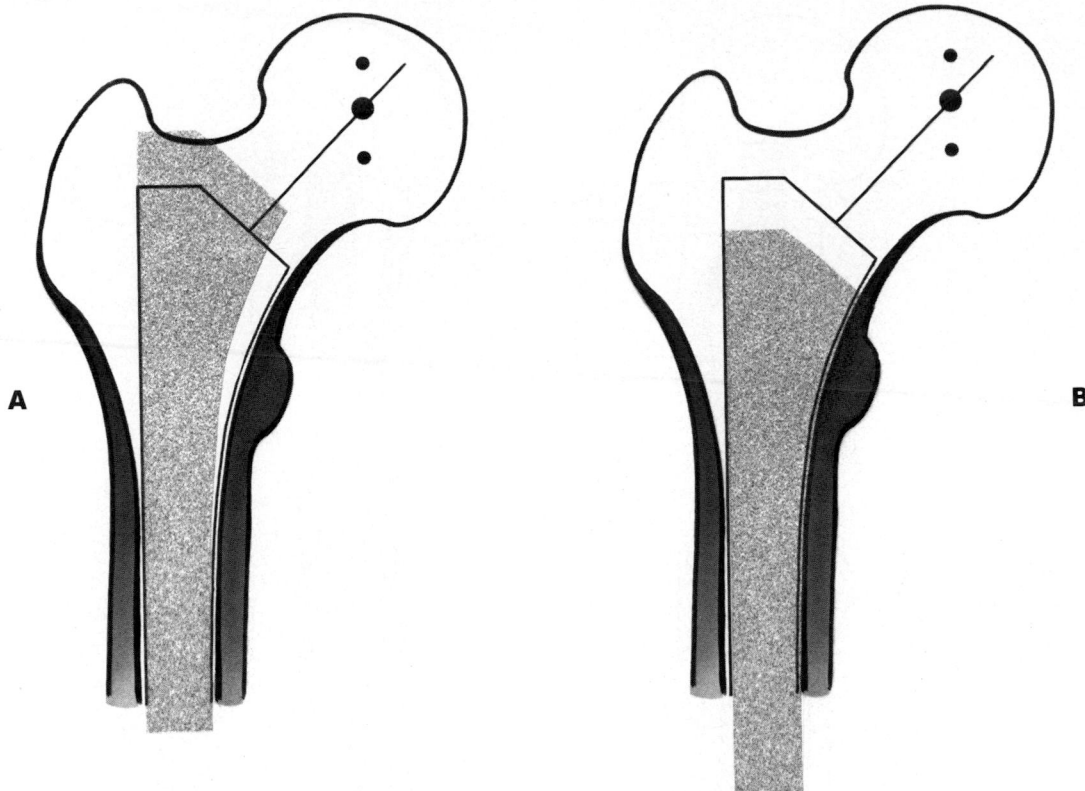

Fig. 6-56. Paradox of fit and fill proximally and distally. **A,** Proximally well-fitted prosthesis distally (diaphysis) may prevent insertion of the tapered segment. **B,** Insertion of both metaphyseal and diaphyseal portions of prosthesis may be only realized if the femoral neck is further sacrificed and a narrow stem for a distal fit is selected. This leads to a tight fit proximally and a loose fit distally (modified from Engh).[54]

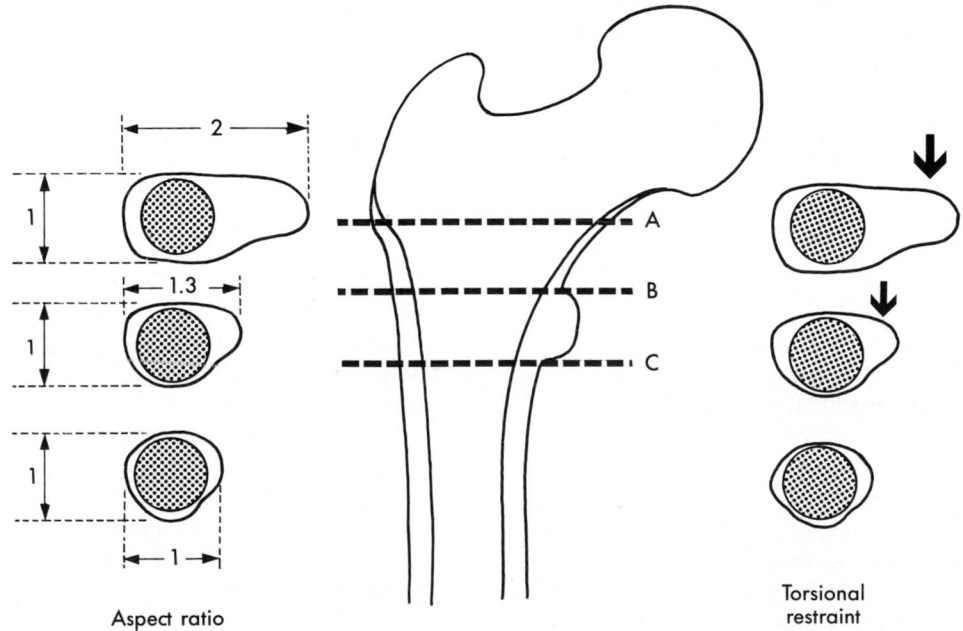

Aspect ratio

Torsional restraint

Fig. 6-57. Maximum rotational stability can be achieved by cutting the neck of the femur as high as possible. *A* to *C* demonstrate a progressive reduction in torsional resistance and compressive forces as the aspect ratio decreases.

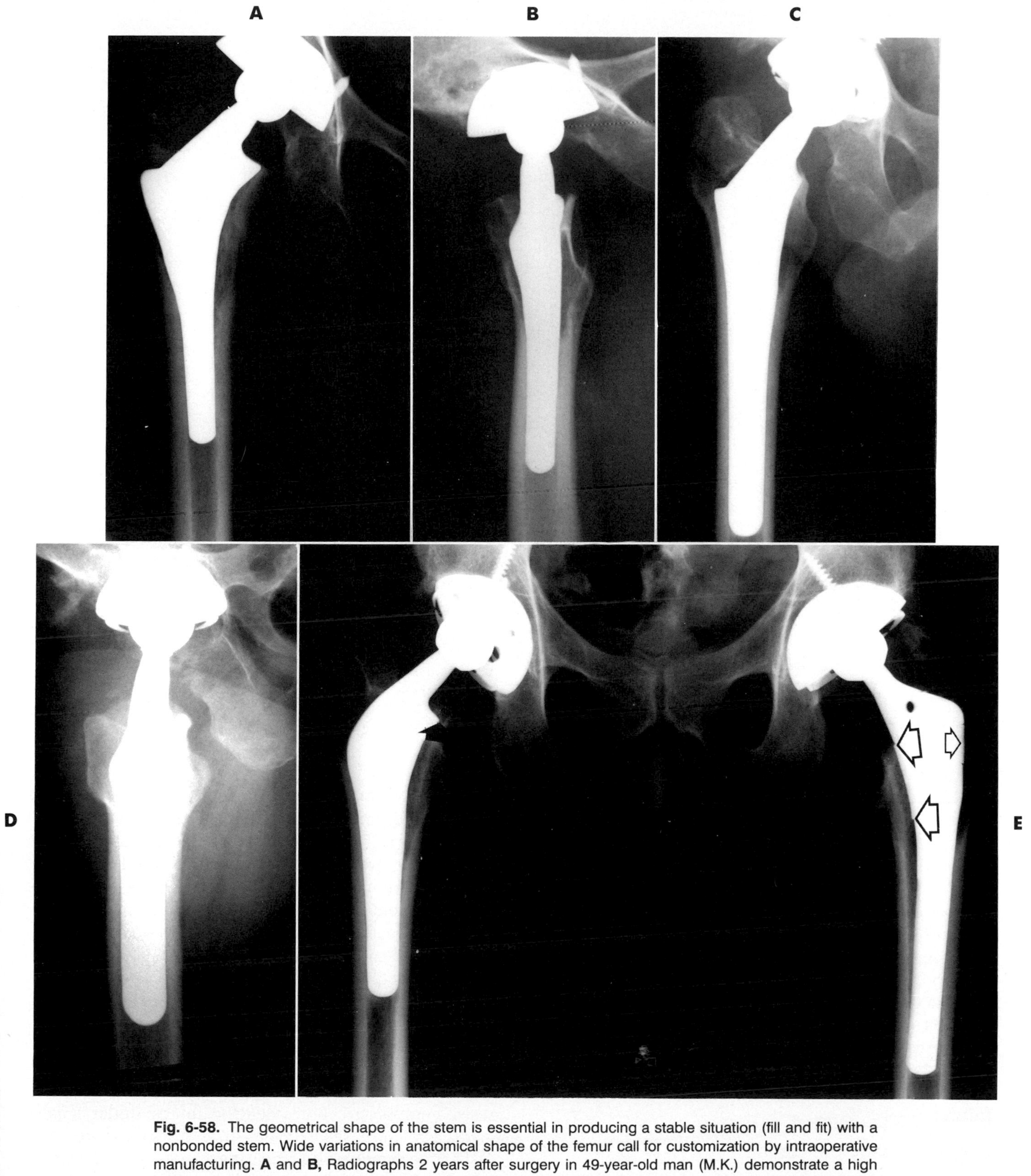

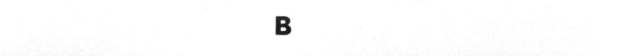

Fig. 6-58. The geometrical shape of the stem is essential in producing a stable situation (fill and fit) with a nonbonded stem. Wide variations in anatomical shape of the femur call for customization by intraoperative manufacturing. **A** and **B,** Radiographs 2 years after surgery in 49-year-old man (M.K.) demonstrate a high Noble's femoral index (champagne flute). **C** and **D,** Radiographs 2 years after surgery in 51-year-old man (E.R.) with a low femoral index (stovepipe) demonstrate an excellent fit and fill of the stems. Both hips score 6,6,6. Both patients weigh over 120 kg. **E,** A small amount of subsidence in a nonbonded stem may occur and is compatible with good clinical results (*right hip, solid arrow*), whereas a well bonded proximally coated stem may not prevent thigh pain. This patient, a 35-year-old man (S.B.) who weighs 80 kg and is extremely active, prefers the nonbonded stem (*right*) and has intermittent pain (*let*), despite evidence of osteointegration (*hollow arrows*). Hip scores B: right 6,6,6 and left 5,6,6.

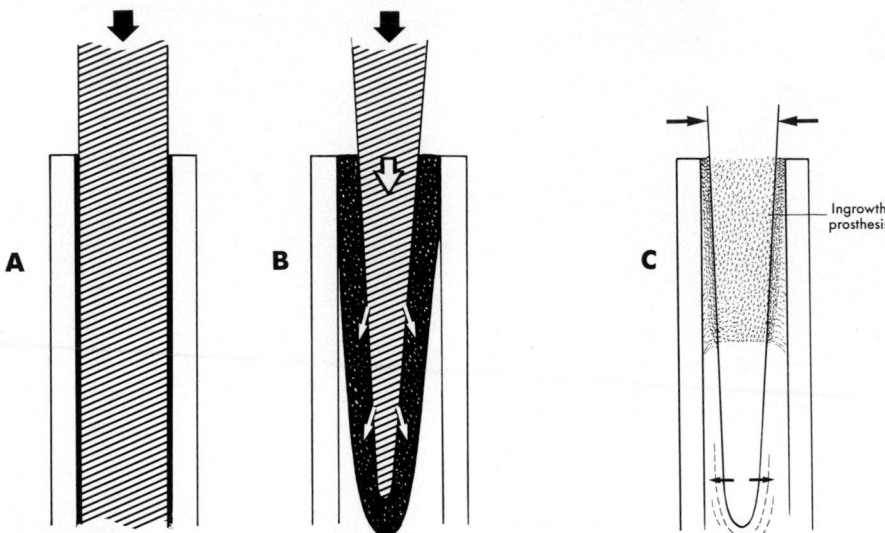

Fig. 6-59. Comparative mechanism of fixation by glue, **A,** and by grouting materials, **B. A,** Adhesive mating parts must be tightly conjoined with thin layer of adhesive between them. When grouting material such as acrylic cement is used, cavity is broached oversized and filled with doughlike material that makes accurate cast or mold of rough interior surface of bone. Thus inserted prosthesis acts as an integral part of cement, that is, "cement-prosthesis unit." Increased external surface area and greater resistance against compressive and shearing forces can be achieved, **B. C,** Proximal bonding (by ingrowth) of porous-coated surface and press-fit of distal prosthesis producing disproportional strain by varied stress in bone. Arrows indicate the relative motion distally.

soluble to allow chemical interaction between the substance and the bone; many available adhesives have allergic and toxic effects that prohibit their use; and adhesive mating parts must be tightly conjoined with a thin layer of adhesive between them, but the variation in sizes of human bones makes it impossible to mate the prosthetic and bone surfaces precisely (Fig. 6-59, *A*). Progressive chemical interaction would ultimately end in absorption of the adhesive material. Living osseous tissue would replace or insulate the adhesive with fibrous tissue, causing the chemical bond to fail. Some experiments currently in progress suggest that materials known as *bioglasses,* which form a direct bond to both soft and hard tissues, will be used in the future.

Acrylic Cement for Fixation

Cemented fixation, in contrast to glue, involves interposing an inert material (such as quick-setting acrylic cement) in bulk between the two parts, where it acts as a "grout" or "filler." This method involves no chemical interaction between the cement and the bone. A thin layer of fibrous acellular-like base membrane or fibro-

cartilaginous membrane ultimately acts as a weight-bearing medium. The biological characteristics of this interposed layer may be altered by load bearing, but as long as the fixation is optimal between bone and cement, it remains noninvasive (Fig. 6-59, *B*). With acrylic cement, the bone cavity does not have to be shaped perfectly to accommodate the prosthesis; instead, it is broached "oversize" and then filled with the doughlike cement, which makes an accurate cast or mold of the rough interior of the bone. The inserted prosthesis acts as an integral part of the cement, forming a cement-prosthesis unit and increasing the total surface area of the cement (exterior). The larger surface area of the cement-prosthesis unit can better resist compressive and shearing forces under axial loads. The increased external surface area and greater resistance against the shearing forces are ideal in treating elderly patients with severe osteoporosis. Undoubtedly, because of differences in the moduli of elasticity of bone and prosthesis (including cement), there must be a relative movement (no matter how minuscule) between the cement and bone. When fixation of the cemented stem is nonuniform, it causes

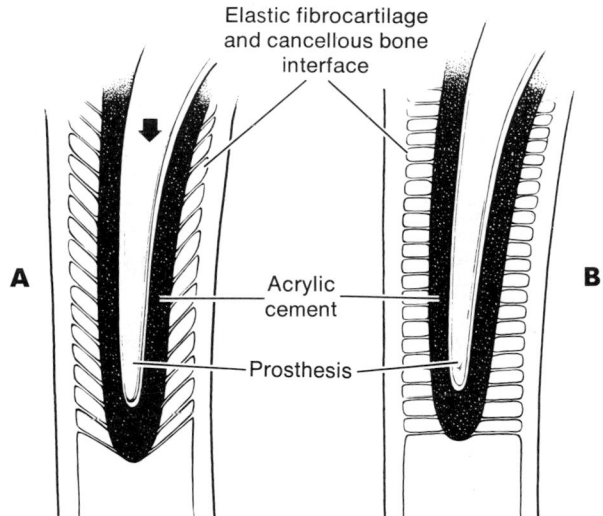

Elastic fibrocartilage
and cancellous bone
interface

Acrylic
cement

Prosthesis

A

B

Fig. 6-60. Elastic fibrocartilaginous bone layer works intimately at interface to produce excellent medium for transmission of load when cement is used. Successful fixation via such a medium will be permanent providing it acts as elastic system at that level allowing only controlled motion under, **A,** loading and, **B,** unloading. Energy must be dissipated in viscoelastic elements of interface or it will destroy bone. **A,** Schematic drawing of elastic behavior of loaded prosthetic cement interface. **B,** The recoile (system unloaded).

a nonuniform pattern of stress distribution (Fig. 6-59, C). However, the amplitude of the movement (coupled with the elastic behavior of the layer of bone) is of such a small degree that it has no deleterious effects (fretting) on the bond (Fig. 6-60). The rough exterior of the "cement-prosthesis unit" might be expected to rasp against the rough interior surface of the bone. This does not occur, however, because the vertical and shearing stresses are neutralized by the very intimate "keying" of the direct bone-cement contact or by the fibrous layer filling the space between the two (see Chapter 4).[24,30] Regardless of the type of tissue present at the interface (fibrous or metaplastic cartilage), thin or thick, the bone remains intact because there is no firm attachment between the two parts. Fig. 6-60 illustrates how the elastic behavior of the interface allows recoiling after force is released in a nonconfined space.

The role of fixation via cement has many advantages:

1. It increases the total contact zone between the prosthesis and bone, improving stress distribution from the prosthesis to the bone.
2. Compressive stresses, which approximate the failure limits of compressive bone strength, are considerably reduced.
3. Fretting—the cause of progressive implant loosening—is minimized when cement is used.
4. The elastic bone, bony trabeculae, and fibrous or cartilaginous tissue are excellent mediums for

transmitting a load—providing it acts as an "elastic system" at that level, allowing only "controlled motion" between cement and bone (see Fig. 6-60).

Unless peak energy is dissipated in viscoelastic or elastic elements (dampening effect), it will destroy the bone. The principle is analogous to the use of periodontal ligament to fix a tooth in the bone. The major drawback to cement is that it requires a strict and perfect technique of application at the time of insertion: the bond must be perfect, or the procedure will fail. The bony support must also be adequate to withstand the compressive forces transmitted to it via the cement. Once loosening is initiated, it leads to further bone damage and further loosening, and nonoperative means do not usually improve the fixation adequately.

Optimum Cement Mantle

Based on the available information, osteolysis is commonly attributed to the cement in the femur in conjunction with total hip arthroplasty; it results largely from the surgeon's creation of a defective cement mantle, rather than from failure of the cement. There is ample documentation of cement mantle deficiencies caused by inadequate cement, allowing direct contact between the prosthesis and bone, or malpositioning of the femoral component with resultant elimination of cement from the load-bearing areas of the femur. In one series, 76% of the femurs with a poor cement mantle developed osteolysis.[83] The inherent strength of the cement mantle depends on (1) the strength of the PMMA, (2) the geometry of the cement mantle, which relates largely to the geometry of the stem, and (3) the magnitude and pattern of stress distribution.

Although the strength of PMMA can be improved to some extent (see Chapters 4 and 5), the greatest strength of this method of fixation derives largely from the geometry of the cement mantle. Several clinical and biomechanical studies indicate that the optimum cement mantle is nonuniform, providing strength proximally and medially, distally, and laterally.* It has been suggested that minimal cement stresses occur proximally when the stem occupies from 80% to 90% of the canal and distally when the cavity is filled 70% to 80% with the stem. The ratio of cement thickness to stem cross-section is a compromise to keep the stem strong enough while leaving a minimum cement mantle of about 2 mm for load transfer.[117] While more information is needed to elucidate fully the ideal shape and thickness of the cement mantle, less that 2 mm of

---

*References 15, 86, 117, 151, 163.

cement mantle appears (based on retrospective clinical studies) to coincide with severe bone resorption resulting from fragmentation of the cement, especially in the region of calcar femorale.[15,151,163] Clearly, the geometrical shape of the cement mantle is largely determined by the size and design of the prosthesis and the shape of the femur. The proximal and distal location of the stem in the prepared medullary canal is also a factor in selecting the appropriate thickness for the cement mantle, both proximally and distally. For this reason, proximal and distal stem centralization is of paramount importance, as are the cross-sectional stem size and shape (see Chapters 15 and 19).

Fixation of the Stem by Porous Coating
Comparison of Strain Patterns

Huiskes, using a two-dimensional finite element model, studied load-transfer mechanisms and stress patterns of smooth, press-fitted, cemented, and ingrowth (fully and proximally) stems in total hip arthroplasty.[86] In testing for the effect when identical prostheses were inserted with and without cement, modeled with equal bone properties and loading characteristics, they reached the following conclusions:

1. The load-transfer mechanism was similar in ingrowth and cemented prostheses, but differed dramatically for press-fit designs.
2. In prostheses with fixation by cement or ingrowth (bonded configurations), interface concentrations occurred on the proximal and distal portions; the stress values depended on the stem rigidity.
3. Higher proximal stress occurred in cemented stems, while higher distal stress occurred in noncemented stems. In nonbonded (press-fit) stems, the interface stresses were affected more by the geometrical shape of the stem than by rigidity.
4. The researchers estimated that titanium would produce a more favorable stress pattern in noncemented prostheses and that chromium-cobalt-alloy would be more effective in cemented varieties.
5. Quantitatively, cortical stress shielding can be caused by all stems, especially in the calcar region.
6. Quantitative measurements differ distinctly in the three modes of fixation: severest in the fully ingrown prosthesis, less so in the partially ingrown, and even less with cemented stems.
7. Prostheses fastened to the bone only by press-fit cause calcar stress shielding and provoke greater stresses than those occurring naturally in the cortex at the stem zone.

Walker and colleagues analyzed the strain pattern produced in the femur by an off-the-shelf exactly fitting titanium stem.[166,167] In strain studies, they reported that bone strains in uncemented components were closer to normal than in smaller cemented components of the same design[167]; calcar strains averaged 56% of normal with uncemented, compared to 30% with cemented components. They also concluded that micromotion was slightly greater in cementless than in cemented controls.

BIOMECHANICAL BASIS OF PROSTHETIC DESIGN
Design for Use with Cement

The Charnley low-friction arthroplasty stem was designed to overcome mechanical failures resulting from the use of other prostheses. For example, the original flat-back design derived from the Austin-Moore and Thompson prostheses was modified to a round-back design and then further improved with an additional flange design (Cobra) to enhance load transfer to the cement. Later the femoral head offset was reduced from 45 to 40 degrees, and Ortron (high-nitrogen-content stainless steel) was introduced (see Chapter 11).

The second generation of Charnley stems, which have additional metal on the lateral surface of the stem and an additional dorsal flange to the round back, were considered a significant improvement in cemented stem designs. By the early 1980s most total hip prosthesis designs had adopted a straight, tapered configuration for the stem; larger caliber prostheses were introduced to reduce the incidence of stem fracture. In most cases, improved metallurgical processes and a better choice of metals accompanied the improvements in design. It is important to analyze these factors because the longevity of the replaced hip depends on the stress distribution throughout the prostheses, cement, and hip. Finite element analysis using computer technology to develop data provides helpful predictive values and aids in the manufacture of total hip devices, but the criteria used are often unrealistic; thus, keep in mind that the results obtained by these methods are only as accurate as the proposed model and its limitations.[98]

Geometrical Stem Shape for Use with PMMA

Adhering to the fundamental principles involved in the fixation of cemented prostheses depends on the following factors: (1) the magnitude and pattern of load applied to the upper femur via the femoral prosthesis; (2) the geometry of the prosthesis, which determines the distribution of the load; and (3) the mechanical strength of the cement supporting the prosthesis and thus transferring the load to the upper femur.

To optimize the design, consider four factors:

1. Protect the cement (which is the weakest element in terms of its mechanical properties) by reducing critical stress and keeping cement under compressive forces. Provide a large surface area on the metal transferring the load to prevent splitting of the cement mantle.
2. Promote maximum load transfer to the upper femur via the strong bony trabecula and cortex of the medial neck and calcar femorale.
3. Retain a sufficiently thick and uniform mantle in the areas that are highly stressed by the design of the prosthesis and bone preparation.
4. The magnitude and pattern of loading of PMMA mantle can be significantly improved by modifying its geometry and cross-sectional shape.

Clinical experience supporting this hypothesis is in accord with analytic three-dimensional finite element analysis (Fig. 6-61),[40,106] demonstrating that loss of proximal support is the most common cause of fixation failure. Loss of this support can also cause the stem to fracture.[28] The loss of proximal bone support usually results from excess stress, but it may also result from stress shielding if the bone of the upper femur has not been loaded uniformly. It is necessary to keep in mind that the medial neck must be kept optimally loaded to avert disuse atrophy. Because PMMA is stronger in compression than in tension or shear (by almost three times),[100] it is logical to keep it under constant boundary compression in the heavily loaded area of the femur. To achieve this compression, use a prosthesis design that is broader on the tension side (lateral border) than on the compression side (medial border). Such a design feature transmits compressive forces between the prosthesis and bone. This author agrees with Crowninshield that it is unwise to design a prosthesis that relies heavily on the presence of a good bond between cement and stem in areas of tensile loading in the cement. The mode and magnitude of compression and tension in the cement are affected by the cross-sectional design of the prosthesis, which can be well demonstrated mathematically by three-dimensional stress analysis[38,40] (see Fig. 6-61). The dorsal flange feature of the Charnley Cobra design[29] not only keeps medial cement under compression, but also transmits the load to the cement in front of and behind the stem and thus resists shear forces. The dorsal flange also stiffens the upper half of the prosthesis to prevent elastic deformation of the metal in compression, and it helps the cement-bone interface in the critically heavily loaded upper femur while the hip is being loaded in flexion in activities such as standing from a sitting position or stair climbing, which load the hip heavily.

Dimensional Size and Length
Size

Clinical data[28] demonstrate a positive correlation between the patient's weight and fatigue fracture of the

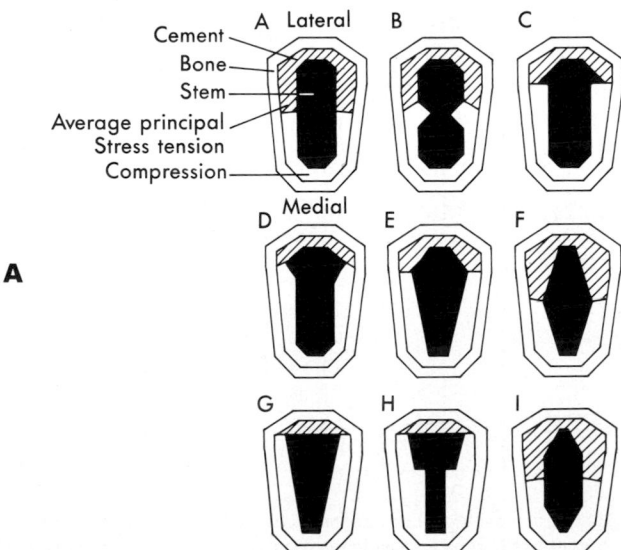

Fig. 6-61. A, The most proximal cross-section of the femur, cement, and prosthesis structure. The shaded portion of the cement represents the region of the cement within which the average principal stress is tensile, within the unshaded portion of the cement the average principal stress is compressive.

Continued.

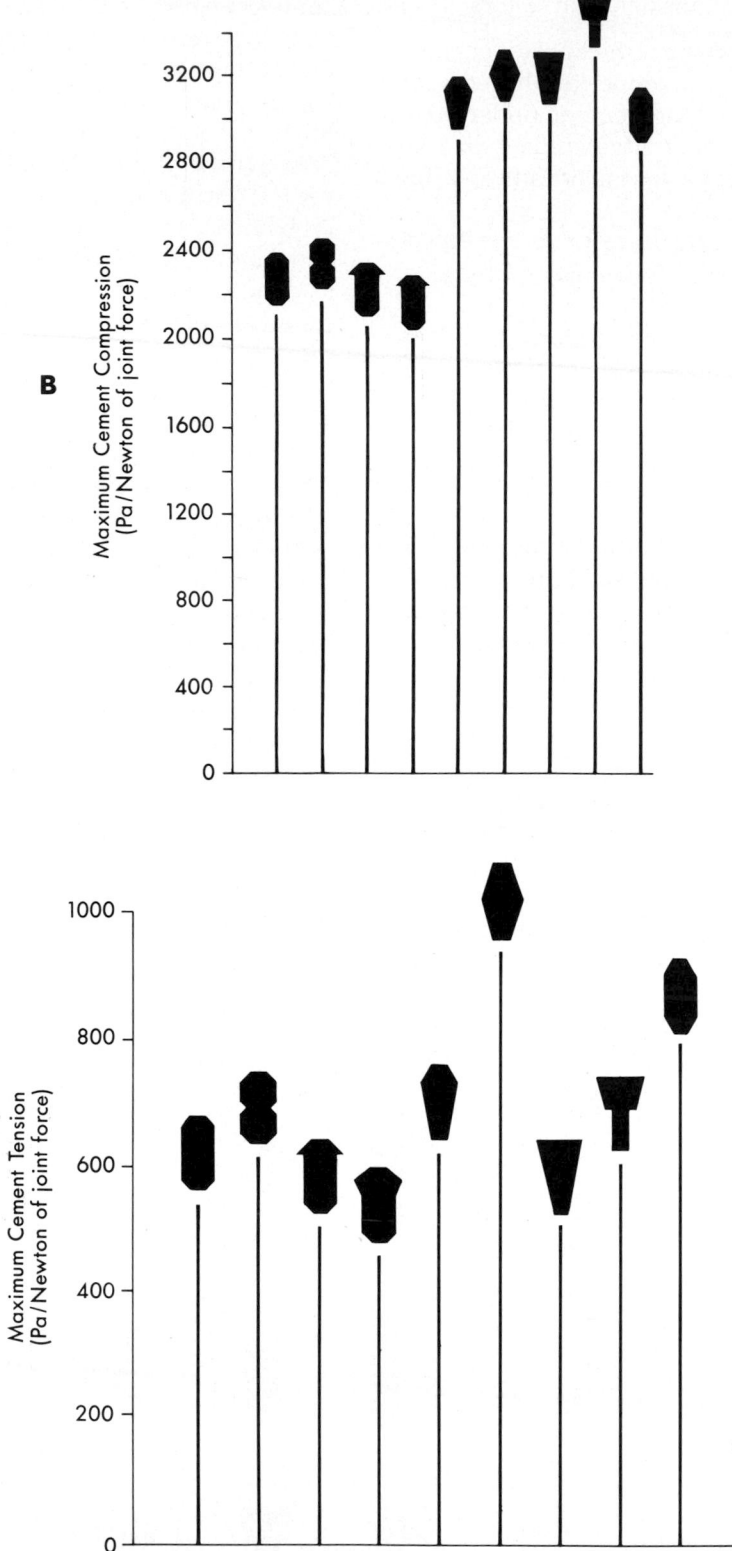

Fig. 6-61—cont'd. B, Maximum cement compression (principal stress) resulting from various stem cross-sectional shapes. Predicted stresses are within the most proximal portion of the structure and result from a one-Newton joint load. **C,** Maximum cement tension (principal stress) resulting from various stem cross-sectional shapes. Predicted stresses are within the most proximal portion of the structure and result from a one-Newton joint load. (From Crowninshield RD, Brand RA, Johnston RC, et al: The effect of femoral stem cross-sectional geometry on cement stresses in total hip reconstruction, *Clin Orthop* 146:71, 1980.

stem independent of all other factors contributing to stem failure. Stem failure also occurs more often in male patients who have achieved an excellent clinical result in function after total hip arthroplasty.[18,28]

Although ideally the size of the prosthesis could be prescribed according to the patient's weight (i.e., the heavier the patient, the stronger the prosthesis), this is not practical, perhaps because of the lack of proportionality between the size of the femur and the patient's weight. Additionally, angular deformities of the upper femur and disproportionality of the metaphysis to the diaphysis of the femur sometimes make it impossible to use the largest possible prosthesis in the heaviest patients. The normal variations in neck length, neck-shaft angle, and femoral offset in the adult femur impose additional difficulties in choosing a large caliber prosthesis for overweight and overly active patients.[34] However, the surgeon must strive to insert the largest caliber prosthesis possible, one that allows enough room to spare for the optimum use of cement and is strong enough to withstand the incumbent forces of heavy individuals. Currently a cementless stem is favored for heavy and active patients.

In striving to insert the largest stem in heavy patients, do not prejudice insertion of the prosthesis either by fracturing the femur or by eliminating the space needed for cement; to do so would prejudice femur insertion by causing direct contact of metal and bone.

In summary, to avoid fatigue fracture of the stem in heavy and active patients, the following mechanical improvements are essential:

1. Within anatomical limits, enlarge the proximal femur to accommodate the prosthesis with maximal cross-sectional dimensions. Increasing the cross-sectional dimension of the stem decreases stress in the stem and in the cement.
2. Improve proximal fixation by using a prosthetic design with a large medial and larger lateral cross-sectional dimension.
3. Produce maximum bone support for cement in the heavily loaded proximal and medial aspects of the femur.
4. Select a prosthesis with a short offset, and maintain the abductor moment arm by lateralizing the greater trochanter.
5. Use prostheses made of high-strength metals and superior surface finish to protect against fatigue cracks. Metals such as cobalt-chromium or high-nitrogen-content steel (Ortron) are preferred to titanium alloys.
6. Use vigorous and diligent technique for proper bone preparation, cement insertion, and alignment of the stem.
7. Elevate the greater trochanter when a good

exposure of the joint is not possible by a nontrochanteric route.

Length

Three-dimensional finite stress analysis suggests that increasing the length of the stem increases stress in the stem while it decreases stress in the cement.[39] This type of analysis shows the "trends" in load distribution in idealized situations. However, in vivo, the pattern of load transfer changes via a long-stem prosthesis because of the geometrical shape of the femur from metaphysis to diaphysis.

The tapered upper femur reverses as it passes beyond the isthmus (the parallel section of the diaphysis). Therefore the parallel segment of the stem does not transfer the load in the same ways to the tapered portion. As a result, the tip of the stem in the cement mantle may become end bearing, placing the cement column under tension and thus fracturing the cement mantle. Mechanically, a standard stem length (i.e., 120 to 160 mm length) seems to be adequate. Increased stem length may in fact increase relative motion between the bone and cement.

Stem Flexibility

Stem flexibility under loading conditions can be influenced by (1) the geometrical size and shape of the stem, and (2) the modulus of elasticity of the metal.

Geometrical Size and Shape of Stem

Stress analysis modeling[40] shows that stem flexibility can be influenced not only by its geometrical shape (design), but by its cross-sectional size. For example, a 20% increase in the stem's cross-sectional size decreases the maximum tensile stress in the stem by 12% and increases the compressive stress in the cement by 5%. Conversely, reducing the cross-sectional size by 20% increases the compressive stress in the cement by 3% and tensile stress in the stem by 14%. Theoretically, it can be argued that a prosthesis with large cross-sectional dimensions can help protect the cement and bone because it produces less deflection than a stem with smaller cross-sectional dimensions. The stiffness of a prosthesis of a given size and shape cannot be increased by using a metal with a greater modulus of elasticity. It can only be achieved by increasing the cross-sectional dimensions of the stem. In theory, a prosthesis made of titanium should have a larger cross-sectional dimension than one made of chromium-cobalt alloy; the modulus of elasticity of titanium is half that of chromium and cobalt.

The issue of size and elasticity also arises in the context of a thin or thick layer of cement, because the elasticity of cement is 100 times that of metal. Most authors propose using more metal (a thicker stem) at the expense of cement (a thin layer), which conflicts with the logic that a thick layer of cement (of low modulus) can absorb energy derived from stress by metal better than a thin layer of cement. Bocco, Langan, and Charnley[15] demonstrated in a radiographic study that a thick layer of cement in the region of the calcar protected the calcar 10 times better than a thin layer of cement.

Modulus of Metal

Analytical studies[39] and practical experience have suggested that lowering stem modulus reduces stress within the stem but increases it within the proximal region of the cement. However, it decreases stress within the distal cement. Conversely, using stiff metal increases stress in the stem, which also reduces stress proximally and increases stress distally. Because of the vast difference in the moduli of elasticity of metal and cement, these studies suggest that stiffer metals with greater moduli of elasticity (such as chromium and cobalt) protect cement better than more flexible metals (such as titanium).

At present, long-term results with cemented titanium are pending. To this author's knowledge, only one study, a non-double-blind, nonrandomized, and noncomparable series, has attempted to compare two stems of different size and geometry, one made of chromium-cobalt and one of titanium[152] based on radiographic performance. When a conventional Charnley 22-mm prosthesis, made of high-modulus chromium and cobalt, was compared with a "similar" 28-mm head size titanium prosthesis, the incidence of calcar absorption and distal cortical hypertrophy fell significantly, but the incidence of bone-cement radiolucency with a titanium prosthesis rose significantly. Overall, however, the straight, narrow stem of titanium performed better when compared with both the curved Charnley prosthesis of chromium and cobalt and the curved titanium prosthesis. According to Sarmiento, the fact that the overall radiographic behavior of the titanium prosthesis was better than that of the curved STH, chromium, and cobalt of the Charnley implant suggests that the geometry of the implant was a more important factor than the metallic composition.[152]

This author believes that high-nitrogen-content steel (high-strength steel) or chromium-cobalt alloy perform equally well in the biological environment when used with cement in total hip arthroplasty.

MODES OF FAILURE

Total hip prostheses are subject to three fundamental types of failure:

1. Biological failure (such as infection and sensitivity)
2. Technical failure (such as poor cement tech-

nique and poor orientation of the components)
3. Mechanical failure (such as loosening, breakage, and defective materials)

Acetabular Loosening

Earlier, we discussed the role of frictional torque in causing acetabular loosening. We suggested that, as a fundamental principle, prostheses must provide the least frictional torque possible at the bone to minimize bond failure and that a good cement technique must be used to ensure adequate and immediate fixation at surgery.[174]

If the radiological demarcation of cemented sockets can be taken as evidence of loosening of the acetabular component, a majority of hip prostheses using HDP sockets and MMA cement for fixation show evidence of loosening. In a study of 141 hips followed over periods of up to 10.1 years[47] the following results were obtained:

1. Sixty-nine percent of 141 hips showed some type of demarcation; 9.2% were thought to be progressive.
2. Radiological demarcation did not always accompany failure, but progressive migration was considered serious.
3. Thirty percent of the cases showed no demarcation even after 10 years, supporting the idea that it is possible to achieve a rigid, permanent fixation by cement.

Paying more attention to technical details can produce a better fixation at surgery, with the hope of eliminating a number of radiolucencies and, more importantly, progressive medial migration.

Recent studies on cemented socket loosening indicate that preservation of the subchondral bone of the acetabulum and the use of a pressure injection cup combined with a meticulous preparation of the acetabulum may improve in both frequency of radiolucencies and loosening of the acetabular cups (see Chapter 28).[97] Our study of the incidence and mechanism of failure of the cemented acetabular cup in various reports in the literature showed that the results vary considerably (from 3% to 32%) based on the clinical series, the type of prosthesis used, and the definitions of loosening.[48] Wroblewski[175] reported late progressive socket loosening associated with linear wear of the HDP (see Chapter 4). This mechanism of fixation failure is also associated with osteolysis and recurrent dislocation of the hip. Radiographic demarcation and loosening occurred most frequently with the use of a large (32-mm) femoral head.[64,113,141]

Generally, the mode of failure of fixation follows one of the following patterns:

1. Acute detachment of the prosthetic socket with complete dislodgement, owing to technical problems related to a poor mechanical fixation at surgery.
2. Acute interpelvic protrusion of the acetabular component (Fig. 6-62), also related to technical errors (excessive deepening or accident).
3. Chronic slow medial or upward migration of the prosthesis, possibly resulting from a technical error, but the presence of infection is also suspected.
4. Possible infection, as indicated by progressive radiological demarcation and alteration in the acetabular orientation with a history of technical difficulties.

Because the thickness of the cement used to fix the socket seems to bear no relation to the frequency of clinical fixation failure, the heat released during polymerization of the cement cannot be incriminated as a cause of loosening, nor does there seem to be any relation between the patient's weight and activities and loosening. Therefore permanent fixation without loosening can only be assured at the initial mechanical fixation by a good surgical technique and by providing a good bony support. Three technical surgical details seem to be most important:

1. Provide adequate bony surface without removing firm subchondral bone from the acetabulum.
2. Pressurize the cement at the time of fixation (Fig. 6-63), and retain cement uniformly between the cup and the bony acetabulum (Figs. 6-64 and 6-65) using a rimmed cup.
3. Provide many small irregular cavities, such as drill holes, in the subchondral bone for "keying"

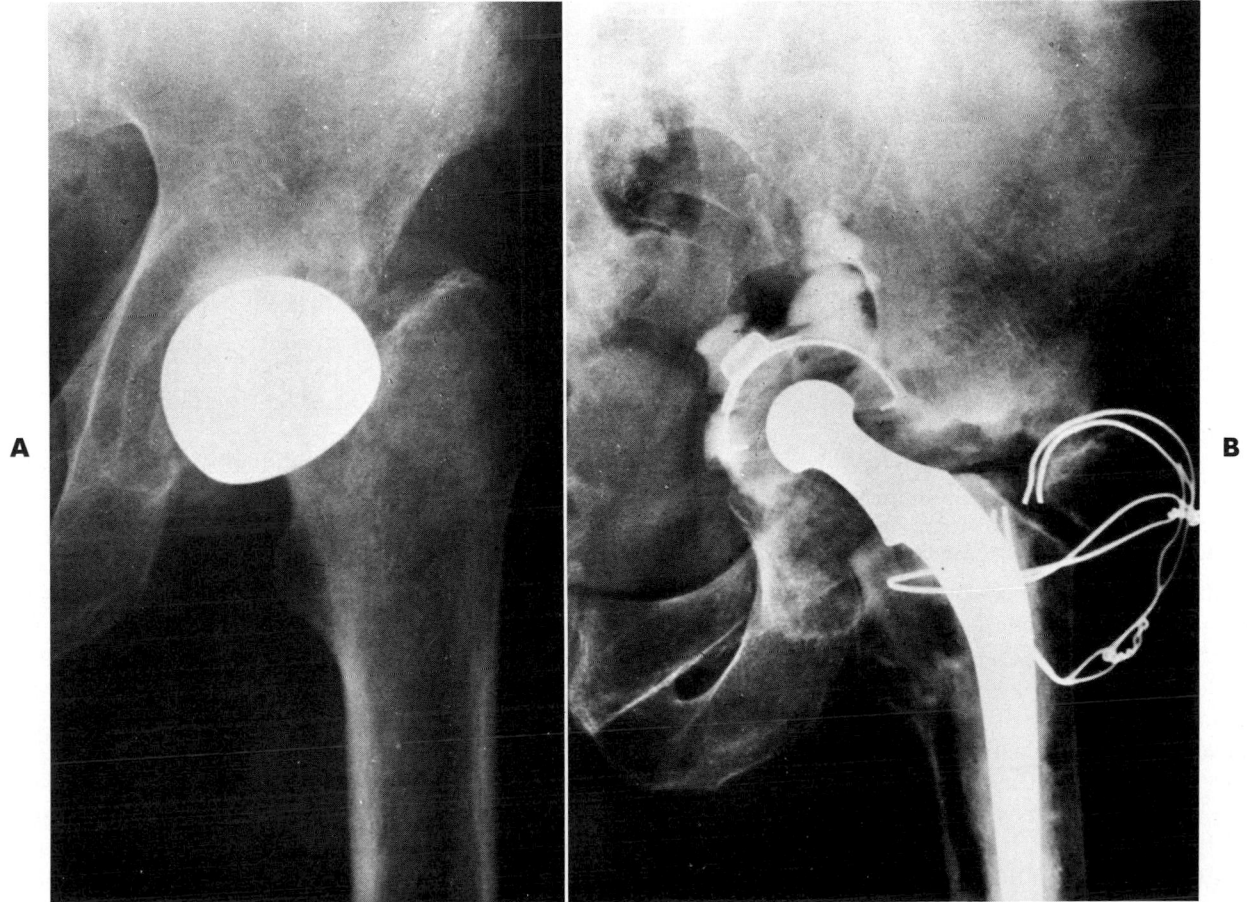

Fig. 6-62. A, Painful left cup arthroplasty originally performed for osteoarthritis in 64-year-old man. **B,** 3-month postoperative x-ray film. Excess deepening of acetabulum leads to fracture of floor, resulting in protrusion of components.

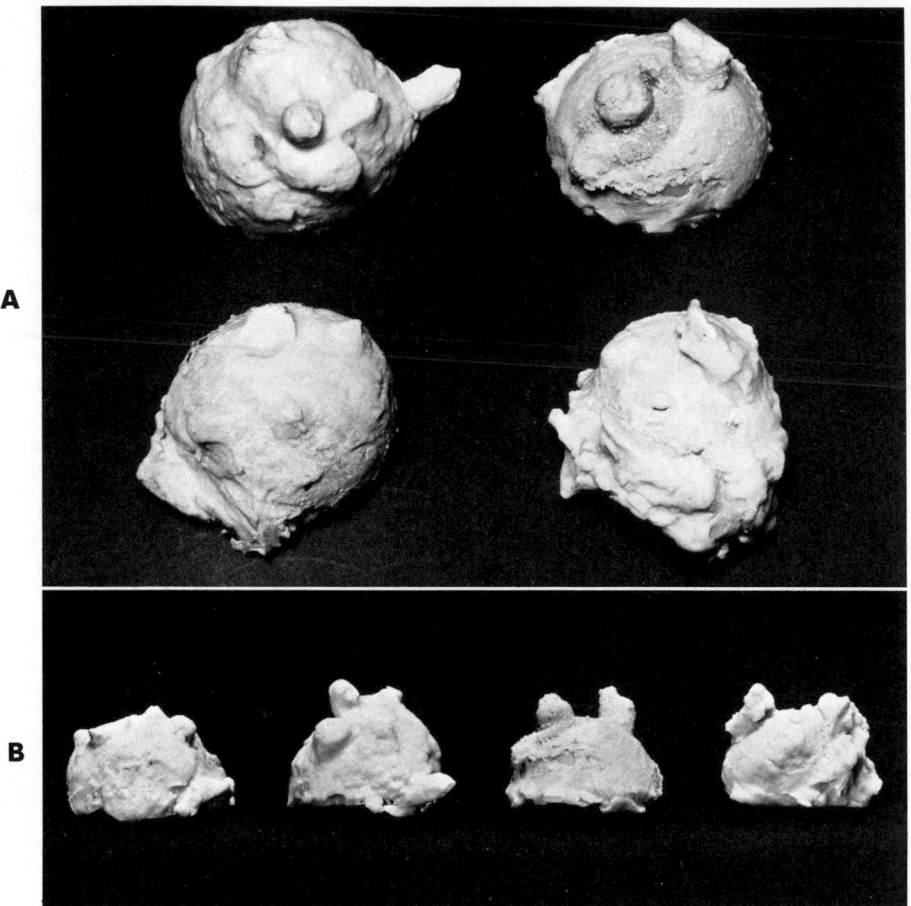

Fig. 6-63. Four failed cemented sockets removed at revision surgery probably share same common cause for loosening. Although considerable thickness of cement is present throughout sphere of acetabular component, smooth surface of exterior of cement indicates possibility of lack of pressure injection by cement or inadequate preparation of acetabulum at time of fixation. All these prostheses were metal-to-plastic type and had been inserted less than 2 years before revision surgery. NOTE: large projections of cement did not prevent loosening. **A,** Top view. **B,** Side view.

of the cement (as stated elsewhere, multiple small holes are better than a few large ones).

Mechanical Failure of the Acetabular Component

Do not dismiss the possibility of degeneration or degradation of the plastic from fatigue (similar to the fatigue of cement exposed to the internal environment under load).

Containing the socket within the acetabulum is important to prevent plastic flow and deformation; this practice contrasts with most designs of total knee arthroplasty prostheses that use unsupported HDP.

Fracture of the polyethylene cup is relatively uncommon but occurs most often in cups with a 32-mm head; it is associated with a thin acetabular cup, that is, a cup with polyethylene less than 8 mm in thickness.* A

classic example of acetabular loosening of the cemented cup arises when thin HDP is used in resurfacing when the retained femoral head requires (1) extensive expansion of the acetabulum beyond subchondral bone, (2) the use of a thin HDP cup, and (3) the use of a thin layer of cement. All of these factors cause deformation of HDP and cement under load, leading to fragmentation, wear, and foreign body response (to debris), resulting in severe osteolysis.[8] Increased acetabular stress may ultimately contribute to fracture.[81] Thick acetabular components (such as Charnley's) are subject to the same mechanical stress and ultimate fracture; the cause is excess wear and possibly degradation of the HDP (delamination), evidenced by radiographic wire marker breakage, wire marker fracture, and florid fractures.[112,164]

Metal-backed acetabular components were designed to prevent loosening. Instead, they have been associ-

---

*References 37, 75, 148, 158, 164.

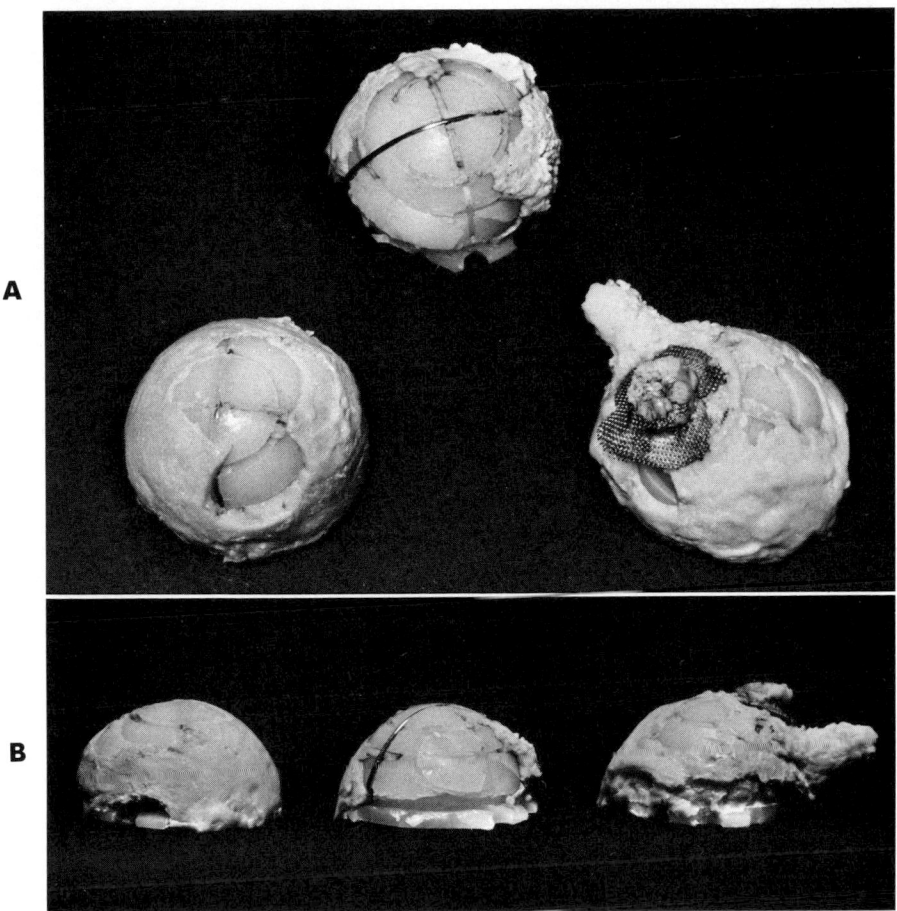

Fig. 6-64. Three loose prosthetic cups removed from patients because of loosening without evidence of infection. NOTE: absence of cement covering cups that were removed with ease at time of surgery: "poor cement technique." **A,** Top view; **B,** side view.

ated with a higher incidence of loosening in clinical practice, as stated earlier in this chapter. Fracture of the metal-backed acetabular components has been rarely reported.[35,69]

Femoral Loosening

Charnley (1969) recognized three forms of cement loosening in bone: (1) loosening of the whole cement mantle in the bone and the loss of intact interface, (2) loosening of the stem inside the cement mantle, but with cement and bone remaining intact, and (3) loosening of the cement (with fragmentation) in the proximal portion of the femur, with the distal portion of the cement-prosthesis complex remaining intact with a sound interface.

Gruen and associates[72] presented a classification of failed cement stems based on a study of radiographs of 56 total hip arthroplasties with progressive loosening. In their study they divided the femur into seven zones: 1, 2, and 3 (lateral); 4 (distal); and 5, 6, and 7 (medial).

They concluded that various mechanisms of loosening caused four modes of failure:

- { IA Pistoning: stem within cement
- { IB Pistoning: stem within bone
- II Medial midstem pivot
- III Calcar pivot
- IV Bending cantilever (fatigue)

Based on his experiences with revision in failed cement total hip arthroplasty and Gruen's classification of classes I and IV, Wroblewski regarded the stem tilt and stem-cement complex tilt as distinct entities. Additionally, Wroblewski observed that the stem complex can pivot within the cement mantle or the cement stem complex can pivot within the femur. Although developing a common language by defining and classifying the failure modes is highly desirable, this author believes two-dimensional radiographs may not be sufficient to illustrate a three-dimensional problem. For example, modes of failure related to torsional

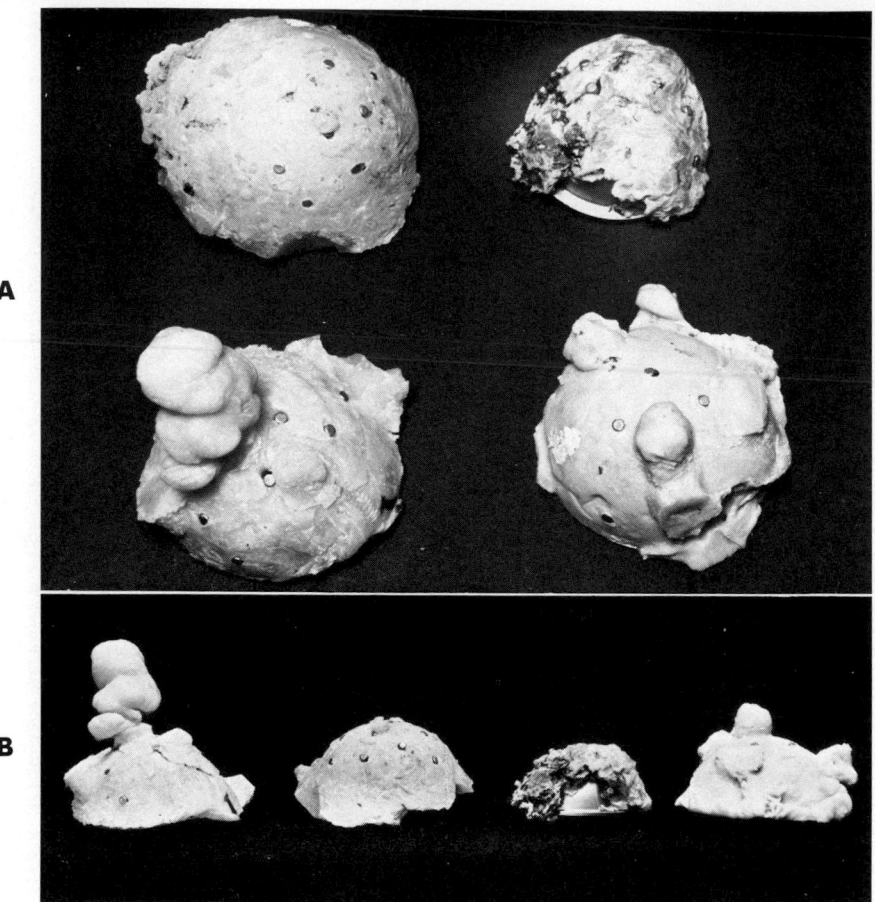

Fig. 6-65. Four acetabular cups removed because of loosening. NOTE: all four prostheses were McKee-Farrar type. Technical defect must have contributed to loosening in addition to high-frictional torque inherent in prosthesis. NOTE: studs of metal cup have protruded through cement mass, and exterior surface of cement is smooth in most areas. This indicates that metal reached bone at insertion obviating pressure injection exerted by operator onto cup. **A,** Top view; **B,** side view.

forces can contribute to failure. This can only be visualized by three-dimensional computerized modeling of the femur. In addition, fixation failures resulting from osteolysis caused by particulate debris have been largely ignored in previous classifications. This is now considered a frequent cause of failure of total hip arthroplasty (cemented or cementless) even when fixation of the prosthesis is sound (see Chapter 4).

Acrylic fractures accompanied by loosening of the femoral component can take the following forms (Fig. 6-66):

1. Subsidence of the entire prosthetic component, moving the cement mantle distally.
2. Pistoning of the stem in the acrylic core without distal migration (Fig. 6-66, *D*) of the stem in relation to the cement core.
3. Sinking of the prosthesis into the cement cone, leaving the cement cone behind; no fracture is

seen in the cement column.
4. Gradual subsidence of the stem in the cement core, fracturing the tip of the cement column without further subsidence.
5. Gradual radiological drift of the stem into a varus position, leaving a gap between the cement and the prosthesis at the convex side of the prosthesis (Fig. 6-66, *E*).
6. Proximal medial drift (migration) of the stem with rigid support distally, leading to plastic deformation or fatigue fracture of the stem produced by increased bending (such as in a cantilever beam) (Figs. 6-66, *F,* and 6-67).

Radiopaque cement allows observation of significant fractures in the cement-bone junction, but, unfortunately, standard x-ray films may not reveal microfractures when they occur; a three-dimensional appearance of the prosthesis does not show up on a single x-ray plane.

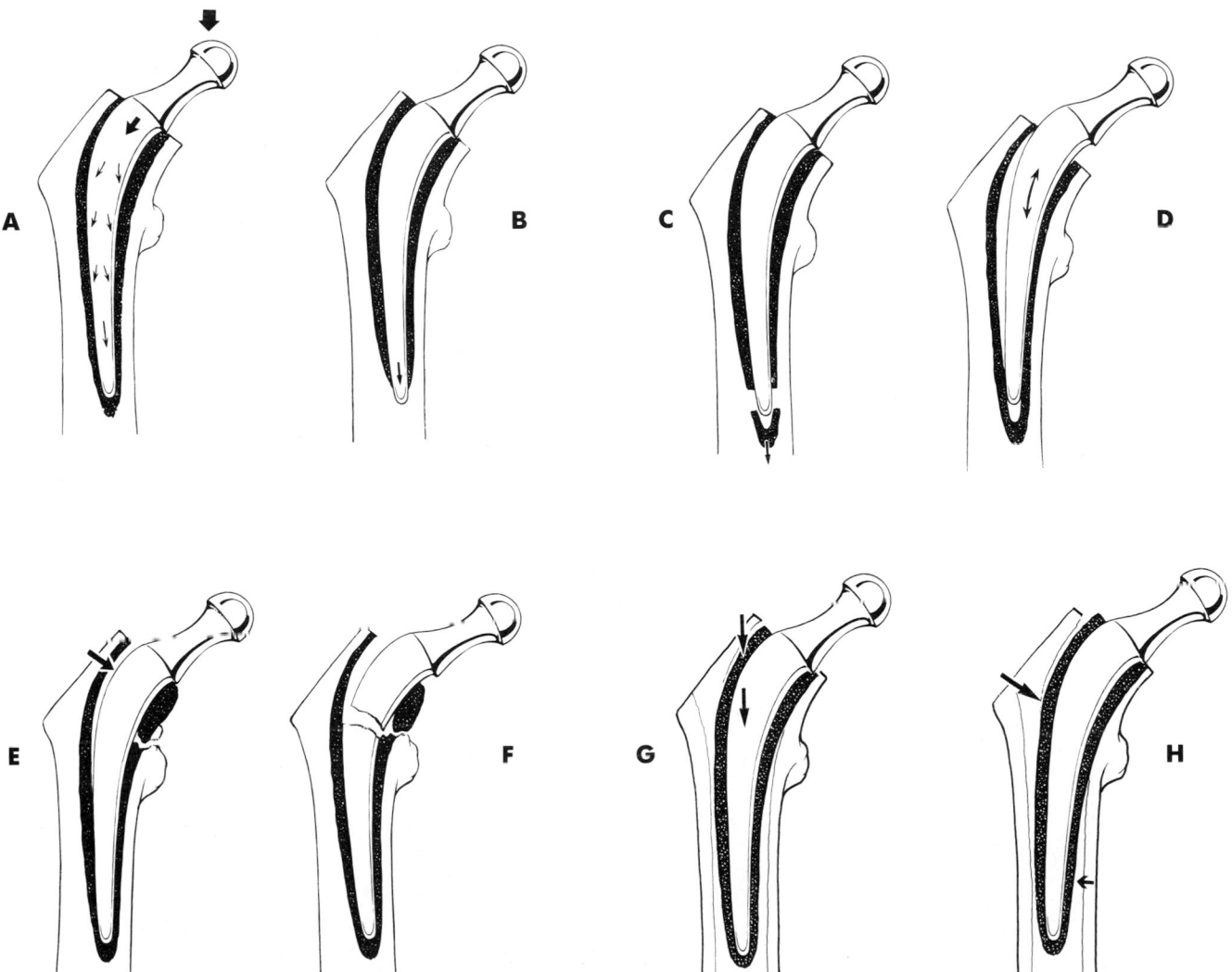

Fig. 6-66. Mode of failure of femoral fixation and stem. **A,** Compressive forces are transmitted via tapered segment of prosthesis onto cement and dissipated over large surface area of bone in this manner. Although distal end of stem conceivably may transmit load, it is far less important than tapered upper segment of stem. **B,** Possibility of minor subsidence of stem inside cement core without any consequence to fixation providing that subsidence is not severe. **C,** Gradual subsidence of stem in cement core resulting in fracture at tip of cement column, but prosthesis is stabilized in new position. This mode of failure of fixation also may remain satisfactory providing that new position of prosthesis inside core of cement is permanent. **D,** Pistoning of stem in acrylic core is possible without being manifested by x-ray films. This mode of failure of fixation is uncommon but may cause cystic erosions of bone without detection of loosening by x-ray films. **E,** Gradual radiological drift of stem into varus position may be documented by radiolucent zone appearing on convex side of upper femur *(arrow)*. This usually coincides with bone absorption or cystic changes in region of calcar. **F,** Loss of proximal fixation after bone absorption at region of calcar leading to fracture of cement. Loss of support in this region leads to plastic deformation of stem (ultimately fatigue fracture). Stem fracture is product of increased bending moment such as in a cantilever beam. Fracture can only occur if distal stem is rigidly fixed in core of cement. **G,** Subsidence of stem and cement inside femur. This type is usually seen in the large medullary canal with the use of an undersize prosthesis with a poorly pressurized cement. **H,** Tilt of stem-cement complex. Inadequate bulk filling of canal and weak bony trabeculae is responsible for this type of failure.

Continued.

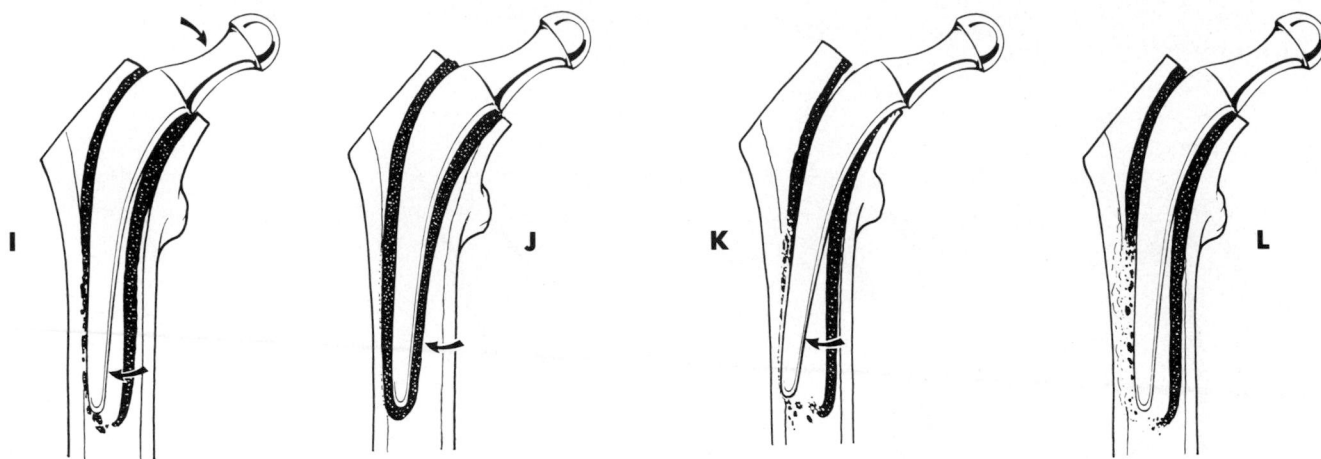

Fig. 6-66—cont'd. I, Calcar pivot shift. Stem separating from cement; breaking the lateral cement (usually thin) while the stem pivots on its medial neck. **J,** Stem-cement pivot shift. The entire stem-cement complex drifts inside the canal, usually toward the lateral cortex pivoting around the medial neck of the prosthesis. **K,** Progressive osteolysis causes bone failure as in calcar pivot shift **I. L,** Progressive osteolysis without visible radiographic evidence of loosening, migration, or fracture of cement mantle.

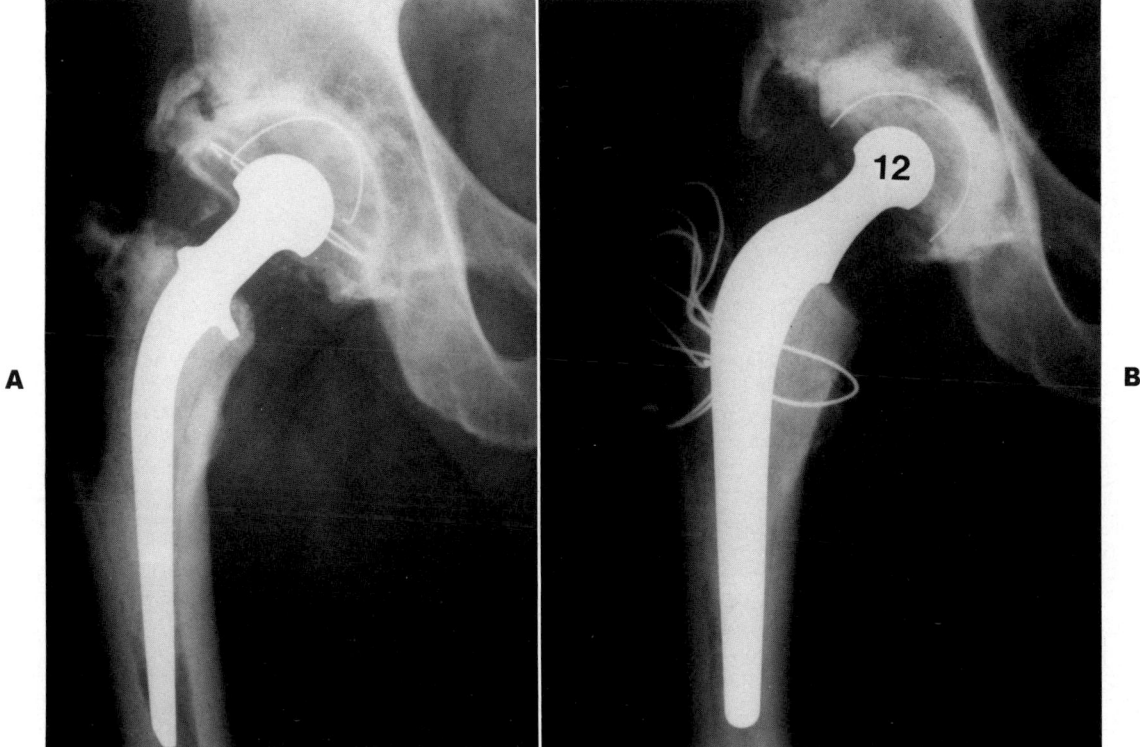

Fig. 6-67. A, Use of undersized stem (T.28) in 60-year-old "large" man (J.P.) (105 kg) failed in less than 2 years. NOTE: severe varus and lack of support for stem. Grade A-2,2,4. **B,** 12 years after revision surgery using a heavy Charnley low-friction arthroplasty. Grade 6,6,6. NOTE: centered stem with mechanical improvement of the abductor moment arm and a lowered position of the socket.

Of the several modes of failure outlined above, the type of cement column fractured at the tip seems unrelated to the inadequate bonding of the cement at the level distal to the stem tip. However, in most instances fracture of the cement column takes place early and in vigorous, healthy individuals. The following may be postulated:

1. The stem has been loose in the cement track.
2. The stem becomes "end-loaded."
3. With end bearing at the stem tip, the acrylic cement is under tension.
4. Acrylic cement is poor in tension.
5. Acrylic cement fractures at the weakest point.
6. The entire stem subsides.
7. The cement track (the whole length) again comes under compression.
8. A new position of stability is achieved.

In the mode of failure that involves radiolucency in the convex side of the stem and a varus drift of the prosthesis, the following causes may be responsible:

1. Cement shrinkage, thus pulling away from the prosthesis.
2. "Stem wobble" during insertion before full polymerization.
3. Uneven distribution of the cement in the canal, leading to fracture of a segment of cement at the lower level in the canal, allowing further subsidence by shifting the entire prosthesis medially.

The idea of cement shrinkage may be eliminated because cement is routinely used and loosening is not observed in most cases. The theory of shrinkage is negated by the negligible volumetric changes occurring in the cement during polymerization (see Chapter 5). Stem wobble and uneven distribution of cement in an unsupported segment of bone remain possible real causes of loosening.

After failure of the cement at the tip of the mantle, subsidence continues until the prosthesis becomes stabilized in the column of cement. This situation is usually accompanied by bone loss in the critical calcar zone. This mechanism does not stabilize the stem; further subsidence causes failure of the prosthesis, additional loosening being inevitable.

Varus loosening is the most serious mode of failure, especially when the upper portion of the prosthesis drifts into a varus position while the distal portion of the stem remains rigidly fixed in the bone. This generates a bending movement at the junction of the rigid column (distally) and a movable segment (proximally), leading to fatigue failure of the metal (Figs. 6-66, E and F, and 6-68) or severe bone loss at the neck region (Figs. 6-69 to 6-71). In this context, plastic deformation of metal to the point of yield (permanent) must be considered before fracture occurs. For technical reasons it is advantageous to revise such a prosthesis before complete fracture, which makes the operation to remove a distal fragment more difficult.

Because porous-coated implants are new, the modes of failure are not as well established as in cemented devices. However, certain failure characteristics attributable to all cementless devices may affect the outcome in short- or long-term stability.

Failure of porous-coated implants may have one or more of the following etiologies:

1. Failure of coating of the implant
2. Stem fracture
3. Loosening
4. Stress shielding (bone resorption)
5. Osteolysis (related to particulate debris)

Failure of Implant
Failure of Porous Surface

To be effective and safe, a porous ingrowth stem must possess a strong coating unaffected by incumbent stresses in the body. Loss of fixation of the porous coating may not only lead to loosening and pain requiring revision surgery, but may also cause osteolysis and severe wear of the joint. Radiographic evidence of separation of coating from the substrate is synonymous with loosening, even in the absence of the clinical symptoms. Many porous-coated implants have had early failure by this mechanism.* Texturing of the implants by nonthermal treatment is advantageous because it produces a high-strength bond between the coating and the substrate. A static bond strength of 8000 to 10,000 PSI has been recommended as application of laser holography has become the state-of-the-art method for applying porous coatings on the prosthesis. It is paradoxical that despite the good strength of coating fixation (static strength and fatigue strength), one can manually separate the coatings from the implants. The metallic surface of unstable implants may abrade against adjacent wires used to fix the trochanter. Occasionally, the abraded material released may not be visualized by x-ray, but radiographic bone erosions adjacent to the implant may appear as evidence of their presence.

Failure of Stem Substrate

Heat treatment of metals is known to reduce their mechanical strength. Since sintering of porous-coated materials requires heat treatment, it may considerably reduce metallic strength. Powder-made porous-coated chromium-cobalt alloy, for example, is subjected to 90% of the melting temperature. Annealing of the substrate by this manner reduces the fatigue strength

---

*References 17, 19, 33, 45, 57, 143.

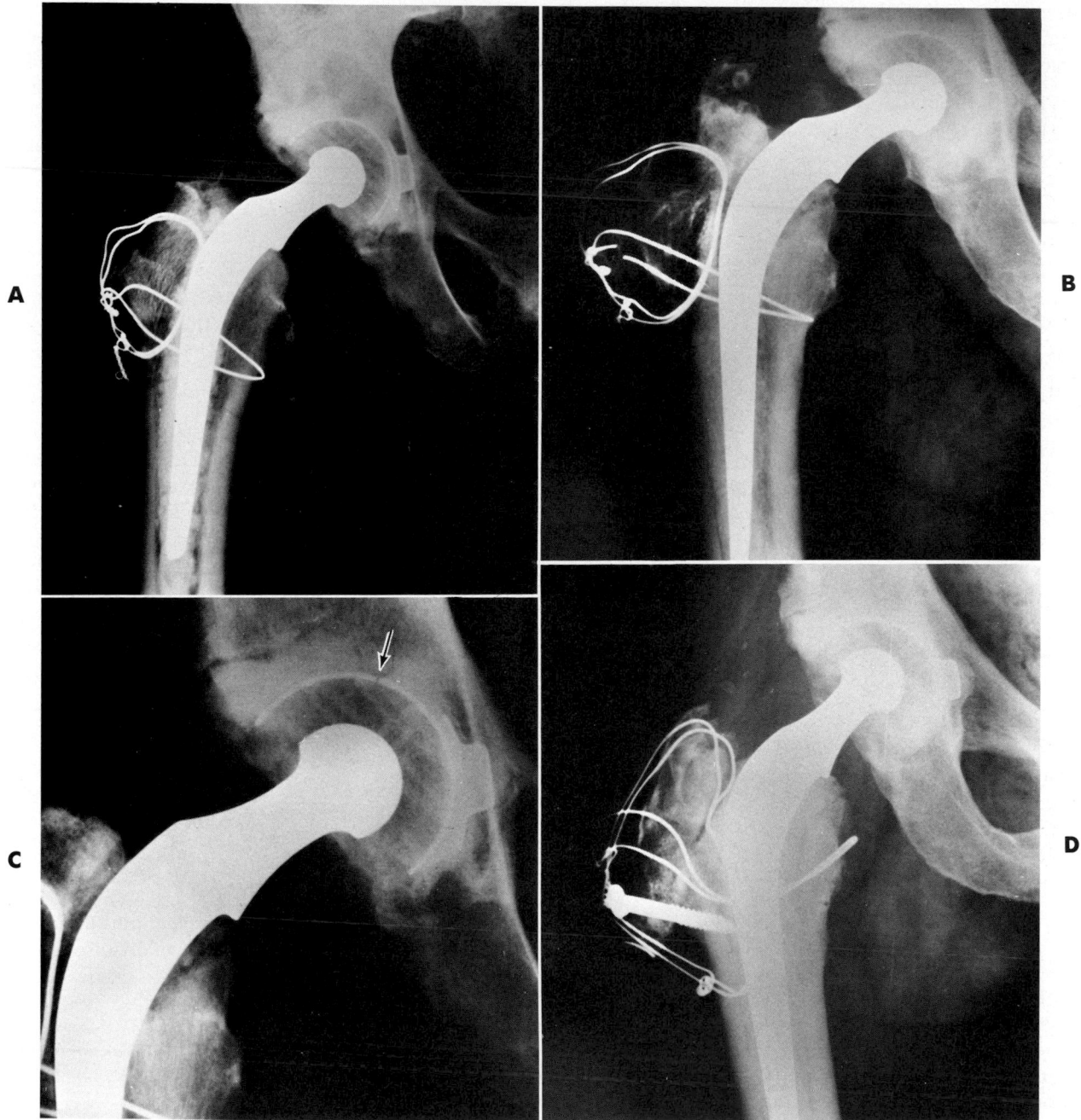

Fig. 6-68. **A,** Sixty-two-year-old man 1 year after low-friction arthroplasty. NOTE: slight varus orientation of stem in shaft. **B,** Loosening of upper end of prosthesis 3 years after surgery. Patient weighed 232 pounds, was extremely active, and played sports competitively. **C,** Close-up of same patient in **B.** NOTE: wire marker on cup is fractured *(arrow),* indicative of possible plastic deformation of wire under excess load. Femoral prosthesis is bent (plastic deformation) but not fractured. **D,** 6 months after revision using heavy stem. Weight reduction succeeded (180 pounds at time of revision surgery).

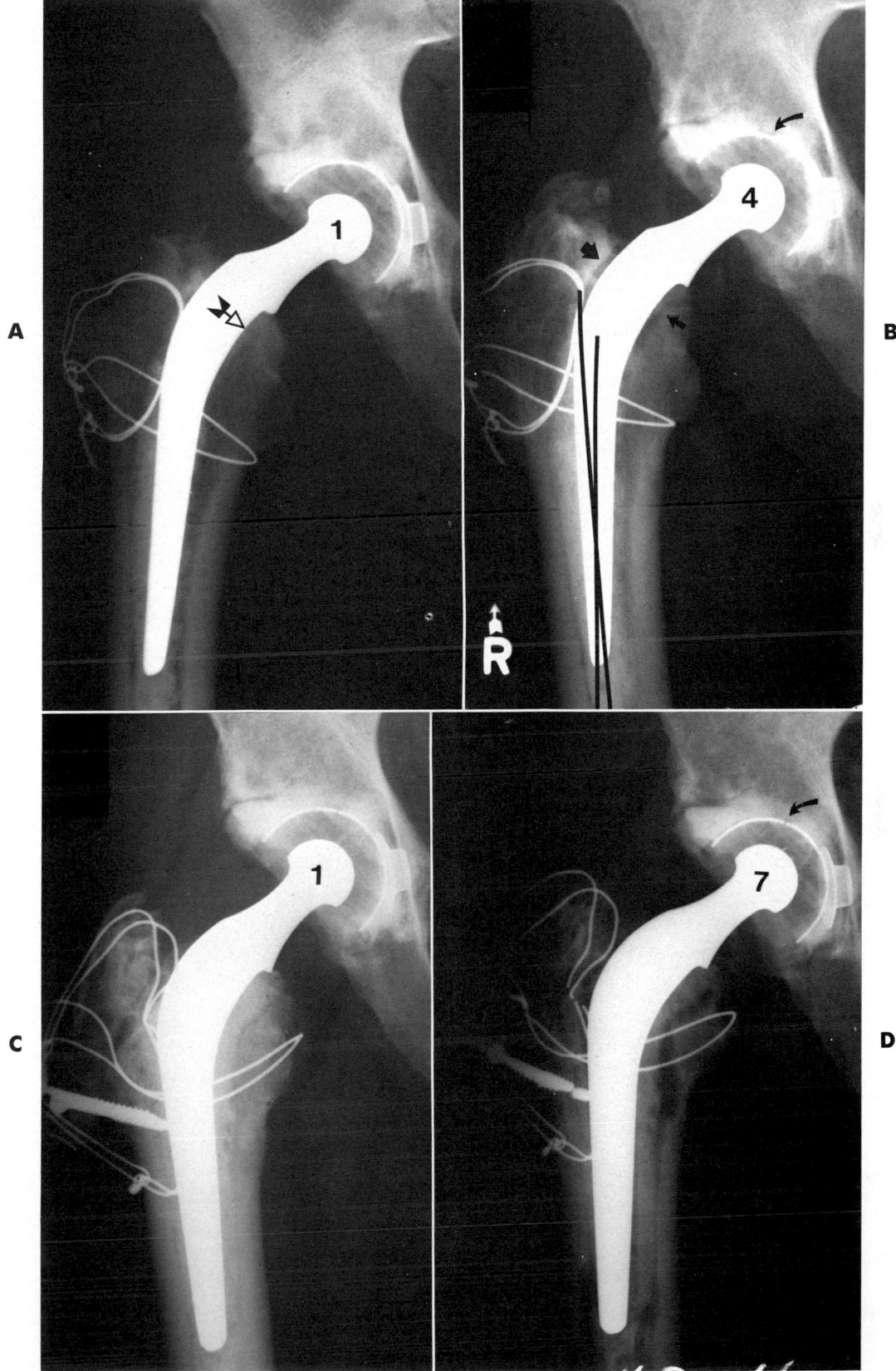

Fig. 6-69. A, Radiograph 1 year after low-friction arthroplasty in 64-year-old man (A.R.) whose weight was 93 kg. A flat-back Charnley's original design was used. NOTE: varus orientation and thin layer of cement proximally and medially *(arrow)*. Patient became very active and participated in sports. **B,** Plastic deformation of stem occurred resulting in fragmentation of cement in proximal and medial neck and calcar region *(arrow)* 4 years after low-friction arthroplasty. Also note fracture of radiographic marker *(curved arrow)*. **C,** 1 year after revision using a heavy stem centered with good support. **D,** Repeat failure caused by osteolysis without loosening 7 years after revision.

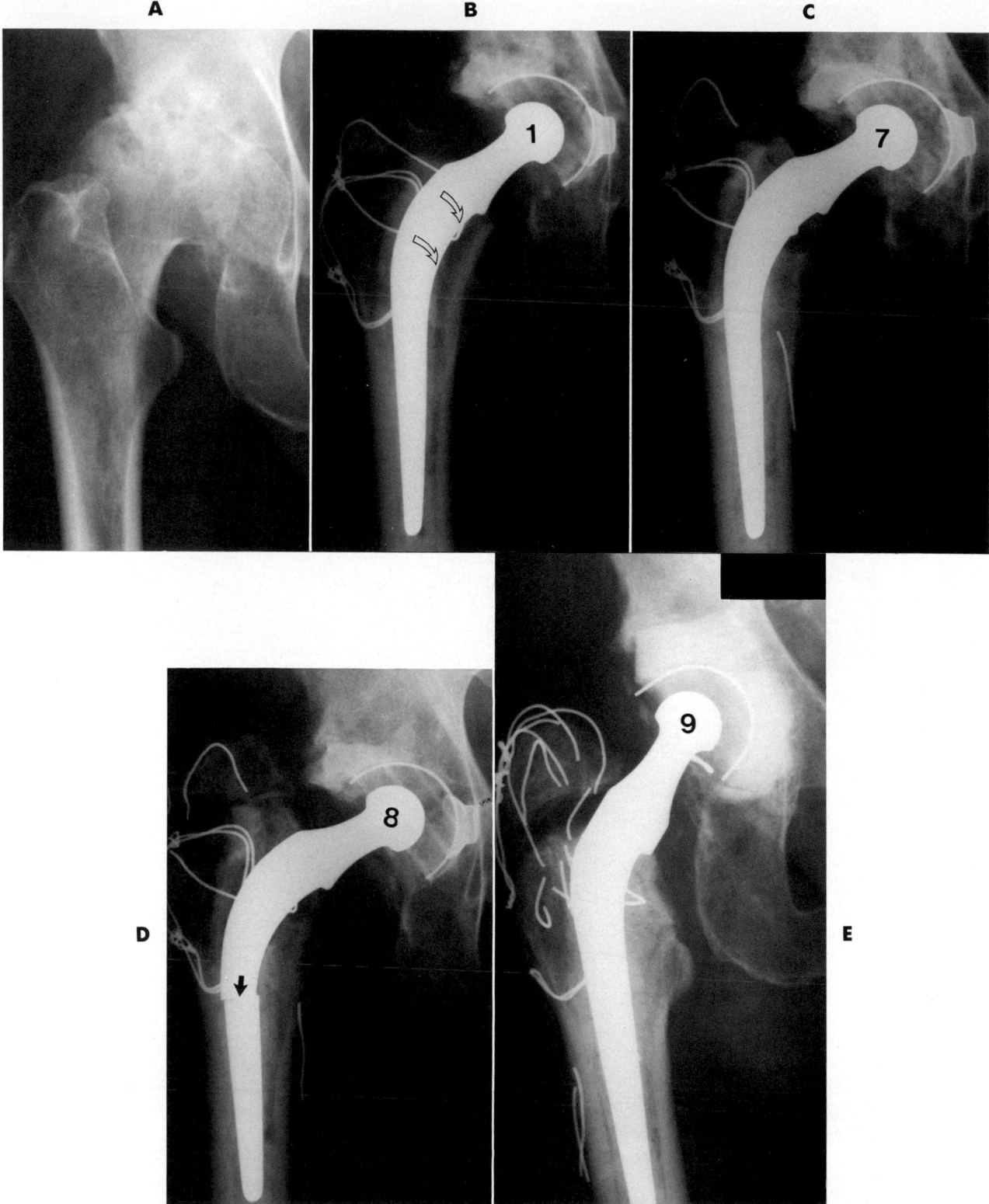

Fig. 6-70. A, Preoperative radiograph in 70-year-old male (J.G.) with osteoarthritis. Patient's weight was 85 kg. **B,** 1 year postoperatively (surgery was performed at another institution). NOTE: absence of cement at the medial and proximal aspects of the femoral stem. **C,** Complete osteolysis and loss of bone support of stem and associated bending of the stem were observed (no fracture has occurred). **D,** Stem fracture occurred at the site *(arrow)* of highest stress (bending moment) and stem defect (notch) caused by longitudinal trochanteric wire. **E,** 9 years after revision, note absence of loosening.

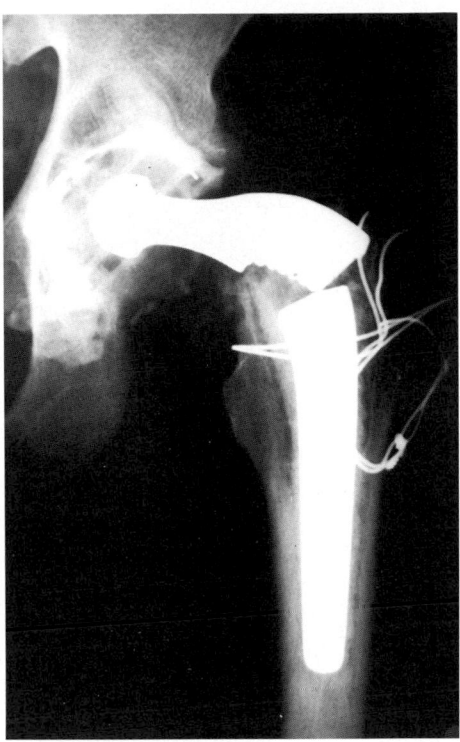

Fig. 6-71. Radiograph of Charnley extra-heavy stem fracture at site of first of serrations on medial aspect of the proximal stem. The design concept was based on the theory that the stem and cement by mechanical bonding would prevent slippage of the stem within the cement mantle which proved to be counterproductive. The patient was a 40-year-old man (P.T.) who sustained a severe fall down several flights of stairs while being chased by police after escaping from prison! Weight was 100 kg.

of the material by a factor of three compared with forged material. Titanium alloy is less likely to be weakened by sintering of fibers or bead porous-coating because sintering can occur at a lower temperature than with chromium-cobalt alloys. However, as stated in Chapter 4, the strength of titanium implants can be markedly reduced by surface imperfections, and prostheses made of titanium alloys are accordingly more notch-sensitive than other metallic alloys used for orthopaedic implants.[134,135,176] Because of fatigue fractures of implants (especially in femoral stems), most manufacturers are unwilling to produce prostheses below certain sizes; the geometrical shape and size determine the strength of the implants. Fractures of fully coated implants are seen increasingly because fatigue is time dependent and because prostheses fail in a cantilever-beam mode (distal fixation and loss of proximal fixation). Surgical treatment of these fractured stems is exceedingly difficult; the surgeon must cut the ingrown metals out of bone without fracturing it.[35,67]

Failure of Morstaper

Failure of the modular head/neck junction has been reported in early designs of cementless devices, espe-

cially those that use dissimilar metals (chromium-cobalt head and titanium stem). While the scope of this problem has not been fully established, manufacturing failures have been implicated as the common cause (see Chapter 4). A perfect fit of the taper-lock and careful handling at surgery are important to reduce complications of this nature. Osteolysis related to the particles released from taper-lock has been reported.

Failure Caused by Osteolysis

Cementless devices were favored in the 1980s and 1990s because severe osteolysis was frequently seen in association with loose cemented prostheses.[83,96] However, recent observations suggest that all particles generated by implants cause osteolysis, including particles from metals and plastics.[150] Granuloma from bead loss, metal fretting, and progressive femoral cortical osteolysis in association with cementless devices is currently cited frequently.[12,17] As noted in Chapter 4, HDP wear debris may travel along the cemented or cementless implants and cause osteolysis. This mode of failure may be a permanent factor in the success of total hip arthroplasty. It has been suggested (although not proven) that the presence of ingrowth may prevent egress of the particulate matter, and thus may partially prevent osteolysis. However, some early enthusiasts of porous-coated stems changed the design for nonporous prostheses because the problem related to long-term osteolysis has not been circumvented entirely.[101,102]

Regarding osteolysis caused by particles, the following conclusions can be drawn:

1. Osteolysis, once thought to be unique to cement, is now seen as associated with cementless devices as well.
2. Metallic debris can cause severe osteolysis.
3. A metallic prosthesis can produce particles by fretting, metallic sintering, beads or wire fiber release, or excess wear of titanium femoral heads against HDP. Fretting between the metallic screw heads of fixed titanium cups also produces particles and osteolysis.
4. Abrasion of metallic components against bone has also been reported.
5. Osteolysis occurs earlier in hips that are stable and fixed without cement (porous-ingrowth or press-fit) than those that are stable but fixed with cement.
6. Osteolysis occurs more in prostheses that are unstable (loose) than in those that are stable.
7. Once osteolysis appears on x-rays it is likely to progress with time.
8. Progression of osteolysis around the cemented devices appears to be slower than around cementless devices.
9. Femoral osteolysis is a potentially serious complication of total hip arthroplasty, especially with cementless devices. It appears to occur even in hips that were initially fixed.

To reduce the amount of debris, consider the following:

1. Titanium implants become more resistant to wear when nitrogen-iron is implanted into the surface.[16b,173a]
2. Micromotion of rough-matted surface can be improved by polishing the surface of the stem.
3. Titanium femoral heads should not be used because they wear more than other metals.[12] However, McKellop and co-workers[104a], based on the original work of Sarmiento and a recent examination of explanted titanium alloy femoral component and histological studies, concluded that in the absence of acrylic or metallic abrasive particles, the wear properties of well-fixed titanium alloy prostheses were comparable with those materials made of stainless steel or cobalt-chromium alloy.
4. HDP wear can be reduced by use of a highly polished ball and a small head (22 or 26 mm).

5. Ceramics may be associated with less wear against HDP.
6. It is possible that "sealing" an interface by cement or fully ingrown interface prevents debris from entering the interface. This has not, however, been well documented in clinical practice.
7. Modularity, allowing attachment of multisegment prostheses, offers a distinct advantage in revision and anatomically difficult situations.[20] However, these designs (similar to modular systems currently routinely used for acetabular and tibial components) are likely to cause fretting and generate particles leading to osteolysis and granulomas.

Stress Protection and Bone Resorption

It is a well-established mechanical fact that when bone and metals (with different moduli of elasticity) are loaded in conjunction to each other, the stiffer implant bears the majority of the load. Such preferential load transfer through the metal seems to be proportional to its increasing stiffness.

Engh and Bobyn showed semiquantitatively that marked femoral resorption occurred in 20% of cementless AML prostheses.[56] The stress shield phenomenon was greatest with stiffer and larger implants.

The mostly coated stems are also associated with the greatest amount of stress shielding and bone resorption. In fact, to reduce stress shielding, the lesser amount of ingrowth should be used on the prosthesis (the lesser amount of ingrowth is paradoxically associated with a lower hip score).[14] To prevent stress shielding, the following must be considered: the prosthesis must be designed with an optimal geometrical shape because the bone remodeling of a cementless-device (nonbonded) prosthesis is affected more by its geometrical shape than by its stiffness. In a bonded prosthesis (ingrowth or cemented), flexibility is more important than geometrical shape, so titanium alloy and a smaller-caliber prosthesis are more desirable.

LOOSENING

Loosening of cementless devices and associated early failure caused by pain are one of the most frequent complications of these prostheses. Loosening of the femoral or acetabular cementless components is related to failure of initial fixation and subsequent abnormal bone remodeling. Initial stability is crucial for clinical and radiographic success. After failure these prostheses exhibit a pattern similar to that of a prosthesis fixed with cement, including radiographic signs of widening radiolucencies around the stem with progressive endosteal enlargement and subsidence. In general, late loosening of the cementless prosthesis is caused by failure of biological fixation, as in cemented devices, where loosening is related to failure of cement mantle, bone, or both to support the prosthesis in long term. The modes of failure of cementless devices are not well established although radiographic representation of bone remodeling has been described by several authors.[55] Failure and the radiographic representation of various prostheses depend largely on design considerations, size variations, the extent of fit and fill, and the amount and location of porous-ingrowth surfaces of the stem and biological environment into which the prosthesis has been implanted.

FATIGUE FAILURE OF METAL (STEM BREAKAGE)

The problems of loosening and fatigue failure of the stem are closely interrelated. Fatigue failure of the stem is the product of repetitive cyclic load, which is normally initiated at a site of high tensile stress that usually resides at the lateral surface of the stem. Cracks are initiated and grow slowly across the stem until not enough metal is available to support the body weight, at which point the stem fractures at a fast pace. Cracks usually start at places where the stress is concentrated, that is, at a defect such as a scratch, notch, or void. Fig. 6-72 illustrates the cross-section of a fractured prosthesis and shows the areas of slow and fast propagation

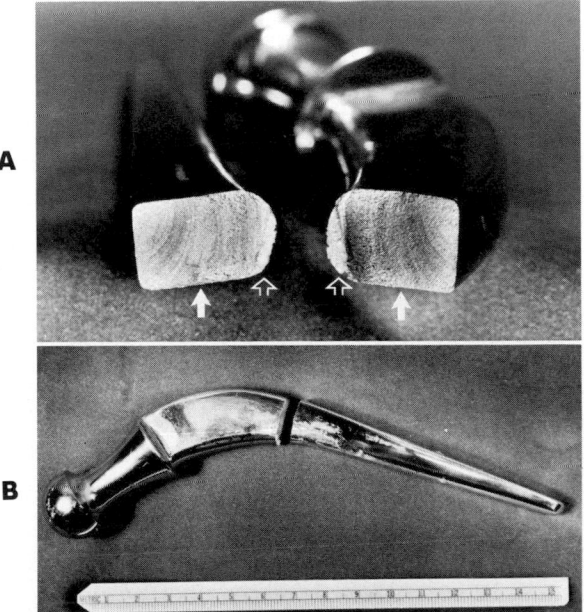

Fig. 6-72. Fatigue failure of stem is product of repetitive cyclic load usually initiated at site of high-tensile stress, which usually resides at lateral surface of stem. NOTE: cross-sectional area of fractured prosthesis that was removed in 215-pound male patient who enjoyed successful total arthroplasty for 5 years. Prosthesis had been inserted in varus orientation. **A,** Areas of slow and fast propagation of crack (slow, solid arrow; fast, hollow arrow). **B,** Level of fractured stem (same prosthesis as shown in **A**).

of the crack.

Fracture waves are similar to tide marks. As one might expect, they occur during different fatigue phases of the metals. They begin at the anterolateral surface of the metal, that is, the anterolateral square edge of the retangular cross section and end with a fracture "lip." The most medial part of the fracture represents the sudden failure.

Since the fracture is the result of "excessive tensile stress" at the lateral surface of the prosthesis owing to the bending moment* and the load (patient's weight and activities), it is important to consider the factors that may contribute to its appearance (Fig. 6-73). They are as follows:

1. The neck shaft angle of the prosthesis; that is, the smaller the neck shaft angle, the greater the stress.
2. The neck length; that is, the longer the neck, the greater the stress (Fig. 6-74).
3. The orientation of the stem in the canal; that is, the greater the angle of varus, the greater the stress (Fig. 6-75).

One must recognize that metallic devices with unlimited "fatigue life" (over 80,000 to 100,000 PSI) have replaced weaker ones to circumvent the problem of fatigue fractures. Accordingly, loosening should be considered the most important problem in tracing the initiation of a failure. Loosening is the result of motion between two dissimilar materials, such as cement and metal or cement and bone, which creates a stress fracture leading to further loosening. In a three-dimensional finite-element analysis, Crowninshield and associates concluded that the basic questions concerning bone are the level of interface shear stress and the degree of protection against slippage.[39,40] From their studies it became obvious that maximum interface shear occurs on the inferior surface of the stem-neck region and over the distal lateral surface at the tip of the stem; within these zones, the largest concentration of values was predominantly in the calcar zone. These values of shear stress would be the minimum that could prevent bond failure, but since impact forces could easily double these values, the bond strength between the stem and the acrylic cement should be at least 35 N-mm.[2] Although this is a good engineering bond (the same level as the ultimate shear stress of acrylic cement), in practice such a bond between metal and cement would make subsequent removal of the prosthesis impossible.

In a similar two-dimensional stress analysis, the effect of some of the factors leading to early fatigue failure of the femoral stem in total hip arthroplasty was

---

*Bending moment: M, force; F, distance from D, line of action, M = F × D.

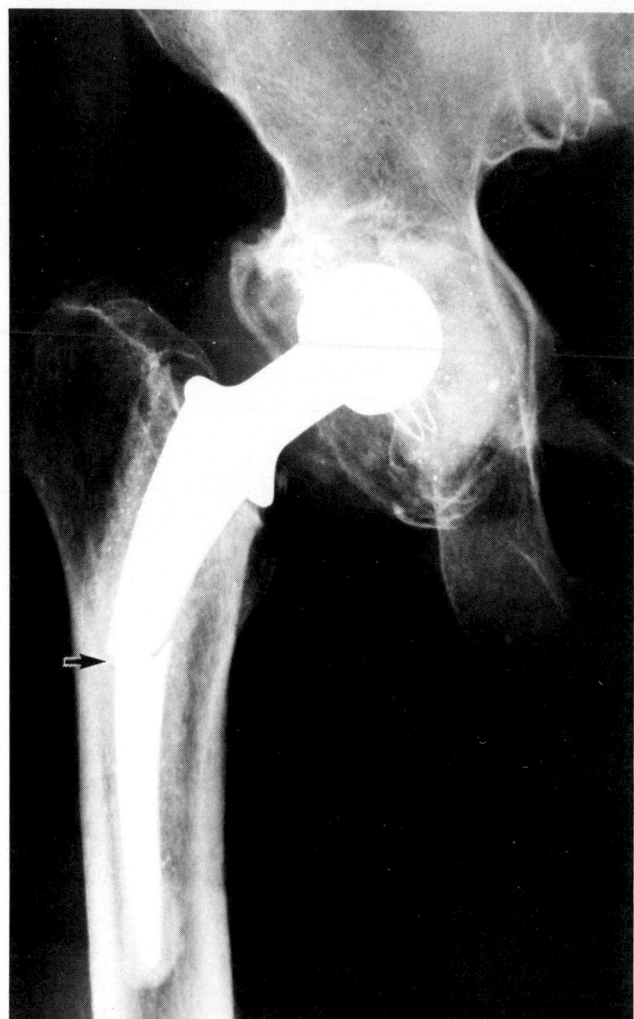

Fig. 6-73. X-ray film of typical patient who sustained fractured stem. Prosthesis is drifted into varus direction, neck is markedly absorbed, radiolucent zone has appeared on lateral upper aspect of prosthesis between bone and stem, distal stem is rigidly fixed in bone. Patient's weight was 245 pounds at time of fracture, 3 years after surgery (arrow shows fracture site).

studied.[4,65] This led to a similar conclusion: loss of proximal stem support at the level of the calcar femorale resulted in a level of stress on the stem that led to fatigue failure. The load (body weight) and the range of cyclic stress played an important part in fatigue life under test conditions. Increasing the stem dimension at the middle-third level of the stem (the critical level, where maximum tensile forces are found) was suggested, although it should be emphasized that static testing in laboratories might oversimplify the three-dimensional geometry of the stem and the forces applied to it as they occur in the body. So this model would only partially explain the early failure of the metal.

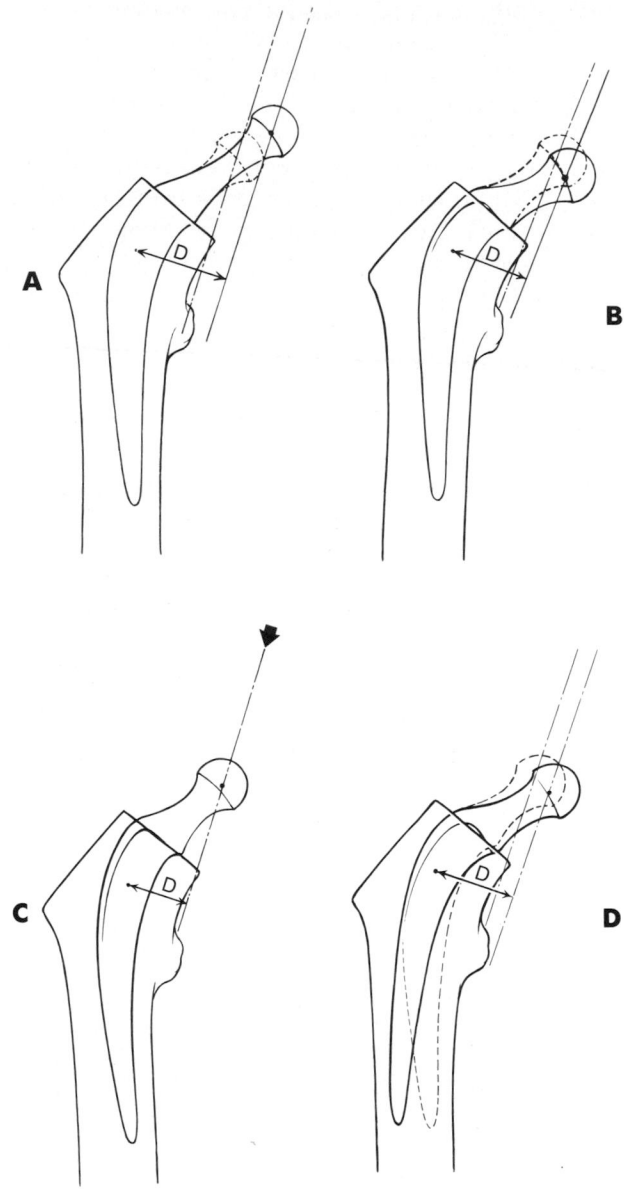

Fig. 6-74. A, Longer the neck of prosthesis, greater the distance, *D,* thus greater bending moment. **B,** Smaller the neck shaft angle, greater the distance, *D,* greater the bending moment on stem. **C,** Slight vagus orientation of stem in shaft; less distance, *D,* thus less bending moment on stem. **D,** More varus orientation of stem the more distance, *D,* thus increased bending moment on stem.

Many unresolved problems besides a failure-free stem must be considered for research. The unknown factors are basically related to the metallic alloy, design features, and lack of understanding of the complex mechanism of weight bearing in the upper femur, which is subjected to many stresses. It is also important to develop techniques for adequate anchoring of the prosthesis into the shaft of the femur. Basically none of the studies so far has been directed toward equalizing the moduli of elasticity between the prosthetic com-

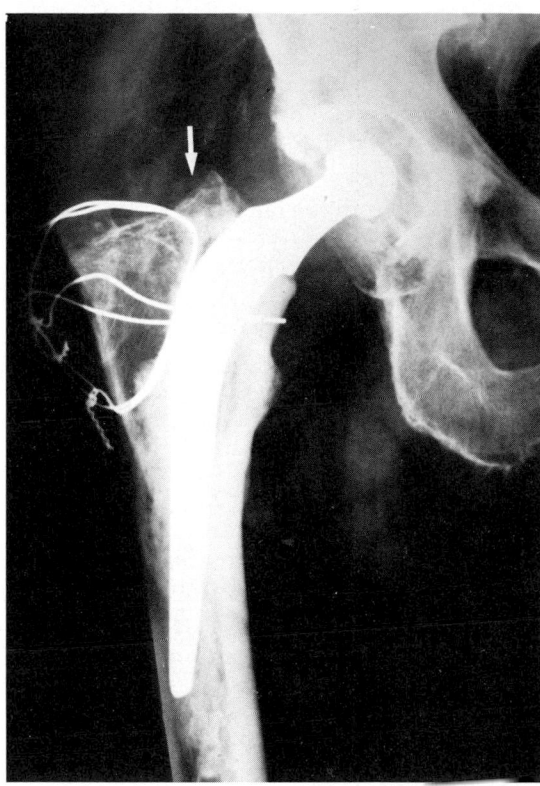

Fig. 6-75. Avoidable complication of varus orientation is demonstrated; greater trochanter is osteotomized, but prosthesis is inserted in marked varus orientation. By removal of bridge between bed of trochanter and neck, prosthesis could have been conveniently inserted without varus orientation. Arrow indicates bone bridge between trochanter and neck (see Chapter 12).

ponents and their fixation and bone, which may be equally important in the future design of the stem.

Based on the clinical analysis of stem failures today, one may search for the cause of failure in the following categories: excessive load, failure of support by the bone, loss of fixation at the cement-bone-metal interface, uneven stress distribution throughout the cement column, metallurgical causes, and failure of surgery.

Excessive Load

Fatigue fracture of the femoral prosthesis is the product of a "successful arthroplasty" in a heavy, athletic, active patient in which the dimensions of a standard prosthesis have been used (see Fig. 6-68). The valgus position of the prosthesis, while important in reducing bending stresses, does not eliminate the fracture. The support of the prosthesis by the cement on the medial aspect is most important; use of an extremely heavy stem in the upper portion automatically reduces the amount of cement used, inviting further loosening problems that can initiate fatigue fractures. The anatomical advantages of a 130-degree

shaft-neck angle are great enough to warrant its sole use in patients with a huge bony structure, to allow clearance between the neck and rim of the acetabulum. Obviously, heavier prostheses have now been designed for people who anticipate excess load from their weight or excess stress from the degree of their activities.

Based on clinical examination of 17 fractures, the especially high-risk patients are males weighing over 170 pounds, especially those with a standard prosthesis whose early design (original flat-back standard stems) was not adequate. The situation is compounded in most cases by inadequate cement support at the concavity of the upper femur. Charnley attributed the low incidence of fracture of the stem in long-term follow-up results to a good cementing technique.[28] The highest-risk patients are those who are physically active, but because of their small bone size (narrow medullary canal) cannot have a large stem inserted. Patients with a severe disability in the opposite extremity are also at risk because of the likelihood of increased loads on the arthroplasty side.

Overactive patients should be warned to reduce their participation in certain kinds of activities, such as contact sports. Technically, especially in large, bony men, the large-sized prosthesis, which can be accommodated in a neutral or slight valgus attitude, should be used. One should avoid using long-necked prostheses (whenever possible) and a varus orientation at surgery. The cement technique for the upper femur is demanding, and good fixation at the calcar level seems to be essential. Manufacturing control in the production of prostheses with a high-strength and highly fatigue-resistant metal has virtually eliminated stress fracture of cemented stems.

Failure of Support by Bone

There is now substantial evidence that the loss of support by the bone is a fundamental cause of the failure of cement fixation in the calcar region, leading to eventual failure of fixation at the concave side of the stem. Therefore from histological evaluation of the calcar region, it seems reasonable to suggest that the cystic erosion of bone in this region is caused by slight movement between the cement and the bone. With the stress concentration at the calcar region and cement fragmentation causing tissue reaction such as bone resorption and necrosis, further varus subsidence of the prosthesis follows; the similarity between the periodontal disease and bone necrosis with the loosened cemented prosthesis is striking. In both instances, once loosening begins, a vicious cycle is created. The cement loses support and permits increased motion in the upper end of the prosthesis between the bone and the calcar at the concave side of the prosthesis, while the remainder of the prosthesis (the distal portion) may remain fixed in the bone (see Fig. 6-66). To solve the problem, it seems reasonable to suggest a surgical technique that should include, in addition to a slight valgus orientation for the prosthesis, removal of the loose cancellous bone of the calcar region to provide strong support by the cement. Poor support by the bone, despite a valgus orientation of the stem, has been occasionally observed.[28]

Loss of Fixation

As indicated earlier, the most important cause of stem failure is initiation of the loosening of the prosthesis in the shaft, especially in the upper region (with the medial side of the prosthesis at the calcar region). Although most loosening may not terminate in failure by stem fracture, retrospective examination of most cases reveals early loosening before stem fracture (see Fig. 6-68). Improper cementing, that is, varus orientation of the stem and lack of support by the cement at the concave side of the prosthesis (in the compression side), increases stresses on the metal and the cement as well as the bone, leading to failure of fixation in this region.

Experimental studies coupled with studies of clinically failed prostheses can help determine the area of high-stress concentration and the location of the fracture. In both clinical and laboratory situations, loss of fixation by the cement precedes failure of metals; therefore it seems reasonable to assume that paying attention to the technical details of insertion and producing adequate support for the prosthesis at the calcar region to eliminate loosening are the first lines of defense against fatigue fracture.

Uneven Stress Distribution (Malposition)

It is commonly agreed that most stems fail from loosening, improper cementing, and inadequate calcar support, but in most cases a varus positioning of the stem has also been noted, although it must be emphasized that support conditions provided by the cement and the bone are more important than simple orientation in the canal. In other words, a valgus orientation of the stem in the canal, and inadequate support by cement and bone medially would not prevent fracture when excess stress is imposed. In an experimental model prediction, a Charnley prosthesis was instrumented with foil strain gauges.[28] The instrumental prosthesis was implanted into a cadaveric femur in a valgus orientation; after the cement had set, static loads were applied, and the resulting strength was recorded, the computed stresses were found to be quite comparable and consistent with a theoretical model. In the finite-element analysis, the stem was in neutral position. If these experimental analyses are representative of conditions in the clinical situation,

efforts must be made at surgery to avoid any degrees of varus orientation of the stem in the shaft; it follows that a stem that is well centered in the shaft is mechanically superior to a valgus-oriented stem.

Wroblewski examined 70 stem fractures (flat-back original of Charnley's design) and noted that when stem was viewed from the lateral side, the fracture line was never exactly transverse but always at an oblique angle to the long access of the stem. This angle varied from 2 to 20 degrees. The obliquity of fracture line implied that a torsional force must have operated to produce fracture. In most if not all fractures, bending to a lesser or larger degree occurred before actual stem fracture.

Metallurgical Causes

Fatigue is an engineering term used to describe the failure of materials by a fluctuating stress, which if applied a sufficient number of times, produces failure in the material. The stress required to produce failure is often much lower than that required to fracture the same material on a single application. While this principle is applicable to most machine elements and laboratory tests may produce the basic information regarding fatigue properties of the materials, the stress cycles that cause fatigue failure in biological situations are usually extremely complex. The gross appearance of a fatigue-fractured surface of a metallic component such as the stem of a total hip prosthesis shows two distinct regions: (1) a relatively smooth surface area with concentric markings described as clamshell, beach, or ripple markings, and (2) a surface area of rough granular appearance with the appearance of a cross-section of a multifilament cord. The smooth area indicates slow propagation of the fatigue cracks, and the rough zone indicates the brittle, ruptured final fracture zone (see Fig. 6-72).

Most femoral components of total hip prostheses are made of annealed stainless steel, chromium-cobalt alloy, or titanium. Annealed stainless steel, cast chromium-cobalt alloys, and titanium have similar ultimate tensile strengths, but the "yield stress" is much lower in annealed stainless steel than in chromium-cobalt or titanium. To avoid plastic deformation (permanent) in annealed stainless steel, the stem must have a greater dimension than a similar design made of chromium-cobalt or titanium alloy.

A new alloy used in Europe and the United States is a combination of cobalt, nickel, chromium, and molybdenum known as *Protosul 10* or *MP36N*. This alloy is made in a "multiphase" state. The mechanical properties of this alloy are outstanding with a yield strength of 60,000 psi when fully annealed with elongation of 70%. With work, hardening, and heat treatment, the yield strengths rise to 300,000 psi with only 10% elongation. These characteristics make MP35N an ideal alloy, combining the good properties of stainless steel and chromium-cobalt.

A study of 35 stainless-steel and chromium-cobalt-molybdenum alloy devices showed that a very large number were defective or deficient; the effects were caused by the presence of delta-ferrite in 315 L stainless steel, porosity in the cast-chromium alloy, and the presence of cracks and pits and in some instances a low molybdenum content in the steel. A number of other mechanical explanations have been proffered for the failure of metal in orthopaedic surgery: a brittle fracture owing to stresses exceeding the ultimate strength of the material, the use of an alloy not resistant to corrosion,[36] brittle fractures as the result of combined mechanical and electrochemical defects,[85] impact loading, fatigue tract propagation of 316 L stainless steel,[169] and weakness of the bone in the region of the femoral calcar.[169] The effect of grain size on the fatigue life of 315 L stainless steel has not been established, but it may be a significant factor in determining the strength of the stainless steel used for the stem of the femoral component. It is possible that a fine grain size is preferable and that a fine and

uniform grain size could be maintained by manufacturers. Galante and associates[66] feel that strings of shrinkage porosity in cast chromium and cobalt alloy should be considered flaws. When string length approaches an appreciable fraction of a millimeter, it must be considered as a progenitor of early failure, and large amounts of shrinkage porosity could impair the strength of the metal. Obviously, maintaining the highest standards of microstructural quality in the metal used in the stem of the prosthesis is imperative.

In regard to metallurgical studies, the main morphological characteristic of most of these fractures is obviously fatigue failure, but in most of the cases examined so far, a premature fatigue failure has occurred, probably because of a combination of circumstances (Fig. 6-76). These include inadequate quality controls in manufacture and flaws in the metallic structures; for example, 316 annealed stainless steel is unsuitable for a femoral stem, since this material can be expected to weaken under loading conditions; wrought cold-worked 316 stainless steel should be the material of choice when stainless steel is used.

One must be skeptical of the estimated fatigue limits

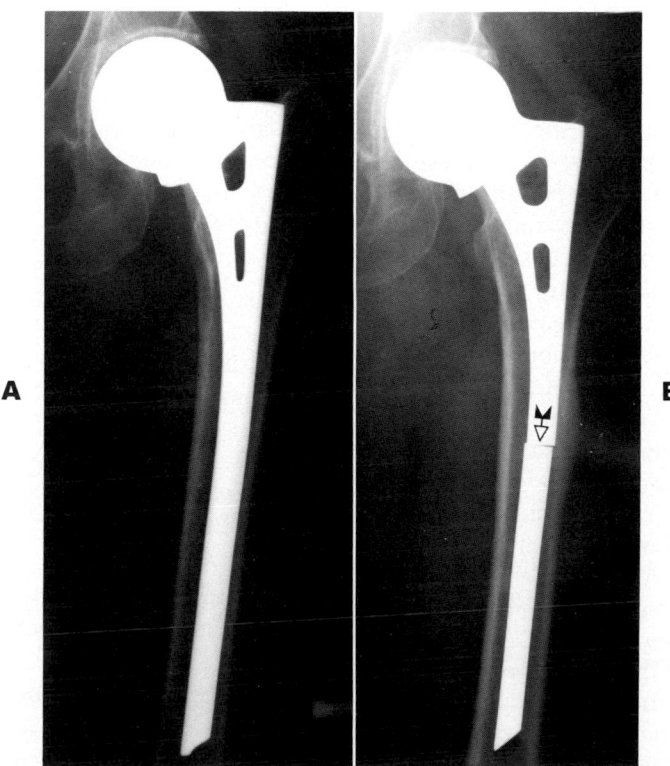

Fig. 6-76. A, The exact mechanism of fracture of long-stem Austin-Moore prosthesis in this patient (F.H.) cannot be determined since there appears to be no evidence of distal fixation of stem to cause the fracture. **B,** Fracture at mid-stem *(arrow)* with lateral cortical hypertrophy denoting stress transfer to the femur. The long stem had caused stress shielding in this noncemented, poorly fit stem.

of surgical metals[71]; exposure to the internal milieu of the body could significantly degrade fatigue strength and lead to corrosion fatigue much more readily than occurs in air-tested specimens.

From a clinical standpoint, the patients most susceptible to stem fractures are those who weigh over 180 pounds and are frequently active in vigorous athletic activities; they are usually careless in lifting heavy objects or participating in sports that cause the prosthesis to be loaded beyond its fatigue endurance limit. The previous designs of prostheses (standard type up to 1973) were generally small, making them inadequate for large bony men. Patients whose bone size is too small for a heavy prosthesis and those who will not limit their activities are considered high-risk. Educating patients in this regard is essential. The cementing technique should include forceful packing of the canal after removal of all loose bony trabeculae and fatty marrow. In preparing the canal in the region of calcar femorale, special attention should be paid to packing the cement well within the concave side of the prosthesis and femur. No "jarring" or "wobbling" is permitted when the prosthesis is being inserted, because this produces a track in the cement that is larger than the size of the stem and initiates a piston action of the stem in the canal.

Any degrees of varus orientation of the stem expose it to excessive load (see Fig. 6-75). Extreme valgus orientation is just as disadvantageous as extreme varus orientation, although a slightly valgus position allows insertion of a thick layer of cement in the calcar region at the concave side of the prosthesis. Excavating the lesser trochanter and filling it with cement creates a good thick support for the stem. A fully ingrowth prosthesis also creates a hazard of fracturing since the distal end of the stem becomes bound to the bone and proximally the stem becomes unstable.

Fractures of Ring prostheses (without the use of cement) and Austin-Moore prostheses used for fractured hip are of special interest because these prostheses are not fixed well distally and most of the results are not in vigorous patients with an athletic gait. Wroblewski observed that fracture sites in these prostheses are toward the opposite side of those found in cemented stems.

Ideally, a prosthesis should possess a shorter neck in valgus position (small center shaft offset) with an increased section modulus. An extremely large stem occupying the main space in the canal is not attractive since it obviates the thickness of cement in the calcar region, which is so essential for support of the prosthesis under compressive load.

SUMMARY OF ESSENTIALS

- Assuming that maximum wear of the artificial joint occurs at the maximum force location, it is calculated that the actual resultant force occurs between 10 and 15 degrees from midaxis of the body. Although the variation may be as much as ±20 degrees toward or away from the midline, the forces acting on the hip joint are influenced considerably by the pelvic angle and the position of the trunk and limbs.

- With the pelvis in a normal walking attitude and the limbs symmetrically disposed, muscle forces range from 1.0 to 1.8 times body weight and joint forces from 1.8 to 2.7 times body weight; even small changes in the positions of the lever arms of the muscles involved alter these forces considerably.

- The forces generated in the hip as a result of muscle action must be kept in mind when planning for postoperative rehabilitation. With simple calculations it has been shown that the load on the hip joint, when the patient lies supine and raises a leg 5 cm off the ground, is approximately twice that of body weight. The clinical implication is a paradox: keep a patient "nonweight bearing" while emphasizing active straight leg-raising exercises.

- While static force is considerably greater than body weight, an even greater force is generated in dynamic situations, such as acceleration and deceleration. Data collected telemetrically by an instrumented prosthesis in the human body indicate that muscle contractions play an important role in creating forces of varying degrees during walking, sitting, standing, and other normal daily activities, such as stair climbing and rising from a chair. The last function creates a much higher force on the posterior acetabular wall than had previously been estimated.

- Instrumented prostheses have also shown that joint reaction force increases to 2.1 times body weight during one-legged stance with the subject using contralateral hand support. Walking between parallel bars produces a maximum joint reaction force of 2.4 times body weight. Load-bearing force also increases progressively with time elapsed from the operation.

- The data on joint reaction force collected from instrumented prostheses in humans are somewhat lower than estimates based on mathematical calculations because the patients with artificial joints have uneven gaits and may take smaller steps.

- Dynamic data obtained using a force plate to determine ground reaction indicate that during the stance phase of gait, forces on the femoral head may be approximately five or six times the body weight; they are at least equal to body weight during the swing phase of gait. Joint reaction forces increase considerably during stair climbing.

- Ascending and descending stairs requires a larger range of hip and knee motion than walking, and although stair climbing creates high joint moments, the highest moment occurs during descent.

- Human hip joint forces can be altered by various methods; a simple way to reduce forces in the hip is by having the patient lean over the affected hip. The hip center of gravity moves laterally toward the center of the femoral head, shortening its lever arm. This simple action reduces the magnitude of forces needed in the abductor muscle for balance and thus reduces the net force across the hip joint. Similarly, joint force can be reduced by increasing the weight-bearing surface of the joint, by reducing weight, by using a cane in the opposite hand, and by slowing the walking speed.

- In reconstructive surgery, loads on the hip joint can be significantly reduced by placing the center of the acetabulum (the center of hip rotation) as far medially, inferiorly, and anteriorly as possible. A prosthesis with a shorter offset and reduced neck shaft angle lowers the moment of force on the prosthesis and the femur. Lateral transfer of the trochanter (abductor moment arm), although desirable, has a less significant effect. In summary, then, the shorter the body-weight moment arm, the less the pull of the abductors required to balance the pelvis; conversely, lengthening the abductor moment arm reduces the gluteal tension required to balance the pelvis and in this way reduces the total load on the hip joint.

- The frictional forces acting on the acetabular component of the total hip prosthesis depend on several factors: the magnitude of the resultant compressive forces, the direction of the forces, the frictional moment and the axes around which they act, the geometry of the prosthesis, and the coefficient of friction between the mating surfaces.

- Using photoelastic methods, Charnley demonstrated that when the diameter of the head of the prosthesis was reduced from 50 mm to 22.5 mm, the frictional torque decreased by a factor of 1.5.

- It is now established that the frictional torque of prostheses is proportional to the diameter of femoral heads, but the relationship is not linear; for a head of a given size, thick HDP effectively lowered the frictional torque. The greater frictional torque was generated when contact was more peripheral than when it was polar.

- Among other variables, the materials used in the components affect frictional resistance and wear in total hip prostheses. Ceramics produce the lowest frictional moment compared to metal heads against HDP. Among metals, cobalt-chromium heads produce lower values than those made of stainless steel or titanium alloy.

- Regarding methods of acetabular cup fixation in clinical practice, it appears that acrylic cement and porous-coated acetabular components are most successful for a long-lasting result.

- The strength of fixation of the acetabulum by acrylic cement can be greatly influenced by the method of acetabular preparation at surgery and the method of cup fixation. Several studies clearly demonstrate that preservation of subchondral bone is advantageous and the use of a thin plastic cup is undesirable, regardless of whether it is supported by bone or by a metal shelf.

- Clinical practice supports the laboratory conclusion that a small femoral head against a thick plastic cup provides the least frictional torque and the smallest volumetric wear, both of which help delay acetabular component failure. Established data indicate that demarcation between cement and bone in the acetabulum is time dependent but depends largely on a good structural bone support and a microinterlock between cement and bone. The cup must remain contained within the acetabular cavity, and cement must be pressurized to produce microinterlock. A thin cup or a thin layer of cement produces "high spots" at the cement-bone interface that might precipitate minute, localized movement between cement and bone. This movement in turn might lead to histiocytic reaction, bone cavitation, and loosening. A thicker component, on the other hand, reduces the stress, but a thick socket can be used if the femoral head prosthesis is small, that is, 22 or 26 mm, for articulation.

- Stiffening of the HDP by a metal backing of the component was favored analytically, but clinical practice has shown that its disadvantages outweigh its advantages. In fact, there is no clinical evidence to support its use. To the contrary, additional metal thickness (1) mandates use of a thinner HDP component, possibly increasing the formation of particles and wear; (2) forces the use of a thin layer of cement because of reduced availability of space; (3) can cause stress shielding because of excess stiffness; and (4) can produce wear of HDP over the convex surface.

- Clinical results of threaded acetabular cups, despite their successful initial fixation in the laboratory, have been disappointingly poor. The high rigidity of the implant overstresses the acetabular bone, causes stress shielding of the trabecular bone, transfers the load through the cortical bone, limits the area of load-bearing, causes significant peak stresses in subchondral bone, and generates a high medial acetabular wall strain at insertion.

- Porous-coated metallic shells with an HDP insert have been favored because of rapid ingrowth onto the hemispherical shell. The acetabular component liner is also extractable for revision, and any size of femoral component can be used to revise failed cemented hips. Assessment of the long-term clinical effectiveness of these devices is awaited.

- Porous-coated hemispherical shells must be fixed rigidly to bone to promote osteointegration. Use of additional screws to fix the porous-coated acetabular shell can result in osteolysis or damage to the polished femoral head because of the potential of fretting between screw heads and the metal shell. Stress shielding of the pelvis can also occur because incorporated bone around the screws absorbs some of the stresses, thus affecting a uniform stress transfer through the cup.

- The biomechanical behavior of the stem and adaptive bone changes are significantly influenced by the geometrical design of the stem, its modulus of elasticity, and the method of fixation, which may determine its immediate and long-term durability. Additionally, the stem's permanent success depends not only on the immediate fixation but on the future maintenance of normal strain patterns to allow continuously favorable adaptive changes in bone.

- Femoral stem fixation by interference fit is an old engineering discipline that requires line-to-line or surface-to-surface contact under loading conditions. A perfect self-locking system provides stability from ever-increasing friction between the prosthesis and bone caused by the applied load.

- In the press-fit stem, stresses are affected more by the geometrical shape of the stem than by stem rigidity. In nonbonded stems, concerning mechanical properties, titanium is expected to produce more favorable results than chromium-cobalt-molybdenum alloys.

- A nonbonded press-fit stem provokes only calcar stress shielding but creates more stress in the midstem region. The lack of uniformity between the bone of the upper femur (metaphysis) and the lower femur (diaphysis) causes a nonuniform progressive stress pattern in the femur.

- The criteria for creating a suitable nonbonded stem include maximizing fit and fill to stabilize the prosthesis to optimize stress distribution; eliminating micromotion; using a feasible surgical technique; and providing an optimal choice of materials. Regarding the fill and fit, at present the only press-fit prosthesis that might achieve this goal is an intraoperatively manufactured prosthesis based on mea-surements made on the mold obtained from the interior of the femur. An off-the-shelf prosthesis will not provide adequate fill or fit.

- Regarding fit and fill of the prosthesis, one should also consider the pattern of stress distribution and alterations in the strain pattern in the femur in response to a stiff material such as the metallic stem, as a long-term limit to their use. The prosthesis must be inserted in such a way that undersizing and oversizing are avoided.

- It has been well established that an undersized, nonbonded stem is likely to produce micromotion leading to thigh pain, subsidence, or loosening, eventually requiring revision surgery. Conversely, an oversized mismatch of stem and femur causes fracture of the trochanter or the femoral shaft.

- Anatomical studies indicate that every femur is unique, and it would be exceedingly difficult to create a fit with any prefabricated prosthesis if no mismatch between the prosthesis and femur is acceptable. When the medial and lateral endosteal contours of the proximal femur and defined to an accuracy of ± 1 mm, no prosthesis is available today with the variations in size or shape to satisfy the need. Therefore the "press-fit" prosthesis by definition cannot be made even if ± 1 mm mismatch is accepted.

- The fit and fill of the prosthesis affect the degrees of micromotion occurring between implant and bone. It can be argued that when materials of dissimilar moduli of elasticity are put in conjunction, micromotion always occurs between them when they are placed under cyclic loads, even if this motion is so minuscule that it cannot be seen or measured by ordinary devices.

- The lock-wedge action, which also causes micromotion under cyclic load, can be minimized only by making the radius of the tapered angle of the wedge so large that it reduces the load transfer to a level that the bone can tolerate. Therefore in the design of a press-fit nonbonded prosthesis, the widest possible angle customized to the shape of the femur and without a collar may achieve the best results for loading the femur, provided there is no mismatch between the bone and the prosthesis.

- Studies have demonstrated that when prosthesis mismatch results from undersizing, a load of four times body weight produced a relative motion of more than 200 μm. When the endosteal cortical bone is in direct contact with the prosthesis, micromotion is remarkably reduced. Also, it has been documented that micromotion values can be indeed small and reversible using 1000-newton vertical force. However, adding rotational forces of 100 newtons about the vertical axis creates a significant degree of stem-bone displacement. To achieve the best results for a poorly fitted intramedullary stem such as an Austin-Moore prosthesis, transmission must be shared by the collar and the tip of the stem as well as the bone in the fenestration. This optimal situation usually results when the prosthesis drifts into a varus or valgus orientation.

- To maximize fixation, one popular method is to use a longer stem for the prosthesis, but because the collar is the main weight-bearing region in a poorly fitted stem of the common device, elongation of the stem offers no added advantage. However, with an extremely elongated stem, the amplitude of fretting movement at the tip of the stem is increased.

- Regarding the collar of a nonbonded prosthesis, bone absorption occurs under the cut surface of the neck routinely, but strengthening of the bone might occur, thus preventing continuous subsidence. The inclination of the ideal collar on the neck of the prosthesis depends on the force generated by the abductor muscles. For example, if the abductor muscles and their force angle are normal, the plane of the collar should be at 90 degrees to the resultant forces, but as the abductor system becomes more defective, the collar must be inclined at a more horizontal angle.

- It has been demonstrated that after the femoral component is inserted into the femur, the pattern of strain in the proximal femur changes dramatically compared with that of the intact femur. In the cemented prosthesis, the pattern of stress is reversed, stress is decreased massively in the calcar region, and maximum strain becomes focused around the tip of the stem. Transferring the load via a collar restores the strain toward normal by shifting 30% to 40% of the normal strain to the collar. These laboratory experiments demonstrate conclusively that use of a collar improves the load distribution pattern in the femur. However, in cemented fixation, the collar must load the top of the femur to be effective. This effect can be negated either by bonding the stem to the cement or by removing the contact between the collar and the bone. The latter situation commonly occurs after replacement by thorough absorption of the bone at the cut surface of the calcar.

- It has been shown that collar contact with the upper femoral cortex and control of stem subsidence have beneficial effects: collar seating substantially decreases subsidence and increases axial load to failure.

- Using a nonbonded prosthesis to achieve distal fixation minimizes micromotion distally and proximally and allows the collar to primarily control axial load transfer. The lateral toggle of the stem has been suggested as a cause of failure in most prostheses resulting from loss of proximal support by bone.

- Distal stem fit is the most significant factor in achieving rigidity against toggle in cementless total hip prostheses. It is most effective in reducing and abolishing micromotion. Although a collar cannot prevent distal micromotion, a well-fixed distal stem can. The main disadvantage of a tight permanent distal fit is the possibility of unloading of the proximal femur, causing stress shielding in that region.

- The criteria for selecting the materials with which to manufacture the stem include strength, corrosion resistance, and biocompatibility. All three metals used in manufacturing total hip prostheses — stainless steel, chromium and cobalt, and titanium alloy — meet these criteria. The stiffer metals, such as chromium and cobalt alloy and stainless steel, are favored for use with cement. The stiffer metal increases stress within the stem but decreases stress in the cement mantle. On the other hand, cementless devices require materials with a reduced modulus of elasticity to reduce stresses from surrounding bone. Reducing the modulus of elasticity is especially important in the large-caliber prosthesis commonly used in a large and heavy individual, because the stiffness increases with the diameter of the femoral stem.

- The biological characteristics of the interface between the cement and bone in the femur have been favorable over a long period. Such an interface tissue is subject to qualitative and quantitative changes based on the applied load. With the use of acrylic cement, the bone cavity need not be shaped perfectly to accommodate the prosthesis; instead it is prepared oversized and filled with a doughlike cement, which makes an accurate cast or mold of the interior of the bone. Thus, the larger surface areas of the cement-prosthesis unit can better resist compressive and shearing forces under axial load. The increased external surface areas and greater resistance to the shearing forces are ideal in treating elderly patients with osteopenia.

- The advantages of the use of cement for stem fixation include increased total contact zone between the prosthesis and bone, improved stress distribution from prosthesis to bone, and reduced compressive stresses and fretting movements. The elastic bone, including the interface tissue, constitutes an excellent medium for load transfer. The strength of the cement mantle depends on (1) the strength of the polymer methacrylate itself, (2) the geometry of the cement mantle, which relates largely to the geometry of the stem, and (3) the magnitude and pattern of stress distribution.

- Clinical and biomechanical studies indicate that the optimum cement mantle is generally nonuniform, providing strength proximally, medially, distally, and laterally. The minimum cement stresses occur proximally when the stem occupies from 80% to 90% of the canal and distally when the cavity is filled 70% to 80% with the stem. The ratio of cement thickness to stem cross-section is a compromise to keep the stem strong enough while leaving a minimum cement mantle of about 2 mm available for load transfer.

- In a comparison of load-transfer mechanisms of cemented, ingrowth, and press-fit prostheses, interface concentrations occurred on the proximal and distal portions of the prostheses with fixation by cement or ingrowth (bonded); the stress values depended on the stem rigidity. The higher proximal stress occurred in cemented stems, while higher distal stress occurred in noncemented stems. In nonbonded press-fit stems, the interface stresses were affected more by the geometrical shape of the stem than by rigidity.

- Titanium appears to produce a more favorable stress pattern in noncemented prostheses. The chromium-cobalt alloy appears to be more effective in cemented prostheses. Press-fit prostheses caused calcar stress shielding and provoked more stress than those occurring naturally in the cortex at the midstem zone.

- To optimize design, four factors must be considered: (1) Protect the cement by reducing critical stress and keeping cement under compressive forces. Provide a large surface area of the metal transferring the load to prevent splitting of the cement mantle. (2) Promote maximum load transfer via the strong bony trabeculae and cortex of the medial neck and calcar femorale. (3) Retain a sufficiently thick and uniform mantle in the areas that are highly stressed by the design of the prosthesis and bone preparation. (4) The mode and magnitude of compression and tension in the cement mantle are affected by the cross-sectional design of the prosthesis, which can be improved by a dorsal flange feature. A dorsal flange not only keeps the medial cement under compression, but also transmits the load to the cement in front of and behind the stem and thus resists shear forces. The dorsal flange also stiffens the upper half of the prosthesis to prevent elastic deformation of the metal in compression and improves the cement-bone interface in the critical heavily loaded upper femur while the hip is being loaded in flexion in such activities as standing from a sitting position or stair climbing, which load the hip heavily.

- To avoid fatigue fracture of the stem in heavy and active patients, one should (1) enlarge the proximal femur to accommodate a prosthesis with maximal cross-sectional dimensions, (2) improve the proximal fixation by using a large medial and a larger lateral cross-sectional dimension, and (3) provide maximum support for cement in heavily loaded proximal and medial aspects of the shaft. Meeting these goals entails selecting a prosthesis with short offset and maintaining the abductor moment arm by lateralization of the greater trochanter. In addition, use prostheses made of high-strength metals, and apply vigorous and diligent technique for proper bone preparation, cement insertion, and alignment of the stem.

- Mechanically, a standard stem length, that is, 120 to 160 mm, is adequate. Increased stem length may increase relative motion between the bone and cement, although it may reduce some stresses within cement by increasing the stress within the stem itself.

- Stem flexibility under loading conditions depends on the geometrical size and shape of the stem and the modulus of elasticity of the metal. For a prosthesis of a given size and shape, the stiffness cannot be increased by using a metal with a greater modulus of elasticity.

- Regarding the modulus of elasticity of the metal used for cemented stems, practical experience suggests that lowering stem modulus reduces stress within the stem but increases it in the proximal region in the cement. However, it decreases stress within the distal cement. Conversely, using stiff metal increases stress in the stem, which reduces stress proximally and increases stress distally. It is commonly agreed now that a stiffer metal with a greater modulus of elasticity may protect cement better than more flexible metals. The long-term comparison studies of the use of high-modulus and low-modulus stems are awaited. High-nitrogen-content steel and chromium-cobalt alloy have performed equally well in the biological environment when used with cement in total hip arthroplasty.

REFERENCES

1. **Albrektsson T, Branemark P, Hansson HA, et al:** The interface zone of inorganic implants in vivo: titanium implants in bone, *Ann Biomed Eng* 11:1, 1983.
2. **Andersson GBJ, Freeman MAR, Swanson SAV:** Loos-

ening of the cemented acetabular cup in total hip replacement, *J Bone Joint Surg* 54[Br]:590, 1972.

3. **Andriacchi TP, et al:** A study of lower-limb mechanics during stair-climbing, *J Bone Joint Surg* 62:749, 1980.

4. **Andriacchi TP, Galante JO, Belytschko TB, et al:** A stress analysis of the femoral stem in total hip prostheses, *J Bone Joint Surg* 58:618, 1976.

5. **Apel DM, Smith DG, Schwartz CM, et al:** Threaded cup acetabuloplasty, *Clin Orthop* 241:183, 1989.

6. **Atkinson PJ, Woodhead C:** The development of osteoporosis. A hypothesis based on a study of human bone structure, *Clin Orthop* 90:217, 1973.

7. **Bartel DL, Johnston RC:** Mechanical analysis and optimization of a cup arthroplasty, *J Biomech* 2:97, 1969.

8. **Bell RS, Schatzker J, Fornasier VL, et al:** A study of implant failure in the Wagner resurfacing arthroplasty, *J Bone Joint Surg* 67:1165, 1985.

9. **Benjamin JB, Gie GA, Lee AJ, et al:** Cementing technique and effects of bleeding, *J Bone Joint Surg* 69[Br]:620, 1987.

10. **Bergmann G, Moessner U, Rohlman A:** *Stresses in a femur with a close fit stem hip prosthesis.* Trans. 30th annual meeting of the Orthopaedic Research Society, Atlanta, Georgia, Feb. 6–9, 1984.

11. **Bergmann G, Siraky J, Rohlmann A:** A comparison of hip joint forces in sheep, dog and man, *J Biomech* 17:907, 1984.

12. **Black J, Sherk H, Bonini J, et al:** Metallosis associated with a stable titanium-alloy femoral component in total hip replacement. A case report, *J Bone Joint Surg* 72:126, 1990.

13. **Blount WP:** Don't throw away the cane, *J Bone Joint Surg* 38:695, 1956.

14. **Bobyn JD, Pilliar RM, Cameron HU, et al:** The optimum pore size for the fixation of porous surfaced metal implants by the ingrowth of bone, *Clin Orthop* 150:263, 1980.

15. **Bocco F, Langan P, Charnley J:** Changes in the calcar femoris in relation to cement technology in total hip replacement, *Clin Orthop* 128:287, 1977.

16. **Bombelli R, Santore RF:** Cementless isoelastic total hip prosthesis: preliminary report on the first 215 consecutive cases. In Morscher E, editor: *The cementless fixation of hip endoprostheses,* Berlin, 1984, Springer-Verlag.

16a. **Bressler B, Frankel JP:** The forces and moments in the leg during level walking, *Trans ASME* 48A:62, 1950.

16b. **Buchanan RA, Rigney ED Jr, Williams JM:** Ion implantation of surgical Ti-6Al-4V for improved resistance to wear-accelerated corrosion, *J Biomed Mater Res* 21:355, 1987.

17. **Buchert PK, Vaughn BK, Mallory TH, et al:** Excessive metal release due to loosening and fretting of sintered particles on porous-coated hip prostheses. Report of two cases, *J Bone Joint Surg* 68:606, 1986.

18. **Callahan:** Fracture of the femoral component, *Orthop Clin North Am* 19(3):637, 1988.

19. **Callaghan JJ, Dysart SH, Savory CG:** The uncemented porous-coated anatomic total hip prosthesis. Two-year results of a prospective consecutive series, *J Bone Joint Surg* 70:337, 1988.

20. **Cameron HU:** Recent advances in artificial hip-joint replacement, *Can Fam Physician* 33:649, 1987.

21. **Carter DR, Vasu R, Harris WH:** Stress distribution in the acetabular region. II. Effects of cement thickness and metal backing of the total hip acetabular component, *J Biomechanics* 15:165, 1982.

22. **Carter DR, Vasu R, Harris WH:** Periacetabular stress distributions after joint replacement with subchondral bone retention, *Acta Orthop Scand* 54:29, 1983.

23. **Charnley J, Ferreira A:** Transplantation of the greater trochanter in arthroplasty of the hip, *J Bone Joint Surg* 46[Br]:191, 1964.

24. **Charnley J:** The bonding of prostheses to bone by cement, *J Bone Joint Surg* 46[Br]:518, 1964.

25. **Charnley J:** Total hip replacement by low-friction arthroplasty, *Clin Orthop* 72:7, 1970.

26. **Charnley J:** *The moments of force about the hip joint mechanism of the low friction arthroplasty,* internal publication no. 40, Wigan, England, 1972, Centre for Hip Surgery, Wrightington Hospital.

27. **Charnley J:** Biomechanical considerations in total hip prosthetic design. In The Hip Society: *The hip: proceedings of first open scientific meeting of The Hip Society.* St Louis, 1973, Mosby–Year Book.

28. **Charnley J:** Fracture of femoral prosthesis in total hip replacement. A clinical study, *Clin Orthop* 111:105, 1975.

29. **Charnley J:** *Low-friction arthroplasty of the hip. Theory and practice,* New York, 1979, Springer-Verlag.

30. **Charnley J, Kettlewell J:** The elimination of slip between prosthesis and femur, *J Bone Joint Surg* 47[Br]:56, 1965.

31. **Charnley J, Pusso R:** The recording and the analysis of gait in relation to the surgery of the hip joint, *Clin Orthop* 58:153, 1968.

32. **Chen SC, Lowe SA, Scales JT, et al:** An in vitro experiment to determine the efficiency of fixation of the McKee-Farrar acetabular component in relation to torsional force, *Acta Orthop Scand* 45:429, 1974.

33. **Cheng CL, Gross AE:** Loosening of the porous coating in total knee replacement, *J Bone Joint Surg* 70[Br]:377, 1988.

34. **Clark JM, Freeman MAR, Witham D:** The relationship of neck orientation to the shape of the proximal femur, *J Arthroplasty* 2:99, 1987.

35. **Cohen MG, Hays MB, Garcia JJ, et al:** Fracture of a metal-backed acetabular cup. A case report, *J Arthroplasty* 3:263, 1988.

36. **Colangelo VJ, Greene ND:** Corrosion and fracture of type 316 S.M.O. orthopedic implants, *J Biomed Mater Res* 3:247, 1969.

37. **Collins DN, Chetta SG, Nelson CL:** Fracture of the acetabular cup: a case report, *J Bone Joint Surg* 64:939, 1982.

38. **Crowninshield R:** An engineering analysis of total hip component design, *Orthop Rev* vol 11, 1983.

39. **Crowninshield RD, Brand RA, Johnston RC, et al:** An analysis of femoral component stem design in total hip arthroplasty, *J Bone Joint Surg* 62:68, 1980.

40. **Crowninshield RD, Brand RA, Johnston RC, et al:** The effect of femoral stem cross-sectional geometry on cement stresses in total hip reconstruction, *Clin Orthop* 146:71, 1980.

41. **Crowninshield RD, Brand RA, Pedersen DR:** A stress analysis of acetabular reconstruction in protrusio acetabuli, *J Bone Joint Surg* 65:495, 1983.

42. **Crowninshield RD, Johnston RC, Andrews JG, et al:** A biomechanical investigation of the human hip, *J Biomech* 11:75, 1978.

43. **Crowninshield RD, Pedersen DR, Brand RA, et al:** Analytical support for acetabular component metal backing. In The Hip Society: *The hip: proceedings of the*

eleventh open scientific meeting of The Hip Society, St Louis, 1983, Mosby–Year Book.

44. **Davidson JA, Brasher T:** *Technical memo OR-90-130,* Memphis, 1990, Smith and Nephew Richards.

45. **Davey JR, Harris WH:** Loosening of cobalt chrome beads from a porous-coated acetabular component: a report of ten cases, *Clin Orthop* 231:97, 1988.

46. **Davy DT, Kotzar GM, Brown RH, et al:** Telemetric force measurements across the hip after total arthroplasty, *J Bone Joint Surg* 70:45, 1988.

47. **DeLee JG, Charnley J:** Radiological demarcation of cemented sockets in total hip replacement, *Clin Orthop* 121:20, 1976.

48. **Eftekhar NS, Nercessian O:** Incidence and mechanism of failure of cemented acetabular component in total hip arthroplasty, *Orthop Clin North Am* 19:557, 1988.

49. **Eftekhar NS, Pawluk RJ:** Role of surgical preparation in acetabular cup fixation. In The Hip Society: *The hip: proceedings of the eighth open scientific meeting of The Hip Society,* St Louis, 1980, Mosby–Year Book.

50. **Elson RA, Charnley J:** The direction of the resultant force in total prosthetic replacement of the hip joint, *Med Biol Eng* 6:19, 1968.

51. **Engelhardt A:** Causal histogenesis and related biomechanical discoveries as a basis for the cementless fixation of hip endoprostheses. In Morscher E, editor: *The cementless fixation of hip endoprostheses,* New York, 1984, Springer-Verlag.

52. **Engh CA:** *Porous coated hip replacement. Five-year follow-up study.* Presented at the 50th annual meeting of the American Academy of Orthopaedic Surgeons, Anaheim, Calif., March 1983.

53. **Engh CA:** Hip arthroplasty with a Moore prosthesis with a porous coating: a five year study, *Clin Orthop* 176:52, 1983.

54. **Engh CA:** Instructional manual, 1989.

55. **Engh CA, Bobyn JD:** *Biological fixation in total hip arthroplasty,* Thorofare, NJ, 1985, Slack.

56. **Engh CA, Bobyn JD:** The influence of stem size and extent of porous coating on femoral bone resorption after primary cementless total hip arthroplasty, *Clin Orthop* 231:7, 1988.

57. **Engh GA, Bobyn JD, Petersen TL:** Radiographic and histologic study of porous-coated tibial component fixation in cementless total knee arthroplasty, *Orthopedics* 11:725, 1988.

58. **Engh CA, Griffin WL, Marx CL:** Cementless acetabular components, *J Bone Joint Surg* 72[Br]:53, 1989.

59. **English TA, Kilvington M:** In vivo records of hip loads using a femoral implant with telemetric output (a preliminary report), *J Biomed Eng* 1:111, 1979.

60. **Etienne A, Cupic Z, Charnley J:** Postoperative dislocation after Charnley low-friction arthroplasty, *Clin Orthop* 132:19, 1978.

61. **Finlay JB, Bourne RB, Landsberg RPD, et al:** Pelvic stresses in vitro. II. A study of the efficacy of metal-backed acetabular prostheses, *J Biomech* 19:715, 1986.

62. **Frankel VH:** The femoral neck: function, fracture mechanism, internal fixation; an experimental study, Springfield, Ill., 1960, Charles C Thomas.

63. **Frankel VH:** Biomechanics of the hip. In Tronzo RG, editor: *Surgery of the hip joint,* Philadelphia, 1973, Lea & Febiger.

64. **Frankel A, Balderston RA, Booth RE Jr, et al:** Radiographic demarcation of the acetabular bone-cement interface, *J Arth* 5(suppl):1, 1990.

65. **Galante JO, Andriacchi T, Rostoker W, et al:** Femoral stem failures in total hip replacements. In The Hip Society: *The hip: proceedings of the third open scientific meeting of The Hip Society,* St Louis, 1975, Mosby–Year Book.

66. **Galante JO, Rostoker W, Doyle JM:** Failed femoral stems in total hip prostheses, *J Bone Joint Surg* 57:230, 1975.

67. **Glassman AH, Engh CA, Griffin WL:** Removal of porous coated femoral hip stems. In *Transactions of the 57th annual meeting of the American Academy of Orthopaedic Surgeons,* 1990.

68. **Goel VK, Valliappan S, Svensson NL:** Stresses in the normal pelvis, *Comput Biol Med* 8:91, 1978.

69. **Gonzalez MH, Glass RS, Mallory TH:** Fracture of a metal-backed acetabular component in total hip arthroplasty. A case report, *Clin Orthop* 232:156, 1988.

70. **Griffith MJ, Seidenstein MK, Williams D, et al:** Eight year results of Charnley arthroplasties of the hip with special reference to the behavior of cement, *Clin Orthop* 137:24, 1978.

71. **Grover HJ:** Metal fatigues in some orthopedic implants, *J Materials* 1:412, 1966.

72. **Gruen TA, McNeice GM, Amstutz HC:** "Modes of failure" of cemented stem-type femoral components. A radiographic analysis of loosening, *Clin Orthop* 141:17, 1979.

73. **Haboush EJ:** A new operation for arthroplasty of the hip based on biomechanics, photoelasticity, fast-setting dental acrylic, and other considerations, *Bull Hosp J Dis* 14:242, 1953.

74. **Hardt DE:** Determining muscle forces in the leg during normal human walking—an application and evaluation of optimization methods, *J Biomech Eng* 100:72, 1978.

75. **Harley JM, Boston DA:** Acetabular cup failure after total hip replacement, *J Bone Joint Surg* 67[Br]:222, 1985.

76. **Harris WH:** Advances in total hip arthroplasty, *Clin Orthop* 183:4, 1983.

77. **Harris WH:** The porous total hip replacement system: surgical technique. In Harris, WH, editor: *Advanced concepts in total hip replacement,* Thorofare, NJ, 1985, Slack.

78. **Harris WH, Penenberg BL:** Further follow-up on socket fixation using a metal-backed acetabular component for total hip replacement, *J Bone Joint Surg* 69:1140, 1987.

79. **Harris WH, White RE Jr:** Socket fixation using a metal-backed acetabular component for total hip replacement. A minimum five-year follow-up, *J Bone Joint Surg* 64:745, 1982.

80. **Hodge WA, Fijan RS, Carlson KL, et al:** Contact pressures in the human hip joint measured in vivo, *Proc Natl Acad Sci USA* 83:2879, 1986.

81. **Hoeltzel DA, Walt MJ, Kyle RF, et al:** The effects of femoral head size on the deformation of ultrahigh molecular weight polyethylene acetabular cups, *J Biomech* 22:1163, 1989.

82. **Holmberg PD, Bechtold JE, Sun BN, et al:** Strain analysis of a femur with long stem press-fit prosthesis, *Proc Orthop Res Soc* New Orleans, 1986.

83. **Huddleston HD:** Femoral lysis after cemented hip arthroplasty, *J Arthroplasty* 3:285, 1988.

84. **Huggler AH, Jacob HAC:** The uncemented thrust plate hip prosthesis in the cementless fixation of hip and prostheses. In Mosher E, editor: Berlin, New York, 1984, Springer-Verlag.

85. **Hughes AN, Jordan BA:** Metallurgical observations on some metallic surgical implants which failed in vivo, *J*

Biomed Mater Res 6:33, 1972.

86. **Huiskes R:** Some fundamental aspects of human joint replacements: analyses of stresses and heat conduction in bone-prosthesis structures, *Acta Orthop Scand* 185:109, 1980.

87. **Huiskes R, Weinans H, Dalstra M:** Adaptive bone remodeling and biomechanical design considerations for noncemented total hip arthroplasty, *Orthopedics* 12:1255, 1989.

88. **Huiskes R, Boeklagen R:** Mathematical shape optimization of hip prosthesis design, *J Biomech* 22:793, 1989.

89. **Huiskes R, Chao EYS:** A survey of finite element methods in orthopaedic biomechanics, *J Biomech* 16:385, 1983.

90. **Inman VT:** Functional aspects of the abductor muscles of the hip, *J Bone Joint Surg* 29:607, 1947.

91. **Jacob HAC, Huggler AH, Dietschi C, et al:** Mechanical function of subchondral bone as experimentally determined on the acetabulum of the human pelvis, *J Biomech* 9:625, 1976.

92. **Jasty M, Harrigan TP, Henshaw RO, et al:** Residual strains produced in the proximal femur during rasping and during the insertion of uncemented metal femoral components, *Trans Orthop Res Soc* 12:399, 1987.

93. **Jasty M, Henshaw RM, O'Connor DO, et al:** Strain alterations in the proximal femur with an uncemented femoral prosthesis emphasizing the effect of component fixation, *Proc Orthop Res Soc,* 1988.

94. **Johnston RA, Brand RA, Crowninshield RD:** Reconstruction of the hip: a mathematical approach to determine optimum geometric relationships, *J Bone Joint Surg* 61:639, 1979.

95. **Johnston RC, Larson CB:** Biomechanics of cup arthroplasty, *Clin Orthop* 66:56, 1969.

96. **Jones LC, Hungerford DS:** Cement disease, *Clin Orthop* 225:192, 1987.

97. **Kobayashi S, Eftekhar NS, Terdyama K:** Predisposing factors in radiological failure of the femoral prosthesis following primary Charnley low-friction arthroplasty, a 10-20 year follow-up study, submitted for publication 1992.

98. **Lee AJC:** Finite element analysis and its significance in total hip replacement. In Stillwell WT, editor: *The art of total hip arthroplasty,* Orlando, 1987, Grune & Stratton.

99. **Lee AJ, Ling RS:** A device to improve the extrusion of bone cement into the bone of the acetabulum in the replacement of the hip joint, *Biomed Eng* 9:522, 1974.

100. **Lee AJC, Wrighton JD:** Some properties of polymethylmethacrylate with reference to its use in orthopedic surgery, *Clin Orthop* 95:281, 1973.

101. **Lord G, Hardy JR, Kummer FJ:** An uncemented total hip replacement. Experimental study and review of 300 madreporique arthroplasties, *CORR* 141:2, 1979.

102. **Lord G, MaRotte JH, Guillamon JL, et al:** Cementless revisions of failed aseptic cemented and cementless total hip arthroplasties: 284 cases, *CORR* 235:67, 1988.

103. **Ma SM, Kabo JM, Amstutz HC:** Frictional torque in surface and conventional hip replacement, *J Bone Joint Surg* 65:366, 1983.

104. **McKellop H, Ebramzadeh E, Sarmiento A, et al:** Stem-bone micromotion in non-cemented hip prostheses. Presented at the Proceedings of the European Congress on Biomaterials, Bologna, Italy, September 1980.

104a. **McKellop HA, Sarmiento A, Schwinn CP, et al:** In vivo wear of titanium-alloy hip prostheses, *J Bone Joint Surg* 72:512, 1990.

105. **McLeish RD, Charnley J:** Abduction forces in the one legged stance, *J Biomech* 3:191, 1970.

106. **McNeice GJ, Gruen TA:** Mechanical failure modes of femoral components — radiographic examination of total hip replacement, *Trans 22nd Annual Orthop Res Soc* 1:6, 1976.

107. **Markolf KL, Amstutz HC:** Compressive deformations of the acetabulum during in vitro loading, *Clin Orthop* 173:284, 1983.

108. **Markolf KL, Amstutz HC, Hirschowitz DL:** The effect of calcar contact on femoral component micromovement, a mechanical study, *J Bone Joint Surg* 62:1315, 1980.

109. **Miller GJ, Petty RW, Piotrowski G:** A comparison of acetabular strain changes following Ti6A14V and CoCr metal-backed component implantation, *Trans Orthop Res Soc* 32:469, 1986.

110. **Mikosz RP, Andriacchi TP, Hampton S, et al:** *The importance of limb segment inertia on joint loads during gait.* Read at the annual meeting of the American Society of Mechanical Engineers, San Francisco, December 1978.

111. **Mizrahi J, Solomon L, Kaufman B, et al:** An experimental method for investigating load distribution in the cadaveric human hip, *J Bone Joint Surg* 63[Br]:610, 1981.

112. **Moreland JR, Jinnah R:** Fracture of a Charnley acetabular component from polyethylene wear, *Clin Orthop* 207:94, 1986.

113. **Morrey BF, Ilstrup D:** Size of the femoral head and acetabular revision in total hip arthroplasty, *J Bone Joint Surg* 71:50, 1989.

114. **Morscher EW, Dick W:** Cementless fixation of "isoelastic" hip endoprostheses manufactured from plastic materials, *Clin Orthop* 176:77, 1983.

115. **Murphy SB, Schneeweis D, Walker PS:** *Strain distribution and micromotion in press-fit and cemented hip prostheses.* Trans. 31st Annual Meeting of the Orthopaedic Research Society, Las Vegas, Jan. 21–24, 1985.

116. **Noble PC, Alexander JW, Lindahl LJ, et al:** The anatomic basis of femoral component design, *Clin Orthop* 235:148, 1988.

117. **Noble PC, Tullus HS, Landon GC:** The optimum cement mantle for total hip replacement: theory and practice, *Instructional course lectures,* vol 30, St Louis, 1991, Mosby–Year Book.

118. **O'Connor DO, Burke DW, Harris WH:** Bone-implant micromotion in titanium ingrowth hip stems, *Trans Soc Biomater* 10:97, 1987.

119. **Oh I:** a comprehensive analysis of the factors affecting acetabular cup fixation and design in total hip replacement arthroplasty: a series of experimental and clinical studies. The Hip Society: *The Hip: proceedings of the eleventh open scientific meeting of The Hip Society,* St Louis, 1983, Mosby–Year Book.

120. **Oh I, Harris WH:** Proximal strain distribution in the loaded femur: an in vitro comparison of the distributions in the intact femur and after insertion of different hip replacement femoral components, *J Bone Joint Surg* 60:75, 1978.

121. **Oh I, Merckx DB, Harris WH:** Acetabular cement compactor: an experimental study of pressurization of cement in the acetabulum in total hip arthroplasty, *Clin Orthop* 177:289, 1983.

122. **Oh I, Sander TW, Treharne RW:** Acetabular cup groove and pod design and its effect on cement fixation in total

hip arthroplasty, *Clin Orthop* 189:308, 1984.

123. **Oh I, Sander TW, Treharne RW:** Total hip acetabular cup flange design and its effect on cement fixation, *Clin Orthop* 195:304, 1985.

124. **Oh I, Treharne RW, Sanders TW:** Acetabular cement strain for different cement thicknesses and shapes of the cement mantle. In vitro strain gauge study, *Trans Biomat* 9:95, 1983.

125. **Paul JP:** Biomechanics. The biomechanics of the hip joint and its clinical relevance, *Proc R Soc Med* 59:943, 1966.

126. **Paul JP:** *Forces at the human hip joint,* Thesis, University of Chicago, 1967.

127. **Paul JP:** Forces transmitted by joints in the human body, *Proc Inst Mech Eng* 181:8, 1967.

128. **Paul JP:** Force actions transmitted by joints in the human body, *Proc R Soc Lond* [Biol] 192:163, 1976.

129. **Pauwels F:** *Der Schenkelhalsbruch, ein Mechanisches Problem,* Stuttgart, 1936, Ferdinand Enke Verlag.

130. **Pawluk RJ, Tsitzikalikas G, Eftekhar NS:** The effect of surgical preparation on acetabular cup fixation. In *Transactions of the twenty-sixth annual Orthopaedic Research Society meeting,* Atlanta, 1980.

131. **Pedersen DR, Crowninshield RD, Brand R, et al:** An axisymmetric model of acetabular components in total hip arthroplasty, *J Biomech* 15:305, 1982.

132. **Petty W, Miller GJ, Piotrowski G:** In vitro evaluation of the effect of acetabular prosthesis implantation on human cadaver pelves, *Bull Prosthet Res* 17:80, 1980.

133. **Petty W, Piotrowski G, Miller GJ:** In vitro evaluation of the effect of acetabular prosthesis implantation on human cadaver pelves, *Trans Orthop Res Soc* 27:73, 1981.

134. **Pilliar RM:** Porous-surfaced metallic implants for orthopaedic applications, *J Biomed Mater Res Appl Biomater* 21[suppl]:1, 1987.

135. **Pilliar RM, Weatherly GC:** Developments in implant alloys. In *Critical reviews in biocompatibility,* Boca Raton, Fla, 1986, CRC Press.

136. **Ponseti I:** Pathomechanics of the hip after the shelf operation, *J Bone Joint Surg* 28:229, 1946.

137. **Poss R, Walker P, Spector M, et al:** Strategies for improving fixation of femoral components in total hip arthroplasty, *Clin Orthop* 235:181, 1988.

138. **Reichelt A, Blasius K:** First experience with the PM prosthesis. In Morscher E, editor: *The cementless fixation of hip endoprostheses,* New York, 1984, Springer-Verlag.

139. **Ring PA:** Five to fourteen year interim results of uncemented total hip arthroplasty, *Clin Orthop* 137:87, 1978.

140. **Ring PA:** Ring UPM total hip arthroplasty, *Clin Orthop* 176:115, 1983.

141. **Ritter MA, Campbell ED:** Long-term comparison of the Charnley, Müller, and Trapezoidal-28 total hip prostheses, *J Arthroplasty* 2:299, 1987.

142. **Röhrle H, Scholten R, Sigolotto C, et al:** Joint forces in the human pelvis-leg skeleton during walking, *J Biomech* 17:409, 1984.

143. **Rosenqvist R, Bylander B, Knutson K, et al:** Loosening of the porous coating of bicompartmental prostheses in patients with rheumatoid arthritis, *J Bone Joint Surg* 68[Am]:538, 1986.

144. **Ruff CB, Hayes WC:** Subperiosteal expansion and cortical remodeling of the human femur and tibia with aging, *Science* 217:945, 1982.

145. **Rydell MW:** Forces in the hip joint. In *Biomechanics and related bioengineering topics,* London, 1964, Pergamon Press.

146. **Rydell MW:** Forces acting on the femoral head prosthesis: a study on strain gauge supplied prostheses in living persons, *Acta Orthop Scand* 88[suppl]:1, 1966.

147. **Saejong S, Hirano S, Granholm JW, et al:** The influence of the interface on bone strains and stem-bone micromotion in press-fit total hip stems, *Trans Orthop Res Soc* 12:484, 1987.

148. **Salvati EA, Wright TM, Burstein AH, et al:** Fracture of polyethylene acetabular cups. Report of two cases, *J Bone Joint Surg* 61:1239, 1979.

149. **Salzer M, Knahr K, Frank P:** Radiologic and clinical follow-ups of uncemented femoral endoprostheses with and without collars. In Morscher E, editor: *The cementless fixation of hip endoprostheses,* New York, 1984, Springer-Verlag.

150. **Santavirta S, Hoikka V, Eskola A, et al:** Aggressive granulomatous lesions in cementless total hip arthroplasty, *J Bone Joint Surg* 72[Br]:980, 1990.

151. **Sarmiento A, Gruen TA:** Radiographic analysis of a low-modulus titanium-alloy femoral total hip component: two to six-year follow-up, *J Bone Joint Surg* 67:48, 1985.

152. **Sarmiento A, Natarajan V, Gruen T, et al:** Radiographic performance of two different total hip cemented arthroplasties. A survivorship analysis, *Orthop Clin North Am* 19:505, 1988.

152a. **Schneider E, Eulenberger J, Steiner W, et al:** In vitro testing of the initial stability of uncemented hip joint prostheses, *Trans Orthop Res Soc* 12:403, 1987.

153. **Seirig A, Arkivar RJ:** Prediction of muscular load sharing and joint forces in the lower extremities during walking, *J Biomech* 8:89, 1975.

154. **Shelley P, Wroblewski BM:** Socket design and cement pressurization in the Charnley low-friction arthroplasty, *J Bone Joint Surg* 70[Br]:358, 1988.

155. **Simon SR, Paul IL, Rose RM, et al:** "Stiction-friction" of total hip prostheses and its relationship to loosening, *J Bone Joint Surg* 57:226, 1975.

156. **Simon SR, Radin EL:** Lubrication and wear of the Charnley, Charnley-Müller, and McKee-Farrar prostheses with special regard to their clinical behavior. The Hip Society: *The Hip: proceedings of the first open scientific meeting of The Hip Society, 1973,* St Louis, 1973, Mosby–Year Book.

157. **Steinmann SC, Eulenberger J, Maeusli PA, et al:** Adhesion of bone to titanium. In Christel P, Meunier A, Lee AJC, editors: *Biological and biomechanical performance of biomaterials,* Amsterdam, 1986, Elsevier.

158. **Stout SY, Marsh HO:** The broken acetabular wire sign, *Orthop Rev* 10:135, 1981.

159. **Sutherland CJ, Wilde AH, Borden LS, et al:** A ten-year follow-up of one hundred consecutive Müller curved-stem total hip-replacement arthroplasties, *J Bone Joint Surg* 64[Am]:970, 1982.

159a. **Tullos HS, McCaskill BL, Dickey R, et al:** Total hip arthroplasty with a low-modulus porous-coated femoral component. Progress report, *J Bone Joint Surg* 66:888, 1984.

160. **Van Gerven DP, Armelagos GJ, Bartley MH:** Roentgenographic and direct measurement of femoral cortical involution in a prehistoric Mississippian population, *Am J Phys Anthropol* 31:23, 1983.

161. **Van Syckle PB, Walker PS:** Parametric analysis of design criteria for acetabular components of surface replacement hip devices, *Trans ORS* 26:292, 1980.

162. **Vasu R, Carter DR, Harris WH:** Stress distributions in the acetabular region. I. Before and after total joint replacement, *J Biomech* 15:155, 1982.

163. **Vives P, de Lestang M, Jarde O, et al:** Intérêt du contact direct entre la tige fémorale et l'os diaphysaire dans les prosthèses totales cimentees, *Rev Chir Orthop* [suppl] 2:218, 1987.

164. **Volz RG:** Fracture of the bony acetabulum following total hip replacement: significance of broken acetabular wire sign, *Orthop Rev* 9:91, 1980.

165. **Volz RG, Wilson RJ:** Factors affecting the mechanical stability of the cemented acetabular component in total hip replacement, *J Bone Joint Surg* 59:501, 1977.

166. **Walker PS, Robertson DD:** Design and fabrication of cementless hip stems, *Clin Orthop* 235:25, 1988.

167. **Walker PS, Schneeweis D, Murphy S, et al:** Strains and micromotions of press-fit femoral stem prostheses, *J Biomech* 20:693, 1987.

168. **Weightman B, Isherwood DP, Swanson SAV:** The fracture of ultrahigh molecular weight polyethylene in the human body, *J Biomed Mat Res* 13:669, 1979.

169. **Wheeler KR, James LA:** Fatigue behaviour type 316 stainless steel under simulated body conditions, *J Biomed Mater Res* 5:267, 1971.

170. **Whiteside LA, Amador DD, Russell K:** The effects of the collar on total hip femoral component subsidence, *Clin Orthop* 231:120, 1988.

171. **Whiteside LA, Easley JC:** The effect of collar and distal stem fixation on micromotion of the femoral stem in uncemented total hip arthroplasty, *Clin Orthop* 239:145, 1989.

172. **Wiles P:** The surgery of the osteoarthritic hip, *Br J Surg* 45:488, 1958.

173. **Williams JL:** Biomechanics of total hip replacement. In Steinberg ME, editor: *The hip and its disorders,* Philadelphia, 1991, WB Saunders.

173a. **Williams JM, Buchanan RA:** Ion implantation of surgical Ti-6A1-4V alloy, *Mater Sci Eng* 69:237, 1985.

174. **Wilson JA, Scales JT:** Loosening of the total hip replacements with cement fixation, *Clin Orthop* 72:145, 1970.

175. **Wroblewski BM:** *Revision surgery in total hip arthroplasty,* New York, 1990, Springer-Verlag.

176. **Yue S, Pilliar RM, Weatherly GC:** The fatigue strength of porous-coated Ti-6% Al-4% V implant alloy, *J Bio Mater Res* 18:1043, 1984.

177. **Zweymuller K:** First clinical experience with an uncemented modular femoral prosthesis system with a wrought Ti-6A1-4V a stem and an A1₂O₃ ceramic head. In Morscher E, editor: *The cementless fixation of hip endoprostheses,* Berlin, 1984, Springer-Verlag.

178. **Zweymuller K:** A cementless titanium hip endoprosthesis system based on press-fit fixation: basic research and clinical results. In *AAOS instructional course lectures,* vol 35, St Louis, 1986, Mosby–Year Book.

ADDITIONAL READINGS

Agins HJ, Alcock NW, Bansal M, et al: Metallic wear in failed titanium-alloy total hip replacements. A histological and quantitative analysis, *J Bone Joint Surg* 70:347, 1988.

Amstutz HC: Practical considerations in the selection of materials and design for total hip replacement. In *American Academy of Orthopaedic Surgeons instructional course lectures,* vol 23, St Louis, 1974, Mosby–Year Book.

Amstutz HC, Lodwig RM, Schurman DJ, et al: Range of motion studies for total hip replacements. A comparative study with a new experimental apparatus, *Clin Orthop* 111:124, 1975.

Amstutz HC, Markolf KL: Design features in total hip replacement. The Hip Society: *The hip: proceedings of the second open scientific meeting of The Hip Society,* St Louis, 1974, Mosby–Year Book.

Averill RG, Pachtman N, Jaffe WL: A basic dimensional analysis of normal human proximal femora. In *proceedings of the eighth annual Northeast Bioengineering Conference,* Cambridge, Mass, 1980.

Baker AS, Bitounis VC: Abductor function after total hip replacement. An electromyographic and clinical review, *J Bone Joint Surg* 71[Br]:47, 1989.

Bartel DL, Bicknele VL, Wright TM: The effect of conformity, thickness, and material on stresses in ultra-high molecular weight components for total joint replacement, *J Bone Joint Surg* 68:1041, 1986.

Bartel DL, Wright TM, Edwards D: The effect of metal backing on stresses in polyethylene acetabular components. In The Hip Society: *The Hip: proceedings of the eleventh open scientific meeting of The Hip Society,* St Louis, 1983, Mosby–Year Book.

Bell RS, Schatzker J, Fornasier VL, et al: A study of implant failure in the Wagner resurfacing arthroplasty, *J Bone Joint Surg* 67:1165, 1985.

Bobyn JD, Pilliar RM, Cameron HU, et al: The optimum pore size for the fixation of porous-surfaced metal implants by the ingrowth of bone, *Clin Orthop* 150:263, 1980.

Bousquet G, Bornand F: A screw-anchored intramedullary hip prosthesis. In Morscher E, editor: *The cementless fixation of hip endoprostheses,* Berlin, 1984, Springer-Verlag.

Cahoon JR, Paxton HW: A metallurgical survey of current orthopedic implants, *J Biomed Mater Res* 4:223, 1970.

Cameron HU, Pilliar RM, MacNab I: The effect of movement on the bonding of porous metal to bone, *J Biomed Mater Res* 7:301, 1973.

Cameron HU, Pilliar RM, MacNab I: The rate of bone ingrowth into porous metal, *J Biomed Mater Res* 10:295, 1976.

Carter DR: Finite-element analysis of a metal-backed acetabular component. In The Hip Society: *The hip: proceedings of the eleventh open scientific meeting of The Hip Society,* St Louis, 1983, Mosby–Year Book.

Chandler DR, Glousman R, Hall D, et al: Prostetic hip range of motion and impingement. The effects of head and neck geometry, *Clin Orthop* 166:284, 1982.

Charnley J: The lubrication of animal joints in relation to surgical reconstruction by arthroplasty, *Ann Rheum Dis* 19:10, 1960.

Charnley J: *Factors in design of hip arthroplasty.* Symposium on lubrication and wear and living artificial human hip joints, vol 6, London, 1968, Institution of Medical Engineers.

Charnley J: The fixation of prostheses in living bone. In Simpson DC, editor: *The modern trends in biomechanics,* vol 1, New York, 1970, Appleton-Century-Crofts.

Charnley J, editor: Total hip replacement (Symposium), guest *Clin Orthop* 72:1, 1970.

Charnley J: Comparison of dynamic frictional torque in different total hip implanting by a pendulum method, internal publication no. 35, Wigan, England, 1971, Centre for Hip Surgery, Wrightington Hospital.

Charnley J: Low friction arthroplasty of the hip joint. In Proceedings and Reports of Universities, Colleges, Council and Associations: British Orthopaedic Association, *J Bone Joint Surg* 53[Br]:149, 1971.

Charnley J: The status of research into the wear of high molecular weight polyethylene in total hip replacement as of Jan. 1974, Internal publication no. 49, Wigan, England, 1974, Centre for Hip Surgery, Wrightington Hospital.

Charnley J, Eftekhar N: Postoperative infection in total prosthetic replacement arthroplasty of the hip joint with special reference to the bacterial content of the air of the operating room, *Br J Surg* 56:641, 1969.

Charnley J, Halley DK: Rate of wear in total hip replacement, *Clin Orthop* 112:170, 1975.

Charnley J, Halley DK: Rate of wear in the total hip replacement, *Orthop Dig* 2:13, 1976.

Charnley J, Kramanger A, Longfield MD: The optimum size of prosthetic heads in relation to the wear of plastic sockets in total replacement of the hip, *Med Biol Eng* 7:31, 1969.

Chen SC, Badrinath K, Pell LH, et al: The movements of the components of the Hastings bipolar prosthesis, A radiographic study in 65 patients, *J Bone Joint Surg* 71[Br]:186, 1989.

Christel P, Meunier A, Lee AJC, editors: *Biological and biomechanical performance of biomaterials,* Amsterdam, 1986, Elsevier.

Cohen MG, Hays MB, Garcia JJ, et al: Fracture of a metal-backed acetabular cup. A case report, *J Arthroplasty* 3:263, 1988.

Collins DN, Chetta SG, Nelson CL: Fracture of the acetabular cup. A case report, *J Bone Joint Surg* 64:939, 1982.

Crowninshield RD, Brand RA, Johnston RC, et al: An analysis of femoral prosthesis design: the effects on proximal femur loading. In The Hip Society: *The hip: proceedings of the ninth open scientific meeting of The Hip Society,* St Louis, 1981, Mosby–Year Book.

Dall D, Charnley J: Comparison of the lever systems in low friction arthroplasty and the McKee-Farrar arthroplasty, internal publication no. 34, Wigan, England, 1971, Centre for Hip Surgery, Wrightington Hospital.

Dewey JR, Bartley MH Jr, Armelagos GJ: Rates of femoral cortical bone loss in two Nubian populations. Utilizing normalized and non-normalized data, *Clin Orthop* 65:61, 1969.

Dickenson RP, Hutton WC, Stott JRR: The mechanical properties of bone in osteoporosis, *J Bone Joint Surg* 63[Br]:233, 1981.

Dorr L, Bloebaum R, Emmanual J, et al: Histologic, biochemical, and ion analysis of tissue and fluids retrieved during total hip arthroplasty, *Clin Orthop* 261:82, 1990.

Duff-Barclay I, Spillman DT: Total human hip joint prostheses; a laboratory study of friction and wear, *Inst Mechn Eng Proc* 181:104, 1966.

Eftekhar NS: Mechanical failure in low-friction arthroplasty. In *American Academy of Orthopaedic Surgeons instructional course lectures,* vol 23, St Louis, 1974, Mosby–Year Book.

Engh CA: Cementless total hip with the AML—an update on the femoral side. In *proceedings of the 19th annual Harvard course on total hip replacement,* Boston, 1989.

Engh CA, Bobyn JD: The influence of stem size and extent of porous coating on femoral bone resorption after primary cementless hip arthroplasty, *Clin Orthop* 231:7, 1988.

Engh CA, Bobyn JD: Results of porous-coated hip using the AML prosthesis. In Fitzgerald R Jr, editor: *Non-cemented total hip arthroplasty,* New York, 1988, Raven Press.

Engh CA, Bobyn JD, Glassman AH: Porous-coated hip replacement. The factors governing bone ingrowth, stress shielding, and clinical results, *J Bone Joint Surg,* 69[Br]:45, 1987.

Finlay JB, Rorabeck CH, Bourne RB, et al: In vitro analysis of proximal femoral strains using PCA femoral implants and hip-abductor muscle simulator, *J Arthroplasty* 4:335, 1989.

Frankel A, Balderston RA, Booth RE Jr, et al: Radiographic demarcation of the acetabular bone-cement interface. The effect of femoral head size, *J Arthroplasty* 5(suppl):51, 1990.

Freeman MAR, McLeod HC, Levai JP: Cementless fixation of prosthetic components in total arthroplasty of the knee and hip, *Clin Orthop* 176:88, 1983.

Galante JO: Overview of current attempts to eliminate methylmethacrylate. The Hip Society: *The hip: proceedings of the eleventh open scientific meeting of The Hip Society,* St Louis, 1983, Mosby–Year Book.

Galante JO, Andriacchi T, Rostoker W, et al: Femoral stem failures in total hip replacements. In The Hip Society: *The hip: proceedings of the third open scientific meeting of The Hip Society,* St Louis, 1975, Mosby–Year Book.

Galante JO, Rostoker W, Doyle JM: Failed femoral stems in total hip prostheses, *J Bone Joint Surg* 57:230, 1975.

Galante JO, Rostoker W, Lueck R, et al: Sintered fiber metal composites as a basis for attachment of implants to bone, *J Bone Joint Surg* 53:101, 1971.

Gold BL, Walker PS: Variables affecting the friction and wear of metal-on-plastic total hip joints, *Clin Orthop* 100:270, 1974.

Gonzalez MH, Glass RS, Mallory TH: Fracture of a metal-backed acetabular component in total hip arthroplasty. A case report, *Clin Orthop* 232:156, 1988.

Goodman SB, Carter DR: Acetabular lucent lines and mechanical stress in total hip arthroplasty, *J Arthroplasty* 2:219, 1987.

Goto H, Bobyn JD, Usui T, et al: Effect of femoral implant stiffness and threaded acetabular cup design on non-cemented fixation and bone remodeling: a canine total hip model, *Trans Biomat* 15:70, 1989.

Greenwald AS, Nelson CL: Biomechanics of the reconstructed hip, *Orthop Clin North Am* 4:435, 1973.

Haddad RJ, Cook SD, Thomas KA: Biological fixation of porous-coated implants, *J Bone Joint Surg* 69:1459, 1987.

Hardcastle P, Nade S: The significance of the Trendelenburg test, *J Bone Joint Surg* 67[Br]:741, 1985.

Harley JM, Boston DA: Acetabular cup failure after total hip replacement, *J Bone Joint Surg* 67[Br]:222, 1985.

Harris WH, Schiller AL, Scholler J, et al: Extensive localized bone resorption in femur following total hip replacement, *J Bone Joint Surg* 58:612, 1976.

Henrichsen E, Jansen K, Krogh-Poulsen W: Experimental investigation of the tissue reaction to acrylic plastics, *Acta Orthop Scand* 22:141, 1952.

Hieokazu: Socket location in total hip replacement, *Acta Orthop Scand* 59:1, 1988.

Hodgkinson: Assinister bias in hip socket wear, *J Bone Joint Surg* 71[Br]:143, 1989.

Hoeltzel DA, Walt MJ, Kyle RF, et al: The effects of femoral head size on the deformation of ultrahigh molecular weight polyethylene acetabular cups, *J Biomech* 22:1163, 1989.

Hofmann AA, Bigler GT, France ER, et al: Increased endosteal bone loss after hip arthroplasty, *Trans Orthop Res Soc* 11:470, 1986.

Hoopes JE, Edgerton MT, Shelley W: Organic synthetics for augmentation mammoplasty: their relation to breast cancer, *Plast Reconstr Surg* 39:263, 1967.

Hudack S: High chromium, low nickel steel in the operative fixation of fractures, *Arch Surg* 40:867, 1940.

Hughes AN, Jordan BA: Metallurgical observations on some metallic surgical implants which failed in vivo, *J Biomed Mater Res* 6:33, 1972.

Huiskes R: Finite element analysis of acetabular reconstruction. Noncemented threaded cups, *Acta Orthop Scand* 58:620, 1987.

Huiskes R, Peeters H, Sloof TJ: Biomechanical analysis of stem, *Trans ORS* 33:507, 1987.

Hungerford DS, Kenna RV: Preliminary experience with a total knee prosthesis with porous coating replacement used without cement, *Clin Orthop* 176:95, 1983.

Jasty M, Rogers SP, Weinberg EH, et al: The role of uniform surgical fit on bone ingrowth into porous coated canine acetabular replacements (abstract), Harvard Hip course, Boston, October 1989.

Judet R, Siguier M, Brumpt B, et al: A noncemented total hip prosthesis, *Clin Orthop* 137:76, 1978.

Lachiewicz PF, Suh PB, Gilbert JA: In vitro initial fixation of porous-coated acetabular total hip components. A biomechanical comparative study, *J Arthroplasty* 4:201, 1989.

Lanyon LE, Paul IL, Rubin CT, et al: In vivo strain measurements from bone and prosthesis following total hip replacement. An experimental study in sheep, *J Bone Joint Surg* 63:989, 1981.

Lewis JL, Askew MJ, Wixson RL, et al: The influence of prosthetic stem stiffness and of a calcar collar on stresses in the proximal end of the femur with a cemented femoral component, *J Bone Joint Surg* 66:280, 1984.

Leyshon RL, Matthews JP: Acetabular erosion and the Monk "hard top" hip prosthesis, *J Bone Joint Surg* 66[Br]:172, 1984.

Ling RSM: Observations on the fixation of implants to the bony skeleton, *Clin Orthop* 210:80, 1986.

Lionberger D, Walker PS, Granholm J: Effects of prosthetic acetabular replacement on strains in the pelvis, *J Orthop Res* 3:372, 1985.

Lombardi AV ,Jr, Mallory TH, Vaughn BK, et al: Aseptic loosening in total hip arthroplasty secondary to osteolysis induced by wear debris from titanium-alloy modular femoral heads, *J Bone Joint Surg* 71:1337, 1989.

Loomis LK: Internal prosthesis for upper portion of the femur, case report, *J Bone Joint Surg* 32:944, 1950.

Maistrelli, et al: The inclination of the weight bearing surface in the hip joint, *Orthop Rev* 15:271, 1986.

Mallory TH: Femoral component geometry. A factor in total hip arthroplasty durability, *Clin Orthop* 223:208, 1987.

Markolf KL, Amstutz HC: Compressive deformations of the acetabulum during in vitro loading, *Clin Orthop* 173:284, 1983.

Mattingly DA, Hopson CN, Kahn A, et al: Aseptic loosening in metal-backed acetabular components for total hip replacement, *J Bone Joint Surg* 67:387, 1985.

McNeice GJ, Eng P, Amstutz HC: Finite element studies in hip reconstruction. *Biomechanics* V-A:394, Baltimore, 1976, University Press.

Miller J, Burke DL, Stachiewicz JW, et al: Pathophysiology of loosening of femoral components in total hip arthroplasty. Clinical and experimental study of cement fracture and loosening of the cement-bone interface. In The Hip Society: *The hip, proceedings of the sixth open scientific meeting of The Hip Society*, St Louis, 1978, Mosby–Year Book.

Mittelmeier H: Anchoring hip endoprosthesis without bone cement. In Schaldach M, Hohmann D, editors: *Advances in artificial hip and knee joint technology*, New York, 1976, Springer-Verlag.

Mjöberg E, Selvik G, Hansson LI, et al: Mechanical loosening of total hip prostheses. A radiographic and roentgen stereophotogrammetic study, *J Bone Joint Surg* 68[Br]:770, 1986.

Moore AT: The self-locking metal hip prosthesis, *J Bone Joint Surg* 39:811, 1957.

Moore AT, Bohlman HR: Metal hip joint; a case report, *J Bone Joint Surg* 25:668, 1943.

Moreland JR, Jinnah R: Fracture of a Charnley acetabular component from polyethylene wear, *Clin Orthop* 207:94, 1986.

Morrey BF, Ilstrup D: Size of the femoral head and acetabular revision in total hip replacement arthroplasty, *J Bone Joint Surg* 71:50, 1989.

Morscher E, Masar Z: Development and first experience with an uncemented press-fit cup, *Clin Orthop* 232:96, 1988.

Morscher EW: Cementless total hip arthroplasty, *Clin Orthop* 181:76, 1983.

Murphy SB, Walker PS, Schiller AL: Adaptive changes in the femur after implantation of an Austin-Moore prosthesis, *J Bone Joint Surg* 66:437, 1984.

Noble PC, Lindahl LJ, Jay JL, et al: *Femoral anatomy and the design of total hip replacements.* Proc. 32nd annual meeting of the ORS, Las Vegas, February 17–20, 1986.

Nunn D, Freeman MA, Tanney KE, et al: Torsional stability of the femoral component of hip arthoplasty. Response to an anteriorly applied load, *J Bone Joint Surg* 71[Br]:452, 1989.

Oh I, Bushelow M, Sander TW, et al: An in vitro strain gauge study of metal-backed acetabular cups, *Trans Biomat* 10:148, 1984.

Oonishi H, Isha H, Hasegawa T: Mechanical analysis of the human pelvis and its application to the artificial hip joint—by means of the three dimensional finite element method, *J Biomech* 16:427, 1983.

Pacheco V, Shelley P, Wroblewski BM: Mechanical loosening of the stem in Charnley arthroplasties. Identification of the "at risk" factors, *J Bone Joint Surg* 70[Br]:596, 1988.

Pilliar RM, Cameron HU, MacNab I: Porous surface layered prosthetic devices, *J Biomed Eng* 10:126, 1975.

Poss R, Staehlin P, Larson M: Femoral expansion in total hip arthroplasty, *J Arthroplasty* 2:259, 1987.

Poss R, Walker P, Spector M, et al: Strategies for improving fixation of femoral components in total hip arthroplasty, *Orthop Clin North Am* 19:591, 1988.

Ritter MA, Fechtman RW: Distal cortical hypertrophy following total hip arthroplasty, *J Arthroplasty* 3:117, 1988.

Ritter MA, Stringer EA, Littrell DA, et al: Correlation of prosthetic femoral head size and/or design with longevity of total hip arthroplasty, *Clin Orthop* 176:252, 1983.

Rubin CT, Lanyon LE: Regulation of bone formation by applied dynamic loads, *J Bone Joint Surg* 66:397, 1984.

Ruff CB: Allometry between length and cross-sectional dimensions of the femur and tibia in *Homo sapiens sapiens, Am J Phys Anthropol* 65:347, 1984.

Ruff CB, Torchia ME: *Diaphyseal involution in femora with prosthetic hip implants.* Trans. 33rd Annual Meeting of the Orthopaedic Research Society, San Francisco, Jan. 19–22, 1987.

Seedhom BB, Dowson D, Wright V: Wear of solid phase formed high density polyethylene in relation to the life of artificial hips and knees, *Wear* 24.35, 1973.

Skinner NB: The effect of abductor forces on femoral stem stresses in cemented prosthetic hip replacement, *J Orthop* 6:55, 1983.

Skinner HB, Cook SD, Weinstein AM, et al: Stress changes in bone secondary to the use of a femoral canal plug with cemented hip replacement, *Clin Orthop* 166:277, 1982.

Smith JW, Walmsley R: Factors affecting the elasticity of bone, *J Anat* 93:503, 1959.

Smith RW Jr, Walker RR: Femoral expansion in aging women: implications for osteoporosis and fractures, *Science* 145:156, 1964.

Soballe K, Christensen F: Calcar resorption after total hip arthroplasty, *J Arthroplasty* 3:103, 1988.

Sumner DR Jr: Postembryonic dimensional allometry of the human femur, *Am J Phys Anthropol* 64:69, 1984.

Tarr: Total hip femoral component design, *Orthop Rev* 11:23, 1982.

Thirupathi RG, Husted C: Failure of polyethylene acetabular cups. Two case reports, *Clin Orthop* 179:209, 1983.

Treharne: Review of Wolff's law and its proposed means of operation, *Orthop Rev* 10:35, 1981.

Turner TM, Sumner DR, Urban RM, et al: A comparative study of porous coatings in a weight-bearing total hip arthroplasty model, *J Bone Joint Surg* 68:1396, 1986.

University of California: *Fundamental studies of human locomotion and other information relating to design of artificial limbs,* Berkeley, California, 1947.

Walker PS, Bullough PG: The effects of friction and wear in artificial joints, *Orthop Clin North Am* 4:275, 1973.

Walker PS, Erkman MJ: Metal-on-metal lubrication in artificial human joints, *Wear* 21:377, 1972.

Walker PS, Onchi K, Kurosawa H, et al: Approaches to the interface problem in total hip joint arthroplasty, *Clin Orthop* 182:99, 1984.

Weber BG: Total hip replacement: rotating versus fixed and metal versus ceramic heads. In The Hip Society: *The hip: proceedings of the ninth open scientific meeting of The Hip Society,* St Louis, 1981, Mosby–Year Book.

Weber BG: Pressurized cement fixation in total hip arthroplasty, *Clin Orthop* 232:87, 1988.

Weber FA, Charnley J: A radiological study of fractures of acrylic cement in relation to the stem of the femoral head prosthesis, *J Bone Joint Surg* 57[Br]:297, 1975.

Weightman BO, Paul IL, Rose RM, et al: A comparative study of total hip replacement prostheses, *J Biomech* 6:299, 1973.

Wheeler KR, James LA: Fatigue behavior of type 316 stainless steel under simulated body conditions, *J Biomed Mater Res* 5:267, 1971.

Williams DF, Roaf R: *Implants in surgery,* Philadelphia, 1973, WB Saunders.

Wilson JA, Scales JT: Loosening of the total hip replacements with cement fixation, *Clin Orthop* 72:145, 1970.

Wroblewski BM: The mechanism of fracture of the femoral prosthesis in total hip replacement, *Int Orthop* 3:137, 1979.

Wroblewski BM: Direction and rate of socket wear in Charnley low-friction arthroplasty, *J Bone Joint Surg* 67[Br]:757, 1985.

Yamamoto: The effect of hydroxyapatite coating on bone growth into porous titanium alloy implants, *J Bone Joint Surg* 71[Br]:213, 1989.

Zweymüller K, Lintner FK, Semlitsch MF: Biologic fixation of a press-fit titanium hip joint endoprosthesis, *Clin Orthop* 235:195, 1988.

See Chapters 4, Biomaterials: Compatibility and Wear; 5, Acrylic Cement: Properties and Application; and 28, Results in Primary Total Hip Arthroplasty for additional information.

PART THREE

GENERAL SURGICAL PRINCIPLES

CHAPTER SEVEN

Preoperative Planning

■ A patient who is to have an elective surgical operation could do no better than to deposit a week or two before the ordeal a pint of blood in the bank to have it available in case it is needed during or after the operation.
B. Fantus

The orthopaedic surgeon performing hip arthroplasty is bound — like all surgeons — by principles that require careful evaluation of the whole patient, well-founded indications for the specific surgical intervention, aseptic technique, and absolute precision if the result is to be successful. Complications after total hip arthroplasty are at times disastrous to the patient, and a total failure (possibly caused by an infected total hip arthroplasty or iatrogenic pathology of the pelvis or femur after the procedure) may require a resection pseudarthrosis. Because of the magnitude of the problem, when serious complications arise, prevention, not salvage after complications, must be emphasized, and the surgeon must pay special attention to all the detailed specifics of technique including the preoperative and postoperative care of the patient. (For specifics, see Chapters 8 to 14). This chapter is designed to assist in preparing the patient for surgery.

SURGICAL AND NURSING CARE OF ELDERLY PATIENTS

Unlike traumatic cases, patients being considered for major elective surgery are not particularly high surgical risks, but they do have special needs. Despite these needs, however, the orthopaedic literature has seldom emphasized the importance of preoperative nursing care for elderly patients scheduled for elective surgery. Most patients undergoing total hip arthroplasty are in their sixties and seventies; some are in their eighties. These patients have many psychological and physical problems that demand special attention.[1,2,26,102] Wilder and Fishbein[105] followed 207 surgical patients who were over 80 years of age for 30 days and found the overall mortality rate to be 33.3%. They also found that mortality varied among specialties; in orthopaedic surgery, for example, the mortality was 31.7%. In a study of 1300 major operations on patients over 70 years of age, Scott[89] and associates found an overall mortality rate of 13.8%; however, the rate dropped to 6.5% when patients at risk for operative complications were excluded from surgery. This high mortality rate is unacceptable in elective surgery (such as total hip arthroplasty) and is obviously related to preexisting conditions in the elderly that affect surgery, to serious complications that may occur postoperatively in abdominal or neurological operations, or to both. Lack of preoperative preparation and diagnostic errors have at times been blamed for the high mortality rate in elderly patients. The mortality in patients undergoing total hip arthroplasty is estimated to be about 1%.

Clearly, the excessively high mortality rate in older patients can be reduced if the surgeon and others address all aspects of their medical care before surgery, performing systemic review and proper consultations. Anesthesia management and rehabilitation programs, for example, must be planned with care; a very old patient should begin ambulation earlier after surgery than is routinely required. When the surgeon considers a severely debilitated patient for surgery, the first step is to identify the patient's needs and then to render the appropriate special care. Although older patients generally tolerate the stress of surgery better than younger patients, this initial tolerance soon gives way to the dangers of shock and death, unless certain precautions are taken. For example, an older patient may not complain as much as a younger patient after hip fracture, but if the fracture is not immobilized, the older patient may soon lapse into shock.

Social factors related to health concern patients greatly. The surgeon and staff can greatly augment the patient's confidence if they address the following issues before surgery:

1. The patient's desire to return home as soon as possible after surgery
2. The patient's loneliness while in the hospital
3. The patient's worries about a spouse or other relatives left alone at home
4. The patient's resentment about loss of self-sufficiency during confinement in bed (for example, being unable to reach for the telephone, pick up eyeglasses, etc.)
5. The absence of useful or familiar objects — either because the hospital does not furnish them or because of inadequate preparation for the hospital stay

In treating elderly patients it is essential to adhere to the many details of patient-centered surgical nursing care. For example, the surgeon must communicate cheerful confidence when answering the patient's questions about what to expect from surgery. Listen carefully and be sensitive to what may seem like minor details but are obviously important to the elderly patient. By treating the elderly patient with respect and remaining aware of his or her great sense of vulnerability, the surgeon comes to understand the patient's demands and the sources of the patient's antagonism. Try to ignore personal feelings about the patient's requests. It is more productive to cheerfully honor a request for a specific type of breakfast cereal (or a particular type of vitamin or drinking water, etc.) than to withhold it arbitrarily or antagonistically. If possible, do not alter the medications the patient customarily takes, even providing the familiar brand name. If a confined older patient does not quickly receive the help he or she requests, it can be terrifying because of the patient's powerlessness to act for himself or herself. Remember that elderly patients are often short-tempered, mentally confused, agitated, and unable to cooperate; do not allow these qualities to provoke argumentative struggles between the patient and the nursing staff.

Educating the patient about the rehabilitation process (including the details of transfer from bed, use of a bedpan, and other assisting devices) must begin upon admission. Anticipate postoperative needs; back care is most essential. To protect the elderly patient's sensitive skin, a pneumatic alternating pressure mattress or an egg-crate foam mattress may be needed after surgery; during the early postoperative days, wrinkles in bed sheets at contact areas, particularly at the heels and elbows, may cause skin breakage. Patients with back pain require regular changes in position. A trapeze and overhead frame are essential for older patients to lift themselves to use the bedpan and for back care.

Breathing exercises, basic arm and leg exercises, and tightening of the abdominal and gluteal muscles (fanny clapping) are both useful in themselves and psychologically important to patients, who expect to assist actively in their quick recovery from their surgery. On the other hand, no carefully planned or regimented physiotherapy program is needed (see Chapter 13). The general strengthening exercise program should include methods of turning and lifting up for positioning, as well as a demonstration of how to sit out of bed postoperatively. After surgery, the physiotherapy department will be unable to attend the patient beyond the regular twice-a-day visits. To supplement the rehabilitation program, the patient should be taught to use a walker or crutches, which will elevate the patient's confidence and allow the patient to establish relationships with other patients. Generally, it is better for older patients to resume ambulation with a walker, which is more stable and provides better confidence than crutches; using a walker will not keep the patient from subsequently mastering a cane.

Make long-range home transfer plans before surgery. In making these plans, it is important to realistically assess several factors, including (1) the patient's views, (2) the feasibility of second institutional care, and (3) the possibility of home care with housekeeping assistance. Every older patient has individual needs, and an experienced senior nurse in charge of the ward must have the greatest responsibility in identifying these needs. If the patient's hearing or vision is impaired, make sure the patient's chart says so and that all nurses are informed of proper individual care. House staff and the attending physician must visit the patient daily, particularly the elderly patient; an early perfunctory visit by an inexperienced staff member will not meet the patient's needs. Ideally, the surgeon should do rounds to see older patients later in the day, when questions and problems about routine activities will have arisen. It is important for the surgeon to explain in advance if he or she will not visit for 1 or 2 days or if another surgeon will be covering his or her service. The surgeon should perform daily neurological evaluation of the elderly patient's lower extremities to detect footdrop or thromboembolism, because elderly patients might not be aware of relevant symptoms.

Elderly patients usually need more reassurance than younger patients. Prepare them for what to expect after surgery, explaining the difference between incision pain and actual hip pain. Many patients expect total freedom from pain immediately after surgery and worry about any postoperative pain.

Many older patients develop some degree of psychosis or respond uncharacteristically to their relatives and friends after surgery; others may be extremely confused for a few days, experiencing memory loss or a lack of awareness of the time or date. It is often disturbing to the patient if such changes are brought to his or her attention by visitors. Reassure these patients and their families, and institute supportive treatment.

During daily visits, be sure to examine the position of the operated hip, because the patient may not complain of any hip pain associated with dislocation; the surgeon can only detect this complication by examining the knee position and extremity length. Occasionally, for example, a patient discards the abduction brace and even ignores the details of postoperative management. In such a case, empathy and proper psychology are more effective than dogmatism and threats. Patients thrive on praise for their good performance rather than criticism of what they have done incorrectly; criticism can be nonconstructive and even dangerous.

Urinary or fecal incontinence occurring in an older patient after surgery can be extremely embarrassing. If it occurs, an experienced nurse should handle it supportively rather than critically. An indwelling catheter controls urinary incontinence and is convenient for the patient. Examine the dressing daily; if adhesive tape causes itching, it must be adjusted. Lightheadedness and dizziness are quite natural after the first attempt at ambulation; prepare the patient for the possibility so that he or she will not be discouraged from further attempts at ambulation.

When you first interview the patient, before he or she has made the decision about surgery, provide the patient with basic information about surgery, the potential risks, and the complications that might arise. It is a good idea to have the family present while discussing the proposed operation. Older persons, who often have deep-seated fears about the procedure, may not be inquisitive about the details of surgery. Do not overemphasize the potential side effects of drugs or surgery. In general, tell the patient as much as he or she wishes to know — but no more. Do not overstate the risks and agitate the patient by describing the worst possible outcome only to advise the patient to go ahead with surgery. If a cardiopulmonary or systemic condition places the patient at high risk, the patient should be fully informed and guided with relatives in deciding whether to undergo surgery. It is not enough to expose all the possible hazards, then leave an older person on his or her own to make a decision. It can be helpful for the surgeon to express what he or she would recommend if the patient were the surgeon's relative. Introducing a fearful patient to one or two other older patients who have undergone the same kind of surgery provides an opportunity to discuss the details.

CHOICE OF ANESTHESIA

The choice of anesthesia involves the anesthesiologist, the patient, and the surgeon and is based on the anesthetist's preoperative evaluation. The anesthesiologist makes the final recommendation and also partic-

ipates in recommending postoperative pain control medication.

The safety of the patient is the prime consideration in choosing anesthesia.[89,102] There are basically three ways to approach the problem of anesthesia for patients undergoing total hip arthroplasty: (1) normotensive standard techniques, (2) hypotensive anesthesia, and (3) regional anesthesia. In most of our cases, general anesthesia (normotensive) and endotracheal intubation are recommended by the anesthesia team after reviewing the patient. An expert anesthesia team is invaluable in dealing with older patients, who may have some cardiopulmonary compromise.

Normotensive General Anesthesia

The normotensive method is used frequently and provides safe and reliable anesthesia with a great deal of flexibility. General anesthesia is delivered by endotracheal intubation. Careful monitoring of the patient should include continuous ECG observation, continuous monitoring of heartbeat and breath sounds with an esophageal stethoscope, and monitoring of central venous and arterial blood pressure, as indicated. The patient's temperature is monitored with an esophageal probe, and arterial blood gas and hematocrit levels are measured intraoperatively as required. After induction with a barbiturate, diazepam, or ketamine, anesthesia is maintained with nitrous oxide (N_2O) in combination with narcotics, neuroleptics, or halogenated inhalation agents and muscle relaxants. Precise attention to blood and fluid replacement is essential. The method and details of anesthesia will be selected by the anesthetist according to the patient's physical examination and individual history.

Hypotensive Anesthesia

Since its inception, controversy has surrounded the use of controlled hypotensive anesthesia. In its developmental years, this method was accompanied by considerable increased morbidity,[8,9,24] but in subsequent studies Bodman[9] and Larson[64] have concluded that most of the complications resulted from technical flaws in anesthesia delivery and were not inherent in the technique. Davis and associates[23] used pentolinium tartrate to lower the systolic blood pressure to 65 to 75 mm Hg, a method previously used by others.[31-33,41] Controlled hypotensive anesthesia has recently been accepted enthusiastically at several centers. Although previously accepted in such surgical areas as neurosurgery, plastic surgery, and general surgical procedures where copious blood loss is anticipated, only recently has its use spread to orthopaedic surgery, particularly total hip arthroplasty. Several reports support its validity and cite its advantages, including decreased blood loss and consequently decreased need for blood replacement, improved operative technique, and decreased operative time. Some also claim improved wound healing.[25,41,53,66]

Charnley used hypotensive anesthesia extensively at Wrightington Hospital with remarkable success and minimal morbidity. Mallory[69] and Harris have also used it successfully and encountered no major complications. Some patients, however, do not qualify for hypotensive anesthesia: those with severe hypertension, obstructive pulmonary disease, cerebrovascular disease, a history of arteriosclerotic heart disease, or a history of renal conditions. Mallory and his associates did not exclude patients with a history of myocardial infarction, providing there was no history of coronary ischemia within 6 months before the time of anesthesia. They explicitly emphasized the need for careful patient selection for this method to succeed and urged that the decision to use this method on an individual patient be mutually agreed upon between the anesthesiologist and the internist. In their series, 80% of the patients qualified. In all cases, they found successful anesthesia with minimum morbidity, reduced operative time, reduced operative blood loss, and subsequent blood replacement. Balanced anesthesia was used in conjunction with trimethaphan camsylate (Arfonad).[69]

In a study of 253 total hip arthroplasty patients anesthetized by induced hypotensive anesthesia, no lasting complications could be attributed to the technique. As in earlier studies, blood loss was considerably reduced, and procedures were performed more easily than under normotensive anesthesia. However, the technique is demanding and requires a highly competent anesthesia staff.

In summary, although induced hypotension during anesthesia has been recommended in total hip arthroplasty, there is insufficient in-depth evidence of its usefulness and related morbidity. Its proper place in general surgery without a skillfully trained team of anesthesiologists has not yet been well defined. In addition, the best overall method of lowering the blood pressure during anesthesia is disputed. The recent use of nitroprusside to produce hypotension seems to offer some advantages, but this author believes that this type of anesthesia should not be used in total hip arthroplasty, despite the unquestionably important dividends attributed to it, unless the anesthesia team is prepared to accept full responsibility for selecting patients and monitoring them precisely during surgery.

Regional Anesthesia (Spinal and Epidural)

Spinal and epidural anesthesia have been accepted in general surgery and in urological and gynecological procedures. In those procedures, operative blood loss

and cardiopulmonary complications have decreased; in addition, a smoother postoperative course has been attributed to it.[10,27,55,68]

Sculco and Ranawat[90] compared the effect of spinal versus general anesthesia in a study of 234 total hip arthroplasties performed by one surgeon (in 199 patients). Thiopental sodium (Pentothal Sodium) was used for the induction of all patients undergoing general anesthesia, which was maintained with N_2O (nitrous oxide in combination with fentanyl, thiopental sodium, or droperidol O fentanyl citrate [Innovar]) or nitrous oxide in combination with halothane. Spinal anesthesia was performed with 10 to 15 mg of 0.5% tetracaine injected in the interspace of the third and fourth lumbar vertebrae, achieving anesthesia below the tenth thoracic vertebra. In addition, most patients were sedated with diazepam (Valium) during the procedure. In these patients, blood loss was reduced by an average of 600 ml, and the amount of blood lost during postoperative suction was also reduced significantly. Because there were fewer postoperative complications in the spinal anesthesia group, the investigators concluded that spinal anesthesia is preferable. This author's own experience supports their view; spinal anesthesia, when indicated, seems to be superior to normotensive general anesthesia in performing total hip arthroplasty. However, we have encountered some practical difficulties: (1) fixed deformities and a painful hip, which make it difficult to position the patient on the table, and (2) the presence of associated arthritis of the lower lumbar spine in most patients with arthritic hips, which makes a spinal tap difficult. In our experience, epidural anesthesia is quite satisfactory for total hip arthroplasty. Epidural or spinal anesthetics may be given by catheter with continuous medication as needed to prolong anesthesia.

One major advantage of regional anesthesia during hip arthroplasty is the lowering of intraoperative bleeding.[77] Also, regional anesthesia is possibly associated with a lower incidence of venous thrombosis than general anesthesia.[76]

These advantages of regional anesthesia, however, can be offset by its failure rate (up to 10%) and by the patient's preference for general anesthesia. Despite the higher success rate of spinal over epidural anesthesia, several contraindications for regional anesthesia are common to both methods; one is the tendency to bleed because of coagulopathy (although patients on low-dose Coumadin or heparin qualify for the procedure). It is essential to obtain a bleeding profile just before the planned surgery. Suspend the patient's use of all antiinflammatory medication 24 hours before a planned epidural or spinal anesthesia. One infrequent but troublesome complication is headache. Undeniably, some patients with spinal anesthesia suffer from postural postanesthetic headache; the headache is worse when the patient sits and occurs with greatest frequency among women and younger patients and when a large-gauge spinal needle has been used. The anesthetist must choose between spinal and epidural anesthesia. In either case, it is preferable to continue an infusion via a catheter to sustain the anesthetic effect throughout the procedure rather than to inject a single dose of anesthesia. Reports reflect a more rapid recovery and an increased success rate with spinal anesthesia as compared with epidural anesthesia, because of the finite duration of spinal anesthesia; however, a vasoconstrictor and local anesthetic agent are commonly used as well.

Selection and Differences

Patients vary regarding whether they wish to know what is happening during surgery. Most patients prefer to be put to sleep for the operation. When using regional anesthesia, spinal or epidural, it is preferable to place the patient in a supine position, which is more comfortable for long periods than lying on one side. Because the patient must remain still during the procedure, he or she must be sedated with general anesthesia. The patient is unconscious but requires analgesics immediately upon recovering from the anesthesia.

The patient's position alters the ventilation-perfusion pattern in the lungs. For example, the supine position shifts the diaphragm in a cephalad direction, whereas the lateral decubitus position produces a shunt and compresses the dependent lung, allowing better ventilation in the nondependent lung and predisposing the patient to hypoxemia resulting from a shunt effect.[14,39,48,111] Using the lateral decubitus position in combination with regional anesthesia and spontaneous ventilation leads to a lesser degree of atelectasis of the dependent lung.[47]

Reports have documented a significant decrease in blood loss (up to 30%) after regional anesthesia. This decrease possibly results from lower arterial and blood pressure caused by the sympathectomy effect that occurs in regional anesthesia but not in general anesthesia. Unfortunately, studies on blood loss during total hip arthroplasty with hypotensive anesthesia have failed to demonstrate significant blood savings.[96,107] On the other hand, intraoperative blood loss is strongly correlated with venous pressure measured in the wound.[77] Onset and recovery from anesthesia are faster with general than with regional anesthesia. Success with general anesthesia is 100% (no failure), but regional anesthesia has a failure rate of up to 10%. Myocardia and ventilation are depressed in general

anesthesia but not with regional anesthesia. Regional anesthesia has the sympathectomy effect already mentioned, which is not present with general anesthesia. And as stated before, both intraoperative and postoperative bleeding and thrombolysis are reduced with regional anesthesia.

Contraindications for Anesthesia in Elective Surgery

At times it may be necessary to call off the planned surgical procedure either temporarily or permanently because of medical conditions that render the risk of anesthesia unacceptably high. The conditions often are correctable upon a full evaluation and appropriate treatment. They are rarely so serious that plans for the surgical procedure must be permanently abandoned.

These associated conditions include recent pulmonary embolism; history of angina pectoris or myocardial infarction; hypertension; congestive heart disease, and asthma. Although other conditions, such as coexisting diabetes, ankylosing spondylitis, rheumatoid arthritis, nephropathy, and the chronic use of steroids or other drugs, may increase the anesthesia risk, none disqualifies the patient for elective surgery. If surgery on one hip has been complicated by a pulmonary embolism, the patient must not be considered for total hip arthroplasty of the other hip for at least 6 months because of the high risk of recurrence (see Chapter 9). It has not yet been clearly demonstrated that a history of myocardial infarction within 6 months before surgery is a contraindication for elective total hip arthroplasty; nonetheless, a high rate of reinfarction of up to 37% has been documented, especially if the surgery is performed soon after myocardial infarction.[88] Despite modern advances in the care of cardiac patients, mortality following reinfarction during the perioperative course is as high as 30%.[88] However, it is encouraging to note a dramatic decrease in reinfarction rate to 5.8%, 2.3%, and 1.5% at 0 to 3 months, 4 to 6 months, and more than 6 months respectively, without any further decrease thereafter.[88] Patients with a history of angina must be studied by a cardiologist; this study should include stress testing and even coronary artery bypass if indicated; it should precede the elective total hip arthroplasty procedure. Patients with a history of angina, treated or untreated, constitute a high risk for perioperative ischemia and myocardial infarction, even when it exists concurrently with a hemodynamically uneventful anesthetic procedure.[92] Angina at rest and asymptomatic (silent) angina puts those patients at risk; it should be thoroughly evaluated because these conditions may signify a preinfarction state of heart disease.[92]

SPECIFIC CONDITIONS AND CONCERNS
Congestive Heart Failure

Congestive heart failure constitutes the most serious risk for elective surgery. It is mandatory that a patient with this condition be treated before the contemplated hip surgery because of the high perioperative morbidity associated with it. The standard treatment, under the supervision of a medical team that includes a cardiologist, includes administration of inotropic or diuretic agents coupled with careful central venous pressure monitoring during surgery and optimal fluid therapy perioperatively.

Asthma

An asthmatic patient must undergo a full preoperative pulmonary function assessment by a pulmonologist. Wheezing should be improved, if not resolved, before surgery with the appropriate pulmonary treatment, including bronchodilators. Because asthmatic patients are significantly predisposed to bronchospasm after airway manipulation and endotracheal intubation, preoperative anesthetic planning is mandatory.[59] Patients who take theophylline should be maintained at a concentration level of 10 to 20 µg/ml. Asthmatic patients who take corticosteroids must be maintained perioperatively at a dose determined by the preoperative dose.

Diabetes

Most controlled diabetic patients impose little or no difficulty as long as there is no evidence of significant hypoglycemia or hyperglycemia or glycosuria. Most experts agree that it is important to achieve good control of the disease before elective total hip arthroplasty. If the preoperative blood glucose level exceeds 300 mg/dl, postpone surgery. It is far easier to regulate the insulin level in a diabetic patient whose blood and urine glucose levels are controlled before surgery than one whose glucose level is high at the time of surgery. Additionally, wounds heal better and are less likely to develop infection if the diabetes is well controlled.[44] Increased wound infection in diabetic patients is discussed in Chapters 8 and 31.

Hypertension

High blood pressure can also increase risk for total hip arthroplasty patients. Hypertensive patients fall into three groups: (1) those with mildly elevated diastolic pressure; (2) those with diastolic pressure of 90 to 110 mm Hg; and (3) those with sustained high blood pressure above 110 mm Hg. The first group is probably not predisposed to increased risk of complications.[43] If the blood pressure is not fluctuating and there is no history of an associated myocardial infarction, the second group can also be accepted for anesthesia without undue concern. However, patients with labile hypertension (fluctuating blood pressure) and patients with high blood pressure may develop a significant increase in blood pressure during endotracheal intubation.[43] There is general agreement that patients with sustained diastolic blood pressure over 110 mm Hg must be treated before planned total hip arthroplasty.

Inflammatory (Systemic) Arthritis

Patients with chronic rheumatoid arthritis, ankylosing spondylitis, and juvenile rheumatoid arthritis should also undergo a special evaluation for anesthesia. Rheumatoid arthritis patients are at high risk for cardiopulmonary disease and low exercise tolerance resulting from confinement and skin and bone fragility. Therefore, preoperative evaluation and careful anesthesia selection and handling are vital (see Chapter 21). These patients have limited range of motion in the temporomandibular joints, which can make intubation difficult and require the use of fiberoptics for intubation orally or through the nasal passage. Furthermore, endotracheal intubation may be hampered by cervical spine autofusion in ankylosing spondylitis and stiffness or instability of the cervical spine from upper cervical spine involvement with anterior laxity of the atlanto-axial joint, especially in rheumatoid arthritis patients. In any case, cricoarytenoid cartilage involvement and stiffness in the temporomandibular joint or cervical spine can be overcome by being aware of the problem and having an expert anesthesiologist available to perform fiberoptic-guided oral or nasal intubation while the patient is awake. A thorough preoperative evaluation of the cervical spine, including flexion-extension films, must be routine in planning anesthesia for rheumatoid arthritis patients (symptomatic or asymptomatic) to prevent catastrophic complications resulting from spinal cord injury.[93] When flexion/extension lateral projection indicates a distance greater than 2 to 3 mm between the posterior aspect of the anterior arch of Atlas and the anterior aspect of the odontoid process, the cervical spine must be protected during the anesthesia. Additional careful examination by a neurologist and a CAT scan, MRI, and myelography may also be indicated. Subluxation of 6 to 7 mm requires careful consideration for spinal fusion before planned surgery. Young patients with the ankylosing type of arthritis are at special risk because of cervical spine stiffness, recessed jaw, or temporomandibular involvement (see Chapter 21). It has been estimated that a large number of patients with rheumatoid arthritis (up to 70%) develop symptomatic cervical spine arthritis requiring treatment.

Concurrent Medications

Many patients undergoing total hip arthroplasty take medications for coexisting medical conditions; drugs commonly encountered include steroids, antihypertensive medications, cardiac medications, diuretics, digoxin therapy, and antidepressants. In such cases, consult in advance with an internist familiar with the patient's problems, the cardiologist, and the anesthesiologist to ensure an appropriate and safe administration of anesthesia. The relationship between hypocalcemia and arrhythmia is controversial, but most anesthesiologists agree that preoperative potassium replacement is needed when the serum potassium level drops below 3 mEq/L. Because deep anesthesia suppresses the normal surge of glucocorticoids during surgery, supplemental doses of these agents are also necessary. Adrenal deficiency usually manifests after surgery, not during. When supplemental steroids are required, no single formula has been advocated, but because of the potential for adrenal depression, consider using a dose equivalent to the normal daily output of the adrenal glands (i.e., 25 mg/day); in addition, consider using a supplemental dose as high as 300 mg/day. An excess dose of corticosteroids imposes no added risk, but if steroids are replaced at only one tenth of the normal cortisol level, hemodynamic instability will result, causing a higher mortality than when normal levels or even levels 10 times greater than normal are used.[95]

Corticosteroid Coverage

Many patients who undergo total hip arthroplasty have had previous corticosteroid treatment. Prolonged treatment with these drugs can depress the adrenal gland's normal output, leading to dysfunction and atrophy. Consequently, a perioperative course of corticosteroids is required for these patients to cope with the stresses of major surgery. Normally, a considerable increase in the corticosteroid output of the adrenal glands is adequate to cope with surgical shock and stress, but if patients have been on corticosteroids for at least 4 to 5 years (regardless of the dose), they require parenteral steroid coverage during surgery. Another recommendation is to administer a corticosteroid dose of three to four times the normal dose to patients who have received corticosteroids before the time of surgery. As a general rule, this author recommends that the preoperative dosage not be the sole factor in deciding the amount to be given during surgery; the extent of surgery and operative complications must also be weighed.

Begin corticosteroids at least 12 hours before surgery; for example, administer cortisone acetate at 6 PM the night before surgery, followed by 50 to 75 mg intramuscular injections every 6 hours until the patient goes to the operating room. During surgery, 100 mg/L of intravenous fluid hydrocortisone sodium succinate (Solu-Cortef [a water-soluble preparation]) is administered. This dose immediately establishes and maintains a sufficient steroid level for the duration of the surgery, with no need to mobilize Depo forms, even in the presence of hypotension. Fluids lost and replaced during surgery carry adequate corticosteroids until the patient returns to the recovery room. On the day of the operation, the patient should receive 250 to 300 mg cortisone, including the preoperative medication and the intraoperative hydrocortisone sodium succinate (Solu-Cortef).

Upon arrival in the recovery room, the patient should receive a 75-mg injection of cortisone acetate intramuscularly, followed every 8 hours to a total of 225 mg. The subsequent day, the patient should receive 50 mg every 8 hours for a total of 150 mg; then 25 mg every 12 hours to total 50 mg; finally, a single injection of 25 mg precedes a return to a 5-mg recommended daily dose of prednisone.

Chernow and associates[15] recommend another schedule: Morning of surgery, two times the usual glucocorticoid dosage orally if possible or 50 mg intravenous hydrocortisone preoperatively; intraoperatively, 100 mg intravenously; postoperatively, 100 mg intravenously every 8 hours for 24 hours, rapidly tapering over the next 48 to 72 hours to the usual dose if the postoperative course is uneventful. The tapering schedule should stabilize and be maintained when the daily dose reaches the preoperative steroid dose. Do not attempt at this time to diminish the dosage below the preoperative equivalent.

Return to oral administration of steroids only when the patient has resumed dependable gastrointestinal function. Modify the preceding tapering schedule as required to provide higher levels for a longer period of time if the patient's postoperative course so requires. Administer steroid intravenously instead of intramuscularly if shock, relative hypertension, hypotension, or cardiac decompensation ensues. Careful ongoing evaluation should focus on the short-term side effects of steroids, including hypokalemia, alkalosis, hyperglycemia, salt and fluid retention, and psychosis. The schedule presented here is a basic guideline; it must be individualized for each case, weighing the preoperative steroid dosage, the nature of the illness requiring steroid therapy and its activity at the time of surgery, the extent of the surgical procedure contemplated, the relative ease or difficulty of the postoperative course, the complications, the patient's nutritional status, and the postoperative wound-healing process.[26]

Blood Transfusions

The average patient undergoing total hip arthroplasty with normotensive anesthesia requires 2 to 3 units of blood during or after surgery; usually this amount can be reduced by half if hypotensive anesthesia is used. When operative time increases (as in revision surgery or when difficult technical problems occur), anticipate the need for more blood transfusions. Most hospitals use conventional banked blood. Improved blood banking practices now strictly screen donors for blood-transmitted diseases (such as AIDS and hepatitis B and C), and transmission by blood transfusion has almost been eliminated. Antigen/antibody tests are used to detect the two hepatitis viruses, and vigorous screening is used for the HIV virus. Nonetheless, during the past three decades, serious complications related to blood transfusion have been noted in approximately 2% to 3% of cases; in addition, a nonicteric hepatitis may escape diagnosis, with the patient suffering only from minor symptoms such as anorexia or slight chemical changes manifested by serum SMA 12 examinations. It is important to recognize that homologous blood transfusions expose the patient to an appreciable risk.

If hypotensive anesthesia is available and the patient needs only 1 unit of blood, avoid the transfusion in patients who can tolerate the mild degree of anemia. But if transfusion is required, the ideal blood to use is banked autologous blood. In addition to serum hepatitis, dangers inherent in transfusion are mismatched blood, clerical errors, and immunological reactions to blood proteins. According to some studies, as many as 5% of patients receiving homologous blood transfusions may have some type of serious reaction. Problematic blood reactions (in particular, serum hepatitis) present a greater risk in large cities, where unrecognized addicts often participate in blood donor pools. Data collected over the past two decades indicate that for each unit of blood the risk for transmitting hepatitis is approximately 6% to 8%. The advantages of autologous banked blood have been pointed out by Grant,[46] Milles and co-workers,[75] and Newman and co-workers.[87]

Complete cooperation on the part of the surgeon, the patient, and the blood bank is essential when using autologous banked blood. Polefsky[86] has described the technique involved in phlebotomy before surgery. Refer the patient to the blood bank for evaluation approximately 4 weeks before surgery, where they will draw and store 1 unit of blood every 5 to 7 days. A hemoglobin and hematocrit examination must precede each phlebotomy, and the patient must immediately begin iron therapy. Patients should receive oral supplements of iron tablets (300 mg t.i.d.). Both osteoarthritis and rheumatoid arthritis patients are good candidates for this type of blood transfusion. Because blood-freezing techniques permit blood storage for several weeks before surgery, the patient will have time to reestablish a normal hemoglobin-hematocrit level before admission to the hospital for surgery.

The surgeon faced with the problem of transfusion of 3, 4, or more units of blood for elective surgery must consider the risks and potential benefits of banked autologous blood. Some banks are reluctant to perform this service because the special screening necessary for these patients adds to their workload. However, the benefits of this method fully compensate for the inconvenience to the patient and the blood bank. In this author's personal experience with this method, no adverse reactions have arisen.

This author strongly advises against transfusing a single unit of blood postoperatively; if the patient needs as little as 1 unit, he or she may well forgo it and avoid the attendant risk of transfusion complications. However, older patients usually do not tolerate a low hemoglobin-hematocrit level postoperatively; if an elderly patient shows any evidence of restlessness, agitation, or psychosis, transfuse the patient with adequate amounts of packed cells to avoid overloading his or her cardiovascular system.

Blood lost during total hip arthroplasty must be replaced. The amount of blood transfusion required during the procedure varies, depending largely on the pathology of the hip, the type and extent of the preoperative medications taken by the patient, the type of anesthesia employed, the patient's position on the operating room table, the extent of the hip surgery, and other factors. Transfusion can require between 1000 to 2000 ml, so plan to have enough on hand to replace at least a portion of the lost blood. The amount lost in revision surgery is greater by 1000 to 2000 ml. With the exception of those whose religious beliefs preclude blood transfusion, most patients welcome a discussion regarding the possibility of autologous blood transfusion for enhanced safety against acquired blood-transfusion diseases over banked homologous blood.

The most direct way to estimate blood loss is by weighing the blood-soaked sponges, measuring the content of the suction bottles (minus irrigation fluid), and comparing the intraoperative hematocrit level with the preoperative hematocrit level. Bourke and Smith[11] have suggested a formula for allowable blood loss:

$$ABL = EBV \times \frac{H1 - HF}{100} \times \frac{[3 - (H1 - Hf]}{200} *$$

In most instances the goal is to replace enough blood to maintain its oxygen-carrying capacity; this differs

---

* ABL = allowable blood loss; EBV = estimated blood volume; H1 = initial hematocrit level (%); Hf = final lowest hematocrit level (5).

from transfusing the patient to replace lost volume. Although blood volume estimations are complex, the common guide is the surgeon's subjective estimate plus hematocrit determinations. Except for patients with coexisting significant cerebral or myocardial ischemia, most tolerate a hemodilution up to 20%.[40,87] Instead of setting a fixed number below which transfusions must be given, consider many factors, such as the patient's age and preoperative medical status.

Sources of Blood; Conservation and Replacement

Conservation is also an important method commonly used in surgical practice to reduce bleeding or to replace blood. There are several options:

1. Hypotensive anesthesia and epidural or spinal anesthesia to reduce bleeding in general. Although helpful, this method alone will not obviate the need to replace blood lost during total hip arthroplasty.
2. Preoperative acute hemodilution by preoperative phlebotomy; this technique meets the requirements of certain religious sects. This method prolongs the procedure and requires careful perioperative monitoring of the patient's blood volume. To be eligible for this technique, the patient must be healthy and have a hematocrit level of greater than 40%.
3. The use of homologous blood from a blood bank. Using homologous blood exposes the patient to many risks, ranging from minor allergic reactions to death. They include isosensitization, hemolytic reaction, exposure to infectious diseases (i.e., bacterial infections, syphilis, malaria, serum hepatitis non-A and non-B, and HIV virus). Risks are significant enough to warrant seeking an alternative to homologous blood in all nonemergency operative procedures. The incidence of serum hepatitis is 20% to 46% with paid donors and 8% to 13% with volunteers.[30,73] Because most serum hepatitises are nonicteric, they remain unnoticed unless specifically tested for with routine liver function tests and antigen screening. Of 113 fatal homologous blood transfusions reported by the FDA between April 1976 and January 1980, 41% of deaths were related to clerical error, 29% to hepatitis, 7% to laboratory error, and 23% to other causes.[79]
4. Transfusion with autologous blood obtained intraoperatively and postoperatively. This method is an excellent alternative to homologous blood transfusion, particularly in procedures where the surgeon anticipates a large blood loss. It can be used in addition to autologous blood donated preoperatively. The newer Cell Savers are cost effective and safe.
5. Preoperative autologous blood donation of up to 6 to 8 units (2 to 4 frozen). This may eliminate the need for homologous red cell transfusion.

AUTOLOGOUS BLOOD TRANSFUSION The first experimental transfusion of autologous blood in animals was recorded by Blundell[7] in 1818. The first use of blood transfusion in orthopaedics was attributed to Duncan,[28] in 1886. In 1921, Grant first reported using previously deposited blood for transfusion in elective surgery.[46] It is of special interest that more than 50 years ago Fantus wrote "a patient who is to have an elective surgical operation could do no better than to deposit a unit of blood a week or two before the ordeal. A pint of blood in the bank to have it available in case it is needed during or after operation." He advocated having blood banks available in hospitals. Several reports have since documented the effectiveness and safety of autologous autotransfusion in gynecology and cardiology surgery.* Turner[98,99] and others have reported the use of autologous blood in patients undergoing elective orthopaedic procedures.†

Patients undergoing primary total hip arthroplasty may donate up to 4 or 5 units of their blood, but it is often more realistic to plan for 3 or 4 units. The amount of blood that must be transfused during a given procedure varies based on several factors: blood pressure at surgery, intraoperative blood loss, and the accuracy with which the blood loss has been estimated. The patient's age, preoperative hematocrit level, and history of cerebral or cardiovascular status may also influence the decision whether to transfuse donated blood during the operation. After surgery, the decision to transfuse is based on the stability of the patient's hemodynamics and hematocrit level during the first several postoperative days. The effect of hematocrit changes after one to six blood donations for autologous blood transfusion is shown in Table 7-1; it varies according to the donor's age group. It may be necessary to transfuse some or all of the patient's donated blood.

Some surgeons and patients may worry about the idea of donating several units of blood 4 or 5 weeks before major surgery; doing so could predispose the patient to such complications as hypovolemia, anemia, even slower wound healing, and the possibility of infection. Until recent years, most blood banks were reluctant to accept prospective patients for phlebotomy and storage of blood because of the cost (Table 7-2) and a lack of facilities. However, fear of HIV transmission via blood transfusion has reversed that trend, and blood banks now encourage the autologous donation of blood preoperatively. Studies have now abundantly shown that a low hematocrit level (slight anemia) during the perioperative course is often nonconsequential, so

---

* References 3, 22, 57, 71, 96.
† References 5, 6, 13, 19, 20, 21, 29, 30, 34, 35, 65, 71, 73, 78, 82, 109, 110.

Table 7-1 Hematocrit Level after One to Six Blood Donations for Autologous Transfusion, by Age Group

	Mean hematocrit level, by number of donations.*				
Age of donors	1	2	3	4	5
Teenage					
Male	44 (53)	41 (54)	38 (22)	37 (7)	36 (1)
Female	41 (141)	37 (114)	36 (43)	38 (6)	37 (1)
Middle age					
Male	44 (34)	42 (28)	39 (13)		
Female	41 (66)	38 (44)	37 (7)		
Elderly					
Male	43 (47)	41 (36)	42 (5)		
Female	42 (50)	38 (40)	37 (11)		

From Silvergleid AJ: Autologous, directed, and home transfusion programs. In Petz LD, Swisher SN, editors: *Clinical practice of transfusion medicine*, ed 2, New York, 1989, Churchill Livingstone.
*The numbers in parentheses indicate the number of donors in that sample. Hematocrit levels have been rounded to the nearest whole number.

Table 7-2 Blood Transfusion Fee Schedule, Cost for Blood at the Institution

Description	Standard price ($)
Whole blood per unit.....................	105.00
Whole blood (divided unit).............	105.00
Autologous whole blood..................	90.00
Whole blood—within 48 hours of collection.............................	160.00
Red blood cells (single unit)............	90.00
Red blood cells (divided unit)..........	90.00
Red blood cells autologous..............	90.00
Red blood cells—washed cells.........	135.00
Red blood cells—spin/cool process (single unit).............................	100.50
Red blood cells—spin/cool process (multiple unit discount)..............	95.25
Red blood cells—leukocytes removed by centrifugation.......................	105.75
Directed donation surcharge...........	90.00
Autologous donation surcharge........	65.00
Frozen thawed red cells per unit.....	315.00
Frozen thawed RBC (divided unit)...	315.00

Courtesy New York Blood Center.

attempting to equalize the preoperative and postoperative blood levels (Hct/Hgb) by blood transfusion is not necessary in most situations. The investigators found no difference between the perioperative blood level of patients with deposited autologous blood and that of patients who received homologous blood transfusions.[20,95,109] Differences in the hematocrit level between blood donation, subsequent hospitalization, and at discharge were not found to be significant (Fig. 7-1). These studies also show that there is no difference between patients receiving autologous blood transfusion and nondonors in average hospital stay or speed of

recovery from operations.

Enough autologous blood can also be supplied for revision surgery. The patient may donate up to 5 units or more if frozen blood techniques are available and the blood banks will accept predeposited blood up to 5 weeks before surgery. A patient undergoing a revision arthroplasty, for example, may donate 4 or 5 units of blood, 2 or 3 units may be deposited several months before surgery to be frozen, and the remainder can be deposited in liquid form within 35 days before surgery.

When Woolson and associates compared the efficacy in patients undergoing total hip arthroplasty of transfusing previously deposited autologous blood to that of transfusing homologous blood for similar surgery, they found several significant advantages in the group who received autologus blood transfusions.[109] Although patients who deposited autologous blood had a mean preoperative hematocrit level of 36%, as compared with 39% for the control group, the average postoperative hematocrit levels of the two groups (33%) did not differ. Additionally, the two groups showed no significant difference in the average total blood loss or need for blood replacement. Moreover, transfusion-related complications occurred only in two of the patients who had not received autologous blood transfusions.

In a 1987 editorial supporting the use of preoperatively deposited autologous blood for transfusion during surgery, Cowell[19] recommended considering use of autologous blood transfusion in all elective orthopaedic operations because of its safety, simplicity, and effectiveness. Such blood transfusions carry no risk of transfusion reactions or exposure to carrier-transmitted diseases, such as the devastating problem of posttransfusion hepatitis and HIV transmission when homologous banked blood is transfused. In 1989, Cowell stated "at present the ready availability of homologous blood has been used as an excuse by many

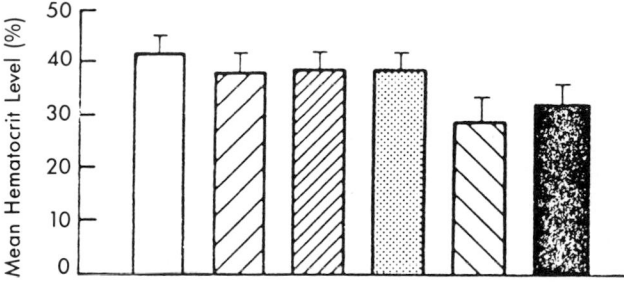

Fig. 7-1. Hematocrit levels during donation and subsequent hospitalization. □ at first donation; ▨ lowest during the donation period; ▨ at last donation; ▦ at time of hospitalization; ◺ lowest during hospitalization; ▩ at discharge. (From Kruskall MS et al: Utilization and effectiveness of a hospital autologous preoperative blood donor program, *Transfusion* 26:335, 1986.)

individuals in the blood-banking industry to avoid the preconceived problems that they believe could be associated with developing an autologous blood-transfusion program." To evaluate whether the use of autologous blood could reduce the need for homologous blood transfusion in total hip arthroplasty, Woolson and others studied a consecutive series of postoperative patients who had undergone this procedure.[65] In their study of 143 patients with 154 primary total hip arthroplasties, they found that the need for homologous blood transfusion was minimized when the use of preoperatively deposited blood transfusions was supplemented with salvage of red blood cells during the intraoperative and postoperative periods. In this study, the sole criterion for using nonautologous blood transfusion was the patient's clinical condition, not hematocrit level. No homologous blood transfusion was necessary in 95% of the total hip arthroplasty procedures for which autologous blood had been previously deposited.[65] Seven of ten patients who had deposited blood preoperatively but also required transfusion of homologous blood had been unable to deposit the recommended number of units before the operation. In 96% of the procedures, blood was salvaged (28% of the total blood lost in the entire series was recovered). In a retrospective study, Thomas and associates[95] studied the use of previously deposited autologous blood at the Walter Reed Army Medical Center; they followed a total of 211 patients undergoing total joint arthroplasty or spinal fusion. Of 159 patients who entered the program, 113 (71%) received only autologous blood. The remaining 46 patients required homologous blood transfusion as well. Only four patients who received homologous blood in this series developed a transfusion reaction. The researchers concluded that the autologous blood program is preferable to all other blood transfusion methods. This study shows a marked improvement on Thompson's

previous study, in which he reported that 64% of 139 patients required predeposited autologous blood transfusion. While many previous studies[30,49,71,96,109] were able to reduce the need for autologous blood transfusion, Wolfson's study was a landmark because he used prospective planning, including all the patients consecutively. Haugen and Hill previously studied the use of autologous blood over a 10-year period (theirs was not a consecutive series); of 1628 patients who had deposited 4 to 6 units of autologous blood that had been frozen, 91% did not require homologous blood.[49]

Reports indicate that the transmission rate of acquired immunodeficiency syndrome (AIDS, caused by the HIV virus) by blood transfusion is extremely low. Fewer than 200 cases were reported by 1984.[85] Nevertheless, fear of such a transmission has reportedly caused tremendous concern among patients undergoing elective hip surgery. Despite the stringent standards applied in selecting homologous blood donors, most patients now prefer to donate their own blood for surgery. Based on this trend, researchers anticipate that HIV transmission through blood transfusion will eventually decrease even more.[22] The fear of HIV and hepatitis transmission persists despite new donor acceptance and screening policies. Policies for donor selections and testing for HIV and hepatitis virus are constantly changing[12]; they include (1) screening for HB_sAG (1972), (2) voluntary exclusion of persons at risk of AIDS (1983), (3) redefinition of high risk (1984), (4) testing for the antibody to HIV (1985), (5) redefinition of high risk for donor transmitting infection, (6) implementation of mechanisms to allow donors to indicate confidentially that their donations shall not be used (1986), (7) testing for apanise aminotransferase (1987), (8) testing for antibody for hepatitis B core antigen (1987), (9) testing for antibody HTLV I/II (1989), and (10) testing for antibody to hepatitis C virus (1990).[12]

In 1988, the risk of AIDS transmission in surgery was estimated to be 1 in 40,000 transfusions[103] and 1 in 36,282 transfusions in cardiac surgery patients.[16] In 1989, this risk was estimated to be decreasing to 1 in 153,000 units of blood components.[74] Screening and testing have significantly reduced the incidence of posttransfusion hepatitis; nevertheless, at present, 1 patient in 1000 who survives one decade after receiving a homologous transfusion will get posttransfusion hepatitis. Such patients will have chemical liver disease, but only a small portion of them will develop liver failure.[61]

One of the difficulties of having patients deposit blood is timing when to transfuse the autologous blood. This author prefers to transfuse 1 or 2 units of blood intraoperatively. But the availability of autologous blood is not a sufficient reason to transfuse. Not uncommonly, the patient's hematocrit level may be low (approximately 35% or lower) at the beginning of the operation; if so, do not transfuse at the outset. To avoid postoperative transfusions, surgical teams tend to transfuse patients injudiciously because their own blood is safe. This practice can be dangerous, causing "overload," pulmonary edema, and even cardiac arrest. Furthermore, the autologous blood technique is vulnerable to the same clerical errors that attend homologous blood banking. Remember, no blood transfusion is entirely safe.[67,104]

Phlebotomies can be performed either at the hospital where the surgery will be performed or at a facility near the patient's home and later shipped to the site of surgery. Blood in liquid form must be used within 5 weeks; blood kept longer than that before surgery requires freezing. Blood banks customarily store the blood at temperatures from 1° to 6° C, using citrate phosphate dextrose adenine solution-1 as an anticoagulant. If it is not frozen within 42 days after donation, the blood will be outdated. Frozen units must be transfused within 24 hours of thawing to avoid the risk of bacterial contamination.

Patients tolerate autologous blood transfusion well, and the program can be well managed by the blood bank staff. It involves no special equipment or undue expense to the hospital and is adaptable to all hospitals with blood banking facilities at their disposal. Autologous blood presents no problems of cross matching and reaction resulting from blood incompatibility, nor will it cause sensitization to antigens or any other allergic reactions. Additionally, prior phlebotomy stimulates the patient's erythropoietic system. Autologous blood transfusion at our institution has been safe, effective, and simple. With few exceptions, we offer preoperative donation of autologous blood as an option for all patients undergoing elective total joint arthroplasty.

INTRAOPERATIVE BLOOD SALVAGE AND TRANSFUSION The procedures for intraoperative blood recovery and autotransfusion during the course of surgery were developed to avoid the need for homologous blood transfusion, and their popularity has increased during the past two decades. While intraoperative autologous blood transfusion has been used extensively and reported in thoracic and general surgical procedures,* the orthopaedic literature contains only a few reports regarding its usefulness, particularly for hip arthroplasty.† With the exception of patients with certain contraindications (such as known malignancy and infection), the process may be carried out for all types of procedures; it is especially suited for primary and revision total hip arthroplasty. The

method should ideally be combined as stated before, ideally, in all cases with preoperative deposit of autologous blood for transfusion.

Goulet and associates[45] justified the cost effectiveness of intraoperative blood collection, which varied significantly from location to location and from patient to patient. This large cost variation depended upon the amount of blood donated preoperatively and recovered intraoperatively. The blood loss ranged from 700 to 7500 ml (see Table 7-2).

In a review of 100 hips of 98 patients undergoing revision total hip arthroplasty, Wilson[106] observed that 50 patients in the study group were transfused during the operation with a mean of 685 ml of autologous blood (47% of the estimated blood loss). In the group studied, the mean total need for homologous blood transfusion was 795 ml in 39 patients; this amount compared favorably with a mean of 1160 ml in a group of 46 patients in the control group who did not have intraoperative autologous blood transfusions. This difference is statistically significant (p value less than 0.029). Wilson concluded that the use of intraoperative autologous blood transfusion reduced the total need for homologous blood by 42%.

ALTERNATIVES TO HOMOLOGOUS BLOOD TRANSFUSIONS The Consensus Development Conference, organized and directed by the National Institutes of Health in 1988, released a statement that made several observations and recommendations[81] regarding blood transfusions. The risks of red cell transfusion, including transmission of infection and immunosuppression, are now undeniable. The risk of infection and death associated with transfusion cannot be eliminated with current screening methods.[18,79,94,103]

There is little or no evidence to indicate that a hemoglobin value of 10 gm/dl or a hematocrit value of 30% alone is a sufficient indication for blood transfusion; instead, use a combination of laboratory factors and good clinical judgment as a guide in recommending perioperative blood transfusion. Healthy and younger patients who are not hypovolemic can tolerate some anemia, except those with a history of cardiac disease. Currently no data suggest that proper healing requires a certain hematocrit or hemoglobin level, below which inadequate oxygen transport by red blood cells can cause morbidity or mortality. Neither is there evidence to suggest that severe postoperative anemia increases the risk of postoperative infection.

To obviate the need for homologous blood transfusions, it is necessary to seek alternatives to replace blood lost during surgery. Acceptable alternatives are limited: predeposited autologous blood,[97] intraoperative and postoperative salvage of autologous blood, intraoperative isovolemic hemodilution,[56,58] pharma-

---

* References 5, 29, 42, 51, 54, 60, 84.
† References 36–38, 50, 62, 63, 72.

cological approaches to blood loss, and designated donors. Designated donors are recruited by the patient from among family and friends. This process of direct donation is in increasing demand by patients who fear blood contamination with hepatitis, HIV, and other viruses. In general, the blood-banking community considers blood from the designated donor to be no safer than blood procured from regular donors. Keep two factors in mind when considering this option: (1) designated donation must never replace autologous blood donation when the latter is possible, and (2) the designated donor must be as rigorously screened as regular homologous blood donors.

Compared with the use of autologous blood, the use of reinfused, washed autologous red cells reclaimed by using a Cell Saver does not increase the risk of viral hepatitis and HIV virus or have any other deleterious effects.[82] In addition, this method of blood replacement seems to be acceptable to patients whose religious beliefs oblige them to consider homologous blood donation unacceptable. In a study of 175 consecutive orthopaedic operations, blood Cell Saver was used at a mean rate of 60% overall. In all groups, mean transfusion requirements were lower than in procedures that only used autotransfusion (p value < 0.001). Using prebanked autologous blood further reduced the mean requirement for homologous blood from 2.4 to 0.8 units per patient (p value 0.005) in patients who had undergone revision total hip arthroplasty.[45]

Semkiw and associates studied the effect of using the Cell Saver during the period immediately after total hip arthroplasty.[91] They used a Cell Saver after wound closure; the drainage tubes remained connected to the Cell Saver in the recovery room for a mean of 2.9 hours. The salvaged blood was processed and transfused to the patient in a manner similar to intraoperative blood collection. In 76 consecutive total hip arthroplasties and total knee arthroplasty procedures, the amount of blood varied from 100 to 2385 ml (average 428 ml). Interestingly, cemented acetabular components in primary arthroplasty were associated with less postoperative blood loss than cementless components (p value equal to 0.018). As expected, during the postoperative course in the recovery room, revision total hip arthroplasty was associated with more blood loss than the primary procedure (p value equal to 0.03), especially when using a cementless total hip arthroplasty (p value less than 0.001).[91]

For cost-effectiveness, others have suggested that this procedure is best reserved for when the blood loss is expected to exceed 1500 ml.[34,78]

Total Hip Arthroplasty Without Blood Transfusion

Major surgical procedures are performed without transfused blood on patients whose religious convic-

tions prohibit them from receiving blood and blood products (such as plasma or albumin),[4,17,83] because such patients accept any and all of the blood substitutes, including dextran, glucose, lactated Ringer's solution, saline solutions, etc. Some sects believe that the prohibition lies within a specific passage in the *Bible*, Leviticus 17:10: "And I will turn my face against anyone, whether an Israelite or a foreigner living among you who eats blood in any form. I will excommunicate him from his people." These groups also prohibit use of an individual's own blood, either stored or frozen, so they usually reject autologous blood transfusion programs. Surgeons who plan to perform surgery without blood replacement on patients with such beliefs must adhere to the following discipline:

- Maintain absolute respect for the patient's belief and rules.
- Study the extensive data available on similar surgery performed successfully without blood.
- Obtain informed surgical consent and a blood release form signed by both husband and wife, if married.
- Evaluate the patient meticulously and fastidiously, including a coagulation screening and hematological consultation as needed.
- Use hypotensive anesthesia after prior consultation with a well-trained anesthesiologist familiar with this technique.
- Plan the surgery carefully in advance to minimize operative time.
- Use meticulous surgical technique, including careful hemostasis.

Nelson reviewed a series of 100 patients undergoing total hip arthroplasty whose religious beliefs precluded using blood transfusion. In 89 of the procedures, hypotensive anesthesia was used (65 of 89 patients underwent primary total hip arthroplasty). The total blood loss was estimated to be 450 ml—a 43% reduction below the level lost in the control group, who received normotensive anesthesia. Only one patient experienced an episode of acute tubular necrosis, which was thought to be related to ischemia; there was no single myocardial infarction in the entire series.[80] The hypotensive agent used in all but four operations was sodium nitroprusside; for those four, halothane was used. Two other methods of induced hypotensive anesthesia have been used for patients with these beliefs: (1) a lumbar plexus block[100] and (2) a combination of hemodilution with induced hypotension.[108]

OPERATIVE TIME VS. SURGICAL SKILL

With increased surgical experience, the beginning surgeon learns to minimize time wasted and increase the speed of surgery. Beginners tend to attempt to set time records for a given surgical procedure or to use shortcuts, but nowhere in orthopaedic surgery is meticulous attention to technical details more important than in total hip arthroplasty. Adequate preparation of the bones of the femur and acetabulum is essential to achieve proper orientation of the components for good functional performance and a long-lasting fixation. "Shortcutting" to gain time during any vital part of the operation produces poor or even catastrophic results, which might require further surgical intervention and add to the misery of the patient. With modern anesthesia and adequate operative care of the wound, there is no justification for shortening the operative period by 15 to 30 minutes at the risk of compromising technique. In older patients whose functional life expectancy is relatively short, performing a less-than-perfect operation is totally unjustifiable, especially because these older patients may not be able to withstand a second corrective procedure. In younger patients, the lengthy period of physiological demand leaves no room for compromise.

In general, operative time for a primary total hip arthroplasty should be between 90 to 120 minutes in a well-equipped and organized center, assuming a standard uncomplicated anatomy exists, that is, a straightforward osteoarthrosis. Depending on the severity of the case and the difficulty of technical problems, operative time may extend to 180 minutes. Radiographs do not necessarily predict the ease or difficulty of a case; however, they may point out the pace, and operative time should be planned accordingly. A standard rule and lesson for the beginner is to emphasize skill and proper execution of technique rather than shorten operative time.

PROPER PREPARATION OF THE BONE AND INSERTION OF THE COMPONENTS

The details of technique are discussed in later chapters. At this point it is essential to emphasize that the artificial hip joint will provide lifetime service to the patient only if properly implanted and rigidly fixed to the bone. Excessive scrupulousness or gentleness in preparing the bone may be ineffective and time-consuming; on the other hand, excessive boldness and inadvertent trauma to the tissue may lead to serious complications, such as femoral fractures or perforation of the pelvis, producing catastrophic results. Common sense is the key to surgical technique; it is important to evaluate difficulties at each step and to redirect the approach if necessary. It is useless to insert a prosthesis that could later become loose or fracture as a result of defective technique; only meticulous attention to all details ensures permanent

fixation. A surgeon must be certain that any modification of a time-tested procedure at any stage is for technical improvement and does not violate the previously stated principles.

IRRIGATION, SUCTION, AND DEBRIDEMENT

Generally, irrigation might be of value during the operation (1) to keep the tissue moistened and to remove debris from the wound, (2) after cementing of each of the components, and (3) at the time of wound closure. Debridement of the muscle fibers (usually the gluteus maximus if detached and devitalized) may be indicated. While irrigation is useful to remove the particles and cement fragments mechanically, swabbing the wound throughout is the most effective way to keep it clean. A strong suction tip inserted into the femoral canal and acetabulum might be useful; however, tight packing of the interior of the bone with dry swabs (both in the femur and the acetabulum) at the final stage provides a dry "bed" for fixation of the cement. Antibiotic deposit into the bed of the bone before cement insertion is not recommended; although irrigation with an antibiotic solution has been used as a "rational exercise" its effectiveness has not been proven (see Chapter 8). Contemplate copious irrigation with large amounts of solution with caution: "oversaturation" may soak the draping, thereby adding more contamination risks than benefits.

DRAINAGE OF THE WOUND AND HEMATOMAS

A Hemovac draining tube inserted at surgery is removed 48 to 72 hours after surgery. While drains are routinely used deep to the fascia, it is also suggested that they be used superficial to the fascia. Do not change the dressing postoperatively for at least 4 or 5 days, unless for a specific reason. Do not disturb clinically diagnosed hematomas (indicated by fullness of the thigh) that are not draining, but curtail the patient's activities until the hematoma subsides. Ice packs to the hip region will make the patient comfortable; needling is not indicated.

Spontaneous draining of a hematoma into the wound is best handled by reoperation and evacuation in the operating room under general anesthesia in absolutely sterile conditions. If anticoagulants are the causative agent, treatment must be reversed at once and the patient's activities stopped until the hematoma has completely dissolved. A draining (leaking) hematoma is a potentially dangerous problem from the standpoint of infection; it is inadequate simply to place the patient on antibiotics and observe the wound. After diagnosing the hematoma, cover the wound with a sterile dressing and prepare the patient for evacuation and closure of the wound under anesthesia. If the fascia is sealed off and not disturbed, it is essential to perform a careful, formal draping technique, similar to that used in total hip arthroplasty. Irrigate the wound copiously, remove all clots, and close the wound carefully (using retention sutures).

STUDY OF ANATOMY AND REHEARSAL

The surgeon must have a detailed knowledge of the surgical anatomy of the hip to comprehend the different ways of approaching the hip joint, choose the appropriate route for a specific procedure, and minimize damage to the patient's vital structures; it is also imperative to avoid damaging the muscles, which basically provide hip function. Because the abductor mechanism is the key source of power in the hip, it is mandatory to protect its fibers, and the surgeon must understand the relationship of these muscles to the anterior and posterior groups of muscles. Surgeons learn the anatomy by several routes: by studying the normal anatomy, by evaluating pathological conditions at surgery, by using their sense of touch and the appropriate surgical instrument, and most importantly, by appraising difficult situations. For example, when a maximum exposure cannot be obtained, sometimes all that is required is altering flexion of the hip by 10 or 15 degrees; in another case, delivery of the upper femur out of the wound by a lever might be the solution. Throughout surgery, the surgeon must reexamine the possibility of improving the exposure. This can be done in several ways: by removing the assistant's fingers from the wound; by adjusting the self-retaining retractors; by swabbing the blood from the surface; by stabilizing the limb in a certain degree of abduction, adduction, or rotation; or by having the table leveled to a more convenient position.

By continuous study of the surgical wound and surgical anatomy, the surgeon can eliminate obstacles and unpredicted nuisances (such as fractures of the femur and pelvis). This helps the surgeon develop surgical "common sense," which will inspire the confidence to advance or retreat when necessary. The surgeon's actions must be based on knowledge, not on fear. As a general rule, remove no tissue unnecessarily during wound exposure. However, excise as much capsule of the joint as necessary to obtain maximum exposure; with the exception of the abductor mechanism, it is safe to release any muscle to achieve a fully mobile hip without residual deformity. Although using a bony skeleton and dissecting a cadaveric hip are important exercises for the beginner, having the surgeon assist in several operations before performing the first total hip arthroplasty is possibly even more valuable. Several factors help the inexperienced surgeon learn how to place the incision correctly along the lines of approach to the joint: study of the surface anatomy of the hip joint; observation of the bony prominences of the anterosuperior spine, the crest of the ilium, and the location of the greater trochanter; palpation of the abductor muscles (gluteus medius and minimus); and orientation of the gluteus maximus from the sacrum investing the buttock into the lateral aspect of the shaft. These anatomical relations may be appraised and compared with those of the opposite side before surgical draping.

SKIN INCISION AND WOUND EXPOSURE

Numerous methods for skin preparation have been recommended; select one that is practical and applicable to the immediate surgical environment. Because the patient is usually in the hospital only briefly before surgery, it is advisable that he or she wash the surgical area with hexachlorophene or a similar antiseptic soap during showers at least twice the day before admission, to combat the general bacterial population of the skin (see Chapter 8). On the night before surgery, the groin should be washed and the pubic hair clipped (shaving often scratches the skin, enhancing colonization of organisms); it is best to remove hair from the entire extremity—from groin to foot. The toenails are clipped and all nail polish removed. It is sensible, although not essential, to towel the hip area and lower extremity before moving the patient to the operating room. It is of paramount importance to defat the skin with ether (or a similar defatting agent, such as Freon) and apply 2% tincture of iodine before draping. Performing an iodine patch test the night before surgery will indicate a possible allergic reaction to iodine; such reactions must be extremely uncommon, because we have rarely observed them. Leave the painted iodine on the skin rather than removing it; this practice has not caused skin burn in our experience, although burning may occur in areas of pooling (such as the buttocks) if the patient lies in it. Often "frictional burns," caused by careless removal of the "transfer sheet," have been mistaken for iodine burns.

During surgery, handle skin edges with care and take care to achieve a perfect skin closure. Insulation by towels will help eliminate trauma to the skin edges and prevent surface contamination by skin contaminants. Using the towel clip method with Turkish towels is effective, but do not cut the incision short by application of the distal and proximal towel clips; the clips should not crush the skin edges. To avoid contact with skin bacteria, we soak the towels at the skin edge with Betadine solution to keep the wound sterile.

Be sure to make the skin incision adequately long; in addition, remember that it is psychologically important to the patient that the surgeon produce symmetrical incisions in bilateral replacements. Correct placement of the incision is of great value in producing maximum exposure with the minimal length incision; however, if the incision is misplaced, make it long enough to prevent undue trauma during surgery. Prolonged heavy retraction of the skin over the corners by additional instrumentation may cause skin ischemia and delay healing; it is always advisable to make a longer incision to avoid having to struggle for a better exposure. It is worth remembering that post-operatively a patient does not discuss the length, location, or type of approach to his or her joint; patients do complain, however, about an operation that failed as a result of complications such as femoral shaft fractures occurring during surgery or infections and hematomas resulting from the excessive struggle involved when surgery is performed through a limited exposure.

It is advisable for the novice to use a longer incision (with experience, he or she will know enough to make it shorter). It is better to have a longer incision from the beginning than to add to its length during the procedure. Also, use a longer incision when you anticipate surgical difficulty; the entire length of the skin incision must be used when the deeper layers are incised. If an adhesive plastic drape has been used, it is advisable to reapply 2% tincture of iodine to the skin before closing the fat retention sutures because bacteria of the deep layers may have been brought to the surface during surgery when removing the adhesive plastic drape. Previous operative scars in close proximity to the hip joint create a nuisance, but they must be handled intelligently; this pitfall occurs commonly when correcting a previously failed surgery. To avoid previous incisions, which are almost, but not precisely, the perfect location for the second surgery, the surgeon may often cut the incision too anteriorly or posteriorly. Although in principle it is advisable to ignore old scars about the hip, the final decision on where to cut the new incision must be based on where it will best expose the hip. Whenever we have placed a new incision in the vicinity of an old incision—at almost any angle or location—it has been safe; no ischemic necrosis has developed about the hip, which sometimes occurs when incisions cross each other. A good supply of skin flaps and abundant anastomotic circulation about the hip allow the surgeon to make almost any type of incision (from the anterior ilioinguinal ligament to the region of the ischium) without fear of necrosis. Avoid cauterizing bleeders close to the epidermis because of the danger that skin edge necrosis will develop; bleeders close to the epidermis are usually controlled by towel clips applied to the skin edges. A continuous running mattress stitch with 3-0 nylon is adequate for closure; however, the surgeon may also use subcuticular closure and interrupted mattress sutures. Be sure to achieve a good approximation of the skin edges, without tension, during skin closure.

SUBCUTANEOUS FAT

When entering the subcutaneous fat along the incision, it is essential to apply skin towels before entering deeper layers of fat. Constantly check against the greater trochanter and midlateral shaft as you deepen the incision in the fat. Do not undercut the fat or separate it from fascia; appropriate cutting of the fat layer can eliminate much of the error in misplacing the skin incision. Occasionally irrigating the fat keeps the tissue from drying out and may minimize cell death. A thin person may be in just as much danger of infection as a very obese person who has heavy deposits of adipose tissue in the hip region. In both extreme cases, a meticulous approximation of subcutaneous fat and retention of the tension within this tissue are essential to prevent accumulation of seroma or production of fat necrosis, which may evacuate into the dressing, a common source of wound contamination. While interrupted 2-0 catgut may be adequate to close the fat layer, retention sutures fastened over thick foam pads (popularized by Charnley) have proved to be superior for closure after total hip arthroplasty (see Chapter 15). Apply fat sutures and tighten them over the sponges after closure of the skin edges. Regardless of fat thickness, it is advisable to apply a separate drain tube superficially to the fascia in the fat layer. The fat layer should be considered as a separate compartment from the hip joint; therefore wound closure technique must focus on a tight fascial closure and elimination of dead space. This important part of the operation should under no circumstances be relegated to an inexperienced resident or student.

FASCIA AND TENDONS

Because of the importance of the abductor muscle function, its tendinous attachment to the greater trochanter must never be removed without a bony fragment. There is only one circumstance when it can be removed without a bony fragment: in the transgluteal approach, reattaching tendon by itself is unsatisfactory and will lead to a defective result. To reattach the greater trochanter (to restore a good and powerful abductor mechanism for the hip), carefully consider technique and apply it meticulously.

Respect the importance of the deep fascia of the thigh, a deep envelope that separates the skin from the hip joint proper. Open this fascia at midline with reference to the iliotibial tract and repair it carefully after surgery to stabilize the hip and separate the superficial inflammatory process and drainage from the deep structures. Place special emphasis on proximal closure of this structure. The gluteal fascia is often thin, and its exposure generally requires considerable retraction of the fat by an assistant. Hematomas commonly form at this site; using nonabsorbable suture material gives the fascia a chance to heal completely. If the fascia has been incised in a T shape, be sure to repair it carefully before closing the remainder of the fascia. To correct fixed deformities during total hip arthroplasty, release the tendinous insertion of the iliopsoas, adductor, and external rotator muscles; to minimize bleeding, disinsert these tendons next to the bone. Like the adductors and rotators, the iliopsoas tendon may be released from the lesser trochanter. Cauterize the blood supply or accompanying vessels after removing these tendons from their insertions. When the short rotator or anterior portion of the gluteus medius and gluteus medius or gluteus maximus tendons are detached as a routine to enhance the exposure, they must be firmly repaired. Commonly, the artery accompanying the piriformis may retract and cause a hematoma. The iliopsoas tendon can be readily visualized by external rotation and thus removed from the lesser trochanter and its vicinity. The adductus longus and brevis may be disinserted from the pubis by subcutaneous tenotomy. As stated, none of the tendons about the hip require resuturing (unless the gluteus medius has been inadvertently disinserted without bone) because tenotomies about the hip are performed during the construction to release the contracture and to correct the deformity. A compression dressing applied to the groin area will assist in tamponade of the bleeders after adductor tenotomy.

HANDLING OF OTHER SOFT TISSUES

Retracting the planes of the muscles and fascia to allow insertion of instruments and placement of the prosthetic components may require considerable force, especially in large and muscular males and when the greater trochanter has not been removed as part of the routine surgical technique. Excessive retraction of the anterior structure can produce femoral nerve palsy, especially if the anterior wall of the acetabulum is defective, as in a dysplastic hip. The sciatic nerve may also be in danger if there is marked anatomical distortion and an excessive posterior scar. For example, in severe protrusion of the head and neck into the pelvis, the greater trochanter is displaced medially and within the vicinity of the sciatic nerve; thus a careless osteotomy of the greater trochanter endangers the sciatic nerve. In such cases, palpate the nerve or be guided by the fat surrounding the nerve. Be careful not to damage the anterior or posterior fibers of the very important gluteus medius when exposing the hip joint without removing the greater trochanter in difficult anatomical situations; such damage would cause scar formation and weaken the abductor mechanism. Avoid excessive retraction or trauma at the interval between

the tensor fascia femoris, which would eliminate an important, yet less appreciated, structure of the hip joint. If the muscle bundles of the gluteus maximus (which are occasionally detached from their parent bundles) appear devitalized, they must be excised. Since cement particles are potential irritants if deposited loosely in the soft tissue about the hip, be sure to irrigate with isotonic solution. It seems advisable to irrigate the muscles and other soft tissue deep to the fascia during at least two stages of the operation: before closure and after cementing the acetabular cup and the femoral component.

HANDLING OF THE GREATER TROCHANTER

When osteotomizing the greater trochanter, be sure to do it at the appropriate level to obtain the optimal size. An excessively large trochanter carries the vastus lateralis ridge with it, thus producing a large bump on the outer aspect of the femur; occasionally it is difficult to reattach onto the lateral aspect of the shaft. On the other hand, an excessively small trochanter may be difficult to handle and produce less than optimal coaptation of the surfaces for union, thereby escaping through the wires provided for its fixation. Handle the trochanter gently from the time of its removal to the final stage of its reattachment. The greatest degree of fixation will only result when it is removed at an optimal size and shape. A fragmented trochanter is not only difficult to reattach but may also disengage from its fixation wires, weakening the abductor mechanism and inviting prosthesis dislocation. Many patients require an undesirably lengthy rehabilitation period to achieve trochanteric healing. If excessively osteoporotic (as in rheumatoid arthritis), remove a larger size trochanter and take special care when retracting and reattaching it. Reattachment of the greater trochanter requires attention to details; orient the fibers of the gluteus medius appropriately to preserve its fiber length and direction. Furthermore, it is essential to obtain a maximum coaptation between the inner surface and the outer aspect of the shaft of the femur; handling will be discussed in detail later. Achieving a firm reattachment is essential to successful hip arthroplasty through a lateral approach. Be sure that the wires used for reattachment are not scarred or nicked; practice rewiring on a model or bone before attempting to do so at surgery. If surgery reveals that the fixation to the trochanter is inadequate, make sure to protect the patient postoperatively with 2 to 3 weeks of bed rest (see Chapters 13 and 37) or by the use of a cast or a brace (see Chapters 13 and 37).

SHAFT OF THE FEMUR AND THE ACETABULUM

Later chapters discuss the details of handling the shaft and the acetabulum; however, it is essential to regard the bony structures as supportive devices; damaging them could cause the prosthetic components to fail. Replacing the bony structure may be compared to embedding a flagpole in concrete. If the surrounding ground is weak, the flagpole will fail despite the strength of its materials; similarly, if the bony structures are weakened, the prosthesis may fail. Removing a previously inserted nail and plate or prosthesis may weaken the femoral shaft, requiring special attention; it may be necessary to retreat if removal of the previously inserted device induces excessive trauma. Excessive damage to the acetabular floor may allow the entire component to migrate medially; at this time, there is no solution available for such migration. Using the reamers carelessly or eccentrically or using drills inappropriately may fracture or remove a part of the bony acetabulum, leading to loosening of the components. Paying special attention to the preparation details of the upper femur and acetabulum is the sine qua non of good replacement surgery. While it is essential to preserve as much bony stalk as possible, remove osteophytes carefully so they cannot function as a fulcrum on the periphery of the acetabulum and upper femur, facilitating dislocation. Bleeding, both in the upper femur and in the acetabulum, is best controlled by tightly packing the canal or the acetabular cavity with a large swab of gauze. This procedure resembles the way a dentist packs cavities before applying the filling material. Maintaining pressure on these swabs for a period of only 1 to 2 minutes will dry the surface almost entirely, which is very important for cement application. A swab soaked in 2% tincture of iodine may be used in the bone cavities from which previous prostheses have been removed; use this surgical disinfectant if you suspect low-grade subclinical infection.

A maximum exposure is absolutely essential. Nowhere in the practice of orthopaedic surgery is "keyhole surgery" more dangerous than in total hip arthroplasty. When the surgeon must struggle throughout the procedure to obtain exposure, he or she loses more time than would have been spent obtaining good exposure at the time of incision. Inadequate exposure is also associated with more blood loss and is never efficient. It is far better to lose time while exposing the hip joint adequately than to be forced to sacrifice it during the actual implantation. As a working rule, in performing this operation routinely we allocate two thirds of the working time for exposure and closure of the wound and only one third to preparing the bone and actually implanting the prosthesis.

ORGANIZATIONAL FACILITIES TO PERFORM TOTAL HIP ARTHROPLASTY

To this author's knowledge, Sir John Charnley was the only proponent of specialized centers for total hip surgery. His enthusiasm stemmed from his experience with the evolution and growth of the Centre for Hip Surgery at Wrightington Hospital.

Despite his great contributions and success, not only in Great Britain, but throughout the world, only a few other centers have been organized for dealing exclusively with surgery of the hip joint. Obviously, to duplicate such a center would require comprehensive geographical planning and devotion of a great deal of time to leadership. Surgeons' concern about the economic impact on private practice is perhaps why no one has attempted to organize such a center in the United States.

There are probably between 700,000 and 1,000,000 people with osteoarthritis, plus those with degenerative disease of the hip joint resulting from trauma, rheumatoid arthritis, and a variety of other afflictions. Half of them may require reconstructive surgery at some point. Some estimate that one third of the major reconstructive surgery in orthopaedic practice is related to the hip.

Since life expectancy has increased to 72 years for males and 78 years for females and approximately 30,000,000 Americans are now over 65, it is clear that the number of potential candidates for total hip surgery is increasing rapidly. According to Kelgren and Lawrence's field sampling in Great Britain, probably 100,000 to 200,000 people have arthrosis of the hip requiring arthroplasty. Therefore we have come to recognize that the heavy load created by total hip arthroplasty (not counting total joint arthroplasty in shoulders, knees, and elbows) calls for definite institutional reform. Furthermore, future repair or maintenance work imposed by the failure of total hip arthroplasties will probably add to the number of patients requiring hip surgery.

Many older people living out the last decade of their lives could benefit from treatment of their hip disabilities. From a humanitarian point of view alone, they should have access to greater mobility and less confinement in their advanced years; it is inhumane to refuse them surgery because we lack the organizational facilities and hospitals to accommodate them. In some areas of Great Britain and in nonprivate institutions in the United States, elderly people must wait for many months to be admitted for this type of elective surgery.

Among the many advantages of a highly centralized and specialized facility for surgery are lower costs, reduced frequency of surgical complications, and above all, improved quality of care associated with technical surgical perfection and minimum morbidity. These achievements would result from optimal productivity provided by maximum use of facilities; they would allow an economy of effort on the part of the surgeon when he or she performs these operations daily. In a unit such as the Wrightington Centre for Hip Surgery, 6 hip arthroplasties are performed in one operating room each workday—18 arthroplasties in three operating rooms. Minimal numbers of staff are required because the routine is not interrupted by unexpected work, such as trauma. Still, the staff can provide excellent patient care and render adequate clinical and basic research in the field. A vivid example of this maximum efficiency is that bilateral operations are performed during the same anesthesia, which is practical because superior organization provides a quick turnover. Two operations may be performed during the same anesthesia without undue strain on the patient or the surgical staff.[52]

The reputation of such a center would attract patients from a wide geographical area. Because this type of surgery is elective and patients are not forced to accept a "compromise solution" to their problems, they are willing to travel to obtain the best possible care. Practitioners and other sources of referral would be encouraged by consistently good results and excellent care to refer patients to such a center.

Total hip arthroplasty is now estimated to be one of the most commonly performed elective orthopaedic procedures in most parts of the world, including the current estimate of 100,000 per year in the United States. Yet despite the frequency of these operations, there has been no trend toward specialization, which would provide continuous care and service. Charnley stated that "to consider the insertion of a total hip replacement into a patient 25 years of age in 1971, without having a 'service station' provided and organized for 1986, is like selling motorcars without providing mechanics and workshops." We have reviewed the experiences of some surgeons who, having performed such operations in community hospitals, later find themselves under considerable pressure to deal with complications such as infections and technical problems. It is obvious that patients referred to the centers for corrective surgery are resentful: revision surgery is of much greater magnitude than the original procedure, and the help available is limited because of the technical complexity of the problems.

Despite the increased need for patient care imposed by the number of total hip operations being performed, major universities and medical centers, because of their patient load and the need to reorganize their staffing, have evidently been unwilling to devote a portion of their postgraduate training in this area.

While it would be impossible to perform all total hip arthroplasties in centers, centers located in major cities could conceivably not only reduce the hospital workload but also provide "training grounds" for orthopaedic surgeons at the postgraduate level; these centers would attract surgeons willing to acquire superior skills to devote their future work (or at least a major portion of it) to this type of surgery. Such centers would also free community hospital facilities for other types of work, provide better overall patient care, and, naturally, guarantee future "repair work."

It is this author's impression that if a center cannot be devoted exclusively to this type of practice, then "pooling" of patients among a group of orthopaedic surgeons practicing in one hospital would be a reasonable compromise. Members of such a group would learn from each other how best to cope with potential complications and failures and be able to offer better total patient care. Rather than groups being hospital-oriented, the popular trend of the so-called group practice in the United States may be the model for "pooling" among practicing orthopaedic surgeons.

It would be regrettable if a university or hospital were to use a procedure such as total hip arthroplasty only to attract residents to their training program (with the promise that they would do a guaranteed number of total hip arthroplasties by the time they were through with training). Since total hip surgery constitutes a large portion of surgical procedures, the young physician eager to enter a training program in orthopaedic surgery might consider it attractive. But operations of this magnitude should not be performed by a junior resident who has devoted insufficient time to the procedure and does not yet understand the scope of the problems, which lie beyond the mere technical ability to perform an operation.

At the New York Orthopaedic Hospital at the Columbia-Presbyterian Medical Center, a junior resident in our training program is in charge of preoperative and postoperative patient care (under the supervision of the senior resident on the hip service). The residents also act as assistants at all operations. The attending physician is responsible for overall supervision and conduct of the surgery. Routine orders are established in the preoperative and postoperative periods, and a medical consultant evaluates the patient daily. This general pattern provides the junior resident with an opportunity to become familiar with preoperative and postoperative management of the patient; thus the daily resident's rounds are bound to be extremely helpful in identifying, documenting, and managing complications.

A senior resident spends a period of 6 weeks exclusively and 6 weeks partially on the hip service; on completing a residency in the third year, he or she will have performed from 20 to 30 technically uncomplicated total hip procedures, assisted in all of them by an experienced attending surgeon. (Even in the final year of training, we discourage the resident from performing more complex procedures.) The resident has also acquired experience through rotation and by having assisted in all cases during this period. By the end of the residency we believe the resident is qualified to select appropriate patients for total hip procedures and can recognize his or her limitations in taking up more technically complicated cases.

We offer basic training to one or two postgraduate trainees, who have a fellowship for the entire year. These fellows are usually the mainstay of the organization of postgraduate training. They not only participate in most operations but also conduct daily rounds with the senior and junior residents. Supervised and assisted, they perform between 200 and 300 arthroplasties during the year and also supervise and assist in operations performed by the staff or residents; they have generally become qualified to perform complicated procedures toward the end of their fellowship.

It would be a great advantage to have all hip patients located in one special area of the hospital, which promotes efficiency, better staff training, and psychological well-being for ambulatory patients, who benefit from sharing accounts of similar experiences with others. One or more operating rooms should be devoted to performing only this type of surgery to provide maximum speed and efficiency.

In summary, this author supports the concept of superspecialization whenever possible, as advocated by Charnley. If we consider the frequency of such operations, the basic need for technical excellence, and humanitarian considerations for older people, the necessity of a team approach is readily recognized and should be acknowledged by authorities in the field of orthopaedic education. Furthermore, establishing such a center would minimize costs and complications, and the staff could devote adequate time to documentation and cooperating with the mechanical engineering staff in developing practical solutions to technical and mechanical problems. We further believe that this system would offer superior training in orthopaedic surgery at both the pregraduate and postgraduate levels, and, above all, provide better patient care and assure that further treatment is available in the future if it becomes necessary.

SUMMARY OF ESSENTIALS

- Because complications after total hip arthroplasty can be disastrous and failure of the operation results in severe disability, more attention must be directed to prevention than to treatment of complications. The surgeon must keep possible complications constantly in mind and carefully plan the preoperative, operative, and postoperative management of elderly patients.

- As surgeons, orthopaedists are bound by principles requiring them to carefully evaluate each patient as a whole, not as a problematic hip; to base decisions

for each specific surgical intervention on well-established indications; and to perform the procedure with aseptic technique and absolute precision.

- It is imperative to recognize and attend to the special needs of elderly patients undergoing total hip arthroplasty when planning preoperative and postoperative nursing, which should be handled by an experienced staff. Obviously, older people are more prone to operative and postoperative complications; the latter can be reduced by quality postoperative care.

- Errors in preoperative preparation and diagnosis have been blamed in part for the high rate of surgical mortality in elderly patients. This mortality rate can be lowered by paying detailed attention to all medical aspects of the patient, especially to the systemic review and proper consultations required in planning anesthetic management and appropriate rehabilitation programs.

- In general, older patients tolerate the pain and stress of operation better than young patients, but the dangers of shock and death are greater for them. Therefore prompt rectification of the complications of surgery in this age group must be emphasized.

- Before major elective surgery, work out the social and psychological issues facing patients and the details of postoperative accommodations. Many details of surgical nursing care must be considered, including the importance of communicating cheerful confidence to the patient when explaining the details of what to expect from surgery.

- On admission, teach the patient the details of rehabilitation, including how to transfer from the bed and how to use assistive devices to ensure smooth and uncomplicated postoperative management. Do not excessively emphasize the side effects of drugs or the potential complications of the operation. Use medications judiciously for pain relief and the patient's comfort, especially during the postoperative course.

- During daily visits, the surgical team should attend not only to the patient's physical disabilities but also to his or her mental attitude toward the progress of the postoperative course. Criticizing patients is not constructive and can be dangerous. Urinary or fecal incontinence, an extreme embarrassment to older patients, should be handled without amplification and with support rather than criticism. An indwelling catheter controls urinary incontinence and is a convenience for the patient.

- It is a good idea to have the family present in the original interview while discussing the proposed operation. Tell the patient as much as he or she wishes to know, but only discuss relevant matters. Older persons often have deep-seated fears and may not be inquisitive about the details. Do not run the risk of agitating the patient by overstating the hazards of the operation. It is essential to communicate cheerful confidence.

- The choice of anesthesia involves the anesthesiologist, the patient, and the surgeon and is based on the anesthetist's preoperative evaluation. The anesthesiologist makes the final recommendation and also participates in recommending postoperative pain control medication.

- Of three methods of anesthesia — the normotensive standard general anesthesia, general hypotensive anesthesia, and regional anesthesia — regional anesthesia, particularly continuous epidural anesthesia, seems to be most advantageous for patients undergoing total hip arthroplasty.

- Recent pulmonary embolism, history of angina pectoris or myocardial infarction, hypertension, congestive heart disease, and asthma are relative contraindications to anesthesia. Before a patient is selected for anesthesia, all of these conditions must be evaluated and anticipated. Other conditions, such as coexisting diabetes, ankylosing spondylitis, rheumatoid arthritis, nephropathy, and chronic use of steroids or other drugs, may increase the anesthesia risk. None disqualifies the patient for elective surgery.

- Patients whose hip surgery is complicated by a pulmonary embolism or myocardial infarction must not be considered for arthroplasty of the other hip for at least 6 months. A high risk of reinfarction and mortality has been documented for both conditions when operations on the second hip were carried out before 6 months had passed. Patients with a history of angina must be studied by a cardiologist. The evaluation should include stress testing. Even coronary artery bypass may be indicated before elective total hip arthroplasty procedures.

- Patients with a history of angina, treated or untreated, constitute a high risk for perioperative ischemia and myocardial infarction, even when it is concurrent with a hemodynamically uneventful anesthetic procedure. Angina at rest and asymptomatic (silent) angina must also be considered as putting those patients at risk and should be evaluated before surgery.

- Many surgeons have used hypotensive anesthesia extensively in doing total hip arthroplasty to reduce blood loss and operative time and to reduce local bleeding, which is detrimental for a cement fixation.

- Although induced hypotensive anesthesia has been recommended for total hip surgery, there is insufficient in-depth evidence of its usefulness and related morbidity. The best overall method of lowering the blood pressure during anesthesia is also disputed.

- The use of hypotensive anesthesia in hip arthroplasty unquestionably has important dividends. However, unless the anesthesia team is prepared to accept full responsibility for selecting the patients and for precise monitoring during surgery, this type of anesthesia might carry added risks for the patient.

- Spinal and epidural anesthesia have been favored by many surgeons and anesthetists for hip arthroplasty. However, patients receiving this type of anesthesia must also be put to sleep for comfort. At our institution, the preferred method is to use epidural anesthesia with a supplemental general anesthesia with endotracheal intubation. This combined anesthesia offers distinct advantages in that the patient's pulmonary function remains intact while the need for medication decreases, since the pain is eliminated by the successful epidural anesthesia. There are practical difficulties in routine use of regional anesthesia. Fixed deformities and painful hips make it difficult to position the patient for insertion of the spinal or epidural anesthetic. The major advantage of regional anesthesia is the reduction in intraoperative bleeding and the patient's ease of recovery postoperatively, which surpass the disadvantages. There are several contraindications for regional anesthesia, including tendency to bleed because of coagulopathy, use of antiinflammatory medications, easy bruisability, and history of postural postanesthetic headaches.

- Congestive heart failure is the most serious risk for elective surgery. Because of the high perioperative morbidity associated with this condition, it is mandatory that it be treated before the contemplated hip surgery.

- An asthmatic patient must undergo a full preoperative pulmonary function assessment by a pulmonologist. Appropriate pulmonary treatment, including bronchial dilators, should be used to improve or resolve wheezing before surgery.

- Most controlled diabetic patients present little or no difficulty as long as there is no evidence of significant hypoglycemia, hyperglycemia, or glycosuria. Most experts agree that it is important to achieve good control of the disease before elective total hip arthroplasty.

- Although patients with mildly elevated diastolic pressure and diastolic pressure of 90 to 110 mm Hg may be accepted for anesthetic without undue concern, patients with labile hypertension and high blood pressure may develop a significant increase in blood pressure during endotracheal intubation. There is general agreement that patients with sustained diastolic blood pressure over 110 mm Hg must be treated before planned total hip arthroplasty.

- A thorough preoperative evaluation of the cervical spine including standard radiographs and flexion-extension views must be routine before surgery on patients with rheumatoid arthritis, ankylosing spondylitis, or juvenile rheumatoid arthritis. When severe C1/C2 instability is encountered or a subluxation of 6 to 7 mm is present, careful consideration of spinal fusion before planned total hip arthroplasty may be indicated. With lesser degrees of displacement by flexion-extension lateral projection of the cervical spine (greater than 2 to 3 mm between the posterior aspect of the anterior arch of atlas and the anterior aspect of the odontoid), the cervical spine must be protected during anesthesia.

- Concurrent medications such as steroids, antihypertensive medications, cardiac medications, diuretics, digoxin therapy, and antidepressants must be adjusted. The internist familiar with the problem must be consulted, and a cardiology anesthesiologist might be specially called in to administer anesthesia.

- The advantages of autologous banked blood have been established. It remains the blood source of choice for transfusions required during or after total hip arthroplasty procedures.

- Several conservation methods and blood replacement procedures are currently practiced in total hip arthroplasty. Conservation accomplished by the use of hypotensive anesthesia and spinal and epidural anesthesia can often eliminate the need to replace blood lost during routine primary total hip arthroplasty. Preoperative acute hemodilution can be used in patients whose religious beliefs prohibit blood transfusions. However, this method has not been universally accepted. The use of homologous blood from blood banks exposes the patient to many risks, ranging from minor allergic reactions to death. They include isosensitization, hemolytic reaction, exposure to infectious diseases (bacterial infections, syphilis, malaria, serum hepatitis non-A and non-B, and HIV). Risks are significant enough to warrant seeking an alternative method to homologous blood in all nonemergency operative procedures.

- Transfusion with autologous blood obtained intraoperatively and postoperatively in addition to preoperative autologous blood donation of up to 6 to 8 units (2 to 4 may be frozen) may eliminate the need for homologous red cell transfusion.

- The risk of AIDS transmission in surgery has been estimated as 1 in 40,000 transfusions and 1 in 36,282 transfusions in cardiac surgery patients. In 1989, estimates indicated that this risk had decreased to 1 in 153,000 units of blood components. At present, screening and testing have reduced the incidence of posttransfusion hepatitis, but the risk remains 1 in 1000 in patients who survive one decade after receiving a homologous transfusion. Such patients will have chemical liver disease, but only a small portion will develop liver failure.

- A patient undergoing a revision arthroplasty may donate 4 or 5 units of blood, 2 or 3 units of which may be deposited and frozen several months before surgery, the remainder being deposited in liquid form within 35 days before surgery. In practice, patients who have donated their own blood for banking commonly have a low hematocrit level at the time of surgery, requiring blood transfusion at the outset. However, a lower hematocrit level may be accepted postoperatively if the medical condition of the patient permits.

- Intraoperative and postoperative blood collection is cost effective and should be supplemented in operations in which autologous blood is insufficient. To be cost effective, intraoperative saving of blood must be limited to patients who either were unable to donate sufficient blood or are expected to lose more than 1500 ml of blood during their surgery.

- Major surgical procedures are performed without transfusion of blood and blood products on patients whose religious convictions prohibit them from receiving such substances. These patients accept any and all blood substitutes including dextran, glucose, lactated Ringer's solution, saline solutions, etc. Respect absolutely the patient's beliefs and restrictions. Study the extensive data available on similar surgery performed successfully without blood. Evaluate the patient meticulously and fastidiously. Perform a coagulation screening and hematologic consultation, and use hypotensive anesthesia. Plan for surgery carefully in advance to minimize operative time, and use meticulous surgical technique, including careful hemostasis.

- The surgeon's ability to minimize wasted time improves with experience. Beginners tend to attempt to break the time record for a given surgical procedure. It is imperative to resist this temptation in performing total hip arthroplasty. A perfect technique is the goal, not a fast technique. Taking shortcuts to gain time for the vital part of the operation produces poor or even catastrophic results requiring further surgical intervention with added misery to the patient.

- Gear the speed during surgery to the circumstances, including the surgical facilities, the experience of the surgeon performing the operation, and any anatomical abnormalities requiring specific attention.

- Being too scrupulous or gentle in preparing the bone may be ineffective and time consuming. On the other hand, being too bold and inadvertently traumatizing the tissue may lead to serious complications. Modify time-tested procedures only on the basis of good logic. The surgeon must bear in mind that the violation of established principles is a grave responsibility.

- Handle the tissue gently, and keep in mind maximizing the life of the repair. Irrigate with isotonic solutions, and remove debris and necrotized tissue per the principles of successful surgery.

- Routinely drain the wound with a suction drain both deep and superficial to the fascia. Never drain or aspirate a hematoma at the bedside. Spontaneous drainage of a hematoma into the wound should be handled by reoperation and evacuation in the operating room under general anesthesia in absolutely sterile conditions.

- A draining (leaking) hematoma is potentially dangerous from the standpoint of infection and must be treated vigorously as an emergency situation.

- The study of anatomy and rehearsal before surgery are essential for the beginner. Participation in several surgical procedures as an assistant not only familiarizes the surgeon with the procedure but gives him or her a better understanding of the unpredicted difficulties that may arise during this operation.

- Preparing the skin before surgery with surgical soap and meticulous clipping of the hair must be supervised. The use of 2% tincture of iodine and proper draping techniques is of paramount importance in performing the operation. The skin incision must be adequate and carefully placed. Correct placement of the incision is of great value, as is good closure of the skin to prevent infection.

- The use of retention sutures has dramatically improved the quality of wound healing after total hip arthroplasty. When handling the wound closure, the surgeon must consider that a thin person is potentially as susceptible to infection as an obese person. In both extreme cases, approximate the fat and retain sutures to prevent the accumulation of seroma or hematoma. It is bad practice to relegate the wound closure to the most junior member of the operating team.

- Handle the greater trochanter with care, and apply meticulously detailed technique for its reattachment. Never remove the tendon of the abductor partially or totally without a bony fragment, because repair would be impossible.

REFERENCES

1. **Aufranc OE:** Preoperative and postoperative treatment of the patient with reconstructive surgery of the hip, *Clin Orthop* 38:40, 1965.
2. **Aufranc OE:** *Constructive surgery of the hip,* St Louis, 1962, Mosby–Year Book.
3. **Ascari WQ, Jolly PC, Thomas PA:** Autologous blood transfusion in pulmonary surgery, *Transfusion* 8:111, 1968.
4. **Andrews, Roelofs, Schwarts:** Legal, ethical, and medical guidelines for Jehovah's Witnesses in surgery, *Anesth Rev* 5:1052. 1979.
5. **Brener BJ, Raines JK, Darline RC:** Intraoperative autotransfusion in abdominal aortic resections, *Arch Surg* 107:78, 1973.
6. **Blaise G, Jackmuth R:** Preoperative autotransfusion for total hip prostheses, *Acta Anaesth Belgi* 30:175, 1979.
7. **Blundell J:** Experiments on the transfusion of blood by the syringe, *Medico-Chir Trans* 9:56, 1818.
8. **Bodman RI:** Death after anesthetic with hypotension, *Lancet* 11:1085, 1952.
9. **Bodman RI:** Controlled hypotension, *Int Anesth Cltn* 5:90, 1967.
10. **Bond AG:** Conduction anaesthesia, blood pressure and haemorrhage, *Br J Anaesth* 41:942, 1969.
11. **Bourke DL, Smith TC:** Estimating allowable hemodilution, *Anesthesiology* 41:609, 1974.
12. **Bove JR:** Transfusion-associated hepatitis and AIDS: what is the risk? *N Engl J Med* 317:242, 1987.
13. **Cain JL:** Autologous transfusion in elderly total joint replacement patients. A review of blood replacement methods, *J Fla Med Assoc* 66:35, 1979.
14. **Capan LM, Turndorf H, Patel C, et al:** Optimization of arterial oxygenation during one-lung anesthesia, *Anesth Analg* 59:847, 1980.
15. **Chrenow B, Alexander HR, Smallridge RC, et al:** Hormonal responses to graded surgical stress, *Arch Intern Med* 147:1273, 1987.
16. **Cohen, ND, Muñoz A, Reitz B, et al:** Transmission of retroviruses by transfusion of screened blood in patients undergoing cardiac surgery, *N Engl J Med*, 320:1172, 1989.
17. **Cooley DA, Crawford ES, Howell JF, et al:** Open heart surgery in Jehovah's Witnesses, *Am J Cardiol* 13:779,
18. **Cowell HR:** Perioperative red blood-cell transfusion, *J Bone Joint Surg* 71:1, 1989 (editorial).
19. **Cowell HR:** Prior deposit of autologous blood for transfusion, *J Bone Joint Surg* 69:319, 1987 (editorial).
20. **Cowell HR, Swickard JW:** Autotransfusion in children's orthopaedics, *J Bone Joint Surg* 56:908, 1974.
21. **Csencsitz TA, Flynn JC:** Intraoperative blood salvage in spinal deformity surgery in children, *J Fla Med Assoc* 66:39, 1979.
22. **Curran JW, Lawrence DN, Jaffe H, et al:** Acquired immunodeficiency syndrome (AIDS) associated with transfusions, *N Engl J Med* 310:69, 1984.
23. **Davis NJ, Jennings JJ, Harris WH:** Induced hypotensive anesthesia for total hip replacement, *Clin Orthop* 101:93, 1974.
24. **Davison MHA:** Pentamethonium iodide in anaesthesia,

Lancet 1:252, 1950.

25. **Ditzler JW, Eckehoff JE:** Comparison of blood loss and operative time in certain surgical procedures completed with and without controlled hypotension, *Ann Surg* 143:289, 1956.

26. **Dolkart RE:** Medical considerations of orthopaedic surgery in the elderly patient, *J Bone Joint Surg* 47:1041, 1965.

27. **Donald JR:** The effect of anaesthesia, hypotension and epidural analgesia on blood loss in surgery for pelvic floor repair, *Br J Anaesth* 41:155, 1969.

28. **Duncan J:** On re-infusion of blood in primary and other amputations, *Br Med J* 1:192, 1886.

29. **Duncan SE, Klebanoff G, Rogers W:** A clinical experience with intraoperative autotransfusion, *Ann Surg* 180:296, 1974.

30. **Eckardt JJ, Gossett TC, Amstutz HC:** Autologous transfusion and total hip arthroplasty, *Clin Orthop* 132:39, 1978.

31. **Enderby GEH:** Controlled circulation with hypotensive drugs and posture to reduce bleeding in surgery; preliminary results with pentamethonium, *Lancet* 1:1145, 1950.

32. **Enderby GEH:** Pentolinium tartrate in controlled hypotension, *Lancet* 21:1097, 1954.

33. **Enderby GEH:** A report on mortality and morbidity following 9107 hypotensive anaesthetics, *Br J Anaesth* 33:109, 1961.

34. **Evarts CM:** Intraoperative autotransfusion in surgery for scoliosis. A preliminary report. In Proceedings of the Scoliosis Research Society, *J Bone Joint Surg* 56:1764, 1974.

35. **Flynn JC, Csencsitz TA:** Present status of intraoperative blood recovery during orthopaedic surgery, *Jefferson Orthop J* 8:22, 1979.

36. **Flynn JC, Metzger CR, Csencsitz TA:** Intraoperative autotransfusion (IAT) in spinal surgery, *Spine* 7:432, 1982.

37. **Flynn JC, Ray JM, Bierman AH:** Intraoperative autotransfusion. A five-year update of its use (in vivo survival study of processed RBC's during major orthopaedic procedures using IAT), *Orthop Trans* 8:500, 1984.

38. **Flynn JC, Ray JM, Bierman AH:** Erythrocyte survival following intraoperative autotransfusion in spinal surgery. An in vivo comparative study, *Orthop Trans* 9:119, 1985.

39. **Froese AB, Bryan AC:** Effects of anesthesia and paralysis on diaphragmatic mechanics in man, *Anesthesiology* 41:242, 1973.

40. **Gaehtgens P, Benner KU, Schickendantz S:** Effect of hemodilution on blood flow, O_2 consumption, and performance of skeletal muscle during exercise, *Bibl Haematol* 41:54, 1975.

41. **Gardner WJ:** The control of bleeding during operation by induced hypotension, *JAMA* 132:572, 1946.

42. **Gillott A, Thomas JM:** Clinical investigation involving the use of the haemonetic Cell Saver in elective and emergency vascular operations, *Am Surg* 50:609, 1984.

43. **Goldman L, Caldera DL:** Risks of general anesthesia and elective operation in the hypertensive patient, *Anesthesiology* 50:285, 1979.

44. **Goodson WH III, Hunt TK:** Studies of wound healing in experimental diabetes mellitus, *J Surg Res* 22:221, 1977.

45. **Goulet JA, Bray TJ, Timmerman LA, et al:** Intraoperative autologous transfusion in orthopaedic patients, *J Bone Joint Surg* 71:3, 1989.

46. **Grant FC:** Autotransfusion, *Ann Surg* 74:253, 1921.

47. **Gravenstein N:** Anesthesia for joint replacement surgery. In Petty W, editor: *Total joint replacement*, Philadelphia, 1991, WB Saunders.

48. **Hedenstierna G, Löfström J:** Effect of anaesthesia on respiratory function after major lower extremity surgery: a comparison between bupivacaine spinal analgesia with low-dose morphine and general anaesthesia, *Acta Anaesthesiol Scand* 29:55, 1985.

49. **Haugen RK, Hill GE:** A large-scale autologous blood program in a community hospital. A contribution to the community's blood supply, *JAMA* 257:1211, 1987.

50. **Iannacone WM, Heppenstall RB, Steinberg ME, et al:** Intraoperative autologous transfusion in adult orthopaedic surgery of the hip and femur. Poster exhibit at the annual meeting of the American Academy of Orthopaedic Surgeons, New Orleans, Louisiana, 1986.

51. **Jacobs LM, Hsieh JW:** A clinical review of autotransfusion and its role in trauma, *JAMA* 215:3283, 1984.

52. **Jaffe WL, Charnley J:** Bilateral Charnley low-friction arthroplasty as a single operative procedure. A report of fifty cases, *Bull Hosp Joint Dis* 32:198, 1971.

53. **Janecki CJ, DeHaven KE, Benton JW:** Preoperative and postoperative management in total hip reconstruction, *Orthop Clin North Am* 4:523, 1973.

54. **Jurkovich GJ, Moore EE, Medina G:** Autotransfusion in trauma. A pragmatic analysis, *Am J Surg* 148:782, 1984.

55. **Kallos T, Smith TC:** Continuous spinal anesthesia with hypobaric tetracaine for hip surgery in lateral decubitus, *Anesth Analg* 51:766, 1972.

56. **Kafer ER, Isley MR, Hansen T, et al:** Automated acute normovolemic hemodilution reduces blood transfusion requirements for spinal fusion, *Anesth Analg* 65:S76, 1986.

57. **Katz AR, Walker WA, Ross PJ, et al:** Autologous transfusion in obstetrics and gynecology, *Int J Gynecol Obstet* 16:354, 1979.

58. **Khine HH, Naidu R, Cowell H, et al:** A method of blood conservation in Jehovah's Witnesses: in-circulation diversion and refusion, *Anesth Analg* 57:279, 1978.

59. **Kingston HGG, Hirshman CA:** Perioperative management of the patient with asthma, *Anesth Analg* 63:844, 1984.

60. **Klebanoff G:** Early clinical experience with a disposable unit for the intraoperative salvage and reinfusion of blood loss (intraoperative autotransfusion), *Am J Surg* 120:718, 1970.

61. **Koretz RL, Stone O, Mousa M, et al:** Non-A, non-B posttransfusion hepatitis — a decade later, *Gastroenterology* 88:1251, 1985.

62. **Kruger L, Colbert J:** Intraoperative autologous transfusion in children undergoing spinal surgery, *Orthop Trans* 7:571, 1983.

63. **Kruger LM, Colbert JM:** Intraoperative autologous transfusion in children undergoing spinal surgery, *J Pediatr Orthop* 5:330, 1985.

64. **Larson AG:** Deliberate hypotension, *Anesthesiology* 25:682, 1964.

65. **Lehner JT, Van Peteghem PK, Leatherman KD, et al:** Experience with an intraoperative autologous blood recovery system in scoliosis and spinal surgery, *Spine* 6:131, 1981.

66. **Little DM Jr:** Induced hypotension during anesthesia and surgery, *Anesthesiology* 16:320, 1955.

67. **Love TR, Hendren WG, O'Keefe DD, et al:** Transfusion of predonated autologous blood in elective cardiac

surgery, *Ann Thorac Surg* 43:508, 1987.

68. **Madsen RE, Madsen PO:** Influence of anesthesia form on blood loss in transurethral prostatectomy, *Anesth Analg* 46:330, 1967.

69. **Mallory TH:** Hypotensive anesthesia in total hip replacement, *Orthop Rev* 4:21, 1975.

70. **Mallory TH:** Hypotensive anesthesia in total hip replacement, *JAMA* 224:248, 1973.

71. **Mallory TH, Kennedy M:** The use of banked autologous blood in total hip replacement surgery, *Clin Orthop* 117:254, 1976.

72. **Marmor L, Berkus D, Robertson JD, et al:** Banked autologous blood in total hip replacement, *Surg Gynecol Obstet* 145:63, 1977.

73. **McMurray MR, Birnbaum MA, Walter NE:** Intraoperative autologous transfusion primary and revision total hip arthroplasty, *J Arthroplasty* 1:61, 1990.

74. **Menitove JE:** The decreasing risk of transfusion-associated AIDS, *N Engl J Med* 14:966, 1989.

75. **Milles G, Langston H, Dalessandro W:** Experiences with autotransfusions, *Surg Gynecol Obstet* 115:689, 1962.

76. **Modig J, Borg T, Karlström G, et al:** Thromboembolism after total hip replacement: role of epidural and general anesthesia, *Anesth Analg* 62:174, 1983.

77. **Modig J:** Regional anaesthesia and blood loss, *Acta Anaesthesiol Scand* 32(suppl 89):44, 1988.

78. **Moller K, Steady HM, Korten KW, et al:** Blood conservation in revision arthroplasty. In Turner RH, Scheller AD, editors: *Revision total hip arthroplasty*, New York, 1982, Grune & Stratton.

79. **Myhre BA:** Fatalities from blood transfusion, *JAMA* 244:1333, 1980.

80. **Nelson CL, Bowen WS:** Total hip arthroplasty in Jehovah's Witnesses without blood transfusion, *J Bone Joint Surg* 68:350, 1986.

81. **Office of Medical Applications of Research, National Institutes of Health:** Consensus conference. Perioperative red blood cell transfusion, *JAMA* 260:2700, 1988.

82. **Orr MD, Blenke JW:** Autotransfusion of concentrated selected washed red cells from the surgical field: a biomechanical and physiological comparison with homologous cell transfusion. Proceedings of the Blood Conservation Institute, 1978.

83. **Ott DA, Cooley DA:** Cardiovascular surgery in Jehovah's Witnesses. Report of 542 operations without transfusion, *JAMA* 238:1256, 1977.

84. **Ottesen S, Froysaker T:** Use of Haemonetics Cell Saver for autotransfusion in cardiovascular surgery, *Scand J Thorac Cardiovasc Surg* 16:263, 1982.

85. **Peterman TA, Jaffe HW, Feorino PM, et al:** Transfusion-associated acquired immunodeficiency syndrome in the United States, *JAMA* 254:2913, 1985.

86. **Polesky HS:** Autologous transfusion, *Lab Med* 5:37, 1974.

87. **Rao TLK, El-Etr AA, Montoya A:** Hemodynamic changes due to normovolemic anemia in coronary artery disease patients, *Anesthesiology* 51:S164, 1979.

88. **Rao TLK, Jacobs KH, El-Etr AA:** Reinfarction following anesthesia in patients with myocardial infarction, *Anesthesiology* 59:499, 1983.

89. **Scott DL:** Anaesthetic experiences in 1300 major geriatric operations, *Br J Anaesth* 33:354, 1961.

90. **Sculco TP, Ranawat C:** The use of spinal anesthesia for total hip replacement arthroplasty, *J Bone Joint Surg* 57:173, 1975.

91. **Semkiw LB, Schurman DJ, Goodman SB, et al:** Postoperative blood salvage using the Cell Saver after total joint arthroplasty, *J Bone Joint Surg* 71:823, 1989.

92. **Shah KB, Kleinman BS, Rao TLK, et al:** Angina and other risk factors in patients with cardiac disease undergoing noncardiac operations, *Anesth Analg* 70:240, 1990.

93. **Smith PH, Sharp J, Kellgren JH:** Natural history of rheumatoid cervical subluxations, *Ann Rheum Dis* 31:222, 1972.

94. **Stevens CE, Aach RD, Hollinger FB, et al:** Hepatitis B virus antibody in blood donors and the occurrence of non-A, non-B hepatitis in transfusion recipients. An analysis of the transfusion-transmitted viruses study, *Ann Intern Med* 101:733, 1984.

95. **Thomas JD, Callaghan JJ, Savory CG, et al:** Prior deposition of autologous blood in elective orthopaedic surgery, *J Bone Joint Surg* 69:320, 1987.

96. **Thornburn J:** Subarachnoid block and total hip replacement: effect of ephedrine on intraoperative blood loss, *Br J Anaesth* 57:290, 1985.

97. **Toy PT, Strauss RG, Stehling LC, et al:** Predeposited autologous blood for elective surgery. A national multicenter study, *N Engl J Med* 316:517, 1987.

98. **Turner RS:** Autologous blood for surgical autotransfusions, *J Bone Joint Surg* 50:834, 1968.

99. **Turner R, Steady HM:** Cell washing in orthopedic surgery. Presented at the First International Autotransfusion Symposium, 1980.

100. **Twyman R, Kirwan T, Fennelly M:** Blood loss reduced during hip arthroplasty by lumbar plexus block, *J Bone Joint Surg* 72[Br]:770, 1990.

101. **Udelsman R, Ramp J, Galluci WT, et al:** Adaptations during surgical stress. A reevaluation of the role of glucocorticoids, *J Clin Invest* 77:1377, 1986.

102. **Viikari S, Vaalasti T:** Surgery in aged persons, *Ann Chir Gynecol Fenn* 48:19, 1959.

103. **Ward JW, Holmberg SD, Allen JR, et al:** Transmission of human immunodeficiency virus (HIV) by blood transfusion screened as negative for HIV antibody, *N Engl J Med* 318:473, 1988.

104. **Wasman J, Goodnough LT:** Autologous blood donation for elective surgery, *JAMA* 258:3135, 1987.

105. **Wilder RJ, Fishbein RH:** Operative experience with patients over 80 years of age, *Surg Gynecol Obstet* 113:205, 1961.

106. **Wilson WJ:** Intraoperative autologous transfusion in revision total hip arthroplasty, *J Bone Joint Surg* 71:8, 1989.

107. **Wittmann FW:** Blood loss associated with uncemented total hip replacement: hypotension does not affect blood loss, *J R Soc Med* 80:213, 1987.

108. **Wong KC, Webster LR, Coleman SS, et al:** Hemodilution and induced hypotension for insertion of a Harrington rod in a Jehovah's Witness patient, *Clin Orthop* 152:237, 1980.

109. **Woolson ST, Marsh JS, Tanner JB:** Transfusion of previously deposited autologous blood for patients undergoing hip-replacement surgery, *J Bone Joint Surg* 69:325, 1987.

110. **Woolson ST, Watt JM:** Use of autologous blood in total hip replacement: a comprehensive program, *J Bone Joint Surg* 73:76, 1991.

111. **Wulff KE, Aulin I:** The regional lung function in the lateral decubitus position during anesthesia and operation, *Acta Anaesthesiol Scand* 16:195, 1972.

ADDITIONAL READINGS

Brzica SM Jr, Pineda AA, Taswell HF: Autologous blood transfusion, *Mayo Clin Proc* 51:723, 1976.

Bunch WH: Posterior fusion for idiopathic scoliosis. In Instructional Course Lectures, the American Academy of Orthopaedic Surgeons, vol 34, St Louis, 1985, Mosby–Year Book.

Charnley J, Specialization or superspecialization in surgery? *Br Med J* 2:719, 1970.

Charnley J, The organization of a special centre for hip surgery, *Br J Hosp Med* 9:389, 1973.

Chaplin H Jr: Frozen blood, *N Engl J Med* 298:679, 1978.

Fantus B: Therapy of Cook County Hospital: blood preservation, *JAMA* 109:128, 1937.

Jones RB, Propst-Proctor SL, McDougall IR, et al: Erythrocyte survival following intraoperative autotransfusion in orthopaedic surgery, *Orthop Trans* 8:381, 1984.

Kobrinsky NL, Letts RM, Patel LR, et al: 1-Desamino-8-D-Arginine vasopressin (desmopressin) decreases operative blood loss in patients having Harrington rod spinal fusion surgery. A randomized double-blinded controlled trial, *Ann Intern Med* 107:446, 1987.

Kruskall MS, Glazer EE, Leonard SS, et al: Utilization and effectiveness of a hospital autologous preoperative blood donor program, *Transfusion* 26:335, 1986.

National Institutes of Health Consensus Conference: Office of Medical Applications of Research. Perioperative red blood cell transfusion, *JAMA* 260:2700, 1988.

Newman MM, Hamstra R, Block M: Use of banked autologous blood in elective surgery, *JAMA* 218:861, 1971.

North ER, Nelson CL, Lawson NW: Prevention of blood loss in total hip replacement surgery by hypotensive anesthesia and intraoperative autotransfusion, *Surg Forum* 26:517, 1975.

Rab GT, Gorin LJ, Eisele JH: Bilateral total hip arthroplasty in a Jehovah's Witness with chronic anemia, *Clin Orthop* 163:134, 1982.

Steen PA, Tinker JH, Tarhan S: Myocardial reinfarction after anesthesia and surgery, *JAMA* 239:2566, 1978.

Silvergleid AJ: Autologous, directed, and home transfusion programs. In Petz LD, Swisher SN, editors: *Clinical practice of transfusion medicine*, ed 2, New York, 1989, Churchill Livingstone.

Zuck TF: Greetings—a final look back with comments about a policy of a zero-risk blood supply, *Transfusion* 27:447, 1987.

See Chapters 8, Prevention of Infection; 9, Prevention of Thromboembolic Complications; 13, Postoperative Management; 15, Principles Common to all Surgical Approaches; 21, Inflammatory, Metabolic, and Hereditary Bone Disorders; 31, Postoperative Wound Infection; and 37, Trochanteric Osteotomy Complications for additional information.

CHAPTER EIGHT

Prevention of Infection

■ But when the surgeon operates on a previously unbroken integument, he
has the opportunity of preventing the septic particles from entering.
Lord Lister

A HISTORICAL REVIEW

During the nineteenth century, the science of surgery progressed tremendously because anesthesia and aseptic technique were introduced. These innovations also permitted surgery to advance as an art.

The concepts of "clean" and "unclean" have been key to developing surgical awareness of aseptic technique. To prevent surgical infection, operating room personnel must practice aseptic technique with regard to themselves, the patient, the operative instruments, and the architecture of the operating room. Robert Koch popularized the concept that bacteria cause infection, based on earlier work by Cestoni, Delpech, Olivier, Bassi, Ehrenberg, Kirchner, van Leeuwenhoeck, and Henle.* Before Koch developed his postulates regarding development of infections, Louis Pasteur disproved the spontaneous regeneration theory of bacteria with his classic studies on fermentation. Spallanzini had previously done similar studies, but Pasteur's were better publicized and hence had a greater impact on science.[100,247] Pasteur believed that infection resulted when an open wound was contaminated by invisible airborne living organisms that could reproduce the signs and symptoms of infection.[189,247]

Once the theory of spontaneous regeneration of bacteria had been disproved and the bacteriological etiology of exogenous infection accepted, medical science was able to accept the results of clinical studies. Oliver Wendell Holmes in 1842 and Ignaz P. Semmelweiss[258] in 1847 supported the earlier laboratory work with experiments on women in a clinical setting. As they demonstrated, the incidence of puerperal infection could be reduced by using the aseptic techniques of hand and instrument cleansing coupled with intravaginal introduction of chlorinated lime.[200]

Expanding these studies beyond gynecology, August Nelaton used alcohol-soaked dressings on open wounds in 1855, and in 1867, Lord Joseph Lister placed carbolic compresses on open fractures as recommended by Jules Lemaire in 1860. Both Nelaton and Lister[182] reported a decreased incidence of infection.[1,242] In 1870, Lister introduced antiseptic preparation of the skin before elective incision.[258] Lister soon extended the use of carbolic acid to all fields of surgery, calling his new principle the antiseptic discipline. The classic Listerian procedure involved spraying the instruments, the wound, and the surgeon with carbolic acid. In 1866, Lister's methods were supplemented by the introduction of steam sterilization, by Schimmelbusch in Von Bergmann's clinic in Berlin and by Octave Terrillon in Paris.[1,89] Subsequent publications contained descriptions of the practical means to implement these findings by using sterile gowns for the surgeons, sterile drapes for the patient, and masks and gloves for the operating team.[200,242]

Lister's report and the application of aseptic technique produced dramatic clinical benefits. Using aseptic methods, isolation methods, and antimicrobial agents, the surgeon could strengthen the body's natural defenses against bacterial infection. Subsequently, investigators have made extensive attempts to trace the causes of infections occurring in clean surgical operations performed in ultramodern operating rooms. Although listerism abolished fulminating and epidemic hospital sepsis, such as clostridial infections ("hospital gangrene"), infections caused by mildly pathogenic organisms such as staphylococci have remained common.

At present, the literature on wound infection and preventive operating room techniques is voluminous in both general surgical and orthopaedic literature. Pro-

---

* References 78, 149, 189, 210, 219, 247.

gress in bacteriology and the use of antibiosis over the past three decades (since the advent of the use of antibiotics for prevention of infection in surgery) has considerably reduced mortality from postoperative infections. Likewise, in certain operations such as those considered "highly susceptible" to infection, the role played by antibiotics to prevent infection is now well recognized. Continuous changes in bacterial ecology and the increasing incidence of gram-negative organisms not previously considered pathogenic have emerged. Fulminating infections caused by fungi have also appeared, at times resulting in the patient's death.[35,86]

This chapter considers the highlights of studies and their role in preventing sepsis in major reconstructive surgery such as total hip arthroplasty.

BACTERIAL INVASION VS. HOST RESISTANCE

Two groups of factors play a part in the critical "disease-producing dose" of organisms: (1) the number of infecting organisms at the site of the wound, and (2) the virulence of organisms in relation to the host or to a given tissue. This time-honored explanation may be considered from another angle: a given host's ability to deal effectively with a certain number of bacteria within a given space. Burke[54,55] has emphasized that the actual number of organisms within a unit of tissue does not matter; what matters, rather, is the number of organisms that the host's defense mechanisms can effectively deal with during a given period of time. Disease develops when the local concentration of bacteria exceeds the level with which the body can deal. Therefore development of postoperative wound infection depends not only on the number of bacteria that enter the wound during surgery and on the exact physiological state of the patient and the wound itself, but also on the "chance association" of bacteria landing on an area with sufficiently reduced resistance to produce infection. Localized reduction in host resistance is at least as important as bacterial contamination, and it might therefore be suggested that the number of wound infections after surgery would not fall to zero in clinical medicine until bacterial contamination is completely eliminated. Consequently, any efforts aimed at further reducing postoperative infection must concentrate on host responses, while still holding down bacterial contamination and recognizing that almost any bacterium may become pathogenic under certain circumstances.[98] It follows that one no longer can identify a harmless saprophyte merely by its morphological characteristics.

In 1957, Elek and Conen[98] reported that it takes more than a million viable pathogenic staphylococci to produce infection by intradermal injection in human volunteers. However, the infection-causing number

was reduced to 100 viable organisms (a 10,000-fold decrease) when a silk stitch was inserted at the same time.

Charnley's[64] earlier experiences suggested that in total hip arthroplasty the wound could be infected with a far lower dosage of organisms than previously imagined; for example, one infected dust particle may be adequate to produce infection (Fig. 8-1). The massive foreign body introduced as an integral feature of total hip arthroplasty procedure is believed to contribute to the development of postsurgical wound infections.

In addition to the "dose-related" virulence of bacterial infection, failure of the body's defense mechanisms that upsets the bacteria-host equilibrium must be seriously considered as a fundamental factor in producing infection. As a rule, the first line of defense against invading organisms is the "operative condition" of the "portal of entry." Once the organism reaches beyond this point, the body fluid and cells dynamically produce defense mechanisms against the invasion.[114] Among these defenses are the condition of surfaces and cavities, cell type, nature of local secretion, drainage, pH, dryness, and so on. Quantitatively, local defense systems destroy a great proportion of bacteria; the number of viable bacteria reaching the bloodstream is approximately 10,000 times lower than the number that reaches and is controlled at the portal of entry. Possibly the number of organisms destroyed at the site is even greater, since Alexander and co-workers[9] have shown that bacteria may survive and even multiply after phagocytosis within the leukocytes. Wandering macrophages and fixed macrophages of the reticuloendothelial system penetrate the defense system and act where leukocytes have failed. Any bacteria not eliminated at this point will enter the lymph nodes and bloodstream, but macrophages in the spleen (or Kupffer's cells) may eliminate them from blood circulation. During the battle between the invading organisms and cellular response, the host's humoral defense system is activated. This is the final and most decisive element in controlling the invading organisms.[7]

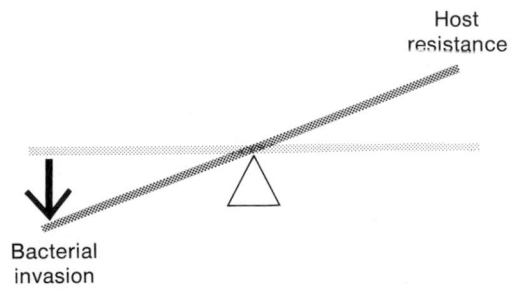

Fig. 8-1. Clinical infection is imminent when host resistance is too weak to repel bacterial invasion. Loss of balance in favor of invading organism is shown.

SURGICAL TREATMENT BY MASSIVE IMPLANTATIONS

Experiments such as those by Elek and Conen[98] classically demonstrate a causal relationship between foreign materials in the surgical wound, added risk, and greater extent of infection. Contamination of the surgical wound sites by only a few bacteria is sufficient to produce infection in an experimental model (that is, a rabbit). It is considerably more difficult to induce infection if the operation does not include a prosthetic implant.[261] Edlich and co-workers have unequivocally documented the role of percutaneous sutures in causing infection.[90] It has been shown that taping skin (rather than suturing) reduces the wound infection rate in experimental animals.[73] It is of special interest that not only the presence of foreign material but also certain of its physical characteristics[8,100,183] reduce the level of host response in experimental wound infection studies.

Early experiences with implanting artificial joints proved that these surgical conditions are particularly favorable to infection, as evidenced by a high incidence of infection in the developmental era of total joint arthroplasty. Charnley and Eftekhar,[64] Wilson and co-workers,[291] Amstutz,[15] and others reported a high incidence of wound infection when they exercised no extra precautions in the ordinary operating room environment. These surgeons had not experienced a comparable increase when dealing with ordinary operations.

The effect of polymethylmethacrylate (PMMA) on phagocytosis of white blood cells was discussed in Chapter 5.

Although it has been recognized that the large mass of foreign body implanted during total hip arthroplasty predisposes the patient to infection, PMMA seems to be an especially sensitive facilitator of infection. Infection in cemented implants has certain characteristics not found in infections of noncemented implants: (1) infection inevitably is diagnosed, even if it takes months or years to appear, (2) infection appears radiologically as "osteitis," and (3) PMMA especially attracts mildly pathogenic organisms (previously known as nonpathogens), for example, *Staphylococcus epidermidis*.

TERMINOLOGY OF SEPSIS

Conventionally, operative wounds are classified as clean, clean contaminated, and dirty, depending on the extent to which intrinsic or extrinsic bacteria enter the wound. In this regard, a total hip arthroplasty is considered a clean (or ultraclean) operation, an appendectomy is a clean-contaminated procedure, and a mutilating, grossly contaminated barnyard accident is a dirty wound.

It may be impossible to determine the true incidence of infection in surgery because there is no standard definition of infection. For example, positive cultures may be obtained from wounds that heal primarily without drainage; likewise, heat, redness, and swelling may be present in a postoperative wound, even with some purulent exudate from which no organism can be cultured. Therefore a workable definition of wound infection applicable to the clinical situation is one that partly disregards the bacteriology but greatly emphasizes the clinical situation:[94,238] (1) *uninfected wound*—heals primarily without drainage, (2) *definitely infected wound*—discharge pus, although culture may be negative, and (3) *possibly infected wound*—inflamed but without drainage or a positive culture (may show nonpurulent drainage).

Confusion has arisen in the past over the statement that an organism must be a pathogen to cause disease, and nonpathogens or saprophytic organisms are merely contaminants. One commonly finds the term *contaminants* in bacteriological reports. Confusion has also arisen about defining infection according to the organism found in the wound. This problem is compounded by use of the term *virulence*, as measured by the number of organisms required to kill members of a particular animal species under standardized conditions in a definite period of time. Since the so-called nonpathogenic organisms have not been incriminated and yet are frequently seen in the wounds, surgeons have often discussed the question of rejection of the plastics without infection. This author has concluded that rejection of or sensitivity to the acrylic cement must be exceedingly rare and that an infected wound without a positive culture from the wound is not related to the cement reaction but rather to a failure of "bacteriological methods" to identify the organism. Many so-called nonpathogenic organisms appear in an infected total hip arthroplasty; in the future, surgeons may require vast knowledge to deal with these organisms. They are usually of low virulence and often are difficult to culture by routine bacteriological methods.

One study of 85 infected total hip arthroplasties determined that 33 were caused by *Staphylococcus aureus*, 4 by *Staphylococcus albus*, 1 by *Pseudomonas* organisms, 6 by *Proteus* bacilli, and 5 by coliform bacilli.[62] As indicated, *S. aureus* coagulase-positive remains the most common offending organism in infected total hip arthroplasties. *S. aureus* also is responsible for both early and late infection. In 18% of early cases the wound has been "sterile" despite the presence of clinical infection.[62,65] Infections produced by coliform bacilli (12%) usually occurred in the early group; in late infections, however, 41% of the infections were caused by a sinus or organisms of low pathogenic nature. These factors are important to consider in planning antibiotic prophylaxis in total hip arthroplasty.

SOURCES OF SURGICAL INFECTION AND PROPHYLAXIS

Because of the numerous factors that contribute to infections, surgeons must consider methods of prophylaxis and treatment separately, choosing different means based on the different etiological factors. Only by understanding all the factors contributing to surgical infections can the surgeon intelligently choose the appropriate means of prophylaxis[94] (Figs. 8-2 and 8-3).

The Patient's Sources

The surgeon must give equal consideration to patient-related factors and those related to the environment. One cannot deny that total arthroplasty involving massive implantation of a foreign body into a 65-year-old woman with rheumatoid disease, severe debility, and previous steroid therapy carries a much higher risk for surgical sepsis than an appendectomy on an otherwise healthy 12-year-old girl. Without adequate statistical proof, authors have suggested that old age, obesity, and diabetes favor infection in general surgical experiences.[202,238]

A poor state of nutrition and previous steroid therapy are important factors to consider. So too are alternate sources of infection such as skin, urinary tract, and pulmonary lesions. The surgeon should attempt to isolate the organisms from the joints of patients who have previous evidence of infection, repeated aspiration, or injections with corticosteroids.

Experimentally, Krizek and Davis have shown that wound infections can result from infections elsewhere in the body[161] (Fig. 8-4). Although this is not a common cause of postsurgical wound infection, the surgeon should keep the possibility in mind.

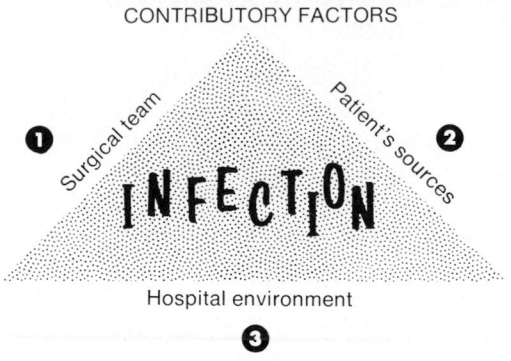

Fig. 8-3. All factors that contribute to surgical infection—surgical team, patient's own sources, and hospital environment—must be considered to find a means of prophylaxis.

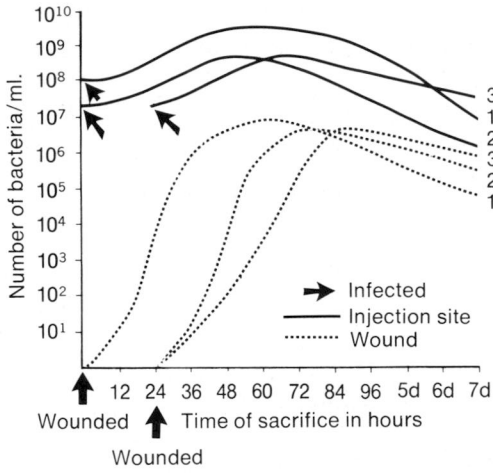

Fig. 8-4. Wounds may become infected from infection elsewhere. Quantitative distribution of staphylococci after subcutaneous injection with wounding of animal: (1) simultaneous wounding with injection, (2) 24 hours after injection animal was wounded, and (3) 24 hours after wounded animal was injected. (From Krizek TJ, David JH: Endogenous wound infection, *J Trauma* 6:239, 1966.)

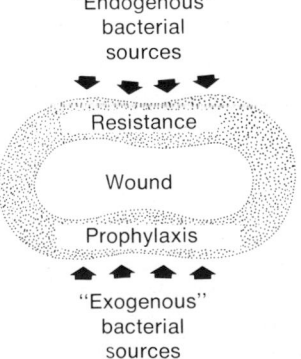

Fig. 8-2. In multifactorial sources of infection, both endogenous and exogenous sources of bacteria must be considered. By increasing local resistance of tissue and prophylactic measures, wounds may be protected from those bacterial sources.

Patients can bring bacteria to the operating room. For example, the bacterial content of psoriatic lesions can be high and varied. Other lesions include draining sores, pilonidal cysts, and infected Bartholin's cysts. Sinuses remote from the site of surgical incision can disperse organisms into the air that can subsequently seed into the wound. It is mandatory therefore that the surgeon treat all skin lesions, including psoriatic, before surgery.

A genitourinary consultation is at times essential; a symptomatic prostate gland should be evaluated preoperatively. Because many patients require postoperative catheterization, prophylactic urinary antibiotics may be indicated in patients with a previous history of urinary tract infection. Urinary tract infection can be one of the most significant sources of infection before and after total hip arthroplasty.[17,144] Postoperative urinary retention must be treated by in-dwelling catheterization performed by trained personnel adequately instructed in aseptic techniques. Suppressive antibiotic therapy has been recommended. The patient's fluid intake has to be maintained at a high level, and when the catheter is removed, cultures and sensitivities should be obtained; if any evidence of active urinary tract infection is found, the operation must be postponed, and appropriate antibiotics should be administered.

Theoretically, chronic obstructive pulmonary disease may be a source of infection. In practice, however, it is not easy to identify the active stage of a chronic lung disease; if any evidence of exacerbation of chronic pulmonary disease exists, surgery must be postponed until the pulmonary state has been fully evaluated. General surgical experiences have suggested that hospitalized patients become colonized with antibiotic-resistant staphylococci.[259]

Studies have also linked an increased staphylococcal infection rate to a lengthy preoperative stay[259] and have shown that the increase is proportional to the length of the stay.[290] Although a lengthy preoperative stay is not common in total hip arthroplasty surgery, it is required for certain patients, such as the elderly and those with debilitating soft-tissue atrophy, rheumatoid arthritis, and diabetes. Such patients have a complex range of susceptibilities predisposing them to infection. It should be noted that transferring a rheumatoid arthritic patient from a medical ward for surgery undoubtedly carries the added risk outlined above.

Previous Hip Surgery and Remote Infection

The incidence of infection is higher after revision surgery than in primary operations, despite conscientious efforts to detect infection; this increase may indicate a high percentage of preexisting infection at the time of revision. All previous wounds must be considered infected unless proven otherwise. Particularly suspect are wounds with an implant. Procedures that require revision may have failed because of undetected infection in the initial procedure. Before total hip arthroplasty the surgeon must evaluate the hip for the presence or history of previous infection. A high rate of positive cultures and an increased rate of sepsis in revision surgery confirm the possibility of preexisting infection in most failed procedures. Several diagnostic measures are used to detect infection: white

blood cell count, erythrocyte sedimentation rate, appearance of infection on radiographs, radionuclide studies, gross appearance of infection at surgery, a smear (made at surgery), and, finally, cellular morphology at operation[96] (see Chapter 4).

For reliable bacterial identification, all antibiotics are discontinued before a revision surgery. Multiple tissue biopsies with four, five, or more specimens are obtained. Each specimen is taken with a separate, sterile forceps not previously used during the operation. Cultures must be taken immediately to the bacteriology laboratory, where they are processed for cultures of aerobic and anaerobic bacteria. Meticulous care reduces to a very low level the number of so-called sterile infections (infections from which no organisms are cultured) (see Chapter 31).

Metastatic (Hematogenous) Source

Although the risk of transient bacteremia leading to metastatic (hematogenous) infection remains unknown, it has been well established that hematogenous seeding of bacteria from a distant primary source can lead to clinical infection in joint arthroplasty.[40] Such seeding is rare but can occur at any time after a clean operative procedure (early or late). While various protective measures (such as routine use of perioperative antibiotics) have reduced the incidence of early seeding, frequent reports seem to indicate that late hematogenous seeding of the joint prosthesis is increasing. At least three clinical modes exist: (1) A healthy patient with a prior successful total hip arthroplasty develops a febrile episode after which the total hip arthroplasty becomes symptomatic because of infection. The source of infection remains unknown. (2) A healthy patient's hip arthroplasty becomes symptomatic because of concurrent infection elsewhere in the body; the same organism is recovered from the hip and is the source of the presenting infection. (3) Hematogenous infection can be documented easily in host-compromised individuals, that is, patients with debilitating rheumatoid arthritis or patients receiving immunosuppressive drugs. To determine the risk of hematogenous infection in total joint arthroplasty surgery, Ainscow and Denham studied 1000 patients with 1112 arthroplasties for an average follow up of 6 years. They identified only three cases of hematogenous infection, all thought to be related to infected skin lesions producing chronic bacteremia. Interestingly, 284 of these patients underwent other surgical procedures in a variety of sites, such as abdominal, orthopaedic, and gynecological; 284 also developed urinary tract, respiratory tract, and other focal infections; none of these patients, however, developed hematogenous infection.[5] These observations suggest that transient bacteremia is not likely to infect total joint prostheses in otherwise healthy individuals.

Proper documentation is necessary to prove unequivocally that an infected hip was seeded hematogenously by a remote source. The infective organism in the joint must be the same as in the primary site; the clinical history must also be appropriate.[4,19] Often such a route is suggested "after the fact," when either a remote source of infection is discovered or an unusual organism is recovered from the joint and the source. Except when unusual organisms appear, this author considers it important to be able to document accurately that the same organism has been cultured from the primary source, the blood, and the joint arthroplasty. Because common organisms must be identified by their phage typing, the most sensitive and accurate method of identifying common strains of staphylococci, it is often difficult to prove that organisms at the joint are the same as those at the primary source. Because this method is expensive and cumbersome, it is not performed routinely on all specimens. A less precise but acceptable way to document hematogenous infection is by detecting similar antibiotic sensitivity patterns in the bacteria recovered from both the hip and the source. Although this method does not provide absolute proof, it offers the next best alternative. Only appropriate cultures for both aerobic and anerobic organisms and expert handling of certain obscure organisms reveals the correct type of organism. For instance, in the author's experience, *Aeromonas hydrophila* and *Peptostreptococcus* have been difficult to isolate, unless the laboratory uses special techniques.

Obviously, the primary focus of infection predates the infection developed in the joint arthroplasty; thus it remains obscure. The bacteremia stage that precedes joint pain also goes unnoticed. Only a retrospective search for the focus of infection may document whether the same offending organism has caused both the primary site infection and the secondary (that of the joint arthroplasty). Many instances of hematogenous infections have not been properly documented, possibly because the history regarding the port of entry is inadequate or because the surgeon is uninterested or unaware. Additionally, although skin is the most common site for the primary source of hematogenous infection, it can be difficult to document minor skin lesions or the presence of cellulitis.

Sources and Types of Organisms in Hematogenous Infection

A vast variety of species has been reported in hematogenous infections of implants. In a review of the literature, Bigliani[40] noted that gram-positive organisms were four times more common than gram-

Table 8-1 Organisms Isolated in 40 Hematogenous Infections

Organism	Type	Number
Staphylococcus aureus	(+)	20
Staphylococcus epidermidis	(+)	2
Streptococcus group A	(+)	6
Streptococcus group G	(+)	1
Pneumococcus	(+)	3
Escherichia coli	(−)	2
Proteus mirabilis	(−)	2
Salmonella typhimurium	(−)	1
Bacteroides fragilis	(−)	1
Aeromonas hydrophila	(−)	1
Pasteurella multocida	(−)	1

From Bigliani LU, Stinchfield FE: Hematogenous infection of total joint replacement. In Eftekhar NS, editor: *Infection in joint replacement surgery, prevention and management*, St Louis, 1984, Mosby–Year Book.

Altered flora of hospitalized patients

ORAL-RESPIRATORY
Enteric bacilli: *Klebsiella, Escherichia coli, Pseudomonas*
Staphylococcus aureus
Candida species

URINARY TRACT IF CATHETERIZED
Enteric bacilli of more antibiotic-resistant types: *Enterobacter, Serratia, Pseudomonas*

From Bigliani LU, Stinchfield FE: Hematogenous infection of total joint replacement. In Eftekhar NS, editor: *Infection in joint replacement surgery, prevention and management*, St Louis, 1984, Mosby–Year Book.

---

negative organisms (Table 8-1). Many organisms in hematogenous infections of the hip joint are common to the human bacterial flora. The box presents the more prevalent flora of the human body. Enteric bacilli are commonly detected, including those in the oral and respiratory cavities (*Klebsiella, Escherichia coli, Pseudomonas, S. aureus, Candida* species) and those in the urinary tract, all of which resist antibiotics: (*Enterobacter, Serratia, Pseudomonas*). Unusual organisms this author has encountered include *Pasteurella multocida, Aeromonas hydrophila,* and *Peptostreptococcus*. Others have reported finding *Bacteroides fragilis* (anaerobic gram-negative bacillus), *Propionibacterum acnes,** *Pasteurella multocida,* and *Aeromonas hydrophila* (the last two are both gram-negative bacilli), especially in

*References 4, 62, 153, 154a, 167, 264, 294.

Table 8-2 Primary Sites of 45 Hematogenous Infections

Site	Number
Skin	15
Urinary tract	9
Throat and respiratory tract	9
Teeth	7
Gastrointestinal tract	3
Parotid gland	1
Ear	1

From Bigliani LU, Stinchfield FE. Hematogenous infection of total joint replacement. In Eftekhar NS, editor: *Infection in joint replacement surgery, prevention and management*, St Louis, 1984, Mosby–Year Book.

immune-compromised individuals. These organisms are extremely unusual but are well known to produce infection from a distant source in total hip arthroplasties.*

Bigliani and Stinchfield noted that the skin is the most common primary site of hematogenous infection, followed by the urinary tract, throat, and respiratory tract. They collected information concerning the origin of the infecting organism in 45 of the 55 reported cases (Table 8-2). Although skin obviously is subjected to repeated trauma and infection, it seems to be too frequently overlooked as a possible source of infection in patients with joint arthroplasty surgery. Patients with dystrophic ulcers caused by venous insufficiency or diabetes need special attention when planning antibiotic prophylaxis. It seems logical to postpone surgery until skin lesions are completely healed. Simply using antibiotics is not sufficient to prevent infection in these patients. Similarly, the surgeon should not consider joint arthroplasty and skin grafting as a combined procedure in these patients.

Patients scheduled for total hip arthroplasty are often elderly and undergo frequent dental manipulation and periodontal work, leading to gum inflammation or infection. Studies have shown an incidence of transient bacteremia as high as 40%. However, only a few bonafide cases of hematogenous seeding caused by dental manipulation have been reported in total hip arthroplasty patients.[40,66,267] Although there is no controlled study available on the subject, the risks of infection are so serious that this author urges antibiotic prophylaxis during danger periods of dental manipulation, such as when inflammation and abscess are present; others consider it unnecessary.[5,137,146]

Distant infections such as in the urinary tract,[118,243] upper respiratory tract,[1,33,73] and the foot,[40,74,115,221] are commonly considered to be potential sources of metastatic infection. Some experts in the field of infection recommend prophylaxis against seeding of organisms in total hip arthroplasty.

Postoperative wound discharge also seems to be a risk factor for infection; Surin and co-workers[268] found that a large number of infected arthroplasties were associated with an early discharge, even if the wound had completely healed by the time the patient left the hospital.

Not surprisingly, a nationwide survey of 1600 orthopaedic surgeons indicated that fewer than half (41%) believed that any relationship existed between the joint infection and a remote source of infection (such as dental manipulation). Nevertheless, 93% of the surgeons responding to the questionnaire recommended antibiotic prophylaxis against infection of the joint arthroplasty. On the choice of antibiotics, 73% recommended first-generation cephalosporins. However, for dental manipulation and prophylaxis against implant infection, a recent editorial recommended penicillin V as the antibiotic of choice and erythromycin as an alternative drug for patients who are allergic to penicillin.[217]

Lowered Resistance to Infection

Earlier in this chapter we advanced the idea that implantation of the foreign body in total hip arthroplasty may lower resistance to infection, making patients who have this procedure especially vulnerable to infection. Evidently, the situation may be further exacerbated if a patient has a lowered systemic resistance to infection caused by diabetes[245] or steroid therapy for rheumatoid arthritis. Several studies, including one multicenter study,[202] identified high-risk groups for total hip and total knee arthroplasty. Rheumatoid patients were found to be at 2.6 times greater risk than those with osteoarthritis; total hip arthroplasty revision patients were at 8 times greater risk than patients undergoing primary surgery.[110]

After seeding of an organism that normally is no threat, rapid dissemination can occur in a compromised host. Such seeding in patients with bacterial endocarditis or with artificial heart valves is a well-known phenomenon.[35,55,68] A compromised host usually is unable to respond even against infection produced by common organisms indigenous to the normal body flora. In one study of 48 patients who developed hematogenous infections of their total hip arthroplasty, 23 had a diagnosis of rheumatoid arthritis[2,65,238]; others have found that the infection rate is also increased in diabetic patients after total joint arthroplasty.[293] Other factors known to lower the host's resistance to infection are such conditions as leukemia and Hodgkin's disease. The use of radiation, antiembolites, alkylating agents, steroids, and immunosup-

*References 104, 129, 156, 224, 264, 273.

pressives are commonly known risk factors in lowering the host's resistance to infection. The effect of surgery, reduced vascularity of bone, and the presence of a massive foreign body also provide ideal circumstances for seeding and colonization of bacteria from other sources.

According to Geddes and Davey,[117] infections at the early stages of immunosuppression are caused by well-recognized and common organisms, such as *E. coli* and *S. aureus*. However, late in treatment, when immunosuppressive drugs are used, rare opportunistic species are common.

Lowered local and systemic resistance may be responsible when patients develop infection from mildly pathogenic organisms or unusual species not commonly colonized in a clean surgical wound; in such patients these pathogens may cause infection in total hip arthroplasty. Several unusual organisms have been cultured in association with deep infection in total hip arthroplasty: *Mycobacterium tuberculosis,** *Candida parapsilosis,*[207] *Peptostreptococcus magnus,*[42] *Propionibacterium acnes,*[41,142] *Mycobacterium fortuitum,*[43,135] *Pasteurella multocida,*[121] *Actinomyces israelii,*[266] miscellaneous anerobic organisms,[128] and others. Therefore early and aggressive treatment is a rational discipline to prevent the spread of these minor infections in patients who develop them. Massive allograft implantations are known to be associated with a high incidence of postoperative infection. Only 30% of infected cases had no predisposition to infection; two thirds had undergone prior extensive surgery, multiple operations, or concomitant chemotherapy, x-ray studies, or both in addition to implantation of massive allografts. Although gram-positive microbes were the most common cause of infection, six patients had gram-negative organisms and nine had mixed organisms in their infections.

Biomaterials

Biomaterials play a major role in the development of infection because of the way the body responds to their chemical and physical characteristics. For example, in-vitro tests of the macrophagic activity of white blood cells have shown that PMMA inhibits phagocytosis of *Candida albicans*. Leak and associates[172] have demonstrated that macrophages become spherical as they come in contact with PMMA in the presence of glass, stainless steel, and Vitallium. They spread out, a feature that is essential to the normal function of the macrophages in combating infection. These investigators suggest that this difference may explain why macrophagic activity is reduced in the presence of PMMA but not these other materials.[172]

Several studies have documented the influence of surgical implants in producing infection. Implants made of stainless steel, cobalt-chromium alloys, HDP, polymerized PMMA, and in-vivo polymerized PMMA were compared with a control (no implant) using *S. epidermidis, S. aureus,* and *E. coli*. All the implants and in-vivo polymerized PMMA were significantly more likely to be associated with infection than the controls with no implant. This association was especially strong for *S. epidermidis* and *E. coli*. The phagocytic action against strains of *S. epidermidis, S. aureus,* and *E. coli* in particular was compromised in the presence of PMMA concentrations as low as 0.156% (Figs. 8-5 and 8-6.) These studies suggest that surgeons must make a particularly great effort to reduce bacterial contamination during implant surgery using acrylic cement.*

The Operating Room and Surgical Environment
Conventional Operating Rooms: Surface Contamination vs. Wound Colonization

Most species of bacteria isolated from infected total hip arthroplasties are of low pathogenic nature and are generated by people present during the surgery, including the patient. Although prophylactic antibiotics reduce the rate of such infections, the antibiotics are ineffective against "gut" organisms. By isolating strains of *S. aureus* from nasal swabs (from patients and operating room staff) and by phage typing and antibiotic sensitivity studies, Lidwell and co-workers found carriers to be the source for 7 of 14 infections and possibly for another 5. They concluded that very small numbers of staphylococci could initiate infection in total joint arthroplasty.[179]

There is some doubt that bacteria are ever freely suspended in the air; it is generally accepted that they are airborne on particles of dust or on desquamating epithelium shed from the skin. The airborne particles most likely to contaminate a wound are those that are heavy enough to settle in less than 1 hour; these particles are usually over 10 μm in size and frequently carry clusters of organisms. Particles as small as 1 μm (the size of bacterial spores) remain suspended in the air for a long time and are less likely to seed a wound in large numbers and cause infection.[14,92,95]

The cost of installing and maintaining an air filtration unit for an operating room therefore can be minimized without sacrificing efficiency simply by filtering air for particles no smaller than 1 μm.[60,62,91,92] Some particles that carry bacteria are generated during the operation. Infected dust particles are principally epithelial scales shed from the skin of personnel; they come from body areas such as the perineum, exposed

---

* References 25, 76, 133, 148, 196.

* References 228, 229, 230, 231, 232.

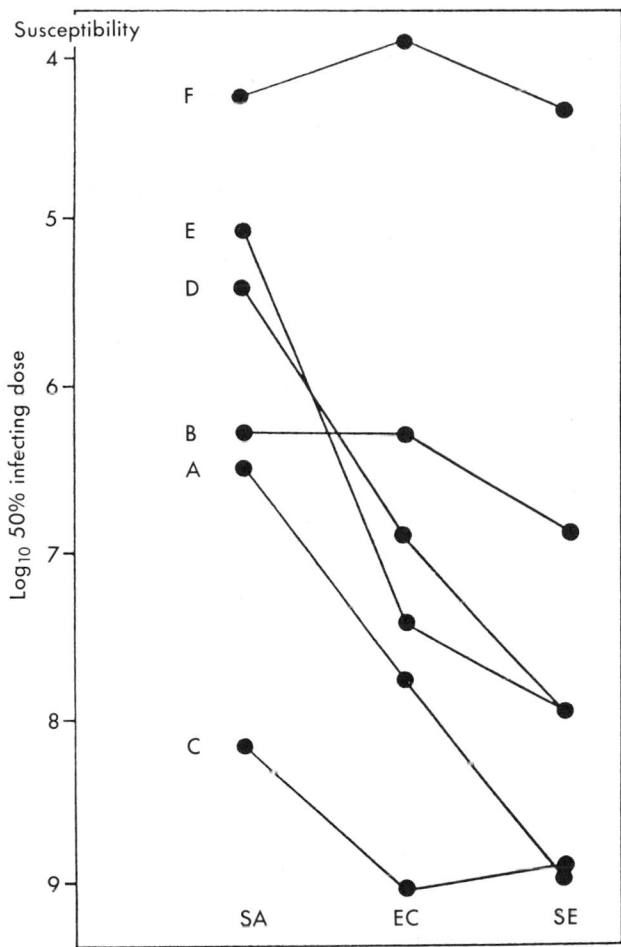

Fig. 8-5. Enhanced susceptibility to bacterial infection associated with an implant. The vertical scale shows the size of the bacterial inoculum ($\log_{10}$ units), which resulted in infection in 50% of the implants in dog femurs. The three vertical rows correspond to infection with SA, *Staphylococcus aureus*; EC, *Escherichia coli*; SE, *Staphylococcus epidermidis*. The lowest group on the figure, *C*, gives the results without any implant. *A, B, D*, and *E* correspond to uncemented implants of cobalt-chromium alloy, machined fully PMMA, stainless steel, and polyethylene, respectively. The uppermost values, *F*, are for an implant cemented with methylmethacry-late cement. The numerical values shown are log means for each group deduced from the data of Petty and associates.[234] (From Lidwell OM: Air, antibiotics, and sepsis in replacement joints, *J Hosp Infection* 11[suppl C]:18, 1988.)

parts of the body such as the face, or, a very obvious source, the nasopharynx (Fig. 8-7). Obviously, conventional ventilation systems do not control the infected dust particles generated in the operating room. The greater the number of persons in the operating room, the greater the emission rate of infected particles. To dilute the concentration of infected dust particles, the volume of filtered air entering the room should be commensurate with the number of persons and the total rate of particle emission.

The surgical environment includes gowns, masks, and gloves, as well as the surgical facilities, including the structure of the operating room and its ventilation system. Air contamination in the operating room can be substantially reduced by prohibiting ward clothes and bedding from entering the room and by preventing unnecessary movements of the staff.[87,92,237,238]

A small proportion of S. *aureus* carriers have been identified as "dispersers," or "spreaders," who may be particularly dangerous on a surgical team if the organisms they shed are highly virulent. Unfortunately, the method of detecting dispersers is too complicated for routine use. Moreover, since "carrier" and "disperser" functions are not consistent and since frequent tests would be necessary to find all dispersers in the team, it is not always possible to prevent sporadic

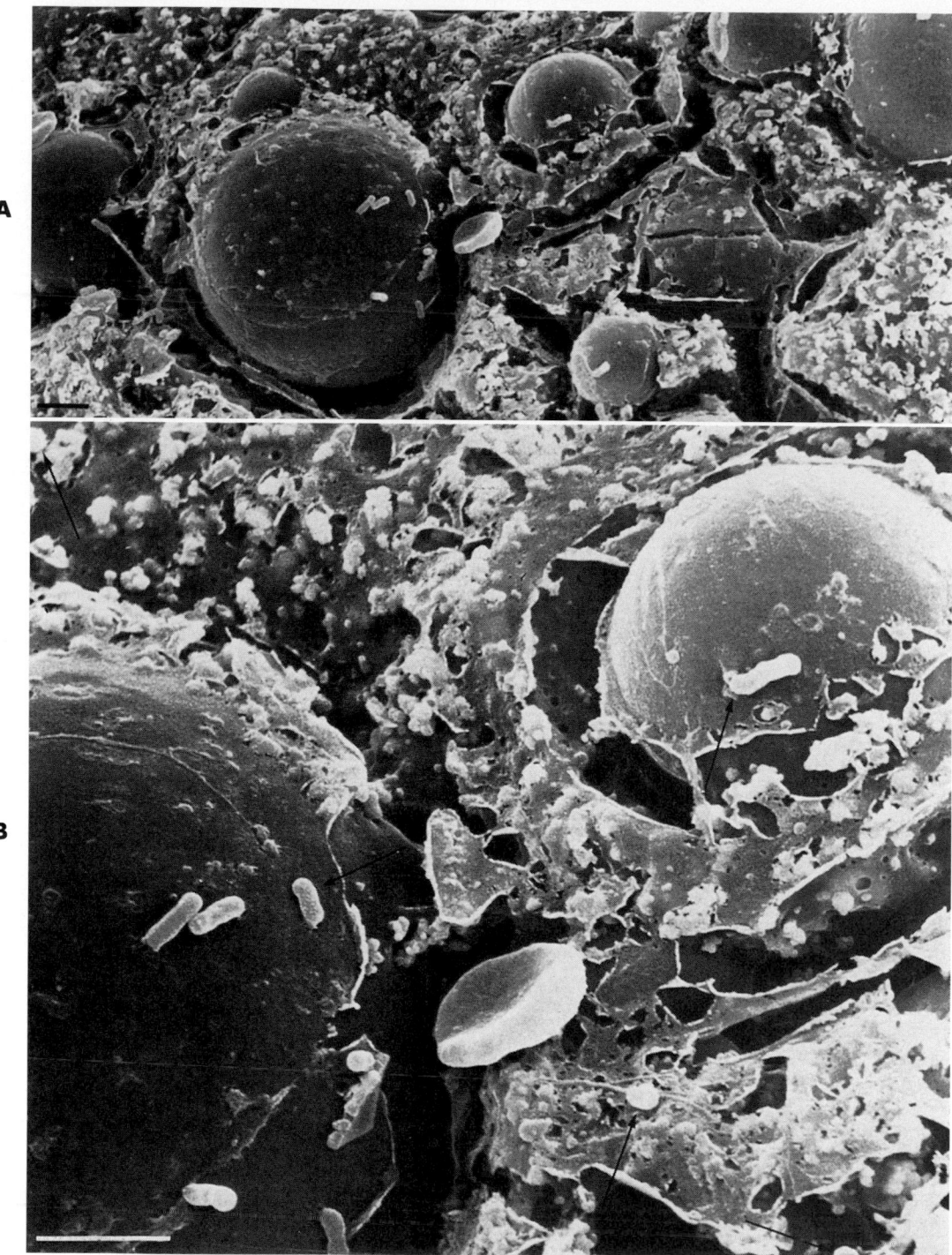

Fig. 8-6. A, Scanning electron micrograph of the intramedullary methylmethacrylate from an infected and loosened total hip joint, showing the surface of the biomaterial to be partly occluded by an extensive biofilm that shows shrinkage damage caused by dehydration in preparation for scanning electron microscopy. Bar = 5 μm. **B,** Higher magnification of the control area of **A,** showing the presence of rod-shaped bacterial cells *(arrows)* in association with and often partly buried in the extensive biofilm on the surface of this biomaterial. *Pseudomonas aeruginosa* was isolated from this specimen. Bar = 5 μm.

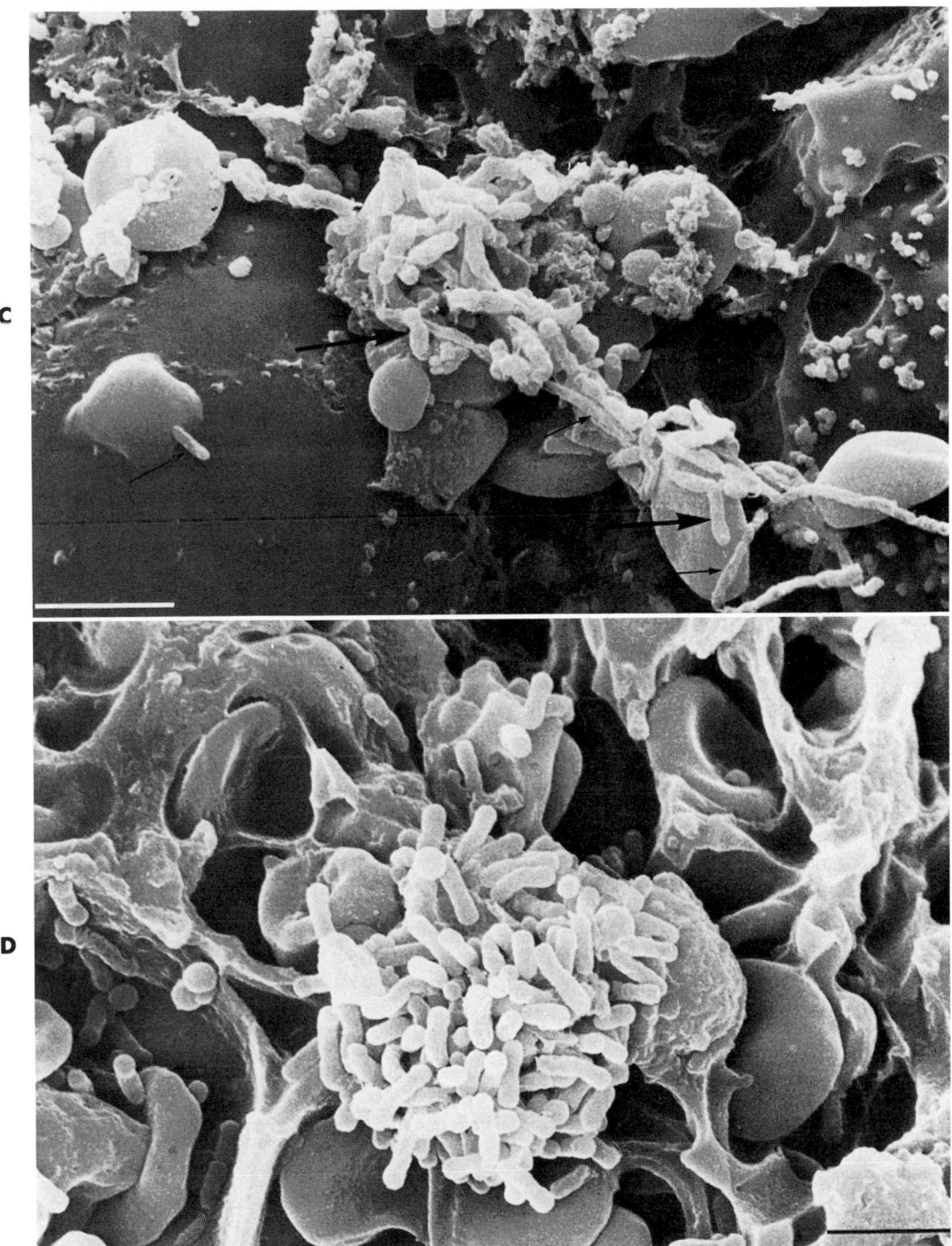

Fig. 8-6—cont'd. C, Scanning electron micrograph of rare areas of the intramedullary methylmethacrylate surface where the biofilm was incompletely formed and individual adherent bacterial microcolonies could be discerned. This microcolony is composed of two bacterial morphotypes: cells 0.5 μm in width *(small arrows)* and cells 1.0 μm in width *(large arrows)* that are partly embedded in the amorphous dehydrated residue of their exopolysaccharides. Bar = 5 μm. **D,** Scanning electron micrograph of the surface of bone from the infected total hip joint, showing the development of discrete adherent microcolonies in which bacteria of a single morphotype (1.0 μm in width) are partly surrounded by amorphous condensed material. Bar = 5 μm. (From Gristina AG, Costerton JW: Bacterial adherence to biomaterials and tissue, *J Bone Joint Surg* 67:264, 1985.)

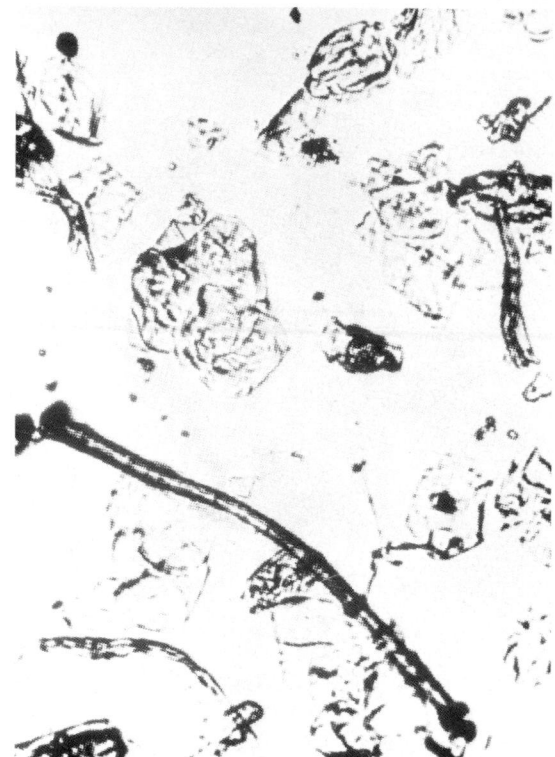

Fig. 8-7. Shape and size of most particles found in conventional operating rooms. The most frequent and dangerous particles are those shed from personnel within the operating room, which at times may contain viable organisms.

Table 8-3 Microorganisms Associated with Wound Colonization

Organism	Number of procedures in which organism was isolated
Staphylococcus epidermidis	129
Streptococcus viridans group	44
Corynebacterium sp.	37
Staphylococcus aureus	7
Group D streptococci	4
Bacillus sp.	5
Micrococcus sp.	1
Propionibacterium acnes	77
Peptococcus magnus	5
Bacteroides melaninogenicus	2
Clostridium ramosum	1
Flavobacterium sp.	5
Acinetobacter calcoaceticus	6
Neisseria sp.	3
Alcaligenes sp.	2
Escherichia coli	2
Enterobacter cloacae	1
Proteus mirabilis	1
Aspergillus sp.	26
Penicillium sp.	12
Cladosporium sp.	4
Neurospora sp.	1
Alternaria sp.	1
Streptomyces sp.	1
Rhodotorula sp.	1

From Fitzgerald RH Jr, Peterson LFA: Wound colonization and deep wound sepsis. In Eftekhar NS, editor: *Infection in joint replacement surgery, prevention and management*, St Louis, 1984, Mosby–Year Book.

dispersers from entering the operating room environment. Reducing the number of people in the room, however, reduces the odds. Thus, when a clean air room and isolation are not used, the surgical team must be kept as small as possible, and no one whose presence is not essential should be admitted to the operating room.

The microorganisms associated with wound colonization (Table 8-3) are predominantly the same organisms found on the skin and in the infected postoperative total hip arthroplasty wound. They include *S. epidermidis*, *S. aureus*, members of the *Streptococcus viridans* group, and other miscellaneous organisms. A highly significant direct correlation between the presence of wound colonization and the development of deep-wound sepsis has been reported.

Conventional (standard) operating rooms are those not modified to produce a unidirectional airflow; also, they commonly have a low air-exchange rate of 25 to 30 times per hour. In contrast, a clean-air operating room has a positive-pressure zone of unidirectional airflow that generates an exchange rate of 300 to 400 times per hour, as well as a highly efficient filtration of 2 μm or less.

Operating rooms with a lower rate of exchange per minute have a higher level of airborne bacterial contamination.[106] These rooms are cleanest when empty (early morning), so this author recommends that surgery be scheduled as early as possible in the day (Fig. 8-8).

CLEAN-AIR OPERATING ROOMS

Transforming a conventional operating room into a clean-air room requires more subtle planning than simply installing a high-quality ventilation system based on conventional methods. Doubling or tripling the rate of air exchange or installing air filters that remove all particles of any size is not sufficient; those changes raise the cost but do not prevent airborne contamination of an open wound.

Within an operating "enclosure" it is possible to bacteriologically isolate personnel who are in direct contact with the open wound without inhibiting their communication with others in the room (Fig. 8-9). In an enclosure, clean air can be admitted at a rate that

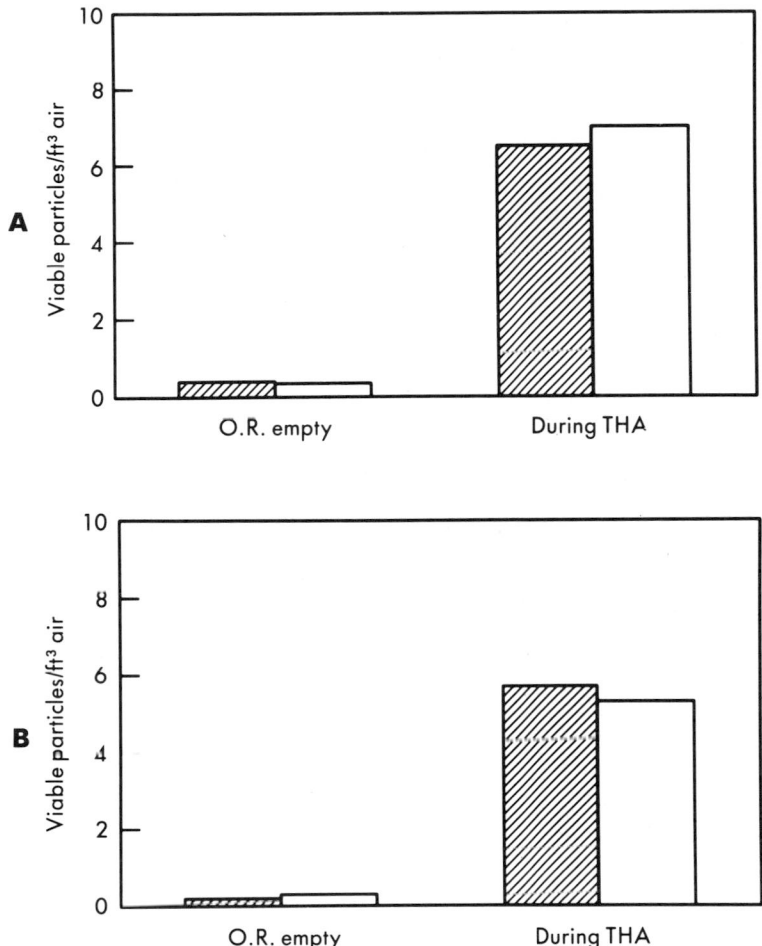

Fig. 8-8. Comparison of airborne bacterial contamination in two conventional operating rooms. **A,** Operating rooms with low rates of room-air exchange (12 to 14 times per hour) evaluated when room was not in use and during total hip arthroplasty. Data are mean numbers of viable particles per cubic foot obtained with a Casella air sampler during 16 procedures in each room. **B,** Operating rooms with high rates of room-air exchange (28 to 32 times per hour) evaluated when room was not in use and during total hip arthroplasty. Data are mean numbers of viable particles per cubic foot obtained with a Casella air sampler during 20 separate procedures in each room. (From Fitzgerald RR Jr, Peterson FA: Wound colonization and deep wound sepsis. In Eftekhar NS, editor: *Infection in joint replacement surgery,* St Louis, 1984, Mosby–Year Book.)

produces a positive movement of air in a predetermined direction (laminar airflow), but the ideal in laminar-flow ventilation is difficult to achieve in practice. The major obstacle is turbulence, which occurs when air strikes stationary objects; the higher the flow, the greater the turbulence. A very fast airflow may also cause other problems, including inordinate cooling of wounds from evaporation; anesthetized patients must be protected from hypothermia by using warming blankets or other measures. Because of these practical problems, it has been suggested that clean air should be admitted to the enclosure at the lowest rate needed to produce a positive movement of air strong enough to prevent air from rising toward the ceiling by thermal convection.

After developing a prototype for a clean-air enclosure, Charnley[60] proposed a permanent installation made of glass, approximately 7 × 7 feet, with a ceiling height of 10 feet. Clean air enters the enclosure through High Efficiency Particulate Air (HEPA) filters from an opening in the ceiling; HEPA filters, also known as absolute filters, are 99.97% effective. The bottom edges of the enclosure rest on metal feet, leaving a space for air to escape to the surrounding room at the floor level. The vertical edges of the glass plate forming the enclosure are separated by gaps of ⅛ inch to facilitate escape of used air and to abolish dead air space in corners. He considered an enclosure measured 7 × 7 feet to be the smallest space needed to perform hip joint surgery conveniently (see Fig.

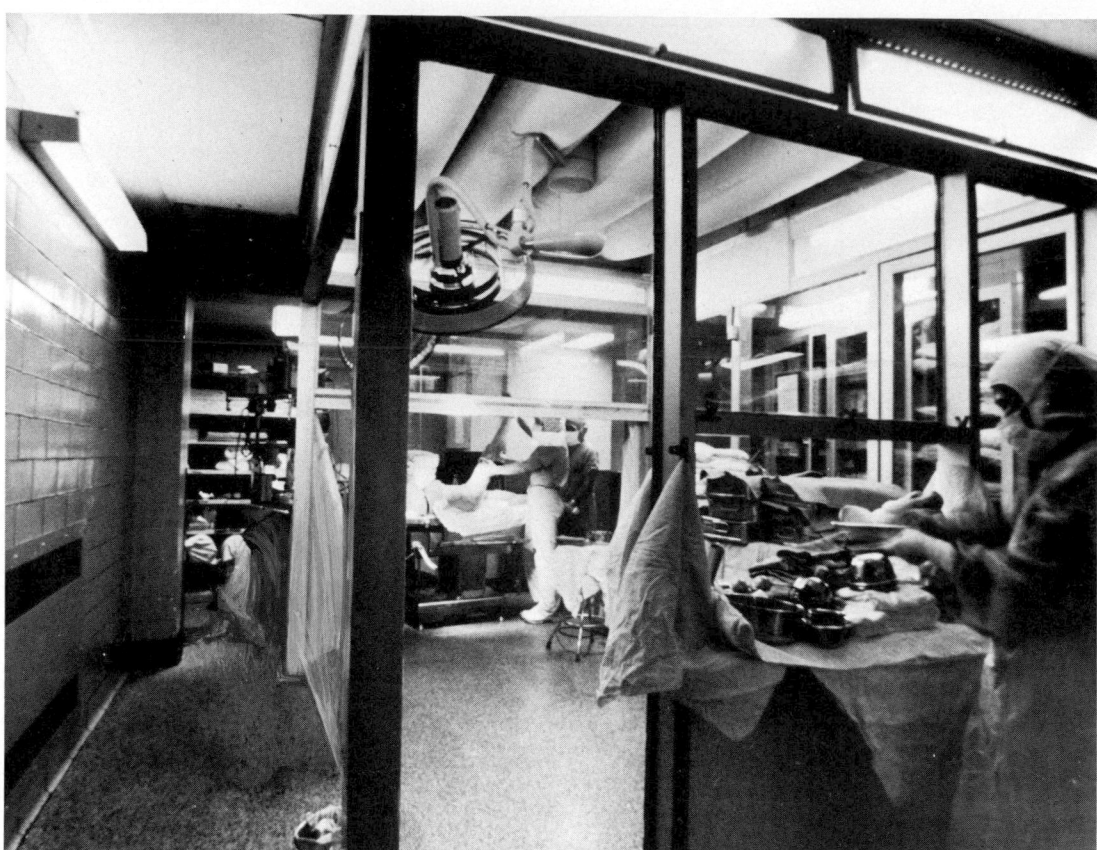

Fig. 8-9. Vertical flow enclosure within standard operating room. NOTE: post filter cloth tubes suspended from ceiling and special light to produce minimal obstruction of airflow. In background, induction room is shown where patient is anesthetized and prepared for surgery before entry to enclosure. (Operating room K at Presbyterian Hospital, Columbia Presbyterian Medical Center, New York, N.Y.)

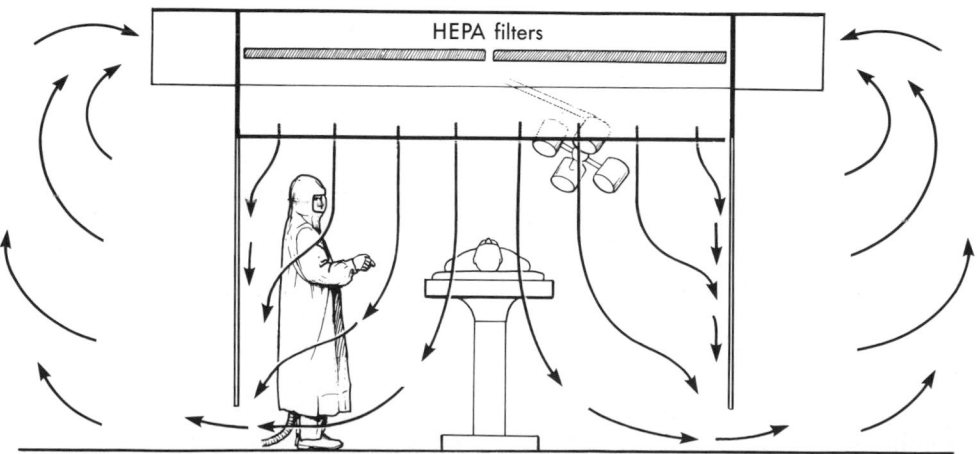

Fig. 8-10. Schematic of the function of a clean air enclosure illustrating the pattern of air circulation in a vertical laminar (unidirectional) airflow room. Note that air movement does not remain truly laminar—it is reflected by hitting objects but remains unidirectional. The air spills under the opening of the glass walls and is recirculated through the HEPA filters.

8-9). However, if the size of the operating room allows, a larger enclosure might be preferable; it would accommodate a larger surgical team or additional equipment for total hip arthroplasty and could also be used for other procedures. Vertical unidirectional "wall-less" enclosures are attractive for their versatility, permitting universal application and the possibility of using portable walls (Figs. 8-10 to 8-13).

To create positive pressure inside the enclosure that

forces air out through its open service hatch at the foot of the enclosure, the entrance is covered by sterile curtains, and the vertical air speed is increased to a maximum. Surgical instruments needed for each operation are planned carefully before surgery and divided into separate trays that are prewrapped and autoclaved inside cloth bags; when needed the contents are inserted through the service hatch of the enclosure.

Clearly, the effectiveness of a unidirectional air

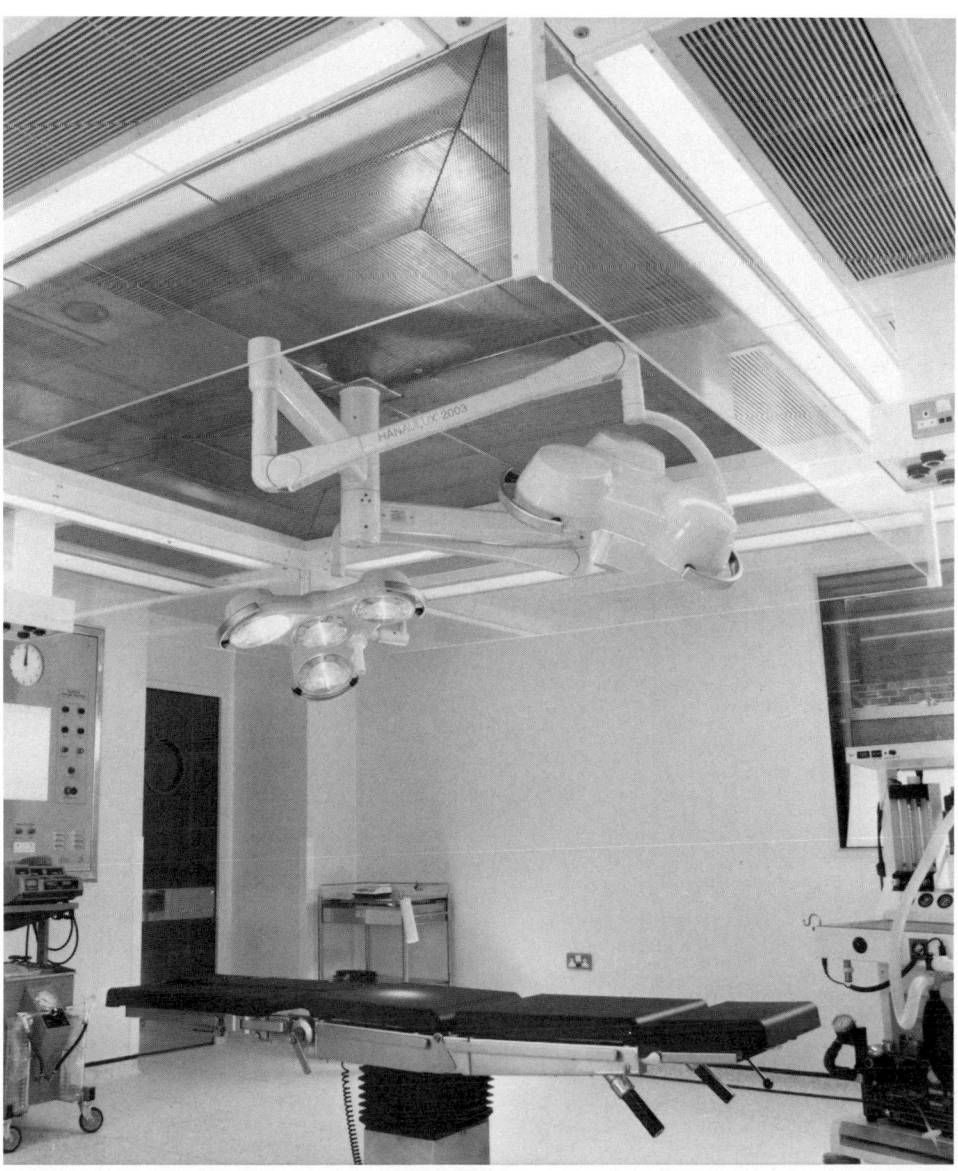

Fig. 8-11. A wall-less vertical laminar airflow room. Note the glass canopy, which directs the air flow maximally to the site of operating table. Cluster lights are desirable with this system because they do not obstruct the air movements or create severe turbulence. (Courtesy Howorth Air Engineering, Bolton, England.)

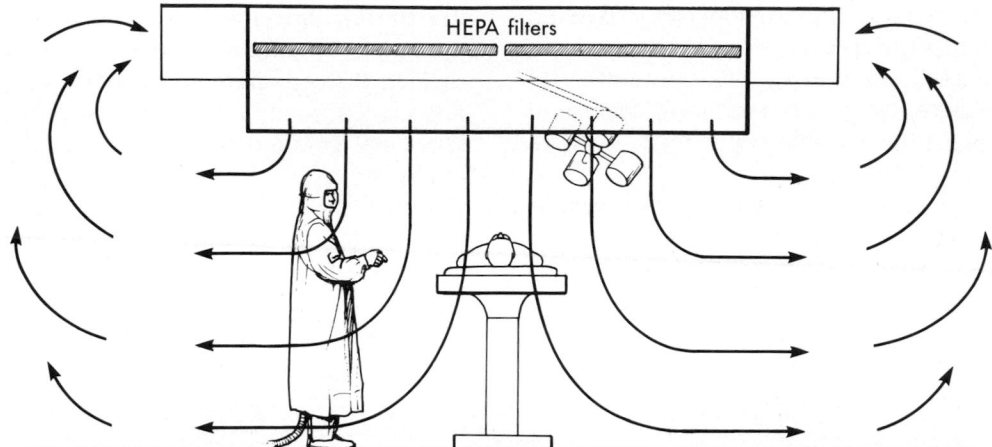

Fig. 8-12. Airflow pattern in a wall-less clean air room. While the air exchange in the room is less frequent than in clean air rooms with an enclosure, the air exchange is still effective because of the large size of the operating room. However, personnel traffic is not controlled as well in rooms without an enclosure (see Figs. 8-9, 8-10, and 8-16).

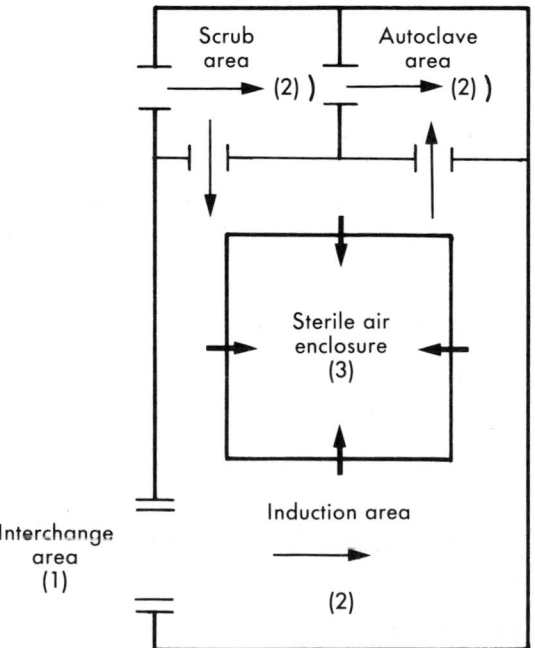

Fig. 8-13. Traffic flow within surgical suite. *1,* Interchange area open to operating room personnel; *2,* restricted area to which only properly attired personnel are admitted; and *3,* sterile work area of vertical laminar airflow (clean-air enclosure) occupied by surgical team. (From Ayer M, Stone R, Eftekhar NS: Operating room asepsis and sterilization techniques. In Eftekhar NS: *Infection in joint replacement surgery,* St Louis, 1984, Mosby–Year Book.)

conditioning system — and the amount of air conditioning needed for a given situation — depends not only on the amount of air entering the enclosure, but also on the number of bacteria-laden particles generated by personnel within the room. Studies have shown that a person may shed from 100,000 to 30,000,000 particles per minute and from 3000 to 5000 microorganisms per minute, depending on the activity level and how effectively clothing contains the shedding particles.* By attacking airborne bacteria directly (listerian concept) and sterilizing equipment, one study reduced wound infection to 1.9% in an uncomplicated operation (such as herniorrhaphy).[235] While this rate of infection might be satisfactory to some surgeons performing herniorrhaphy, it is totally unacceptable to surgeons performing total hip arthroplasty. This author considers it imperative to prevent all bacteria from entering the wound. In conventional operating rooms, airborne bacteria are still a large part of the inoculum of open wounds. In such rooms, 30,000 to 60,000 organisms per hour may sediment into the 3- × 4-mm sterile field of a major operation.[260]

EXTREME AIR FILTRATION AND WOUND INFECTION

It is of historical interest that in 1930 the United States Chemical Warfare Service consigned refinements of earlier models of air filters to be used in masks designed to protect against newer types of chemical and biological warfare. During the early 1950s, the Atomic Energy Commission further refined these filters to make them effective in ridding air of radioactive submicrometer particles[22,283]; their results led to the development of HEPA filters.

The principle of laminar airflow was proposed by Whitfield in 1962 and subsequently used by the National Aeronautics and Space Administration to protect microelectronics and spacecraft components.[103,282,283] Turner has summarized the development and evaluated the clinical results of clean-air laminar-airflow rooms used during surgery. The prototype laminar-airflow room has been in use at Batta Memorial Hospital, Albuquerque, New Mexico, since January 1966.[271]

After extensive bacteriological study of air-sampling techniques and colony counts on settle plates, several investigators have demonstrated the effect of clean-air systems on the bacterial content of air in the surgical enclosure and associated degrees of wound contamination.†

In 1964, Charnley[60,61,65] pioneered the modern concept of surgical environmental control after a continuous surveillance of case studies at Wrightington Hip Centre and studies designed to correlate air cleanliness with infection rates. To control the environment, he devised an insulator "enclosure," which kept the air separate from the environment within the main part of the operating room. Only members of the surgical team were allowed within this enclosure; the anesthetist and other personnel were excluded from the vicinity of the wound. The surgical instruments were presented following a preprogrammed pattern; they were not exposed to the external air in the operating room. Air exhaled by members of the surgical team was drawn away by a suction system fitted inside ordinary masks.[61] Early results indicated that use of this improved operating room reduced infection.

In 1969, a controlled study confirmed the favorable outcomes resulting from the improved air cleanliness that the enclosure provided.[65] It also provided a unique set of data for investigation: (1) The degree of air contamination was controlled and recorded. (2) One operation was repeatedly performed by a team of surgeons following the same protocol throughout. (3) Most of the patients were in good health and in their sixties and seventies. (4) No prophylactic antibiotics were used throughout the study. (5) Last, and perhaps most important, the entire environment could be controlled, including traffic and other variables that undoubtedly were not controlled in other studies.

DILEMMA OF STATISTICS AND THEIR INTERPRETATION

The effectiveness of clean air or antibiotics in preventing infection in total hip surgery has been an extremely controversial issue in recent years.* No significant data indicate that one method of prophylaxis is superior to another. (The emotionalism of surgeons advocating either method often compounds the controversy.) Reasoning is based on several criteria:

1. The multifactorial nature of infection.
2. Definition of clinical infection and clean air in the operating room.
3. Inadequate statistical interpretation of results.
4. Development of late wound infections.
5. Use of antibiotics for prophylaxis in combination with clean-air rooms.
6. Introduction of protective measures in the operating room such as the body exhaust system, special masks, and gowns.

The debate is further exacerbated by the lack of information on the true incidence of infection after

---

* References 8, 22, 70, 77, 83, 112, 212, 218, 239.

†References 3, 15, 16, 47, 49, 50, 68, 69, 107, 108, 113, 122, 123, 125, 141, 143, 192, 197, 210, 225, 241, 244, 245, 252, 256, 257, 284, 285, 286, 288.

---

* References 115, 162, 163, 164, 165.

total hip arthroplasty in general practice in a conventional operating room.

Perhaps the greatest difficulty in judging the efficacy of antibiotics versus clean air lies in how the statistics are evaluated, the size of the sample, and the lack of conformity in defining "wound infection." (This last problem is further confounded because infections may not present until years after surgery.) According to Lidwell and others[178] and Lindbom and Laurell,[180] to demonstrate a significant reduction in the infection rate (from 3% to 1.5%), a study would have to follow 800 operations in a control group and 800 operations in an experimental group. To prove the significance of one factor for a rate below 1.5%, a sample of 5000 operations of precisely the same type is essential. As a practical demonstration, a series of 1750 operations grouped in blocks of 100 was studied. The rate of infection in these blocks varied from 0% (ninth block) to 6% (third block).[65] No obvious reasons could explain these differences. It is therefore imperative to ignore statistics from studies with fewer than 5000 samples to track an infection rate of less than 3%.

Late Appearance of Infection

Interpretation of the infection rate in total hip arthroplasty is made especially difficult by the high incidence of late-occurring infection appearing months or even years after surgery. Of the five infections that appeared in the first 1500 total hip arthroplasties at the New York Orthopaedic Hospital, one manifested itself in less than 3 months, another in 14 months, and a third at 18 months; the remaining two infections appeared 4 years after implantation of the prosthesis. Because of late-appearing infection, figures from this institutional sample could not be validated until several years later.[62,65]

To determine the effectiveness of ultraclean-air rooms and antibiotics three independent studies are considered.

Study I: Multicenter Study, The Hip Society

A multicenter retrospective study of the report by the members of The Hip Society was presented by this author at the second open scientific meeting of The Hip Society.[93]

To identify the scope of the infection problem and document it statistically, this author distributed a questionnaire to members of The Hip Society requesting the following information:

1. Number of total hip procedures performed.
2. Number of operations with a minimum of 1-year follow up.
3. Respective rate of infection.
4. Use of systemic or local antibiotics.

5. Opinions on the necessity of a clean-air room in total hip arthroplasty procedures.

To summarize, these cooperative statistical data, based on the experience of 17 major training institutions and 21,903 total hip arthroplasties, were inconclusive in proving the advantages of clean air over antibiotics or vice versa. However, they do indicate a low infection rate when both were used. Eight of the 17 institutions used a special clean-air room and 9 did not; 14 used systemic antibiotics and 3 did not; 11 used local antibiotic irrigations and 6 did not; 9 believed a special clean-air room was essential and 8 believed it was not.

It is apparent that with the advent of total hip arthroplasty, orthopaedic surgeons have become more aware of the relationship between environmental control and wound infection. This study indicated that those using a clean-air room and prophylactic antibiotics had the lowest rate of infection.

If the figures of the six institutions that had performed more than 1000 total hip arthroplasties can be taken as evidence, the infection rate was lower than 1% at 1 year after surgery; perhaps it would not have been more than 4% if a longer follow-up study had been done. There was no difference in the infection rate between users and nonusers of clean-air rooms; all nonusers, however, routinely used systemic and local antibiotics. The significance of this fact in relation to late-appearing infections could not be determined from available data. The size of the sample is the most significant factor in interpreting the incidence of wound infection—keeping in mind that only 40% to 50% of the total number of infections appeared within a year.[62,65,93]

The view expressed on the questionnaire by members of The Hip Society led to the conclusion that the clean-air room was considered a "rational discipline"—and "essential" if the surgeon did not use prophylactic antibiotics. This is especially true in the institutions in which it is difficult to control traffic in the operating room, especially in teaching hospitals. The respondents thought, however, that further clinical investigation would be necessary to prove the absolute necessity of a clean-air room and of the use of local or systemic prophylactic antibiotics alone. In this study, although the beneficial effects of clean-air rooms and antibiotics were demonstrated, the role played by each in lowering the infection rate could not be documented independently.

Study II: Report of the Medical Research Council of Great Britain: A Prospective (Randomized) Study

In view of the continuing controversy over the beneficial effect of clean-air operating rooms, especially in connection with major joint arthroplasty surgery, the Infection Committee of the Medical Research Council recommended a controlled study of clean-air rooms in Great Britain. OM Lidwell, EJL Lowbury, W Whyte, R Blowere, SJ Stanley, and D Lowe reported the result of this multicenter prospective study, which appeared in the *British Medical Journal* in 1982.[174] In this multicenter study, operations were randomized between control and ultraclean-air operating rooms. The results relate to over 8000 operations and were conducted by 19 participating hospitals over a period of 3 years. Although a strictly controlled study of the use of prophylactic antibiotics was not included, the use of these agents during the operations was recorded as a "variable."

To establish the difference between an infection rate of 2% in the control series and 1% in clean-air rooms at the 95% confidence level, it was estimated that 2500 operations would be needed in each series.[174] Further, it was considered that if, in addition to the ultraclean-air groups, the study included one group that used body exhaust for every group that did not use it, 7500 operations would be required. The reader is referred to recent publications by Lidwell and associates[174] for the details of the plan and conduct of the investigation.

In this study, bacterial counts were recorded at the operative site using a slit sampler or Sartorius gelatin filters. The level of bacterial contamination varied from hospital to hospital; the results are shown in Tables 8-4 and 8-5. The operating facilities for this study included conventional (turbulent air), Allander system, horizontal-airflow rooms, vertical-airflow rooms without walls, vertical-airflow rooms with walls,

and a Trexler isolator (Table 8-4). In over 3000 operations, wound wash samples were collected during the operations in 16 hospitals included in the study. A correlation of the various ventilation systems with bacterial contamination is shown in Table 8-4.

The study clearly demonstrated that the incidence of infections after total joint arthroplasty was dramatically reduced at a high confidence level after the use of the ultraclean-air rooms. Deep wound infection developed after 63 out of 4133 operations in the control group (1.5%) and in 23 out of 3922 operations in the ultraclean-air groups (0.6%; this is a ratio of 2.6%, 95% confidence at 1.6% to 4.2%, P less than 0.001%). Table 8-5 demonstrates the relationship of the operating room condition to the rate of infection of the control series with ultraclean-air series.

In this study, the use of prophylactic antibiotics was associated with a lower incidence of sepsis than that in patients who had not received prophylactic antibiotics. The evaluation of the influence of prophylactic antibiotics on postoperative wound infection is summarized in Table 8-6.

To summarize the evaluation of the British study conducted by Lidwell and associates, their results are strong evidence that use of ultraclean-air rooms during total joint arthroplasty surgery reduced postoperative wound infection involving an implant. Use of a whole-body exhaust suit increased protection against infection (as reflected by the statistics). This study produced evidence that the airborne route of surgical infection may be controlled by the use of clean-air operating rooms.

Although this study was not set up to evaluate the effect of prophylactic antibiotics in preventing infection, the data suggested that prophylactic antibiotics produced a substantial benefit. About four times as many cases of postoperative sepsis occurred in patients who had not received prophylactic antibiotics as in those who had received them. These data suggested that ultraclean air and antibiotic prophylaxis had an independent but cumulative effect in preventing postoperative joint infection. Ultraclean air led to a twofold reduction in infection, and antibiotic prophylaxis led to a fourfold reduction, so the combined use of the clean-air room and antibiotics produced an eightfold reduction in the infection rate.

From this valuable contribution (published in the *British Medical Journal*, vol. 285) it emerges with great clarity that the standard environment of the operating theatre is unacceptable without some additional protection against infection.[168]

Study III: Salvati's Report on Airflow and Infection

In 1982, Salvati investigated the effect of a horizontal laminar airflow ventilation system on the infection

Table 8-4 Air Contamination in Relation to Ventilation and Clothing

Ventilation system	Median number of bacteria-carrying particles m³ (number of hospitals) for operations performed with:	
	Conventional-pattern clothing	Body-exhaust suits
Conventional (turbulent)	164 (15)*	51 (1)*
Allander	49 (3)*	14 (3)†
Horizontal flow	22 (3)†	1 (1)†
Downflow without walls	10 (3)†	—
Downflow with walls	2 (4)†	0.4 (6)†
Trexler isolator	0.5 (3)†	

From Lidwell OM: Effect of ultra-clean air in operating rooms on deep sepsis in the joint after total hip or knee replacement: a randomised study, *Br Med J* 285:10, 1982.
*Values from operating rooms regarded as controls.
†Values with ultraclean-air systems.

Table 8-5 Sepsis in Relation to Operating Room Conditions

Hospital group (number of hospitals)	Conditions in ultraclean-air series	Air contamination	Control series		Ultraclean-air series		Ratio‡ control: ultraclean	P (95% confidence limits)
			Number of operations*	Number (%) septic	Number of operations*	Number (%) septic †		
1 (n = 6)	Conventional-pattern clothing	Low	1252	28 (2.2)	1058	11 (1.0)	2.2	<0.05
2a (n = 3)	Body-exhaust suits	Very low	832	6 (1.0)	954	1 (0.1)	6.9	<0.05
2b (n = 3)	Trexler isolator	Very low	411	9 (2.2)	338	3 (0.9)	2.5	0.2–0.1
2a + 2b (n = 6)		Very low	1243	15 (1.2)	1292	4 (0.3)	3.9	<0.01
3 (n = 4)	Conventional-pattern clothing	Low	1392	19 (1.4)	546	5 (0.9)	1.5	0.5–0.3
	Body-exhaust suits	Very low			841	2 (0.2)	5.7	<0.01
4 (n = 3)	Body-exhaust suits	Moderately low	246	1	185	1	–	–
1 + 3 (n = 10)	Conventional-pattern clothing	Low	2644	47 (2.0)§	1604	16 (1.0)	2.0	<0.02 (1.1–3.6)
2 + 3 (n = 10)	Body-exhaust suits or isolator	Very low	2635	34 (1.3)§	2133	6 (0.3)	4.5	<0.001 (1.8–11.0)
All groups (n = 19)		Very low	4133	63 (1.5)	3922	23 (0.6)	2.6	<0.001 (1.6–4.2)

From Lidwell OM: Effect of ultra-clean air in operating rooms on deep sepsis in the joint after total hip or knee replacement: a randomised study, *Br Med J* 285:10, 1982.
*For insertion of prosthesis.
†Sepsis (category 3) confirmed after reoperation on joint.
‡Sepsis rate in control series/sepsis rate in ultraclean-air series.
§Weighted for contribution made to comparison by the two groups.

Table 8-6 Influence of Prophylactic Antibiotics on Sepsis

Operating conditions	Without antibiotics		With antibiotics		Ration without:with antibiotics	P (95% confidence limits)
	Number of operations*	Number (%) septic†	Number of operations*	Number (%) septic†		
Control	1161	39 (3.4)	2968	24 (0.8)	4.2	<0.001
Ultraclean:						
Low	516	8 (1.6)	1279	9 (0.7)	2.2	0.1
Very low	544	5 (0.9)	1584	1 (0.06)	14.5	0.001
All ultraclean	1060	13 (1.2)	2863	10 (0.3)	3.5	<0.01
All groups	2221	52 (2.3)	5831	34 (0.6)	4.0	<0.001 (2.6-6.2)
Selected hospitals‡	1049	33 (3.2)	1129	14 (1.2)	2.5	<0.01 (1.4-4.8)

From Lidwell OM: Effect of ultra-clean air in operating rooms on deep sepsis in the joint after total hip or knee replacement: a randomised study, *Br Med J* 285:10, 1982.
*For insertion of prosthesis.
†Sepsis (category 3) confirmed after reoperation on joint.
‡Five hospitals at which prophylactic antibiotics given to between 38% and 58% of patients. Note the data on antibiotics were not obtained on a fully controlled comparison as were those in Tables 8-4 and 8-5.

rate of 3175 single-stage total hip and knee arthroplasties.[250] He found that the infection rate after total hip arthroplasty dropped from 1.4% to 0.9%. However, at the same time and using the same ventilation system, the infection rate in total knee arthroplasties rose from 1.4% to 3.9%. The differences were statistically significant in both groups; Salvati attributed the discrepancy to the position of the patient and operating team in relation to the airflow, hypothesizing that a horizontal airflow was beneficial when used correctly but had an adverse effect when the theory of unidirectional airflow systems was not observed during the surgical procedure.

QUALITATIVE BACTERIOLOGY VS. WOUND SEPSIS

Commonly, the types of organisms found in the total hip arthroplasty wound when the procedure is conducted in conventional operating rooms are similar to those generated by the operating team and personnel within the vicinity of the wound. In 273 of 320 tissues submitted for culture during total hip arthroplasty, Nelson found a single isolate; he recovered two isolates from 36 specimens, and three from 11 specimens. S. epidermidis is most commonly found. S. aureus and gram-negative bacilli are recovered infrequently (Table 8-7). In his studies, Nelson isolated gram-positive organisms from settle plates from the wound 81.7% to 95.1% of the time. He observed a striking similarity in the frequency of S. epidermidis isolates, closely followed by diphtheroids, in the air of the operating room, on sterile surfaces, and in the wound.[215] A small, persistent number of S. aureus and gram-negative organisms have been reported, affecting intraoperative

contamination significantly (see Table 8-7). The bacteriology of infected total hips shows that most infections are caused by organisms similar to those found in the operating room environment.

Until recently, much controversy and at times confusion existed regarding the relationship of positive wound cultures and the actual wound sepsis rate. There is a saying that all wounds are contaminated at the end of a procedure, but only a few become infected. This argument is often offered to excuse the surgeon's ineffectiveness in preventing ultraclean operations from becoming contaminated. Several important studies now point to a contrary view, that the presence of wound colonization is directly correlated with the development of wound sepsis. Fitzgerald found that 6% of wounds with positive cultures isolated from tissue specimens obtained at surgery developed deep wound infection, while only 0.6% of wounds with sterile tissue cultures became infected. The difference was significant (P value less than 0.001).[106]

Nelson summarized data relating the degree of airborne contamination using a regular operating room and an ultraclean-air room with and without personnel isolators.[215] He observed a progressive reduction in airborne bacterial contamination with the use of clean air and personnel isolators. Similarly, he reported a definite reduction in surface contamination when he introduced the clean-air room and improved barrier techniques (Tables 8-8 to 8-10).

SURGICAL SUITE AND PERSONNEL

For purposes of aseptic technique, the surgical suite may be located on any hospital floor; however, to ease handling of emergency cases, it is best to quarter the

Table 8-7 Comparative Airborne, Wound, and Deep Infection Bacteriology

Organism	Airborne (active) Number of isolates	%	Airborne (settle) Number of isolates	%	Wound Number of isolates	%	Sepsis (384 cases) Number of isolates	%
Gram-positive	1779	88.2	6599	95.1	264	81.7	246	62.8
Staphylococcus epidermidis	784	38.9	2591	37.4	129	39.9	84	21.4
Staphylococcus aureus	12	0.6	31	0.4	6	1.9	109	27.8
Micrococcus	0	0	1571	22.6	3	0.9	13	3.3
Diphtheroid	291	14.4	1007	14.5	92	28.5	3	0.8
B. subtilis	515	25.5	1350	19.5	3	0.9	0	0
Other	134	6.6	112	1.6	31	9.6	37	9.4
Gram-negative	112	5.6	51	0.7	9	2.8	80	20.4
E. coli							30	7.7
Proteus							21	5.4
Other							29	7.4
Other	169	8.4	286	4.1	49	15.2	0	0
Mixed							4	1.0
Sterile							34	8.7
Not valid							27	6.9
Aerobic							309	78.8
Anaerobic							18	4.6
TOTAL	2017	100.0	6936	100.0	323	100.0	392	100.0

From Nelson JP: Operating room environment: clean rooms and personnel-isolator systems. In Eftekhar NS, editor: *Infection in joint replacement surgery, prevention and management*, St Louis, 1984, Mosby–Year Book.

Table 8-8 Summary of Airborne Bacterial Contamination at or Near Wound

Reports	Type of operating room*	Garment†	Average bacteria/m³
9	Reg	Reg	190.7
5	CR (H)	Reg	21.2
2	CR (V)	Reg	10.6
4	CR (H)	P-I	7.1
2	CR (V)	P-I	0.7

From Nelson JP: Operating room environment: clean rooms and personnel-isolator systems. In Eftekhar NS, editor: *Infection in joint replacement surgery, prevention and management*, St Louis, 1984, Mosby–Year Book.
*Reg, Regular; CR, clean room; H, horizontal airflow; V, vertical airflow.
†Reg, Regular; P-I, personnel-isolator.

Table 8-9 Summary of Settle-Plate Bacterial Fallout at Wound

Reports	Type of operating room*	Garment†	Average bacteria/m²/hr
6	Reg	Reg	1143.1
2	CR (H)	Reg	322.9
2	CR (H)	P-I	271.3
1	CR (V)	P-I	32.3

From Nelson JP: Operating room environment: clean rooms and personnel-isolator systems. In Eftekhar NS, editor: *Infection in joint replacement surgery, prevention and management*, St Louis, 1984, Mosby–Year Book.
*Reg, Regular; CR, clean room; H, horizontal airflow; V, vertical airflow.
†Reg, Regular; P-I, personnel-isolator.

Table 8-10 Summary of Wound Contamination Rates

Number of reports	Type of operating room*	Garment†	Number of cultures	Number positive	%
5	Reg	Reg	3532	881	24.9
2	CR	Reg	705	33	4.7
3	CR	P-I	533	21	3.9

From Nelson JP: Operating room environment: clean rooms and personnel-isolator systems. In Eftekhar NS, editor: *Infection in joint replacement surgery, prevention and management*, St Louis, 1984, Mosby–Year Book.
Reg, Regular; *CR*, clean room.
†*Reg*, Regular; *P-I*, personnel-isolator.

operating rooms on a low floor in close proximity to such support services as laboratories and x-ray facilities and to surgical patient floors to expedite patient transport. The operating room should have only one access door, equipped with a foot-pressure panel or a photoelectric opening mechanism. Of course, emergency exits are necessary; however, having one access point provides maximum protection from contamination and limits traffic flow. The surgical suite should be arranged to keep traffic flow of personnel and equipment to a minimum and to encourage the flow of air, personnel, and equipment from clean to dirty. This flow provides maximum protection from contamination in an operating room unit composed of a scrub room, induction room, vertical laminar-airflow operating room, and sterilization room (see Fig. 8-8).

With a wall-less vertical laminar-airflow room, solid marking of the floor to correspond to the canopy (area of air delivery) is a good practice and serves as a reminder to avoid contamination of the team by unsterile individuals moving about the room.

There is no concrete evidence that one surgical suite design holds any demonstrable advantage over any other in the control of infection.[14,164,165]

Air contaminants can enter the wound by two routes—directly, by settling in the wound, or indirectly, through the use of contaminated instruments and contaminated air in the operating room. These bacteria (whether alone or adhering to inorganic particles) either are shed by the surgical team or are present in the ambient air entering the operating unit. Aseptic technique to ameliorate shedding by the surgical team is discussed elsewhere.

Particulate matter in the ambient air can be reduced to less than 1% of all particles larger than 3 μm by using HEPA filters.[14] However, because the significant bacteria carrying particles are usually larger than 10 μm, the cost and maintenance of an air filtration unit for the operating room can be minimized without sacrificing efficiency by filtering particles no smaller than 1 μm.[60,62,91,95] Despite adequate air filtering, however, larger particles shed by the surgical team contaminate

the air, having escaped masks, gowns, and gloves. Studies have shown that the particles containing *S. aureus* have an average diameter of 12 μm. These particles make 8 to 12 traverses in a room with turbulent ventilation before discharging through the exhaust vents. Particles usually traverse a laminar- or mass-airflow room once before discharging.[14] Quick particulate settling is aided by gravity. Use of a vertical laminar-airflow room reduces by over 88% the chance that a given particle will contaminate the wound. Thus laminar airflow reduces contamination from particles in filtered air and particles shed by the operating room team.

Because operating room personnel are the greatest source of contamination since they shed bacteria from the skin, hair, perineum, and nasopharynx,* their health is very important. Employees with respiratory tract infections, skin lesions, or local infections should be restricted from the operating room, and personnel working in the operating room should practice good personal hygiene.[14,184]

All personnel should observe a prescribed dress code to present a clean barrier to contamination. The dress code should cover all clothing worn above underwear, since underwear removal is not necessary.[184] Scrub suits are not worn outside of the operating room. Legs must be covered with pantyhose or scrub pants. There is no advantage to one-piece over two-piece scrub suits with respect to preventing contamination.[184] Fingernails should be clipped short and should be smooth and free of polish because chipped nail polish may harbor bacteria.[184]

Use of disposable head covering is preferable. All head and facial hair, including sideburns, should be covered. Inadequately covered hair presents a hazard, since hair is known to shed bacterial particles.†

All personnel should wear high-filtration masks inside the operating room and surgical suite. Masks

---

* References 7, 21, 62, 67, 71, 98, 181, 186, 206.
† References 21, 67, 71, 98, 181, 186, 206.

should be securely fastened, completely covering the nose and mouth with no venting at the sides. Masks should not be saved by hanging them around the neck or tucking them into a pocket for future use. They should be removed and disposed of at the end of each surgical procedure.[20,71]

Shoes should be made of a durable substance and kept clean.[184] Shoe covers should be worn when entering the surgical suite and removed when leaving the suite. Clean covers should be put on when returning.[20]

ULTRAVIOLET LIGHT*

In an attempt to provide clean air in the operating room at Duke University, Hart installed ultraviolet lights in early 1936. Since their introduction, the number of airborne bacteria collected during the surgical procedure has been reduced.[130,132] Eliminating 75% to 90% of viable bacteria by the settle-plate method reduced the wound infection rate in ultraclean cases.†

Referring to Hart's work, Goldner concluded that the use of ultraviolet light in operating rooms is the simplest, most economical, and least-involved means to obtain a relatively clean air environment in surgery. He and his associates have produced evidence suggesting favorable results when ultraviolet lights are used during total hip arthroplasty.[119,120] Lowell[184,185] has also demonstrated a marked reduction in bacterial contamination with the use of ultraviolet lights, but as in other studies, his statistical results suffer because he failed to use controls in gathering his clinical data.

A National Research Council study evaluating ultraviolet light reported a statistically significant reduction of postoperative wound infections after clean, refined operations; the average postoperative infection rate was reduced from 3.8% to 2.9%. Nonetheless, the main body of this report did not encourage the use of ultraviolet light for this purpose. Although this average drop might not have been impressive, it represented a 24% improvement for the five hospitals participating in the study; at one hospital, the range of improvement was a high 44%.

Ultraviolet radiation is the segment of the electromagnetic spectrum ranging between 150 and 4000 Å, just below the visible spectrum. The peak of bactericidal activity is at 2630 Å; the maximum erythema peak at approximately 3000 Å. Mercury vapor lamps have a resonance line at 2537 Å, which is sufficiently close to the bactericidal peak to make them germicidally

effective. The recommended intensity of radiation is 25 to 30 $\mu W/cm^2/sec$ at the level of the operative field. The lamps must be used at a relative humidity of 60% or below; their effectiveness drops dramatically about this level, rendering them almost ineffective at 70% humidity.

Ultraviolet lights are relatively inexpensive and convenient to install. However, there are hazards to their use. The most unpleasant is conjunctivitis, which develops when the eyes are exposed to direct rays of the radiation for more than 2 to 3 minutes at a time; the second, modest erythema of the skin after a 20-minute exposure; and the last, possible increase in the drying rate of the surgical wound. All of these problems are preventable by simple measures: the first, by using industrial goggles or eye shields to prevent both reflected and direct radiation from reaching the eyes; the second by using a benzophenone-containing sunscreen; and the last by using an irrigating solution to keep the wound moist during surgery. Radiation from the ultraviolet lights is sufficiently strong to destroy microorganisms that are airborne or resting on exposed flat surfaces by penetrating them and destroying their DNA; however, it is not strong enough to penetrate the cornea, to damage the retina, or to produce tanning or blistering. And although it penetrates distilled water, it does not penetrate body fluids or exudates. Nor can it decontaminate or sterilize a wound.[184]

The protocol for using ultraviolet radiation requires that all personnel wear goggles of a standard industrial type, eye shades similar to those used by the proverbial croupier in a gambling house, or some form of side shield on ordinary eyeglasses. Radiation at 2537 Å does not penetrate ordinary eyeglasses or industrial goggles. Contact lenses, which cover only the cornea, do not, of course, suffice. Paper hoods that cover the neck and are inserted inside the operating gown protect the neck area; alternatively, an application of benzophenone-containing sunscreen over exposed skin surfaces ordinarily remains effective for 4 hours. Surgical drapes, including plastic, protect the patient's skin, but the patient's face should be shielded by extending the drapes over an anesthesia screen.

The Peter Bent Brigham Hospital installed ultraviolet lamps in its operating rooms in 1973. Studies were carried out at that time to assess their effectiveness, and a careful follow-up study of the patient population undergoing total joint arthroplasty has been maintained since. The lamps were installed on 10-foot ceilings with proper spacing to distribute radiation throughout the room. Settle-plate studies indicated that four to eight viable particles settled over every square foot of surface during each minute the room was occupied when no ultraviolet radiation

---

* Adapted from Lowell JD: Use of ultraviolet radiation in total hip replacement surgery. In Eftekhar NS, editor: *Infection in joint replacement surgery: prevention and management*, St Louis, 1984, Mosby–Year Book.

† References 12, 39, 70, 139, 238.

was present. Illuminating the lamps produced a 20-fold decrease, to 0.2 viable particles/ft^2/min. Studies showed that using a Wells air centrifuge without radiation reduced the viable particles to seven particles per 5 feet^3 of air; when both the centrifuge and the radiation were used, the level dropped to one viable particle per 5 ft^3. Viable particle counts of rodac contact plates pressed against numerous flat surfaces in the operating room (such as the top of the operating room lamp, the floor, the anesthesiologist's cart, the electrodesiccating unit, the top of an oscilloscope, and the top of a Mayo stand) ranged before surgery from zero on top of a Mayo stand to highs of 23 and 26 per 25 cm^2 on top of an operating room lamp and an open shelf. The floor had organisms too numerous to count, which easily became airborne if scuffed by shoes. With the lamps illuminated, only the surfaces shielded from the radiation (such as the foot of an operating room lamp covered by an overhanging surgical drape) supported more than one or two organisms, and most areas supported none; no viable organisms were recoverable from the floor. The top of the Mayo stand remained sterile.

According to Lowell and collaborators, "from the time of lamp installation to the present, deep wound infection rate has remained satisfactorily low. For primary total hip arthroplasty, the rate has dropped from 2.1% to 0.4%; for all total hip surgery, from 3.06% to 0.53%."[184]

SURGICAL MASKS AND THEIR EFFECTIVENESS

Surgical masks are intended to prevent bacteria-laden particles generated by the nasopharynx and face from spreading to the environment; they have become an absolute requirement in operating rooms throughout the world. Wound-contaminating bacteria are carried on droplets approximately 25 μm in diameter.[126,289] Spraying the face with microspheres of human albumin reveals the route and potential degree of contamination from the nasopharynx.[126,289] Using this technique and the standard surgical face mask* in a simulated surgical condition, investigators found most airborne organisms to be gram-positive cocci, gram-negative cocci, or gram-positive bacilli. They also observed a positive correlation between the number of organisms in the wound and the length of time the masks were worn. This phenomenon was thought to be caused by microspheres escaping around the mask. Because masks cannot totally eliminate bacterial escape, the nasopharynx remains a source of infection; thus conventional surgical masks may have very little or no influence on the overall surgical environment.[241]

Sompolinsky and co-workers conclusively demonstrated that the nasopharynx can occasionally serve as a source of wound infection, though not commonly.[260] Masks may decrease contamination of the wound by as much as 90%. Ritter has shown that the filter efficiency of most disposable masks is greater than 95%.[241] Dineen,[82] like others,[111] has shown that cloth masks are inefficient and that thin ones allow bacteria to escape easily; however, moistened disposable masks tested for up to 8 hours of continuous use were found to be effective filters.[82] Improper use of masks and excessive conversation in a simulated surgical situation increased the number of microspherule-containing organisms that escaped to the environment and entered the wound.[173]

Direct transference of organisms from the nasopharynx is a rare cause of exogenous infection in the operating room. It is impossible to detect all carriers, so some carriers may be among operating room personnel; consequently, routine use of conventional double masks or masks installed with a vacuum system is a rational discipline for the operating room. Combining the use of an all-investing gown and mask with the use of suction respirators has become increasingly popular since originally advocated by Charnley.[61] Several models of these units are available; some carry their own communication system for teaching purposes. Although these units are initially somewhat cumbersome and complicated for personnel not adequately trained in total hip arthroplasty, they are cool despite the impermeable material used in their design.[199]

Surgeons traditionally are accustomed to wearing a head cover and a face mask, but they often are unaware of their ineffectiveness in preventing bacterial dispersion into the wound and the surgical environment. Fig. 8-14 shows various methods of wearing masks and their level of effectiveness. A properly worn head cover and mask is shown in Fig. 8-14, C.

SCRUB SUITS AND HEAD GEAR

The reason all members of the surgical team and all personnel entering the operating room suite must wear scrub suits and head gear is to create a barrier between the individual's "particle-generating surfaces" and the surgical environment. However, this barrier is only theoretical and is ineffective in preventing microbial contamination. Several factors explain this failure: (1) standard scrub suits are not impervious to particles generated by the body (shedding), so bacteria do not remain contained within the suit; (2) the effective alternative, an all-investing hood and pants with occlusive neck and ankles, becomes so hot from trapped body heat that some operating room personnel find it intolerable.

Shedding caused by clothing worn under the scrub suits can be even harder to control. For example,

---

* Manufactured by Johnson and Johnson.

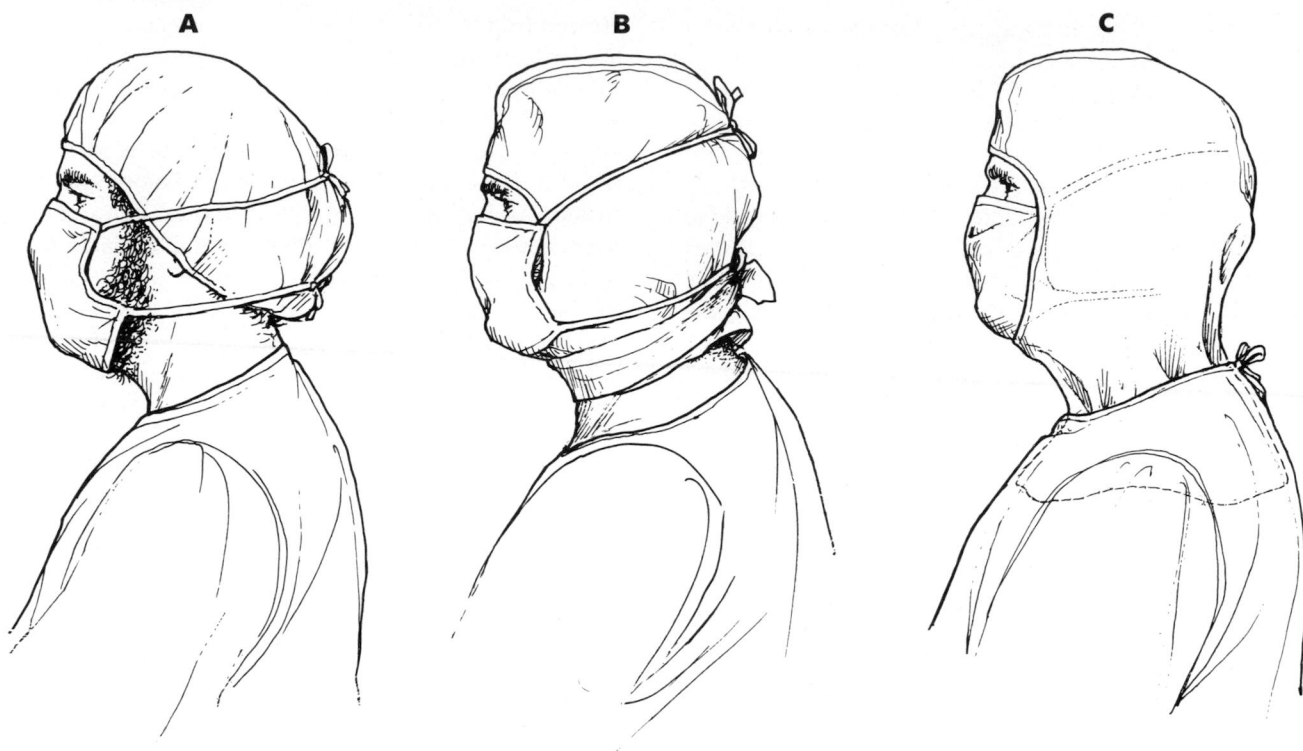

Fig. 8-14. Conventional face masks and head covers are not effective in reducing bacterial contamination unless they are made of impervious materials and used properly. **A,** "Traditional practice," a bad way to use a head cover and mask in the operating room. Note exposed hair and skin. **B,** A somewhat better coverage of the face and the neck by an extension of the hood over the neck. **C,** The right way to cover head and neck; note that the "apron" position of the head gear is long enough to reach the shoulders. The mask is put on first, and the head gear covers the head. The gown has closed up the neck circumferentially.

Table 8-11 Microbiological Comparison of Surgical Head Coverings Used in Conjunction with Hair Spray

Type of head covering	Without hair spray	With hair spray	Reduction (%)	Significance
No head covering	336	228	32	$P < 0.05$
Caps	462	162	65	$P < 0.02$
Hoods	214	168	21	$P < 0.02$

From Ritter MA, Eitzen HE, Hart JB: The surgeon's garb, *Clin Orthop* 153:204, 1980.
All figures are in colony-forming units/ft^{2n}/h.

studies have shown that wearing impervious bathing trunks reduces shedding by 90% or more when no clothing is covering them.[139,204] But wearing a scrub suit negates their effectiveness, and shedding returns to normal levels. A one-piece suit of impermeable fabric (bunny-type or boiler suit) controls shedding, especially for men, who shed more than woman.[204] Scrub suits that have shirttails that hang out or can be tucked in prevent all but minor environmental contamination; they are designed for men and women.[46] Hairspray was also found to reduce bacterial shedding into the environment (Table 8-11).

In another display of how clothing affects bacterial dispersion, Ritter noted a 51% reduction (*P* value less than 0.05) when all personnel in a simulated operating room setting wore a Tyvec wrap-around gown instead

Table 8-12 Comparisons of Different Types of Surgical Garb

Comparison	Reduction (%)	Significance
Scrub clothes (661) *vs.* wraparound gown (325)	51	$P < 0.05$
Wraparound gown (325) *vs.* helmet and exhaust equipment (201)	38	$P < 0.05$
Scrub clothes (661) *vs.* helmet and exhaust equipment	69	$P < 0.01$

From Ritter MA, Eitzen HE, Hart JB: The surgeon's garb, *Clin Orthop* 153:204, 1980.
Numbers in parentheses indicate colony-forming units/ft²/h.

of scrub clothes. Bacterial dispersion was reduced even further when personnel wore an all-investing gown/helmet/aspirator (reduction to 69.5% [*P* value less than 0.01]) (Table 8-12).[242] Despite previous studies documenting contamination associated with woven fabrics and demonstrating their ineffectiveness in preventing bacterial shedding,* these materials are currently used in operating room surgical gowns. Ritter found an all-investing gown/helmet/aspirator to be the most efficient means of controlling bacterial shedding from the head and neck, particularly when all operating room personnel wore such systems. However, Ritter's study[242] reported no significant difference in environmental contamination between laminar-airflow operating rooms where an inclusive gown/helmet/aspirator was used and those where it was not.

SURGICAL GOWNS

Wearing surgical gowns made of permeable textile can compromise assiduous application of the clean-air room theory; the wound can be contaminated by direct contact no matter how effectively the air route has been controlled.[11,62,64,166]

In an early study, we found that the cloth used for the conventional surgical gown was inadequate for controlling infection.[64] Light microscopy revealed perforations of 1 to 50 μm, large enough for particles and bacteria to pass through (Fig. 8-15). This route of infection is considered particularly significant in operations like total hip arthroplasty when an instrument frequently comes in contact with the surgeon's gown (especially at the time of manipulation of the limb and reduction of the prosthesis). In a later study, we examined the front of the gown bacteriologically at the end of each operation. Tables 8-7 and 8-8 demonstrate

---

* References 11, 32, 65, 82, 127.

the results of these studies and indicate the type and frequency of organisms recovered by this method.[64] On the basis of these findings, we considered gowns designed with impermeable material. Although we found them to be undoubtedly superior, the buildup of body heat made them almost intolerable to wear during surgery. After considering ways to overcome this serious drawback, we installed a ventilation system within the gown that produced a considerably cooler environment.

In studies similar to those by Charnley and Eftekhar,[64] Dineen and Ritter[81,84,242] demonstrated that the exterior of gowns made with occlusive fabric remains sterile throughout surgery if the air in the operating room remains sterile. Disposable synthetic fiber gowns are the first choice for surgery and should be used at all times. These gowns are resistant to water and totally impervious to bacterial penetration.

DESIGN OF ALL-INVESTING GOWN/HELMET/ PERSONNEL ISOLATORS

A good personnel isolator provides a complete barrier between the surgical personnel (surgeon, assistants, and nurses) and the wound. A cooling system is essential to the design of the isolator; the buildup of body heat otherwise makes it intolerable.

As mentioned earlier, gowns and hoods have been created using a wet-resistant, impervious material of a tightly woven texture (such as tightly woven polymers and a variety of paper materials—if they provide air circulation. The gown should be loose-fitting to permit air circulation and comfort; the helmet supports the weight of the gown and allows full visibility. Communication and visibility, essential in performing the procedure, are achieved with the improved headpieces now available that are delivered sterile to the surgeon and worn over the headpiece vacuum tubing. The head-neck junction of the gown should not be constricted. A negative air pressure allows cooling and removal of the bacteria generated (shed) by the body. This design eliminates bacteria at the source and reduces the number of bacteria reaching the wound because of the impervious material used in its design (Figs. 8-16 to 8-18).

SURGICAL SCRUB AND GLOVING

Most surgeons accept the surgical scrub as a routine practice fundamental to prophylaxis against infection—an additional protective step in preparing for surgery. Because gloves may be torn or punctured during an operation, the added protection of a high-quality surgical glove (or a double pair of gloves) is essential in handling surgical wounds involving instrumentation and soft tissue and bone. It has been established that the 10-minute hand scrub is an

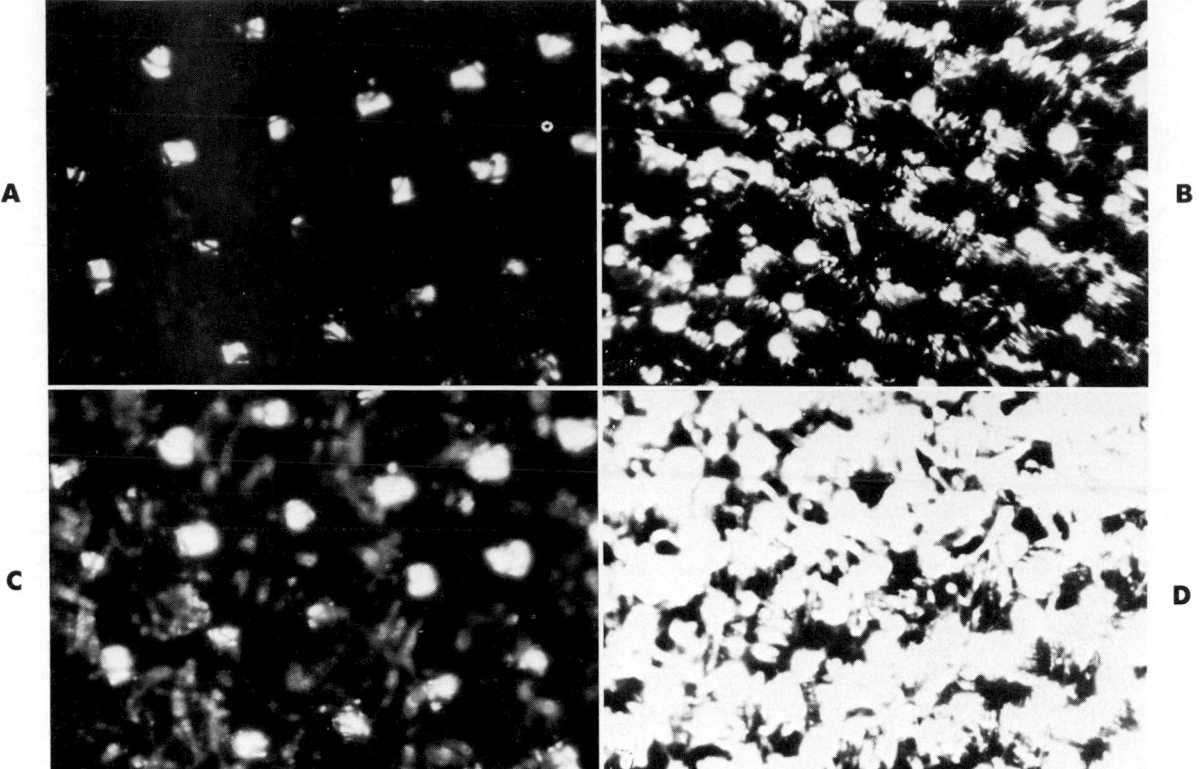

Fig. 8-15. A, Gown material (conventional balloon cloth) of excellent quality with tightly woven texture under light microscope. **B,** Same material as **A** but different brand showing less tightness of texture, thus allowing greater penetration. **C,** Conventional balloon cloth gown material before laundering. Perforation size ranging from 1 to 50 μm. **D,** Same material as in **C** after heavy laundering. Size of apertures now ranging from 100 to 1000 μm. (From Eftekhar NS: The surgeon and clean air in the operating room, *Clin Orthop* 96:188, 1973.)

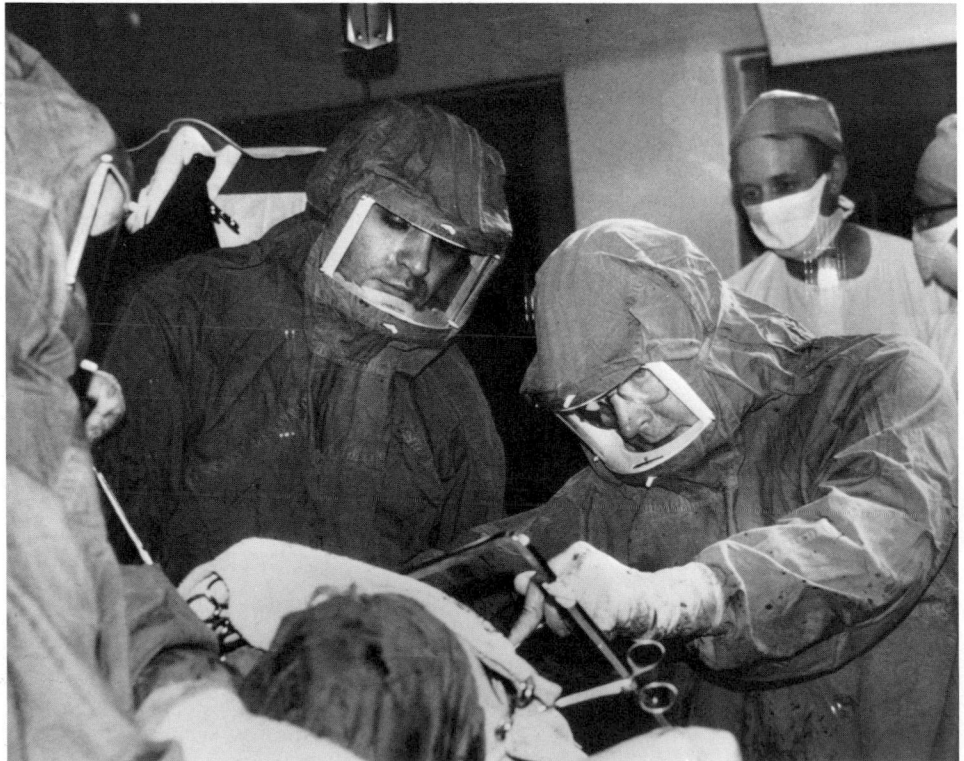

Fig. 8-16. The first use of a personal isolator (the so-called space suit developed by Sir John Charnley in 1967). In his design the head and body sections are in continuity (without separating them into two compartments), and the headpiece is closely applied to the face. The gown is made of impervious cloth and is laundered.

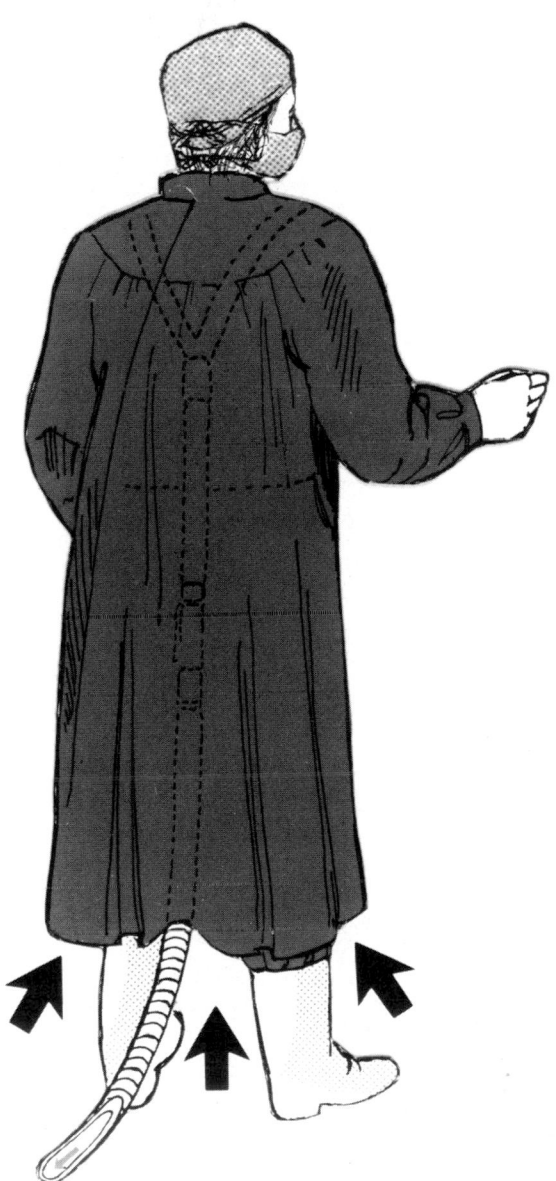

Fig. 8-17. A conventional disposable gown may be worn with an exhaust system (without a hood with suction). This system does not offer a great deal of protection because the route of contamination from head and neck has not been eliminated. It may provide some cooling effect and reduce the total bacterial contamination in the operating room environment.

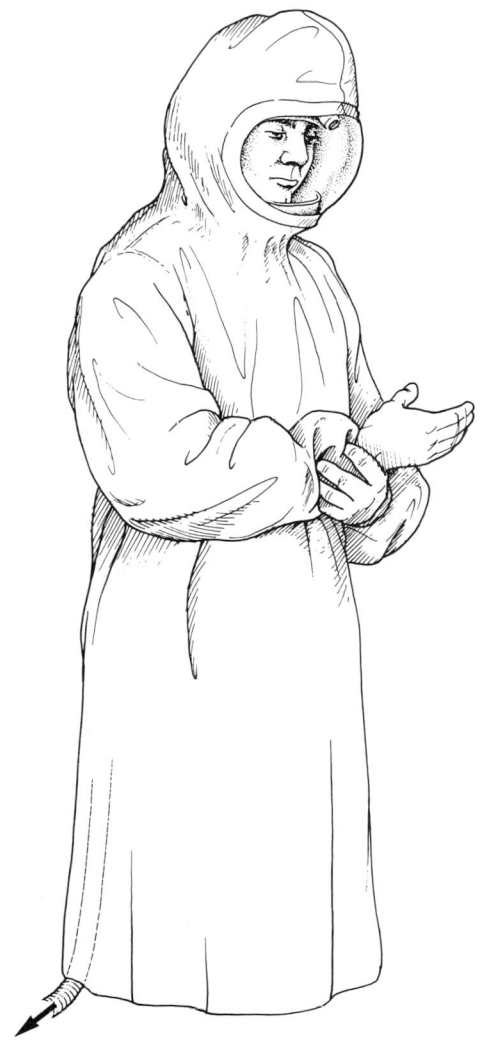

Fig. 8-18. A two-piece "space suite" with a visor similar to a "fish bowl" can include a head light. Such a system has become popular because it can be used with disposable paper gowns. The source of air suction may be a fixed outlet within the operating room, or members of the surgical team may wear battery-operated units on their waists, which enables them to move about freely.

unnecessary ritual, although in comparing several cleansing agents, Dineen[80] showed differences between 5- and 10-minute scrubs (Fig. 8-19). Some have suggested that a 1-minute scrub may be adequate because of the slight difference in bacterial count of fingertips examined after 1 minute of scrubbing and up to 2 hours after scrubbing. Bernard[37] has also shown no difference in reducing bacterial counts with 3-, 5-, or 10-minute scrubs.

Most gloves have been punctured by the end of an operation, so it is essential to check them frequently throughout the operation for obvious tears and perforations. The practice of changing gloves frequently during surgery is a good and rational discipline (Fig. 8-20). In a study of 100 operative procedures,[57] Butterfield noted that one or more glove punctures occurred in 70% of the operations.

Other investigators[67] have also documented the frequent puncture of gloves, as evidenced by blood seeping through the puncture site; they have even demonstrated bacterial counts of S. aureus reaching as high as 18,000.

With regard to this mode of bacterial transmission, no scientific report has proved that the punctured glove is the source of postsurgical infection. Nonetheless, it

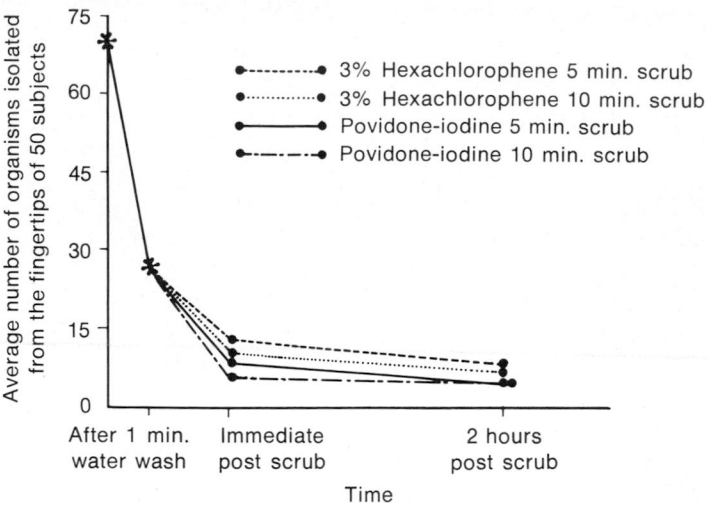

Fig. 8-19. Comparison of 5- to 10-minute surgical scrub on skin counts obtained from 50 subjects using different agents. * — Indicates drop in bacterial population after 1-minute wash. (From Dineen P: An evaluation of the duration of surgical scrub, *Surg Gynecol Obstet* 129:1181, 1969.)

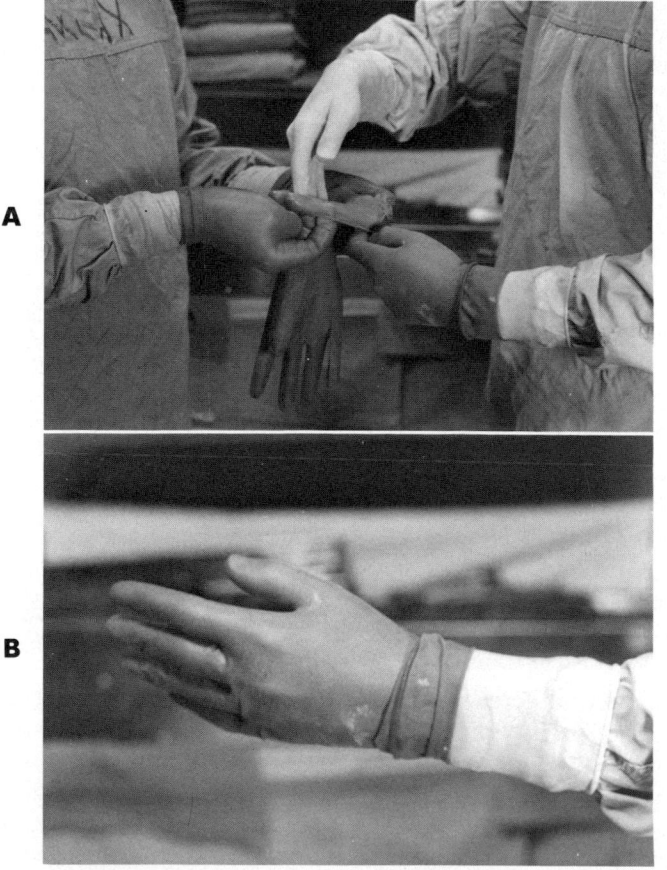

Fig. 8-20. A, Gloving technique. **B,** Second pair of gloves is pulled only to the wrist to facilitate their subsequent exchange and to avoid contaminating outer gloves with elastic cuff of gown. (From Ayer M, Stone R, Eftekhar NS: Operating room asepsis and sterilization techniques. In Eftekhar NS, editor: *Infection in joint replacement surgery*, St Louis, 1984, Mosby–Year Book.)

is a rational discipline to avoid puncturing gloves during surgery and to replace them immediately if any puncture is detected. Regardless of the sterility of the surgeon's hands at the end of the scrub period, the chances remain remarkably high that they will become contaminated by the end of the operation because of sweating and self-contamination within the surgical gloves. The practice of leaving some surgical antiseptic soap on the hands at the end of the scrub period may produce some disinfecting effect. Surgeons must insist that all surgical team members wear two pairs of high-quality gloves.

McCue has demonstrated that the outer gloves are the pair most often punctured and also that they are contaminated after performing a draping procedure.[195] After 10 total hip arthroplasties, he tested 275 outer and inner gloves, both mechanically and bacteriologically. The surgeons who used their hands most strenuously developed more holes in their gloves than those who did not. Paradoxically, the greatest number of colonies (44%) grew from the gloves used for draping, although they had no holes and had only been used for a few minutes. These findings confirm that changing gloves after draping and frequently during surgery are ways to prevent contamination.

In addition to wound contamination via the surgeon's hands, soiling of the wound by contamination during postoperative recovery is an important source of exogenous infection. The first 24 hours after surgery seems to be the most critical period in terms of direct contamination; once natural epithelial formation has begun at the end of this period, it provides a barrier and the skin is self-protected. In a primary wound closure without drainage, from the purely bacteriological point of view, a dressing may be unnecessary after a few hours of skin closure.[134] Nevertheless, total hip arthroplasty wounds are subject to considerable movement; elderly patients are commonly restless after surgery, and the chances of self-inoculation are high. A logical solution is to seal the wound after the operation to prevent self-induced traumatic lesions or contaminations, as well as contamination of superficial minor hematomas during the early postoperative course.

SKIN DISINFECTION

Hair at the site of the operation has been incriminated as an important source of surgical contamination; the method of hair removal and the time elapsed before surgery affect the rate of bacterial colonization at the site. Razor preparation of the operative site presents a potential danger of skin contamination. Seropian and Reynolds[258a] found an infection rate of 3.1% when routine razor preparation was scheduled less than 24 hours before the operation, and the rate rose to 20% when razor preparation was more than 24 hours before

surgery. The use of a chemical depilatory (Surgex) reduced the infection rate to 1.6% compared to 5.6% using a razor for control.

Cruse,[72] in a series of 20,105 operations, found that clipping the hair at the surgical site reduced wound infection; the rate when the site had been shaved was 2.3%; when clipped, it was 1.9%, and it was 0.9% when no attempt had been made to remove the hairs. He concluded that the differences were caused by razor-induced trauma, which created a port of entry for exogenous bacteria, the injured tissues serving as a culture medium for bacterial growth.

In preparing the surgical site in the operating room, Fitzgerald[108] has shown that it is better to use a soap that leaves a residual bactericidal barrier than an ordinary detergent soap. He suggests removing the chemical soap left on the skin the night before surgery and reapplying 2% tincture of iodine after defatting the skin, followed by alcohol and then freon. Zdeblick has proved the effectiveness of replacing the patient's preoperative scrub with a hexachlorophene shower.[295] Further, applying a hexachlorophene compound as a foam provides an excellent bactericidal and bacteriostatic effect; additionally, it takes less time than a scrub and is easier to apply.[97]

SURGICAL DRAPES

Bacteria from the surface of the skin can migrate during surgery and infect the wound. To reduce this type of contamination, use plastic adhesive drapes, such as Steri-drapes (Table 8-13).[116,131,240] To determine the percentage of positive deep-wound cultures colonized during total hip arthroplasty, a contamination level was obtained from the surface of plastic and linen drapes (Table 8-14). As the tables indicate, plastic drapes efficiently control bacterial contamination of the wound from the patient's skin surface. Bacterial sampling of the wound after the application of an

Table 8-13 Contamination Levels of Surface Plastic and Linen Drapes Obtained During Total Hip Arthroplasty Surgery

Time of sampling (minutes)	Colony-forming units/Rodac plates (4 in²)	
	Plastic	Linen
T = 0	0.14	0.0
T = 15	1.3	0.27
T = 30	3.98	10.3
T = 45	0.97	27.7
T = 60	2.4	20.3

From Ritter MA: The effect that time, touch, and environment have upon bacterial contamination of instruments during surgery, *Ann Surg* 184:46, 1976.

Table 8-14 Percentage of Positive Deep Wound Cultures During Total Hip Arthroplasty

	Plastic	Linen
Opening	2%	27%
Closing	6%	60%

From Ritter MA: The effect that time, touch, and environment have upon bacterial contamination of instruments during surgery. *Ann Surg* 184:46, 1976.

Idophore-impregnated plastic adhesive drape dramatically reduced wound contamination by skin bacteria from 15% to 1.6%. This reduction may be significant for patients undergoing total joint arthroplasty.[102] One caution: gloves frequently become contaminated during removal of these drapes at the end of an operation. This author routinely places a sterile sponge inside the hip and applies 2% tincture of iodine to the skin after removing the plastic drape, then exchanges the outer glove for a new one after removing the drape.

INSTRUMENTS, INSTRUMENT TABLES, AND SPLASH BASIN
Instruments

Studies of surface contamination indicate that contaminated surfaces remain contaminated, although the degree of contamination eventually reaches an equilibrium with the environment. In one study, Ayliffe[23] concluded that disinfectants had little effect on the equilibrium of bacteria on the contaminated surface and that bacteria did not disperse. Furthermore, contamination from surfaces occurred only by direct contact.[23] Other authors have studied the surfaces of many instruments, such as surgical knife blades, equipment, sponges, and so on, and have cultured various common organisms from these surfaces exposed to the operating room air.[311,314] In a study of knife blades, there was no statistical difference between the "skin knife" and "deep knife," but most surgeons exchange the first knife for a fresh one after cutting the skin. Significantly, the investigators recovered a statistically greater number of bacteria in cultures from knife blades used in conventional rooms

than from those used in laminar-flow rooms (Table 8-15).

Instrument Tables

The traditional back instrument tables are a notorious source of contamination in the operating room. Bacterial contamination of the air occurs before the procedure begins. Airborne organisms settle on the tables and instruments as they would on an exposed culture plate. Thus, organisms may enter the wound via instruments or the hands of operating team personnel. Fitzgerald noted the mean number of colony-forming units per square foot per hour as 121 CFU/foot^2/hour with 12 to 14 room air exchanges per hour and 48 CFU/foot^2/hour with 28 to 32 room air exchanges per hour.[106] Thus unidirectional airflow rooms are essential when instrument tables in the operating room remain exposed throughout the procedure.

Splash Basin

Most scrub nurses and surgeons consider it essential to use a splash basin in the operating room during surgery. Such a basin, filled with sterile water or saline solution, sits on the instrument table so that blood-soaked instruments can be immersed in it for a temporary wash and cleansing before being returned to the surgical field. Additionally, the contents furnish a solution for irrigating the wound by rubber syringe. The same solution can be used throughout the procedure, or sterile water can be added as needed to replenish the supply used in irrigation and in soaking sponges.

These splash basins, however, can serve as a breeding ground for bacteria because their large surface area acts as a settle plate.[24] The high incidence of positive cultures in these basin solutions indicates that the contaminants are similar to most bacteria found in the operating room environment. In one study, for example, Baird and associates[24] showed that 74% of 78 splash basins contained positive cultures and that only 26% of these 78 cultures remained negative at the end of the operation. *S. epidermidis* was the most common among all positive cultures (45%), and 88% of the positive cultures contained *S. epidermidis, S. aureus,*

Table 8-15 Microbial Contamination of Knife Blades

	Laminar-airflow cases			Conventional operating room cases			
	Number tested	Number contaminated	%	Number tested	Number contaminated	%	Probability
Skin	102	3	3	106	16	15	$P<0.005$
Deep	209	9	4	165	33	20	$P<0.005$

From Ritter MA et al: Bacterial contamination of the surgical knife; *Clin Orthop* 108:158, 1975.

or other gram-positive cocci; 34% of the positive cultures also grew multiple organisms.[24] Other organisms included gram-negative rods, *Bacillus* species, diphtheroids, *Pseudomonas*, and more.

SUCTION TIPS

Because reusable suction tubing cannot be sterilized easily,[106] disposable suction tubing and tips are preferred. The collecting containers must be sterilized before use. At the end of surgery, the drainage tubes are connected to a temporary vacuum container as the patient leaves the operating room. In the recovery room, the tubes are connected to a wall suction system that uses a similar disposable tubing and connecting system. The sterile containers are used when transferring the patient to his or her room. The tubes are then connected to the wall suction.

Investigators have also described contamination of suction tips occurring independent of surgical wound contamination. Such contamination comes from air sucked in via the suction tip; it can increase with time during the course of an operation.[125,265] The organisms recovered most frequently from suction tips are coagulase-negative staphylococcus (S. *epidermidis*) and other bacteria commonly cultured from operating room air. Some 80% of infections in total hip arthroplasty are caused by such airborne bacteria.[159] The large volume of air drawn from the operating room environment through the suction tip may partly account for the high rate of bacterial colonization reported in wounds during total hip arthroplasty.[201] Because aerobic organisms are prevalent in delayed appearing infections and also at revision surgery, some authors have suggested a causal relationship with air contamination in the operating room during revision surgery.[18,125] It may be concluded that a high rate of bacterial colonization reported in the wounds during total hip arthroplasty may be caused in part by wound contamination by the suction tip, which contains a large number of operating room bacteria. Therefore the greater the level of air contamination and the greater the volumetric air suction by the suction tip, the larger the number of bacteria in both the suction tip and the wound. Several preventive measures protect the wound from contamination via the suction tip: (1) exchange the old suction tip for a new one during the course of the operation (i.e., use a new one in preparing the medullary canal); (2) shut off the suction tip when not in use; and (3) protect the suction tip in a container hidden in a large sponge soaked with Betadine solution.

GURNEY

Fitzgerald[106] noted that gram-negative bacteria are rarely isolated from the operating room environment.

However, a large number of these organisms can be found in the operating room environment, apparently introduced when the patient is transferred directly from the hospital room environment to the operating room. To prevent these bacteria from entering the operating room, patients should be taken from their hospital rooms to a holding area where they are transferred onto a sterile gurney. This fresh gurney is then used to transfer them to the operating room.

After surgery, the total hip arthroplasty patient should be moved as little as possible. With this in mind, it is wise to transfer the patient to his or her sterile hospital bed after surgery. The transfer to the bed takes place in the corridor immediately outside the operating room, thus minimizing opportunities for introducing bacteria. If this is done, the bed remains outside in the corridor, and the operating table is moved outside the operating room for patient transfer. An alternative is to use a canvas that is placed on the operating table during the procedure. After surgery, the patient can be moved out of the operating room without moving the operating table.

Table 8-16 Contamination of Operating Room

Source	CFU/ft²/hr	Organism isolated
Patient's gown	84	*Escherichia coli*
Sheet	190	*Enterobacter aerogenes*
Gurney	1037	*Acinetobacter calco-aceticus,* *Pseudomonas aeruginosa,* *Staphylococcus epidermidis*

From Fitzgerald RH Jr: In *The American Academy of Orthopaedic Surgeons instructional course lectures*, vol 26, St Louis, 1977, Mosby–Year Book.

Table 8-17 Airborne Bacterial Contamination in Corridors and Cast Room

Location and activity level	Viable particles /ft³ air
Corridor	
Mild	16.3
Moderate	20.3
Maximum	24.9
Cast room	
Mild	6.0
Moderate	10.8

From Fitzgerald RH Jr: In *The American Academy of Orthopaedic Surgeons instructional course lectures*, vol 26, St Louis, 1977, Mosby–Year Book.

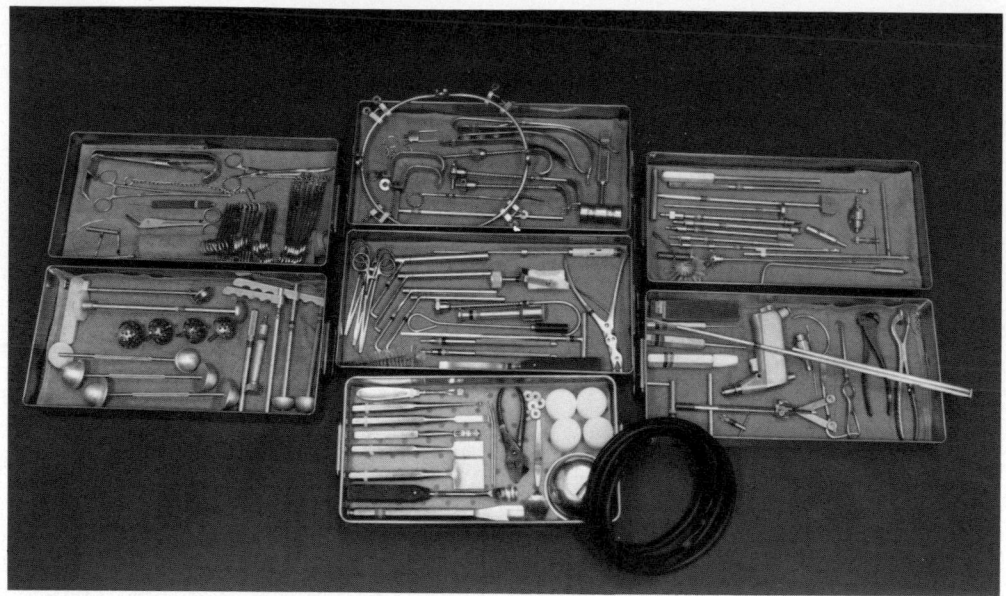

Fig. 8-21. Preprogrammed and selected instruments for total hip arthroplasty (author's method) are shown before wrapping and sterilization. The wrapped trays are delivered individually to the field according to the phases of operation in progress (see Chapters 15, 18, and 19). (From Ayer M, Stone R, Eftekhar NS: Operating room asepsis and sterilization techniques. In Eftekhar NS, editor: *Infection in joint replacement surgery*, St Louis, 1984, Mosby–Year Book.)

If the operating table or gurney has been wheeled out of the operating room, it must be cleansed before return to the operating enclosure. If it is not, it can introduce considerable contamination into the operating room (Tables 8-16 and 8-17).[106]

STERILIZATION

Sterilization of instruments and implants entails destroying all living organisms and may be accomplished by the following methods: steam, ethylene oxide (gas), and gamma radiation.

The most dependable and economical method of sterilization is steam under pressure.[226] Most instruments are prearranged in various trays and wrapped before sterilization (Fig. 8-21). Basically, all steam sterilizers function the same way. Water is heated to the boiling point and converted into steam. In the outer chamber of the sterilizer, the steam temperature is elevated by increased pressure. The sterilizing cycle is then activated, and the steam enters the inner chamber of the sterilizer. The cooler air, which is heavier than the incoming steam, is forced to the bottom of the inner chamber and removed via a steam trap. At this point, a temperature gauge is located in the discharge line. The gauge indicates increasing temperature readings, which means the air is being effectively removed from the inner chamber. When the correct temperature is achieved in the chamber, the sterilizing cycle proceeds to the timing phase. When the proper time elapses, the chamber pressure exhausts, and the cycle is completed. The effectiveness of the sterilization process is directly related to direct steam contact with the article being processed.[226]

Not all delicate equipment and prostheses are stable at the temperatures necessary to achieve steam sterilization, so a cold sterilization method using gas and often chemicals was developed. Ethylene oxide is the gas most often chosen for this purpose because of its easy availability and low toxicity compared to other gases. However, plastic material such as HDP and PMMA monomer absorbs ethylene oxide, which damages the materials and burns the tissue. Therefore radiation or gamma sterilization, which was developed for sterilizing tissues for banking, is the method of choice for sterilizing these materials. For gamma sterilization, an electron beam from a Van de Graaff or other accelerator is directed downward onto sterilizable items moving at a prescribed speed so that an amount of radiation appropriate for the thickness and size of the material may be absorbed.[30]

Sterilizers also require monitoring and daily biological testing with *Bacillus stearothermophilus* spore strips for steam sterilizers; *Bacillus subtilis* strips are suggested for ethylene oxide and gamma sterilizers.

Regardless of the method of sterilization, all sterile instruments and supplies used in the sterile area of the operating room are covered by two layers of wrapping that are sterilized with the instruments and supplies.

After use in the operating room, the instruments are taken to the autoclave area and washed free of debris in the washer-sterilizer, which is similar in appearance to the autoclave but is never used for the sterilization of packs. This process is called *decontamination* and prevents cross-contamination. Once the instruments are decontaminated in the washer-sterilizer, they are ready for ultrasonic processing. Ultrasound waves passing through the water remove or dissolve organic matter adhering to the instrument. Ultrasonic cleaning keeps the box locks and movable parts of the instruments free of debris and in good working condition.

After the instruments have been processed, they must be rinsed and thoroughly dried. The instruments are now ready for arranging into sets for sterilization. It should be noted that ultrasound processing is not a substitute for decontamination. The instrument set should be wrapped after being arranged (in open position), autoclaved, and stored in a room near the operating room suite.

SYSTEMIC USE OF ANTIBIOTICS
Historical Review

A review of early surgical experiences that explored the role of antibiotics in preventing wound infection supports the possibility that antibiotics lower the incidence of postoperative infection. In sharp contrast, however, some experiences yielded unsatisfactory results. Even some contemporary reviews have suggested that the widespread use of prophylactic antibiotics may be more harmful than beneficial, and some have suggested that their use increases the chance of infection. These reports in the early days of total joint arthroplasty unfortunately caused surgeons to be reluctant to use these agents as a prophylactic measure. In most cases, antibiotics were not administered during the perioperative period, and the times when antibiotics should be administered were not well defined. In some cases, antibiotics were used indiscriminately, for instance, only during the postoperative course.*

Early use of antibiotics, whether prophylactic or therapeutic, is important for the successful control of infection and has been well established both clinically and in laboratories.[53] If prophylactic antibiotics are to be used, the first few hours after contamination seem to be critical.[203] In fact, according to Burke's observations, to be most effective the antimicrobial agent must

* References 26, 38, 56, 79, 154, 188, 220, 236, 248, 251, 263.

be present before bacterial lodgment takes place.[53] The effectiveness of antimicrobial agents depends largely not only on the bacterial sensitivity to them but also on the presence of adequate levels of these agents in serum and tissue. In many retrospective studies[79,220,238] in which the prophylactic benefits of antibiotics were debated, the time at which the antibiotic was administered was not known or the antibiotic was not administered during the critical period as outlined by Burke. In most instances it actually was given after bacterial lodgment.

There are surprisingly few prospective studies of a random selection of patients after the administration of antibiotics. The study by Bernard and co-workers demonstrated the value of short-term prophylaxis in patients with a high-risk of infection.[38] Their work included potentially contaminated wounds (including abdominal surgery); the infection rate was lowered from 27% to 8% when chloramphenicol and penicillin were used as the prophylactic agents. Experimental studies by Alexander and co-workers,[10] Burke,[53] Bowers and co-workers,[44] and Polk and Lopez-Mayor[235] have shown that antibiotics may reduce infection during bacterial contamination of the wound. Wilson[290a] concluded that a hematoma can be penetrated by antibiotics if they are administered as late as 4 days after its formation. Others have also shown that antibiotics are capable of penetrating the interstitial fluid and even "clots" if given at the bactericidal level. Nelson and co-workers[213] have shown the ability of antibiotics to penetrate a hematoma and thereby play an important role in preventing infection during the first few hours after surgery. The extent of penetration and the efficacy of antibiotics in hematomas, wound fluids, and bone depends on the type of antibiotic and the mode of its administration.

The studies of Nelson and colleagues[213] found that both lincomycin hydrochloride and sodium oxacillin are capable of penetrating the area of the aspirating tubes within the depth of the wound, and they are found in measurable quantities regardless of the size and depth of the wound. This finding correlates well with previous studies that have shown that antibiotics are capable of penetrating interstitial fluid, wound fluid, and fibrin clots at bactericidal levels.[27–29,149,198] The Nelson and co-workers studies also substantiate the importance of antibiotics by intermittent intravenous administration over a 48-hour period.

Several studies favor the use of systemic antibiotics in orthopaedic surgery: Fogelberg and colleagues,[110] Boyd and colleagues,[45] Pavel and co-workers,[223] Erickson and colleagues,[99] and Welch and co-workers.[281a] However, because of flaws in their design, many surgeons do not consider these studies conclusive. These flaws include inadequacies of sample size or follow-up time, comparison of dissimilar clinical situations, and failure to use controls. Many other studies, however, support the systemic use of antibiotics; these conclusions were based on a large series of total hip arthroplasty cases performed by this author and by Lidwell.[174] Most surgeons in the United States (more than 87%) observed encouraging results from using antibiotic prophylaxis when performing total hip and total knee arthroplasty.[157]

An increasing number of observations in the literature indicate that hematogenous seeding of the implant occurs. Only occasionally is the same organism identified in the "source," the blood, and the joint. Nevertheless, the sudden onset of pain in a previously pain-free joint when there is evidence of infection elsewhere in the body strongly suggests hematogenous infection. Long-term antibiotic prophylaxis is justified only during a "danger period." Danger periods occur when an area of the body is obviously infected or when bacteremia is present, releasing large numbers of bacteria into the bloodstream; bacteremia results when body areas that have bacterial flora suffer trauma or substantial manipulation. The choice of antibiotics, of course, depends on the particular lesion or flora.

Time of Delivery

Although a single bacterium can produce infection in a patient whose natural resistance is sufficiently reduced, Schurman[255] found that it takes an inoculation of at least 1000 S. aureus bacteria to cause an infection in a healthy animal (a rabbit knee). Ordinarily the animal's defense mechanisms destroy smaller amounts of bacteria, restoring the animal to a "disease-free" state about 2 hours after inoculation. These 2 hours after bacterial inoculation are the *decisive period*. If large numbers of bacteria survive this period, a *stand-off* period follows when the host's defense mechanisms continue to destroy the bacteria. The body destroys bacteria at a rate similar to the reproduction rate of the surviving bacteria. This stand-off, called the *golden period*, continues for about 6 hours. When the golden period ends, the surviving bacteria reproduce exponentially, and tissue contamination grows quickly into an established infection.

It is important to note that antibiotics given in divided doses are as effective as those given continuously, because bacteria do not reproduce during their stationary growth period.[253] Antibiotics do not kill bacteria instantaneously on contact; rather their effect accumulates over a considerable time. Conversely, bacteria do not immediately resume their productivity as soon as antibiotics are withdrawn; they remain stationary for a variable number of hours, depending on the type of bacteria and the antibiotic used. After this stationary growth period, the bacteria once again resume their exponential growth.

Large doses of intravenous antibiotics are no more effective than smaller doses given at intervals in reaching tissue concentration levels adequate to kill bacteria. Additionally, large doses of antibiotics may be toxic without producing any added therapeutic effect.

The *Physician's Desk Reference* recommendations for "serious infections" are the best guide for the use of antibiotics. Although a single dose of a penicillin-like drug given at the time of bacterial inoculation annihilates a thousand times more S. aureus organisms than host defenses normally destroy, multiple doses of antibiotics started at the optimal time are more effective than a single prophylactic dose. Starting antibiotics later is less efficient and less likely to produce a good result than starting them earlier so they can be present in the tissue at the time of bacterial inoculation. They are still effective if they are begun 6 hours after the onset of bacterial contamination and continued over a period of time.

The *Physician's Desk Reference* gives the maximum effective dose of preferred antibiotics. In prescribing the loading dose (bolus) given the first time antibiotics are administered, the surgeon should follow the recommended usage. Peak antibiotic concentration in bone lags behind the serum concentration by 15 minutes or so. Antibiotics need not be started the night before surgery because adequate blood and bone concentrations will result if the medication is administered immediately before surgery.[109,223,254]

The practice of administering antibiotics much before the actual start of an operative procedure has two potentially serious disadvantages: (1) If a patient who has been administered an antibiotic on-call to the procedure develops an anaphylactic reaction, there may be no one in attendance to witness the problem, or the person in attendance may be unable to handle the problem effectively. (2) Early administration may theoretically cause propagation of antibiotic-resistant organisms.

Selecting an Antibiotic

Three factors guide the selection of prophylactic antibiotics:

1. The organism's susceptibility to common pathogens in the operating room (airborne bacteria) environment.
2. The ability of the antibiotic to affect the broadest spectrum of bacteria.
3. The bactericidal and bacteriostatic properties of the antibiotic.

Burke[53] has demonstrated that the most propitious time to administer intravenous antibacterial agents is 3 to 4 hours before bacterial lodgment occurs.

There is some concern about the wisdom of using antibiotics widely as a prophylaxis. One fear is that it will allow the bacteria responsible for nosocomial infections to change their structure and allow previously benign bacteria to mutate into virulent species.[2,147] Furthermore, they could increase the danger to a patient sensitive enough to develop a toxic reaction.[193] Altemeier[13] based his criticism of the widespread use of antibiotics on his observation of changes in the pattern of infecting organisms arising from their use:

1. Increased incidence of gram-negative infections.
2. Superimposed infections developing during the use of antibiotics.
3. Increased incidence of gram-negative infections by bacteria of low virulence.
4. Mixed bacterial infections.
5. Infections by *Candida albicans*.

Prophylaxis Against Skin Bacteria

Gram-negative organisms and other aerobic and anaerobic organisms are commonly present both in the patient's skin and in operating room air (S. *aureus* and S. *epidermidis*, for example). Thus antibiotics must be aimed at all common offenders. Studies have shown that skin normally possesses up to 1 million bacteria per square centimeter. Paradoxically, the surgeon's glove may be in greater danger of contamination from the patient's wound than the patient's wound from the surgeon's glove.

S. *aureus* coagulase-positive and S. *epidermidis* are the most common offending organisms, so prophylaxis against them is essential. S. *aureus* is the most commonly encountered organism; S. *epidermidis* accounts for a third of joint arthroplasty infections.

Although S. *epidermidis* rarely causes infection after normal operative procedures (and when it does, they are transient and insignificant), its association with infection in implant surgery is well established. Prophylaxis against this bacterium is difficult because it is resistant to several familiar and safe antibiotics: penicillin, erythromycin, clindomycin, chloramphenicol, and semisynthetic penicillins (the rates of resistance are 83%, 40%, 29%, 15%, and 15% respectively).

However, cephalosporin has been found 99% effective in routine laboratory sensitivity testing. This semisynthetic antibiotic's structure is closely related to that of penicillin and it acts by inhibiting cell-wall synthesis. It is the logical choice, being bactericidal, broad-spectrum, and relatively safe and effective against many pathogens commonly encountered in joint arthroplasty.

Surgeons have documented a significant reduction in the infection rate when cephalosporin is used in total hip arthroplasty patients. Except for the rare instance of anaphylaxis, their toxicity level is very low when used for short-term prophylaxis.

Several first-generation versions of this drug are on the market: cephalothin, cephapirin, cephradine, and cefazolin. Cefazolin, because of its higher serum peak and lower half-life, is less costly than the other first-generation drugs, requiring lower doses at less frequent intervals. Both cephazolin and cephalothin are effective against gram-positive cocci such as S. *aureus* (including penicillinase-producing strains), streptococci (except for enterococcus), and S. *epidermidis* (except some resistant strains). They are also active against gram-negative bacilli (E. *coli*, K. *pneumoniae*, P. *mirabilis*, and so on). However, they are not active against enterococci, *Enterobacter*, *Serratia*, *Pseudomonas*, *Bacteroides fragilis*, or indole-positive *Proteus* organisms.

The second generation of cephalosporins—cefamandole and cephoxitin—is less effective against staphylococci but more effective against gram-negative bacilli; cefamandole has the longest half-life in this group.

The third generation—moxalactam and cefaperazone—are especially active against P. *aeruginosa* but less effective against gram-positive cocci.

This author recommends using first-generation cephalosporins as the first line of defense; they are more effective against gram-positive cocci. The second and third generations of these antibiotics, which are effective against gram-negative organisms, should be reserved to treat organisms resistant to the first-generation cephalosporins. A single intravenous dose of 1 gm cefazolin had a half-life of 1.8 hours for normal volunteers and 48 patients undergoing total hip arthroplasty. The mean concentration in bone was 5.7 μg/gm of bone and that of synovial fluid was 24.4 μg/ml.[255]

One study found coagulase-positive S. *aureus* and S. *epidermidis* to be the most common organisms responsible for late infection in total joint arthroplasty (54%). Since the three most common organisms of late infections were from the skin (45%), dental area (15%), or urinary tract (13%), Maderazo and co-workers concluded that prophylaxis against staphylococci and E. *coli* is advisable; they are the most common pathogens when the urinary tract is the source of infection. They advocate using first-generation cephalosporins to prevent delayed infections from remote sources in total hip arthroplasty.[187]

A prospective, randomized, double-blind study comparing cefazoline with cephamandole showed that cefazolin, given at half the dose of cephamandole, appeared to be equally safe and effective despite the lower bone concentration of antibiotic.[48]

In a study of nearly 1000 total hip arthroplasties,[101] Evrard and colleagues compared the prophylactic effect of a 5-day course of cefazolin with a 2-day regimen of cephamandole. They judged the relative prophylactic effects by the degree of bacterial colonization on drains. They found no significant difference between the two groups in the percentage of infected drains. They concluded that a 2-day prophylaxis with cephamandole is effective in preventing infection in total hip arthroplasty procedures.[101] Once again, we can conclude that first-generation cephalosporins are adequate for prophylaxis; the second and third generations may be used to treat resistant infections.[85, 254]

Thus adequate serum and bone concentration can be achieved with antibiotics given in conjunction with anesthesia in the operating room.

The optimum dose and duration for prophylactic antibiotics postoperatively have not been fully established. In making this decision, the surgeon must consider the many side effects linked to lengthy trials of antibiotics. They include allergic reaction, thrombophlebitis, superimposed infection, resistant organism emergence, and drug fever; in addition, these medications can be costly. Empirically, this author advises administering antibiotics between 48 and 72 hours after primary total hip arthroplasty surgery, to continue for a minimum of 48 hours (until wound drains have been removed) and for no longer than 72 hours postoperatively. Revision surgery mandates continuing the trial of antibiotics until 5 to 7 days after the procedure, when permanent cultures have been processed and subcultures evaluated.

Two practical problems must be considered in designing a plan for antibiotic prophylaxis: (1) patient allergy to penicillin, requiring the use of alternative antibiotics, and (2) spiking fever occurring in a patient receiving antibiotics for which no cause other than infection can be found. Penicillin-allergic patients whose reaction is only a rash or an itch should be treated with cephalosporins. However, cephalosporins should be used only with caution for patients with mild delayed reaction; a safe alternative is to use vancomycin, clindamycin, or tetracycline for prophylaxis. Do not use cephalosporins on patients with a history of penicillin-induced anaphylactic shock. For such patients, short-term parenteral administration of aminoglycosides may be a good alternative.

When a patient develops a high fever while receiving antibiotic prophylaxis during the postoperative period and there is reason to suspect infection, discontinue the antibiotics to evaluate the patient for infection. If an infection is causing fever, the infecting organism is evidently invulnerable to the antibiotic, so discontinuing it will not harm the patient.

Antibiotic diarrhea is an unpleasant side effect when systemic antimicrobial agents are taken for more than 48 hours; it develops after a latency period of at least 3 days after administration. Use of cephardin, particularly when prolonged, was implicated in 16 cases of severe antibiotic-induced diarrhea. In 5 of 16 cases reviewed in one study, *Clostridium difficile*[58] caused a cross infection (clustering) among patients in the hospital. This author also observed during 1 week of his practice four patients with concurrent infection by *Clostridium difficile* caused by cephalosporin. The most serious complication of antibiotics is pseudomembranous colitis. Roberts has reported death as a complication of antibiotic prophylaxis (cephardin) for joint arthroplasty.[246]

Induced Hypotension and Antibiotic Prophylaxis

Hypotensive anesthesia is now commonly used during total hip arthroplasty, raising the question of whether it reduces the beneficial effects of antibiotics by lowering their tissue concentration. Current data suggest that while tissue concentration is reduced, the effect is not critical. Ritter and co-workers correlated the degree of tissue perfusion (soft tissue and bone) with the serum concentration of cephalosporin during total hip arthroplasty sampling. Patients received either cephalothin or cefamandole and hypotensive anesthesia using nitroprusside. Tissue concentrations of the drugs were not significantly altered compared with those in patients receiving normotensive anesthesia.

In one study, Patel and colleagues[222] determined the concentration of cephalosporin after intravenous injection in 48 patients with and without deliberately induced hypotensive anesthesia. In this way they could monitor the concentration of cephalosporin during operations, early versus late. They found that trimethaphan did not lower cephalothin concentration in serum, bone, or muscle as compared with control normotensive patients. However, when they used pentolinium as a hypotensive agent, the late serum concentration and early bone cephalothin concentrations were lowered.

LOCAL DELIVERY OF ANTIBIOTICS VIA CEMENT
Historical Review

Buchholz and Gartmann first reported the use of antibiotic-impregnated acrylic cement for prophylaxis.[51] They compared the use of systemic penicillin or erythromycin for prophylaxis in 1409 patients (with a deep wound infection rate of 3%) with a subsequent series of 2928 patients using gentamicin in the cement (with a deep wound infection rate of 0.99%). Although this was not a controlled study, the authors thought the gain from the use of gentamicin-loaded cement was significant. Buchholz and colleagues concluded that gentamicin-loaded acrylic cement may be used for prophylaxis in all cases of total hip arthroplasty where infection is present at the time of revision surgery (see Chapter 26) and that gentamicin is the preferred antibiotic for prophylaxis in primary and revision surgery.

In a prospective, controlled, and randomized (not double-blind) multicenter study of 939 patients, Josefsson investigated the prophylactic effectiveness of systemic antibiotics using gentamicin-loaded cement with a follow up of 1 year.[150] Using pain, elevation in sedimentation rate of greater than 33 mm/hour, and progressive radiographic bone resorption (not bacteriological proof) as criteria for infection, he found 13 deep infections in the systemic antibiotic group and 3 in the gentamicin-loaded acrylic cement group (P value less than 0.01).

It has been shown that acrylic cement without antibiotics had no bacteriostatic effect on S. aureus, E. coli, and Pseudomonas. Hessert and Ruckdeschel[137] showed that ampicillin and gentamicin added to methylmethacrylate were released in effective quantities, but tetracycline lost its antibacterial properties when added to methylmethacrylate cement. Also, these investigators showed that acrylic cement had no bactericidal or bacteriostatic action against S. aureus, B. cereus, E. coli, and Pseudomonas. Studies by Marks and co-workers[191] clearly demonstrated that oxacillin, gentamicin, and cefazolin are stable in both types of cement (Simplex or Palacos) and diffuse from the cement in an active form over a prolonged period. Oxacillin, cefazolin, and gentamicin were stable in acrylic cement and were released in a microbiologically active form. The three antibiotics diffused from the Palacos in larger amounts daily and for a significantly longer time than from the Simplex, indicating that the type of cement used in combination with antibiotics is very important. Palacos may be preferred because of its larger pore size in comparison with Simplex as demonstrated by scanning electron microscopy.

Bacteriostatic concentrations of oxacillin in wound hematomas were measured for 14 days after implantation of an oxacillin-Simplex combination in dogs. A high bactericidal concentration of antibiotics was measured in the surrounding bone for 21 days after implantation; the highest level (127 μg/gm) was observed 24 hours after implantation. It decreased over the 3-week experimental period but continued to be bactericidal up to 52 μg/gm of bone. In a separate study by Kolczun and co-workers[158,159] after infusion of 2 gm oxacillin, the concentration was 7.66 μg/gm; therefore this study indicates that concentrations of antibiotics observed in surrounding bone are many times greater than the level that can be achieved by intravenous infusions.

One objection to the use of antibiotic-loaded cement is the possible alteration of the mechanical properties of cement when mixed with antibiotics. Tests have shown that the addition to cement of powdered oxacillin, cefazolin, or gentamicin had no significant influence on the compressive or tensile strength either at the time of mixture or after 40 days of waterbath treatment. However, adding aqueous solutions of antibiotics to acrylic cement not only interfered with the early prepolymerizing process during mixing but also resulted in mechanically weakened cement. It was demonstrated that the alteration is caused by the water and not the antibiotic.

The theoretical objection to using an antibiotic-cement combination is the possibility of serious complications from an allergic reaction to these materials, which may eventually necessitate removing the entire combination of the cement and antibiotics, with obvious consequences. These aspects have not been studied or reported at the present time.

In evaluating the comparative role of prophylaxis by antibiotics, Petty and associates[233] used a canine model and S. aureus, S. epidermidis, and E. coli after joint arthroplasty surgery with and without bone cement. In this study, they used the antibiotics via (1) intraoperative irrigation (normal saline solution for control), (2) perioperative administration of antibiotics systemically, and (3) the addition of an antibiotic to the acrylic cement. They found that irrigation with normal saline solution did not reduce the incidence of infection. They noted a slight reduction after neomycin irrigation, but the use of bone cement containing gentamicin significantly reduced the rate of infection; no infection developed in animals treated with gentamicin-loaded acrylic cement. In an independent study on the use of gentamicin (by irrigation of the wound during total hip arthroplasty in one group and implanted in the cement in another), Sorensen also found a very high and effective concentration of antibiotic when he inserted it with cement as opposed to irrigation solution.[262] Antibiotic-loaded cement has been used for prophylaxis in Europe.[52,151,152] Investigators have reported a very low incidence of deep wound infection (0.4%) using PMMA mixed with erythromycin, collistin, and gentamicin.[145,211]

Experimental work suggests that an antibiotic-PMMA compound is capable of preventing osteomyelitis in a canine tibial model. By using gentamicin-impregnated PMMA (Palacos) cement and Palacos in bulk alone (for control using S. aureus), Fitzgerald demonstrated the ability of such compounds to prevent osteomyelitis.[105] Although gentamicin-loaded PMMA has not been approved by the Food and Drug Administration for general use at this time, using a mixture of antibiotics with cement at the surgeon's discretion is an acceptable practice.[211] Although the mechanical properties of antibiotic-loaded cement (2 gm of antibiotic added to 40 gm polymer) do not significantly reduce the mechanical strength of acrylic cement,[150,281] the fatigue life (strength) decreases considerably. The excretion pharmacokinetics of gentamicin-released cement after total hip arthroplasty show a very high concentration in urine collected for up to 60 days after surgery. Data obtained 2 years after operation suggest that the half-life of the terminal phase was much longer than calculated from data obtained during the first 60 days; the half-life was more than 240 days.[270]

Antibiotic Concentrations' Pharmacokinetics

Controversial data have been published concerning the amount of antibiotics that can elute as well as the duration of elution of antibiotics from cement. Different antibiotics and cements exhibit curious and somewhat puzzling behavior vis-à-vis how their combinations affect elution of these agents from the acrylic cement. After early in-vitro studies, Wahlig and Buchholz[275] and Nelson and Bergman[214] reported the following results:

1. Gentamicin was released in microbiologically active form from cement.
2. In-vitro release of gentamicin depended almost solely on the surface area of the mass as opposed to the volume or weight of specimens used for elution studies; adding either 0.5 or 2 gm gentamicin did not significantly affect the amount of antibiotic released, but significant antibiotics were released if the amount of antibiotic added was increased to 5 gm.
3. Release of gentamicin also depended on the amount of fluid used. Thus antibiotics were released from the outer layer of the synthetic substance; the antibiotics initially were high level and decreased in concentration within the first 3 days. The amount of gentamicin could be detected after an incubation period of 70 weeks.
4. After 1 year, the center of the cement specimen showed approximately 90% of the original amount of antibiotics, and 75% of the antibiotic was present 1 mm from the surface of the cylindrical specimen. This finding indicated that elution of antibiotics was a surface phenomenon.

Wroblewski performed a simple elution test, using salt and acrylic cement, that suggested that the elution from cement composite was entirely a surface elution phenomenon that negates the long-term effectiveness of antibiotic by prolonged leaching of the antibiotic from the acrylic cement.[292] Most studies indicate that most leaching of the antibiotic takes place within the first 24 to 72 hours and that only approximately 10% of the antibiotic is eventually released by the composite. Varying quantities of residual drug reportedly are found in the cement after antimicrobial activities have been completed. Further slow release indicates that antibiotics do not remain fixed in PMMA. They can be released at such a slow rate by a process of "perfusion," which cannot be determined by serial plate transfer tests.[214] However, a very high concentration of antibiotic can be obtained in a hematoma after surgery if the antibiotic-cement composite is used. An antibiotic delivered in this manner in high concentration is capable of saturating the surrounding tissues for a long period; even small quantities can be detected for up to 6 months. This contrasts with intravenous administration of antibiotics (in therapeutic doses) as detected in the hematoma at the operative site; intravenous delivery of antibiotics yields a greater tissue concentration than can be achieved by their maximum serum concentration in the circulating blood.[255]

Alterations in Mechanical Properties of Cement

Several investigators have shown alterations in the mechanical properties of cement, that is, the tensile, shear, and fatigue strength of PMMA.[136,205,287] It is now universally agreed that the use of antibiotic in aqueous form adversely affects the mechanical properties of the antibiotic-cement composite to a significant degree. Various investigators[169,170,274-278] agree that although detectable changes in the mechanical properties of cement occur with the addition of antibiotics, these changes are not significant when the amount of antibiotic does not exceed 2 gm per 40-gm packet of bone cement. This range alters the mechanical properties of cement far less than technical imperfections, such as admixture of blood during insertion of cement. No significant changes occurred from storing antibiotic-impregnated cement for a long period,[169,170] and only minor weaknesses resulted from elution of antibiotic from antibiotic-acrylic cement deposit.[281]

Emergence of Antibiotic-Resistant Bacteria

Concern has been expressed regarding the emergence of gentamicin-resistant coagulase-negative organisms. In a study of 91 patients with deep wound infection of a cemented total hip arthroplasty caused by coagulase-negative staphylococci, 27 showed multiple strains of coagulase-negative staphylococcus, many of which were resistant to previously used antibiotics. Hope and co-workers[140] concluded that the use of gentamicin-loaded cement in the primary operation was significantly associated with the emergence of gentamicin-resistant, coagulase-negative staphylococci.

LOCAL DELIVERY OF ANTIBIOTICS VIA IRRIGATING SOLUTIONS

Investigators have demonstrated that irrigating the wound with saline solution is inconsistent and ineffective in reducing or eliminating bacteria from the wound.[34,249,269] The theoretical advantage of using a topical antibiotic is that local application can achieve a concentration level far in excess of that achieved by other routes.[6]

Although much evidence supports the effectiveness of systemic antibiotic administration, no clinical studies substantiate the usefulness of local antibiotic application. Despite the experimental work supporting its effectiveness in the context of total joint arthroplasty, the effectiveness of local antibiotic application has never been proven. In early reports of a local deposit of antibiotic powder into the bone before the insertion of cement, there was no evidence of effectiveness.[65]

Initially, penicillin G was widely used locally. In recent years, however, antibiotics that give a broader spectrum of bacterial coverage have become more popular. Spraying the wounds during surgery with a mixture of neomycin, bacitracin, and polymyxin has been suggested to reduce the incidence of staphylococcal infections; the use of this method in neurosurgery was followed by a reduction of major infection.

Benjamin and Volz[34] observed a significant reduction in bacterial colony count by using a simple in-vitro test with saline solution as the control. Use of saline solution (without antibiotics) reduced bacterial count by 12% to 56%, but inconsistently, while use of a topical antibiotic solution (bacitracin/neomycin) was effective against S. aureus, S. epidermidis, and E. coli. Antibiotic irrigation prevented growth in all organisms tested except for persistent colonization by Pseudomonas organisms in a single plate. Samples of fat and muscle and bone assays suggest that an effective level of these antibiotics is absorbed during the course of irrigation.

Lazansky[171] and Müller[209] were early advocates of irrigating the wounds with local antibiotics in total hip arthroplasty. However, I believe that further experience is required to evaluate the role of local prophylactic antibiotic solutions and to compare their effectiveness with that of electrolyte solutions without added antibiotics in total joint arthroplasty.

Any useful prophylactic antibiotics must combat S. aureus, the most common cause of orthopaedic wound infections. In operations of long duration with considerable deep-tissue necrosis and a high frequency of deep-seated hematomas from the bone, an effective concentration of antibiotics in the wound might provide an additional margin of safety to the patient who is also receiving antibiotics systemically.

Risk of toxicity by systemic absorption of antibiotics can occur in patients whose wounds are irrigated with antibiotic solutions during surgery. Systemic neomycin absorption, with the risk of nephrotoxicity, occurred in 10 patients undergoing total hip arthroplasty.[280] In all cases of ototoxicity, nephrotoxicity, or neurotoxicity, patients had received a large amount of neomycin by continuous irrigation for a prolonged period or a single large bolus of more than 6 gm.[75,155,194] Benjamin and co-workers, in experience with more than 1000 total hip arthroplasties using a bacitracin/neomycin solution, reported none of these side effects.[34]

ECONOMIC CONSIDERATIONS

The cost of infection and the resultant disability, both to the patient and to society, is so great that every effort should be made toward sound prevention rather than treatment after the fact. In Altemeier's[13] 1967 study of 1,391,200 patients with infection, the estimated cost was $7000 per patient for each infection, a total of $9.8 million in that year. These costs are for minor infections reflecting general surgical experiences; the cost of each infected total hip must be well above $50,000 and perhaps 10 times as much in certain difficult and complex infections (see Chapter 31). Beyond the financial cost to the patient and the social impact, the misery and resulting lifelong disability are of the greatest concern.

A number of factors may influence increased capital investment in special air-handling systems and the maintenance of such equipment. This is especially important if the number of total joint operations in a given hospital is fewer than 200 per year.

A logical solution is to design an enclosure that isolates the surgical team from circulating personnel and spectators. The air entering the enclosure would be free of particles greater than 2 to 3 μm in diameter. Air pressure would be slightly positive and relatively unidirectional. Even if turbulence occurs within the enclosure, it would be acceptable since it is relatively clean. The surgical team does not contribute much to air contamination since they use impermeable all-investing gowns and hoods and a body-exhaust system. This, then, would be a "nonlaminar-flow," slightly "turbulent" but unidirectional enclosure, without the expensive equipment necessary for ultrafiltration and laminar-flow maintenance. Filtration of air particles smaller than 1 to 2 μm is not necessary because smaller particles do not appear to carry organisms, and bacteria do not suspend in air by themselves. Similarly, a horizontal-flow room may be designed to be installed in a conventional operating room without the necessity of altering the existing structure of the room. The walls may be removable (for surgeons who prefer to work without them), and existing operating lights may be used.[212,216]

While the cost and "scientific proof" of the value of air cleanliness have been challenged, if we surgeons accept aseptic techniques as essential, the concept of exposing the surgical wound only to sterile air is a fundamental principle in surgery. Despite early opposition, especially from hospital administrators and general surgeons who usually do not deal with ultraclean cases involving massive implantation of foreign bodies, the use of clean-air technology continues to grow in joint arthroplasty surgery, where infection could bring about the most catastrophic results. Abundant literature now demonstrates that the use of clean-air systems results in a marked reduction of wound contamination and a very low incidence of wound infections (0.5%) in large series of total hip procedures.[63] This reduction occurred while more than 6000 total hip arthroplasties were performed by various surgeons, including a large number of residents in training, which counters the argument that the skill of the surgeon is linked to postoperative wound infection rates. Charnley considered the cost of construction and operation of three clean-air rooms at Wrightington an effective barrier against infection.[65]

Cost of Clean-Air Systems

Obviously, the cost effectiveness of prophylaxis against infection depends on the number of arthroplasties performed each year[227] and how long that system has been in use.[138] Many surgeons have expressed concern about the cost of clean-air room systems, and indeed, some institutions have ignored the surgeons' demands on economic grounds alone. When the surgeon is doing only a small number of total hip arthroplasty operations, the difference between a low and very low rate of infection cannot be detected, especially with the often delayed appearance of infection. However, when hundreds and thousands of these operations are performed, the accumulated results of a high rate of infection can be a tremendous burden to health-care providers and institutions.

Lidwell[175] points out the accumulated cost/benefit ratio of the use of clean-air rooms, body-exhaust systems, and antibiotics. These data indicate that the hospital costs for any or all of these preventive measures (clean-air room, exhaust body suit, and prophylactic antibiotics) in avoiding sepsis are several times lower than the cost of treating a septic joint.[175–177]

Ultraviolet lights are relatively inexpensive, but they are not as effective as ultraclean air rooms, which offer no-colony-forming units/cubic meter.[174] Ultraviolet lights can produce bacterial counts of 15 CFU/m^3. In an operating room with an ordinary ventilation system, the rate is about 100 CFU/m^3. However, a justifiable cost/benefit ratio could be calculated if 200 operations are performed per year.[36]

Cost of Antibiotics

In a randomized study that followed 466 total hip arthroplasty patients for more than 4 years, Heydemann and Nelson found no difference in the infection rate related to the duration of antibiotic prophylaxis; patients received antibiotics on one of four schedules: intraoperatively only, for 48 hours, for 3 days, or for 7 days. For 100,000 patients taking antibiotics on these schedules, the savings of using antibiotics intraoperatively rather than for 48 hours would have been $7,700,000; the reduction from 7-day to one-dose antibiotics would have saved $29,700,000.[138] As stated previously, it is extremely difficult to judge the efficacy of a prophylactic antibiotic protocol when the infection rate is so low (less than 1%). Therefore this author believes that until a more comprehensive study in a large population is available, a one-dose antibiotic prophylaxis should not be considered safe or effective. This author continues to give antibiotics with administration of anesthesia and intraoperatively and for 48 hours postoperatively until the wound drains and urinary catheter have been removed.

SUMMARY OF ESSENTIALS

- Concerning infection control, three factors must be considered: (1) the number of infecting organisms at the site of the wound, (2) the virulence of the organisms, and (3) the chance association of bacteria with an area of sufficiently reduced host resistance.

- Localized or systemic reduction in host resistance is at least as important as bacterial contamination. Consequently, with the recognition that almost any bacteria may become pathogenic under certain circumstances, any effort to reduce postoperative infection must concentrate on host responses, as well as reducing bacterial contamination. Thus, one can no longer identify a harmless saprophyte merely by its morphological characteristics.

- A sound prophylaxis must address the patient's sources of contamination, environmental sources of contamination, and contamination of the wound by the surgical team.

- Among other things, old age, obesity, diabetes, poor state of nutrition, and steroid therapy increase the chances of infection.

- Above all, the urinary tract, pulmonary lesions, and silent sources of infection, especially skin, must be examined and treated before total hip arthroplasty. In this regard, a history of previous infection in the hip joint must be verified and evaluated before contemplated surgery.

- There is a causal relationship between foreign materials in the surgical wound and added risk of infection. In the presence of a foreign material, contamination of surgical wound sites by only a few bacteria is sufficient to produce infection in an experimental model.

- Infection in cemented total hip arthroplasty has certain characteristics not found in infections of noncemented implants in that infection is inevitably diagnosed even if (1) the diagnosis is not established for many months or years; (2) infection appears on x-ray film; and (3) PMMA has an affinity for attracting mildly pathogenic organisms not previously considered pathogens.

- Although the risk and scope of transient bacteremia leading to metastatic infection remain unknown, a seeding of bacteria from a distant primary source into the implanted joint can lead to a clinical infection after joint arthroplasty. Although such seeding is rare, it can occur at any time after a clean operative procedure. It generally occurs in a healthy patient with a prior successful total hip arthroplasty. A healthy patient's hip arthroplasty can become symptomatic without injury or mechanical failure. An unusual organism can be cultured from aspirate of the hip when the patient has been receiving immunosuppressive drugs. Proper documentation of hematogenous infection is necessary to prove unequivocally that an infected hip was seeded hematogenously by a remote source. The active organism in the joint must be the same as in the primary site; the clinical history must also be appropriate.

- Review of the literature indicated that gram-positive organisms were four times more common than gram-negative organisms. Many organisms in hematogenous infections of the hip joint are common in the human bacterial flora. The enteric bacilli commonly detected include those found in the oral and respiratory cavities. Others are unusual organisms not commonly found in standard forms of infections.

- There are a few bonafide cases of hematogenous seeding caused by dental manipulation. A distal infection in the foot also has been incriminated for hematogenous infection of the ipsilateral hip.

- It has been established that patients with lowered resistance to infection, particularly those with diabetes and those receiving immunosuppressive drugs, must be especially protected against postoperative infection. Other conditions that may be consistent with lowered resistance to infection include leukemia, Hodgkin's disease, rheumatoid arthritis, and systemic embolizing conditions, such as sickle cell disease. Also, massive allograft implantations are associated with a high incidence of postoperative infection.

- Biomaterials play a major role in developing infection because of the way bone responds to their chemical and physical characteristics. For example, in-vitro tests of the macrophagic activity of white blood cells have shown that PMMA inhibits phagocytosis of *Candida albicans*. All the implants and in-vivo polymerized PMMA were significantly more likely to be associated with infection than the controls, even with no implant. This association was especially strong for *S. epidermidis* and *E. coli*.

- Because bacteria are generated by and their numbers are proportional to the number of personnel within the room, bacteria-containing particles may be kept to a minimum by the use of a clean-air enclosure. The volume of filtered air entering the enclosure should be commensurate with the number of persons present and their rate of particle emission. The surgical environment should provide a positive unidirectional movement of air in a predetermined direction. The laminar nature of the flow can be disregarded because turbulence results from the air striking stationary objects.

- The use of a surgical enclosure improves discipline in operating room traffic patterns. This is critical in eliminating unnecessary, uncontrollable traffic in teaching institutions.

- Microorganisms associated with wound colonization are found on the skin and in the infected postoperative total hip arthroplasty wound. They include *S. epidermidis*, streptococcus, members of the viridans group, *S. aureus*, and other miscellaneous organisms. The direct correlation between the presence of wound colonization and the development of deep wound sepsis is highly significant.

- Operating rooms with a lower rate of exchange per minute have a higher level of airborne bacterial contamination. These rooms are cleanest when empty, so in the absence of a clean-air enclosure, surgery must be performed early in the morning when the rooms are the cleanest.

- Air contamination in the operating room may also be substantially reduced when the personnel use an all-investing hood and masks with a sectioned system (personal isolator). Ultraviolet lights can also substantially reduce air contamination in the operating room. However, the use of an enclosure seems to be a superior method because it separates the surgical wound and the team physically and it is not necessary to protect the operating personnel from the side effects of ultraviolet lights.

- Bacterial dispersion is considerably reduced (by 51%) when all personnel in the operating room wear a wraparound impervious gown instead of scrub clothes. Bacterial dispersion is reduced even further when personnel wear an all-investing gown/helmet/aspirator combined with a suction respirator. The latter is the most efficient means of controlling bacterial shedding from the head and neck, particularly when all operating room personnel wear such systems.

- It has been established that the 10-minute hand scrub is an unnecessary ritual; studies have shown that there is no difference in reducing bacterial counts with 3-, 5-, or 10-minute scrubs. The 3- to 5-minute scrub is commonly accepted.

- Most gloves have been punctured by the end of an operation, so it is essential to check them frequently for obvious tears and perforations.

- It is rational to avoid puncturing gloves during surgery and to replace them frequently. Leaving some surgical antiseptic soap on the hands at the end of the scrub period may produce some disinfecting effect, thus controlling self-contamination within the surgical gloves resulting from sweating. Surgeons must insist that all surgical members wear two pairs of high-quality gloves.

- Paradoxically, the greatest number of colonies can be cultured from the gloves used for draping, although they have no holes and have been used only for a few minutes. Therefore gloves should be changed after draping.

- Hair at the operative site should be shaved with a razor in the operating room just before the final preparation and making the incision.

- Disposable synthetic fiber gowns are the first choice for surgery and should be used at all times if available. These gowns are resistant to water and totally impervious to bacterial penetration.

- One common flaw in the operating room is the practice of exposing the instruments to the dirty air in rooms without laminar air-flow ventilating systems. These systems are most effective in eliminating surface contamination.

- Plastic drapes efficiently control bacterial contamination of the wound from the patient's skin surface.

- Splash basins serve as a breeding ground for bacteria because their large surface area acts as a settle plate. Their high incidence of positive cultures indicates that they should be eliminated from the operating room.

- A study of knife blades shows that there is no difference in the degree of contamination between the first knife and the one used after cutting the skin. More bacteria can be cultured from knives left

on the Mayo stand in conventional operating rooms than from those used in a clean-air operating room.

- To prevent bacterial contamination, the patient should be brought into the operating room on a sterile gurney. If the gurney leaves the operating room area, it must be cleaned before it is returned.

- Traditional back instrument tables are a notorious source of contamination in the operating room. Unidirectional-airflow rooms are essential when instrument tables remain exposed throughout the procedure.

- Because reusable suction tubing cannot be sterilized easily, disposable suction tubing tips are preferred.

- The large volume of air drawn from the operating room environment through the suction tip may account partly for the high rate of bacterial colonization reported in wounds during total hip arthroplasty. To prevent this contamination (1) exchange the old suction tip for a new one during the course of the operation, and (2) shut off the suction tip, and protect the suction tip in a container with a filtration system.

- The use of chemoprophylaxis in total hip arthroplasty has become an accepted practice. Transient bacteremia is not uncommon, and hematogenous seeding of organisms in a patient with low resistance is a real possibility. The choice of a specific antibiotic must be based on the prevalence of organisms in a given institution and the type of organisms commonly found in infected total hip arthroplasties.

- A combination of antibiotics effective against both gram-negative and gram-positive organisms should be selected. It should affect the broadest spectrum of bacteria, bactericidally and bacteriostatically. It has been suggested that the most propitious time to administer antibacterial agents is 3 to 4 hours before bacterial lodgement occurs. The first dose of antibiotics may be given when anesthesia is induced. The effectiveness of antimicrobial agents depends largely not only on the bacteria's sensitivity to the agents, but also on the presence of adequate levels in serum and tissue. Large doses of intravenous antibiotics are no more effective than smaller doses given at intervals in reaching tissue concentration levels adequate for bactericidal purposes. Additionally, a large dose of antibiotic may be toxic without producing any added therapeutic effect.

- Multiple doses of antibiotics started at the optimal time are more effective than a single prophylactic dose. Antibiotics are less efficient and less likely to produce a good result when they are started later than when they are present in the tissue at the time of bacterial inoculation. However, they are still effective if they are begun 6 hours after the onset of bacterial contamination and continued over time.

- Adequate bone and blood concentration results if antibiotics are administered immediately before surgery. The practice of administering them the night before an operative procedure has two serious disadvantages: (1) possible anaphylactic reaction at a time when no one is present to witness the problem; (2) early administration may produce organisms resistant to antibiotics.

- Because they are more effective against gram-positive cocci, first-generation cephalosporins are the first line of defense. The second and third generations of these antibiotics are not commonly used for prophylaxis. They should be used cautiously and only for organisms that are resistant to first-generation cephalosporins. Except for rare instances of anaphylaxis, their toxicity level is very low when used for short-term prophylaxis. Antibiotics should be discontinued 48 to 72 hours after primary total hip arthroplasty. In the case of revision surgery, antibiotics should be continued for 5 to 7 days after permanent cultures have been processed and subcultures evaluated.

- Widespread and prolonged use of antibiotics can lead to (1) increased incidence of gram-negative infections; (2) superimposed infections; (3) increased incidence of gram-negative infections by bacteria of low vigilance; (4) mixed bacterial infections; (5) infections by *Candida albicans*; (6) an increased number of infections from L-forms and other atypical bacterial forms.

- Antibiotic diarrhea is an unpleasant side effect when systemic antimicrobial agents are taken for more than 48 hours; it develops after a latency period of at least 3 days after administration of the antibiotics.

- Hypotensive anesthesia may reduce antibiotic tissue concentration, but the effect is not critical and not significantly different from the tissue concentration associated with normotensive anesthesia. However, it has been found that patients taking trimethaphan did not have lower cephalothin concentration in serum, bone, or muscle compared with controlled normotensive patients. However, use of pentolinium as a hypotensive agent produced late serum concentration and lowered early bone cephalothin concentration.

- At this time, no definitive data support the effectiveness of cement in combination with antibiotics in preventing infection, although this has been suggested by a few centers. The type of cement used in combination with antibiotics is very important. Palacos may be preferred over Simplex because of its larger pore size as demonstrated by scanning electromicroscopy.

- A theoretical objection to using an antibiotic-cement combination is the possibility of serious allergic reaction and the emergence of antibiotic-resistant organisms. In practice, an allergic reaction has not been reported. Nevertheless, the emergence of a strain of S. *epidermidis* resistant to antibiotics has been reported.

- Routine use of gentamicin-loaded cement in the primary operation is significantly associated with emergence of gentamicin-resistant, coagulase-negative staphylococci.

- Much evidence supports the effectiveness of systemic antibiotic administration, but no clinical studies have substantiated the usefulness of irrigating the wounds with a local antibiotic. Evidently, further experience is required to evaluate the place of local prophylactic antibiotic solutions and to compare their effectiveness to electrolyte solutions without antibiotics in total joint arthroplasty.

- Systemic neomycin absorption, with the risk of nephrotoxicity, can occur in patients undergoing total hip arthroplasty when wounds are irrigated by a combination of neomycin and other antibiotics. In all cases of autotoxicity, nephrotoxicity, or neurotoxicity, patients received a large amount of neomycin by continuous irrigation for a prolonged period or a single large bolus of more than 6 gm. None of the above complications have been reported when using bacitracin-neomycin solutions.

- The cost of clean-air rooms, body-exhaust systems, and antibiotics is several times lower than the cost of treating a septic joint, provided that 200 operations are performed per year. The cost of using antibiotics perioperatively for a short duration is quite small, and the gain is significant compared with any other method.

- Prevention of infection is a multifaceted and complex problem. A germ-free human is not healthy; a germ-free wound may not be possible. No single technique, prophylaxis measure, or germicide can produce an effective "infection-free" situation. Attention to countless details is necessary to minimize postoperative wound infection.

REFERENCES

1. **Ackerknecht EH**: *A short history of medicine*, Baltimore, 1982, Johns Hopkins University Press.
2. **Adler JL, Burke JP, Finland M**: Infection and antibiotic usage at Boston City Hospital, January, 1970, *Arch Intern Med* 127:460, 1971.
3. **Aglietti P, Salvati EA, Wilson PD Jr, et al**: Effect of a

surgical horizontal unidirectional filtered air flow unit on wound bacterial contamination and wound healing, *Clin Orthop* 101:99, 1974.

4. **Ahlberg A, Carlsson AS, Lindberg L**: Hematogenous infection in total joint replacement, *Clin Orthop* 137:69, 1978.

5. **Ainscow DA, Denham RA**: The risk of haematogenous infection in total joint replacements, *J Bone Joint Surg* 66[Br]:580, 1984.

6. **Alexander JW, Alexander NS**: The influence of route of administration on wound fluid concentration of prophylactic antibiotics, *J Trauma* 16:488, 1976.

7. **Alexander JW, Good RA**: *Immunobiology for surgeons*, Philadelphia, 1970, WB Saunders.

8. **Alexander JW, Kaplan JZ, Altemeier WA**: Role of suture materials in the development of wound infections, *Ann Surg* 165:192, 1967.

9. **Alexander JW, Meakins JL**: Natural defense mechanisms in clinical sepsis, *J Surg Res* 11:148, 1971.

10. **Alexander JW, Sykes NS, Mitchell MM, et al**: Concentration of selected intravenously administered antibiotics in experimental surgical wounds, *J Trauma* 13:423, 1973.

11. **Alford DJ, Ritter MA, French MLV, et al**: The operating room gown as a barrier to bacterial shedding, *Am J Surg* 125:589, 1973.

12. **Allen BL Jr, Higgins MV, Goldner JL**: Current status of ultraviolet radiation in operating room. In The Hip Society: *Proceedings of the second open scientific meeting of The Hip Society*, St Louis, 1974, Mosby–Year Book.

13. **Altemeier WA**: The significance of infection in trauma, *Bull Am Coll Surg* 57:7, 1972.

14. **American College of Surgeons**: *Manual on control of infection in surgical patients*, Philadelphia, 1976, JB Lippincott.

15. **Amstutz HC**: Treatment of sepsis in total hip replacement. In *American Academy of Orthopaedic Surgeons instructional course lectures*, vol 23, St. Louis, 1974, Mosby–Year Book.

16. **Amstutz HC**: High velocity directional air flow systems (HVDAFS). Status of "clean air rooms," *West J Med* 122:154, 1975.

17. **Amstutz HC, Irvine R, Johnson BL Jr**: The relationship of genitourinary tract procedures and deep sepsis after total hip replacements, *Surg Gynecol Obstet* 139:701, 1974.

18. **Andersen AA**: A new sampler for the collection, sizing, and enumerations of viable airborne particles, *J Bacteriol* 76:471, 1958.

19. **Andrews HJ, Arden GP, Hart GM**: Deep infection after total hip replacement, *J Bone Joint Surg* 63[Br]:53, 1981.

20. **Association of Operating Room Nurses**: AORN standards for OR wearing apparel, draping, and gowning material, *AORN J* 21:1223, 1975.

21. **Association of Operating Room Nurses**: AORN standards for OR surgical hand scrub, *AORN J* 21:594, 1976.

22. **Austin PR**: *Design and operation of clean rooms*, rev ed, Detroit, Detroit Business News Publishing.

23. **Ayliffe GA, Collins BJ, Lowbury EJL, et al**: Ward floors and other surfaces as reservoirs of hospital infection, *J Hyg* (Camb.) 65:515, 1967.

24. **Baird TV, Nickel FR, Thrupp LD, et al**: Splash basin contamination in orthopaedic surgery, *Clin Orthop* 187:129, 1984.

25. **Baldini N, Tuni A, Greggi T, et al**: Deep sepsis from *Mycobacterium tuberculosis* after total hip replacement, case report, *Acta Orthop Trauma Surg* 107:186, 1988.

26. **Barnes J, Pace WG, Trump DS, et al**: Prophylactic postoperative antibiotics, *Arch Surg* 79:190, 1959.

27. **Barza M, Brusch J, Bergeron MG, et al**: Penetration of antibiotics into fibrin loci in vivo. III. Intermittent vs. continuous infusion and the effect of probenecid, *J Infect Dis* 129:73, 1974.

28. **Barza M, Samuelson T, Weinstein L**: Penetration of antibiotics into fibrin loci in vivo. II. Comparison of nine antibiotics: effect of dose and degree of protein binding. *J Infect Dis* 129:66, 1974.

29. **Barza M, Weinstein L**: Penetration of antibiotics into fibrin loci in vivo. I. Comparison of penetration of ampicillin into fibrin clots, abscesses, and interstitial fluid, *J Infect Dis* 129:59, 1974.

30. **Bassett CAL, Packard AG Jr**: A clinical assay of cathode ray sterilized cadaver bone graft, *Acta Orthop Scand* 28:198, 1959.

31. **Bayston R, Milner RDG**: The sustained release of antimicrobial drugs from bone cement, *J Bone Joint Surg* 64[Br]:4, 1982.

32. **Beck WC, Collete TS**: False faith in the surgeon's gown and surgical drape, *Am J Surg* 83:125, 1952 (editorial).

33. **Beckenbaugh RD, Ilstrup DM**: Total hip arthroplasty, *J Bone Joint Surg* 60:306, 1978.

34. **Benjamin JB, Volz RG**: Efficacy of a topical antibiotic irrigant in decreasing or eliminating bacterial contamination in surgical wounds, *Clin Orthop* 184:114, 1984.

35. **Benner EJ**: The use and abuse of antibiotics—1967, *J Bone Joint Surg* 49:977, 1967.

36. **Berg M, Bergman BR, Hoborn J**: Shortwave ultraviolet radiation in operating rooms, *J Bone Joint Surg* 718:483, 1989.

37. **Bernard HR**: The effect of scrub time on hand antisepsis using povidone-iodine surgical scrub for 3-, 5-, 10- minute scrubs. In Polk HC, Ehrenkranz NJ, editors: *Therapeutic advances and new clinical implications: medical and surgical antisepsis with Betadine microbicides*, Norwalk, Conn, 1972, Purdue Frederick.

38. **Bernard HR, Cole WR**: The prophylaxis of surgical infection: the effect of prophylactic antimicrobial drugs on the incidence of infection following potentially contaminated operations, *Surgery* 56:151, 1964.

39. **Bernard HR, Cole WR, Gravens DL**: Reduction of iatrogenic bacterial contamination in operating rooms, *Ann Surg* 165:609, 1967.

40. **Bigliani LU, Stinchfield FE**: Hematogenous infection of total joint replacement. In Eftekhar NS, editor: *Infection in joint replacement surgery: prevention and management*, St Louis, 1984, Mosby–Year Book.

41. **Blomgren G, Lundquist H, Nord CE, et al**: Late anaerobic haematogenous infection of experimental total joint replacement: a study in the rabbit using *Propionibacterium acnes*, *J Bone Joint Surg* 63[Br]:614, 1981.

42. **Blomgren G, Svensson O, Nord CE**: *Peptostreptococcus magnus* does not cause hematogenous infections in experimental arthroplasties, *Clin Orthop* 241:248, 1989.

43. **Booth JE, Jacobson JA, Kurrus TA, et al**: Infection of prosthetic arthroplasty by *Mycobacterium fortuitum*, *J Bone Joint Surg* 61:300, 1979.

44. **Bowers WH, Wilson FC, Greene WB**: Antibiotic prophylaxis in experimental bone infections, *J Bone Joint Surg* 55:795, 1973.

45. **Boyd RJ, Burke JF, Colton T**: A double-blind clinical trial of prophylactic antibiotics in hip fractures, *J Bone Joint Surg* 55:1251, 1973.

46. **Bradburn NC, French MLV, Ritter MA**: Dress combinations and laminar flow as they relate to contamination at wound height, *Surg Team* 4:30, 1973.

47. **Brady LP, Enneking WF, Franco JA**: The effect of operating-room environment on the infection rate after Charnley low-friction total hip replacement, *J Bone Joint Surg* 57:80, 1975.

48. **Bryan CS, Morgan SL, Caton RJ, et al**: Cefazolin versus cefamandole for prophylaxis during total joint arthroplasty, *Clin Orthop* 228:117, 1988.

49. **Buchberg H**: Management of the air environment of operating rooms. In *American Academy of Orthopaedic Surgeons instructional course lectures*, vol 23, St Louis, 1974, Mosby–Year Book.

50. **Buchberg H, Amstutz HC, Wright JD, et al**: Evaluation and optimum use of directed horizontal filtered air flow for surgeries, *Clin Orthop* 111:151, 1975.

51. **Buchholz HW, Gartmann HD**: Infektionsprophylaxe und operative Behandlung der schleichenden tiefen Infektion bei der totalen Endoprothese, *Chirurg* 43:453, 1972.

52. **Buchholz HW, Elson RA, Heinert K:** : Antibiotic loaded acrylic cement: current concept, *Clin Orthop* 190:96, 1984.

53. **Burke JF**: The effective period of preventive antibiotic action in experimental incisions and dermal lesions, *Surgery* 50:161, 1961.

54. **Burke JF**: Identification of the sources of staphylococci contaminating the surgical wound during operation, *Ann Surg* 158:898, 1963.

55. **Burke JF**: Factors predisposing to infection in surgical patients. In Maibach III, Hildick-Smith G, editors: *Skin bacteria and their role in infection*, New York, 1965, McGraw-Hill.

56. **Busch H, Lane M**: *Chemotherapy*, Chicago, 1967, Year Book Medical Publishers.

57. **Butterfield WC**: Puncture wounds in surgical gloves, *Conn Med J* 34:180, 1970.

58. **Cannon SR, Dyson PHP, Sanderson PJ:** Pseudomembranous colitis associated with antibiotic prophylaxis in orthopaedic surgery, *J Bone Joint Surg* 70[Br] 600, 1988.

59. **Carpendale MT, Sereda W**: The role of the percutaneous suture in surgical wound infection, *Surgery* 58:672, 1965.

60. **Charnley J**: A sterile-air operating theater enclosure, *Br J Surg* 51:195, 1964.

61. **Charnley J**: *Instructions for using the Charnley ventilated operating gown and mask*, internal publication no. 22, Wrightington, England, 1969, Centre for Hip Surgery, Wrightington Hospital.

62. **Charnley J**: Postoperative infection after total hip replacement with special reference to air contamination in the operating room, *Clin Orthop* 87:167, 1972.

63. **Charnley J**: *Low-friction arthroplasty of the hip: theory and practice*, New York, 1979, Springer-Verlag.

64. **Charnley J, Eftekhar N**: Penetration of gown material by organisms from the surgeon's body, *Lancet* 1:172, 1969.

65. **Charnley J, Eftekhar N**: Postoperative infection in total prosthetic replacement arthroplasty of the hip-joint. With special reference to the bacterial content of the air of the operating room, *Br J Surg* 56:641, 1969.

66. **Cioffi GA, Terezhalmy GT, Taybos GM**: Total joint replacement: a consideration for antimicrobial prophylaxis, *Oral Surg* 66:124, 1988.

67. **Cole WR, Bernard HR**: Inadequacies of present methods of surgical skin preparation, *Arch Surg* 89:215, 1964.

68. **Cook R, Boyd NA**: Reduction of the microbial contamination of surgical wound areas by sterile laminar air flow, *Br J Surg* 58:48, 1971.

69. **Coriell LL, Blakemore WS, McGarrity GJ**: Medical applications of dust free rooms. II. Elimination of airborne bacteria from an operating theater, *JAMA* 203:1038, 1968.

70. **Cown WB, Kethley TW**: In *proceedings, Fifth Annual Technical Meeting*, Boston, Mass, 1966.

71. **Crooks LC, editor**: *Operating room techniques for the surgical team*, Boston, 1979, Little Brown.

72. **Cruse PJE**: *Postoperative study of 20,105 surgical wounds with emphasis on use of topical antibiotics and prophylactic antibiotics*. Paper presented at the fourth symposium on control of surgical infection, Washington DC, November 10, 1972.

73. **Cutcher JL, Goldberg JR, Lilly GE, et al**: Control of bacteremia associated with extraction of teeth. II. *Oral Surg* 31:602, 1971.

74. **D'Ambrosia RD, Shoji H, Heater R**: Secondarily infected total joint replacement by hematogenous spread, *J Bone Joint Surg* 58:450, 1976.

75. **Davis JE, Siemsen AW, Anderson RW**: Uremia, deafness, and paralysis due to irrigating antibiotic solutions, *Arch Intern Med* 125:135, 1970.

76. **Davies PD, Humphries MJ, Byfield SP, et al**: Bone and joint tuberculosis. A survey of notifications in England and Wales, *J Bone Joint Surg* 166[Br]:326, 1984.

77. **Davies RR, Noble WC**: Dispersal of bacteria on desquamated skin, *Lancet* 2:1295, 1962.

78. **Delpech JM**: *Memoire sur la complication des plaises et das ulceres, commue sous le nom de pourriture d'hospital: suive du rapport fait à la premier classe de L'Institut royal de Francii par M.M. Portal et Deschamps, le 31 Octobre, 1814*, Paris, 1815, Meguignon-Maruig.

79. **Derian PS, Green BM**: Postoperative wound infections— 5-year review of 1,163 consecutive operative orthopaedic patients, *Am Surg* 32:388, 1966.

80. **Dineen P**: An evaluation of the duration of the surgical scrub, *Surg Gynecol Obstet* 129:1181, 1969.

81. **Dineen P**: Penetration of surgical draping material by bacteria, *Hospitals* 43:931, 1969.

82. **Dineen P**: Microbial filtration by surgical masks, *Surg Gynecol Obstet* 133:812, 1971.

83. **Dineen P**: The role of impervious drapes and gowns in preventing surgical infection, *Clin Orthop* 96:210, 1973.

84. **Dineen P, Drusin L**: Epidemics of postoperative wound infections associated with hair carriers, *Lancet* 2:1157, 1973.

85. **DiPiro JT, Record KE, Bivins BA**: Evaluation of new cephalosporins for prophylaxis of surgical infection, *Clin Pharmacol* 1:135, 1982.

86. **Drill VA**: *Pharmacology in medicine, a collaborative textbook*, ed 2, New York, 1958, McGraw-Hill.

87. **Duguid JP, Wallace AT**: Air infection with dust liberated from clothing, *Lancet* 2:845, 1948.

88. **Dupont JA**: Significance of operative cultures in total hip arthroplasty, *Clin Orthop* 211:122, 1986.

89. **Earle AS**: The germ theory in America: antesepsis and asepsis (1867–1900), *Surgery* 65:508, 1969.

90. **Edlich RF, Tsung MS, Rogers W**: Studies in management of the contaminated wound. I. Technique of closure of such wounds together with a note on a reproducible experimental model, *J Surg Res* 8:585, 1968.

91. **Eftekhar NS**: Operating room design, ventilation, and clothing as factors in infection control, *Hosp Top* 50:69, 1972.

92. **Eftekhar NS**: The surgeon and clean air in the operating room, *Clin Orthop* 96:188, 1973.

93. **Eftekhar NS**: Controversy of clean air and total hip replacement. In The Hip Society: *the hip: proceedings of the second open scientific meeting of The Hip Society*, St Louis, 1974, Mosby–Year Book.

94. **Eftekhar NS**: Sepsis in total hip replacement: prevention and management. In *American Academy of Orthopaedic Surgeons instructional course lectures*, vol 23, St Louis, 1974, Mosby–Year Book.

95. **Eftekhar NS**: *Principles of total hip arthroplasty*, St Louis, 1978, Mosby–Year Book.

96. **Eftekhar NS, Smith DM, Henry JH, et al**: Revision arthroplasty using Charnley low-friction arthroplasty technic. With reference to specifics of technic and comparison of results with primary low friction arthroplasty, *Clin Orthop* 95:48, 1973.

97. **Eitzen HE, Ritter MA, French MV, et al**: A microbiological in-use comparison of surgical hand-washing agents, *J Bone Joint Surg* 61:403, 1979.

98. **Elek SD, Conen PE**: The virulence of *Staphylococcus pyogenes* for man. A study of the problems of wound infection, *Br J Exp Pathol* 38:573, 1957.

99. **Erickson C, Lidgren L, Lindberg L**: Cloxacillin in the prophylaxis of postoperative infections of the hip, *J Bone Joint Surg* 55:808, 1973.

100. **Everett WG**: Suture materials in general surgery, *Progr Surg* 8:14, 1970.

101. **Evrard J, Duyon F, Acar JF, et al**: Two-day cefamandole versus five-day cephazolin prophylaxis in 965 total hip replacements. Report of a multicentre double blind randomised trial, *Int Orthop* 12:69, 1988.

102. **Fairclough JA, Johnson D, Mackie I**: The prevention of wound contamination by skin organisms by the preoperative application of an iodophor-impregnated plastic adhesive drape, *J Int Med Res* 14:105, 1986.

103. **Favero MS, Puleo JR, Marshall JH, et al**: Comparison of microbial contamination levels among hospital operating rooms and industrial clean rooms. *Appl Microbiol* 16:480, 1968.

104. **Finegold SM, George WL, Mulligan ME**: Anaerobic infections, II. In Cotsonas NJ, editor: *Disease-a-month*, vol 31, Chicago, 1985, Year Book Medical Publishers.

105. **Fitzgerald RH Jr**: Experimental osteomyelitis: description of a canine model and the role of depot administration of antibodies in the prevention and treatment of sepsis, *J Bone Joint Surg* 65:371, 1983.

106. **Fitzgerald RH Jr, Peterson LF**: Wound colonization in deep wound sepsis. In Eftekhar NS, editor: *Infection in total joint replacement surgery: prevention and management*, St Louis, 1984, Mosby–Year Book.

107. **Fitzgerald RH, Peterson LF, Washington JA II, et al**: Bacterial colonization of wounds and sepsis in total hip arthroplasty, *J Bone Joint Surg* 55:1242, 1973.

108. **Fitzgerald RH Jr, Washington JA II**: Contamination of the operative wound, *Orthop Clin North Am* 6:1105, 1975.

109. **Fitzgerald RH Jr, et al**: (M. J. Patzakis, moderator): The use of antibiotics, *Contemp Orthop* 2:348, 1980.

110. **Fogelberg EV, Zitzmann EK, Stinchfield FE**: Prophylactic penicillin in orthopaedic surgery, *J Bone Joint Surg* 52:95, 1970.

111. **Ford CR, Peterson DE, Mitchell CR**: An appraisal of the role of surgical face masks, *Am J Surg* 113:787, 1967.

112. **Ford CR, Peterson DE, Mitchell CR**: Microbiological studies of air in the operating room, *J Surg Res* 7:376, 1967.

113. **Fox DG, Baldwin M**: Contamination levels in a laminar flow operating room, *Hospitals* 42:108, 1968.

114. **Francis T**: Response of the host to the parasite. In Dubos RJ, editor: *Bacterial and mycotic infections in man*, ed 2, Philadelphia 1962, JB Lippincott.

115. **Friedman RJ**: Infection in total joint arthroplasty for distal intravenous lines. A case report, *J Arthroplasty* 35:69, 1988.

116. **French ML, Eitzen HE, Ritter MA**: The plastic surgical adhesive drape: an evaluation of its efficacy as a microbial barrier, *Ann Surg* 184:46, 1976.

117. **Geddes AM, Davey PG**: The compromised host and antibacterial treatment, *Scand J Infect Dis* 23(suppl): 161, 1980.

118. **Glynn MK, Sheehan JM**: The significance of asymptomatic bacteriuria in patients undergoing hip/knee arthroplasty, *Clin Orthop* 185:151, 1984.

119. **Goldner JL, Allen BL Jr**: Ultraviolet light in orthopedic operating rooms at Duke University, thirty-five years' experience, 1837 to 1973, *Clin Orthop* 96:195, 1973.

120. **Goldner JL, Lowell JD**: *Ultraviolet light in orthopaedic operating suites*, presented at American Academy of Orthopaedic Surgeons' Meeting, scientific exhibit, 1975.

121. **Gomez-Reino JJ, Shah M, Gorevic P, et al**: *Pasteurella multocida* arthritis. A case report, *J Bone Joint Surg* 62:1212, 1980.

122. **Goodrich EO Jr, Whitfield WW**: Air environment in the operating room, *Bull Am Coll Surg* 55:7, 1970.

123. **Goodrich EO Jr, Whitfield WW, Blakemore WS, et al**: Laminar clean air flow in operating rooms, *Bull Am Coll Surg* 58:9, 1973.

124. **Gould JC, Bone FJ, Scott JH**: The bacteriology of surgical theatres with and without unidirectional airflow, *Bull Soc Int Chir* 33:53, 1974.

125. **Greenough CG**: An investigation into contamination of operative suction, *J Bone Joint Surg* 68[Br]:151, 1986.

126. **Ha'eri GB, Wiley AM**: The efficacy of standard surgical face masks: an investigation using "tracer particles," *Clin Orthop* 148:160, 1980.

127. **Ha'eri GB, Wiley AM**: Wound contamination through drapes and gowns. A study using tracer particles, *Clin Orthop* 154:181, 1981.

128. **Hall BB, Fitzgerald RH Jr, Rosenblatt JE**: Anaerobic osteomyelitis, *J Bone Joint Surg* 65:30, 1983.

129. **Hanson PG, Standridge J, Jarrett F, et al**: Freshwater wound infection due to *Aeromonas hydrophila*, *JAMA* 238:1053, 1977.

130. **Hart D**: Sterilization of the air in the operating room by special bactericidal radiant energy. Results of its use in extrapleural thoracoplasties, *J Thorac Cardiovasc Surg* 6:45, 1936.

131. **Hart JB, French ML, Eitzen HE, et al**: Rodac plate-holding device for sampling surfaces during surgery, *Appl Microbiol* 26:417, 1973.

132. **Hart D, Nicks J**: Ultraviolet radiation in the operating

room. Intensities used and bactericidal effects, *Arch Surg* 82:449, 1961.

133. **Hecht RH, Meyers MH, Thornhill-Joynes M, et al**: Reactivation of tuberculosis infection following total joint replacement. A case report, *J Bone Joint Surg* 65:1015, 1983.

134. **Heifetz CJ, Richards FO, Lawrence MS**: Comparison of wound healing with and without dressings; experimental study. *AMA Arch Surg* 65:746, 1952.

135. **Herold RC, Lotke PA, MacGregor RR**: Prosthetic joint infections secondary to rapidly growing *Mycobacterium fortuitum, Clin Orthop* 216:183, 1987.

136. **Hessert GR**: Bruchfestigkeit und Struktur des Knochemzementes Palacos nach Zusatz von Gentamycin-Sulfat, *Arch Orthop Unfallchir* 69:289, 1971.

137. **Hessert GR, Ruckdeschel G**: Antibiotiche Wirksamkeit von Mischungen des Polymethylmethacrylates mit Antibiotica, *Arch Orthop Unfallchir* 68:249, 1970.

138. **Heydemann JS, Nelson CL**: Short-term preventive antibiotics, *Clin Orthop* 205:184, 1986.

139. **Hill J, Howell A, Blowers R**: Effects of clothing on dispersal of *Staphylococcus aureus* by males and females, *Lancet* 2:1131, 1974.

140. **Hope PG, Kristinsson KG, Norman P, et al**: Deep infection of cemented total hip arthroplasties caused by coagulase-negative staphylococci, *J Bone Joint Surg* 71[Br]:851, 1989.

141. **Hopton DS**: Investigation of wound protection by a sterile laminar air curtain, *J R Coll Surg Edinb* 19:98, 1974.

142. **Inman RD, Gallegos KV, Brause BD, et al**: Clinical and microbial features of prosthetic joint infection, *Am J Med* 77:47, 1984.

143. **Irvine RD, Amstutz HC**: Studies of airborne bacteria in the operating room, *Surg Forum* 23:457, 1972.

144. **Irvine R, Johnson BL Jr, Amstutz HC**: The relationship of genitourinary tract procedures and deep sepsis after total hip replacement, *Surg Gynecol Obstet* 139:701, 1974.

145. **Isacson J, Collert S**: Renal impairment after high doses of dicloxacillin-prophylaxis in joint replacement surgery, *Acta Orthop Scand* 55:407, 1984.

146. **Jacobson JJ, Matthews LS**: Bacteria isolated from late prosthetic joint infections: dental treatment of chemoprophylaxis, *Oral Med Oral Pathol* 63:122, 1987.

147. **Johnson BL Jr**: Prevention and treatment of sepsis: bacteriologic analysis of "laminar flow" operating room and the use of antibiotics. In *American Academy of Orthopaedic Surgeons instructional course lectures*, vol 23, St Louis, 1974, Mosby–Year Book.

148. **Johnson R, Barnes JK, Owen R**: Reactivation of tuberculosis after total hip replacement, *J Bone Joint Surg* 61[Br]:148, 1979.

149. **Joos RW, Kading WH, Hall WH**: Effect of antibiotics on growth of staphylococci in plasma clots, *Am J Med Sci* 253:305, 1967.

150. **Josefsson G**: Gentamicin-impregnated bone cement in total hip replacement: prevention and treatment of deep infection. Dissertation. Gävle, 1980, Westlund & Söner Boktryckeri AB.

151. **Josefsson G**: Prevention and treatment of deep infection following total hip replacement, *Can J Surg* 26:405, 1983.

152. **Josefsson G, Lindberg L, Wiklander B**: Systemic antibiotics and gentamicin-containing bone cement in the prophylaxis of postoperative infection of total hip arthroplasty, *Clin Orthop* 159:194, 1981.

153. **Kamme C, Lindberg L**: Aerobic and anaerobic bacteria in deep infections after total hip arthroplasty: differential diagnosis between infectious and non-infectious loosening, *Clin Orthop* 154:201, 1981.

154. **Karl RC, Mertz JJ, Veith FJ, et al**: Prophylactic antimicrobial drugs in surgery, *N Engl J Med* 275:305, 1966.

154a. **Kellgren JH, Ball J, Fairbrother RW, et al**: Suppurative arthritis complicating rheumatoid arthritis, *Br Med J* 1:1193, 1958.

155. **Kelly DR, Nilo ER, Berggren RB**: Brief recording: deafness after topical neomycin wound irrigation, *N Engl J Med* 280:1338, 1969.

156. **Ketover BP, Young LS, Armstrong D**: Septicemia due to *Aeromonas Hydrophila*: clinical and immunologic aspects, *J Infect Dis* 127:284, 1973.

157. **Kittay W, editor**: O.R. survey signs most orthopaedic surgeons use regularly, *Orthop Rev* 3:56, 1974.

158. **Kolczun MC, Nelson CL**: Antibiotic concentration in human bone. In The Hip Society: *Proceedings of the second open scientific meeting of The Hip Society, 1974,* St Louis, 1974, Mosby–Year Book.

159. **Kolczun MC, et al**: Antibiotic concentration in human bone, a preliminary report, *J Bone Joint Surg* 56:305, 1974.

160. **Krizek TJ, Davis JH**: The role of the red cell in subcutaneous infection, *J Trauma* 5:85, 1965.

161. **Krizek TJ, Davis JH**: Endogenous wound infection, *J Trauma* 6:239, 1966.

162. **Laufman H**: The surgeon views environmental controls in the operating room, *Hosp Top* 47:73, 1969.

163. **Laufman H**: Current status of special air-handling systems in operating rooms, *Med Instrum* 7:7, 1973.

164. **Laufman H**: Surgical hazard control. Effect of architecture and engineering, *Arch Surg* 107:552, 1973.

165. **Laufman H**: Architectural and engineering aspects of the operating room environment, *Bull Soc Int Chir* 33:1, 1974.

166. **Laufman H, Eudy WW, Vanderroot AM, et al**: Strikethrough of moist contamination by woven and nonwoven surgical materials, *Ann Surg* 181:857, 1975.

167. **Launder WJ, Hungerford DS**: Late infection of total hip arthroplasty with *Propionibacterium acnes*: a case and review of the literature, *Clin Orthop* 257:170, 1981.

168. **Laurence M**: Ultra-clean air, *J Bone Joint Surg* 65[Br]:375, 1983.

169. **Lautenschlager EP, Jacobs JJ, Marshall GW, et al**: Mechanical properties of bone cements containing large doses of antibiotic powders, *J Biomed Mater Res* 10:929, 1976.

170. **Lautenschlager EP, Marshall GW, Marks KE, et al**: Mechanical strength of acrylic bone cements impregnated with antibiotics, *J Biomed Mater Res* 10:837, 1976.

171. **Lazansky MG**: Complications revisited. The debit side of total hip replacement, *Clin Orthop* 95:96, 1973.

172. **Leak ES, Wright JG, Gristina AG**: Comparative study of the adherence of alveolar and peritoneal macrophages, and of blood monocytes to methyl methacrylate polyethylene, stainless steel and Vitallium, *J Reticuloendothelial Soc*, 30:403, 1981.

173. **Letts RM, Doermer E**: Conversation in the operating theater as a cause of airborne bacterial contamination, *J Bone Joint Surg* 65:357, 1983.

174. **Lidwell OM, Lowbury EJ, Whyte W, et al**: Effect of

ultra-clean air in operating rooms on deep sepsis in the joint after total hip or knee replacement: a randomised study, *Br Med J* 285:10, 1982.

175. **Lidwell OM**: The cost implications of clean air systems and antibiotic prophylaxis in operations for total joint replacement, *Infect Control* 5:36, 1984.

176. **Lidwell OM**: Air, antibiotics and sepsis in replacement joints, *J Hosp Infect* 11(suppl C):18, 1988.

177. **Lidwell OM**: The economics of sepsis control, *J Hosp Infect* 11:97, 1988.

178. **Lidwell OM, William REO, Schuter RA, editors**: Methods of investigation and analysis of results—infection in hospitals. Symposium of UNESCO and the WHO, Oxford, 1963, Blackwell Scientific Publications.

179. **Lidwell OM, Lowbury EJL, Whyte W, et al**: Bacteria isolated from deep joint sepsis after operation for total hip or knee replacement and the sources of the infections with *Staphylococcus aureus*, *J Hosp Infect* 4:19, 1983.

180. **Lindbom G, Laurell G**: Studies on the epidemiology of staphylococcal infections. 4. Effect of nasal chemotherapy on carrier state in patients and on postoperative sepsis. *Acta Pathol Microbiol Scand* 69:237, 1967.

181. **Lindsey D, Nava C, Marti M**: Effectiveness of penicillin irrigation in control of infection in sutured lacerations, *J Trauma* 22:186, 1982.

182. **Lister J**: On a new method of treating compound fracture, abscess, etc., with observations on the condition of suppuration, *Lancet* 1:326, 1867.

183. **Localio SA, Casale W, Hinton JW**: Wound healing: experimental and statistical study; bacteriology and pathology in relation to suture material, *Surg Gynecol Obstet* 77:481, 1943.

184. **Lowell JD**: Use of ultraviolet radiation in total hip replacement surgery. In Eftekhar NS, editor: *Infection in joint replacement surgery: prevention and management*, St Louis, 1984, Mosby–Year Book.

185. **Lowell JD, Kundsin RB**: Ultraviolet radiation: its beneficial effect on the operating room environment and the incidence of deep wound infection after total hip and total knee arthroplasty. In *The American Academy of Orthopaedic Surgeons instructional course lectures*, vol 26, St Louis, 1977, Mosby–Year Book.

186. **Lowell JD, Kundsin RB, Schwartz CM, et al**: Ultraviolet radiation and reduction of deep wound infection following hip and knee arthroplasty, *Ann N Y Acad Sci* 353:285, 1980.

187. **Maderazo EG, Judson S, Pasternak H**: Late infections of total joint prosthesis. A review and recommendation for prevention, *Clin Orthop* 229:131, 1988.

188. **Maguire WB**: The use of antibiotics, locally and systemically, in orthopaedic surgery, *Med J Aust* 2:412, 1964.

189. **Major RH**: *A history of medicine*, Springfield, Ill, 1954, Charles C Thomas.

190. **Maki DG, Goldman DA, Rhame FS**: Infection control in intravenous therapy, *Ann Intern Med* 79:867, 1973.

191. **Marks KE, Nelson CL, Lautenschlager EP**: Antibiotic-impregnated acrylic bone cement, *J Bone Joint Surg* 58:358, 1976.

192. **Marsh RC, Nelson JP**: Comparing surgical clean room filters, *Contemp Surg* 7:33, 1975.

193. **Martin WJ**: Complication of antibiotic therapy in the management of bacterial infections, *Lancet* 86:159, 1966.

194. **Masur H, Whelton PK, Whelton A**: Neomycin toxicity revisited, *Arch Surg* 111:822, 1976.

195. **McCue SF, Berg EW, Saunders EA**: Efficacy of double-gloving as a barrier to microbial contamination during total joint arthroplasty, *J Bone Joint Surg* 63:811, 1981.

196. **McCullough CJ**: Tuberculosis as a late complication of total hip replacement, *Acta Orthop Scand* 48:508, 1977.

197. **McDade JJ, Whitcomb JG, Rypka EW, et al**: Microbiological studies conducted in a vertical laminar air flow surgery, *JAMA* 203:125, 1968.

198. **McFadden HW Jr**: *Assay of antibiotic levels in body fluids. Antimicrobial susceptibility testing*. Commission on Continuing Education, Council on Microbial Microbiology, American Society of Clinical Pathology, 1971.

199. **McLauchlan J, Pilcher MF, Trexler PC, et al**: The surgical isolator, *Br Med J* 1:322, 1974.

200. **Meade RH**: *An introduction to the history of general surgery*, Philadelphia, 1968, WB Saunders.

201. **Meals RA, Knoke L**: The surgical suction tip: a contaminated instrument, *J Bone Joint Surg* 60[Am]:409, 1978.

202. **Medical Research Council Report**: Aseptic methods in the operating suite, *Lancet* 1:705, 1968.

203. **Miles AA, Miles EM, Burke J**: The value of duration of defense reactions of the skin to the primary lodgement of bacteria, *Br J Exp Pathol* 38:79, 1957.

204. **Mitchell NJ, Gamble DR**: Clothing design for operating room personnel, *Lancet* 2:1133, 1974.

205. **Moran JM, Greenwald AS**: *Mechanical properties of Palacos with varying amounts of gentamicin*, Res. Rep. 044-77, Cleveland, 1979, Cleveland Clinic Foundation Biomechanics Laboratory.

206. **Moran JM, Greenwald AS, Matejczyk MB**: Effect of gentamicin on shear and interface strengths of bone cement, *Clin Orthop* 141:96, 1979.

207. **Morley DC Jr, Patterson A**: *Candida parapsilosis* infection of total hip replacement: a case, *Orthop Rev* 12:61, 1983.

208. **Moylan JA, Balish E, Chan J**: Intraoperative bacterial transmission, *Surg Gynecol Obstet* 141:731, 1975.

209. **Müller ME**: Total hip prosthesis, *Clin Orthop* 72:46, 1970.

210. **Murray WR**: Total hip replacement in non-specialized environment. In The Hip Society: *Proceedings of the second open scientific meeting of The Hip Society, 1974*, St Louis, 1974, Mosby–Year Book.

211. **Murray WR**: Use of antibiotic-containing bone cement, *Clin Orthop* 190:89, 1984.

212. **Nelson CL**: Clean air and the total hip arthroplasty, *Orthop Clin North Am* 4:533, 1973.

213. **Nelson CL, Bergfeld JA, Schwartz J, et al**: Antibiotics in human hematoma and wound fluid, *Clin Orthop* 108:138, 1975.

214. **Nelson CL, Bergman BR**: Antibiotic-impregnated acrylic composites. In Eftekhar NS, editor: *Infection in joint replacement surgery: prevention and management*, St Louis, 1984, Mosby–Year Book.

215. **Nelson JP**: Operating room environment: clean rooms and personnel-isolator systems. In Eftekhar NS, editor: *Infection in joint replacement surgery: prevention and management*, St Louis, 1984, Mosby–Year Book.

216. **Nelson JP, Glassburn AR Jr, Talbott RD, et al**: Horizontal flow clean room. Bacteriologic studies, *Rocky Mt Med J* 72:243, 1975.

217. **Nelson JP, Fitzgerald RH Jr, Jaspers MT, et al**: Prophylactic antimicrobial coverage in arthroplasty patients (editorial), *J Bone Joint Surg* 72:1, 1990.

218. **Noble WC, Lidwell OM, Kingston D**: The size distribution of airborne particle carrying micro-organisms, *J Hyg (Camb)* 61:358, 1963.

219. **Olivier AF**: *Traité Expérimenta du typhyus traumatique. Gangréne Ou pouriture des hôpitaux*, Paris, 1822, Seignott.

220. **Olix ML, Klug TJ, Coleman CR, et al**: Prophylactic penicillin and streptomycin in elective operations on bones, joints and tendons, *Surg Forum* 10:818, 1960.

221. **Passick J, Hirsch DM**: Recurrent infection of a total hip arthroplasty associated with radiation-induced ulcerative colitis, *J Arth* 4:87, 1989.

222. **Patel D, Moellering RC Jr, Thrasher K, et al**: The effect of hypotensive anesthesia on cephalothin concentrations in bone and muscle of patients undergoing total hip replacement, *J Bone Joint Surg* 61:531, 1979.

223. **Pavel A, Smith RL, Ballard A, et al**: Prophylactic antibiotics in clean orthopaedic surgery, *J Bone Joint Surg* 56:777, 1974.

224. **Pearson TA, Mitchell CA, Hughes WT**: *Aeromonas hydrophila* septicemia, *Am J Dis Child* 128:579, 1972.

225. **Peers JG**: Cleanup techniques in the operating room, *Arch Surg* 107:596, 1973.

226. **Perkins JJ**: *Principles and methods of sterilization in health sciences*, ed 2, Springfield, Ill, 1969, Charles C Thomas.

227. **Persson U, Montgomery F, Carlsson A, et al**: How far does prophylaxis against infection in total joint replacement offset its cost? *Br Med J [Clin Res]* 296:99, 1988.

228. **Petty RW**: The effect of methylmethacrylate on chemotaxis of polymorphonuclear leukocytes, *J Bone Joint Surg* 60:492, 1978.

229. **Petty W**: The effect of methylmethacrylate on the bacterial inhibiting properties of normal human serum, *Clin Orthop* 132:266, 1978.

230. **Petty W**: Evaluation of the efficacy of topical antimicrobial solutions in reducing bacterial contamination in an experimental wound, *Orthop Trans* 3:132, 1979.

231. **Petty W**: Methylmethacrylate concentrations in tissue adjacent to bone cement, *J Biomed Mater Res* 14:427, 1980.

232. **Petty W, Caldwell JR**: The effect of methylmethacrylate on complement activity, *Clin Orthop* 128:354, 1977.

233. **Petty W, Spanier S, Shuster JJ**: Prevention of infection after total joint replacement. Experiments with a canine model, *J Bone Joint Surg* 70[Am]:536, 1988.

234. **Petty W, Spanier S, Shuster JJ, et al**: The influence of skeletal implants on incidence of infection: experiments in a canine model, *J Bone Surg* 67:1236, 1985.

235. **Polk HC Jr, Lopez-Mayor JF**: Postoperative wound infection—a prospective study of determinant factors and prevention, *Surgery* 66:97, 1969.

236. **Prothero SR, Parkes JC, Stinchfield RE**: Complications after low-back fusion in 1,000 patients. A comparison of two series one decade apart, *J Bone Joint Surg* 48:57, 1966.

237. **Ravitch MM, editor**: *Current problems in surgery—biology of surgical infection*, Chicago, 1973, Year Book Medical Publishers.

238. **Report of Ad Hoc Committee of the Committee on Trauma, Division of Medical Sciences, National Academy of Sciences–National Research Council**: Postoperative wound infection; the influence of ultraviolet irradiation of the operating room and of various other factors, *Ann Surg* 160:1, 1964.

239. **Riemensnider DK**: Spacecraft sterilization technology, *NASA SP* 108:97, 1966.

240. **Ritter M**: Ecology of operating room. In Eftekhar NS, editor: *Infection in total joint replacement surgery: prevention and management*, St Louis, 1984, Mosby–Year Book.

241. **Ritter MA, Eitzen HE, French ML, et al**: The operating room environment as affected by people and the surgical face mask, *Clin Orthop* 111:147, 1975.

242. **Ritter MA, Eitzen HE, Hart JB, et al**: The surgeon's garb, *Clin Orthop* 153:204, 1980.

243. **Ritter MA, Fechtman RW**: Urinary tract sequelae: possible influence on joint infections following total joint replacement, *Orthopaedics* 10:467, 1987.

244. **Ritter MA, French MLV, Eitzen HE**: Bacterial contamination of the surgical knife, *Clin Orthop* 108:158, 1975.

245. **Ritter MA, French MLV, Hart JB**: Microbiological studies in a horizontal wall-less laminar air-flow operating room during actual surgery, *Clin Orthop* 97:16, 1973.

246. **Roberts AP, Hughes AW**: Complications with antibiotics used prophylactically in joint replacement surgery: a case report of Cephardine-induced pseudomembranous colitis, *Int Orthop* 8:299, 1985.

247. **Robinson MC, Krizek TJ, Heggers JP**: *Biology of surgical infections of current problems in surgery*, Chicago, 1973, Year Book Medical Publishers.

248. **Rocha H**: Postoperative wound infection. A controlled study of antibiotic prophylaxis, *Arch Surg* 85:456, 1962.

249. **Rodeheaver GT, Smith SL, Thacker JG, et al**: Mechanical cleansing of contaminated wounds with a surfactant, *Am J Surg* 129:241, 1975.

250. **Salvati EA, Robinson RP, Zeno SM, et al**: Infection rates after 3175 total hip and total knee replacements performed with and without a horizontal unidirectional filtered air-flow system, *J Bone Joint Surg* 64:525, 1982.

251. **Sanchez-Ubeda R, Fernand E, Rousselot LM**: Complication rate in general surgical cases. The value of penicillin and streptomycin as postoperative prophylaxis—a study of 511 cases, *N Engl J Med* 259:1045, 1958.

252. **Schonholtz GJ**: Maintenance of aseptic barriers in the conventional operating room: general principles, *J Bone Joint Surg* 58:439, 1976.

253. **Schurman DJ**: Use of systemic antibiotics in total joint replacement. In Eftekhar NS, editor: *Infection in joint replacement surgery: prevention and management*, St Louis, 1984, Mosby–Year Book.

254. **Schurman DJ, Hirshman HP, Burton DS**: Cephalothin and cefamandole penetration into bone, synovial fluid, and wound drainage fluid, *J Bone Joint Surg* 62:981, 1980.

255. **Schurman DJ, Hirschman HP, Kajiyama G, et al**: Cefazolin concentrations in bone and synovial fluid, *J Bone Joint Surg* 60:359, 1978.

256. **Scott CC**: Laminar-linear flow system of ventilation. Its application to medicine and surgery, *Lancet* 1:989, 1970.

257. **Scott CC, Guthrie TD**: Environmental tests of linear flow ventilation for an operating theater, *Br J Surg* 62:462, 1975.

258. **Semmelweiss IP**: *Die Aetiologie der Begriff and und die Prophylaxis des Kindbettfiebers*, Pest Wien and Leipzig, 1861, C.A. Hartleben.

258a. **Seropian R, Reynolds BM**: Wound infections after preoperative dipilatory vs. razor preparation, *Am J Surg* 121:251, 1971.

259. **Snider SR**: Clean wound infections: epidemiology and bacteriology, *Surgery* 64:728, 1968.

260. **Sompolinsky D, Hermann Z, Oeding P, et al**: A series of postoperative infections, *J Infect Dis* 100:1, 1957.

261. **Southwood RT, Rice JL, McDonald PJ, et al**: Infection in experimental hip arthroplasties, *J Bone Joint Surg* 67[Br]:229, 1985.

262. **Sorensen TS, Anderson MR, Glenthoj J, et al**: Pharmacokinetics of topic gentamicin in total hip arthroplasty, *Acta Orthop Scand* 55:156, 1984.

263. **Stevens DB**: Postoperative orthopaedic infections. A study of etiological mechanisms, *J Bone Joint Surg* 46:96, 1964.

264. **Stinchfield FE, Bigliani LU, Neu HC, et al**: Late hematogenous infection of total joint replacement, *J Bone Joint Surg* 62[Am]:1345, 1980.

265. **Strange-Vognsen HH, Klareskov B**: Bacteriologic contamination of suction tips during hip arthroplasty, *Acta Orthop Scand* 59:410, 1988.

266. **Strazzeri JC, Anzel S**: Infected total hip arthroplasty due to *Actinomyces israelii* after dental extraction, *Clin Orthop* 210:128, 1986.

267. **Sullivan PM, Johnston RC, Kelley SS**: Late infection after total hip replacement, caused by an oral organism after dental manipulation, *J Bone Joint Surg* 72:121, 1990.

268. **Surin VV, Sundholm K, Bäckman L**: Infection after total hip replacement with special reference to a discharge from the wound, *J Bone Joint Surg* 65[Br]:412, 1983.

269. **Taylor FW**: An experimental evaluation of operative wound irrigation, *Surg Gynecol Obstet* 113:465, 1961.

270. **Torholm C, Lidgren L, Lindberg L, et al**: Total hip joint arthroplasty with gentamicin-impregnated cement. A clinical study of gentamicin excretion kinetics, *Clin Orthop* 181:99, 1983.

271. **Turner RS**: Laminar air flow. Its original surgical application and long-term results, *J Bone Joint Surg* 56:430, 1974.

272. **Ulrich JA**: Microbiology of human skin and its relation to post-surgical infections. In *Workshop on control of operation room airborne bacteria*, Washington, DC, 1976, National Academy of Sciences.

273. **Von Graevenitz A, Mensch AH**: The genus *Aeromonas* in human bacteriology: report of 30 cases and review of the literature, *N Engl J Med* 278:245, 1968.

274. **Wahlig H**: *Antibiotic-loaded acrylic bone cement: experimental and pharmacokinetic studies*, paper presented at the twenty-fourth annual meeting of the Orthopaedic Research Society, Dallas, Feb. 21–23, 1978.

275. **Wahlig H, Buchholz HW**: Experimentelle und klinische Untersuchungen aur Freisetzung von Gentamycin aus einem Knockenzement, *Chirurg* 43:441, 1972.

276. **Wahlig H, Dingeldeine E, Bergmann R, et al**: The release of gentamicin from polymethyl-methacrylate beads. An experimental and pharmacokinetic study, *J Bone Joint Surg* 60[Br]270, 1978.

277. **Wahlig H, Haëister W, Grieben A, et al**: Uber die Freisetzung von Gentamycin aus Polymethylmethacrylat. I. Experimentelle Untersuchungen in vitro, *Langenbecks Arch Chir* 331:169, 1972.

278. **Wahlig H, Schliep HJ, Bergmann R, et al**: Uber die Freisetzung von Gentamycin aus Polymethylmethacrylat. II. Experimentelle Untersuchungen in vivo, *Langenbecks Arch Chir* 331:193, 1972.

279. **Waterman NG, Howell RS, Babich M**: The effect of a prophylactic topical antibiotic (cephalothin) on the incidence of wound infection, *Arch Surg* 97:365, 1968.

280. **Weinstein AJ, McHenry MC, Gavan TL**: Systemic absorption of neomycin irrigating solution, *JAMA* 238:152, 1977.

281. **Weinstein AM, Bingham DN, Sauer BW, et al**: The effect of high-pressure insertion and antibiotic inclusions upon the mechanical properties of polymethylmethacrylate, *Clin Orthop* 121:67, 1976.

281a. **Welch RB, Taylor W, Garnet W**: The prophylactic effect of clean air systems and antibiotics in total hip replacement surgery, *Orthop Rev* 5:27, 1976.

282. **Whitcomb JG, Clapper WE**: Ultraclean operating room, *Am J Surg* 112:681, 1966.

283. **Whitfield WJ**: *A new approach to clean room design*, SC-4673 (RR), 1962, Scandia.

284. **Whyte W, Shaw BH**: Comparison of ventilation systems in operating rooms, *Bull Soc Int Surg* 33:42, 1974.

285. **Whyte W, Shaw BH, Barnes R**: A bacteriological evaluation of laminar flow systems for orthopaedic surgery, *J Hyg (Camb)*71:559, 1973.

286. **Whyte W, Shaw BH, Freeman MA**: An evaluation of a partial-walled laminar flow operating room, *J Hyg (Camb)* 73:61, 1974.

287. **Wilde AH, Greenwald AS**: Shear strength of self-curing acrylic cement, *Clin Orthop* 106:126, 1975.

288. **Wiley AM, Barnett M**: The prevention of surgical sepsis. Clean surgeons and clean air, *Clin Orthop* 96:168, 1973.

289. **Wiley AM, Ha'eri GB**: Routes of infection. A study of using "tracer particles" in the orthopaedic operating room, *Clin Orthop* 139:150, 1979.

290. **Williams RE, Jevons MP, Shooter RA, et al**: Nasal staphylococci and sepsis in hospital patients, *Br Med J* 5153:658, 1959.

290a. **Wilson FC, Worcester JN, Coleman PD, et al**: Antibiotic penetration of experimental bone hematomas, *J Bone Joint Surg* 53:1622, 1971.

291. **Wilson PD Jr, et al**: Total hip replacement with fixation by acrylic cement: a preliminary study of 100 consecutive McKee-Farrar prosthetic replacements, *J Bone Joint Surg* 54:207, 1972.

292. **Wroblewski BM**: Leaching out from acrylic bone cement. Experimental evaluation, *Clin Orthop* 124:311, 1977.

293. **Wroblewski BM, del Sel HJ**: Urethral instrumentation and deep sepsis in total hip replacement, *Clin Orthop* 146:209, 1980.

294. **Young LS**: Infection in the compromised host, *Hosp Pract* 16:73, 1981.

ADDITIONAL READINGS

Altemeier WA, Levenson S: Trauma workshop report: infections, immunology, and gnotobiosis, *J Trauma* 106:108, 1970.

Association of Operating Room Nurses: AORN standards for OR sanitation, *AORN J* 23:976, 1975.

Baker G, Hung TK: Penicillin concentration in experimental wounds *Am J Surg* 115:531, 1968.

Ballinger WF, Treybal JC, Vose AB: *Alexander's care of the patient in surgery*, ed 6, St Louis, 1978, Mosby–Year Book.

Beck WC: Justified faith in surgical drapes. A new and safe material for draping, *Am J Surg* 105:560, 1963.

Beeching NJ, Thomas MG, Roberts S, et al: Comparative in-vitro activity of antibiotics incorporated in acrylic bone cement, *J Antimicrob Chemother* 17:173, 1986.

Bethune DW, Blowers R, Parker M, et al: Dispersal of *Staphylococcus aureus* by patients and surgical staff, *Lancet* 1:480, 1965.

Bourgault AM, Rosenblatt JE, Fitzgerald RH: *Peptococcus magnus*: a significant human pathogen, *Ann Intern Med* 93:244, 1980.

Buchholz HW, Engelbrecht H: Über die Depotwirkung einiger

Antibiotica bei Vermischung mit dem Kunstharz Palacos, *Chirurg* 41:511, 1970.

Buchholz HW, Siegel A: Erfahrungen mit refobacin Palacos in der Prosthesenchirurgie Actuel, *Traumatol* 3:233, 1973.

Buchholz HW, Engelbrecht H, Rottger J, et al: Erkenntnisse nach Wechsel von über 400 infizierten Hüftendoprothesen, *Orthop Praxis* 12:1117, 1976.

Cardenal FA, Aufranc OE: Incidence of wound infection in hip surgery. In proceedings of the American Academy of Orthopaedic Surgeons: *J Bone Joint Surg* 44:1266, 1962.

Carlsson AK, Lidgren L, Lindberg L: Prophylactic antibiotics against early and late deep infections after total hip replacements, *Acta Orthop Scand* 48:405, 1977.

Casten DF, Nach RJ, Spinzia J: An experimental and clinical study of the effectiveness of antibiotic wound irrigation in preventing infection, *Surg Gynecol Obstet* 118:783, 1964.

Chapman MW, Hadley WK: The effect of polymethylmethacrylate and antibiotic combinations on bacterial viability, *J Bone Joint Surg* 58:76, 1976.

Charnley J: The future of total hip replacement, *Hip* 198, 1982.

Committee on Operating Room Environment: Special air systems for operating rooms, *Bull Am Coll Surg* 57:18, 1972.

Committee on Operating Room Environment of American College of Surgeons: Definition of surgical microbiologic clean air, *Bull Am Coll Surg* 61:19, 1976.

Dubuc F, Guimont A, Roy L, et al: A study of some factors which contribute to surgical wound contamination, *Clin Orthop* 96:176, 1973.

Eftekhar NS: Combined use of chemoprophylaxis and ultraclean-air technology in preventing infection. In Eftekhar NS, editor: *Infection in joint replacement surgery: prevention and management*, St Louis, 1984, Mosby–Year Book.

Ehrenberg F: Die Infusions-thierchen asl vollkommene Organismen, Ein Blick in das tie tere organischer, *Leben der Natur*, Leipzig, 1838, L. Voss.

Eitzen HE, et al: The effect of variable human microbial shedding on the control of the contamination in surgical suites. *Proceedings of the International Symposium of Contamination Control, September 1974.*

Elson RA: Prophylactic use of gentamicin-Palacos in the Northern General Hospital, Sheffield, England. In Burri C, Rutter A, editors: *Actual problems in surgery and orthopaedic surgery*, vol 16, Berne, 1979, Verlag Hans Huber AG.

Elson RA, Jephcott AE, McGechie DB, et al: Antibiotic-loaded acrylic cement, *J Bone Joint Surg* 59[Br]:200, 1977.

Elson RA, Jephcott AE, McGechie DB, et al: Bacterial infection and acrylic cement in the rat, *J Bone Joint Surg* 59:452, 1977.

Feigan A: *The case for clean air*. Presented at American Academy of Orthopaedic Surgeons meeting, audiovisual section, 1975.

Forbes GB: Staphylococcal infection of operation wounds with special reference to topical antibiotic prophylaxis, *Lancet* 2:505, 1961.

French ML, Ritter MA, Eitzen HE, et al: Microbial evaluation of reusable and disposable laparotomy sponges, *Surg Gynecol Obstet* 137:465, 1973.

Gingrass RP, Close AS, Ellison EM: The effect of various topical and parenteral agents on the prevention of infection in experimental contaminated wounds, *J Trauma* 4:763, 1964.

Grisyina AG, Costerton JW: Bacterial adherence to biomaterial and tissue, *J Bone Joint Surg* 67:264, 1985.

Henderson ED, Kornblum SS: Studies on the epidemiology of staphylococcal wound infections in previously clean surgical cases on an orthopaedic service. In *American Academy of Orthopaedic Surgeons instructional course lectures*, vol 18, St Louis, 1961, Mosby–Year Book.

Howorth FH: The air in the operating theatre. In Johnson ID, Hunter AR, editors: *The design and utilisation of operating theatres*, London, 1984, Edward Arnold.

Hughes S, Field CA, Kennedy MR, et al: Cephalosporins in bone cement: studies in vitro and in vivo, *J Bone Joint Surg* 61[Br]:96, 1979.

Illingworth CF, editor: Wound healing: a symposium based on the Lister Centenary Scientific Meeting (1965), Boston, 1966, Little, Brown.

Jacobson JJ, Millard HD, Plezia R, et al: Dental treatment and late prosthetic joint infections, *Oral Surg* 61:413, 1986.

James ET, Hunter GA, Cameron HU: Total hip revision arthroplasty: does sepsis influence the results? *Clin Orthop* 170:88, 1982.

Jaspers MT, Little JW: Prophylactic antibiotic coverage in patients with total arthroplasty: current practice, *J Am Dent Assn* 111:943, 1985.

Johnson JE III: Wound infections, *Postgrad Med* 50:126, 1971.

Kamme C, Lidgren L, Lindberg L, et al: Anaerobic bacteria in late infections after total hip arthroplasty, *Scand J Infect Dis* 6:161, 1974.

Knight WE, Long JW: *The use of antibiotic-impregnated bone cement in total joint replacement*. Paper presented at the Arkansas Orthopaedic Association Meeting, Fort Smith, Arkansas, October 1975.

LeMaitre GD, Finnegan JA: *The patient in surgery: a guide for nurses*, ed 4, Philadelphia, 1980, WB Saunders.

Lidwell OM: Apparent improvement in the outcome of hip or knee-joint replacement operations over the period of a prospective study, *J Hyg* (Lond) 97:501, 1986.

Lidwell OM, Lowbury EJL, Whyte W, et al: Extended follow-up of patients suspected of having joint sepsis after total joint replacement, *J Hyg* (Lond) 95:655, 1985.

Louria DB, Brayton RG: The efficacy of penicillin regimens with observations on the frequency of superinfection, *JAMA* 186:987, 1963.

Madsen PO, Madsen RE: A study of disposable surgical masks, *Am J Surg* 114:431, 1967.

Moggio M, Goldner JL, McCollum DE, et al: Wound infections in patients undergoing total hip arthroplasty: ultraviolet light for the control of airborne bacteria, *Arch Surg* 114:815, 1979.

Moore B: Antibiotics in cement, *J Bone Joint Surg* 59[Br]:139, 1977.

Moran JM, Greenwald AS: *The strength of the Palacos-bone interface*, Res. Rep. 045-77, Cleveland, 1979, Cleveland Clinic Foundation Biomechanics Laboratory.

Murray EGD: A synopsis of the history of American bacteriology. In Dubos RJ, Hirsch JG, editors: *Bacterial and mycotic infections of man*, ed 4, Philadelphia, 1965, JB Lippincott.

Nagy R: Application and measurement of ultraviolet radiation, *Am Industr Hyg Assoc J* 25:274, 1964.

Nakata MM, Lewis RP: Anaerobic bacteria in bone and joint infections, *Rev Infect Disc* 6(suppl):165, 1984.

Neer CS II, Watson KC, Stanton FJ: Recent experience in total shoulder replacement, *J Bone Joint Surg* 64:319, 1982.

Nelaton A: *Clinical lectures on surgery*, Philadelphia, 1855, JB Lippincott.

Nelson CL, Evarts CM, Andrish J, et al: Results of infected total hip replacement arthroplasty, *Clin Orthop* 147:258, 1980.

Nelson CL, Marks KE: Antibiotic acrylic composites, unpublished manuscript, 1983.

Nelson JP: Bacterial studies in a horizontal flow operating room clean room. In Proceedings from the Western Orthopaedic Association, *J Bone Joint Surg* 57:137, 1975.

Nelson JP: The prevention of orthopaedic surgical sepsis, *Orthop Dig* 4:14, 1976.

Nelson JP, Glassburn AR Jr, Talbott RD, et al: Horizontal flow operating room, clean rooms, *Cleve Clin Q* 40:191, 1973.

Nelson JP, Glassburn AR Jr, Talbott RD, et al: Clean room operating rooms, Clin Orthop 96:179, 1973.

Nordbring F: Is dicloxacillin nephrotoxic? *Acta Orthop Scand* 55: 405, 1984 (editorial).

O'Connell CJ, Plaut ME: Fibrin penetration by penicillin: in vitro simulation of intravenous therapy, *J Lab Clin Med* 73:258, 1969.

Petty W: The effect of methylmethacrylate on bacterial phagocytosis and killing by human polymorphonuclear leukocytes, *J Bone Joint Surg* 60:752, 1978.

Petty W: Influence of methymethacrylate on quantitative gel diffusion assay of immunoglobulins, *J Biomed Mater Res* 13:645, 1979.

Public Health Laboratory Service Report: Incidence of surgical wound infection in England and Wales, *Lancet* 2:659, 1960.

Queenel LB: The efficiency of surgical masks of varying design and composition, *Br J Surg* 62:936, 1975.

Randall HT, et al: *Manual of preoperative and postoperative care*, Philadelphia, 1978, WB Saunders.

Reichelt A, Wahlig H, Riedl K: Antibiotic prophylaxis in allo-arthroplastic hip joint surgery: concentration assays in the wound exudate after parenteral administration of gentamicin, *Arch Orthop Unfallchir* 84:249, 1976.

Ritter MA, Eitzen HE, French MLV: Comparison of horizontal and vertical unidirectional (laminar) air-flow systems in orthopaedic surgery, *Clin Orthop* 129:205, 1977.

Ritter MA, Eitzen HE, French ML, et al: The effect that time, touch, and environment have upon bacterial contamination of instruments during surgery, *Ann Surg* 184:642, 1976.

Ritter MA, French MLV, Eitzen HE, et al: The antimicrobial effectiveness of operative-site preparation agents: a microbial and clinical study, *J Bone Joint Surg* 62:862, 1980.

Ritter MA, French MLV, Eitzen HE: Evaluation of microbial contamination of surgical gloves during actual use, *Clin Orthop* 117:303, 1976.

Ritter MA, Stringer EA: Intraoperative wound cultures: their value and long-term effect on the patient, *Clin Orthop* 155:180, 1981.

Rubin R, Salvati EA, Lewis R: Infected total hip replacement after dental procedures, *Oral Surg* 41:18, 1976.

Ruedy J: Antibiotics: an overview, *Clin Orthop* 96:31, 1973.

Schentag JJ, Jusko WJ, Plaut ME, et al: Tissue persistence of gentamicin in man, *JAMA* 238:327, 1977.

Scherr DD, Dodd TA, Buckingham WW Jr: Prophylactic use of topical antibiotic irrigation in uninfected surgical wounds: a microbiological evaluation, *J Bone Joint Surg* 54:634, 1972.

Schurman DJ, Burton DS, Kajiyama G: Cefoxitin antibiotic concentration in bone and synovial fluid, *Clin Orthop* 168:64, 1982.

Schurman DJ, Swenson LW Jr, Piziali RL: Bone cement with and without antibiotics: a study of mechanical properties. In The Hip Society: *The hip: proceedings of the sixth open scientific meeting of The Hip Society*, St Louis, 1978, Mosby–Year Book.

Schurman DJ, Trindade C, Hirshman HP, et al: Antibiotic-acrylic bone cement composites. Studies of gentamicin and Palacos. *J Bone Joint Surg* 60:978, 1978.

Selzer R: *Mortal lessons: notes on the art of surgery*, New York, 1977, Simon & Schuster.

Summers MM, Lynch PF, Black T: Hair as a reservoir of staphylococci, *J Clin Pathol* 18:13, 1965.

Tachdjian MO, Compere EL: Postoperative wound infections in orthopaedic surgery. Evaluation of prophylactic antibiotics, *J Int Coll Surg* 28:797, 1957.

Taylor GW: Preventive use of antibiotics in surgery, *Br Med Bull* 16:51, 1960.

Walter CW: *Carriers as a special problem in cross contamination in the operating room*. Presented at the second symposium for control of surgical infections, American College of Surgeons, Washington DC, March 8–9, 1971.

Walter CW, Kundsin RB: The bacteriologic study of surgical gloves from 250 operatings, *Surg Gynecol Obstet* 129:949, 1969.

Walter CW, Kundsin RB: The airborne component of wound contamination and infection, *Arch Surg* 107:588, 1973.

Wangensteen OH, Wangensteen SD: Military surgeons and surgery, old and new: an instructive chapter in management of contaminated wounds, *Surgery* 62:1102, 1967.

Wardle MD, Nelson JP, LaLime P, et al: A surgeon body—exhaust clean air operating room system, *Orthop Rev* 3:43, 1974.

Waterman NG, Kastan LB: Interstitial fluid and serum antibiotic concentrations, *Arch Surg* 105:192, 1972.

Weinstein L, Daikos G, Perrin TS: Studies on the relationship of tissue fluids and blood levels of penicillin, *J Lab Clin Med* 38:712, 1951.

Whitcomb JG, et al: Ultraclean operating rooms, *Lovelace Clin Rev* 2:65, 1965.

Whyte W, Vesley D, Hodgson R: Bacterial dispersion in relation to operating room clothing, *J Hyg* (Camb) 76:367, 1976.

Wigren A, Karlstrom G, Kaufer H: Hematogenous infection of total joint implants: a report of multiple joint infections in three patients, *Clin Orthop* 152:288, 1980.

See Chapters 4, Biomaterials: Compatibility and Wear; 5, Acrylic Cement: Properties and Application; and 31, Postoperative Wound Infection for additional information.

CHAPTER NINE

Prevention of Thromboembolic Complications

■ The possibility of fatal embolism after total hip replacement is a hip
surgeon's constant worry.
Sir John Charnley

Thromboembolic disease is a leading cause of morbidity and mortality after total hip arthroplasty. Better recognition of this problem is rapidly increasing its reported incidence. Increases in elective surgery on older patients and in the extent of surgery performed in the face of underlying cardiovascular abnormalities followed by immobilization will raise the incidence even higher, along with the associated risk of fatal outcome. Consequently, for orthopaedic surgeons performing total hip arthroplasty, this is a critical issue.

It has been estimated that each year there are between 150,000 and 200,000 fatal pulmonary emboli cases[85,137] and 300,000 cases of deep vein thrombosis that require hospitalization in the United States alone. It is the most common complication of lower-extremity surgery in patients over 40 years of age. It has also been estimated that a significant number of these patients (100,000 or more) who die from massive pulmonary embolism in hospitals are normal individuals who undergo major elective surgery.[88] Pulmonary embolism is a preventable cause of death in the hospital. Because of the advent of total joint arthroplasty in the 1960s and 1970s and the large number of such operations performed throughout the world, there has been much interest in preventing the associated complication of thromboembolic disease. This has resulted in better detection, as well as measures for prevention.*

INCIDENCE

In the past, the true incidence of thromboembolic disease was underestimated because investigations were usually based on grossly inaccurate clinical diagnoses. Surgeons' proclivity to deny the high incidence of thromboembolism is directly related to their awareness of and search for this condition. To determine the precise incidence of thromboembolic disease after total hip arthroplasty, the method of diagnosis, the age group (the risk is higher at advanced ages), and methods of prophylaxis must be considered. Death after sudden onset of chest pain has often been attributed to myocardial disease, but in many instances autopsy proved conclusively that death was caused by pulmonary embolism (while the surgeon or internist was concentrating on a cardiac etiology). Autopsy studies of patients who died after a hip fracture, for example, demonstrated that pulmonary embolism was the cause of death in 38% of 247 cases.[189]

Although venous thrombosis is the most common complication of adult hip surgery,* fatal pulmonary emboli, which reportedly occur in 0.5% to 2% of patients undergoing elective total hip surgery, constitute the major concern. Because of this high death rate after total hip arthroplasty, most investigators no longer can justify an untreated control group in an experiment to evaluate drug effectiveness or other methods of prophylaxis.[30,57,159]

---

* References 68, 104, 157, 160–162, 168, 170, 199.

* References 52, 68, 69, 71, 72, 138, 160, 170, 189.

According to a comprehensive study by Salzman and Harris,[159] fatal pulmonary emboli occurred in 1.8% to 3.4% of patients after total hip arthroplasty and in 1.7% to 2.5% after cup arthroplasty and prosthetic replacement; however, after hip fractures the reported rate was 4% to 10% in the absence of preventive measures.

According to Hirsh,[83] the incidence for all deep vein thrombi is 40% to 60% and 20% for proximal deep vein thrombi for western Europeans and North Americans. Proximal deep vein thrombosis has been reported to cause fatal embolism in 75% of the cases detected as such based on autopsy studies.[80]

Sikorski and associates have reported a higher incidence of deep vein thrombosis in patients with osteoarthritis of the hip.[176] A low incidence of deep vein thrombosis in Asian patients after total hip arthroplasty may be related to both genetic and dietary factors that require further investigation.[29,110]

The incidence of fatal pulmonary embolism varies for general surgical patients and is less than 1% (ranging from 0.1% to 0.8%), but for patients undergoing emergency hip surgery the incidence is 4% to 7% and for elective total hip arthroplasty as much as 2% to 3% (without prophylaxis). When surgeons use newer methods of detection, deep vein thrombosis is seen to occur at a rate as high as 45% to 75% after total hip or total knee arthroplasty.

Johnson and Charnley[98,99] and Charnley[29] have produced data on bilateral, simultaneous (during the same anesthesia) total hip arthroplasty. Bilateral operations showed a higher incidence of pulmonary embolism than unilateral operations regardless of whether anticoagulation therapy was given. The incidence of pulmonary embolism for a series of 7959 cases was 1.04% fatal and 7.89% nonfatal pulmonary embolism; in 243 bilateral, simultaneous operations there was an incidence of 1.65% fatal occurrences and 12.8% nonfatal pulmonary emboli. These data can be interpreted as if the patient had undergone two operations and had twice the risk of pulmonary embolism. This also indicates that local trauma to the femoral vein during surgery may play an important part in thromboembolic disease in total hip arthroplasty (see Pathophysiology and Predispositions).

Johnson and Charnley[98,99] determined the risk of pulmonary embolism in sequential bilateral arthroplasty for the second hip when pulmonary embolism did or did not follow the first operation. In 1140 patients undergoing total hip arthroplasty on the second side who had no history of embolism after surgery on the first side, there was no evidence of increased incidence of pulmonary embolism (fatal and nonfatal combined). However, the investigators reported a significant difference in the development of postoperative pulmonary embolism after the second hip surgery if the patient had experienced pulmonary embolism after the first hip operation. Significantly, the chance of this complication increased if the second operation was performed during the same hospitalization. In 61 patients who had pulmonary embolism after the first operation, the risk was significantly reduced when the second operation was performed more than 1 year after the first operation. Deep vein thrombosis is also a contributing ancillary factor in an untold number of deaths.

Until recently, most studies of pulmonary embolism were based partially on clinical assumption and partially on postmortem examinations. Significantly, a large number of pulmonary embolisms go unnoticed because the disease is sometimes silent. In one study, the combined incidence of fatal and nonfatal pulmonary embolism ranged from 4.6% to 19.7%.[63] Routine postoperative lung scans revealed an incidence of pulmonary embolism of 19.7%, almost twice the combined rate (11.4%) of all eight studies in which pulmonary embolism had been diagnosed only clinically.[63]

The peak incidence of clinically evident thromboembolism is between the seventh and fourteenth day postoperatively, but studies using fibrinogen uptake have shown that most thrombi may be initiated within 48 hours after operation; some are present at the end of the operation.

In a study of the natural history of deep vein thrombosis after total hip arthroplasty, Sikorski showed that the peak onset of the thrombosis was on the fourth day after surgery. This peak of onset is later and longer in general surgical patients. In this study, 125-I fibrinogen was used by ascending phlebography in selected patients to elucidate the deep vein thrombosis for a period of 14 to 18 days after surgery. The use of subcutaneous heparin or intermittent pneumatic compression of the calves delayed the appearance of thrombi.[176] My own experience and that of others indicates that there is a higher risk of patients developing thromboembolic complications after surgery if they have had prior thromboembolic disease. In a series studied by Stone,[184] one third of the patients with a history of thromboembolic disease developed thromboembolic disease despite the use of drugs for prophylaxis. Haake and Berkman[63] have suggested that thrombi of the popliteal and other proximal veins carry a 50% risk of pulmonary embolism whereas distal vein thrombi carry a risk as low as 1% to 2%.

PATHOPHYSIOLOGY

Virchow[193] postulated a triad of features leading to the development of thrombosis: (1) stasis, (2) hypercoagulability, and (3) local damage to the vessel walls. One or more of these predisposing factors can always occur in total hip arthroplasty. The horizontal position of the lower extremities allows considerable venous stasis in the calf and thigh.[44] Stasis is usually increased during the operation.[125,140] Blood flow in the external iliac and popliteal veins is reduced 50% during induction of anesthesia with thiopental.[34]

Wessler and his associates[194–196] have clearly shown that hypercoagulability is associated with thrombosis. Their experimental work demonstrated massive thrombosis in vascular segments containing stagnant blood quite far from the site of infusion of thrombi-free serum. The prophylactic effect of low-dose heparin on the state of hypercoagulability occurs through augmentation of the natural anticlotting agents in the blood. Abnormal activation of the coagulation system (caused by trauma of surgery and postoperative immobilization) may be so intense that it cannot be inhibited by natural antithrombin agents of the blood; thus a small amount of an agent, such as heparin, can be helpful. Undoubtedly, platelets play an important role in the production of thrombi; damage to the vessel walls and endothelium may lead to the adhesion and aggregation of platelets, with subsequent thrombus formation.[32,33,132,172]

The distinction between calf and thigh thrombi as potential sources of pulmonary emboli is more sharply defined by accurate diagnostic methods. It is now suggested that although calf thrombi develop frequently, they are not likely to cause embolization unless they extend proximally into the popliteal region and thigh. The major life-threatening emboli are generated in the thigh and pelvis (95% of all pulmonary emboli and 90% of all fatal pulmonary emboli), and detecting these "hazardous thrombi" is most important. However, these thrombi are not thought to be primary lesions, and often they are extensions from a calf thrombus or arise in association with a discontinuous but concomitant calf thrombus. It is suggested that isolated thrombi in the ipsilateral thigh are common and account for at least 20% of all thrombi formed after total hip surgery.[39,43] Salzman and Harris[159] believe this predilection for the operated or injured area is caused by local trauma, and initiation of thrombi preferentially at this hazardous site is responsible for the unusually high risk of fatal pulmonary emboli after total hip surgery. In contrast, celiac and pelvic thrombi after hip surgery are rarely observed. In fact, only one was observed in more than 400 roentgenographic studies after total hip surgery.[159]

Local Damage to the Endothelium

Review of the literature indicates that clinically documented thrombi after total hip arthroplasty occur proximally at the level of the hip joint (lesser trochanter) where the femoral vein is most vulnerable. This correlates well with the occurrence of pulmonary embolism after deep vein thrombosis at a proximal site. In one study, 9 of 16 (56%) patients with proximal (and none with distal) limb thrombosis developed pulmonary embolism. Most studies also suggest a higher incidence of deep vein thrombosis on the operated side (45%) than on the contralateral side (29%).[63]

In Lowe's two post-mortem studies[121] and Stewart's experimental models[183] following arthroplasty of the hip, the investigators observed induced injury in a previously healthy vein distant from the surgical site. The mechanism of clotting distant from the site of surgery is poorly understood.

Venography studies by Stamatikis[180] and Nillus[141] and co-workers found a high incidence (50% and 58% respectively) of deep vein thrombosis after total hip arthroplasty. These authors implicated two types of deep vein thrombosis; the first occurred with equal frequency in both the operated leg and the contralateral extremity, could be attributed to all types of surgery, and could possibly result from a hypercoagulability state caused by activation of coagulation factors and inhibition of fibrinolysis. The second resulted from damage to the wall of the femoral vein during surgery. Intraoperative venography by Stamatikis[180] and Johnson[153] and associates suggests that distortion of the femoral vein during total hip arthroplasty may initiate deep vein thrombosis in the femoral vein.

In an anatomical pathological study of fresh cadavers, Planes and associates[149] demonstrated that placing the limb in certain positions can cause a change in configuration and alignment and even potential injury to the femoral vein. They also observed folding and kinking of the femoral veins for both the supine and lateral decubitus positions using a direct lateral and posterolateral approach to the hip. Internal rotation from 90 to 110 degrees (in the posterior approach) did not induce a fold in the vein. However, with flexion and adduction, a fold appeared with kinking at the extreme position. The kinking disappeared with reversal of the position of the limb to neutral. With the hip adducted and flexed (in the direct lateral approach), placing the leg across the body caused the fold once again to appear and then reverse when the limb was placed in anatomical position.[149] Hampson and co-workers have also suggested intraoperative trauma during hip surgery as the cause of femoral vein thrombi on the operated side when calf clots are evenly distributed in both legs (operated and nonoperated limbs).[67] In one study the posterior approach was responsible for fewer femoral vein thrombi (9%) than the modified Charnley anterior approach.[56] Several studies point to the fact that dangerous thrombi are those generated and released from the proximal limb, that is, the femoral vein, leading to a 7% to 10% incidence of fatal pulmonary emboli (without anticoagulation)[63]; the distal emboli cause an incidence as low as 0.1% to 0.8% in patients receiving anticoagulation treatment.*

State of Hypercoagulability

The state of hypercoagulability can be caused by several inherited or acquired anomalies of elements needed to maintain the balance of hemostasis leading to the state of hypercoagulability. These factors include antithrombin III, heparin factor II, protein C, and protein S. While the state of hypercoagulability can manifest itself spontaneously in various decades of life, it can be exacerbated by trauma, surgery, or pregnancy. Other conditions cited in the predisposition for thrombosis include homocystinuria and deficiency or dysfunction of fibrinogen, plasminogen, or plasminogen activator. Acquired predisposing conditions include ulcerative colitis, Behcet's syndrome, diabetes, adenocarcinoma, and pancreatic carcinoma and other cancer. In addition, estrogen administration and estrogen-containing oral contraceptives have increased risks.†

In studying factors that make total hip arthroplasty patients more susceptible to deep vein thrombosis and pulmonary embolism (other than factors encountered in elective general surgical and orthopaedic procedures), Gitel and associates[59] compared the depletion of antithrombin III as a marker of activation of the coagulation system in two groups of patients. One group included those undergoing general surgical procedures and the other included those undergoing total hip arthroplasty. Their data suggest that total hip arthroplasty patients had a strong system of activation of clotting cascade, which these investigators thought to be associated with local vessel injury and local stasis of the femoral vein. This association is not present in most general surgical procedures.

Venous Stasis

Immobility from osteoarthritis and confinement before surgery, lengthy anesthesia, and postoperative immobilization are compounding factors that lead to a state of hypercoagulability.[193] Heart failure and previous deep vein thrombosis have been implicated as additional factors in increasing the possibility of thromboembolic complications. Cinephlebography techniques have demonstrated that venous stasis occurs in the absence of calf muscle contractions in the calf veins (soleal veins) because of immobilization after surgery. Although studies have shown that elevation of the limb, active and passive pumping action of the calf, and

---

* References 47, 129, 169, 173, 177.
†References 4, 20, 26, 35, 63, 65, 94, 97, 114, 131, 133, 142, 151, 152, 155, 166, 174, 179, 182, 188, 192, 200.

antiembolic stockings help prevent venous stasis, early ambulation is most effective in preventing stasis during the postoperative course of total hip arthroplasty patients.[2,28,45,116]

PREDISPOSITIONS

Several risk factors have been implicated in development of thromboembolic conditions. They include advanced age, prior history of thromboembolic disease, trauma, immobilization, and surgical procedures on the lower extremities, especially the hip and knee.[137] According to the Consensus Development Conference Statement on Prevention of Venous Thrombosis and Pulmonary Embolism,[137] the following inherited risk factors must be considered: antithrombin III deficiency, protein 3 deficiency, protein S deficiency, dysfibrinogenemia, disorders of plasminogen, and plasminogen activation. Acquired risks include lupus anticoagulant, nephrotic syndrome, paroxysmal nocturnal hemoglobinuria, cancer, congestive heart failure and stasis, cardiomyopathy, myocardial infarction, pericarditis, anasarca, sepsis, stroke, polycythemia vera, inflammatory bowel disease, prior vein surgery, and trunk or lower extremity surgery.

Although most studies have included obesity as a risk factor in thromboembolic complications after hip surgery, this risk factor has not been scientifically proven independent of a multitude of other predisposing factors.[139]

DIAGNOSIS OF DEEP VEIN THROMBOSIS

In diagnosing deep vein thrombosis, the four most important diagnostic tools in addition to clinical impression are (1) roentgenographic phlebography, (2) the labeled fibrinogen uptake test, (3) impedance or occlusion plethysmography, and (4) augmented ultrasound techniques based on the Doppler effect. These advanced diagnostic techniques have been developed concurrently with the appearance of excellent clinical studies evaluating the prophylactic efficacy of a variety of older and newer agents. Total hip arthroplasty has offered an opportunity to study thromboembolic disease, not only because it is a commonly performed operation on older patients, but because the operation involves the proximal limb and pelvis and requires postoperative bed rest and produces a high incidence of thromboembolic disease.

As clearly pointed out by many contributors in the field, the clinical signs and symptoms of thromboembolic disease are grossly inadequate for diagnosis. Harris and his associates suggested that physical examination of the extremities fails to detect 50% to 90% of thrombi in deep venous systems. It has also been suggested that when the physical signs are interpreted as indicative of thrombosis, incorrect diagnoses may be made in as many as 34% to 50% of the cases.[87] These observations make it of paramount importance to diagnose deep vein thrombosis only after clinical suspicion is confirmed by objective evidence from newer methods of detection.

Before the use of modern techniques, the only study to diagnose thromboembolic disease by objective means was that of Sevitt and Gallagher,[169] in which the incidence of fatal pulmonary embolism was determined by autopsy. Fortunately, deep venous thrombosis and pulmonary embolism can now be diagnosed with considerable accuracy in living patients. Objective diagnostic tests have radically changed our concepts of the detection, incidence, and prevention of thromboembolic disease. It has been suggested that more than 50% of thromboses are silent. This makes clinical recognition of deep vein thrombosis exceptionally tenuous. Diagnosis based on calf tenderness or Homans' sign is grossly inaccurate and inadequate. In a study in 172 patients who underwent total hip arthroplasty,[72] none of the 52 patients with deep vein thrombosis complained of symptoms at the time the thrombi were first demonstrated by radioactive fibrinogen scan or phlebography, with the exception of 2 patients who had clinical evidence of pulmonary embolism. In a large series of fatal thromboembolic conditions, only 2% of the cases had been diagnosed before death.[52] If one bases the diagnosis of pulmonary embolism on the clinical situation alone, one sees that pulmonary embolism may kill immediately in some instances, before a diagnosis can be made. Consequently, surgeons urgently need accurate, objective, repeatable tests rather than inaccurate clinical evaluations to detect deep vein thrombosis and pulmonary embolism and to thereby guide prophylaxis and effective treatment of established thromboembolic disease. Two thirds of the patients with pulmonary emboli die within 30 minutes of the event.[43] This statistic alone demonstrates that some form of routine effective prophylaxis must be instituted, as opposed to waiting for thromboembolic disease to occur, as recently suggested by some surgeons.[91] Once an embolism has occurred, a fatal outcome may be unavoidable.

Knowledge of anatomical facts in understanding the location of the thrombus and thus its significance is essential for diagnosis and treatment. The three major veins of the lower extremities are the anterior tibial vein, the posterior tibial vein, and the soleal veins (see Chapter 2). The veins drain into the popliteal vein at the popliteal space and become the superficial femoral vein proximal to the popliteal space at the adductor canal. Superficial and deep femoral veins form the common femoral vein in the upper thigh. The external iliac vein is then formed by the junction of the greater saphenous vein and the external iliac vein as it traverses under the iliac vein (see Fig 2-26).

The clinical diagnosis of deep venous thrombosis is based on the presence of several signs and symptoms, including lower extremity pain, tenderness, swelling, erythema, cord formation, increased skin temperature, distended superficial veins, calf fullness, induration, edema, and positive Homans' sign.

Homans' sign, classically and traditionally accepted as a diagnostic clinical test for deep vein thrombosis, is grossly inaccurate because of false positive and false negative tests in the absence or presence, respectively, of deep vein thrombosis. It is falsely positive in more than half of patients suspected of a diagnosis of deep vein thrombosis and in whom the venograms were negative.[64,84] It also can be falsely negative in two thirds of the patients in whom deep vein thromboses are positively diagnosed by venogram.

Some importance has been placed on repeated examination that demonstrates a positive Homans' sign. However, it is now commonly agreed that Homans' sign is of little value in the diagnosis of deep vein thrombosis, as are the signs of superficial vessel engorgement or discoloration of the skin and edema.

In summary, clinical tests are only suggestive or presumptive and not diagnostic of deep vein thrombosis.[112] Therefore venography is the "gold standard," the reliable method to which other diagnostic measures are compared. Its diagnostic accuracy in deep vein thrombosis for proximal and distal venous thrombi is 95%.[109] Other accurate, objective diagnostic tests include 125-I fibrinogen scan and ultrasonic plethysmographic techniques.

Venography

By conventional methods of venography (such as those described by Rabinov and Paulin),[150] the common femoral and iliac veins can be adequately viewed in approximately 70% of the cases, and the muscular veins of the calf can be shown regularly in all cases.[2] As suggested by Salzman and Harris,[159] this technique is without doubt the "diagnostic benchmark" of deep vein thrombosis in the living patient, and in the last analysis it is the final arbiter in areas of dispute. Venography patterns and their usefulness after total hip arthroplasty for normal and pathological conditions of the veins affected by thrombosis have been established.*

Routine Preoperative Venography

Becker and Schampi[10a] and Heatley[81] and their associates described the preoperative, asymptomatic existence of deep vein thrombosis in general surgical patients and estimated its incidence to be 25% (Becker

---

* References 11, 51, 101, 127, 130, 156, 176, 190.

and Schampi) and 62% (Heatley et al). This provocative and interesting concept might be significant in patients with osteoarthritis undergoing total hip arthroplasty, a category of patients with a known high incidence of thromboembolic complications. However, in a preoperative venography study of 93 patients undergoing total hip arthroplasty, Chumas and associates[31] reported abnormal radiographic changes in only four patients. This was not statistically significant when compared with the control group. While there were no complications from the venography, in which new low-osmol, nonionic contrast media agents for venography were used, the investigators concluded that existent, preoperative deep vein thrombosis was not an important predisposing factor. Nonetheless, preoperative venography may be indicated before total hip arthroplasty for high-risk patients with a history of previous thromboembolic complications.

Contraindications

Venography is a painful procedure, and many patients will not permit it to be repeated. Because it is an invasive procedure it is not routinely available to all patients. A skilled radiologist is required, and some discomfort and cost are involved. Furthermore, phlebitis and other complications such as extravasation of dye have been reported in approximately 3% of cases.

Iodine allergies, abnormal renal function, and pregnancy are major contraindications to venography.[19] Allergic reaction to dye occurs in approximately 1 in 5000 cases with occasional death. For patients allergic to iodine, alternative diagnostic tests such as radionucleid venography, impedance plethysmography, Doppler ultrasonography or 125-I fibrinogen scanning, or a combination of leg scanning and impedance plethysmography should be considered.

Radionucleid Venography

Radionucleid venography, also known as thromboscintoscan, has an accuracy of 84% to 100% in proximal thrombosis but is less accurate for distal thromboses.[14,46,86] The test uses radiolabeled macroaggravated albumin. A simultaneous lung scan perfusion is also obtained. When venography is contraindicated this test is an alternative.[14,46,86]

125-I Fibrinogen Test

The 125-I fibrinogen test has been used extensively to detect deep vein thrombosis below the knee. It is based on the incorporation of radioactive fibrinogen into the fibrin clot. Use of this test is beneficial when a clot is anticipated because it requires 24 hours to become positive.[23,58,84,104] Despite the test's high sensitivity for calf thrombi, false positives are possible because of the presence of a fracture, cellulitis, or hematoma.[104,109,123,145] A positive scan is defined as greater

than 20% increased radioactivity compared with adjacent ipsilateral areas corresponding to contralateral areas or the same areas on an earlier occasion persisting over 24 hours. This technique is attractive because it is sensitive, accurate (approximately 90%), noninvasive, repeatable, and painless. In total hip arthroplasty, however, it has been shown by Harris and associates[74] to be inadequate in assessing the thigh and proximal limb for thrombus formation. This failure results because of the postoperative accumulation of fibrinogen in the wound, abrasion, and hematoma proximal to the knee, the area where thrombi-causing pulmonary emboli are usually generated. Therefore 125-I fibrinogen testing should not be used alone despite its high accuracy.[16,73]

Cuff-Impedance Venography

Cuff-impedance phlebography is distinctly more accurate and suitable than the 125-I fibrinogen scanning technique in detecting major thrombi in the thigh after total hip arthroplasty.[73] Cuff-impedance phlebography is of no value in detecting thrombi in the calf. However, as stated before and based on Kakkar's observations,[104] the thrombi formed in and limited to the calf are generally of no consequence and do not cause major pulmonary embolization. Kakkar found the clinical signs or symptoms of venous thrombosis in only 2 of 78 limbs examined, but many of these patients subsequently had some clinical signs. Accurate detection of major thrombi by cuff-impedance phlebography before the signs and symptoms of deep vein thrombosis occur is extremely significant because prophylaxis can be instituted early and exclusively in those with major thigh thrombi.

Doppler Ultrasonography and Plethysmography

With Doppler ultrasonography and plethysmography a flow velocity detector emitting an ultrasound beam is used to detect the flow characteristics of the vein. This method can reliably assess the patency of the popliteal, femoral, and iliac proximal veins.[21,175,185] The main drawback to this technique is the subjective interpretation of an audible signal, which requires an experienced technician, and its insensitivity for below-the-knee clots.

Obstruction to venous flow also can be detected by pneumatic or hydraulic (impedance) plethysmography and Doppler ultrasound methods. Plethysmographic techniques are based either on electrical impedance or on physical volume changes in the blood content of the limb in response to respiration or application of a tourniquet (inflation and deflation). These techniques sometimes are supplemented by assessment of the effect of compression of the calf or the pumping effect of foot movement.[37,197] These methods appear to be most accurate in detecting occlusive thrombi in iliac, femoral, or popliteal veins and are generally ineffective in detecting calf thrombi. Hume and associates[92] have studied both impedance plethysmography and 125-I fibrinogen scanning of the lower extremities in 140 total hip patients. Half of the patients had no evidence of thrombosis, one quarter had moderate or extensive thrombosis, and one quarter had abnormal scans only. In patients with abnormal scans, the condition appeared to resolve spontaneously. Impedance plethysmography differentiated thrombi that would and would not resolve; on this basis the investigators suggested that for some patients a monitoring regimen may be preferentially selected over routine prophylaxis.[92]

During the past few years many advances have been made in ultrasonography. For example, real-time B-mode ultrasound has produced a great degree of accuracy and sensitivity in detecting thrombi in the smaller veins. There are early indications that the results of these techniques may be as good as or superior to those of venography with the obvious advantage of being noninvasive.[55,198] Woolson and associates[201] reported the sensitivity, specificity, and accuracy of this technique to be as high as 89%, 100%, and 99%, respectively, for proximal vein thrombosis and 63%, 100%, and 93%, respectively, for a diagnosis of thrombosis involving the entire lower limb. They performed ultrasonography and venography (for control) in 152 extremities with primary or revision total hip arthroplasties.

These tests are especially useful if the surgeon suspects the patient may develop a recurrence of pulmonary embolism while on adequate anticoagulant treatment. Objective studies must be performed to document the recurrence of pulmonary emboli (while the patient is on adequate anticoagulants) when interruption of the vena cava is being considered.

DIAGNOSIS OF PULMONARY EMBOLISM

The diagnosis of pulmonary embolism is clinically suggested by the presence of pleuritic chest pain, shortness of breath, tachycardia, hemoptysis, diaphoresis, pleuritic friction rub, increased temperature, elevated erythrocyte sedimentation rate, and white blood cells (WBC).

Basing the diagnosis of pulmonary embolism on clinical signs and symptoms alone can be grossly inaccurate. Hemoptysis, for example, occurs in only 17% of the documented pulmonary emboli, and an infarct must be present before hemoptysis is seen. Salzman and Harris[159] state that the risks inherent in prolonged anticoagulation treatment of pulmonary embolism and the inaccuracies of clinical findings suggest that this diagnosis should not be accepted without objective confirmation. This is particularly true if the surgeon suspects recurrent embolization despite adequate anticoagulation, in which case the

surgeon must consider vena cava ligation. Arterial blood-gas changes are a good gross scanning test; diagnosis of pulmonary embolism in a patient with P_{O_2} above 90 mm Hg, breathing room air, is suspect. Abnormal electrocardiograms and consistent chest x-ray films are of diagnostic assistance but are generally nonspecific; on the other hand, a positive lung perfusion scan, a pulmonary ventilation scan, and selective pulmonary angiography[22] are most specific for diagnosis but are not readily repeatable. These tests are especially useful if the patient is apt to develop recurring pulmonary embolism while on adequate anticoagulant treatment.

Pulmonary emboli after total hip arthroplasty can be reliably detected using a serial $C150^2$ pulmonary scan.[77] This readily reproducible and repeatable test is useful in detecting silent emboli and allows evaluation of the efficacy of prophylactic means against pulmonary embolism. Objective studies must be performed to document the recurrence of pulmonary emboli (while the patient is on adequate anticoagulants) when interruption of vena cava is being considered.

PREVENTIVE METHODS

As stated previously, prophylaxis against thromboembolism is necessary in view of the high incidence and suddenness of fatal pulmonary embolism in unprotected patients undergoing total hip arthroplasty.[28,29,40] The surgeon, however, must consider the risk of thromboembolic disease against the risk of bleeding complications and individualize prophylaxis for each patient while considering contraindications to various agents. Bleeding complications from anticoagulation therapy can be of such serious magnitude that some investigators have argued against the routine use of prophylactic anticoagulants and have even debated their role in the treatment of thromboembolic disease.[143,146]

In 1959, Sevitt and Gallagher[167,169,170] published the first study showing the efficacy of oral anticoagulants as prophylaxis in thromboembolic disease in hip fracture patients. Considerable advances have been made since then to define the proper use of these agents as a preventive measure in thromboembolic disease after hip surgery. The prophylactic use of low-dose heparin was first studied by Sharnoff and reported in 1966.[171] Heparin works by augmenting the effect of antithrombin 3 (heparin factor), a potent naturally occurring inhibitor of activated factor X and thrombin, and by decreasing platelet adhesiveness.

Coumadin is a proven antithrombotic, interfering with the hepatic synthesis of clotting factors by depressing vitamin K activity. Dextran, a branched polysaccharide of bacterial origin, alters platelet function and also disturbs the structure of a fibrin clot formed in its presence. Dextran preparations with an average molecular weight of 40,000 to 70,000 are used to prevent deep vein thrombosis and pulmonary embolism; dextran has been reported to be effective in patients with hip fractures and elective hip operations and in general surgical, urological, and gynecological procedures.[1,51] Despite its efficacy, however, routine prophylactic administration has not gained wide acceptance because of the frequent side effects, high cost, and need for intravenous administration. Newer agents that interfere with platelet adhesiveness, such as aspirin, are attractive because they are easy to administer, have few side effects, and cost little. However, aspirin is now considered ineffective in reducing significant deep vein thrombosis after total hip arthroplasty and fatal pulmonary embolism in particular. Hydroxychloroquine has shown promise, but further clinical trials using newer methods of detection are awaited to demonstrate its efficacy as compared with warfarin, which may be considered the "gold standard" for prophylaxis.[1,124,157,159,161]

Besides chemical agents, physical modalities such as external pneumatic compression and electrical stimulation of the calves during operation have been used. Further clinical studies are required to confirm claims that these techniques are efficacious and can feasibly be applied to large numbers of cases to prevent thromboembolic disease.

In practice, several approaches can be taken to prevent thromboembolic disease after total hip arthroplasty. The first is to wait for clinical evidence of embolism or phlebitis and then institute anticoagulation therapy. However, as stated previously, fatal pulmonary embolism is often sudden and unheralded; clinical signs may not appear until it is too late. A second alternative is prophylactic anticoagulation in high-risk patients such as patients who have a history of thromboembolic disease, cardiac disease, or vein surgery or who show significant venous disease. A third approach is routine prophylactic anticoagulation in all patients unless contraindicated by hypertension, bleeding diathesis, liver disease, peptic ulcer, and ulcerative colitis. The fourth is to use the newer objective noninvasive techniques, such as 125-I fibrinogen scanning and impedance plethysmography, switching from prophylactic anticoagulation to therapeutic anticoagulation if fresh thrombi are noted. A fifth approach is to combine objective detection techniques and adjunctive mechanical compression, that is, stockings and intermittent calf compression, and routine administration of low-dose warfarin or high-dose Plaquenil (which has been shown to reduce thromboembolic complications).

Investigators continue to use experimental and trial series of prophylaxis against thromboembolic complications in their search for the "ideal" prophylactic method or agent for prevention.[63,88,187]

The single most common and critical complication associated with anticoagulation is hemorrhage at the surgical site or in a remote area.

Crawford[38] has reported discontinuation of prophylaxis because of complications arising from the treatment itself. He and his co-workers reported a study of 900 total hip arthroplasties in which half the patients received oral anticoagulants and half did not; the death rates in the two groups were approximately the same: 2%. While deaths in the untreated group were caused by fatal pulmonary embolism, deaths in the treated group were related to pulmonary emboli and gastrointestinal bleeding associated with anticoagulants; the study also found a threefold increase in the incidence of deep wound infection and an increased number of hemorrhagic complications in the treated group.

Crawford's criticism of anticoagulation was not related to its efficacy, but focused on its bleeding complications. Oral anticoagulants such as warfarin (Coumadin) have been proven most effective in prophylaxis, but they require careful control and immediate discontinuation should local or remote hemorrhage complications develop.

Precautions

Given the frequency of venous thrombosis and the mortality from pulmonary emboli, the benefits of prophylactics must be considered in all cases (Table 9-1). The choice of the agent or agents must be judged against the danger of complications resulting from prophylaxis.[70,103] The incidence of hemorrhagic complication may be minimized by scrupulous patient selection; patients with hemorrhagic diathesis or thrombocytopenia, coincidental gastrointestinal bleeding, a history of recently active peptic ulcers or ulcerative colitis, diabetic retinopathy, or uncontrolled and severe hypertension would be excluded. It is essential that anticoagulation be well controlled throughout the prophylactic period. Ideally, for safety's sake, only one person should be responsible for the anticoagulation of each patient; this should not be a "rotating task" for the resident or attending physician covering on a particular date. The medical consultant is invaluable in this regard. All noninvasive physical measures are important, such as elevation of the foot of the bed, muscle exercises, and antiembolic stockings. Early ambulation appreciably reduces the threat of thromboembolic disease, and standing and walking should begin as soon as the patient is able after the operation.

Patients receiving anticoagulation treatment require observation for the clinical signs of hematoma: local pain, swelling, fluctuation, warmth, falling hematocrit level, temperature elevation, and occasional spontaneous drainage of dark blood from the

Table 9-1A Incidence of Thromboembolic Disease (Deep Venous Thrombosis or Pulmonary Embolism) After Total Hip Arthroplasty Without Prophylaxis

First author, year of publication, and reference number	All patients with thromboembolic disease		Operative side*		Nonoperative side†		Proximal DVT*	
	TED/patient	%	DVT/patient	%	DVT/patient	%	DVT/patient	%
Morris 1981[128]	17/27	63	—	—	—	—	—	—
Bergquist 1979[17]	32/51	63	28/51	55	19/51	37	14/51	27
Harris 1977[75]	23/51	45	—	—	—	—	14/51	27
Stamatakis 1977[180]	81/160	51	81/160	51	—	—	46/160	29
Sagar 1976[156]	22/32	69	22/32	69	—	—	17/32	53
Schondorf 1976[164]	9/15	60	9/15	60	3/15	20	6/15	40
Bergquist 1976[16a]	6/10	60	5/10	50	3/10	30	2/10	20
Hampson 1974[67]	28/52	54	—	—	—	—	—	—
Morris 1974[127]	16/32	50	—	—	—	—	5/32	16
Evarts 1971[51]	30/56	54	25/56	45	11/56	20	19/56	34
TOTAL	264/486	54	170/324	52	36/132	27	123/407	30
Range (all studies)		45–69		45–69		20–37		16–53

*Some studies did not report the location of deep venous thrombosis.
†Some studies did not report the incidence of deep venous thrombosis in the nonoperative extremity.
TED: Number of patients with thromboembolic disease, including deep venous thrombosis and/or pulmonary embolism. DVT: Number of patients with deep venous thrombosis.

Table 9-1B The Incidence of Pulmonary Embolism after Total Hip Arthroplasty Without Prophylaxis

First author, year of publication, and reference number	All pulmonary emboli		Fatal pulmonary emboli		Percentage of total mortality		Total mortality	
	PE/patient	%	FPE/patient	%	FPE/TM	%	TM/patient	%
Bergquist 1979[17]	14/71	19.7	2/71	2.8	2/2	100	2/71	2.8
Johnson 1977[106]	179/1174	15.2	26/1174	2.3	—	—	—	—
Schöndorf 1976[164]	2/15	13.3	1/15	6.7	1/1	100	1/15	6.7
Sagar 1976[156]	2/32	6.2	1/32	3.1	1/1	100	1/32	3.1
D'Ambrosia 1975[40]	7/99	7.1	1/99	1.0	1/2	50	2/99	2.0
Coventry 1973[36]	3/58	5.2	2/58	3.4	—	—	—	—
Rothermal 1973[153]	4/60	6.7	0/60	0.0	0/1	0	1/60	1.7
Charnley 1972[28]	27/582	4.6	8/582	1.4	8/12	67	12/582	2.1
TOTAL	238/2091	11.4	41/2091	2.0	13/19*	68	19/859*	2.2
Range (all studies)		4.6–19.7		0.06–6.7		0–100		1.7–6.7

*From Haake DA, Berkman SA: Venous thromboembolic disease after hip surgery: risk factors, prophylaxis, and diagnosis, *Clin Orthop* 242:212, 1989.
*Johnson and Coventry studies not included because total mortality was not reported.
PE: Number of patients developing pulmonary embolism. FPE: Number of patients with fatal pulmonary embolism. TM: Total mortality from all causes.

wound. The patient's urine and stool require inspection for evidence of gastrointestinal and genitourinary bleeding.

Thromboembolic complications after total hip arthroplasty are rarely recurrent. Thus long-term prophylaxis is unnecessary. Recovery after thromboembolic disease after total hip arthroplasty surgery is most often complete. Both pulmonary function and swelling of the leg return to normal or near normal.

PHYSICAL AND MECHANICAL PROPHYLAXIS

The noninvasive nature of mechanical and physiological methods makes them extremely attractive; however, none of the mechanical methods have proved to be sufficient, singularly or in combination, in preventing thromboembolic disease after total hip arthroplasty. They must be used as adjuncts to chemical anticoagulation prophylaxis.

Early Ambulation and Elevation of Foot of Bed

One of the most recognized methods of prophylaxis against thromboembolic disease is early postoperative physical activity, including early postoperative ambulation and exercise.[116] In particular, calf, thigh, buttock, and hamstring contractions (isometric) and deep breathing exercises are routinely prescribed. Another physical modality, elevation of the foot of the bed, is also effective.[78]

Compression Stockings

Of various prophylactic methods, compression of the calf by elastic socks and stockings has been most popular, but used alone it is probably the least effective prophylactic method to protect against thromboembolic disease. In one study, Browse and Hall reported no prophylactic benefit from the wearing of elastic stockings.[24] However, other investigators have found graded compression elastic stockings beneficial because of their theoretical ability to provide gradual compression in the calf with decreasing compression proximally. The use of graded compression stockings has been compared with the use of dextran 70 to reduce thromboembolic disease.

Using venography for diagnosis, the incidence of deep vein thrombosis was reduced significantly to 20%, compared to 54% in the control group.[10,13] This author prefers the use of thigh-high stockings in total hip arthroplasty patients, on the assumption that longer sleeves compress a greater muscle mass than short ones. The thigh-high stockings do not interfere with the surgical wound. It may be advantageous to have patients wear them preoperatively to become used to them and because they might offer more protection against deep vein thrombosis as well.

Electrical Stimulation

Electrical stimulation of the calf to prevent thromboembolic disease has been used in neurosurgical patients, but because it causes discomfort and there is little data supporting its efficacy, it is not commonly used in elective surgery.[119]

Intermittent Pneumatic Compression of the Calf

This method uses a pneumatic calf sleeve applied to the legs to create a sequential, cyclic compression. The portable controller attached to the sleeve provides a peak pressure of approximately 45 mm Hg at the ankle and approximately 25 mm Hg at the thigh level. Cyclic compression is applied continuously preoperatively, intraoperatively, and postoperatively, usually until the patient begins ambulation.[79] Current studies of the use of this device suggest different pressures, frequencies of compression, and durations of use, among other variables.[77]

The early use of this device was evaluated by Hartman and associates,[79] who compared the use of pneumatic compression and elevation of the leg with elevation of the leg alone. The investigators studied 52 patients in each group. Support stockings were removed after the compression device was discontinued. Using radionucleid fibrinogen scanning to identify thrombi, the investigators found that a deep thrombosis developed in 19% of the control group, compared with 2% of the group treated with the compression device. In a similar study that used Doppler ultrasound in 100 patients against a control group (wearing stockings), Pedegana and co-workers[147] reported that 17% had deep vein thrombosis, compared with none in the trial group. When Gallus and associates[56] used 125-I fibrinogen scanning and venography to diagnosis deep vein thrombosis, they found that pneumatic compression did not reduce the proximal vein thrombi. The incidence of calf thrombi was decreased 45% in untreated patients versus 16% in the treated group. These studies indicate that although intermittent pneumatic compression seems to be relatively effective in preventing deep vein thrombosis, it is not sufficiently safe to be recommended as the sole source of prophylaxis to prevent deep vein thrombosis after total hip arthroplasty.

Vena Cava Filters

The use of a transvenous filter such as a Greenfield filter in patients with a history of thromboembolic disease who need total hip arthroplasty should definitely be considered, especially if the patient also has a history of active duodenal ulcer bleeding or other contraindications for anticoagulation treatment.[113] This procedure is indicated in patients whose anticoagulation treatment fails to control repeated pulmonary embolism. It can be performed in an angiography suite. The morbidity related to this method is relatively minimal. This author has also advocated use of this protective method in patients who have had repeated pulmonary embolism despite adequate therapeutic anticoagulation treatment.

CHEMICAL PROPHYLAXIS
Warfarin (Crystalline Sodium Warfarin [Coumadin])

Indications and modes of administration for warfarin have varied with investigators. In a Mayo Clinic study[36] anticoagulation with sodium warfarin after 1900 total hip arthroplasties proved safe and effective in preventing fatal thromboembolic disease. The investigators used delayed administration of the drug; that is, anticoagulation did not begin before the fifth postoperative day. Clinical diagnosis of thromboembolic disease was the main criterion for this study. It is of special interest that 50% of all thromboembolic complications occurred during the first 5 days before anticoagulation. Sodium warfarin requires very careful monitoring if hemorrhagic complications are to be avoided, because a 10% to 20% risk of bleeding exists with this drug. However, when carefully and effectively used, sodium warfarin is the best method available for reducing and treating thromboembolic conditions.

In a random prospective study, Harris and associates[72] demonstrated that there was no significant difference in the prophylactic efficacy of warfarin, dextran, and aspirin in reducing the number of patients with fresh thrombi, but warfarin and dextran were superior to aspirin in reducing the number of thrombi formed. However, significantly fewer bleeding complications occurred with aspirin than with warfarin. Those investigators further concluded that prophylactic use of warfarin or aspirin, followed by warfarin therapy whenever a thrombus was detected by phlebography, provided effective protection against pulmonary embolism. They used phlebography to detect venous thrombosis of the lower extremities, because in their view the clinical diagnosis of venous

thrombosis was grossly inaccurate.

A number of clinical investigations have shown that warfarin (crystalline sodium warfarin [Coumadin]) reduces the incidence of postoperative venous thrombi (Table 9-2). Review of the literature regarding the use of warfarin indicates the following facts:

1. Warfarin is a potent anticoagulant that can prevent both distal and proximal deep vein thrombosis.
2. Administration of warfarin for prophylaxis is easy, safe, and effective when it is used at "prophylactic levels." Several studies now have reported no deaths from pulmonary embolism following the use of low-dose warfarin.[3,54,72]
3. With the exception of one study,[9] warfarin has been proven to be more effective than heparin, dextran, and aspirin.
4. Bleeding resulting from warfarin-induced anticoagulation is largely dose-related and can be

Table 9-2 Thromboembolism Prophylaxis Using Oral Anticoagulants in Patients Treated with Total Hip Arthroplasty

First author, year of publication, and reference number	Study type	Diagnostic methods	Oral anticoagulants		Control	
			DVT	PE	DVT	PE
Francis 1983*[54]	Prosp.	CV (all)	8/39	0/39	–	–
	Random.		21%	0%	–	–
Guyer 1982[62]	Prosp.	Clin DX: CV	9/88	6/88	–	–
	Random.	LS (all)	10%	7%	–	–
Barber 1977[9]	Prosp.	FLS	34/58	0/58	–	–
	Random.	LS (all)	59%	05	–	–
Harris 1974*[72]	Prosp.	CV (all)	10/55	0/55	–	–
	Random.		18%	0%	–	–
Hume 1973[89]	Prosp.	FLS (all)	FLS 10/17	–	FLS 8/19	–
	Random.	CV (all)	CV 4/19	–	CV 4/19	–
	Blinded		FLS 59%	–	FLS 42%	–
			CV 21%	–	CV 21%	–
Harris 1972[71]	Prosp.	Clin DX: CV	3/114	6/114	–	–
	Random.	LS, PA	3%	5%	–	–
Salzman 1971[161]	Prosp.	Clin DX:CV	4/43	2/43	–	–
	Random.		9%	5%	–	–
Harris 1967[70]	Prosp.	Clin DX: PA	5/70	0/70	23/67	7/67
	Random.		7%	0%	34%	10%
TOTAL (all studies)			83/484	14/467	31/86	7/67
TOTAL CV			21/111		4/19	
Percent (all studies)			17%	3%	36%	10%
Percent CV			19%		21%	
Range (all studies)			3%–59%	0%–7%	34%–42%	10%
Range CV			18%–21%		21%	

From Haake DA, Berkman SA: Venous thromboembolic disease after hip surgery: risk factors, prophylaxis, and diagnosis, *Clin Orthop* 242: 212, 1989.
*Oral anticoagulants begun preoperatively.
DVT: Incidence of deep venous thrombosis. PE: Incidence of pulmonary embolism. LS: Lung scan. CV: Contrast venography. Clin DX: Clinical diagnosis. PA: Pulmonary angiogram. FLS: Fibrinogen leg scan. Prosp.: Prospective. Random.: Randomized; if controls receiving no prophylaxis are not listed, the study used controls receiving an alternative prophylactic regimen.

minimized if the dose is kept at a low level and not at the therapeutic level. In their study of 3000 consecutive total hip arthroplasties, Amstutz and associates[3] administered low-dose warfarin prophylactically in addition to using elastic stockings and elevating the limb. The administration schedule of warfarin included a first dose the night of the operation and maintenance of the prothrombin time between 16 and 18 seconds. No single fatal pulmonary embolism occurred in the entire series. The 14 nonfatal pulmonary embolisms constituted a rate of 0.5%. Patients experienced 44 hemorrhagic complications (1.5%).

In a period after 1974 during which the protocol just described was strictly maintained, the rate of pulmonary embolism in 2595 patients in the same series was 0.2% and bleeding complications were only 1%. This study parallels this author's experience in more than 700 consecutive operations (primary and revision patients who received low-dose Coumadin as described). My experience includes no fatal pulmonary embolism and only nonfatal embolisms. Discrepancies exist in the literature regarding the incidence of hemorrhagic complications related to this prophylactic agent. These discrepancies stem from the unknown quality of control during the anticoagulation program. Warfarin appears to be most effective when given preoperatively and continued postoperatively while the prothrombin time is maintained at a low level within the range of 1.2 to 1.5 times the patient's control (prior treatment). Warfarin can be used for routine prophylaxis in low- or moderate-risk patients as follows:

1. 10 mg of warfarin given the night before surgery.
2. 5 mg of warfarin given the day of surgery and a daily maintenance dose of 5 to 7 mg of warfarin until the prothrombin time is approximately 1.5 times that of the control value. This level should not be exceeded since hemorrhagic complications may result.

Some authors have suggested that high-risk patients, those with prior thromboembolic disease or heart conditions, should be treated with a "two-step" form of warfarin therapy.[49,54] First, the warfarin is given 14 days before surgery to prolong the prothrombin time from 1.5 to 3 seconds greater than the control level. At the second stage immediately after surgery the dosage is increased to a prothrombin time level of 1.5 times the level of control.[49] Currently we have been using the above regimen but excluded the preoperation dose the night before surgery for patients without prior history of thromboembolic disease.

Contraindications

Contraindications to warfarin are listed in the box.

> ### Relative and Absolute Contraindications to Warfarin (Coumadin)
>
> - All hemorrhagic conditions
> - History of hematoma, melena, or hemostasis
> - History of hemolysis
> - Peptic ulcer
> - Active liver disease
> - Stroke
> - Cerebral insufficiency
> - Concomitant treatment with barbiturates (decreases warfarin's effectiveness), aspirin compounds and other antiinflammatory drugs (increase warfarin's activity)
> - A lack of monitoring (guaiac stool test on alternate days, PT, Hct/Hgb daily while in hospital)

A documented rare but serious complication of Coumadin therapy involves skin and soft tissue. It typically affects obese, middle-aged women on the third to fifth day of Coumadin therapy. Pain, erythema, and ecchymosis are followed by frank necrosis.* The currently acceptable treatment is to immediately discontinue Coumadin therapy and to begin intravenous administration of heparin.[136] Ultimate gangrene may necessitate amputation, skin grafting, or both.

Combined Low-Dose Warfarin and Pneumatic Compressions

A comparison of the use of low-dose warfarin with external pneumatic compression in a prospective randomized study found both methods to be safe and effective.[144] Deep vein thrombosis developed in 12 of 72 in the Coumadin group versus 11 of 66 patients in the external pneumatic compression group. No major bleeding complications occurred in either group.

Heparin

Although low-dose heparin has been found to be a dependable prophylaxis in general surgery, its use in orthopaedic surgery is now in dispute. The bulk of the evidence suggests that it is inadequate for patients undergoing major hip surgery.† On the other hand, several papers document the efficacy of low-dose heparin in cases of hip fracture and elective hip surgery.[42,106,157,161] This method involves 5000 units of aqueous calcium heparin injected subcutaneously 2 hours before surgery and then given postoperatively every 8 hours during the next 10 days. Obviously, full therapeutic doses of heparin are not appropriate for prophylaxis since a considerable risk of associated bleeding exists after surgery.

---

* References 6, 25, 53, 134, 135, 191.
† References 51, 57, 67, 72, 105.

Other investigators have reported that low-dose heparin (5000 units b.i.d. or t.i.d.), although effective in high-risk general surgical patients, is inferior to dextran and Coumadin for prophylaxis in orthopaedic patients.[51,88]

In one study, Planes and co-workers[149] performed routine venography for 12 to 15 days after total hip arthroplasty in 745 consecutive patients, all of whom had received heparin prophylaxis. Eighty-one (10.8%) of the patients in this group showed evidence of deep vein thrombosis. Of these, 23 (3%) were distal, 44 (5.9%) were isolated proximal, and 5 (0.7%) had both a proximal and a distal thrombosis. In addition, 9 (1.2%) had an extension of the thrombosis from calf to thigh. This study also indicated that although heparin reduced the number of distal thromboses and clots in the contralateral limb, it failed to reduce proximal femoral thrombosis.

Low-molecular-weight heparin has been used for prophylaxis for hip surgery. It is an effective anticoagulant that produces less bleeding than regular heparin. In one study using low-molecular-weight heparin in total hip arthroplasty patients, Turpie and associates[190] reported a reduction in incidence of [10.8% of deep vein thrombosis for over 51.3% of the control]; the incidence of proximal limb thrombosis was also reduced from 23.1% to 5.4%. Using an adjusted dose of heparin and the partial thromboplastin time (PTT) at the upper limits of normal with a protocol starting at 3500 units every 8 hours and commencing 2 days before planned surgery, Leyvraz and co-workers[117] significantly reduced deep vein thrombosis after total hip arthroplasty. Venography documented deep vein thrombosis in 5 of 38 patients (13%) with adjusted dose and 16 of 41 patients (39%) with fixed low-dose heparin (*P* value less than 0.01). The incidence of

Table 9-3 Heparin/Dihydroergotamine Thromboembolism Prophylaxis in Hip Surgery

First author, year of publication, and reference number	Operation	Study type	Diagnostic methods	Number prophylaxis DVT	Number prophylaxis PE	DHE/Heparin TID DVT	DHE/Heparin TID PE	DHE/Heparin BID DVT	DHE/Heparin BID PE
Kakkar 1985[107]	THA	Prosp.	CV	—	—	131/500	4/500	—	—
		LS			25%	0.8%			
Laedloff 1984[118]	THA	Prosp.	FLS, CV	—	—			25/100	3/100
		Random.	AT	—	—			25%	3%
Morris 1981[128]	THA	Prosp.	FLS	17/27	6/27	2/27	1/27	—	—
		Random.							
		Blind	LS	63%	22%	7%	4%	—	—
Westermann 1981[196a]	THA	Prosp.	FLS, CV	—	—	16/63	1/63	15/61	0/61
			LS, AT	—	—	25%	2%	25%	0%
Lahnborg 1980[111]	HFX	Prosp.	FLS	28/69	0/69	—	—	12/71	1/71
		Random.							
		Plcbo.	Clin DX	41%	0%	—	—	17%	1%
Bergquist 1980[18]	THA	Prosp.	FLS	—	—	—	—	6/59	5/45
		Random.	LS, AT	—	—	—	—	10%	11%
	HFX	Prosp.	FLS	—	—	—	—	2/25	—
		Random.	AT	—	—	—	—	8%	—
Schondorf 1980[165]	THA	Prosp.	FLS, DU, CV	—	—	2/53	0/53	—	—
		Random.	AT	—	—	4%	0%	—	—
Kakkar 1979[108]	THA	Prosp.	FLS, CV	—	—	10/50	0/50	—	—
		Random.	Clin DX	—	—	20%	0%	—	—
Sagar 1976[156]	THA	Prosp.	FLS, CV	22/32	2/32	4/25	0/25	—	—
		Random.	AT	69%	6%	16%	0%	—	—
	THA	TOTAL		39/59	8/59	165/718	6/718	46/220	8/206
		Percent		66%	14%	23%	0.8%	21%	39%
		Range		63%–69%	6%–22%	4%–26%	0.8%–4%	10%–25%	0%–11%
	HFX	TOTAL		28/69	0/69	—	—	14/96	1/71
		Percent		41%	0%	—	—	15%	1.4%
		Range		41%	0%	—	—	8%–17%	1.4%

From Haake DA, Berkman SA: Venous thromboembolic disease after his surgery: risk factors, prophylaxis, and diagnosis, *Clin Orthop* 242:212, 1989.
CV: Contrast venography. LS: Lung scan. FLS: Fibrinogen leg scan. AT: Autopsy. DU: Doppler ultrasonography. DVT: Incidence of deep venous thrombosis. Clin DX: Clinical diagnosis. THA: Total hip arthroplasty. HFX: Hip fracture surgery. Prosp.: Prospective. Random.: Randomized; if controls receiving no prophylaxis are not listed, the study used controls receiving an alternative prophylactic regimen.

proximal vein thrombosis was significantly reduced for the adjusted-dose group (5% versus 32% for the fixed group [P value less than 0.003]). The superiority of the adjusted over the fixed group was not associated with an increase in hemorrhagic complications. It seems that prophylaxis for total hip arthroplasty by adjusted-dose heparin is safe and effective.

From the bulk of available information it may be concluded that low-dose heparin alone is not as effective in prophylaxis against deep vein thrombosis after total hip arthroplasty as it might be for general surgical, gynecological, neurosurgical, and urological procedures. A therapeutic regimen of heparin after total hip arthroplasty requires extremely careful monitoring, and serious hemorrhagic complications can result from a full therapeutic dose (Table 9-3).

Complications

Complications of heparin used as a prophylactic or therapeutic agent in surgery have been well documented and include serious bleeding from operative wounds and various other sources, thrombocytopenia, and arterial and venous thromboses.* In the treatment of thromboembolic disease in total hip and total knee arthroplasty in 1784 patients, complications occurred as frequently as 30% in 112 patients who were treated with heparin.[146] The frequency of bleeding complications had an inverse ratio to the days lapsed from surgery when treatment was initiated (for example, at 6 days postoperatively the frequency of bleeding was 45%, which declined to 15% when the patients were treated at 7 days after arthroplasty). In addition, thrombocytopenia developed in less than 5% of the patients. The incidence of thrombocytopenia after heparin administration has been reported to be as high as 30% and as low as less than 5%.† This author believes that the use of heparin for minor thromboembolic complications is contraindicated and that the thromboembolic problem and its significance must be fully evaluated by venography, plethysmography, 125-I fibrinogen, and pulmonary angiography before using a full therapeutic dose of this agent.

Combined Heparin and Warfarin

In a study from our institution of thromboembolic disease after total hip arthroplasty,[60] low-dose heparin-warfarin prophylactic anticoagulation afforded significant protection against fatal pulmonary embolism and reduced nonfatal thromboembolic complications, even in patients with venous disease or a history of thromboembolic disease. The inves-

tigators believed the 13.1% hematoma rate (5% major) was a small, nonlethal, and acceptable price to pay for this protection. In this retrospective uncontrolled study, 796 patients satisfied the requirement of having been placed on the prophylactic anticoagulation treatment program during the first 2 postoperative days. (It should be noted that in this series 34% of the patients had evidence of prior venous disease or a history of thromboembolic disease.) The incidences of deep venous thrombosis and pulmonary embolism in the entire group were 1.8% and 3%, respectively. For all patients without a history of thromboembolic disease and without venous disease, the figures were 1.1% and 2.4%, respectively. The incidence of fatal pulmonary embolism was 0.1% for the total population in the study; the single fatality occurred in a patient who had had two episodes of phlebitis.* The investigators concluded therefore that this combined program of low-dose heparin-warfarin anticoagulation treatment was efficacious in preventing thromboembolic disease in the general population and in high-risk patients with prior thromboembolic disease and venous disease.

Complications occurring during the anticoagulation program in this study deserve special comment: 13.1% of the patients in this study developed a wound hematoma. Undoubtedly, such a successful outcome may not be reproducible unless this combination anticoagulation regimen is carefully monitored.

Combined Heparin and Dihydroergotamine

Dihydroergotamine (DHE) is a known vasoconstrictor for venous circulation that has been used in combination with heparin (5000 units of heparin and 0.5 mg of DHE) 2 hours preoperatively and every 2 hours thereafter until the patient is ambulatory. Table 9-3 compares nine trials involving heparin-DHE prophylaxis against thromboembolic complications of hip surgery.[18,165] The combination has been shown to be better than the effect of each substance individually.[107] In a prospective study involving 500 total hip arthroplasties, deep vein thrombosis (diagnosed by venography) developed in 26% of patients. Four patients developed pulmonary embolism (one fatal). Of 25 patients (5.0%) who developed a severe hematoma, 6 required evacuation. A combination of heparin and aspirin has been used for prophylaxis without a significant improvement of the results over the combinations of heparin and Coumadin.[164]

---

* References 5, 7, 8, 12, 61, 122, 126, 146, 148.
† References 5, 8, 66, 120, 146

---

* Patients with venous disease had incidences of deep vein thrombosis and pulmonary embolism of 2.0% and 4.1% respectively; those with a history of thromboembolic disease had incidences of 4.3% and 4.3%. The "prior thromboembolic disease" group had a fatal pulmonary embolism rate of 0.9%.

Table 9-4A Thromboembolism Prophylaxis Using Dextran 70 in Patients Treated with Total Hip Arthroplasty

First author, year of publication, and reference number	Study type	Diagnostic methods	Dextran 70		Control	
			DVT	PE	DVT	PE
Bergquist 1980[18]	Prosp.	FLS (all)	15/56	8/46*	—	—
	Random.	LS	27%	17%	—	—
Bergquist 1979[17]	Prosp.	FLS (all)	27/47	21/70	32/51	20/71
	Random.	LS (all)	57%	30%	63%	28%
Hurson 1979[93]	Prosp.	RV-CV	15/55	9/55	9/51	8/51
	Random.	LS	27%	16%	18%	16%
Barber 1977[9]	Prosp.	FLS (all)	26/51	2/51	—	—
	Random.	AT	51%	4%	—	—
TOTAL			83/209	40/222	41/102	28/122
Percent			40%	18%	40%	23%
Range			27%–57%	4%–30%	18%–63%	16%–28%

From Haake DA, Berkman SA: Venous thromboembolic disease after hip surgery: risk factors, prophylaxis, and diagnosis, *Clin Orthop* 242:212, 1989.
*Lung scan performed in 46/56 patients.
DVT: Incidence of deep venous thrombosis. PE: Incidence of pulmonary embolism. FLS: Fibrinogen leg scan. LS: Lung scan. RV-CV: Radionuclide venography confirmed by contrast venography. AT: Autopsy. Prosp.: Prospective. Random.: Randomized; if controls receiving no prophylaxis are not listed, the study used controls receiving an alternative prophylactic regimen.

Table 9-4B Thromboembolism Prophylaxis Using Dextran 40 in Patients Treated with Total Hip Arthroplasty

First author, year of publication, and reference number	Study type	Diagnostic methods	Dextran 40		Control	
			DVT	PE	DVT	PE
Francis 1983[54]	Props.	CV (all)	11/29	1/29	—	—
	Random.		38%	3%	—	—
Harris 1974[72]	Prosp.	CV (all)	14/61	2/61	—	—
	Random.		23%	3%	—	—
Rothermel 1973[153]	Prosp.	Clin. DX	4/60	3/60	6/60	4/60
	Random.	LS	7%	5%	10%	7%
Harris 1972[71]	Prosp.	Clin. DX	7/113	7/113	—	—
	Random.	CV, LS, PA	6%	6%	—	—
Salzman 1971[161]	Prosp.	Clin. DX	5/49	2/49	—	—
	Random.		10%	4%	—	—
Evarts 1971[51]	Prosp.	CV (all)	5/19	2/19	10/20	2/20
	Random.		26%	11%	50%	10%
	Blinded	LS				
TOTAL			46/331	17/331	16/80	6/80
Percent			14	5.1	20	7.5
Range			6%–38%	3%–11%	10%–20%	7%–10%

From Haake DA, Berkman SA: Venous thromboembolic disease after hip surgery: risk factors, prophylaxis, and diagnosis, *Clin Orthop* 242:212, 1989.
DVT: Incidence of deep venous thrombosis. PE: Incidence of pulmonary embolism. LS: Lung scan. CV: Contrast venography. PA: Pulmonary angiogram. Clin. DX: Clinical diagnosis. Prosp.: Prospective. Random.: Randomized; if controls receiving no prophylaxis are not listed, the study used controls receiving an alternative prophylactic regimen.

Dextran

Of the two different molecular weight dextrans (one with a mean weight of 70,000 [dextran 70] and the other with a mean weight of 40,000 [dextran 40]), dextran 40 is more efficient than dextran 70 in terms of excretion by the kidney. Dextran operates by inhibiting platelet aggregation and coating the vascular endothelium. Its antiembolic action has been extensively studied clinically and experimentally.* After receiving dextran 40, patients have shown increased lysis of thrombin and improved blood flow in addition to platelet reductions and changes in the fibrin structure (Table 9-4).

Several investigators have reported that dextran reduces the incidence of thromboembolic complications.† The agent usually is administered in the operating room at the beginning of surgery, then on a schedule of 500 ml daily for 3 days, followed by 500 ml on alternate days until the patient is discharged.

Studies using either 125-I fibrinogen leg scanning or venography during use of dextran 70 demonstrated no effect on the frequency of deep vein thrombosis and only a slight decrease in pulmonary embolism following total hip arthroplasty[63] (Table 9-4, A). Of interest was a significant decrease in the incidence of deep vein thrombosis and pulmonary embolism (fatal and nonfatal) in patients diagnosed with hip fracture who were treated with dextran 70. However, the literature indicates that dextran 40 is more effective, because it decreases the incidence of deep vein thrombosis and pulmonary embolism after total hip arthroplasty.[63] Nevertheless, it is less beneficial than the protection imparted by the use of warfarin.

In 4096 patients who received intravenous dextran 70 (a standard method at Wrightington Hospital for 3 hours[29] consisting of 500 ml dextran 70 on the day of surgery followed by 500 ml of Macrodex 40 the following day), dextran 70 (Macrodex) was not started until the end of the operation because of the potential for capillary bleeding from the wound. This study included 46 (1.1%) fatal and 339 (8.2%) clinically diagnosed pulmonary embolisms.

A renal profile of the patient must be obtained preoperatively when administration of low-molecular-weight dextran is planned. Patients treated with dextran require careful observation for fluid-electrolyte balance in view of the plasma-extending nature of dextran and the possibility of pulmonary edema, congestive heart failure, and renal failure. The use of dextran as advocated by Evarts[49] entails preoperative, operative, and postoperative administration of low-molecular-weight dextran, which continues for 4 to 5 days postoperatively until the patient is ambulatory. The dose is adjusted on a sliding scale, with a loading dose of 7 to 10 ml/kg infusion given over 12 hours beginning 1 hour before surgery. A maintenance dose of 5 ml/kg is given as a constant infusion. Evarts and co-workers[49] reported the efficacy of treatment with dextran 40, based on the number of deaths after surgery. The rate of fatal pulmonary embolism in 3000 untreated patients was 1.5%, which favorably decreased to 0.4% in 3000 patients treated with dextran.

Complications

Although the anticoagulant effect of dextran is well recognized, like other agents it can cause bleeding. Other possible complications are renal failure and anaphylaxis. Pulmonary edema is another deleterious side effect, which may be caused by erroneous judgment in postoperative fluid therapy.[153] Because dextran must be administered intravenously, its main disadvantage is the potential to produce congestive heart failure by overhydration. Despite its efficacy, it has not gained wide acceptance as a prophylactic agent for routine administration because of its cost, frequent side effects, and the need for intravenous administration. At our institution, dextran used in prophylaxis against thromboembolic disease was less than effective and was accompanied by serious complications.[153]

Allergic reactions to dextran can be minor (cutaneous eruptions), but they can also be serious (anaphylactic shock). The allergic reactions usually occur after the administration of the first few ml.

Contraindications

Contraindications to the use of low-molecular-weight dextran are congestive heart failure, pulmonary dysfunction, chronic kidney disease or failure, and allergic reactions.

Aspirin

Salzman and associates[161] have reported reduction of venous thromboembolism with prophylactic aspirin. This agent is attractive because of its ease of administration and management. On the day before the operation the patient receives 600 mg orally b.i.d., and postoperatively the patient receives 600 mg orally twice a day or 1200 mg twice a day rectally. As previously stated, Harris and associates found warfarin and dextran superior to aspirin in reducing the number of thrombi formed. Based on their early experience, however, they found the three drugs equally effective in reducing the prevalence of thrombi in the thigh. Also of note was the significantly lower rate of bleeding complications associated with aspirin compared with the other two agents. Harris and associates[74,96] concluded that aspirin may be the preferred drug in

---

*References 15, 48, 50, 82, 154.
†References 50, 71, 95, 106, 115, 127.

patients without prior thromboembolic disease or significant venous disease; however, they found aspirin to be less effective in females than in males as a prophylactic against thromboembolic disease.

That several reports would indicate that aspirin was a preferred anticoagulant for prophylaxis in total hip arthroplasty is logical because it is easy to administer and has relatively minor side effects. It operates through antiplatelet action. Unfortunately, the results of clinical trials using aspirin for prophylaxis have been mixed and disappointing.[181] In one study (a double-blind trial), aspirin was effective only in men,[76] but the results of other studies have been disappointingly negative for both sexes.[80,158] In an attempt to show a difference between a low dose and a high dose of aspirin in protection against deep vein thrombosis, Harris and co-workers[76] conducted a randomized trial.

They showed that the higher dose of aspirin was neither more nor less effective than the lower dose. Thus their data continued to support 1.2 gm of aspirin daily in men. In a retrospective study, Stone and associates[184] from our institution showed the value of the protection provided by aspirin against thromboembolic disease to be equal for men and women. Postoperative thromboembolic disease developed in 9 of 218 men (3.6%) and 13 of 254 women (5.1%). This difference was not statistically significant (P value less than or equal to 0.51). Among all patients, bleeding complications occurred in 24 of 481 (5.8%) patients given aspirin and 76 of 479 (16.0%) patients given a heparin-warfarin combination. This difference was statistically significant (P value $\leq$ 0.001). The large number of patients reported here permitted retrospective statistical analysis of prophy-

Table 9-5 Aspirin Thromboembolism Prophylaxis After Total Hip Arthroplasty

First author, year of publication, and reference number	Study type	Diagnostic methods	Aspirin dose (mg)	Control		Aspirin	
				DVT	PE	DVT	PE
Sautter 1983[163]	Prosp. Random. Double Blind	FLS, CV LS, PA	225 q.i.d.*	37/63 59%	5/63 7.9%	21/54 38.5%	2/54 3.7%
Guyer 1982[62]	Prosp.	Clin DX, CV LS (all)	650 b.i.d.	— —	— —	20/96 21%	19/96 20%
Harris 1982[79]	Prosp. Random. Double Blind	FLS, IP, CV LS, PA	300 q.i.d.	— —	— —	36/92 39%	1/92 1.1%
Stulberg 1982[186]	Prosp.	LS (all)	650 b.i.d.†	— —	— —	— —	13/168 7.7%
Westermann 1981[196a]	Prosp.	FLS, CV LS, AT	500 t.i.d.	— —	— —	32/95 35%	3/95 3.1%
Hume 1978[90]	Prosp. Random. Double Blind	FLS, IP, CV LS, PA	600 b.i.d.	9/54 17%	4/54 7.4%	6/58 10%	0/58 0%
Harris 1977[75]	Prosp. Random. Double Blind	FLS, IP, CV LS, PA	600 b.i.d.	22/51 43%	1/51 2%	11/44 25%	0/44 0%
Hume 1977[92]	Prosp.	FLS, IP, CV	650 b.i.d.	4/20 20%	—	2/21 10%	—
Soreff 1975[178]	Prosp. Random. Double Blind	CV (all)	500 q.i.d.	5/14 36%	—	10/21 48%	—
Harris 1974[72]	Prosp. Random.	CV (all)	600 q.i.d.	— —	— —	18/50 36%	0/50 —
TOTAL				77/202	10/168	156/531	38/657
Percent				41	5.9	29	5.8
Range				17%–59%	2%–8%	10%–48%	0%–20%

From Haake DA, Berkman SA: Venous thromboembolic disease after hip surgery: risk factors, prophylaxis, and diagnosis, *Clin Orthop* 242:212, 1989.
*Patients were also given 200 mg q.i.d. of sulfinpyrazone.
†Patients were also given 50 mg t.i.d. of dipyridamole.
DVT: Incidence of deep venous thrombosis. PE: Incidence of pulmonary embolism. Clin DX: Clinical diagnosis. CV: Contrast venography. LS: Lung scan. AT: Autopsy. IP: Impedance plethysmography. FLS: Fibrinogen leg scan. PA: Pulmonary angiography. Prosp.: Prospective. Random.: Randomized; if controls receiving no prophylaxis are not listed, the study used controls receiving an alternative prophylactic regimen.

Table 9-6 **Effect of Gender on Results of Aspirin for DVT Prophylaxis After Total Hip Arthroplasty**

First author, year of publication, and reference number	Males		Females	
	Treated	Untreated	Treated	Untreated
Sautter 1983[163]	11/25	21/34	10/29	16/29
	44%	62%	35%	56%
Harris 1982[76]	13/40	–	23/52	–
	33%	–	44%	–
Hume 1978[90]	4/32	3/25	2/26	6/29
	13%	12%	7.7%	21%
Harris 1977[75]	4/23	14/25	7/21	9/26
	17%	56%	33%	35%
Soreff 1975[178]	2/7	3/8	8/14	2/6
	29%	37%	57%	33%
TOTAL	34/127	41/92	50/142	33/90
Percent	27%	45%	35%	37%
Range	13%–44%	12%–62%	8%–57%	21%–56%

From Haake DA, Berkman SA: Venous thromboembolic disease after hip surgery: risk factors, prophylaxis, and diagnosis, *Clin Orthop* 242:212, 1989.
*Patients were also given 200 mg of sulfinpyrazone.
DVT: Deep venous thrombosis.

lactic effect, bleeding complications, and comparisons of men versus women.[184]

As shown in Tables 9-5 and 9-6, the use of aspirin does not produce a statistically significant reduction in deep vein thrombosis.[42,90,178] In fact, aspirin was inferior to warfarin.[62,72] However, combining the results, the incidence of deep vein thrombosis and pulmonary embolism showed a modest but significant reduction.[90,163] Aspirin being protective only for men against thromboembolic complications has been confirmed by some and disputed by others (Table 9-6).[72,163,184]

From these studies and the bulk of the literature, it may be concluded that using aspirin to prevent thromboembolic disease is less effective than other methods but perhaps better than no anticoagulation regimen at all.

Hydroxychloroquine

Hydroxychloroquine has reduced the incidence of thromboembolic disease[31] after orthopaedic procedures. Charnley demonstrated its effectiveness in patients after total hip arthroplasty. Hydroxychloroquine sulfate (Plaquenil) acts to prevent platelet adhesiveness and to a lesser degree through the aggregation that follows adherence of the platelets to the damaged endothelium.[27]

After much experience and working with various methods of prophylaxis, Charnley favored Plaquenil to other methods for prophylaxis in total hip arthroplasty.[29] Between 1966 and 1973, he reported 4684 total hip arthroplasties with 53 fatal emboli (1.13% ranging from 0.7% to 1.1%) and 381 nonfatal emboli (8.13%, ranging from 6.5% to 9.5%). In 2144 patients treated

with Plaquenil, the rate of fatal embolism was 0.28% (6 patients) and of nonfatal embolism was 4.15% (89 patients). Charnley also compared the efficacy of dextran with Plaquenil on a separate group of low-friction arthroplasties (private clinic at Milhurst). In this study, 344 total hip arthroplasty patients were treated with dextran, and Charnley reported 1 fatal embolism (0.29%) and 40 nonfatal emboli (11.6%). He compared these results with those of 418 patients undergoing low-friction arthroplasty performed under similar circumstances but receiving Plaquenil. There was one fatal embolism (0.23%) and seven nonfatal emboli (1.7%). Charnley concluded that Plaquenil was significantly better than any other agent previously tried.[29,100–102] Complications of Plaquenil were limited to allergic rashes (in 18 cases), temporary blurring of vision (6 cases), genitourinary tract bleeding (5 cases), and gastric dilation (7 cases). All complications subsided once Plaquenil prophylaxis stopped.

Johnson and Loudon have emphasized the usefulness and safety of Plaquenil[102] in total hip arthroplasty. These authors have reported improved results and greater effectiveness with larger doses of Plaquenil than previously reported. As shown in Table 9-5, they compared two large series of arthroplasties that used either 600 mg or 1200 mg of Plaquenil. They found a significant reduction in fatal and nonfatal pulmonary embolism from the use of the higher dose of Plaquenil. Giving 1200 mg of Plaquenil daily and continuing this dose daily until the patient was fully mobile reduced death after low-friction arthroplasty from 23/1000 to 1/1000. Only a few minor complications resulted from this regimen (Table 9-7).[29,102]

Table 9-7 Incidence of Pulmonary Emboli and Complications Using 600 mg vs. 1200 mg of Plaquenil

	600 mg (%)	1200 mg (%)
Nonfatal pulmonary embolism	1.8	2.2
Fatal pulmonary embolism	0.7	0.1
Hematoma	2.3	1.5
Delayed healing	0.5	1.0
Superficial infection	1.0	0.8
Deep infection	0.3	0.1

From Johnson RJ, Loudon JR: Hydroxychloroquine sulfate prophylaxis for pulmonary embolism for patients with low-friction arthroplasty, *Clin Orthop* 211:151, 1986.

As recommended and used by Charnley after total hip arthroplasty, Plaquenil is given over 3 weeks for prophylaxis. The dosage of hydroxychloroquine sulfate given by mouth in 200 mg capsules is as follows: 1200 mg every 24 hours starting 24 hours before surgery and continuing for 2 weeks, whereupon the dosage is reduced to 400 mg every 24 hours for 1 week.

Other Antiplatelet Agents

Carter,[27] using radioactive-tagged fibrinogen and venography for diagnosis, reduced the incidence of deep vein thrombosis from 16% to 5% in general surgical patients, demonstrating the beneficial effect of dipyridamole in reducing the number of deep vein thrombi. Dipyridamole has been ineffective in preventing thromboembolic disease in both general surgical and total hip arthroplasty patients.[23,161]

EFFECTS OF ANESTHESIA ON DEEP VEIN THROMBOSIS

A randomized study of 140 elective total hip arthroplasties compared the effects of spinal and general anesthesia to the development of deep vein thrombosis. This series used an impedance plethysmography and 125-I fibrinogen uptake test for diagnosis. In selected cases the investigators also used venography to diagnose deep vein thrombosis. The overall incidence of deep vein thrombosis was 20%; it was 13% in the spinal anesthesia group and 27% in the general anesthesia group (P value less than 0.05). Less proximal thrombosis and fewer bilateral thrombi occurred in the spinal anesthesia group than in the general anesthesia group.[41]

SUMMARY OF ESSENTIALS

- Thromboembolic disease is considered the leading cause of death in an unprotected patient after total hip arthroplasty. A death rate of 1% to 2% has been attributed to pulmonary embolism after total hip arthroplasty.

- Although venous thrombosis is the most common complication of adult hip surgery, the possibility of fatal pulmonary embolism means that routine prophylaxis against this complication is mandatory. Use of an untreated "control group" in an experimental evaluation of drug effectiveness or other methods of prophylaxis is no longer justifiable.

- Increased elective surgery in older patients, the extent of surgery performed, underlying cardiovascular abnormalities, and immobilization after surgery contribute to pulmonary embolism, the incidence of which is higher than was formerly recognized. Basically, three predisposing factors—stasis, hypercoagulability, and local trauma to the vessels—may occur during total hip arthroplasty. Hypercoagulability is clearly a predisposing factor, which has been proven both clinically and experimentally in patients who develop thromboembolism.

- Of the modern techniques for early detection and proper management of deep vein thrombosis, roentgenographic phlebography, the labeled fibrinogen-uptake test, impedance plethysmography, and augmented ultrasound techniques based on the Doppler effect have been most useful. Total hip arthroplasty has undoubtedly advanced the study of thromboembolic disease.

- Ultrasonography has become an increasingly accurate and popular tool in detecting thrombosis of smaller veins, offering high sensitivity, specificity, and accuracy for the entire lower limb. It may well replace venography because of its accuracy and noninvasiveness.

- In the past, most studies of pulmonary embolism were based on clinical assumption or postmortem studies. Significantly, a large number of pulmonary embolisms went unnoticed because the disease is sometimes silent. Routine postoperative lung scans showed that the incidence of pulmonary embolism was nearly 20%, almost twice the rate found in several studies in which pulmonary embolism was diagnosed clinically.

- There are numerous methods of prophylaxis against thromboembolic disease, each with a specific mechanism against this condition. Heparin works by decreasing platelet adhesiveness and augmenting the effect of antithrombin 3 (heparin factor), a potent naturally occurring inhibitor of activated factor X and thrombin. Coumadin interferes with the synthesis of clotting factors by depressing vitamin K activity. Dextran alters the function of platelets and also disturbs the structure of the fibrin clot formed in its presence.

- In addition to chemical agents, modalities such as early ambulation, external pneumatic compression, electrical stimulation of the calves during operation, and more recently, newer antithromboembolic stockings and medications such as aspirin and hydroxychloroquine (Plaquenil) have been introduced. The role to be played by these modalities awaits adequate clinical documentation.

- Regardless of the method of prophylaxis, the single most critical complication after anticoagulation treatment is hemorrhage at the surgical site or in a remote area. It is essential to minimize this complication by scrupulous patient selection for anticoagulation and well-controlled and balanced management throughout the prophylactic period. It is also essential that one person be responsible for anticoagulation for each patient; the role of the interested medical consultant is invaluable in this regard.

- Reports of the incidence of the thromboembolic condition in the literature have varied considerably, which reflects surgeons' efforts to detect this condition. It is generally felt that the incidence is much greater than clinical diagnosis would suggest. It is now clear that calf thrombi develop frequently but are not likely to cause embolization unless they extend proximally into the popliteal region and thigh. The major life-threatening emboli are generated in the thigh and the pelvis, and the detection of these emboli is most important. However, these thrombi are not primary lesions; most often they are extensions from a calf thrombus or are associated with a discontinued but concomitant calf thrombus.

- Because fatal pulmonary emboli may occur in 1% to 2% of patients in elective total hip surgery, early detection and prophylaxis are essential.

- Substantial evidence now exists that heparin, warfarin, dextran, and aspirin are all effective in preventing thromboembolic complications.

- While the diagnosis of deep vein thrombosis by phlebography is most accurate, this diagnostic test carries considerable morbidity and should be considered invasive, so it should not be routinely used in all cases. On the other hand, the 125-I fibrinogen test and calf-impedance ultrasound plethysmography are sufficiently accurate for routine use. The clinical diagnosis of deep vein thrombosis and pulmonary embolus is grossly inaccurate and underestimates the true incidence.

- Pulmonary embolism can only be clinically diagnosed if the surgeon suspects it and if symptoms such as pleuritic chest pain, shortness of breath, hemoptysis, diaphoresis, and pleuritic friction rub cannot be attributed to other conditions. A good monitoring test for the diagnosis of pulmonary embolism is arterial blood-gas changes. In addition to an abnormal ECG and consistent chest x-ray changes, the most specific means of diagnosis are a positive lung perfusion scan, pulmonary ventilation scan, and pulmonary angiography. No diagnosis of pulmonary embolism should be accepted without objective confirmation.

- Because of the high incidence of fatal pulmonary embolism, most authorities agree that some form of prophylaxis is necessary. Several methods are available, including mechanical methods such as compression of the calf and electrical stimulation; antithrombotic drugs such as warfarin, heparin, dextran, aspirin, and hydroxychloroquine; and early ambulation, antiembolic stockings, and elevation of the foot of the bed.

- At present, a wide range of experiences suggests that although heparin and warfarin are effective and must be used in a therapeutic dose in patients with a history of thromboembolic disease who undergo total hip arthroplasty. A low dose Coumadin is the preferred choice for prophylaxis.

- Aspirin appears to be the drug preferred by some surgeons for patients without prior thromboembolic disease. Aspirin, cuff-impedance phlebography or ultrasound plethysmography (for early detection of thigh and pelvic thrombi), and proper management when thromboembolic disease is detected appear to be a compromise since such methods do not prevent the fatal pulmonary embolism.

- Plaquenil is significantly better than other agents in reducing the incidence of fatal and nonfatal pulmonary embolism. In addition, it has relatively few, minor side effects.

- Warfarin is a potent anticoagulant agent that can prevent both distal and proximal vein thrombosis and thus fatal pulmonary embolism. Its administration is easy, safe, and effective when it is used at prophylactic levels. Warfarin-induced bleeding, which is largely dosage-related, can be negligible if prothrombin time is maintained at a low level, in the range of 1.2 to 1.5 times the patient's control. It is the author's preferred choice for prophylaxis, combined with antiembolic stockings and early postoperative ambulation.

REFERENCES

1. **Ahlberg AKE, Nylander G, Robertson B, et al:** Dextran in prophylaxis of thrombosis in fractures of the hip, *Acta Surg Scand* 387 (suppl):83, 1968.
2. **Almen T, Nylander G:** Serial phlebography of the normal lower leg during muscular contraction and relaxation,

Acta Radiol (Stockholm) 57:264, 1962.

3. **Amstutz HC, Friscia DA, Dorey F:** Warfarin prophylaxis to prevent mortality from pulmonary embolism after total hip replacement, *J Bone Joint Surg* 71:321, 1989.

4. **Atik M, Harkess JW, Wichman H:** Prevention of fatal pulmonary embolism, *Surg Gynecol Obstet* 130:403, 1970.

5. **Babcock RB, Dumper CW, Scharfman WB:** Heparin-induced immune thrombocytopenia, *N Engl J Med* 295:237, 1976.

6. **Bahadir I, James EC, Fedde CW:** Soft tissue necrosis and gangrene complicating treatment with the Coumarin derivatives, *Surg Gynecol Obstet* 145:497, 1977.

7. **Baird RA, Convery R:** Arterial thromboembolism in patients receiving systemic heparin therapy. A complication associated with heparin-induced thrombocytopenia, *J Bone Joint Surg* 59:1061, 1977.

8. **Barber FA, Burton WC, Guyer R:** The heparin-induced thrombocytopenia and thrombosis syndrome. Report of a case, *J Bone Joint Surg* 69:935, 1987.

9. **Barber HM, Feil EJ, Galasko CSB, et al:** A comparative study of dextran-70, warfarin and low-dose heparin for the prophylaxis of thrombo-embolism following total hip replacement, *Postgrad Med J* 53:130, 1977.

10. **Barnes RW, Brand RA, Clarke W, et al:** Efficacy of graded-compression antiembolism stockings in patients undergoing total hip arthroplasty, *Clin Orthop* 132:61, 1978.

10a. **Becker J, Schampi B:** The incidence of postoperative venous thrombosis of the legs. A comparative study on the prophylactic effect of dextran 70 and electrical calf-muscle stimulator, *Acta Chir Scand* 139:357, 1973.

11. **Beisaw NE, Comerota AJ, Groth HE, et al:** Dihydroergotamine/heparin in the prevention of deep-vein thrombosis after total hip replacement. A controlled, prospective, randomized multicenter trial, *J Bone Joint Surg* 70:2, 1988.

12. **Bell WR, Royall RM:** Heparin-associated thrombocytopenia: a comparison of three heparin preparations, *N Engl J Med* 303:902, 1980.

13. **Bell WR, Tomasulo PA, Alving BM, et al:** Thrombocytopenia occurring during the administration of heparin. Prospective study in 52 patients, *Ann Intern Med* 85:155, 1976.

14. **Bentley PG, Hill PL, deHaas HA, et al:** Radionuclide venography in the management of proximal venous occlusion. A comparison with x-ray contrast venography, *Br J Radiol* 52:289, 1979.

15. **Bergentz SE:** Dextran in the prophylaxis of pulmonary embolism, *World J Surg* 2:19, 1978.

16. **Bergquist E, Bergquist D, Bronge A, et al:** Diagnosis of venous thrombosis in the lower limbs, *Ups J Med Sci* 78:191, 1973.

16a. **Bergquist D, Elvelin R, Eriksson U, et al:** Thrombosis following hip arthroplasty, *Acta Chir Scand* 47:549, 1976.

17. **Bergquist D, Efsing HO, Hallbook T, et al:** Thromboembolism after elective and post-traumatic hip surgery—a controlled prophylactic trial with dextran 70 and low-dose heparin, *Acta Chir Scand* 145:213, 1979.

18. **Bergquist D, Efsing HO, Hallbook T, et al:** Prevention of postoperative thromboembolic complications. A prospective comparison between dextran 70, dihydroergotamine heparin and a sulphated polysaccharide, *Acta Chir Scand* 146:559, 1980.

19. **Bettmann MA, Paulin S:** Leg phlebography: the inci-

dence, nature, and modification of undesirable side effects, *Radiology* 122:101, 1977.

20. **Bick RL:** Alterations of hemostasis associated with malignancy: etiology, pathophysiology, diagnosis and management, *Semin Thromb Hemost* 5:1, 1978.

21. **Bolton JP, Hoffman VJ:** Incidence of early post-operative iliofemoral thrombosis, *Br Med J* 1:247, 1975.

22. **Braun SD, Newman GE, Ford K, et al:** Ventilation-perfusion scanning and pulmonary angiography: correlation in clinical high-probability pulmonary embolism, *Am J Roentgenol* 143:977, 1984.

23. **Browse NL, Clapham WF, Croft DN, et al:** Diagnosis of established deep vein thrombosis with the 125 I fibrinogen uptake test, *Br Med J* 4:325, 1971.

24. **Browse NL, Hall JH:** Effect of dipyridamole on the incidence of clinically detectable deep-vein thrombosis, *Lancet* 2:718, 1969.

25. **Campbell R, Clanton TO, Heckman JD:** Necrosis and gangrene as a complication of coumarin therapy, *J Bone Joint Surg* 62:1016, 1980.

26. **Carrell N, Gabriel DA, Blatt P:** Hereditary dysfibrinogenemia in a patient with thrombotic disease, *Blood* 62:439, 1983.

27. **Carter AE, Eban R:** Prevention of post-operative deep venous thrombosis in legs by orally administered hydroxychloroquine sulphate, *Br Med J* 3:94, 1974.

28. **Charnley J:** The long term results of low-friction arthroplasty of the hip performed as a primary intervention, *J Bone Joint Surg* 54[Br]:61, 1972.

29. **Charnley J:** *Low friction arthroplasty of the hip: theory and practice*, Berlin, 1979, Springer-Verlag.

30. **Chrisman OD, Snook GA, Wilson TC, et al:** Prevention of venous thromboembolism by administration of hydroxychloroquine. A preliminary report, *J Bone Joint Surg* 58:918, 1976.

31. **Chumas P, O'Doherty DP, Pearse M, et al:** Preoperative lower limb venography in patients undergoing total hip arthroplasty, *J Arth* 3:225, 1988.

32. **Clagett GP, Salzman EW:** Prevention of venous thromboembolism in surgical patients, *N Engl J Med* 290:93, 1974.

33. **Clagett GP, Salzman EW:** Prevention of venous thromboembolism, *Prog Cardiovasc Dis* 17:345, 1975.

34. **Clark C, Cotton LT:** Blood-flow in deep veins of leg. Recording technique and evaluation of methods to increase flow during operation, *Br J Surg* 55:211, 1968.

35. **Comp PC, Esmon CT:** Recurrent venous thromboembolism in patients with a partial deficiency of protein S, *N Engl J Med* 311:1525, 1984.

36. **Coventry MB, Nolan DR, Beckenbaugh RD:** Delayed prophylactic anticoagulation: a study of results and complications in 2,012 total hip arthroplasties, *J Bone Joint Surg* 55:1487, 1973.

37. **Cranley JJ, Gay AY, Grass AM, et al:** A plethysmographic technique for the diagnosis of deep venous thrombosis of the lower extremities, *Surg Gynecol Obstet* 136:385, 1973.

38. **Crawford WJ, Hillman F, Charnley J:** A clinical trial of prophylactic anticoagulant therapy in elective hip surgery. Internal Publication No. 14. 1968, Centre for Hip Surgery, Wrightington Hospital.

39. **Culver D, Crawford JS, Gardiner JH, et al:** Venous thrombosis after fractures of the upper end of the femur. A study of incidence and site, *J Bone Joint Surg* 52[Br]:61, 1970.

40. **D'Ambrosia RD, Lipscomb PR, McClain EJ, et al:**

Prophylactic anticoagulation in total hip replacement, *Surg Gynecol Obstet* 140:523, 1975.

41. **Davis FM, Laurenson VG, Gillespie WJ, et al:** Deep vein thrombosis after total hip replacement: a comparison between spinal and general anaesthesia, *J Bone Joint Surg* 71[Br]:181, 1989.

42. **Dechavanne M, Saudin F, Viala JJ, et al:** Prevention des thromboses veineuses. Succes de l'heparine a fortes doses lors des coxarthroses, *Nouv Presse Med* 3:1317, 1974.

43. **Donaldson GA, Williams C, Schnnel JG, et al:** A reappraisal of the application of the Trendelenburg operation to massive fatal embolism. Report of a successful pulmonary-artery thrombectomy using a cardiopulmonary bypass, *N Engl J Med* 268:171, 1963.

44. **Doran FSA, Drury M, Sivyer A:** A simple way to combat the venous stasis which occurs in the lower limbs during surgical operations, *Br J Surg* 51:486, 1964.

45. **Dorr LD, Sakimura I, Mohler JG:** Pulmonary emboli following total hip arthroplasty: incidence study, *J Bone Joint Surg* 61:1083, 1979.

46. **Ennis JT, Elmes RJ:** Radionuclide venography in the diagnosis of deep vein thrombosis, *Radiology* 125:441, 1977.

47. **Eskeland G, Solheim K, Skjorten F:** Anticoagulant prophylaxis, thromboembolism and mortality in elderly patients with hip fractures. A controlled clinical trial, *Acta Chir Scand* 131:16, 1966.

48. **Evarts CM:** Low molecular weight dextran, *Med Clin North Am* 51:285, 1967.

49. **Evarts CM:** Prevention of venous thromboembolism, *Clin Orthop* 222:98, 1987.

50. **Evarts CM, Alfidi RJ:** Thromboembolism after total hip reconstruction. Failure of low doses of heparin in prevention, *JAMA* 225:515, 1973.

51. **Evarts CM, Feil EJ:** Prevention of thromboembolic disease after elective surgery of the hip, *J Bone Joint Surg* 53:1271, 1971.

52. **Fitts WT Jr, Lehr HB, Bitner RL, et al:** An analysis of 950 fatal injuries, *Surgery* 56:663, 1964.

53. **Flood EP, Redish MH, Bociek SJ, et al:** Thrombophlebitis migrans disseminata: report of a case in which gangrene of a breast occurred; observations on the therapeutic use of dicumarol (3.3' methylenebis, 4-hydroxycoumarin), *NY State J Med* 43:1121, 1943.

54. **Francis CW, Marder VJ, Evarts CM, et al:** Two-step warfarin therapy. Prevention of postoperative venous thrombosis without excessive bleeding, *JAMA* 249:374, 1983.

55. **Froehlich JA, Dorfman GS, Cronan JJ, et al:** Compression ultrasonography for the detection of deep venous thrombosis in patients who have a fracture of the hip. A prospective study, *J Bone Joint Surg* 71:249, 1989.

56. **Gallus A, Raman K, Darby T:** Venous thrombosis after elective hip replacement—the influence of preventive intermittent calf compression and of surgical technique, *Br J Surg* 70:17, 1983.

57. **Gallus AS, Hirsh J, Tuttle RJ, et al:** Small subcutaneous doses of heparin in prevention of venous thrombosis, *N Engl J Med* 288:545, 1973.

58. **Gallus AS, Hirsh J, Hull R, et al:** Diagnosis of venous thromboembolism, *Semin Thromb Haemost* 2:203, 1976.

59. **Gitel SN, Salvati EA, Wessler S, et al:** The effect of total hip replacement and general surgery on antithrombin III in relation to venous thrombosis, *J Bone Joint Surg* 61:653, 1979.

60. **Goss TT, Stinchfield FE, Cosgriff SW:** The efficacy of heparin-warfarin anticoagulation prophylaxis after hip replacement, Arthroplasty, unpublished data.

61. **Graham B, Loomer RL:** Anterior compartment syndrome in a patient with fracture of the tibial plateau treated by continuous passive motion and anticoagulants. Report of a case, *Clin Orthop* 195:197, 1985.

62. **Guyer RD, Booth RE Jr, Rothman RH:** The detection and prevention of pulmonary embolism in total hip replacement. A study comparing aspirin and low-dose warfarin, *J Bone Joint Surg* 64:1040, 1982.

63. **Haake DA, Berkman SA:** Venous thromboembolic disease after hip surgery: risk factors, prophylaxis, and diagnosis, *Clin Orthop* 242:212, 1989.

64. **Haeger K:** Problems of acute deep venous thrombosis. I. The interpretation of signs and symptoms, *Angiology* 20:219, 1969.

65. **Haim S, Sobel JD, Friedman-Birnbaum R:** Thrombophlebitis. A cardinal symptom of Behcet's syndrome, *Acta Derm Venereol* (Stockholm) 54:299, 1974.

66. **Hammerschmidt DE:** Thrombocytopenia during heparin therapy (correspondence), *N Engl J Med* 295:1200, 1976.

67. **Hampson WGJ, Harris FC, Lucas HK:** Failure of low-dose heparin to prevent deep-vein thrombosis after hip replacement arthroplasty, *Lancet* 2:795, 1974.

68. **Hampton AO, Castleman B:** Correlation of postmortem chest teleroentgenograms with autopsy findings with special reference to pulmonary embolism and infarction, *Am J Roentgenol* 43:305, 1940.

69. **Harris WH:** Thromboembolic disease in elective reconstructive surgery in the adult hip. In American Academy of Orthopaedic Surgeons instructional course lectures, vol 23, St Louis, 1974, Mosby–Year Book.

70. **Harris WH, Salzman EW, DeSanctis RW:** The prevention of thromboembolic disease by prophylactic anticoagulation. A controlled study in elective hip surgery, *J Bone Joint Surg* 49:81, 1967.

71. **Harris WH, Salzman EW, DeSanctis RW, et al:** Prevention of venous thromboembolism following total hip replacement. Warfarin vs dextran 40, *JAMA* 220:1319, 1972.

72. **Harris WH, Salzman EW, Athanasoulis C, et al:** Comparison of warfarin, low-molecular-weight dextran, aspirin, and subcutaneous heparin in prevention of venous thromboembolism following total hip replacement, *J Bone Joint Surg* 56:1552, 1974.

73. **Harris WH, Salzman EW, Athanasoulis C, et al:** Comparison of 125 I fibrinogen count scanning with phlebography for detection of venous thrombi after elective hip surgery, *N Engl J Med* 292:665, 1975.

74. **Harris WH, Athanasoulis C, Waltman AC, et al:** Cuff-impedance phlebography and 125 I fibrinogen scanning vs roentgenographic phlebography for the diagnosis of thrombophlebitis following hip surgery. A preliminary report, *J Bone Joint Surg* 58:939, 1976.

75. **Harris WH, Salzman EW, Athanasoulis CA, et al:** Aspirin prophylaxis of venous thromboembolism after total hip replacement, *N Engl J Med* 297:1246, 1977.

76. **Harris WH, Athanasoulis CA, Waltman AC, et al:** High and low-dose aspirin prophylaxis against venous thromboembolic disease in total hip replacement, *J Bone Joint Surg* 64:63, 1982.

77. **Harris WH, McKusick K, Athanasoulis CA, et al:** Detection of pulmonary emboli after total hip replacement using serial C $^{15}O_2$ pulmonary scans, *J Bone Joint*

Surg 66:1388, 1984.

78. **Hartman JT, Altner PC, Freeark RJ:** The effect of limb elevation in preventing venous thrombosis. A venographic study, *J Bone Joint Surg* 52:1618, 1970.

79. **Hartman JT, Pugh JL, Smith RD, et al:** Cyclic sequential compression of the lower limb in prevention of deep venous thrombosis, *J Bone J Surg* 64:1059, 1982.

80. **Havig O:** Deep vein thrombosis and pulmonary embolism. An autopsy study with multiple regression analysis of possible risk factors, *Acta Chir Scand* 478 (suppl):1, 1977.

81. **Heatley RV, Hughes LE, Morgan A, et al:** Preoperative or postoperative deep-vein thrombosis? *Lancet* 1:437, 1976.

82. **Hirsh J:** The clinical role of antiplatelet agents, *Drug Ther* 11:49, 1981.

83. **Hirsh J, Genton E, Hull R:** *Venous thromboembolism,* New York, 1981, Grune & Stratton.

84. **Hirsh J, Hull R:** Natural history and clinical features of venous thrombosis. In Colman RW, Hirsh J, Marder VJ, et al, editors: *Hemostasis and thrombosis: basic principles and clinical practice,* Philadelphia, 1982, Lippincott.

85. **Hirsh J, Salzman E:** Prevention of venous thrombolism. In Colman RW, Hirsh J, Marder JW, et al, editors: *Hemostasis and thrombosis: basic principles and clinical practice,* Philadelphia, 1982, Lippincott.

86. **Holden RW, Klatte EC, Park HM, et al:** Efficacy of noninvasive modalities of diagnosis of thrombophlebitis, *Radiology* 141:63, 1981.

87. **Hull R, vanAken WG, Hirsh J, et al:** Impedance plethysmography using the occlusive cuff technique in the diagnosis of venous thrombosis, *Circulation* 53:696, 1976.

88. **Hull RD, Raskob GE, et al:** Prophylaxis of venous thromboembolic disease following hip and knee surgery, *J Bone Joint Surg* 68:146, 1986.

89. **Hume M, Kuriakose TX, Zuch L, et al:** 125 I fibrinogen and the prevention of venous thrombosis, *Arch Surg* 107:803, 1973.

90. **Hume M, Donaldson WR, Suprenant J:** Sex, aspirin, and venous thrombosis, *Orthop Clin North Am* 9:761, 1978.

91. **Hume M, Turner RH, Kuriakose TX, et al:** Venous thrombosis after total hip replacement. Combined monitoring as guide for prophylaxis and treatment, *J Bone Joint Surg* 58:933, 1976.

92. **Hume M, Bierbaum B, Kuriakose TX, et al:** Prevention of postoperative thrombosis by aspirin, *Am J Surg* 133:410, 1977.

93. **Hurson B, Ennis JT, Corrigan TP, et al:** Dextran prophylaxis in total hip replacement: a scintigraphic evaluation of the incidence of deep vein thrombosis and pulmonary embolus, *Irish J Med Sci* 148:140, 1979.

94. **Inman WH, Vessey MP, Westerholm B, et al:** Thromboembolic disease and the steroidal content of oral contraceptives. A report to the Committee of Safety of Drugs, *Br Med J* 2:203, 1970.

95. **International Multicentre Trial:** Prevention of fatal postoperative pulmonary embolism by low doses of heparin, *Lancet* 2:45, 1975.

96. **Jennings JJ, Harris WH, Sarmiento A:** A clinical evaluation of aspirin prophylaxis of thromboembolic disease after total hip arthroplasty, *J Bone Joint Surg* 58:926, 1976.

97. **Johansson L, Hedner U, Nilsson IM:** A family with

thromboembolic disease associated with deficient fibrinolytic activity in vessel wall, *Acta Med Scand* 203:477, 1978.

98. **Johnson R, Charnley J:** Treatment of pulmonary embolism in total hip replacement, *Clin Orthop* 124:149, 1977.

99. **Johnson R, Charnley J:** *Hydroxychloroquine in prophylaxis of pulmonary embolism following hip arthroplasty.* Internal Publication No. 74, 1977, Centre for Hip Surgery, Wrightington Hospital.

100. **Johnson R, Green JR, Charnley J:** Pulmonary embolism and its prophylaxis following the Charnley total hip replacement, *Clin Orthop* 127:123, 1977.

101. **Johnson R, Orth MC, Carmichael JHE, et al:** Deep venous thrombosis following Charnley arthroplasty, *Clin Orthop* 132:24, 1978.

102. **Johnson RJ, Loudon JR:** Hydroxychloroquine sulfate prophylaxis for pulmonary embolism for patients with low-friction arthroplasty, *Clin Orthop* 211:151, 1986.

103. **Johnston RC, Larson CB:** Results of treatment of hip disorders with cup arthroplasty, *J Bone Joint Surg* 51:1461, 1969.

104. **Kakkar VV:** The diagnosis of deep vein thrombosis using the 125 I fibrinogen test, *Arch Surg* 104:152, 1972.

105. **Kakkar VV, Field ES, Nicholaides AN, et al:** Low doses of heparin in prevention of deep-vein thrombosis, *Lancet* 2:669, 1971.

106. **Kakkar VV, Corrigan T, Spindler J, et al:** Efficacy of low doses of heparin in prevention of deep-vein thrombosis after major surgery. A double-blind, randomized trial, *Lancet* 2:101, 1972.

107. **Kakkar VV, Fok PJ, Murray WJG, et al:** Heparin and dihydroergotamine prophylaxis against thromboembolism after hip arthroplasty, *J Bone Joint Surg* 67[Br]:538, 1985.

108. **Kakkar VV, Stamatakis JD, Bentley PG, et al:** Prophylaxis for postoperative deep-vein thrombosis. Synergistic effect of heparin and dihydroergotamine, *JAMA* 241:39, 1979.

109. **Kerrigan GNW, Buchanan MR, Cade JF, et al:** Investigation of the mechanism of false positive 125-I labeled fibrinogen scans, *Br J Haematol* 26:469, 1974.

110. **Kim Y-H, Suh J-S:** Low incidence of deep-vein thrombosis after cementless total hip replacement, *J Bone Joint Surg* 70:878, 1988.

111. **Lahnburg G:** Effect of low-dose heparin and dihydroergotamine on frequency of postoperative deep-vein thrombosis in patients undergoing post-traumatic hip surgery, *Acta Chir Scand* 146:319, 1980.

112. **Lambie JM, Mahaffy RG, Barber DC, et al:** Diagnostic accuracy in venous thrombosis, *Br Med J* 2:142, 1970.

113. **Langsjoen P, Murray RA:** Treatment of postsurgical thromboembolic complications, *JAMA* 218:855, 1971.

114. **Lawson DH, Davidson JF, Jick H:** Oral contraceptive use and venous thromboembolism: absence of an effect of smoking, *Br Med J* 2:729, 1977.

115. **Lazansky MG:** Complications revisited. The debit side of total hip replacement, *Clin Orthop* 95:96, 1973.

116. **Leithauser DJ, Saraf L, Smyka S, et al:** Prevention of embolic complications from venous thrombosis after surgery: standardized regimen of early ambulation, *JAMA* 147:300, 1951.

117. **Leyvrza PF, Richard J, Bachmann F, et al:** Adjusted versus fixed dose subcutaneous heparin in the prevention of deep vein thrombosis after total hip replacement, *N Engl J Med* 309:954, 1983.

118. **Liedloff H, Brauckhoff KF, Heerdegen R, et al:** Zur Anwendung von Heparin in Kombination mit Dihydro-ergotamin zur postoperativen Thromboseprophylaxe bei Hüftgelenkoperationen, Z *Gesamte Inn Med* 39:428, 1984.

119. **Lundstrom B, Jonsson O, Petrusson B, et al:** Optimized electrical calf muscle stimulation as prophylaxis against postoperative DVT, *Acta Chir Scand* 493 (suppl):42, 1979.

120. **Lotke PA, Ecker ML, Alavi A, et al:** Indications for the treatment of deep venous thrombosis following total knee replacement, *J Bone Joint Surg* 66:202, 1984.

121. **Lowe LW:** Venous thrombosis and embolism, *J Bone Joint Surg* 63[Br]:155, 1981.

122. **Mandt PR, Robinson CA, Sarnoff RB, et al:** Heparin-associated thrombocytopenia with venous thrombosis. A case report, *J Bone Joint Surg* 67:1123, 1985.

123. **Mavor GE, Walker MG, Dhall DP, et al:** Peripheral venous scanning with 125-I tagged fibrinogen, *Lancet* 1:661, 1972.

124. **Medical Research Council:** Effect of aspirin on postoperative venous thrombosis, *Lancet* 2:441, 1972.

125. **McLachlin AD, McLachlin JA, Jory TA, et al:** Venous stasis in the lower extremities, *Ann Surg* 152:678, 1960.

126. **Moore JR, Weiland AJ:** Heparin-induced thromboembolism. A case report, *J Hand Surg* 4:382, 1979.

127. **Morris GK, Henry APJ, Preston BJ:** Prevention of deep-vein thrombosis by low-dose heparin in patients undergoing total hip replacement, *Lancet* 2:797, 1974.

128. **Morris WT, Hardy AE:** The effect of dihydroergotamine and heparin on the incidence of thromboembolic complications following total hip replacement: a randomized controlled clinical trial, *Br J Surg* 68:301, 1981.

129. **Moser KM, LeMoine JR:** Is embolic risk conditioned by location of deep vein thrombosis? *Ann Intern Med* 94:439, 1981.

130. **Moskowitz PA, Ellenberg SS, Feffer HL, et al:** Low-dose heparin for prevention of venous thromboembolism in total hip arthroplasty and surgical repair of hip fractures, *J Bone Joint Surg* 60:1065, 1978.

131. **Mudd SH, Skovby F, Levy HL, et al:** The natural history of homocystinuria due to cystathionine beta-synthase deficiency, *Am J Hum Genet* 37:1, 1985.

132. **Mustard JF, Packham MA:** Factors influencing platelet function, adhesion release and aggregation, *Pharmacol Rev* 22:97, 1970.

133. **Mustard JF, Packham MA:** Platelets and diabetes mellitus (editorial), *N Engl J Med* 311:665, 1984.

134. **Nalbandian RM, Mader IJ, Barrett JL, et al:** Petechiae, ecchymoses, and necrosis of the skin induced by coumarin congeners. Rare, occasionally lethal complication of anticoagulant therapy, *JAMA* 192:603, 1965.

135. **Nalbandian RM, Mader IJ, Barrett JL, et al:** A rare and striking dermatologic complication of Coumarin congener anticoagulant therapy, including a note on effective treatment, *Dermatol Dig* 5:65, 1966.

136. **Nalbandian RM, Beller FK, Kamp AK, et al:** Coumarin necrosis of skin treated successfully with heparin, *Obstet Gynecol* 38:395, 1971.

137. **National Institutes of Health Consensus Development Conference:** *Prevention of venous thrombosis and pulmonary embolism,* vol 6, no 2, 1986.

138. **Neu LT Jr, Waterfield JR, Ash CJ:** Prophylactic anticoagulant therapy in the orthopaedic patient, *Ann Intern Med* 62:463, 1965.

139. **Nicolaides AN, Irving D:** Clinical factors and the risk of deep venous thrombosis. In Nicolaides AN, editor: *Thromboembolism aetiology: advances in prevention and management,* Lancaster, England, 1975, MTP Press.

140. **Nicolaides AN, Kakkar VV, Field ES, et al:** Venous stasis and deep-vein thrombosis, *Br J Surg* 59:713, 1972.

141. **Nillius AS, Nylander G:** Deep vein thrombosis after total hip replacement: a clinical and phlebographic study, *Br J Surg* 66:324, 1979.

142. **Odegard OR, Abildgaard U:** Antithrombin III: critical review of assay methods: significance of variations in health and disease, *Haemostasis* 7:127, 1978.

143. **Ogilvie JW, Higgins GL:** Physiologically significant thromboembolic disease following total hip arthroplasty: a prospective study, *Clin Orthop* 171:68, 1982.

144. **Paiement G, Wessinger SJ, Waltman AC, et al:** Low-dose warfarin versus external pneumatic compression for prophylaxis against venous thromboembolism following total hip replacement, *J Arth* 2:23, 1987.

145. **Partsch H, Lofferer O, Mostbeck A:** Diagnosis of established deep vein thrombosis in the leg using 131-I fibrinogen, *Angiology* 25:719, 1974.

146. **Patterson BM, Marchand R, Ranawat C:** Complications of heparin therapy after total joint arthroplasty, *J Bone Joint Surg* 71:1130, 1989.

147. **Pedegana LR, Burgess EM, Moore AJ, et al:** Prevention of thromboembolic disease by external pneumatic compression in patients undergoing total hip arthroplasty, *Clin Orthop* 128:190, 1977.

148. **Phelan BK:** Heparin-associated thrombosis without thrombocytopenia, *Ann Intern Med* 99:637, 1983.

149. **Planes A, Vochelle N, Fagola M:** Total hip replacement and deep vein thrombosis: a venographic and necropsy study, *J Bone Joint Surg* 72[Br]:9, 1990.

150. **Rabinov K, Paulin S:** Roentgen diagnosis of venous thrombosis in the leg, *Arch Surg* 104:134, 1972.

151. **Rickles FR, Edwards RL:** Activation of blood coagulation in cancer: Trousseau's syndrome revisited, *Blood* 62:14, 1983.

152. **Rosenberg RD:** Actions and interactions of antithrombin and heparin, *N Engl J Med* 292:146, 1975.

153. **Rothermel JE, Wessinger JB, Stinchfield FE:** Dextran 40 and thromboembolism in total hip replacement surgery, *Arch Surg* 106:135, 1973.

154. **Russell HE Jr, Bradham RR, Lee WH Jr:** An evaluation of infusion therapy (including dextran) for venous thrombosis, *Circulation* 33:839, 1966.

155. **Sack GH Jr, Levin J, Bell WR:** Trousseau's syndrome and other manifestations of chronic disseminated coagulopathy in patients with neoplasms: clinical, pathophysiologic, and therapeutic features, *Medicine* (Baltimore) 56:1, 1977.

156. **Sagar S, Nairn D, Stamatakis JD, et al:** Efficacy of low-dose heparin in prevention of extensive deep-vein thrombosis in patients undergoing total hip replacement, *Lancet* 1:1151, 1976.

157. **Salzman EW:** Prevention of venous thromboembolism with drugs that alter platelet function. In Frantantoni J, Wessler S, editors: *Prophylactic therapy of deep vein thrombosis and pulmonary embolism.* Washington, DC, 1975, US Department of Health, Education and Welfare, Publication (NIH) No 76-866.

158. **Salzman EW:** Progress in preventing venous thromboembolism, *N Engl J Med* 309:980, 1983 (editorial).

159. **Salzman EW, Harris WH:** Prevention of venous throm-

boembolism in orthopaedic patients, *J Bone Joint Surg* 58:903, 1976.

160. **Salzman EW, Harris WH, DeSanctis RW:** Anticoagulation for prevention of thromboembolism following fractures of the hip, *N Engl J Med* 275:122, 1966.

161. **Salzman EW, Harris WH, DeSanctis RW:** Reduction in venous thromboembolism by agents affecting platelet function, *N Engl J Med* 284:1287, 1971.

162. **Sasahara AA:** The diagnosis of pulmonary embolism, current status. In Frantantoni J, Wessler S, editors: *Prophylactic therapy of deep vein thrombosis and pulmonary embolism*, Washington, DC, 1975, US Department of Health, Education and Welfare, Publication (NIH) No 76-866.

163. **Sautter RD, Koch EL, Myers WO, et al:** Aspirin-sulfinpyrazone in prophylaxis of deep venous thrombosis in total hip replacement, *JAMA* 250:2649, 1983.

164. **Schöndorf TH, Hey D:** Combined administration of low dose heparin and aspirin as prophylaxis of deep vein thrombosis after hip joint surgery, *Haemostasis* 5:250, 1976.

165. **Schöndorf TH, Weber U:** Prevention of deep vein thrombosis in orthopedic surgery with the combination of low dose heparin plus either dihydroergotamine or dextran, *Scand J Haematol* 25 (suppl):126, 1980.

166. **Schwarz HP, Fischer M, Hopmeier P, et al:** Plasma protein S deficiency in familial thrombotic disease, *Blood* 64:1297, 1984.

167. **Sevitt S:** Venous thrombosis and pulmonary embolism. Their prevention by oral anticoagulants, *Am J Med* 33:703, 1962.

168. **Sevitt S:** Venous thrombosis in injured patients (with some observations on pathogenesis). In Sherry S, Brinkhaus KM, Genton E, et al: editors: *Thrombosis*, Washington DC, 1969, National Academy of Sciences.

169. **Sevitt S, Gallagher NG:** Prevention of venous thrombosis and pulmonary embolism in injured patients. A trial of anticoagulant prophylaxis with phenindione in middle-aged and elderly patients with fractured necks of femur, *Lancet* 2:981, 1959.

170. **Sevitt S, Gallagher N:** Venous thrombosis and pulmonary embolism. A clinicopathological study in injured and burned patients, *Br J Surg* 48:475, 1961.

171. **Sharnoff JG:** Results in the prophylaxis of postoperative thromboembolism, *Surg Gynecol Obstet* 123:303, 1966.

172. **Sharnoff JG, Rosen RL, Sadler AH, et al:** Prevention of fatal pulmonary thromboembolism by heparin prophylaxis after surgery for hip fractures, *J Bone Joint Surg* 58:913, 1976.

173. **Shepard RM Jr, White HA, Shirkey AL:** Anticoagulant prophylaxis of thromboembolism in post-surgical patients, *Am J Surg* 112:698, 1966.

174. **Sie P, Dupouy D, Pichon J, et al:** Constitutional heparin cofactor II deficiency associated with recurrent thrombosis, *Lancet* 2:414, 1985.

175. **Sigel B, Felix WR, Popky GL, et al:** Diagnosis of lower limb venous thrombosis by Doppler ultrasound technique, *Arch Surg* 104:174, 1972.

176. **Sikorski JM, Hampson WG, Staddon GE:** The natural history and aetiology of deep vein thrombosis after total hip replacement, *J Bone Joint Surg* 63[Br]:171, 1981.

177. **Skinner DB, Salzman EW:** Anticoagulant prophylaxis in surgical patients, *Surg Gynec Obstet* 125:741, 1967.

178. **Soreff J, Johnsson H, Diener L, et al:** Acetylsalicylic acid in a trial to diminish thromboembolic complications after elective hip surgery, *Acta Orthop Scand* 46:246, 1975.

179. **Sproul EE:** Carcinoma and venous thrombosis. The frequency of association of carcinoma in the body or tail of the pancreas with multiple venous thromboses, *Am J Cancer* 34:566, 1938.

180. **Stamatakis JD, et al:** Femoral vein thrombosis and total hip replacement, *Br Med J* 2:223, 1977.

181. **Stamatakis JD, Kakkar VV, Lawrence D, et al:** Failure of aspirin to prevent post-operative deep vein thrombosis in patients undergoing total hip replacement, *Br Med J* 1:1031, 1978.

182. **Stead NW, Bauer KA, Kinney TR, et al:** Venous thrombosis in a family with defective release of vascular plasminogen activator and elevated plasma factor VIII/von Willebrand factor, *Am J Med* 74:33, 1983.

183. **Stewart GJ, Alburger PD, Stone EA, et al:** Total hip replacement induces injury to remote veins in a canine model, *J Bone Joint Surg* 65:97, 1983.

184. **Stone RG, Stinchfield FE, Eftekhar NS:** Clinical comparison of aspirin prophylaxis with heparin and warfarin in patients after total hip arthroplasty, *Orthop Trans* 9:82 1985.

185. **Strandness DE Jr:** Thrombosis detection by ultrasound, plethysmography, and phlebography, *Semin Nucl Med* 7:213, 1977.

186. **Stulberg BN, Dorr LD, Ranawat CS, et al:** Aspirin prophylaxis for pulmonary embolism following total hip arthroplasty. An incidence study, *Clin Orthop* 168:119, 1982.

187. **Swierstra BA, Stibbe J, Schouten HJA:** Prevention of thrombosis after hip arthroplasty: a prospective study of preoperative oral anticoagulants, *Acta Orthop Scand* 59:139, 1988.

188. **Tran TH, Marbet GA, Duckert F:** Association of hereditary heparin cofactor II deficiency with thrombosis, *Lancet* 2:413, 1985.

189. **Tubiana R, DuParc J:** Prevention of thromboembolic complications in orthopaedic and accident surgery, *J Bone Joint Surg* 43[Br]:7, 1961.

190. **Turpie AGGG, Levine MN, Hirsh J, et al:** A randomized controlled trial of a low-molecular-weight heparin (Enoxaparin) to prevent deep-vein thrombosis in patients undergoing elective hip surgery, *N Engl J Med* 315:925, 1986.

191. **Verhagen H:** Local haemorrhage and necrosis of the skin and underlying tissues. During anti-coagulant therapy with dicoumarol or dicumacyl, *Acta Med Scand* 148:453, 1954.

192. **Vessey MP:** Female hormones and vascular disease: epidemiologic overview, *Br J Fam Plan* 6:1, 1980.

193. **Virchow R:** *Thrombose und Embolie* (1846–1856). Leipzig, Germany, 1910, Verlag-von Johann Ambrosius Barth.

194. **Wessler S:** Studies in intravascular coagulation; pathogenesis of serum induced venous thrombosis, *J Clin Invest* 34:647, 1955.

195. **Wessler S:** Venous thromboembolism, scope of the problem. In Frantantoni J, Wessler S, editors: *Prophylactic therapy of deep vein thrombosis and pulmonary embolism*, Washington, DC, 1975, US Department of Health, Education and Welfare, Publication (NIH) No 76-866.

196. **Wessler S, Yin ET:** Theory and practice of minidose heparin in surgical patients. A status report, *Circulation* 47:671, 1973.

196a. **Westermann K, Trentz O, Pretschner P, et al:** Thromboembolism after hip surgery, *Int Orthop* 4:253, 1981.

197. **Wheeler HB, O'Donnell JA, Handerson FA Jr, et al:** Occlusive impedance phlebography. A diagnostic procedure for venous thrombosis and pulmonary embolism. In Sasahara AA, Sonneblick EH, Lesch M, editors: *Pulmonary emboli,* New York, 1975, Grune & Stratton.

198. **White RE, Helpenstell T, Jacob TP:** *Accuracy of evaluation of deep venous thrombosis in the calf following total hip replacement by use of real-time B-mode ultrasound venous imaging.* Paper presented at the Annual Meeting of the American Academy of Orthopaedic Surgeons, New Orleans, 1990.

199. **Williams WJ:** Venography, *Circulation* 47:220, 1973.

200. **Winter JH, Fenech A, Ridley W, et al:** Familial antithrombin III deficiency, *Q J Med* 51:373, 1982.

201. **Woolson ST, McCrory BA, Walter JF, et al:** B-mode ultrasound scanning in the detection of proximal venous thrombosis after total hip replacement, *J Bone Joint Surg* 72:983, 1990.

ADDITIONAL READINGS

Aoki N, Moroi M, Sakata Y, et al: Abnormal plasminogen. A hereditary molecular abnormality found in a patient with recurrent thrombosis, *J Clin Invest* 61:1186, 1978.

Collins DN, Barnes CL, McAndrew MP, et al: *Vena caval filter use in orthopaedic patients with recognized preoperative deep venous thrombosis.* Presented at the Annual Meeting of the American Academy of Orthopaedic Surgeons, New Orleans, 1990.

Dechavenne M, Ville D, Viala JJ, et al: Controlled trial of platelet anti-aggregating agents and subcutaneous heparin in prevention of postoperative deep vein thrombosis in high risk patients, *Haemostasis* 4:94, 1975.

Delen JS, Alpert JS: Natural history of pulmonary embolism. In Sasahara AA, Sonneblick EH, Lesch M, editors: *Pulmonary emboli,* New York, 1975, Grune & Stratton.

Faraci PA, Deterling RA Jr, Stein AM, et al: Warfarin induced necrosis of the skin, *Surg Gynecol Obstet* 146:695, 1978.

Harris WH: The incidence and prevention of thromboembolic disease. In American Academy of Orthopaedic Surgeons: *Instructional course lectures,* vol 19, St Louis, 1970, Mosby–Year Book.

Harris WH, Athanasoulis CA, Waltman AC, et al: Prophylaxis of deep-vein thrombosis after total hip replacement. Dextran and external pneumatic compression compared with 1.2 or 0.3 gram of aspirin daily, *J Bone Joint Surg* 67:57, 1985.

Hull RD, Hirsh J, Sackett DL, et al: Cost-effectiveness of primary and secondary prevention of fatal pulmonary. Embolism in high-risk surgical patients, *Can Med Assoc J* 127:990, 1982.

Koch-Weser J: Coumarin necrosis (editorial), *Ann Intern Med* 68:1365, 1968.

Rosove MH: Hematologic complications of cancer and its treatment. In Haskell CM, editor: *Cancer treatment,* ed 2, New York, 1985, WB Saunders.

Strandness DE Jr, Langlois Y, Cramer M, et al: Long-term sequelae of acute venous thrombosis, *JAMA* 250:1289, 1983.

Stulberg BN, Insall JN, Williams GW, et al: Deep-vein thrombosis following total knee replacement. An analysis of six hundred and thirty-eight arthroplasties, *J Bone Joint Surg* 66:194, 1984.

Szucs MM Jr, Brooks HL, Grossman W, et al: Diagnostic sensitivity of laboratory findings in acute pulmonary embolism, *Ann Intern Med* 74:161, 1971.

Terayama K: Experience with Charnley low-friction arthroplasty in Japan, *Clin Orthop* 211:79, 1986.

Tremaine MD, Choroszy CJ, Gordon G, et al: *Duplex venous venography in the total joint patient: which is the gold standard?* Presented at the Annual Meeting of the American Academy of Orthopaedic Surgeons, New Orleans, 1990.

See Chapter 2, Applied Surgical Anatomy, for additional information.

PART FOUR

PERIOPERATIVE MANAGEMENT

CHAPTER TEN

Indications, Contraindications, and Alternatives

■ The ability of a surgeon to perform a given operation is not, in itself, an indication for that operation.
Robert S. Salter

A PHILOSOPHICAL PERSPECTIVE

The enormous extra workload imposed by total hip arthroplasty in clinics and outpatient offices poses the problem of how to select appropriate patients for this type of surgery. Concerned surgeons have suggested that if in the future this procedure contributes more to misery than to well-being, the failure will not lie with the researchers who developed the device but with surgeons who fail to select patients properly.[33,34] By "promoting the spectacular," the popular press has encouraged floods of prospective patients to seek the procedure, many of them inappropriately. To neutralize any harm that might result, clinicians must fine-tune the diagnostic skills that will allow them to select the patients likely to benefit from the procedure.[33,84]

At a certain stage in developing a new surgical technique or drug, strict criteria for its use must be established. After the development of total hip arthroplasty, considerable caution was exercised in advocating the new procedure over time-tested, conventional operations.[36,38,58] After the failure of Teflon as an appropriate material for arthroplasty, Charnley[33] emphasized the need for caution in using new materials (e.g., high-density polyethylene) in total hip arthroplasty. At the time of this writing, some 30 years after the first insertion of a total hip prosthesis using acrylic cement and high-density polyethylene, it is generally agreed that the operation is suitable for adult patients with advanced degenerative arthritis and rheumatoid arthritis at any age after epiphyseal closure. The procedure remains unchallenged because of its spectacular results: relief of pain, preservation or increase of mobility, and above all, ease of rehabilitation without extensive physiotherapy. These achievements far surpass the results of such conventional operations as osteotomy or cup arthroplasty. In addition, the procedure's high success rate—over 95 percent when the operation is properly performed—bears strong witness to its superiority.

With certain provisions, total hip arthroplasty may be indicated as the method of choice for all kinds of patients in whom the acetabulum and the femoral surfaces are both involved. It is ideally suited for rheumatoid hips in particular, because the prosthesis bonds to porotic bone with cement. In addition, the severe disability of polyarthritis shelters the artificial joint against heavy mechanical stress. However, even patients with rheumatoid arthritis are not totally immune to mechanical failure. Indeed, an increased incidence of socket loosening has been reported after cemented total hip arthroplasty in rheumatoid patients.

Total hip arthroplasty is now regarded to be ideally suitable for older patients. As a general rule, total hip arthroplasty should be reserved for patients over 60 years of age who are retired or close to retirement. However, under certain circumstances a younger patient may be accepted, especially when a coexisting condition leads to a shortened life expectancy. The most common application of total hip arthroplasty by statistical analysis is in primary or secondary osteoarthritis (caused by trauma, congenital dysplasia, or

Text continued on p. 428.

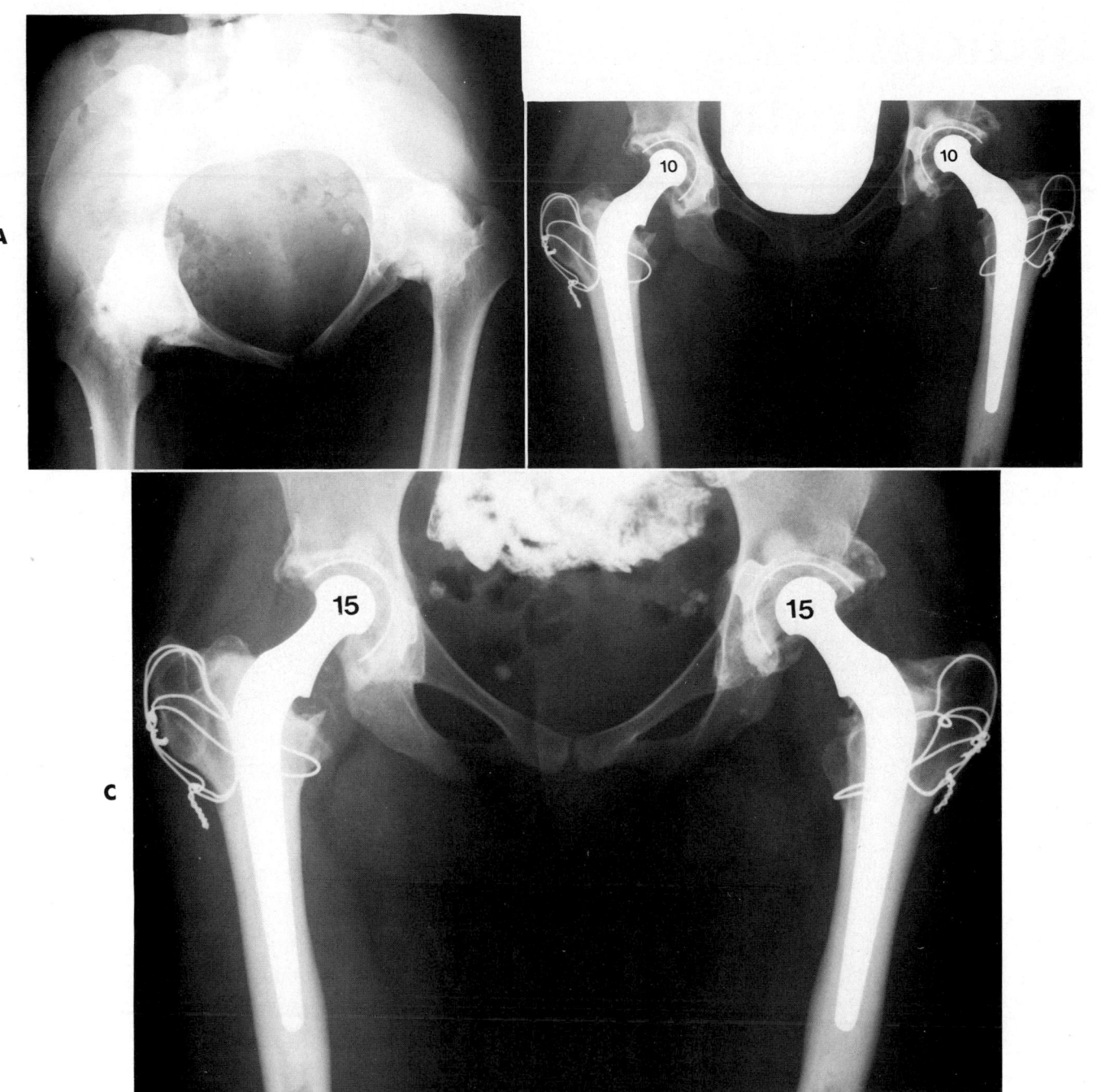

Fig. 10-1. A, Radiograph of a 19-year-old female (C.S.) with a chair- and bed-bound existence (Grade: C-bilateral 2,1,2) shows bilateral flexion contractures with severe shortening of the left lower extremity. **B,** 10 years after low-friction arthroplasty with very satisfactory clinical and radiological results (absence of demarcation). **C,** 15 years after index operation, there is 2 mm linear wear on the left and 1 mm on the right. Grade: C-right 6,5,6 and C-left 6,5,6. (Patient's knees were also replaced with an excellent clinical result.)

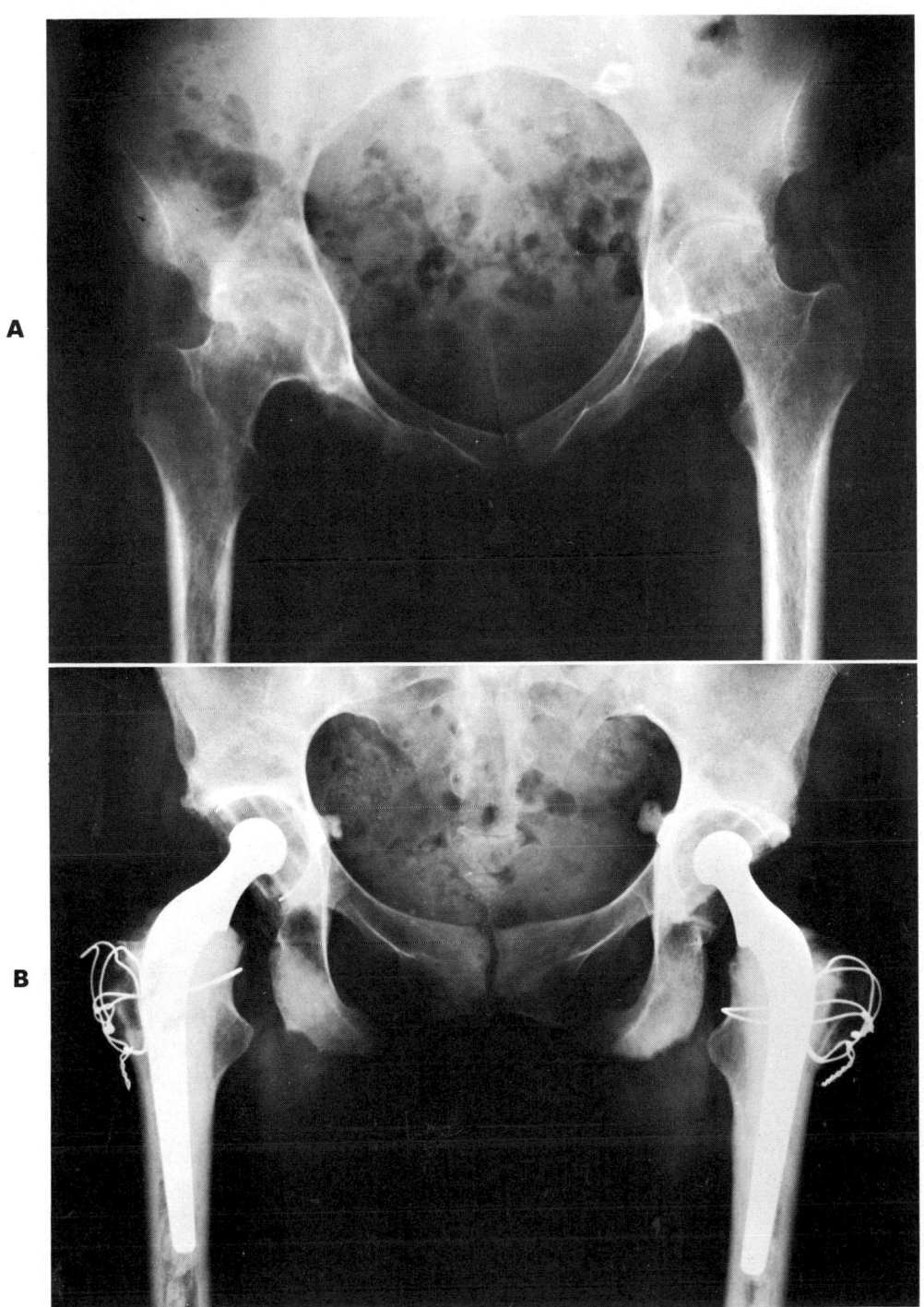

Fig. 10-2. This 31-year-old woman (E.F.) with history of bilateral painful hips of 5 years' duration was to undergo bilateral total hip arthroplasty because of pain and stiffness (preoperative grading of the hips, B-right 3,3,3 and B-left 3,3,3). No conventional operation would be indicated here despite young age of patient for total hip arthroplasty. Obliteration of sacroiliac joints is suggestive of diagnosis of ankylosing spondylitis, although spine and other joints are spared. **A,** Preoperative radiograph. **B,** 3-year postoperative radiograph.

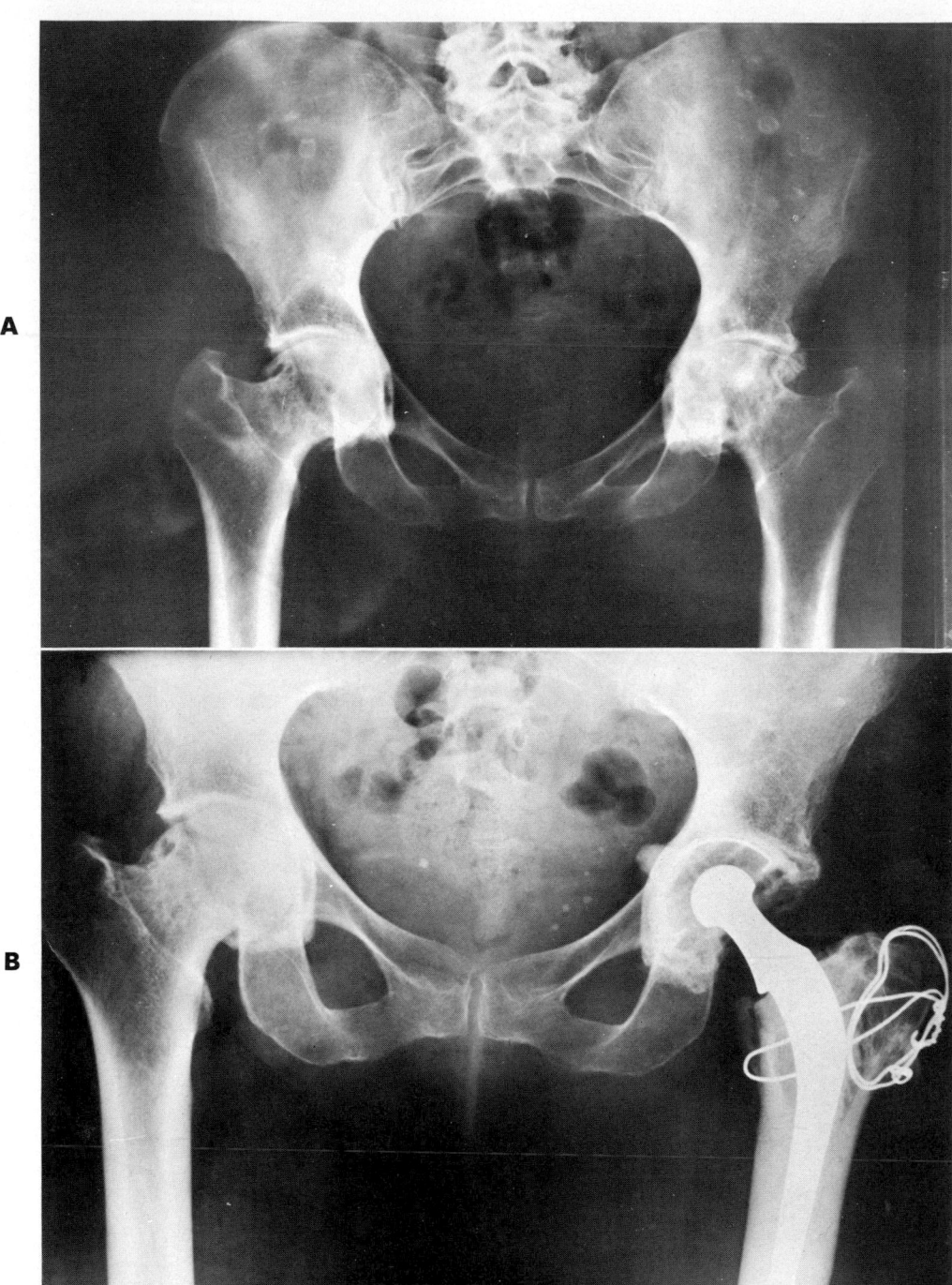

Fig. 10-3. Bilateral degenerative osteoarthritis of hip in 56-year-old housewife. Patient had pain in left hip predominantly, limiting her daily living activities, such as shopping and cleaning. Right hip was somewhat painful, but she could cope well with it. Preoperative grading of hips was B-right 5,3,5 and B-left 3,3,2. **A,** Preoperative status of both hips in 1969. **B,** One year after left total hip arthroplasty, 1970.

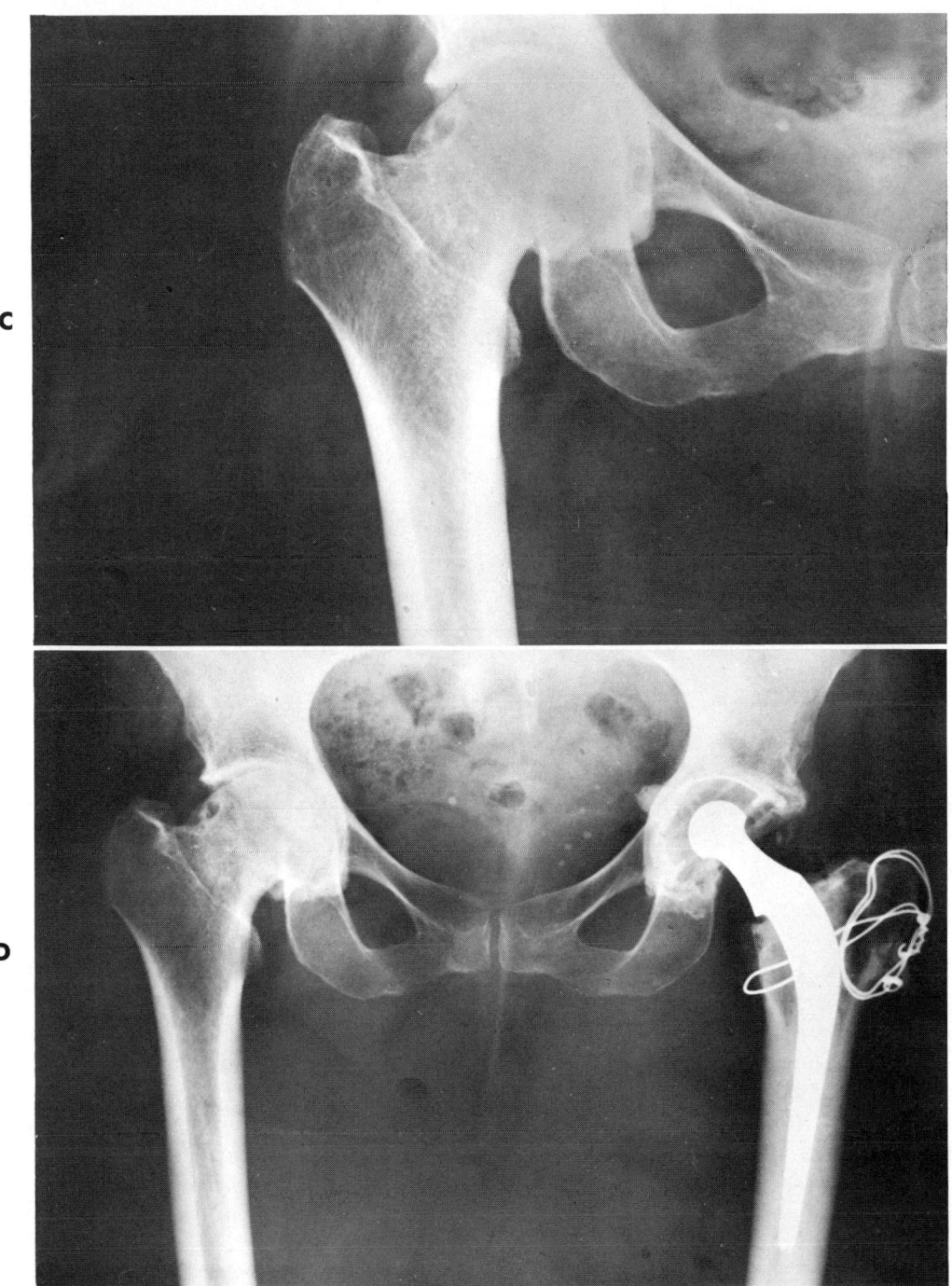

Fig. 10-3—cont'd. C, Status of right hip in 1973. **D,** Status of both hips in 1976. It is of special interest that after total hip arthroplasty of left hip pain from right hip has completely disappeared. There are no material radiological changes of right hip. Final grades B-right 6,6,6 and B-left 6,6,6. Whether this patient might require further surgery in the future on right hip cannot be ascertained, but it is now 7 years after surgery on left hip and she has no pain to justify recommending surgery on right hip.

Continued.

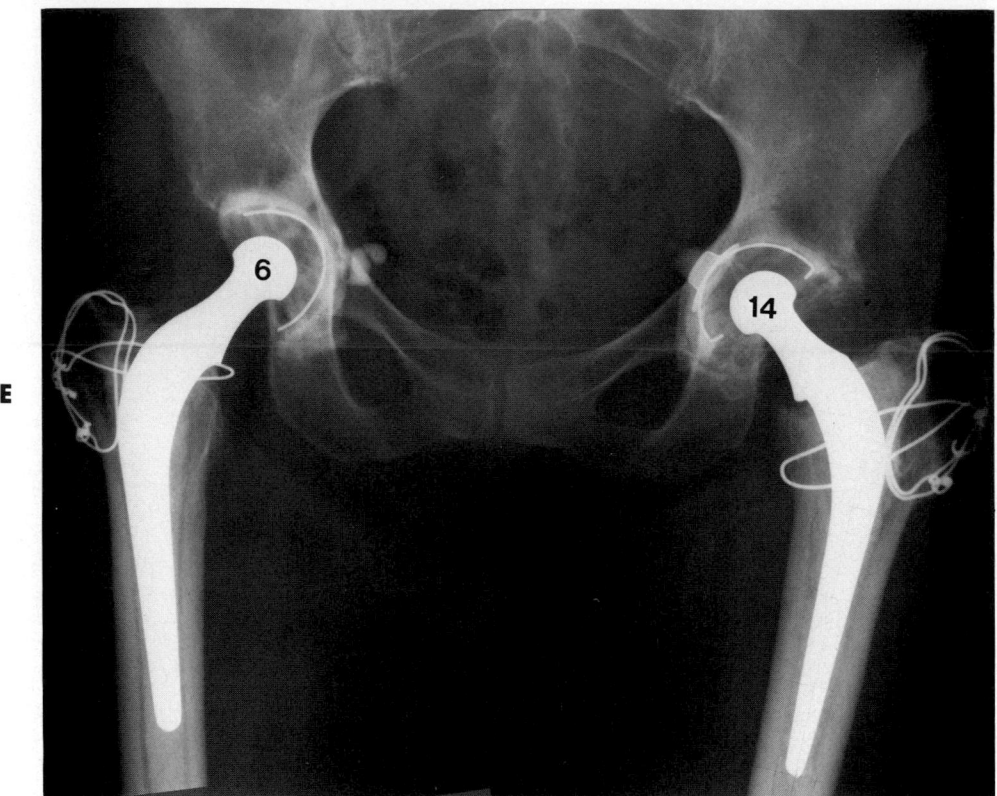

Fig. 10-3—cont'd. E, 6 *(right)* and 14 *(left)* years after surgery. Grades of hip at last follow up, B-right 6,6,6 and B-left 6,6,6.

other conditions). In patients with polyarthritis, such as rheumatoid or ankylosing spondylitis, it can be performed at almost any age, especially if knees and ankles will remain a disabling factor or will need corrective surgery after the hip operation (Fig. 10-1).

It is well known that the most spectacular results are achieved when surgery of both hips is performed. Patients with bilateral hip disease are usually handicapped by lack of mobility and pain. When alternatives to total hip arthroplasty are used instead, rehabilitation is long and tedious, requiring prolonged periods without weight bearing.* But with total hip arthroplasty, mobility is achieved rapidly, and weight bearing is resumed early. Therefore this operation is ideally suited for bilateral hip conditions (Fig. 10-2). Based on these facts, it is appropriate to use total hip arthroplasty on patients of almost any age with bilateral hip disease if the disease is severe and advanced enough.

In planning bilateral surgery, the interval between the two operations should be less than 3 months; in certain circumstances both hips may be done during the same anesthesia or the same hospitalization. In this author's experience, when marked deformity is absent it is best to postpone operating on the less symptomatic side, reconsidering the need at a future date. In some instances, the opposite hip improves after surgery to the point where further operation is not necessary. Early radiological changes of the opposite hip without symptoms do not justify plans for surgery. The second hip may remain unchanged for many years or even indefinitely after arthroplasty of one hip (Fig. 10-3).

There are three instances in which early surgery of both hips is advisable: (1) when treating bilateral disease in patients who are in their seventies, (2) when a severe fixed flexion deformity is present bilaterally, and (3) when a technical failure arises after arthroplasty and the second hip is also arthritic. In the first case, early surgery should be advised because of the possibility that medical complications will develop if the patient waits too long for the operation.[58] If medical complications do arise, one would not want to risk operating on the second hip. In the second instance, a resistant fixed-flexion deformity of the unoperated side would greatly interfere with hip mobility and postoperative rehabilitation (Fig. 10-4). In the third instance, if revision of a failed operation requires prolonged partial or non–weight bearing, operating on the second

* References 10, 49, 89, 90, 93.

Text continued on p. 432.

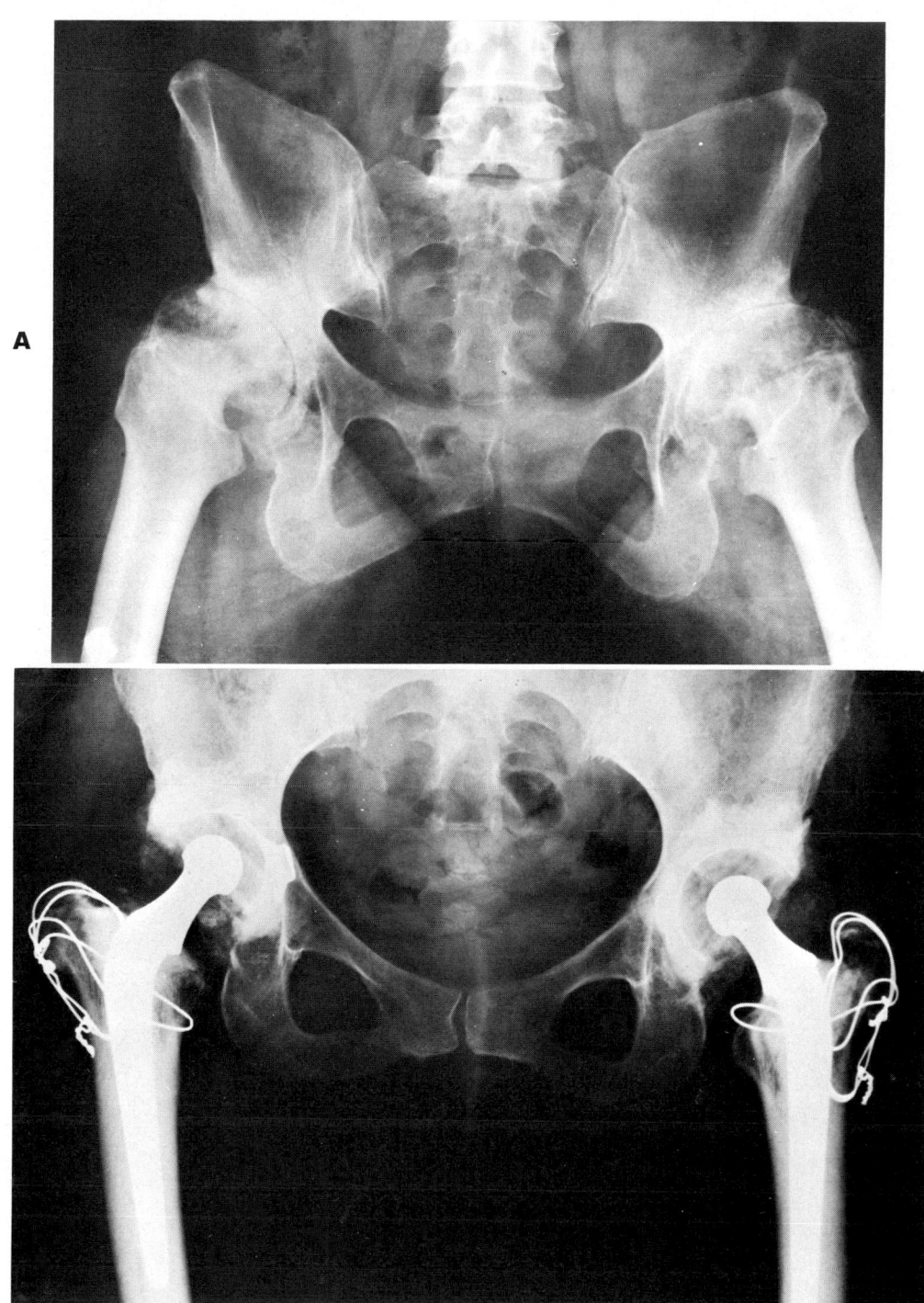

Fig. 10-4. A, Bilateral degenerative osteoarthrosis of hips in 55-year-old female who weighed 205 pounds and was only able to get about with aid of two crutches. She graded C-right 4,2,2 and C-left 4,2,2. NOTE: pelvis deformity as result of bilateral fixed flexion deformity of 65 degrees. After weight reduction before surgery; at surgery weight was 180 pounds. **B,** 5 years after surgery patient grades B-right 6,6,6 and B-left 6,6,6.

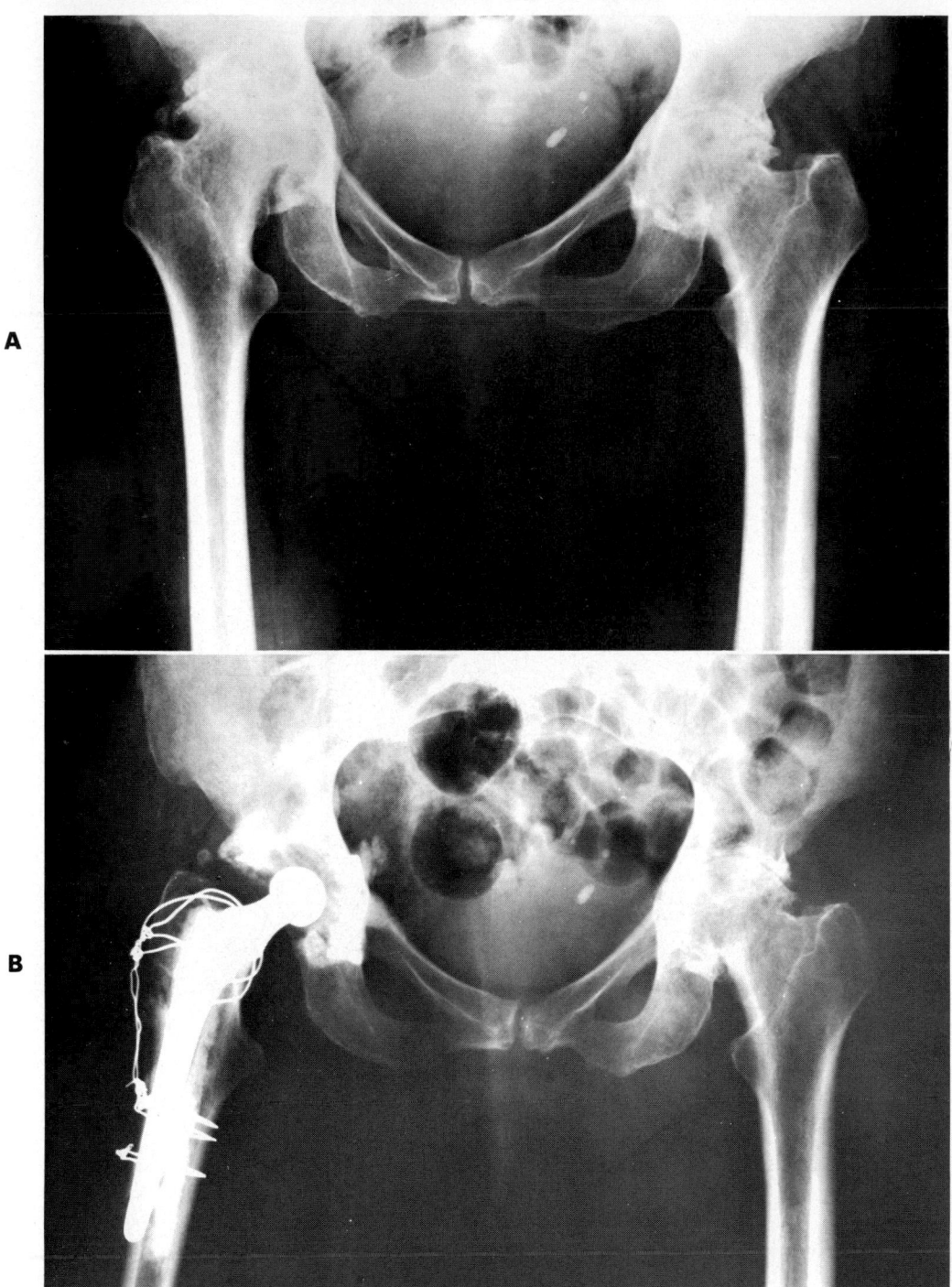

Fig. 10-5. A, Preoperative status of bilateral degenerative osteoarthritis of hips in 66-year-old woman with marked stiffness of both hips. Hip grade B-right 4,3,1; B-left 4,3,1. **B,** 3 months postoperative radiograph of patient with unfortunate complication of fracture of shaft of femur and circlàge wiring of upper femur to rectify problem at surgery. At this point patient was referred to us for treatment of defective surgery.

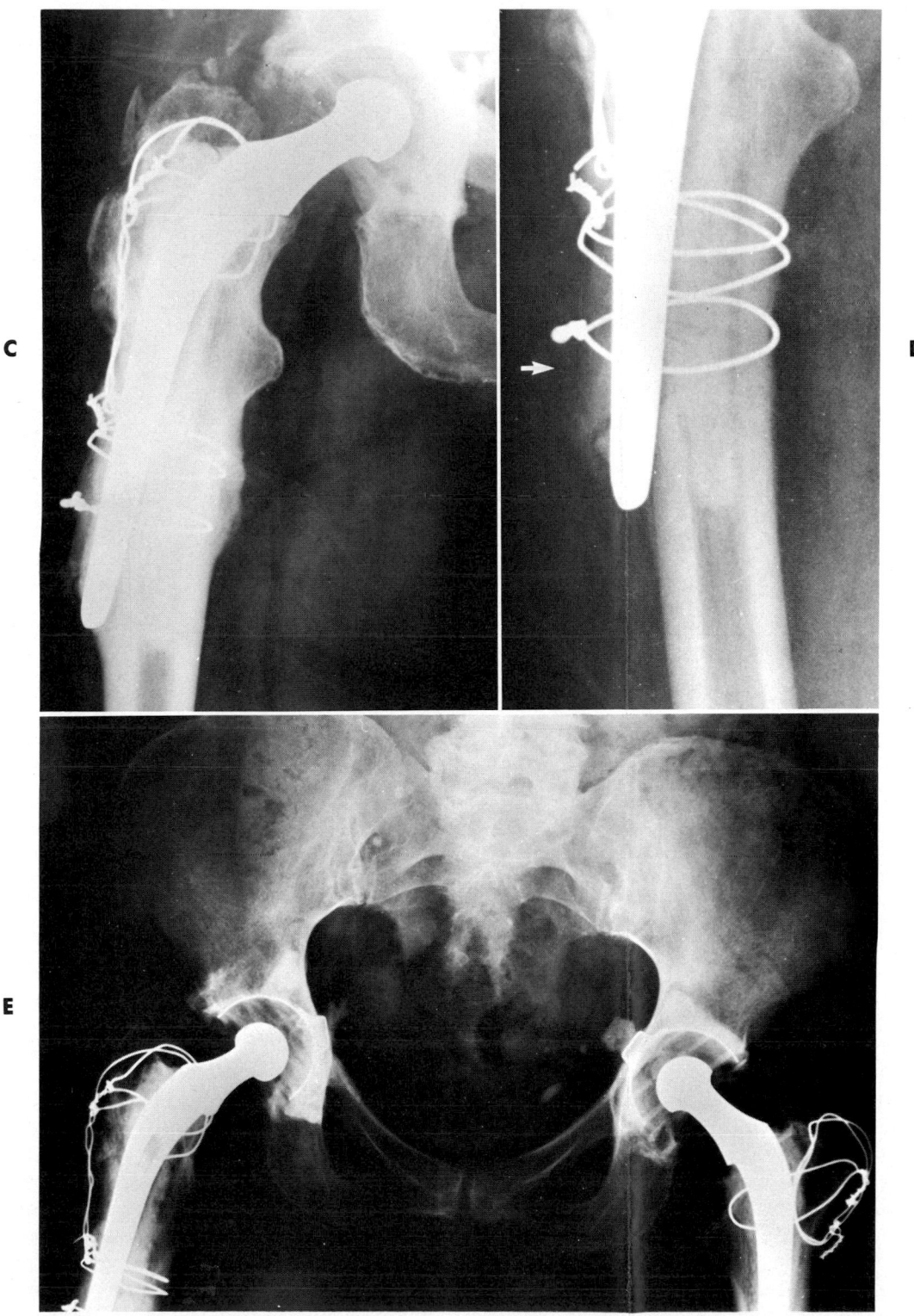

Fig. 10-5—cont.'d. C and **D,** Lateral extrusion of stem. NOTE: callus formation with stability achieved by "nature repair." In **D** arrow shows bone formation at stem tip level. **E,** Instead of revising right hip, it was decided to perform left total hip arthroplasty to provide patient with good and sound weight-bearing joint. After recovery of left total hip arthroplasty, patient did exceptionally well while she remained non—weight bearing on right with gradual increased weight bearing as tolerated. By 6 months after second hip operation patient had no pain in right hip and became functionally satisfactory. Now 6 years after second hip operation, **E,** Patient is totally asymptomatic despite precarious situation of right hip.

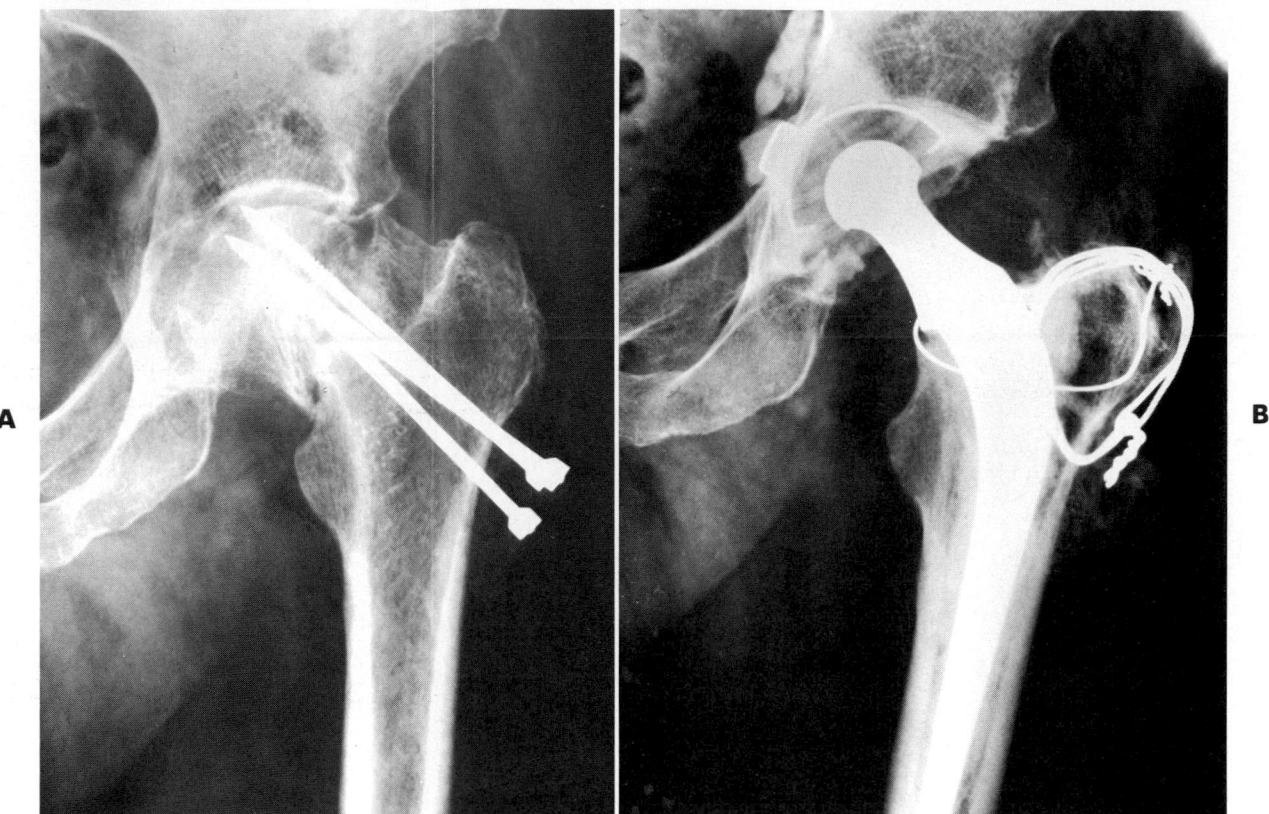

Fig. 10-6. Chronological age alone is not a contraindication to total hip arthroplasty. If patient's physiological age permits and systemic examination reveals no contraindication, total hip arthroplasty will be a great bonus to an invalid aged person. **A,** Anteroposterior view of left hip in an 86-year-old woman who sustained fracture of hip followed by pinning and avascular necrosis and nonunion. Medial migration of pins additionally led to acetabular damage. Hip evaluation revealed A-left 3,3,2. Because of patient's desire despite age, total hip arthroplasty was performed. **B,** Left hip 6 years after total hip arthroplasty. Now at age 92, patient is independent, walks without assistance, and is pleased with decision regarding surgery. She had been denied surgery by three other orthopaedic consultants because of her age.

hip before the revision provides a sound extremity that helps with rehabilitation (Fig. 10-5).

In general, it is not a good idea to plan bilateral surgery for patients in their eighties. Although we no longer maintain the ultraconservative attitude of accepting a chairbound existence for the very old patient, it is best to plan such surgery before age 80. Pain as a result of osteoarthritis may be very intense. A low pain threshold in the aged may cause disability and, when compounded by a narrowing socioeconomic horizon, may result in total confinement for elderly patients. When the operation is used appropriately, an elderly person suffering acute misery from arthritis of the hips can be totally freed from pain and able to function in 2 to 3 weeks (Fig. 10-6). In such cases, the physician is profoundly gratified to see that the decision to operate on this patient was justified. Aged female patients usually recover more durably from this operation than their male counterparts.

A CASE FOR CONSERVATISM

A note of caution when treating a younger patient: the surgeon must not underestimate the possibility that total hip arthroplasty will introduce ultrafine particles of metal or plastic into the tissue, creating as-yet-unknown consequences for the patient in 10 to 20 years. Both the patient and the surgeon are faced with an exceedingly difficult decision: should a young, handicapped patient be advised to postpone surgery for another 5 to 10 years, awaiting long-term results of the safety and effectiveness of recent innovations and hoping new materials will be available? Or should the physician balance the present degree of disability against the worst that could happen if the total prosthesis failed as a result of implantation? Clearly, this decision demands careful clinical judgment, and the patient must be fully familiarized with all the alternatives so he or she can participate knowledgeably in the decision-making process.

Surgeons practicing total hip surgery find themselves under enormous pressure to perform this operation on patients in whom the only indication is the subjective complaint of pain, unsupported by objective signs of crippling disability. As our experience with newer methods of arthroplasty strengthens, doubtless we will find it justifiable to perform this major procedure, with all its theoretical hazards in younger patients, when the precipitating factor is simply a low threshold for pain. The new technologies and materials—porous-coated implants and ceramics—are of more recent vintage and still in the developmental stage. Most early designs have been abandoned and none of the newer ones has passed the 10- to 15-year point, when it will be possible to compare them with the conventional method, cemented total hip arthroplasty.

While awaiting the long-term results of these newer techniques, surgeons would be well advised to ascertain objective signs of disability before deciding to operate. Patients will be grateful for the surgeon's decision to postpone the procedure when it is based on such logical grounds. Although this is elementary advice for experienced surgeons, it bears repeating when we are faced with a patient intoxicated by the news of the spectacular results that often follow this surgery when performed on older and less active adults.

Charnley stated that total prosthetic arthroplasty at any age is indicated when a Girdlestone pseudarthrosis would be beneficial.[33] This is still frequently true today as the newer implants are being tested in young patients.

Total hip arthroplasty can be performed at any age as a salvage procedure to correct a previously unsuccessful operation. When total hip arthroplasty is considered in such a case, the surgeon must first rule out the possibility that infection caused the failure. If infection is present, surgeon and patient must reach a special understanding regarding the magnitude of the problem and the possibility of failure resulting from reoperation.

In the past, total hip arthroplasty was considered inadvisable in patients with previous infection, but recent studies suggest that this type of surgery can succeed in patients with low-grade infection or those with a good bone stock and bacteria sensitive to commonly used antimicrobial agents. It is generally a good policy to advise against total hip arthroplasty in the following conditions:

1. If a patient with unilateral hip disease is under 60 years of age and can continue to work without undue disability.
2. Where the pain or disability is not sufficient to call for pain medications, and the patient's principal motivation is participation in sports.
3. If the patient is obese, a definite relative contraindication. Patients weighing over 200 pounds should not be accepted for surgery without at first making a genuine effort to reduce their weight. In addition to increasing the risks of thrombophlebitis, infection, and so on, obesity makes performing the procedure technically more difficult and increases the likelihood of early mechanical failure of the cemented devices. The long-term results of cementless hip arthroplasty in young and heavy patients remain unknown. Whenever possible, the patient's weight should be reduced to about 176 pounds or less before the planned surgery. Likewise, weight must be monitored postoperatively.
4. In the presence of infections caused by gram-negative organisms or of active infection or osteomyelitis in the upper femur or pelvis.

In general, skilled or unskilled manual laborers under 60 years of age who are still able to work should not undergo total hip arthroplasty. The same applies to a retired 70-year-old person who is able to walk without a cane for unlimited distances. This type of patient is not a good candidate for total hip arthroplasty. Radiological changes alone are never a sufficient criterion for patient selection (Figs. 10-7 and 10-8).

INITIAL PATIENT INTERVIEW

The initial interview is one of the most important steps in selecting patients for total hip arthroplasty. During this interview, the surgeon must evaluate not only the patient's medical and orthopaedic history, but also such psychological factors as intelligence, motivation, and expectations from the surgery. Realistically, a 1-hour exchange is the minimum requirement to unravel some of the complex personal issues that patients often omit, consciously or unconsciously.

In deciding whether to operate, the surgeon should consider the patient as a whole, not just as a hip. Although patients considering total hip arthroplasty have been examined previously by their referring physicians and may be psychologically prepared to undergo surgery, the original interview by the surgeon contemplating the procedure is by far the most important means of evaluation. The surgeon's decision must be completely independent of the recommendations and evaluations of the referring physician.

Although in some cases one interview may be adequate to determine whether total hip arthroplasty is indicated, that is not always true. For example, in considering a patient whose objective findings do not correspond with his or her subjective complaints, a second or third interview might be required, coupled with initial nonoperative recommendations (these may include the use of nonsteroidal antiinflammatory drugs, a cane, etc.).

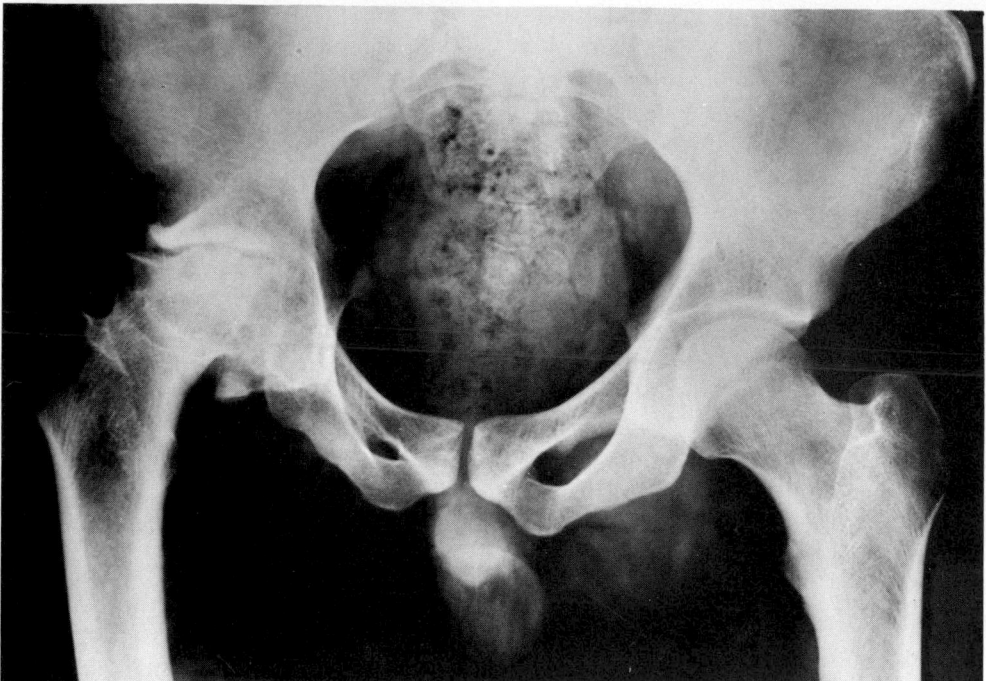

Fig. 10-7. Unilateral degenerative osteoarthritis secondary to childhood septic arthritis in 29-year-old lawyer. Despite extensive radiological changes and evidence of avascular necrosis of femoral head by radiography, patient has minimal discomfort, is able to work without taking medications, and has only minimal limp. Radiological changes alone are not indications for surgery in this patient.

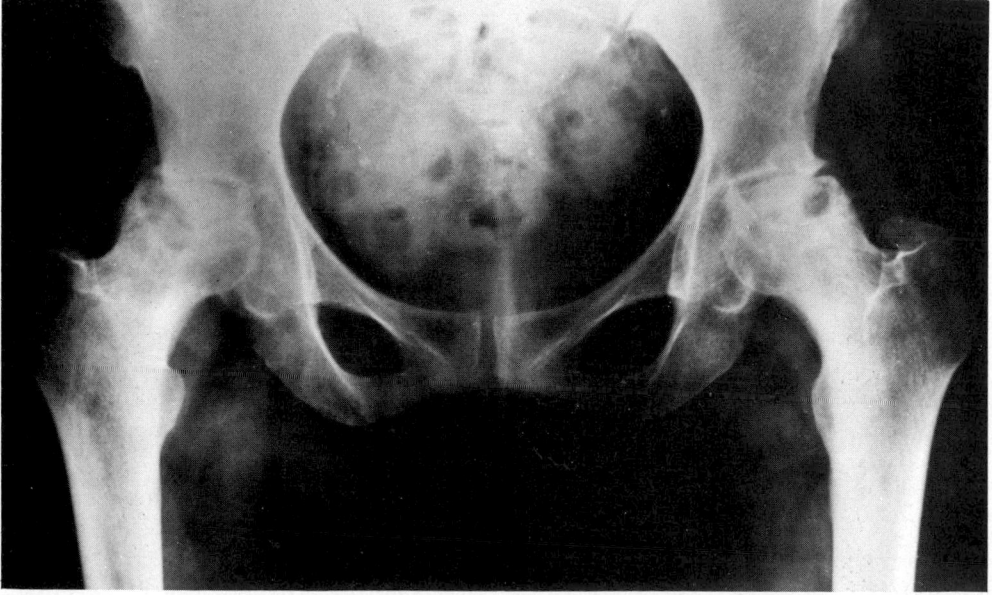

Fig. 10-8. Bilateral avascular necrosis with collapse of femoral head in 19-year-old female with lupus erythematosus. Currently she is taking 40 mg prednisone and weighs 200 lbs. Despite radiological changes, she is able to get about without pain with assistance of cane. Because of history of kidney involvement and absence of pain, despite bilateral hip involvement, no surgery is contemplated, particularly because of her weight and high steroid dosage.

When selecting young and active patients for total hip arthroplasty, this author finds as a general rule that it is best to postpone the decision until a second interview. Preferably, such patients should be asked to return (and I emphasize: no charge for this visit!) with a close family member to emphasize the significance of the surgeon's decision to operate. The patient must understand that commitment to total hip surgery is an entirely irreversible decision and that both surgeon and patient have eliminated all other options.

Whatever the outcome, the first interview and examination greatly influence the surgeon's thinking. It is also where the surgeon inspires the patient's confidence. Therefore it is of paramount importance that the physician answer all questions sincerely. Because it is often difficult to dissuade a patient who wants to have the operation, it is essential to establish a good relationship with him or her during the original interview. Begin by allowing the patient to tell their own story in their own words. Listen attentively, and try not to interrupt until the patient asks for some guidance or direction. After the patient has fully expressed the complaints, the physician can take over the interview, asking the questions that will provide the information he or she needs to evaluate the hip disability, based on what can be learned about the pain and the effect on functional activities. An assessment of the social and personal motivation behind the patient's consultation is essential. Leading questions help the surgeon assess the hip disability's impact on the patient's life in work and social situations and whether the patient is seeking correction primarily to continue certain hobbies and sports. The amount of "pain medication" the patient consumes in 24 hours usually helps determine the intensity of pain. Knowledge of the location and distribution of pain, its type, and duration and the patient's need for medication help the physician define the problem. A polyarthritic patient, for example, may have more disability from related joints, such as the sacroiliac and lumbar spine, than from the hip. Pain stemming from abdominal or gynecological sources is frequently misinterpreted as hip pain. In such instances the pain may be referred and unrelated to the hip joint. It is also essential to consider the source of referral as an important factor in the overall evaluation. Many patients with mild hip disability seek advice because they have read or seen spectacular results in a patient who has undergone such a procedure or because they have been pressured by sympathetic friends or relatives.

PAIN: THE CARDINAL SIGN

The most certain guide in determining the need for total hip arthroplasty is the severity of the pain and the resultant disability. The pain may be described as fatigue, inability to stand on the leg, or inability to function or accommodate certain motions. If it is referred or radiating, the pain may affect the buttock, groin, or upper thigh or may be focused completely in the knee, confounding the patient's ability to explain it accurately. Often a patient's lack of anatomical knowledge may cause him or her to identify the hip as the focus when the principal pain is unrelated to the hip. (For example, patients may point to the greater trochanter or the crest of the ilium.)

More important is the character of the pain, generally mechanical in nature, that is produced by walking, weight bearing, or other physical activities. Some patients with severe hip involvement and severe handicaps resulting from marked destructive changes in their hips have little or no complaint of pain, but with questioning they reveal that their activities have been markedly reduced. Indeed, some may have become housebound to avoid pain. (On occasion, a patient's discomfort disappears when he or she is admitted to the hospital for surgery. After resting for a few days the patient may wonder whether surgery is required after all.) In other instances, the hip joint becomes insensitive after marked absorption of the femoral head or expansion of the acetabulum with reduction of friction in the joint; ankylosis of the hip occasionally reduces the pain at the cost of stiffness. Pain in the osteoarthritic hip is rarely spontaneous, and, when present at night, it usually appears after the patient turns in bed. Pain in rheumatoid arthritis may be severe at times, but the patient rarely describes it as throbbing, burning, or stabbing. It is often coincidental with inflammatory exacerbation of the disease and is similar to the pain of gouty arthritis. Pain is always elicited in the patient's joint with passive movement and is also produced with sharp internal or external rotation.

The location of the pain must be pinpointed from a careful history and physical examination based on normal functional anatomy. This is most important, especially when examining a previously failed hip operation to ascertain its origin. The following locations are used as a guide in determining the specific origin of pain about the hip joint: (1) groin pain, (2) gluteal pain, (3) trochanteric pain, (4) back pain, (5) knee pain, (6) anterior thigh pain, (7) sciatic pain, and (8) abdominal and deep groin pain.

The diffusion of pain about the hip stems from the fact that nerve fibers supplying the hip joint (derived from the femoral obturator and sciatic nerves) also innervate the skin, muscle, and bone in the region. The sympathetic nerve fibers that supply the joint supply the blood vessels and also produce pain. While mechanical arthritic pain is completely eliminated after total hip arthroplasty, minor discomfort from scars of previous surgery or inflammatory response in soft tissue may persist and must be accepted. These responses are generally self-limiting, and the patient with previous surgery and a low pain threshold (especially one who obsessively speaks about his or her scar sensitivity or appearance) should be forewarned of their possibility.

If pain is in the gluteal region, it may originate in the area of the hamstrings or be related to the gluteal bursa. In the trochanteric region the greater trochanteric bursa may be responsible. Pain posterior and deep to the trochanter may originate from the piriformis bursa and occasionally may radiate to the buttock or midposterior thigh. The pain in this area may, indeed, be referred from the hip joint. Pain in the back is usually located in the area of the sacroiliac joint, especially when there is fixed deformity of the hip transmitting motion to this region. When the pain is in the knee, it may be related to the hamstring attachment, to the hip, or to the innervation of the obturator along the adductor muscle. Irradiation of the psoas muscle and its bursa may produce pain radiating toward the inner abdominal region. If the patient has had previous reconstructive surgery of the hip, the pain may be diffused or it may be in more than one of the previously mentioned locations. The patient with hip pain resulting from arthritis is often unable to bear weight fully but feels no pain when at rest. An exception to this rule is pain resulting from avascular necrosis of the femoral head; this pain is intense and unrelated to motion. It is often disproportionate to radiological changes or the range of motion in the affected hip.

It is important to consider the cause of pain in the hip in terms of more remote areas; abdominal tumors, pelvic tumors, or adhesions and infections within the abdomen may refer pain to the region of the obturator nerve, causing pain in the groin. Degenerative disease of the upper lumbar region with femoral nerve irritation or of the sacroiliac joint may lead to pain referred to the hip area. Benign or malignant tumors in the hip region may produce hip pain; occasionally inflamed abdominal viscera including the bladder, bowel, rectal sigmoid colon, prostate, or female genitourinary tract may lead to radiating pain in the area of the hip.

When a hip is fused it is not painful, but often, strain on the sacroiliac or lower lumbar spine produces pain in the hip region. Thorough evaluation of the location and source of pain therefore is of paramount importance, especially when radiological changes of the hip are not consistent with the intensity and location of the pain as described by the patient. Examination of the hip to identify painful points requires gentle expert handling. It is generally best to identify the landmarks on the unaffected or less symptomatic side to assure the patient of the gentleness of the examination and then switch to the affected hip. If the intensity of the pain cannot be determined, the patient can be asked to walk while the physician observes the gait. Many patients can better identify the source of pain produced by walking.[9]

SELECTION BY AGE ALONE

The patient's age and life expectancy compared to the functional life of the total hip arthroplasty are major considerations in selecting a candidate for this procedure. It is now generally agreed that if the patient is close to retirement, 60 or 65 years old, there is less concern about considering him or her for surgery. However, patients in their forties and fifties present the problem of possible mechanical failure and need for reoperations in subsequent years. Fear that one or more of the substances used in total hip arthroplasty may become carcinogenic is a theoretical concern that has not been substantiated based on the reports in the literature. However, the possibility of late manifestation of mutagenic elements, such as plastics and metals in man, cannot be entirely overlooked over a long period. It is also important that the functional age of the patient and his or her general physical condition should be considered rather than chronological age alone. For instance, an otherwise healthy 55-year-old man with unilateral osteoarthritis of the hip may impose greater strain on the hip joint than a 45-year-old woman with rheumatoid arthritis in whom involvement of the other joint may prevent full activity. The 55-year-old man, incidentally, may be a former tennis champion, looking forward to returning to a competitive game, whereas the 45-year-old woman may be seeking limited ambulation and relief of pain.

Perhaps an even more important criterion for determining surgery at any age is the list of alternatives and their ramifications. Considering other methods and age alone, for example, a surgeon must recognize that he or she will never satisfy a 30-year-old man with cup arthroplasty or an osteotomy. This is true in terms of needed rehabilitation, economic implications, and physical demands on the hip itself. With bilateral arthritis, approximately 1 year of rehabilitation might be needed. Often a patient may not be psychologically prepared to undergo surgery on the other side after one operation. Obviously, these criteria must be balanced against the potential risks and worst possible outcomes, as well as the theoretical objections to total hip arthroplasty in a young person. Although we are enjoying an astonishing absence of late defects in surgery performed 10 or 15 years ago, further failures resulting in wear of high-density polyethylene have become a concern frequently associated with socket loosening and migration. Viewing the overall picture optimistically, total hip arthroplasty will succeed in no more than 95% of patients by 10 years and between 85% and 90% between 10 and 20 years.

Only a soundly skilled surgeon who keeps abreast of

new revision techniques should select younger patients for total hip arthroplasty. This author believes that when a surgeon selects a young patient for surgery, the surgeon must acknowledge a threefold responsibility: (1) advising the patient of the potential risks involved including further intervention, if needed; (2) accepting the responsibility of performing a technically perfect operation; and (3) accepting the moral responsibility of an unwritten contract to provide future service should it become necessary. Therefore the surgeon must follow each patient for as long after surgery as the surgeon and the patient believe necessary, to determine whether any technical problems arise and to rectify them accordingly. The ability to recognize the need for revision arthroplasty plays a vital role in the surgeon's decision to concentrate exclusively on this type of practice. It is mandatory that a surgeon involved in total hip arthroplasty commit himself or herself to providing "maintenance operations" as needed.[34–38] As a fundamental principle, young patients undergoing total hip arthroplasty must understand that potential adverse biological reactions may arise, requiring revision. Further, a decision regarding revision might not necessarily be related to the patient's pain and disability but rather to ominous radiological signs of bony erosion resulting from wear or loosening. This intervention may be necessary despite the patient's total satisfaction with the existing clinical condition.

PATIENT'S DEMANDS AND PSYCHOLOGY

When a younger patient consults us about total hip arthroplasty surgery, it is important to elicit the reasons for the consultation. Is it because of anxiety and fear of progressive disability? Or is the existing problem sufficient to justify the present consultation? Often we find that the patient knows of a person who became chairbound a few years after becoming arthritic. Many patients consult us because they have heard that the condition becomes so severe that nothing can be done about it, and they want surgery done now to preserve hip mobility. Some socially active patients in their forties and fifties who have a limp but no severe pain may also seek surgery.

When cautioned against total hip arthroplasty, the patient often challenges the surgeon's reasons for refusing to operate. When confronted with such a situation, the physician can fall back on several cautionary findings. Considering only statistics, there is approximately a 1% death rate from this type of surgery. Mechanical failure occurs in perhaps no more than 5% (in the first 10 years) and about 1% of total hip arthroplasties each year thereafter; infection occurs in not more than 1% of the cases. (These figures are based on results in older patients, whose activities are limited; they would not apply to younger, more active persons.) But the literature has documented an in-

creasing number of young patients requiring revision surgery because of significant wear of the prosthetic materials or tissue reaction to them. Revisions of high-density polyethylene prostheses caused by excessive wear are becoming a prime concern in long-term follow-up of cemented and noncemented prostheses (Figs. 10-9 and 10-10). If ceramics or newer high-density polyethylene shows an improved wear property in vivo, perhaps greater relaxation of the criteria for total hip arthroplasty will be indicated and justifiable in the next 5 to 10 years.

Faced with exciting new technology such as computer/laser-associated designs used for a better fit of the prosthesis, it is imperative that both surgeon and patient be aware of possible negative outcomes. For example, we may find that abnormal bone remodeling and pathological osteolysis and osteopenia may cause permanent limitations, which will only manifest themselves 5 to 10 years after such innovative technology is used.

Surgeons frequently have great difficulty dissuading some patients, who pressure them to go ahead with surgery despite their own misgivings. The physician should candidly cite all the potential risks and complications of the surgery, including the 1% death rate. This information may be adequate to dissuade most patients (Fig. 10-11). Furthermore, the patient may decide to wait if the surgeon helps him or her understand the philosophy behind the postponement and that the operation may be done just as well or with better results in the future, when improved techniques and materials may be available. This author does not advocate temporizing with a conventional operation such as osteotomy or cup arthroplasty and proceeding with total hip arthroplasty at a later date. As a rule, patients treated in this way are dissatisfied with a temporizing operation, forcing the surgeon to perform total hip arthroplasty sooner than previously anticipated.

Patient Cooperation

Another important element to assess in considering a patient for total hip arthroplasty is how cooperative the patient is likely to be after surgery. For example, the patient's cooperation is needed to protect the hip against dislocation (see Chapter 32) and against weight bearing. Also the patient's willingness to maintain optimal body weight and avoid athletic activities after surgery is required for long-term survival of the artificial joint. A patient with a history of drug addiction and alcoholic avascular necrosis accompanied by obesity is not a suitable candidate for total hip arthroplasty. Such individuals are prone to falls and infection that will cause failure of the prosthesis; they might best be treated by consulting a psychiatrist before contemplating hip arthroplasty. We do accept patients

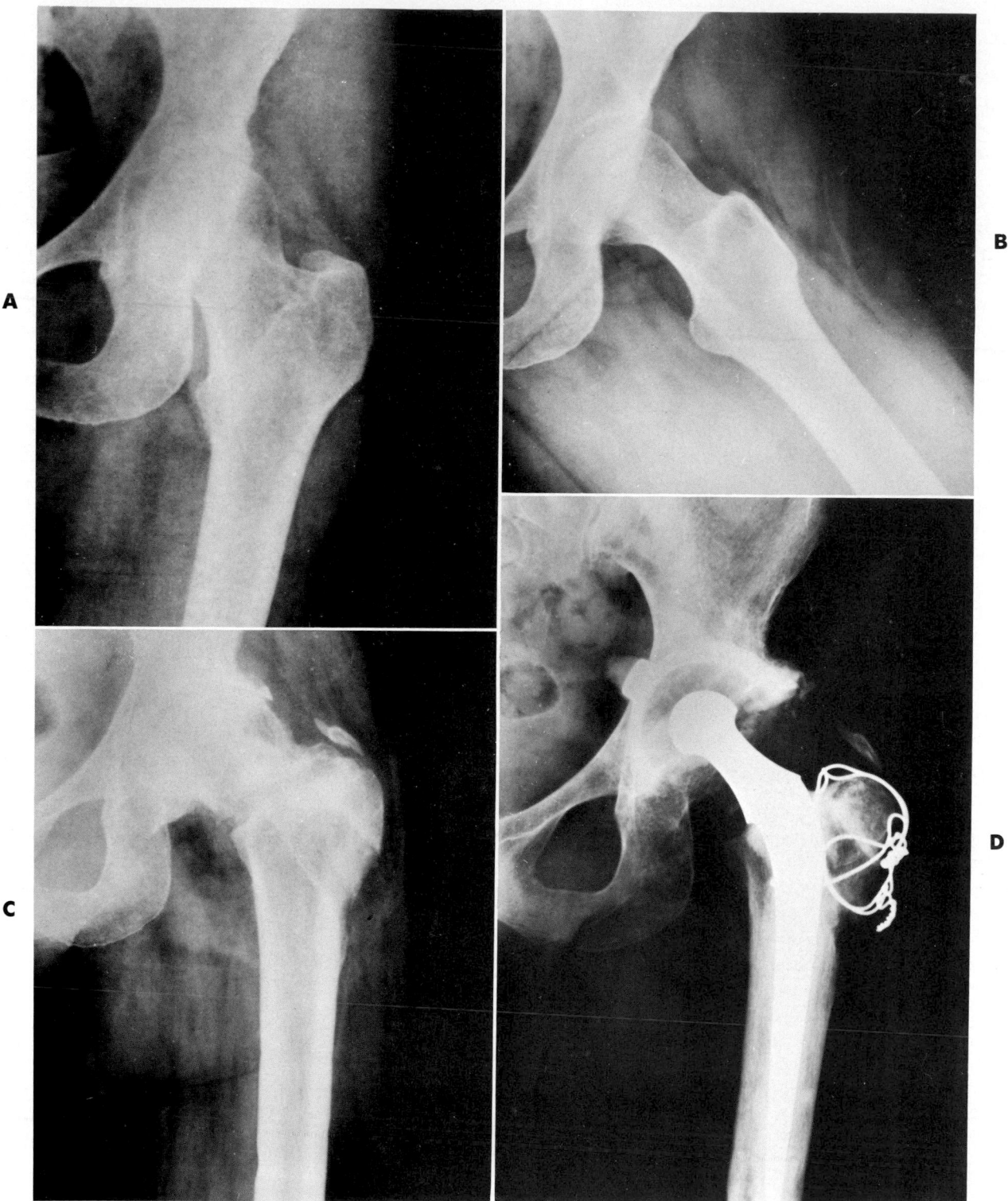

Fig. 10-9. This 34-year-old nurse was subjected to osteotomy of left hip (in another institution) for early signs of degenerative joint disease. At time of osteotomy her range of motion was good, and she had only minimum discomfort necessitating occasional aspirin. **A** and **B,** Anteroposterior and lateral views of hip before osteotomy. Osteotomy had been performed to prevent further progression of osteoarthritis and to achieve better coverage of femoral head. **C,** Same hip 1 year after osteotomy with progression of osteoarthritis despite osteotomy. Patient was indeed worse after osteotomy, which had been done to prevent progression of osteoarthritis. Internal fixation device was removed. **D,** Because of persistent pain and inability to walk patient was forced to have total hip arthroplasty, which successfully relieved her pain (4-year follow-up radiograph after arthroplasty). Patient could have been well treated by conservative treatment originally and perhaps total hip arthroplasty at her age would not have been needed.

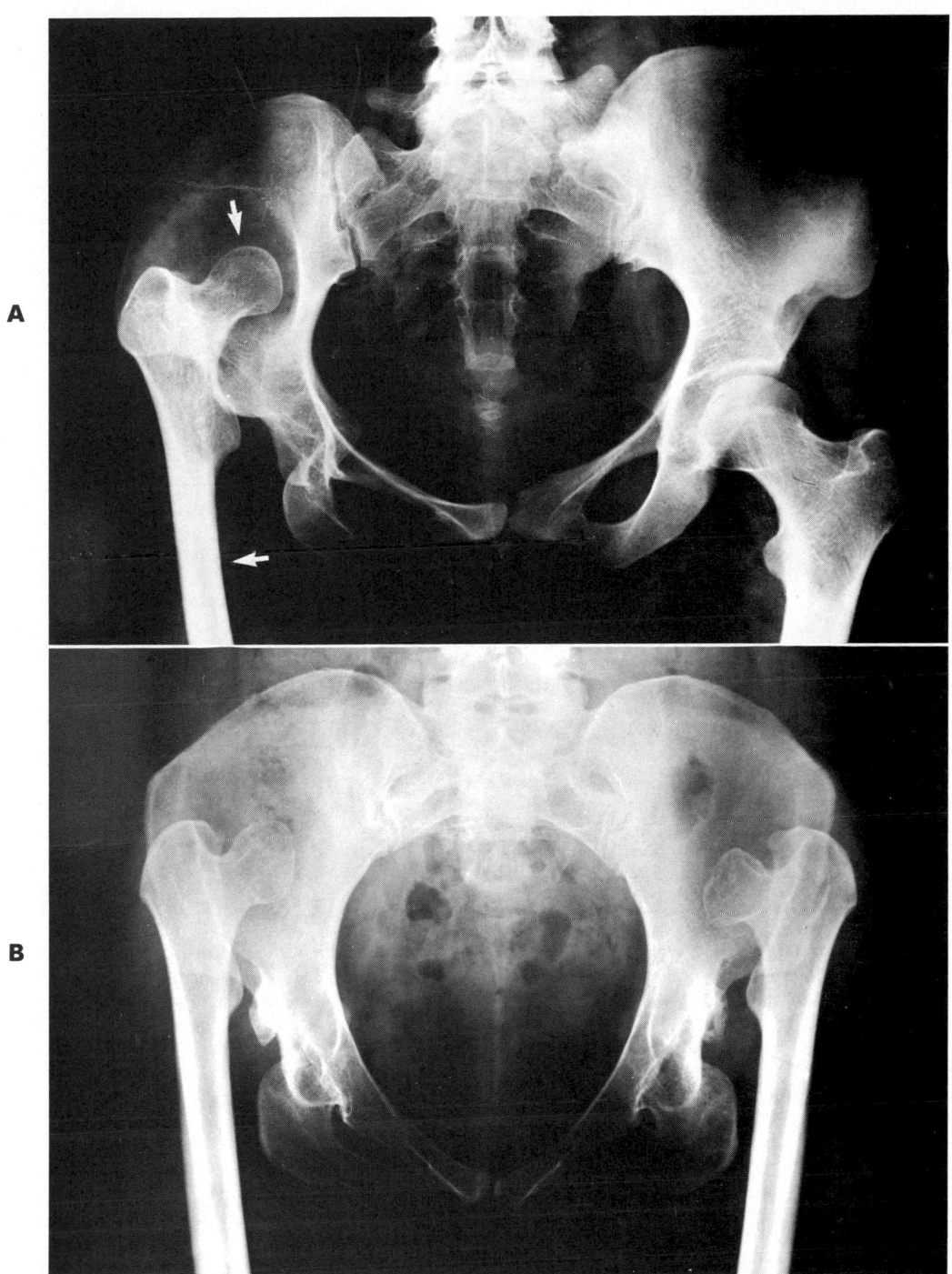

Fig. 10-10. A, Unilateral congenital hip dislocation in 26-year-old graduating medical student who has no pain and can cope well with her disability. She has no pain except for fatigue in hip and mild low back discomfort. No arthritis can be demonstrated by x-ray film *(top arrow).* Three-inch lift is required to compensate for short extremity. Patient is of Mediterranean extraction and seeks improvement in appearance more than relief of pain. Because of extreme dysplasia of hip *(lower arrow),* especially medullary canal of femur, at her active age operation is not performed. **B,** Bilateral congenital dislocations in 32-year-old female who has no leg length discrepancy with excellent range of motion in both hips. She walks unlimited but with bilateral, symmetrical, weak gluteal lurch; she can cope well with daily living activities and is fully gainfully employed as secretary. This clinical picture is contraindication for total hip arthroplasty at this time. Hip grades, B-right 5,5,6 and B-left 5,5,6.

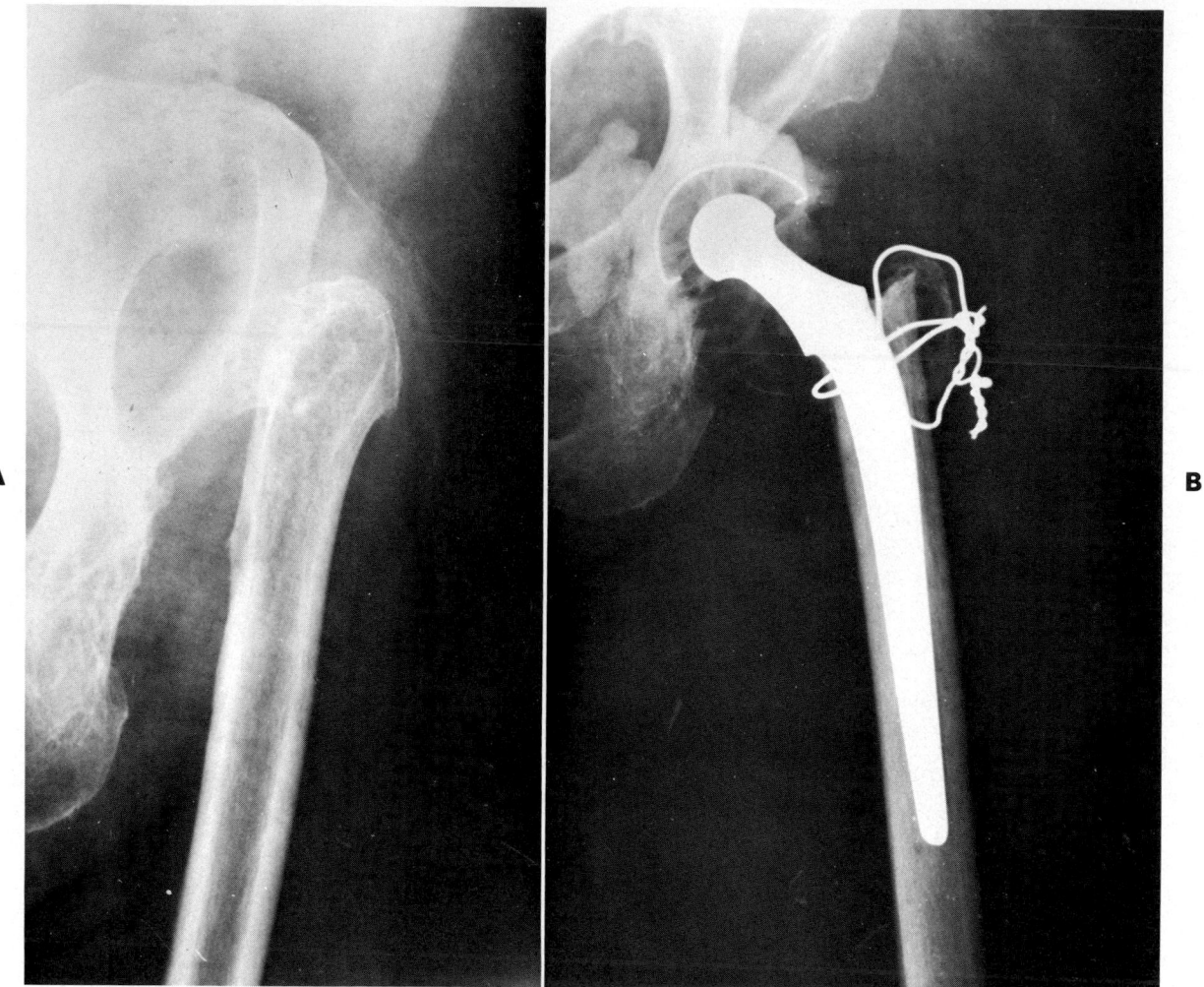

Fig. 10-11. Complete and unreduced congenital dislocation of hip without reconstructive procedures of acetabulum is relative contraindication for surgery. **A,** Unilateral dislocation in 69-year-old female with congenital dislocation of left hip. Hip graded 3,3,5 before surgery and patient had moderate low back pain. **B,** Immediate arthroplasty in which portion of acetabular component was not well seated and remained uncovered because of inadequate bony roof. (Bone graft would have been beneficial.) (Operation was performed by a colleague at our institution.) **C,** Spontaneous detachment of acetabular component 2 months after surgery. **D,** Hip was converted to Girdlestone pseudarthrosis after removal of artificial device.

with mental depression as well as borderline psychotic and neurotic patients; results with these patients are comparable to those with emotionally stable patients. In the past, hysterical or neurotic patients were not recommended for operations such as cup arthroplasty because the procedures often required extensive co-operation but never entirely relieved the pain. However, because it is so successful in eradicating pain, total hip arthroplasty alters the patient's attitude remarkably, and the result is similar to that seen in a nonhysterical patient. Similarly, in senile patients with borderline "senile psychosis" and a low threshold of pain, this operation improves attitudes remarkably and often prevents confinement.

TOTAL HIP ARTHROPLASTY IN VERY YOUNG PATIENTS

Patients under 30 years of age present the greatest difficulty in assessing the use of total hip arthroplasty because of their youth and the risk that they will use the artificial device with excess force. In the United States a healthy 30-year-old white female lives 81½ years and the life expectancy of her male counterpart is only 5 to 6 years less. Based on these figures, it is clear that many patients who undergo total hip arthroplasty at age 30 will need 50 years of service, some of them up to 70 years, from their artificial joint. This simple calculation helps the surgeon see the need to postpone the procedure as long as possible, in the hope that the

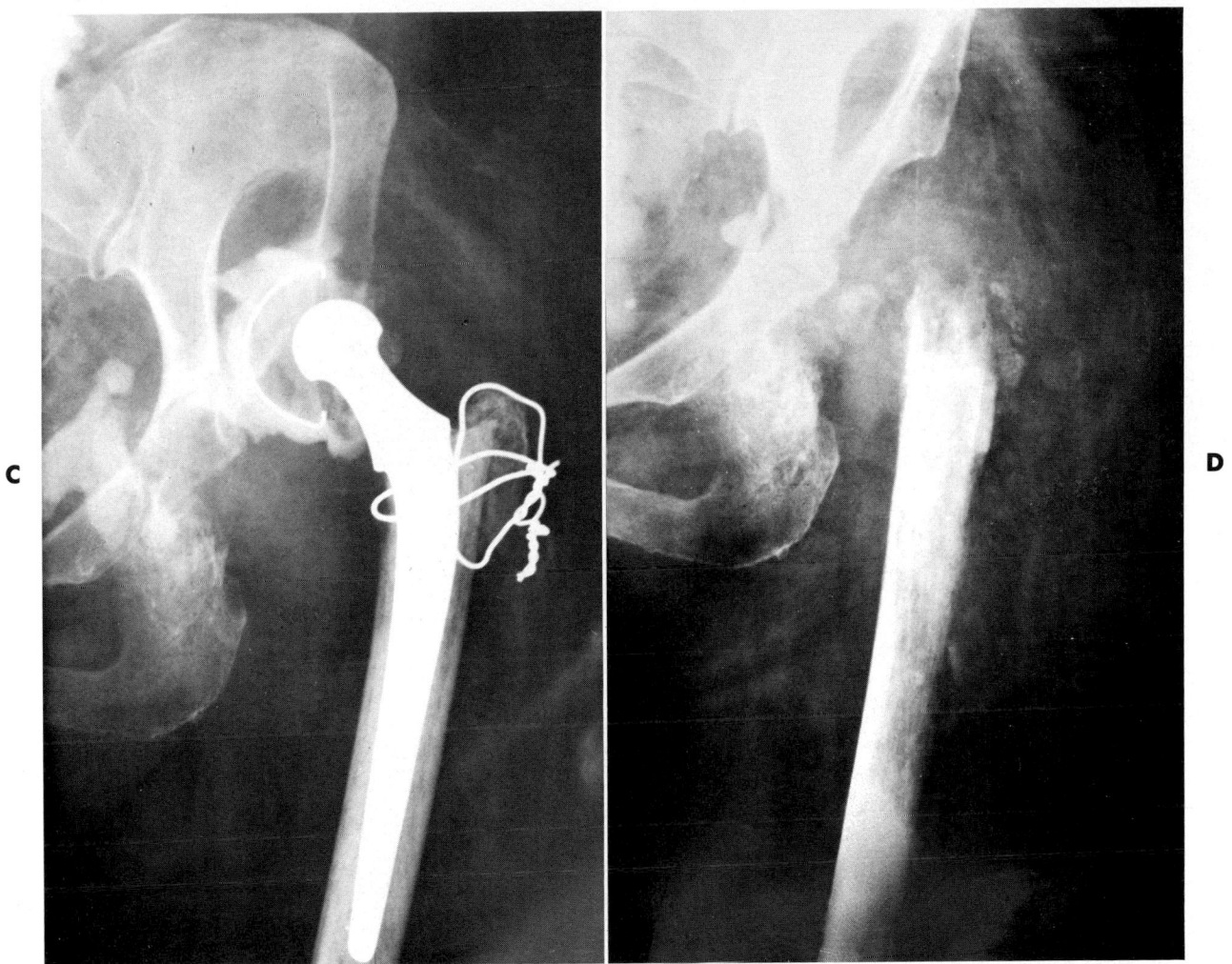

Fig. 10-11—cont'd. See legend on opposite page.

delay will reduce the need for revisionary operations and allow the surgeon to take advantage of improved technology developed in the interim.

This advice does not include patients suffering from juvenile or other diseases where a factor such as short life expectancy precludes excessive or prolonged use of the artificial device. In younger patients with traumatic unilateral disease or a unilateral slipped capital femoral epiphysis with degenerative osteoarthritis, arthrodesis is still an accepted procedure. In such an instance we must be certain that the ipsilateral knee, back, and opposite hip are unequivocally normal. In this author's view, mold arthroplasty or osteotomy has an extremely limited place in these cases because they require lengthy rehabilitation and the results are unpredictable; furthermore, because they involve severe anatomical changes, these operations are not applicable. In addition to a core decompression operation and bone grafting, there are a few rare cases with avascular necrosis (without any degree of collapse of the femoral

head) in which a bipolar prosthetic replacement may be appropriate. However, temporization by the use of cane and analgesics is quite possible for these younger patients who have a limp without sufficient pain to justify surgical intervention. Most patients under age 30 suffering from a unilateral hip disease may be able to get along well with analgesics and the use of a cane for long-distance walking, although the majority must eliminate sports activities. However, because of their critical age, these patients, especially young females, may apply considerable psychological pressure for surgical intervention. At times, pain or deformity will be a determining factor in the decision to proceed with early surgery, especially if the patient has had one or more previous unsuccessful hip operations. There are several conditions for which surgery is indicated: osteoarthritis secondary to slipped femoral epiphysis, traumatic arthritis, congenital subluxation, or dislocation. An aseptic necrosis of the femoral head resulting from previous treatment or such systemic disorders as

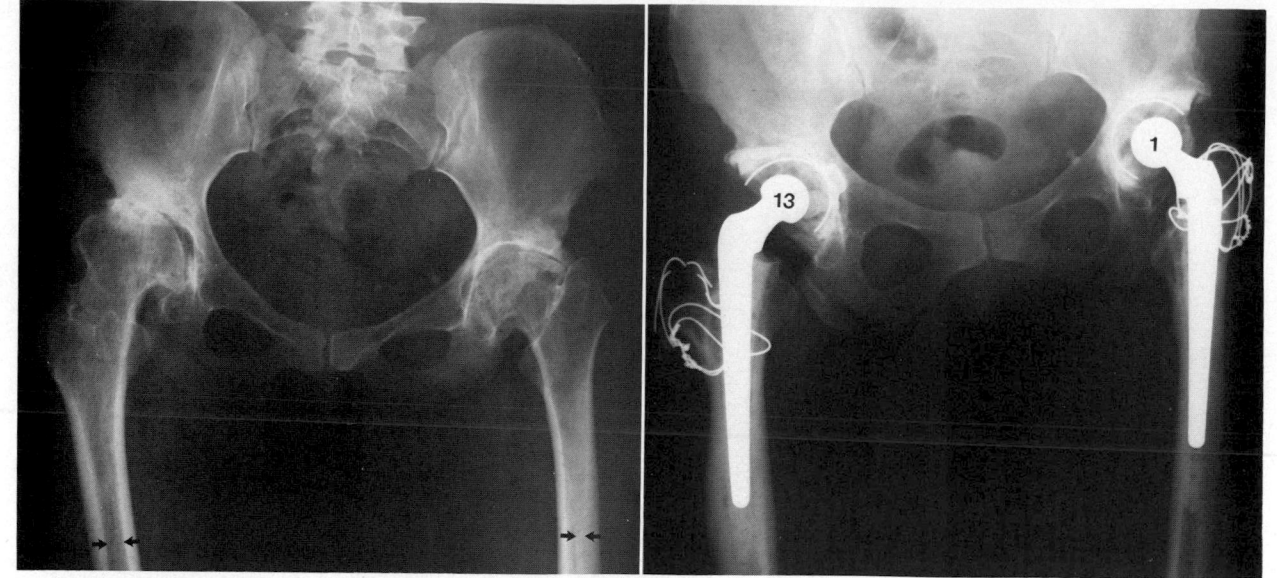

Fig. 10-12. Bilateral hip dislocation treated at early age by open and closed methods; grades B-right 3,2,3 and B-left 3,2,3. **A,** AP radiographs of patient (E.M.), whose age at index operation on the right side was 31 years. **B,** After one hip surgery, patient did well, thus avoiding further surgery for 12 years. Bilateral low-friction arthroplasty was performed using standard and small C.D.H. prostheses. Grade: B-right 5,5,5 and B-left 5,5,5.

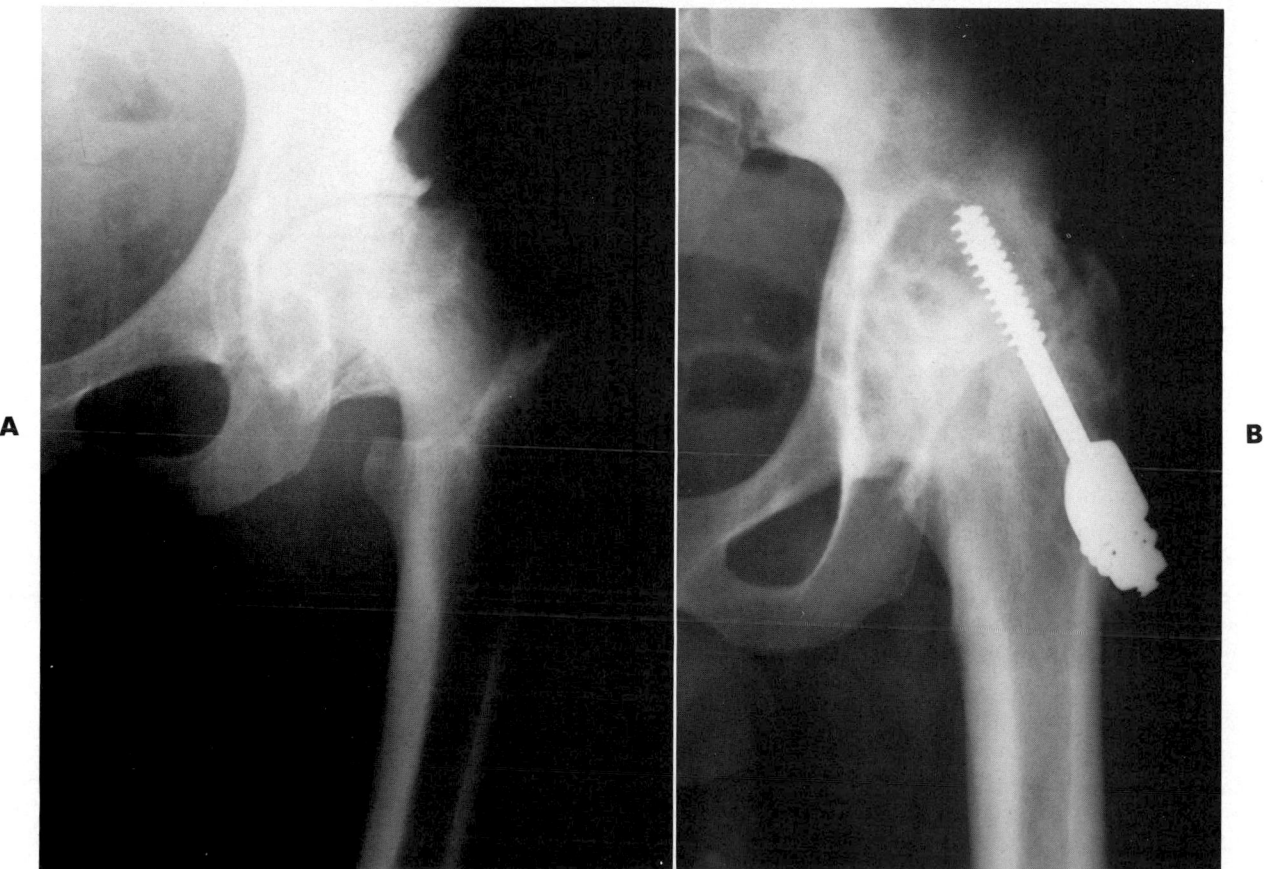

Fig. 10-13. A, Radiograph of unilateral hip degenerative osteoarthritis in a 5'9" college student (M.T.) whose age at the index operation was 19 years. **B,** 10 years after primary hip fusion using Charnley compression arthrodesis, patient works as a banker. Grade: A-6,5,1.

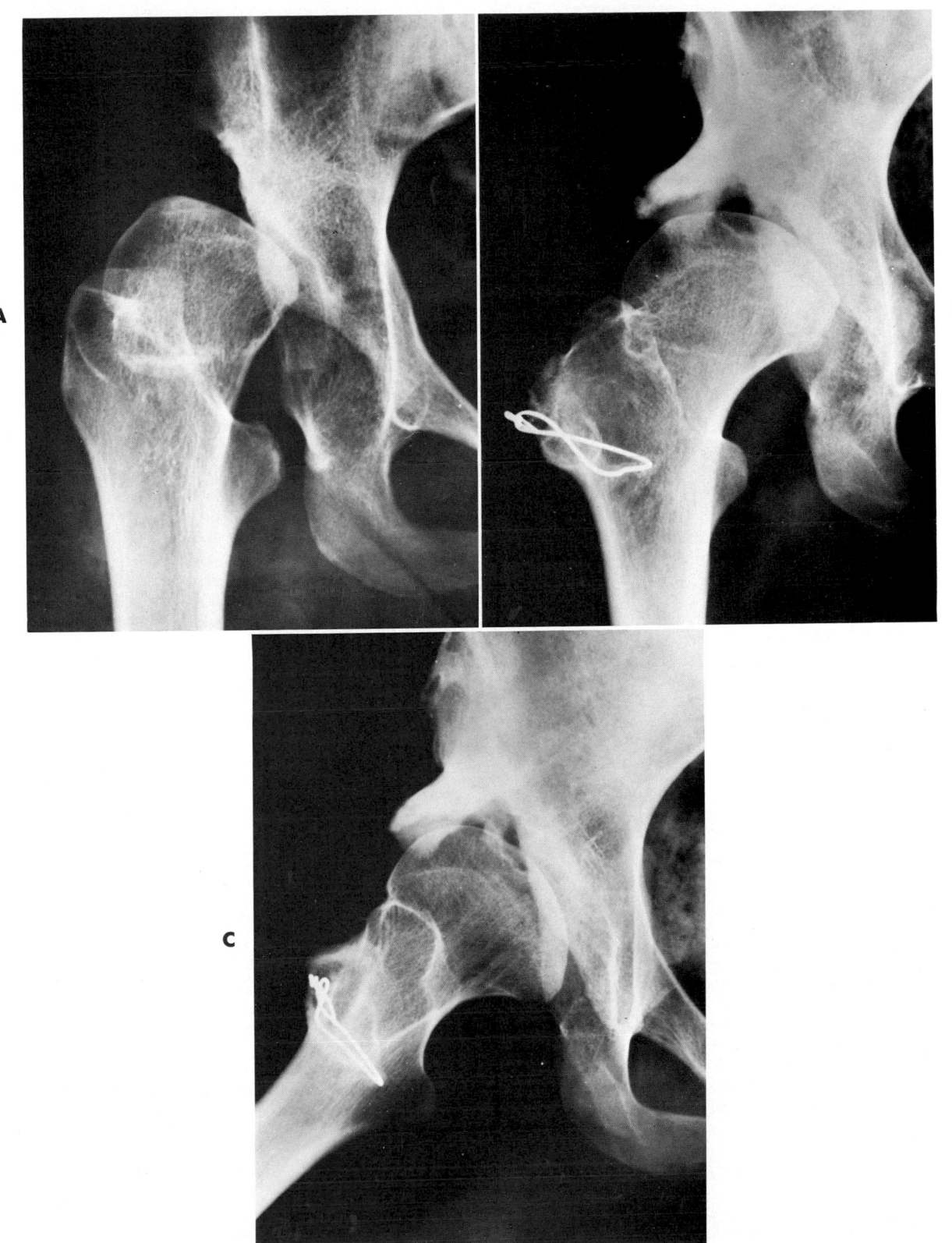

Fig. 10-14. A, Intermediate congenital dislocation in 18-year-old female with marked dysplasia in addition to low back pain, fatigue, and hip pain. Because of back pain and ipsilateral valgus knee, fusion of hip joint is not indicated. **B,** 4 years after shelf procedure. **C,** Lateral view of same hip showing amount of coverage of femoral head after shelf procedure in addition to transfer of abductor muscles. Six months after surgery patient's pain had completely resolved, limp had diminished, and patient at present is very pleased with result. Hip joint has become stable and functional.

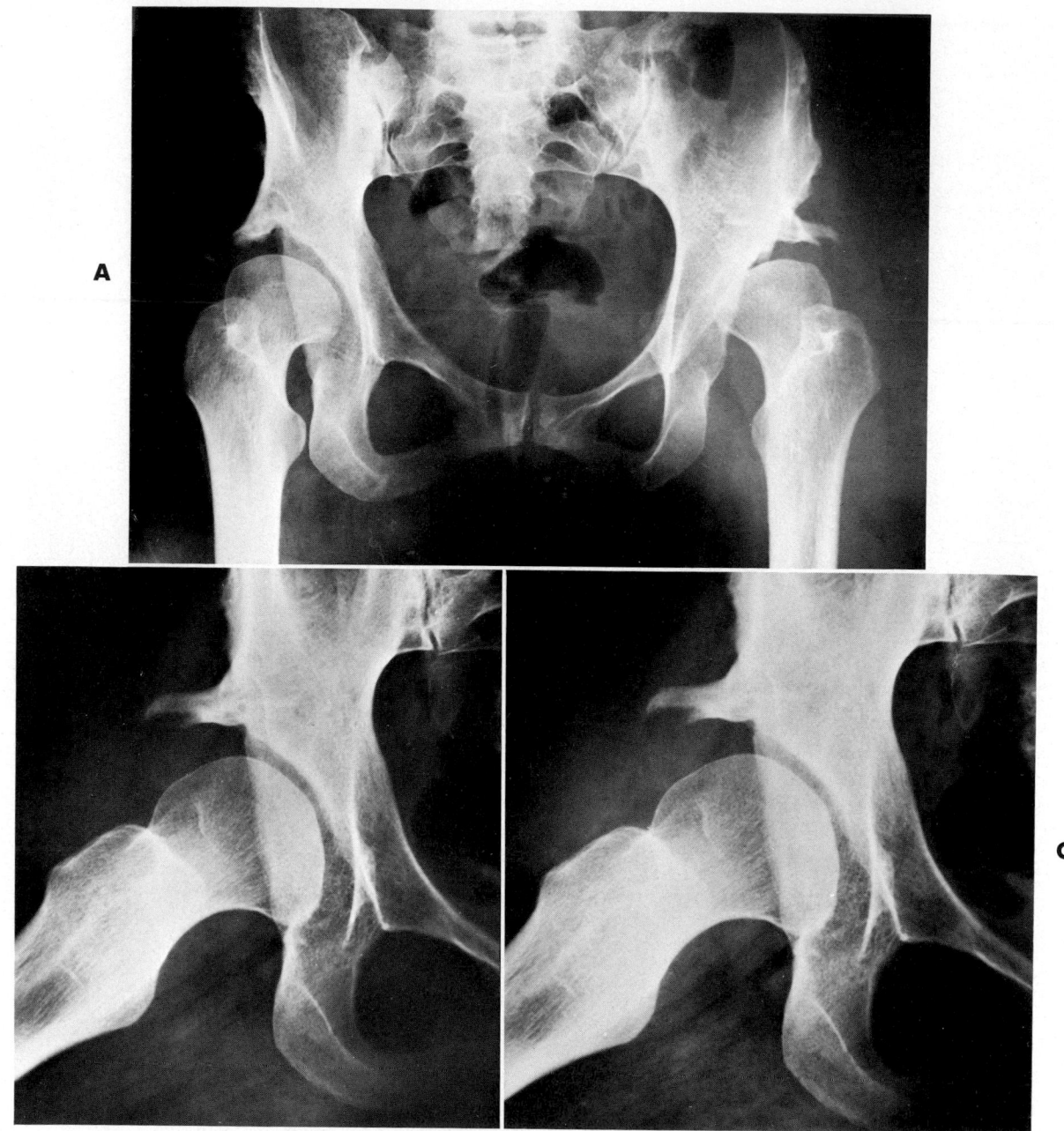

Fig. 10-15. A, Postoperative shelf procedure in 38-year-old school teacher who had her operation at age 28. Now 10 years after bilateral shelf operation, she has only minimal discomfort in hips. She has full range of motion and walks without assistance but with minor bilateral gluteus medius gait. Operation definitely reduced her symptoms and discomfort, especially in reference to fatigue and, obviously, development of degenerative joint disease. **B,** Lateral view of right hip. **C,** Lateral view of left hip.

Gaucher's disease, childhood sepsis in the hip, and failure of previous operations accounts for a large portion of this group.

When surgery is considered in patients less than 30 years of age, Charnley's advocacy of the "pseudarthrosis test" should be applied; that is, if the patient is so disabled that a Girdlestone procedure might help, we may consider total hip arthroplasty. The patient and the surgeon must be reminded that a Girdlestone pseudarthrosis is a salvage procedure that only relieves the pain. After the Girdlestone procedure, the hip remains unstable. The procedure causes a moderate-to-severe shortening of the limb, resulting in an unsightly gait that many patients find unacceptable, and permanent use of a walking aid is required (see Chapter 27).

It is extremely important that the physician discuss all potential risks and complications with the patient and his or her family and that all agree upon the decision. If a patient in this age group has bilateral hip disease, it is advisable to operate on one hip and postpone surgery on the opposite hip as long as possible (Fig. 10-12). The surgeon should not recommend a combination of arthrodesis for one side and total hip arthroplasty for the other. Patients are never satisfied with the functional outcome of the arthrodesis once they have had the arthroplasty.

In patients between 20 and 30 years of age whose arthrosis is caused by conditions such as congenital dysplasia, slipped capital femoral epiphysis, trauma, and so on, a decision regarding advisability of total hip arthroplasty is extremely difficult, because the patient is not necessarily required to restrict his or her activities. With this group of patients, the surgeon should consider the alternatives, advising them to undergo an osteotomy or a hip arthrodesis as an alternative to total hip arthroplasty (Fig. 10-13). On the other hand, in patients with a short life expectancy or polyarthritic rheumatoid or ankylosing spondylitis a total hip arthroplasty may be recommended regardless of the patient's age, because such cases are commonly accompanied by associated joint disability that limits the patient's activities. Here again, in these cases it is essential to consider a pseudarthrosis test when contemplating a total hip arthroplasty.

We hope someday to be able to replace hip joints in young people whose main concern is appearance rather than pain. There are three effective temporizing measures that offer considerable help for patients in their teens and twenties with severe dysplasia: a femoral osteotomy, a pelvic osteotomy, or a shelf procedure (Figs. 10-14 and 10-15). The operations generally reduce the symptoms of fatigue and pain, increase stability, and leave a better bone stock for subsequent arthroplasty.

SPECIFIC CONSIDERATIONS IN TOTAL HIP ARTHROPLASTY
Bilateral Hip Arthroplasty

Bilateral disability usually more than doubles the problems associated with disability in one hip; conversely, after successful unilateral surgery, many patients improve by more than 50%. A patient with one arthritic hip can frequently cope with the stiffness and pain through such conservative means as a cane and analgesics. Similarly a single compromised hip can improve significantly with osteotomy or arthrodesis, but when both hips are involved the compromise resulting from these operations is intolerable. All activities that were possible with one normal hip are now curtailed, and the patient is unable to get about without walking aids. This limitation usually interferes with the patient's ability to travel to work, and he or she becomes housebound. Because motion in one extremity affects the other, resting and sitting (and occasionally even sleeping) become difficult. It is widely known that the results of any surgical reconstructive method other than total hip arthroplasty are poor when both hips are diseased.[89,90,93] Therefore treatment of bilateral hip disability is exigent. Alleviating the affliction and confinement from two arthritic hips is one of the most challenging experiences for the hip surgeon; the decision to operate must always be deliberated—not against the successful outcome, but against the patient's plight if failure occurs. Since loss of motion or fixed deformity may be of more concern than pain, the possibility of total disability must be considered in advising surgery, even in patients in their forties and fifties. Patients with some deformity of one or both hips have complaints of low back pain (Fig. 10-16) and frequently knee pain as well. Although established deformity or pain in the spine and knee often precede the hip involvement, hip surgery should be considered first, because it often reduces disability in the spine or knee.

A combination of bilateral hip disease and back pain caused by spinal stenosis can be extremely disabling. Because of lost mobility in the hips and spine, performing such daily functional activities as dressing and perineal care may become impossible. Frequent falls are common in these patients, because they cannot balance themselves while walking. In cases where spinal surgery is also being contemplated, it is advisable to perform hip arthroplasty first. Bilateral surgery is performed most frequently in the following conditions:

1. Bilateral primary monarticular osteoarthritis.
2. Late involvement of the second hip after total hip arthroplasty.
3. Primary general osteoarthritis.
4. Late results of ischemic necrosis of the femoral

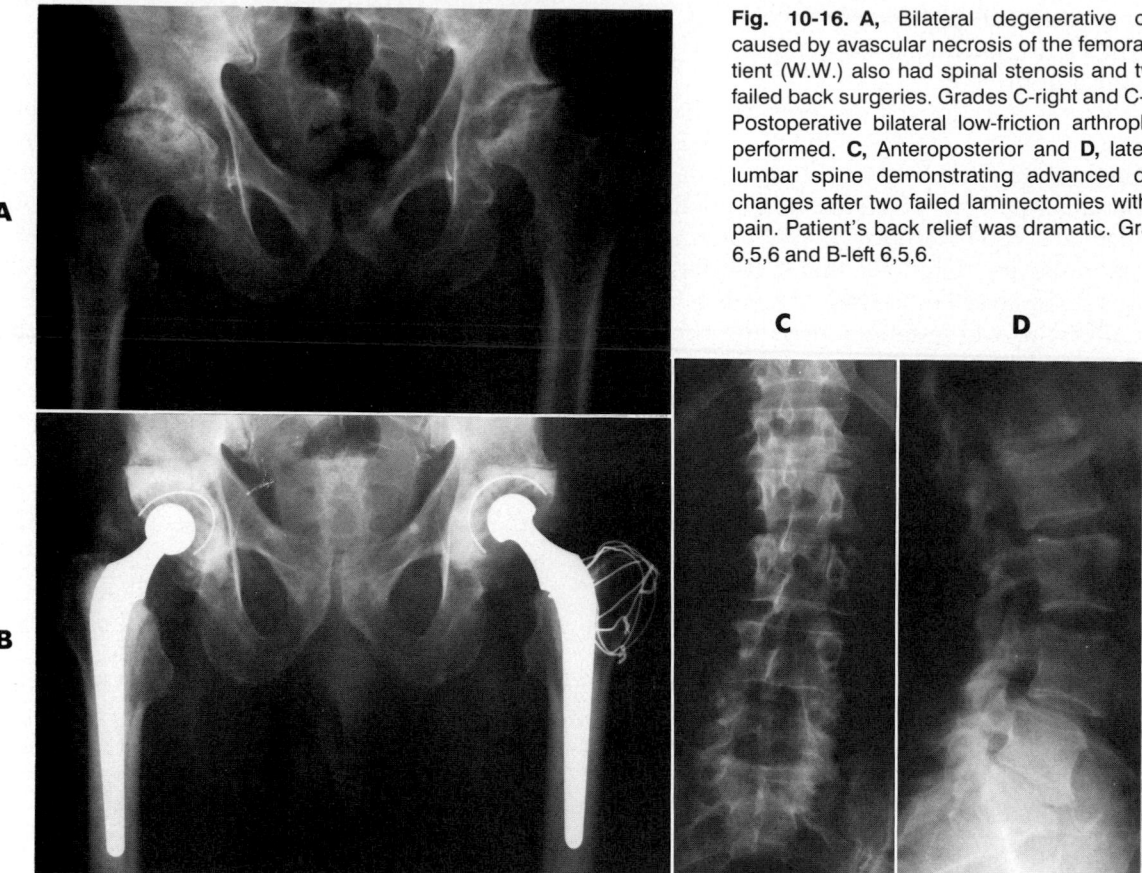

Fig. 10-16. A, Bilateral degenerative osteoarthritis caused by avascular necrosis of the femoral heads. Patient (W.W.) also had spinal stenosis and two previous failed back surgeries. Grades C-right and C-left 2,1,1. **B,** Postoperative bilateral low-friction arthroplasties were performed. **C,** Anteroposterior and **D,** lateral views of lumbar spine demonstrating advanced degenerative changes after two failed laminectomies without relief of pain. Patient's back relief was dramatic. Grades B-right 6,5,6 and B-left 6,5,6.

head with secondary acetabular changes.

5. Bilateral degenerative osteoarthritis of the hip secondary to congenital dysplasia, slipped capital femoral epiphysis, etc.
6. Systemic disease such as rheumatoid arthritis, Paget's disease, and so on.

The plan for bilateral total arthroplasty is a clinical decision, not a radiological one. When the patient has symmetrically advanced degenerative changes with bilateral hip disease, it is only natural to assume that both hips may require surgery. However, statistics show that only about 25% of the patients who have this condition need bilateral hip surgery within the first 5 years (Figs. 10-17 to 10-19). It is advisable to recommend bilateral hip surgery only if these conditions coexist:

1. Hip flexion deformity more than 30 degrees.
2. One hip in fixed adduction, the other in fixed abduction.
3. Marked shortening of one leg or severe lumbar spine deformity with degenerative changes.
4. Bilateral hip disease in older patients (usually over the age of 70).
5. Progressive acetabular protrusion—especially in rheumatoid arthritis (Fig. 10-20).
6. Severe loss of motion as a result of ectopic bone formation after total hip arthroplasty of one hip.
7. Correction of fixed deformity, even if the hip has been surgically arthrodesed and is relatively pain-free but malpositioned.
8. Contemplated bilateral knee surgery.
9. Progressive systemic arthritis, such as rheumatoid or ankylosing spondylitis with flexion deformity of the hips.
10. Low back pain and advanced degenerative osteoarthritis of the lumbar spine.
11. Bilateral hip disease associated with infection in one hip.

If both hips have been immobile for a long time, a good range of motion may not be achieved by only one operation; the unoperated hip may act as a splint, hampering postoperative rehabilitation and interfering with the operated hip's potential to regain motion. It is our policy therefore to do the two hip operations as a single stage (under the same anesthesia) or to schedule the second soon after the first. The same policy applies to revision of only one of the bilateral failed total hip arthroplasties with severe ectopic bone formation.

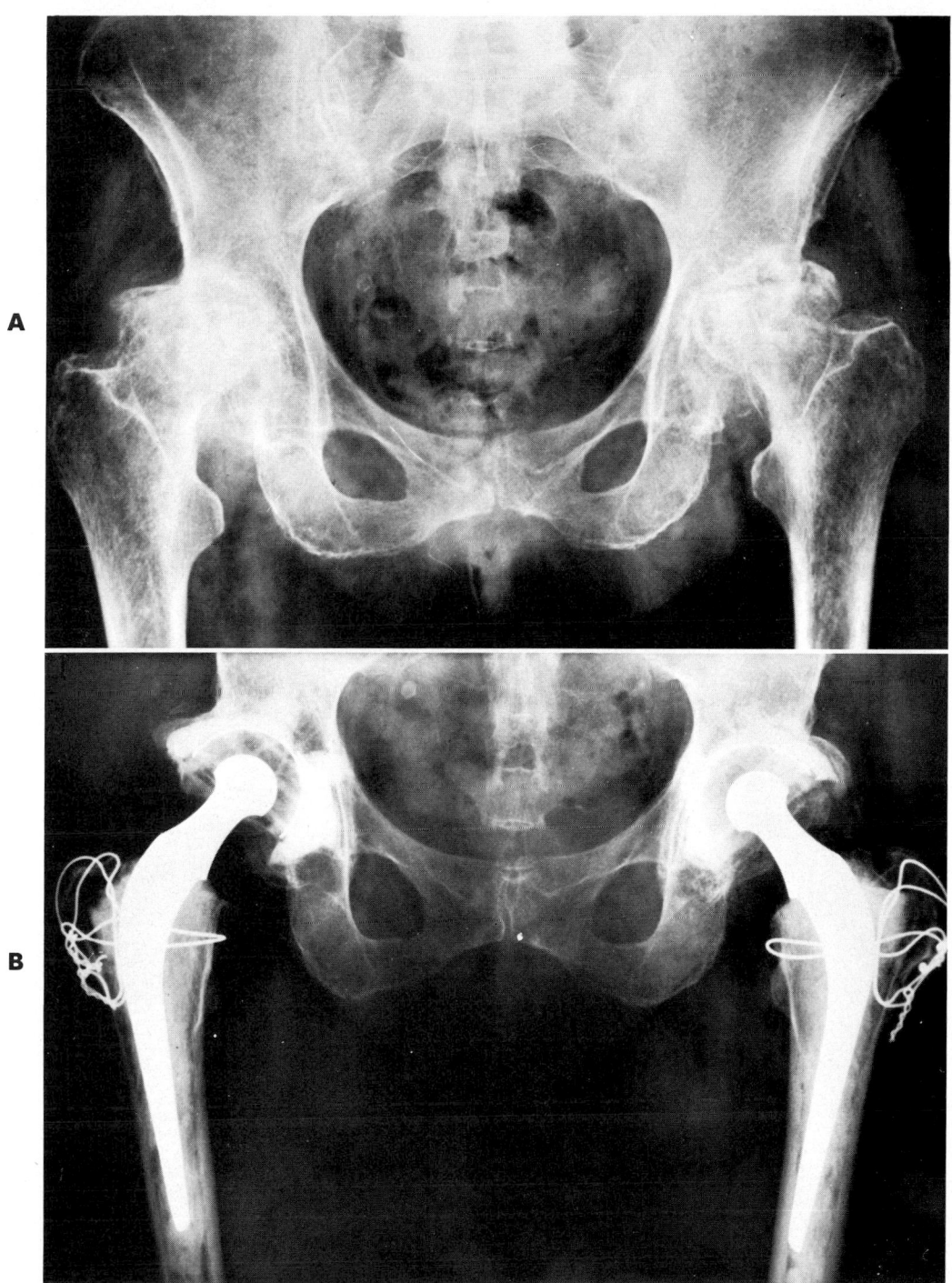

Fig. 10-17. A, This 68-year-old female retired pharmacist coped with her bilateral hip osteoarthritis by continuous intake of steroids to alleviate pain. Preoperative grades of hip were B-right 2,3,4 and B-left 3,3,4. **B,** After accepting surgery, two hip operations were performed within 2 weeks. Right hip (more symptomatic hip) was done first. Postoperative grading at 1 year after surgery was 6,6,6 on right and 6,6,6 on left.

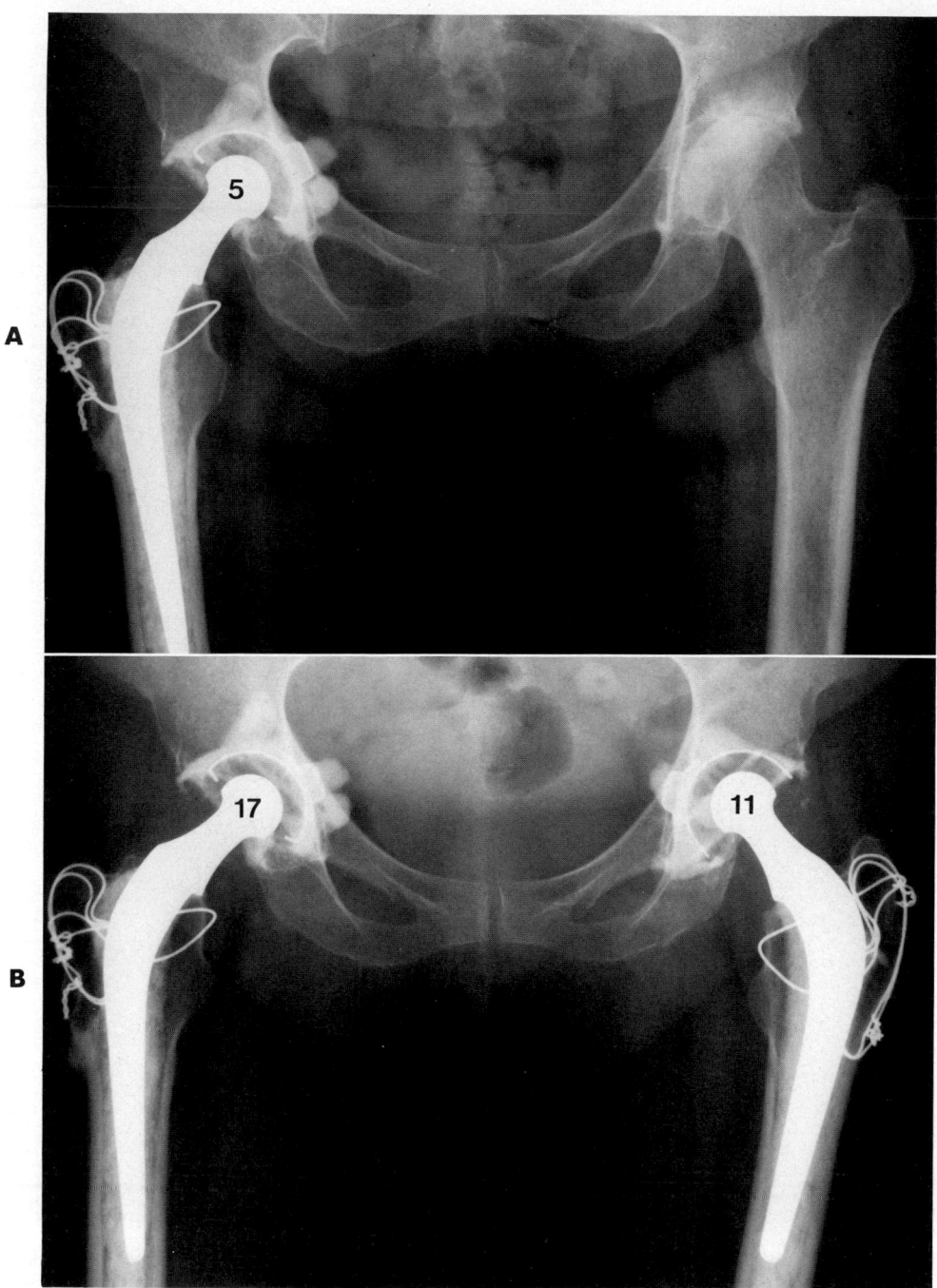

Fig. 10-18. A, Radiograph of a 53-year-old woman (M.L.) with a diagnosis of classic rheumatoid arthritis. She had equal pain in both hips. Grades C-right 3,2,3 and C-left 3,2,3. **B,** After low-friction arthroplasty on the right hip patient became nearly asymptomatic on the opposite hip. The surgery on the opposite hip was performed 6 years later. Grade C-right 6,5,6 and C-left 6,5,6. Radiograph indicates a good bonding between cement and bone.

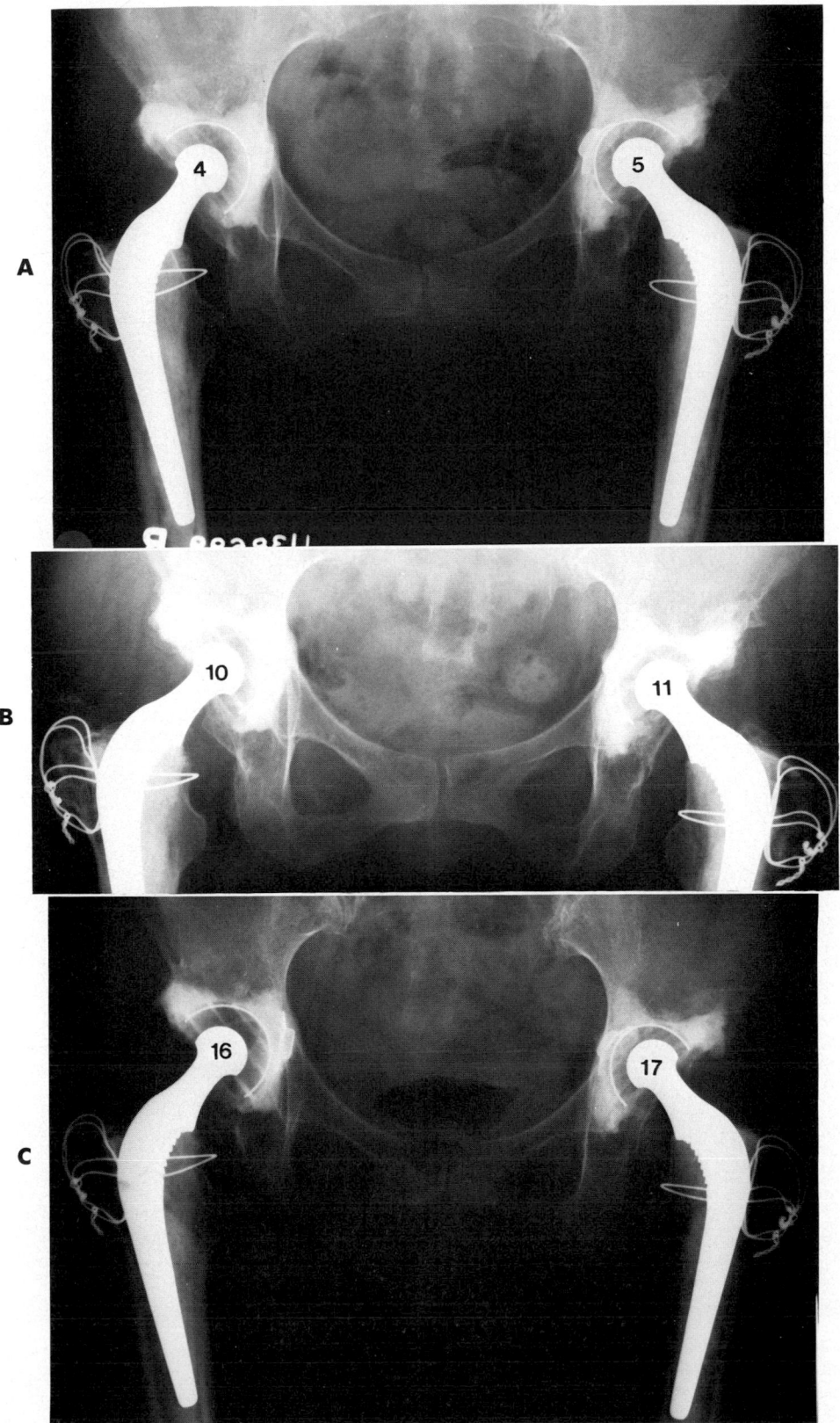

Fig. 10-19. Postoperative radiographs of a 49-year-old (M.S.) with bilateral degenerative osteoarthritis secondary to a mild-to-moderate hip dysplasia. **A,** Radiographs taken at 4 and 5 years after surgery of the right and left hip respectively. **B,** Follow-up radiographs at 10 and 11 years. **C,** Follow-up radiographs at 16 and 17 years. This patient has been very active since surgery. Preoperative grades B-bilateral 3,3,3.

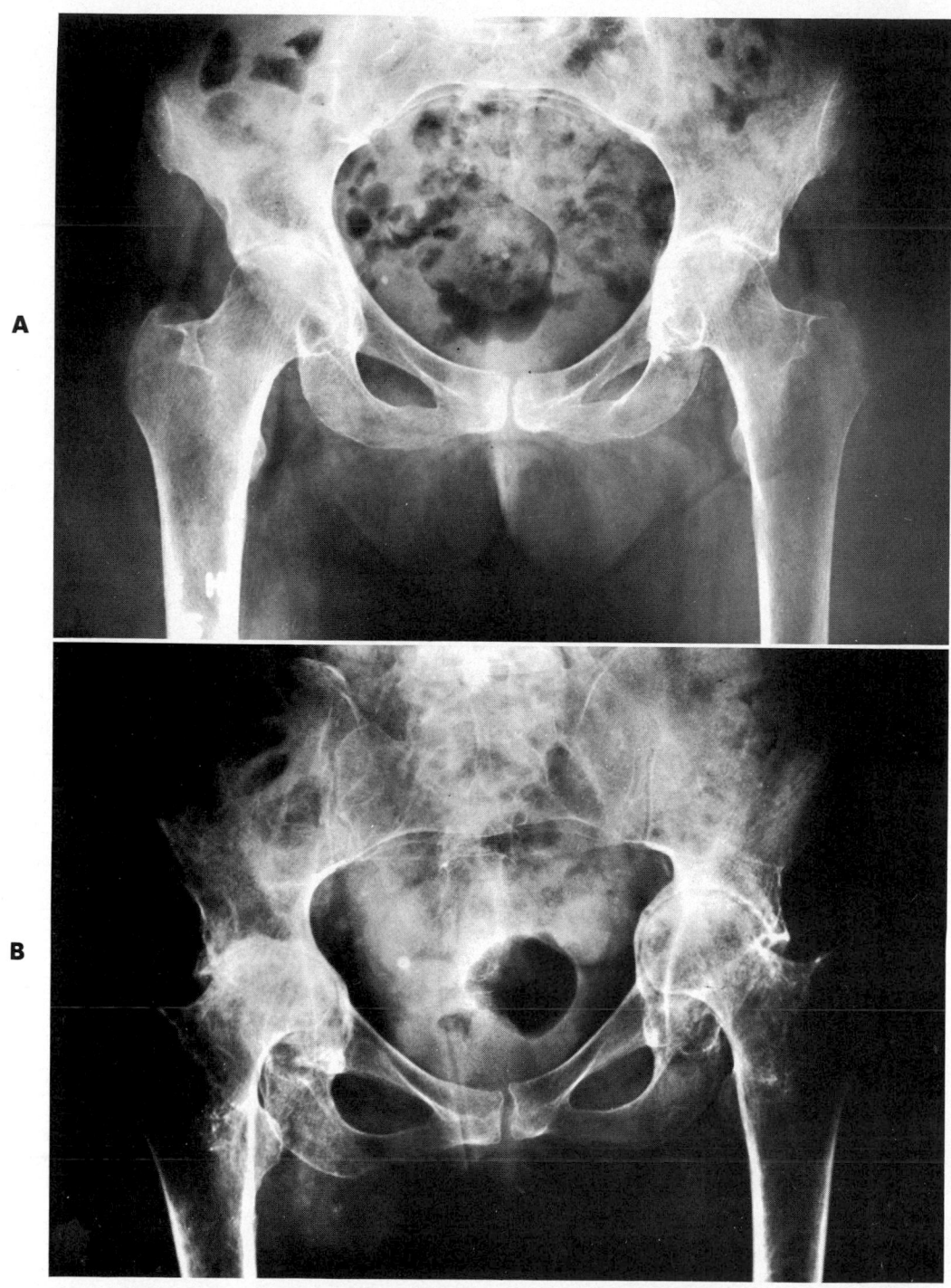

Fig. 10-20. A, Patient with rheumatoid arthritis and bilateral hip involvement. Left hip is already showing evidence of protrusio. **B,** Rapid progression of protrusio acetabuli during period between 1974 and 1975, just before surgery. Hip surgery was procrastinated until 1975. **C,** Preoperative evaluation indicated hip grading C-right 3,2,2 and C-left 3,2,2. Postoperative evaluation 1 year after surgery grading is C-right 6,4,6 and C-left 6,4,6.

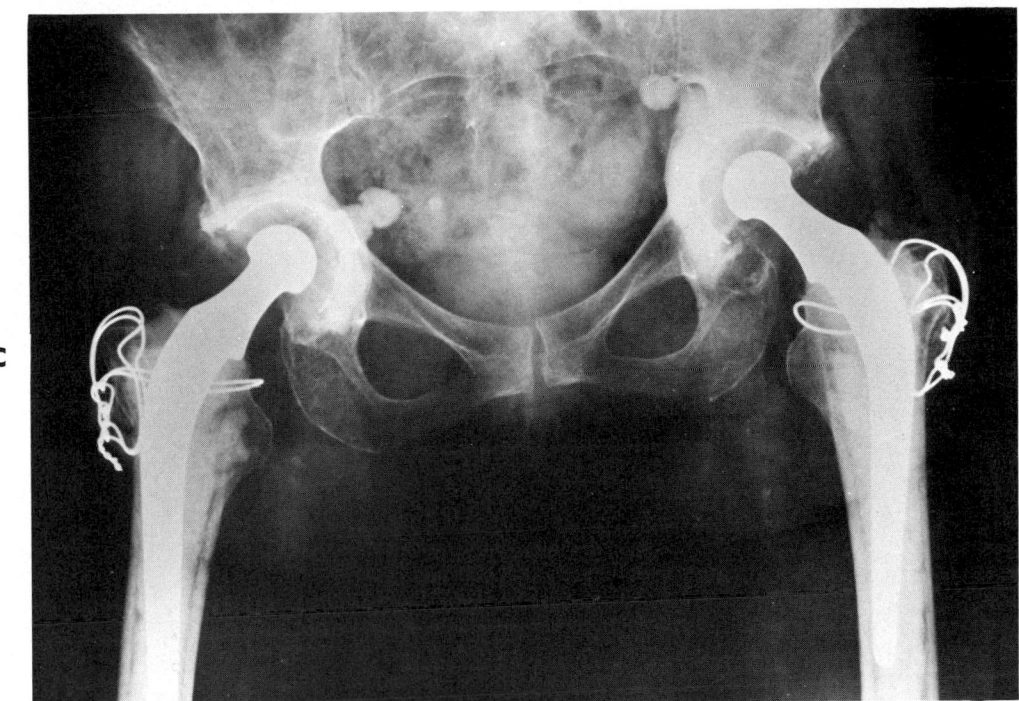

C

Fig. 10-20—cont'd. See legend on opposite page.

Infected Opposite Hip

For a discussion of infected previous surgery and total hip arthroplasty, see Chapter 26.

Total hip arthroplasty may be performed and indeed is advisable in a patient with known infection of the opposite hip.[35] This procedure gives the patient a functional joint, facilitating plans for removal or revision of the infected side. Patients with a documented infection of one joint must not be denied another joint replacement for fear of a blood-borne infection in the new joint. A decision to proceed with the replacement of the hip is not merely of academic interest; it is a practical solution when treating a patient with an infected hip who is also suffering from a painful opposite hip. Clearly, the patient, who fears infection, must be psychologically supported and protected with appropriate antibiotics during and after surgery. As indicated, the infected side should be converted to a pseudarthrosis after complete recovery of the newly replaced hip. This author has performed hip arthroplasty in eight patients whose first hip was infected at the time of the second operation. None of the patients who underwent primary hip operations developed hip infections. The planned resection pseudarthrosis on the infected side was carried out in all patients within 6 weeks to 2 years of the total hip arthroplasty (Fig. 10-21).

The Sequence of Bilateral Hip Operations

As a rule, the most symptomatic hip must always be replaced first. Frequently one hip is less painful than the other, despite equal or near-equal involvement as shown on radiographs. On the other hand, if both hips are equally involved and painful, the surgeon can plan for bilateral operation under the same anesthesia or schedule the second operation later in the same hospitalization. Barring complications after the first operation, the second procedure may be scheduled 7 to 14 days later. Although some patients are eager to schedule the second operation in this way, for others there is less psychological and physical stress if they return 3 to 6 months later for the second operation (Fig. 10-22).

Bilateral Total Hip Arthroplasty as a Single Procedure

Although bilateral operation during the same anesthesia is a practical possibility, it is recommended only in well-organized centers where surgical and anesthesia teams are expert in dealing with the magnitude of operations of this type. One excellent example is the Centre for Hip Surgery at Wrightington Hospital, where bilateral operations are routinely performed during the same anesthesia. Although this method has definite advantages, it should be considered only with

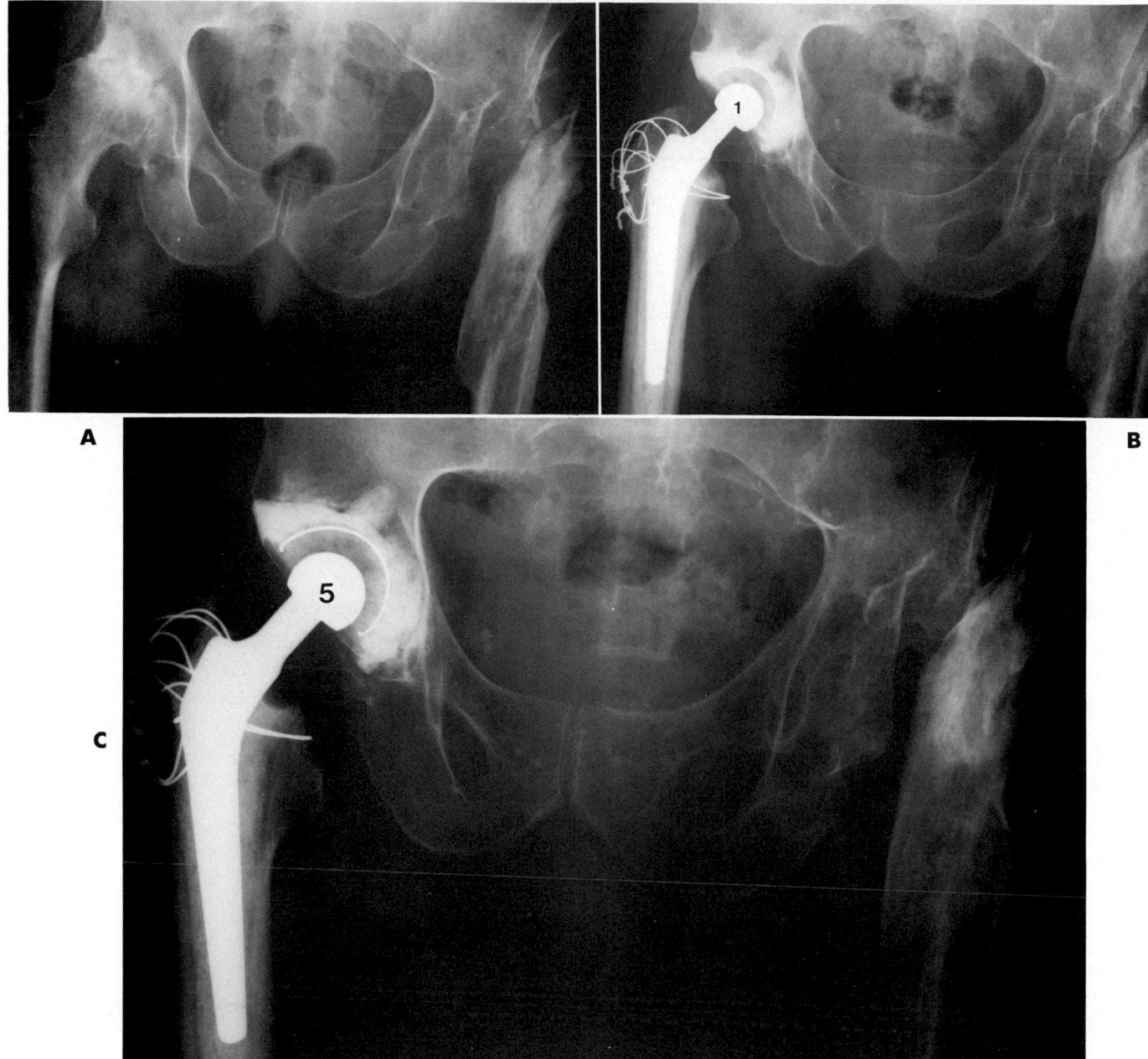

Fig. 10-21. Presence of infection in one hip is not an absolute contraindication for replacing the opposite hip. **A,** Degenerative osteoarthritis of the right hip in this 68-year-old man (W.S.) is associated with proximal femoral osteomyelitis of the left hip. Patient, who had multiple surgical procedures to eradicate left hip infection, was chair-bed-bound. Grades right—3,1,3; left—2,1,4. Note pseudarthrosis and femoral fracture caused 11 cm shortening of the left leg. **B** and **C,** 1 and 5 years after right hip replacement, patient has no pain and walks with one cane. Grades right—6,4,5; left—4,4,4.

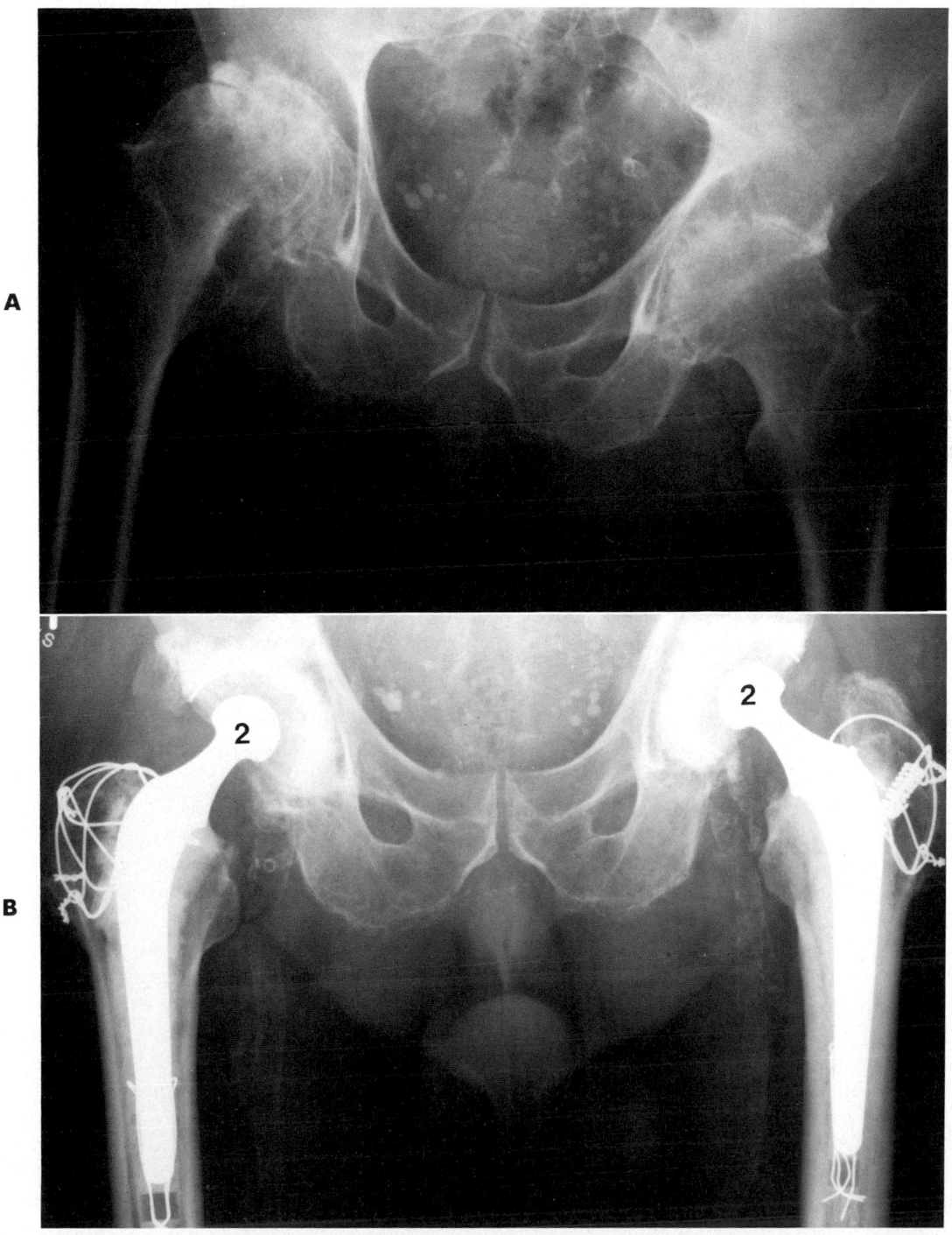

Fig. 10-22. Bilateral total hip arthroplasty in patients over age 80 is relatively contraindicated under the same anesthesia or same hospitalization. The procedures are best staged 3 months apart. **A,** Preoperative bilateral degenerative osteoarthritis in 83-year-old man (B.B.). Grades B-right 3,2,2 and B-left 3,2,2. **B,** Bilateral total hip arthroplasty was performed in preplanned stages 3 months apart. There were no postoperative complications. Grade B-right 6,6,6 and B-left 6,6,6 2 years postoperatively.

great caution in teaching hospitals and community practice; it is better reserved for centers that specialize in total joint arthroplasty.

A study of bilateral low-friction arthroplasty performed at Wrightington Hospital as a single operation found that patients' average length of stay was 30.3 days, only a few days longer than the average stay for patients undergoing unilateral low-friction arthroplasty. The 30.3 day average was also considerably shorter than the average stay for patients undergoing bilateral hip surgery in most other institutions (including our own), where the operations are performed as separate unilateral surgeries. Patients at our hospital undergoing sequential bilateral arthroplasty stay an average of 5 weeks; the second operation is routinely performed 7 to 14 days after the first. In their series, Jaffe and Charnley[83] found that this practice provided minimal risk to the patient and produced very good results. Nevertheless, it must be emphasized that the low risk is largely because of the efficient surgical team developed at a center that specializes in this particular type of hip arthroplasty. At the Centre for Hip Surgery, more than 1000 low-friction arthroplasties were done annually; 10% were bilateral, performed in a single operative session, often with two surgical teams operating successively on the same patient. Speed of surgery, conservation of time, and minimization of blood loss cannot realistically be duplicated in a general teaching hospital setting. In a study of 400 patients having bilateral low-friction arthroplasty with a single anesthesia, 75% had primary osteoarthritis; 8% rheumatoid arthritis; 5% congenital dislocation of the hip; the remainder suffered from miscellaneous conditions.[25] The patients chosen for this procedure were generally younger, free of concurrent medical conditions, and better motivated than the average patient. Because no untreated opposite hip was slowing them down, the patients responded well to early ambulation. An added benefit of the single anesthesia operation is that theoretically the patient is exposed to less risk than he or she would be with repeated anesthetization. However, neither the incidence of infection nor that of thromboembolic disease is lessened by performing both operations under the same anesthesia (see Chapter 9). Patients with severe deformity and distorted anatomy (such as severe protrusio acetabuli) requiring bone graft and revision surgery are not very good candidates for bilateral hip arthroplasty under a single anesthesia.

Although there seem to be definite advantages in bilateral total hip arthroplasty under the same anesthesia (Fig. 10-23), the accurate mortality rate in double operations under single anesthesia remains unknown because of a lack of consistency in reported series, as well as a low incidence of perioperative death in total hip arthroplasty, making it difficult to interpret the results.[83,114,115,197] In Salvati's and Ritter's series the death rates in bilateral operations under single anesthesia were similar to the rates for single operations. Bracy reported 6 deaths in 400 bilateral operations, somewhat higher than the rate for single operations in the same period (although the difference was not statistically significant).

As a principle, the more symptomatic hip should always be done first, in both bilateral operations performed under one anesthesia and those scheduled for two separate dates during the same hospitalization. In bilateral fixed deformity, one in adduction and one in abduction, the abducted hip must be done first. If postoperative complications arise and the second operation cannot be performed, recurrence of fixed adduction deformity of the operated hip will have been avoided. Progressive destructive hip changes in rheumatoid conditions such as protrusio acetabuli must be treated early and without undue conservatism in hopes of stopping these changes. It is important that both hips be considered for early treatment to allow preservation of muscle strength while sparing other joints. This approach also permits a lower maintenance dose of cortisone in patients undergoing steroid therapy because two major sources of inflammation (the hips) have been eliminated.

Combination of Hip Fusion and Knee Disease

In general, when a hip is arthrodesed and in a good position, it must be left alone unless disability of the low back or the ipsilateral knee warrants converting it to a total hip arthroplasty (see Chapter 21).

Conversion of failed hip fusion to total hip arthroplasty is possible with a modest but significant gain in mobility. Naturally, when the opposite side of the fused hip requires total hip arthroplasty, the surgeon is well advised to proceed with arthroplasty of the opposite side, despite a theoretical objection to placing arthroplasty under the risk of loosening. A higher mechanical failure of the hip or knee with ipsilateral total knee or contralateral total hip arthroplasty in a patient with hip fusion has been recorded.[74] The ipsilateral or contralateral knee arthroplasty can also be performed as indicated. Nevertheless, when the hip has been fused in a nonanatomical position, that is, severe adduction or abduction, it is best first to convert the fused hip to a total hip arthroplasty and then to perform an arthroplasty of either the opposite hip or total knee, as indicated.

Congenital Dysplasia and Dislocation

Because of its largely predictable success, total hip arthroplasty has been extended to treating secondary

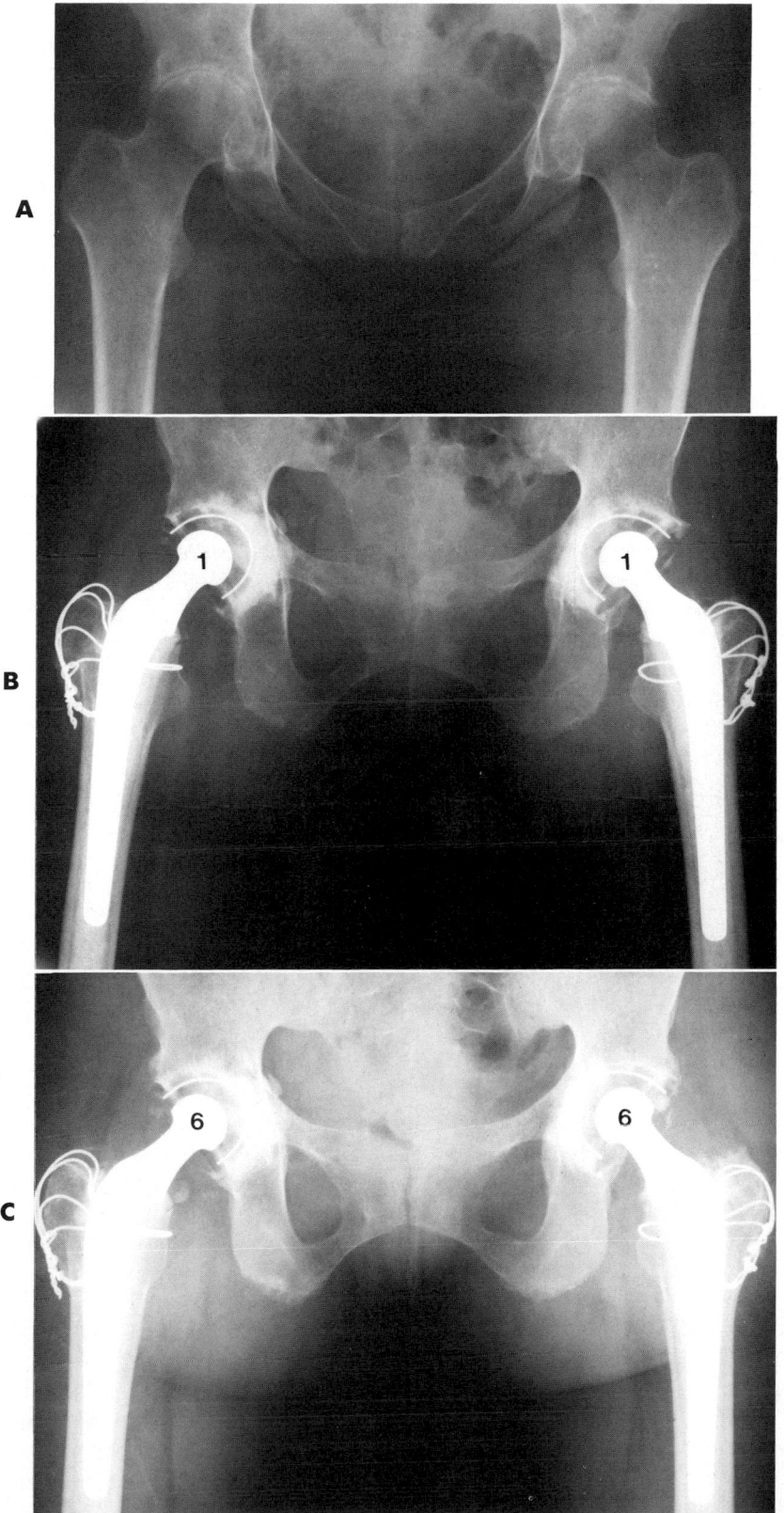

Fig. 10-23. A, Preoperative radiograph of a 23-year-old female medical student (A.G.) with ankylosing spondylitis. **B**, 1 year after bilateral low-friction arthroplasty performed under a single anesthesia. Grades-6,6,6 bilaterally. **C**, Radiograph taken at 6-year follow-up visit, shows excellent bone response. Hip grades C: right–6,6,6; left–6,6,6.

osteoarthritis resulting from congenital dysplasia and dislocation of the hip. Early recognition of congenital dysplasia or dislocation is of paramount importance. Efforts toward treatment and restoration during childhood present distinct advantages. Unrecognized early childhood dysplasia will continue to be a common cause of degenerative osteoarthritis of the hip.[77,78,133,142] A large percentage of idiopathic degenerative osteoarthritis may be caused by insidious dysplasia hidden until much later in life. Therefore only thorough treatment of congenital dislocation of the hip in the newborn is likely to render the hip functional and prevent degenerative osteoarthritis. Even if treatment in childhood fails to achieve perfect results, surgeons must attempt to reduce a completely dislocated hip when bilateral hip disease is present, even in older children. Even a compromised result, marked by a stiff hip (or hips) resulting from late treatment (6 to 8 years), is far better than leaving the hips completely dislocated. A completely dislocated hip remains severely underdeveloped, posing a significant technical problem for reconstruction later in life.

Although the number of completely dislocated hips is diminishing in the Western world, many young patients in their teens and twenties suffer from a limp and fatigue caused by dysplasia and subluxation. They usually do not have a truly painful limp, but rather a weak abductor lurch. On radiographs they may show nothing more than moderate-to-varying degrees of dysplasia of the acetabulum, femur, or both. These young patients should be evaluated for corrective surgery, such as pelvic osteotomy, appropriate upper femoral osteotomies, or both. A number of reports in the literature suggest that these procedures are valuable in reducing the symptoms and providing patients several years of comfort, but there is no guarantee of permanent effects. Another operation this author favors and has performed numerous times is a shelf procedure, which is less radical than the other types of pelvic osteotomy in adults. We have found it very effective in reducing the symptoms of discomfort and fatigue in these young patients (see Figs. 10-13 and 10-14). Rehabilitation is generally quick, and the early results have been rewarding.

In patients 30 to 40 years of age who are still able to walk despite moderate radiological evidence of dysplasia and arthritis, surgery is not indicated. These patients should be encouraged to delay surgery until their disability becomes more severe. This advice applies specifically to young patients who demand surgery for recreational activities or to be rid of a limp. Such patients are likely to be better served by total hip arthroplasty in their 40s than by one or two intermediate operations (such as osteotomies) with no guarantee of a successful outcome.

Generally, intermediate and high dislocations associated with arthritis lend themselves technically well to hip arthroplasty (Figs. 10-24 and 10-25), and where severe disability exists, surgery is indicated. However, reconstruction may be difficult if not formidable on completely dislocated, unreduced hips without evidence of any development of the acetabulum (see Chapter 20). In a high dislocation of the hip, the contact between the upper end of the femur and the acetabulum has fortunately been minimal throughout, because there is no true constrainment or osteoarthritis. The main complaint is shortening of the limb, causing a gross limp, especially in cases of unilateral involvement. When hips have been bilaterally dislocated throughout life and no false acetabulum has formed, leg length is equal and back pain is usually relatively insignificant. This type of patient should be discouraged from early surgery because of obvious technical problems and because of the likelihood that a complex operation will not improve the limp, which is generally related to severely underdeveloped adductor muscles.

Others[78,142] have successfully attempted early reconstruction in cases of untreated complete dislocation of the hips. In my experience, a unilaterally high dislocated hip is a greater problem than bilateral hip dislocations. Therefore, because of disability, early reconstructive surgery may be advisable despite all theoretical objections. Reconstructive surgery in congenital dislocation and dysplasia is not difficult, but the surgeon must be well informed and skilled in performing total hip arthroplasty surgery. Surgeons should postpone performing this type of operation until they are altogether familiar with its details, usually not before they have acquired considerable experience in performing the procedure (see Chapter 20).

With a few exceptions in advanced arthritis associated with congenital hip dysplasia, arthrodesis, osteotomies, or other procedures are not suitable alternatives to total hip arthroplasty. Arthrodesis in women is undesirable, and osteotomy (with some exceptions) may aggravate an already stiff and shortened extremity (see Alternatives to Total Hip Replacement). Mold arthroplasty results are not satisfactory because of the lack of bony stock in the acetabulum and the excessive anteversion of the femoral neck.

Results of total hip arthroplasty for congenital subluxation and dislocation have been extremely encouraging. Nonetheless, patients must be selected judiciously because of the age factor and the possibility of a persistent limp caused by abductor weakness. (For a discussion of technique, see Chapter 20; for a discussion of results, see Chapter 29.)

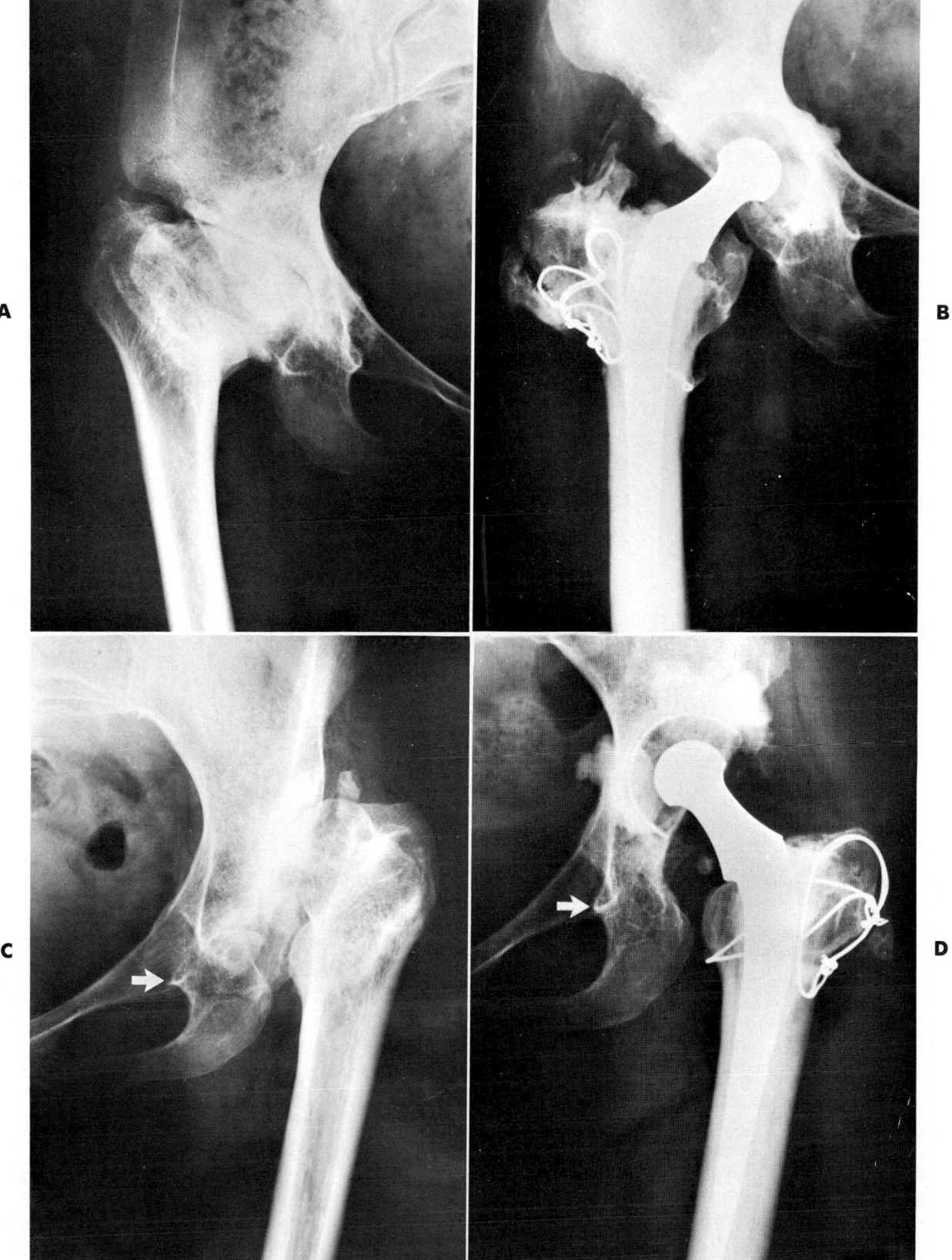

Fig. 10-24. Generally, intermediate and high dislocations technically lend themselves well to total hip arthroplasty despite shallow socket; floor permits adequate deepening, allowing insertion of prosthesis. **A,** Unilateral congenital subluxation of hip with high-riding greater trochanter. **B,** Postoperative view of same patient 5 years after total hip arthroplasty with excellent recovery. Preoperative grading of hip, A-3,4-3; postoperatively, A-6,6,6. NOTE: marked improvement of cortex as result of excellent function. **C,** Preoperative radiograph of unilateral hip dysplasia with marked dysplasia of socket but good bone stock at floor of acetabulum. Arrow points to inner wall of pelvis (teardrop and thickened floor). **D,** Same hip as in **C,** with optimum deepening and seating of acetabulum, component in slightly higher position as compared with **A** and **B** (see Chapter 20). Preoperative grading, A-4,4,3; postoperatively, A-6,6,5.

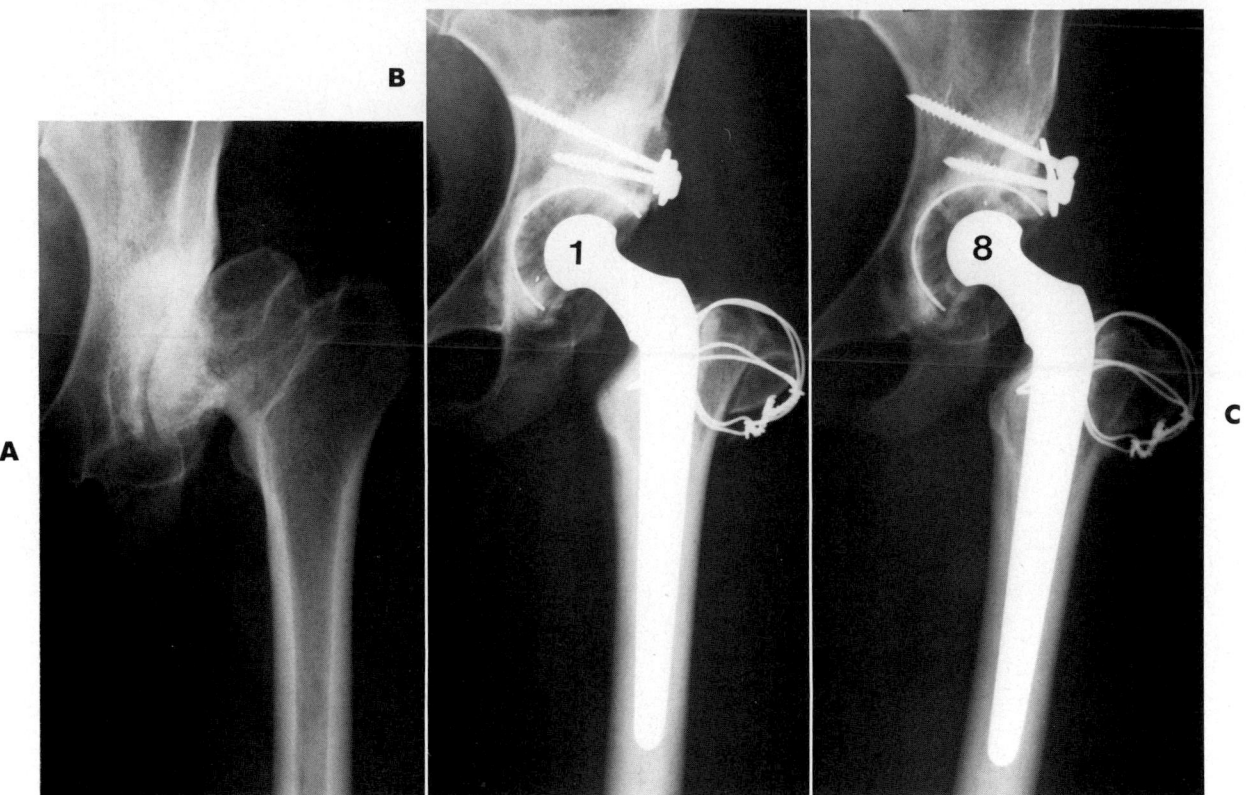

Fig. 10-25. A, Preoperative radiographs of 34-year-old woman (E.C.) with severe dysplasia and osteoarthritis. Patient was followed without surgery for 8 years. At surgery grade A-3,3,4. **B,** Reconstructed hip with low-friction arthroplasty at 1 year and **C,** 8 years postoperatively. Grade A-6,6,6.

Chronic Suppurative and Tuberculous Arthritis

As stated elsewhere (see Chapters 26 and 32), the presence of osteomyelitis is a contraindication to total hip arthroplasty. As a general rule, the maxim is "once the bone has been infected, it will always be infected," and we select cases for total hip arthroplasty with caution, preferring a resection pseudoarthrosis instead. This advice applies particularly in the case of a previously tuberculous hip that has been quiescent for many years. However, at times when the organism is sensitive to antibiotics, it may be justifiable to treat these patients prophylactically with antibiotics by antibiotic-loaded acrylic cement and consider long postoperative treatment by antibiotics.

Patients whose infections occurred in childhood or adolescence with complete resolution may be accepted for total hip arthroplasty. In this regard, old pyogenic arthritis is manifested radiologically as primary osteoarthritis, and only occasionally is there a scar or adherent sinus formation about the hip indicating an early life problem. We perform hip arthroplasties in these patients with no fear that the infection will be reactivated after arthroplasty surgery (Figs. 10-26 and

10-27). However, it is necessary to process cultures carefully intraoperatively for proper management (see Chapter 26).

Scoliosis

Total hip arthroplasty may become necessary in an arthritic hip accompanying an old unrecognized or untreated scoliosis in the lumbar or thoracolumbosacral spine. The preexisting scoliosis may lead to pelvic obliquity, often exaggerating the limp and causing deformity and complete decompensation. Usually the hip disease in these individuals is unilateral. The affected hip is on the concave side of the lumbar or lumbosacral curve and higher than the opposite side. The affective hip consequently assumes the position of adduction with associated subluxation. Treatment is particularly indicated in these individuals because of extreme shortening produced by the fixed adduction deformity, which cannot be compensated because the lumbar spine is fixed by secondary osteoarthritis. Early surgery may be indicated because of difficulty in walking, extreme stress on the lumbosacral spine, or both, which contribute to severe back pain. It is best to

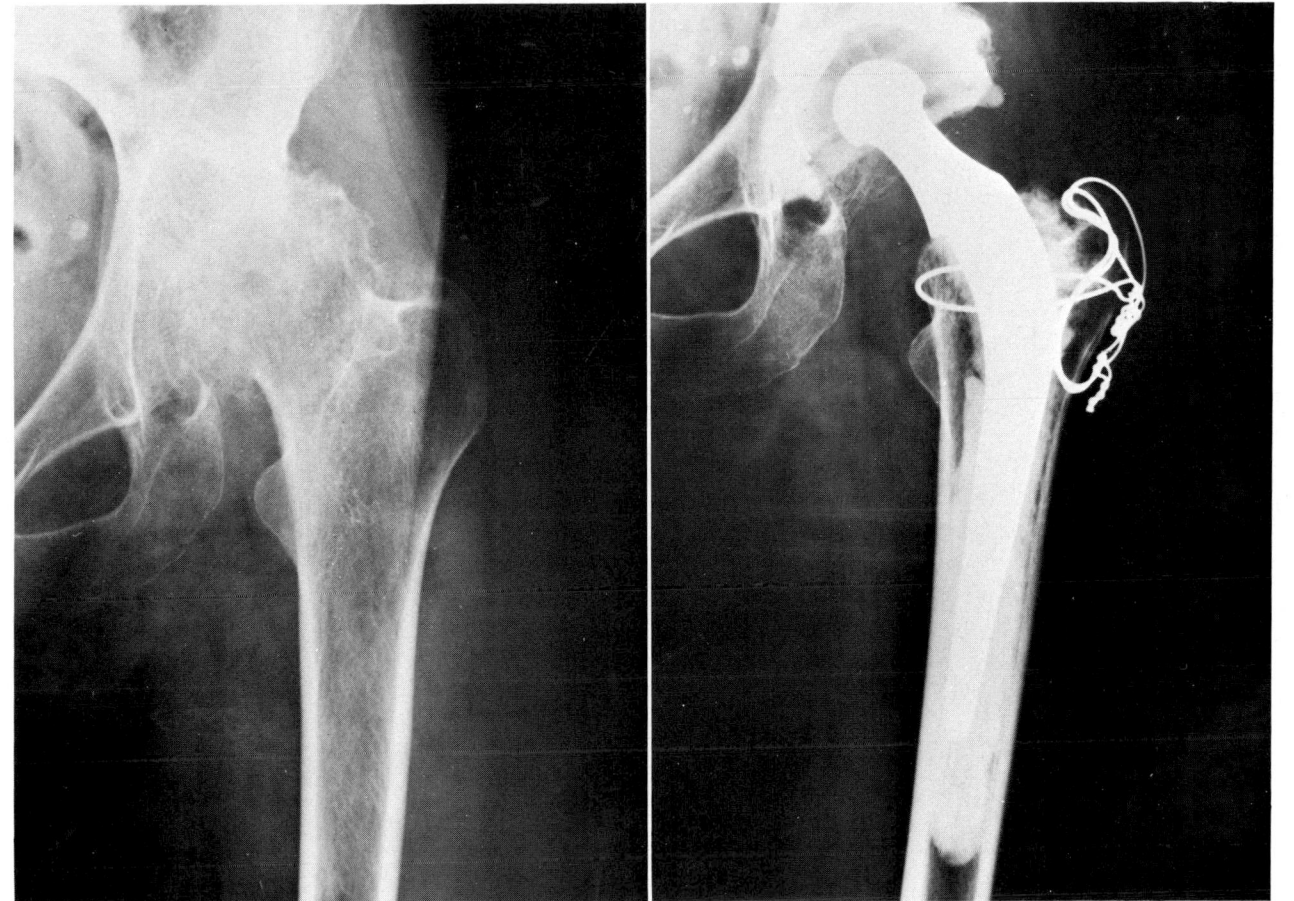

Fig. 10-26. A, Preoperative radiograph of 48-year-old woman with septic hip at age 12. Original infective organism was staphylococci and several scarred chronic sites of drainage from hip were present. Sedimentation rate was within normal range, and there was no evidence of infection for over 36 years. Preoperative grading of the hip was A-3,4,2. **B,** 5-year postoperative radiographic improvement was A-6,6,6. Patient received prophylactic antibiotics during surgery and 3 months postoperatively. No organism was cultured from hip after surgery.

consider arthroplasty without any aim toward equalization, since deformity of the spine is often fixed and further elongation of the limb may place further strain on the lumbar area and thus cause further decompensation. When the accompanying spinal deformity is equally painful to the patient, spinal fusion before hip surgery may be suggested. On the other hand, we often consider surgery of the hip the ultimate solution where spinal strain will be alleviated after total hip arthroplasty.

Systemic Disease

In many conditions, such as sickle cell disease, lupus erythematosus, Gaucher's disease (Figs. 10-28 and 10-29), and disseminated avascular necrosis of the bone, the general systemic disease leads to destructive changes of the hip, necessitating arthroplasty. Because

in most instances life expectancy may be shorter than normal, age is not often a factor in patient selection. However, the outcome of total hip arthroplasty might be somewhat in jeopardy because of abnormal bone, and progressive loosening or persistent pain might occur despite total hip arthroplasty. True indications for surgical procedure are derived when the disability of the patient is weighed against the systemic conditions causing hip impairment.

Rare Congenital and Developmental Conditions

A number of congenital and developmental conditions (such as multiple epiphyseal dysplasia, achondroplasia, congenital coxa vara, and osteopetrosis) may eventually require mechanical replacement because of secondary arthritic changes in the hip. These condi-

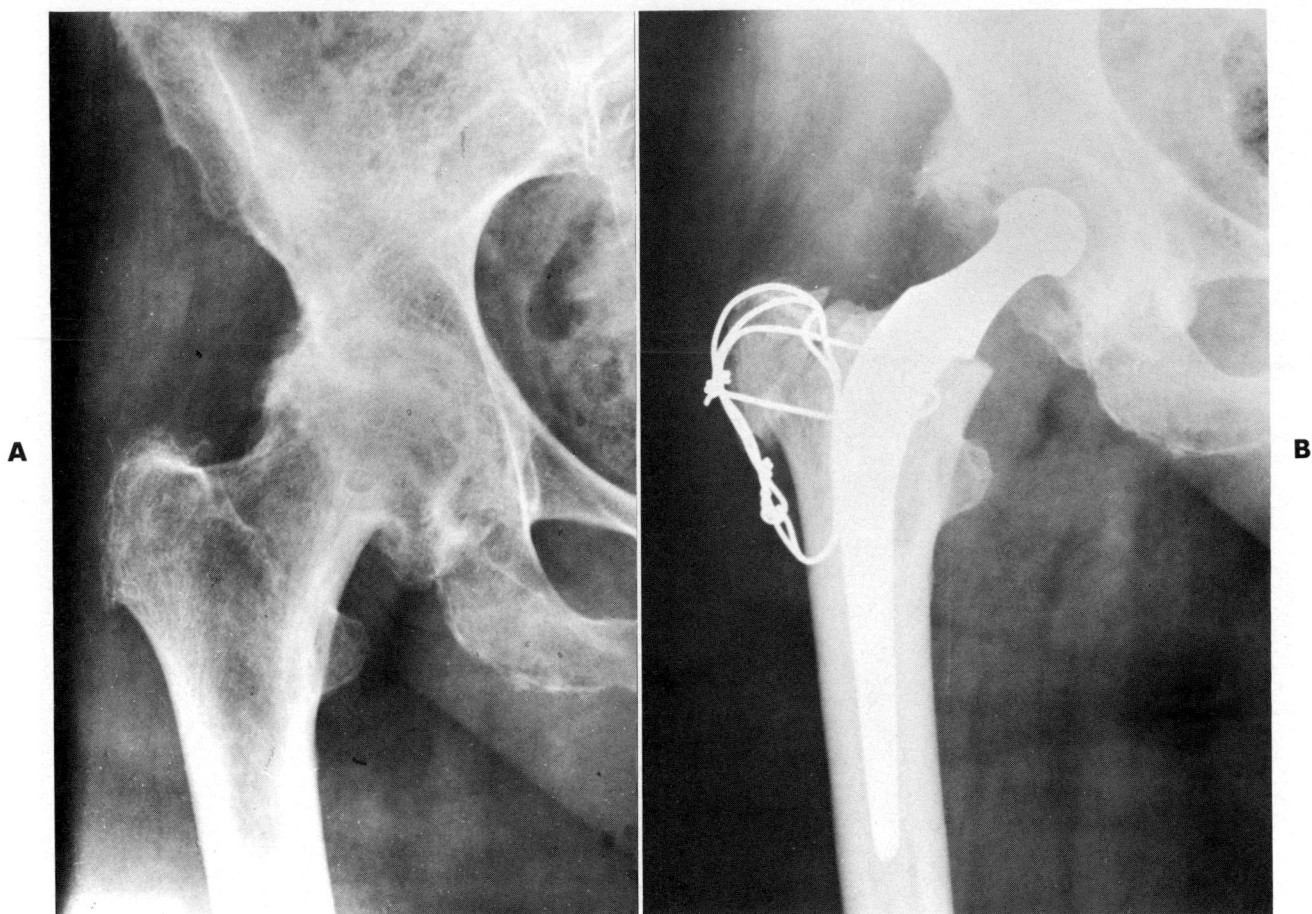

Fig. 10-27. There should be no concern in performing total hip arthroplasty in cases of hematogenous childhood infections. In this 55-year-old woman with drainage at age 2, only small old scar was present posterolateral to greater trochanter. Sedimentation rate was normal without any history of drainage since childhood. **A,** Preoperative radiograph of right hip shows it to be completely ankylosed. Grading A-5,3,1. **B,** 3-year postoperative grading, right hip 6,5,6.

tions are rare but may present idiosyncratic anatomical changes requiring specific preparation and handling at surgery. For example, a patient with coxa vara may present technical problems similar to congenital dysplasia: a shortened femur neck and high-riding of the upper femur. An achondroplastic individual may require a specially designed prosthesis because of the small bone. In instances where multiple joints are involved, the perspective of total function and the patient's activities must also be considered.

Small or Large Patients

As has been indicated in Chapter 15, total hip arthroplasty is not contraindicated in small or extremely large patients. The surgeon should have prostheses available for patients at both ends of the spectrum. The most commonly involved joints in acromegaly syndrome are the hips, shoulders, knees,

hands, and elbows. Marie, in describing acromegaly in 1890, noted the presence of juxtaarticular swelling.[95] The condition is considered noninflammatory mechanical arthritis; it leads to cartilage hypertrophy and hyperplasia, which cause changes in joint geometry and disruption of cartilage metabolism; thus, the degenerative process is secondary.

Bone Tumors

A number of primary and metastatic lesions may involve the hip joint, and part or all of the joint may be replaced after elimination of the tumorous condition. The goal here is to eradicate the tumor with the hope of a permanent cure and hip joint reconstruction for improved function. The former is a lifesaving procedure, and the latter is obviously secondary to the primary goal. In the past, lack of interest in replacing the upper femur was related to difficulty in securing

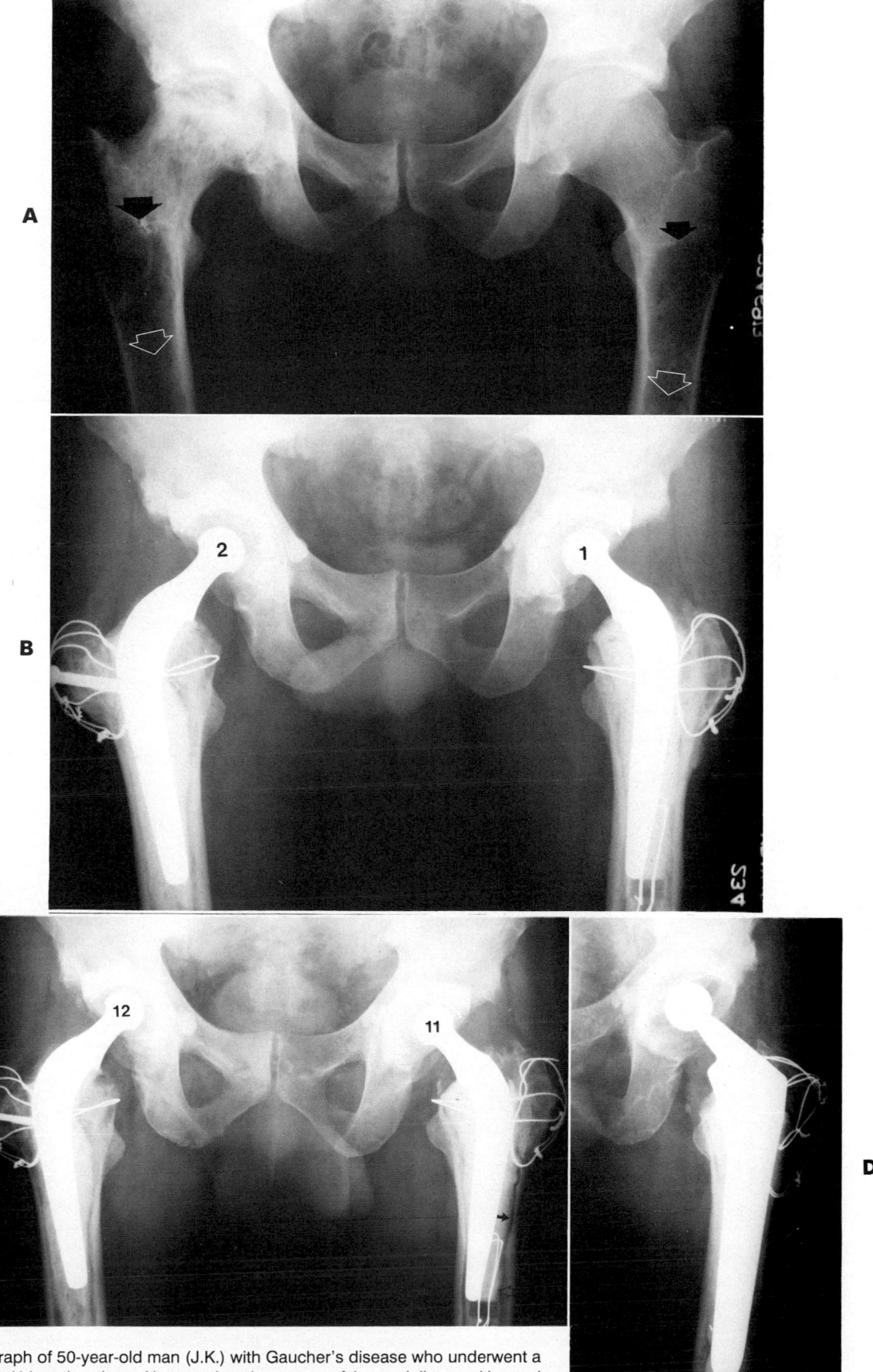

Fig. 10-28. A, Radiograph of 50-year-old man (J.K.) with Gaucher's disease who underwent a splenectomy before total hip arthroplasty. Note cystic enlargement of the medullary cavities and associated cortical thinning of the femur caused by Gaucher's cells. **B,** Radiographs taken 2 years after bilateral low-friction arthroplasty. Preoperative grade was C-bilateral 3,3,3. Grades improved to C-5,5,5 bilaterally. **C,** 12 and 11 years after surgery, note radiolucency at the cement bone interface *(arrows)* in left hip, which is also associated with subsidence of stem. **D,** After revision of the left hip. Note the unusually large size of the upper femur requiring customization of the stem intraoperatively using acrylic cement.

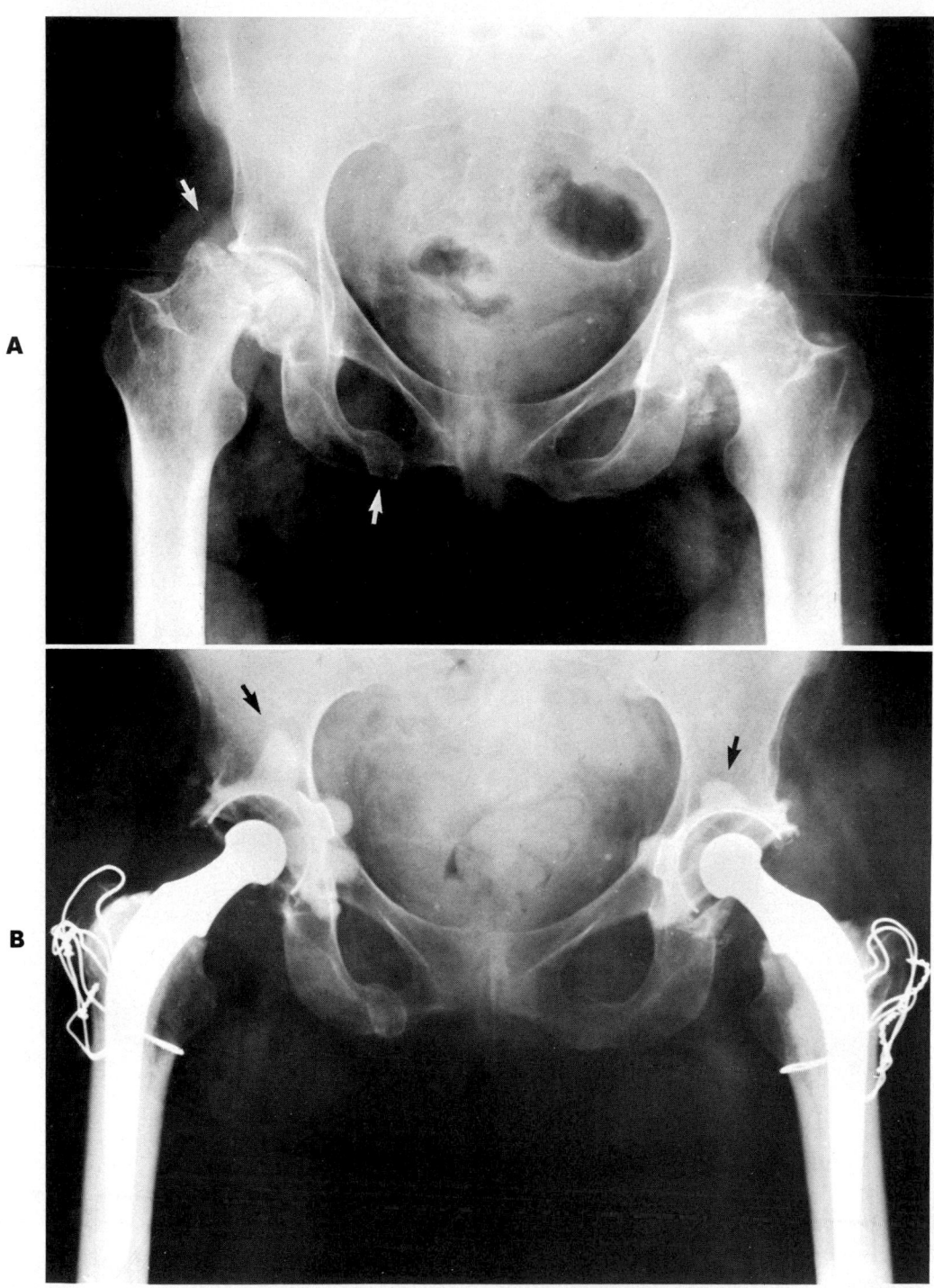

Fig. 10-29. A, Preoperative radiograph of hips in 26-year-old female with sickle cell disease. Patient was chairbound at time of surgery in view of spontaneous fracture of femoral neck. Top arrow shows acute fracture of head. Bottom arrow shows fracture through ilioischial ramus. **B,** Postoperative radiograph showing satisfactory clinical results of arthroplasty despite patient's complaint of pain in both hips. Sedimentation rate was within normal limit, and patient has no indication of infection. It is possible that bone infarction within region of hip and spontaneous microfractures in area of pelvis are cause of pain. Preoperative grades of hip were C-right 1,2,2 and C-left 1,2,2; postoperative assessment, C-right 4,4,6 and C-left 4,4,6.

prosthetic components to the pelvis and femur. Because of advances in total hip surgery and bone grafts to reconstruct the pelvis or upper femur after segmental resection, replacement has become a reality.[118,121] En bloc resection of a tumor (depending upon the aggressiveness of the tumor, the patient's age, the feasibility of resection, and so on) has replaced amputation in most instances. Similarly, a metastatic lesion of the upper femur or pelvis may be satisfactorily replaced by total hip arthroplasty. Alternate modes of treatment are considered based on the nature of the disease, life expectancy, and so on before reconstruction of the upper femur or pelvis and total hip arthroplasty are considered. Periosteal osteogenic sarcoma and low-grade, primary malignant bone tumors (for example, giant cell tumors) may be considered for en bloc resection. Improvement in function makes total arthroplasty an attractive mode of treatment, especially because of quick recovery and relatively short rehabilitation after this procedure (see Chapters 21 to 24).

Neurovascular Conditions

At times a difficult decision must be made about whether a patient with an osteoarthritic hip with vascular compromise of the lower extremity should have a total hip arthroplasty. There are two main concerns: (1) If the patient subsequently becomes more active, the severity of vascular compromise will be enhanced (in effect, removal of the safety valve), and claudication and vascular compromise will prevent use of the corrected hip. (2) If the vascular condition of the extremity is further jeopardized, ischemia may develop and result in loss of the limb. It is of paramount importance that a vascular surgeon be consulted in these situations and that a mature decision be reached based on Doppler studies, angiograms, or both. If a history of intermittent claudication is indeed present despite limited activities, total hip arthroplasty is contraindicated: increased activities after the procedure would only deteriorate the vascular compromise of the limb. On the other hand, when arteriosclerotic disease of the extremity is well tolerated despite absent dorsalis pedis pulse (but with good posterior tibialis pulse) without dystrophy of the skin of the toes, total hip arthroplasty may be considered. At times, vascular repair such as arterial bypass may be performed before the contemplated surgery (Fig. 10-30). Venous flow and venous stasis may present difficulties after total hip arthroplasty, especially in older people and patients with diabetes. This unfortunate situation can compromise the results of arthroplasty because of persistent trophic ulcers of the lower leg after surgery.

Paralytic conditions in an extremity should be carefully evaluated and no arthroplasty contemplated if there are imbalanced muscles or atonia about the hip. A case in point would be a long-standing palsied hip in which the flexors and adductors are overreacting against weak abductors and extensors. Obviously, in these situations instability of the hip and dislocation may be anticipated. In contrast to neurological imbalance of the ipsilateral limb, an affected contralateral hip or knee is no contraindication for hip surgery. Patients with prior poliomyelitis or other peripheral neuropathies may benefit tremendously from total arthroplasty of the opposite hip. However, it must be recognized that the involved opposite hip places a considerable burden on the operated side (Fig. 10-31), and it might be a good idea to suggest continued use of a walking aid for these patients.

Neurotrophic Joints (Charcot's)

The neurological imbalance and lack of sensitivity of these patients make total arthroplasty unsuitable. Frequent complications such as dislocation make this operation a relative contraindication in neurotrophic joints. Isolated reports of arthroplasty with subsequent dislocation support this conclusion.[1] Because they do not experience severe pain, patients with Charcot's joint may be treated nonoperatively in most instances; in fractures of the hip, a simple prosthetic replacement is advantageous and preferable to total arthroplasty. However, the Charcot joint can be a significant disability because of instability, pain, or both. It is not clear why some neurotrophic joints are painful, but impingement of the irregular bone or microfracture has been considered the main cause of pain. Hip involvement was relatively uncommon and occurred in only 7 of 68 patients studied by Eichenholtz.[63] Previously no definitive treatment other than protective methods was recommended for the treatment of Charcot's joint.[82] Because of pain and instability or highly individualized circumstances, the surgeon may elect to perform a total hip arthroplasty in the neurotrophic joints.[129] This author found an indication in four instances when a total hip arthroplasty had to be performed in Charcot's joints (Fig. 10-32).

Hemophilia

Because of recent advances in the management of hemophilia, surgery has become possible for these patients. As cited in the discussion of perioperative management in Chapters 9 and 11, proper indication and care of these individuals must be coordinated with an interested hematologist who can determine the degree of severity and the risks involved. Reported experiences with hemophiliac patients undergoing total hip arthroplasty are most encouraging.[54]

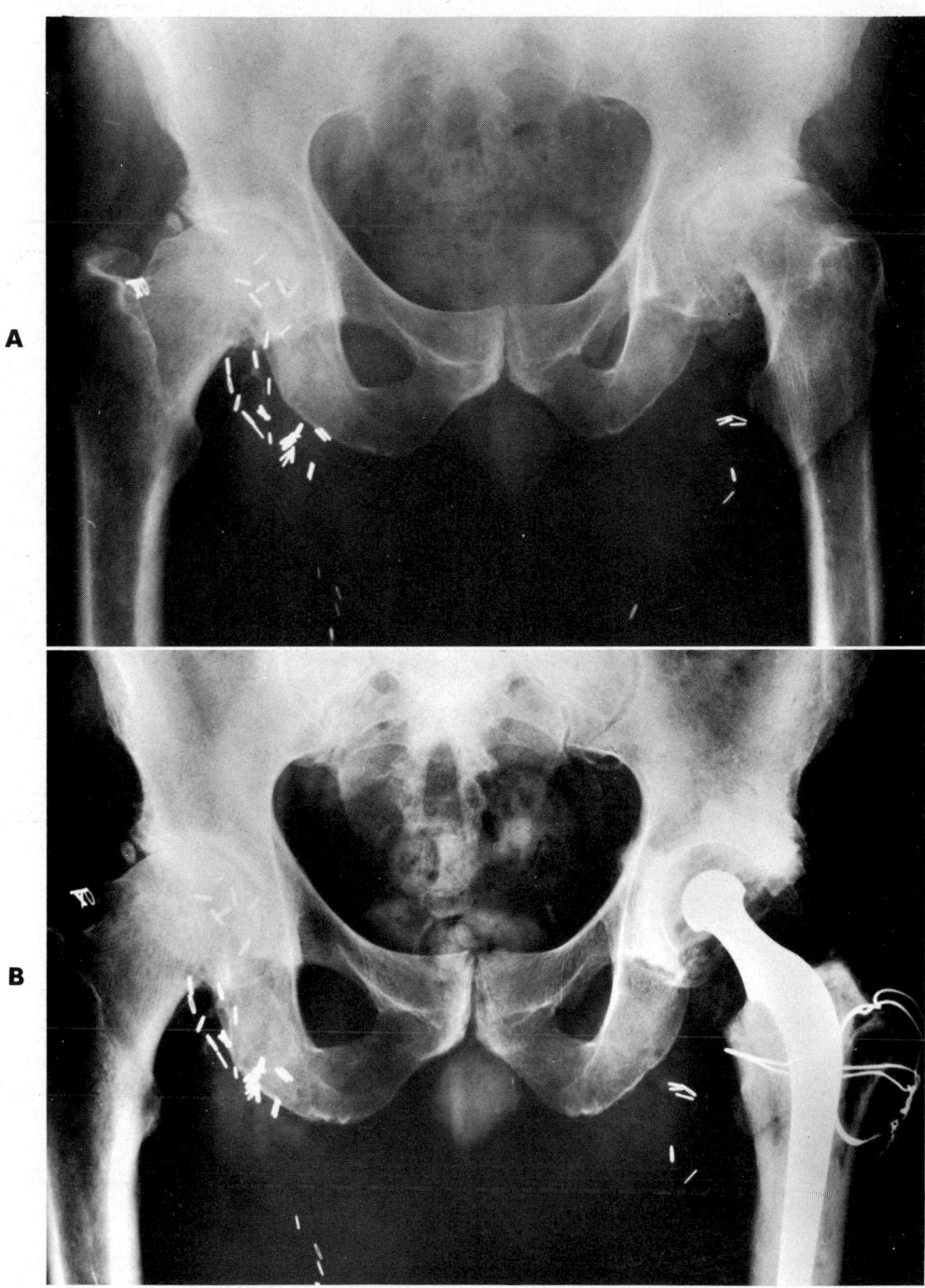

Fig. 10-30. Examples of arterial disease accompanied by degenerative joint disease. **A** and **B,** Preoperative and postoperative radiographs of 64-year-old man with bilateral degenerative osteoarthrosis. When patient was originally seen, he demonstrated bilateral claudication as a result of arteriosclerosis and compromise of blood supply to lower extremities. After bilateral arterial bypass 1 year later, left total hip arthroplasty was performed, which was uneventful postoperatively.

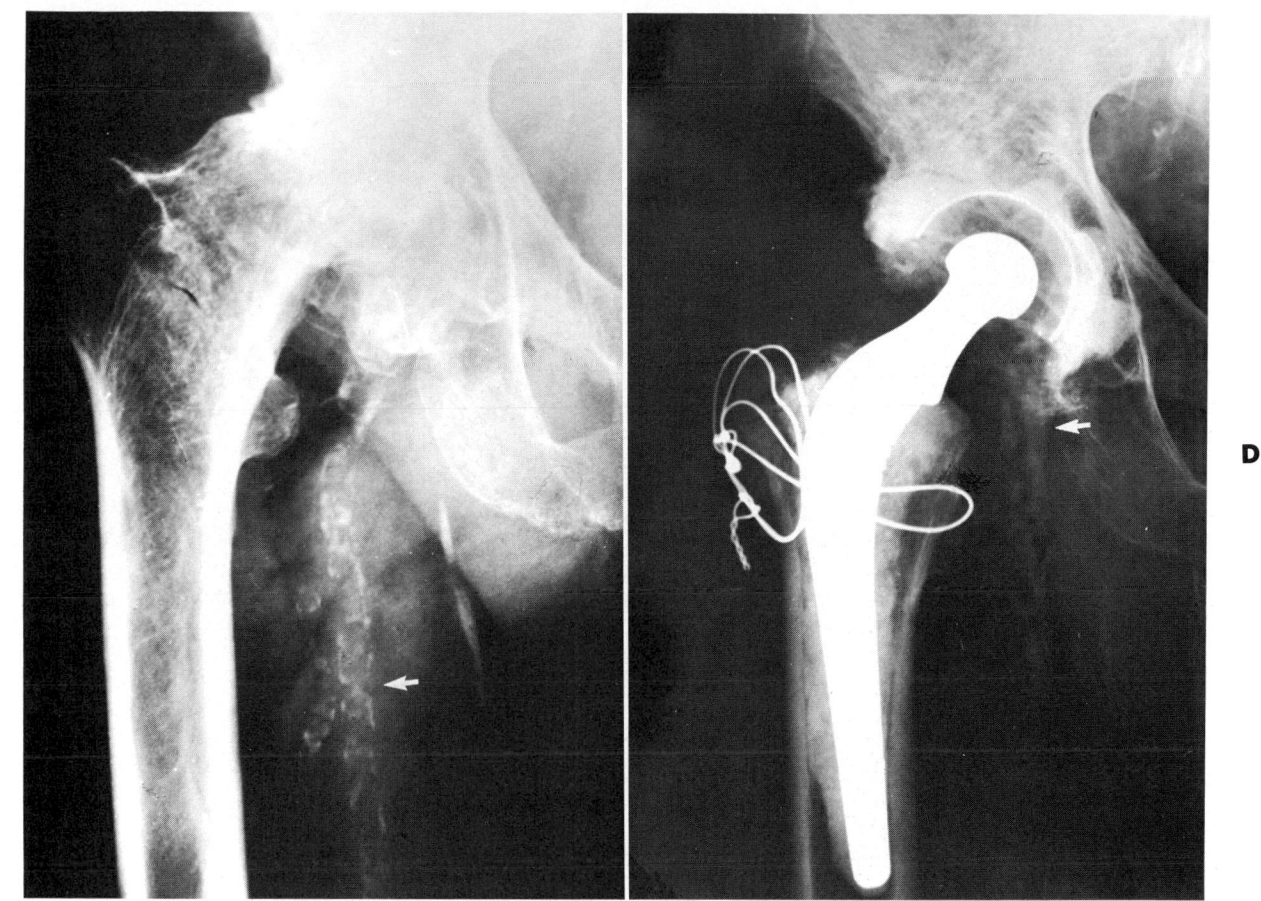

Fig. 10-30 — cont'd. C, Preoperative radiograph of hip in 74-year-old mildly hypertensive patient with extensive atheroma *(arrow)*. **D,** 3-year postoperative radiograph of same patient. Presence of atheroma on radiograph is not contraindication for surgery.

Nonambulatory Patients

At times total hip arthroplasty in patients who have been chairbound or bedbound for several years may be indicated. Patient's desire and motivation are positive factors in reaching a decision. Other joints such as knees and upper extremities may also be a significant factor in determining whether the patient can become ambulatory again. Total hip arthroplasty should also be performed in patients with severe pain whose main concern is relief of pain and not ambulation (see Chapter 21).

Avascular Necrosis

Osteonecrosis of the femoral head resulting from traumatic conditions, such as fracture of the neck of the femur or dislocation of the hip, is a well-known problem; it is observed in many older patients after femoral neck fracture as well as young persons following traumatic dislocations, fracture, and fracture-dislocation.

Patients with nontraumatic avascular necrosis are usually young and suffer from bilateral hip disease. The underlying cause of avascular necrosis may be excess alcohol intake, steroid medications, blood dyscrasia, or maintenance doses of immunosuppressive drugs in patients with renal and cardiac transplants.

Renal Transplantation

One of the common complications of renal transplantation is avascular necrosis of the femoral head. It results from long-term or lifelong chemical immunosuppression (in the form of daily steroids, azathioprine, or both) to prevent allograft rejection (Fig. 10-33). Patients who continue to receive these drugs are prone to develop multiple avascular necroses, commonly in the hips. They are also usually prone to orthopedic complications of chronic hemodialysis, including osteoporosis, osteomalacia, secondary hyperparathyroidism, and peripheral neuropathies.[76] They may also suffer steroid myopathy and pathological fractures.

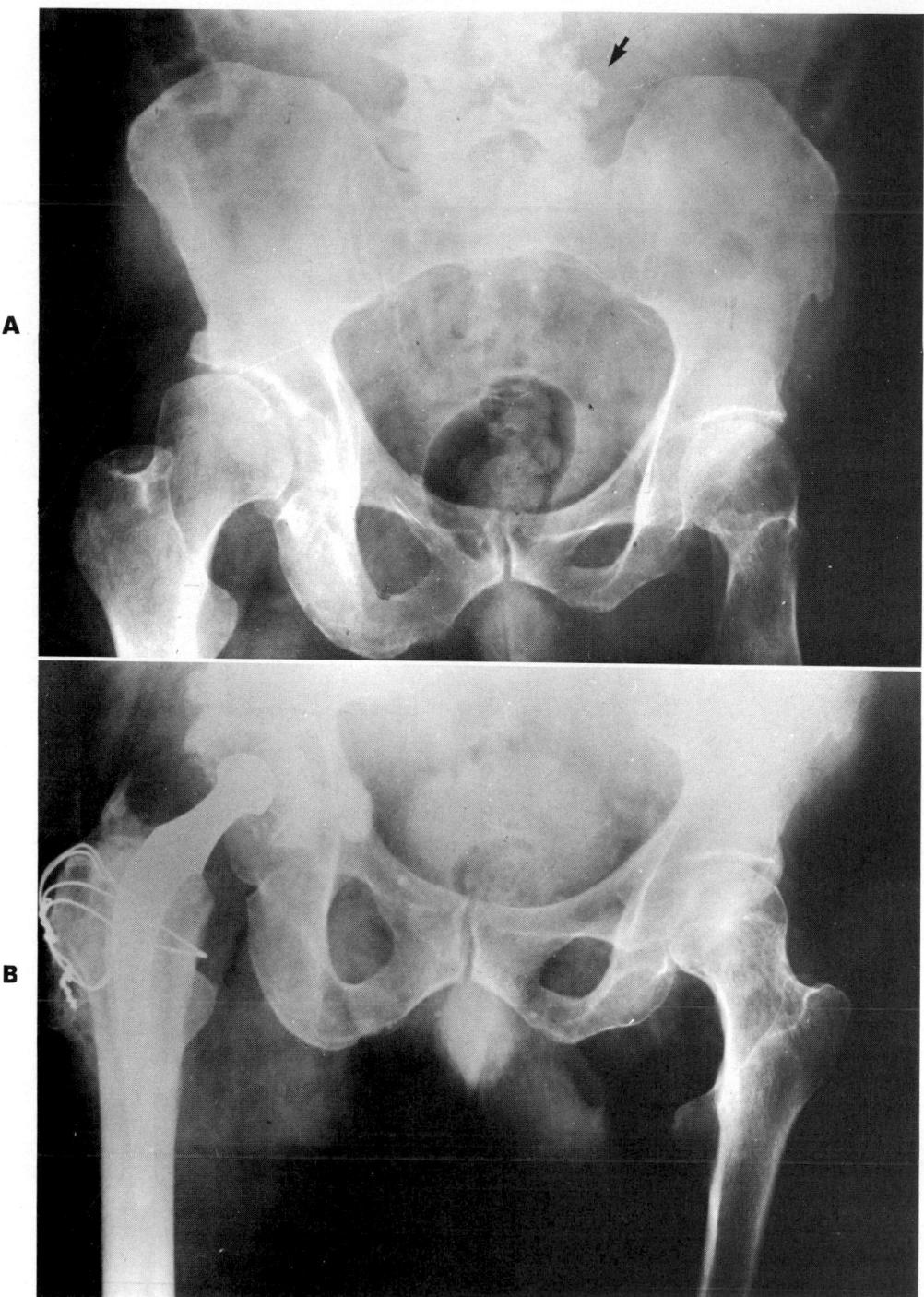

Fig. 10-31. Fifty-six-year-old male with long-standing postpolio paralysis of left lower extremity and marked atrophy. **A,** He developed severe pain in left hip and lumbar spine from scoliosis and degenerative arthritis *(arrow).* Preoperative grading of hips on right was C-3,3,4 but left was C-6,3,6. Two inches of shortening were present on left side. **B,** After total hip arthroplasty patient continued to use cane, but pain was relieved both from hip and back. Postoperative grading was C-6,4,5.

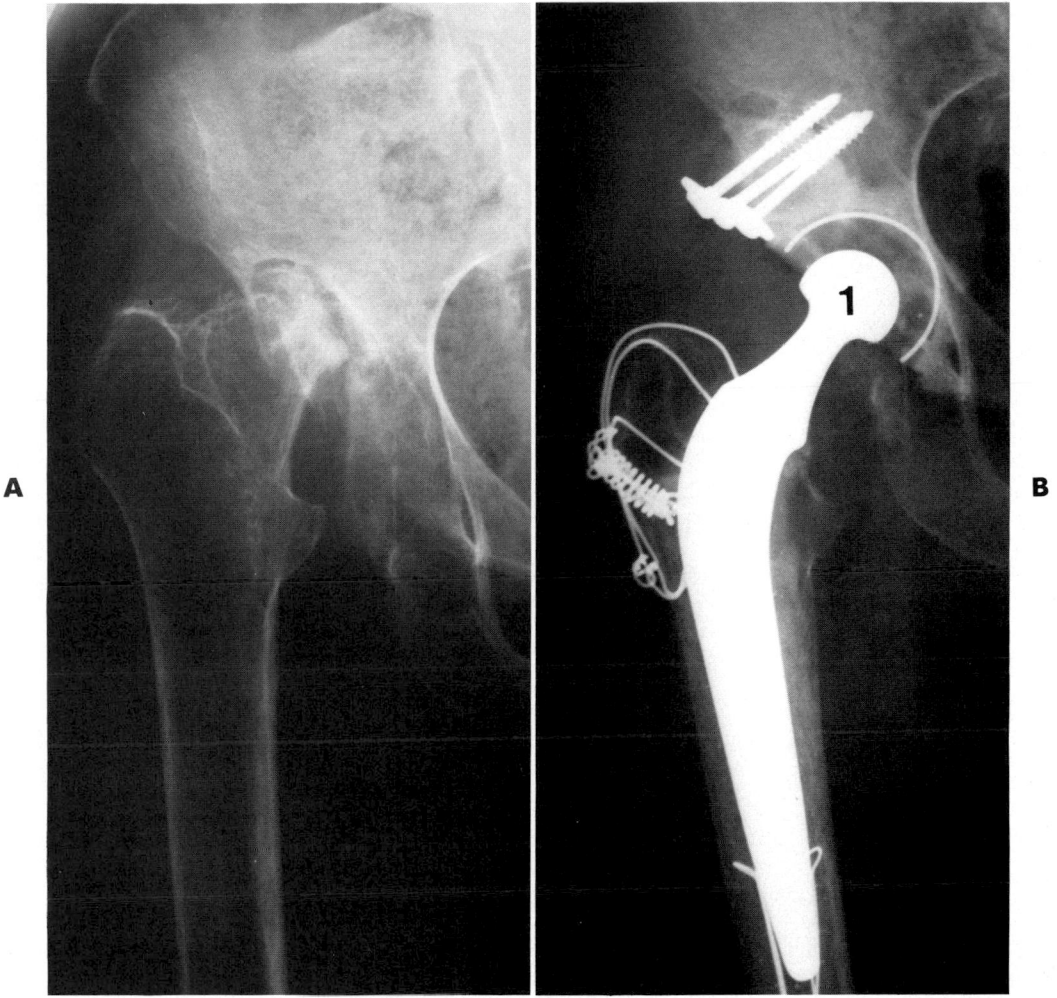

Fig. 10-32. Charcot's joint can be a source of severe disability and at times may be associated with pain. **A,** Preoperative radiograph of 54-year-old woman (M.H.) shows severe destructive changes of a neurotrophic joint (VDRL was positive). Hip grade C-4,2,6. **B,** Postreconstruction by low-friction arthroplasty and allograft. Grade C-6,6,6. Patient was instructed to wear hip brace permanently.

Many reports indicate that total hip arthroplasty is ideally suited for patients with relatively short life expectancies, dramatically improving their condition. It must be recognized, however, that this population of patients presents a relatively high risk of infection because of the systemic immunosuppressive drugs they take and will continue to take postoperatively—in most cases, indefinitely. These cases are also potentially more at risk from the standpoint of anesthesia and postoperative morbidity, especially with reference to urinary tract infections and kidney problems. In many of these patients, chronic renal disease may be responsible for fluid and electrolyte retention and hypertension. In one study by Bradford and associates[26] of 66 hips of renal transplant patients, the average age was 32 years (16 to 54 years). With an average follow-up of 44 months, 9 of 39 patients died after total hip arthroplasty from various causes, ranging from gram-negative sepsis to acute myelogenous leukemia. In addition, a high rate of postoperative dislocation (10 of 66 hips) was observed. Although these patients have a reduced life expectancy, many are young and fully active. Therefore they impose considerable stress on an artificial joint while their bones might not be strong enough to support a prosthesis adequately, possibly causing loosening and fracture of the prosthesis because of vigorous activities.[51,76,85,109] The consensus of surgeons with vast experience is that total hip arthroplasty can be safely performed in this high-risk population of patients with the hope of good early results.[51,76,85,109] It must be recognized, however, that long-term results of a sizable series are not yet

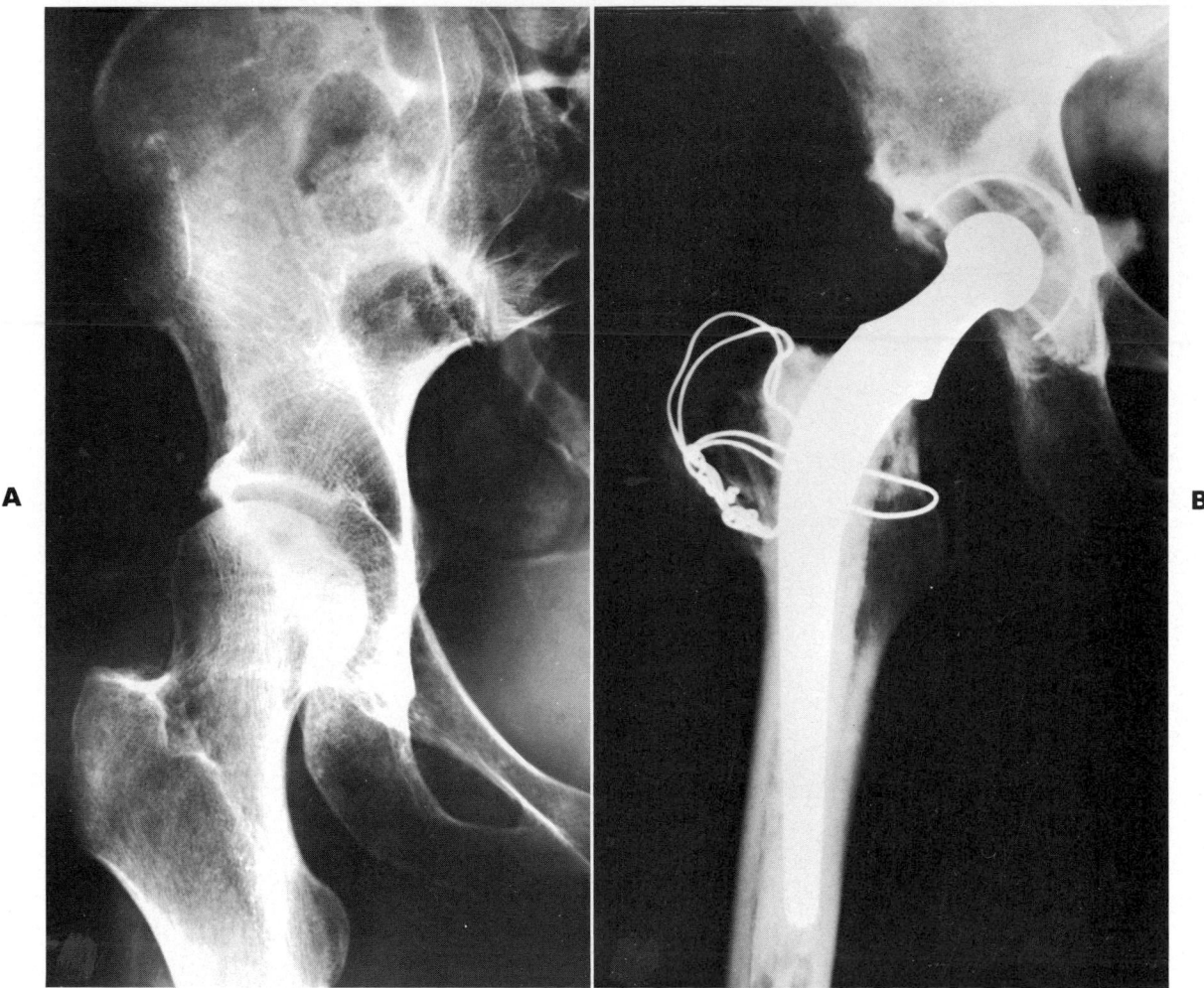

Fig. 10-33. Avascular necrosis of femoral head after kidney transplant and immunosuppressive drugs is now best treated by total hip arthroplasty. **A,** Status of hip in 28-year-old female 6 years after cadaveric kidney transplant. One year, **B,** and 6 years, **C,** after total hip arthroplasty with excellent clinical result. Preoperative grading of hip is C-2,3,4; postoperative grade, C-6,6,6. NOTE: hypertrophy *(arrow)* of femoral shaft at level of tip of prosthesis.

available to make a final judgment in treating this particular condition.

Cardiac Transplantation

Like steroid-induced avascular necrosis after kidney transplant, osteonecrosis developing after cardiac transplantation is on the rise. The first human heart transplantation in the United States was performed at Stanford University Hospital in January 1968.[80] By November 1984, 344 heart-lung transplants had been performed at the same institution, with a longer survival rate (up to 15 years and longer). Many of these patients also require hip arthroplasty. Total hip arthroplasty in cardiac transplant patients is indicated if the patient is severely handicapped by pain and restriction of motion.

Idiopathic Avascular Necrosis

The so-called idiopathic avascular necrosis is commonly bilateral, although it often first manifests itself as unilateral. In some cases there may be a delay of several years before the second hip is affected. In the routine practice of a hip surgeon, a startling number of patients have no evidence of joint narrowing on radiographs and only minimal or no changes of the femoral head but experience extreme pain during rest as well as activity. The problem is often compounded by the lack of underlying conditions and the young age of the person subjected to the treatment, especially when augmented by the absence of symptoms of the opposite hip and an unknown fate regarding development of avascular necrosis of the opposite hip.

When patients are seen early, prevention of sub-

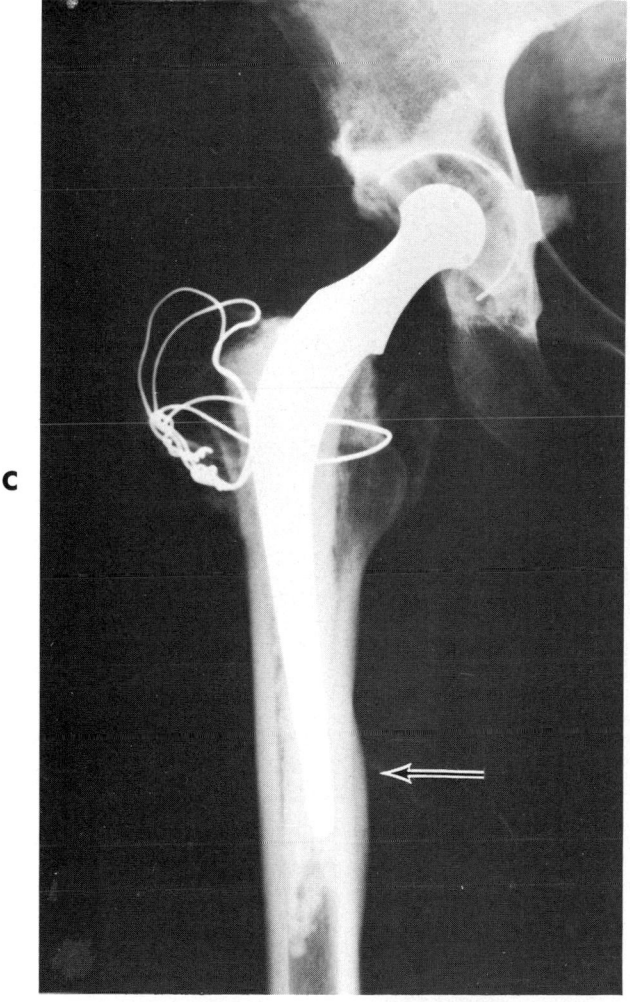

C

Fig. 10-33. See legend on opposite page.

chondral fracture with collapse of the head leading to osteoarthrosis is the prime goal, particularly in young patients. In past attempts, conservative management, including reduction of weight bearing through use of crutches, has rarely been successful. Treatment by core decompression has remained controversial. Bone grafting, or osteotomy, has been reported as having varying success. When there is radiographic evidence of subchondral fracture and loss of sphericity in the femoral head bone, it is now commonly agreed that bone grafting or osteotomy may not restore hip function. On the other hand, in very early stages (stage 1 or 2), especially in very young patients, bone grafting or osteotomy might be of some value and should be considered.[20–22,113,130] However, when subchondral bone fracture and head collapse are seen through routine radiographs, CT scan, or MRI, a total arthroplasty is indicated. The major question often confronting us is whether to replace the femoral head.

This author's experience indicates that hemiarthroplasty by a single-unit prosthesis or a bipolar device has a limited place in reconstruction of the hip after head collapse and acetabular disease. Many surgeons advocate a bipolar prosthesis for end-stage avascular necrosis, an alternative that is more conservative than a total hip arthroplasty. However, a good number of these operations will have to be revised because of short-term failure resulting from degenerative changes occurring in the acetabulum.[59]

The best indication for hemiarthroplasty (by monopolar or bipolar prostheses) is for treating femoral neck fractures in geriatric patients (75 years and older) whose acetabula are normal. There are several other indications: fracture dislocation of the femoral neck, comminuted fractures that cannot be reduced, pathological fractures, fractures poorly reduced at surgery, fractures whose treatment was delayed for several days, and fractures that fell apart after nailing. In addition to these traumatic conditions, patients with Parkinson's disease or severe osteoporosis and patients with a limited life expectancy may also be considered for prosthetic replacement.

Femoral Neck Fractures
Internal Fixation vs. Hemiarthroplasty

Some orthopaedic surgeons have advocated treating all fractures of the femoral neck in patients past 65 years of age by an endoprosthesis. The reason is that a high incidence of nonunion and avascular necrosis often results in these patients when the fragments are fixed internally by nailing. While fracture of the neck of the femur is usually prone to such complications as nonunion and avascular necrosis, especially when there is displacement, in a good many of these cases union is successful after internal fixation and avascular necrosis does not develop. Nor can we overlook the fact that no prosthetic replacement can ever be as good as the patient's own femoral head.[24,102]

This author believes that prosthetic replacement of the femoral head must be reserved for patients whose fractures cannot be reduced, who have conditions that may limit ambulation, or who cannot be satisfactorily treated by internal fixation of their fractures. The prosthesis may be used when a fracture is more than 1 week old or in cases of subcapital fractures in aged patients. In very young and active patients, when closed reduction is not possible, it is advisable to use an open reduction and internal fixation instead of prosthetic replacement. The use of endoprosthesis and bipolar devices should be restricted to fresh femoral neck fractures with a normal acetabular cartilage. A femoral head replacement or a bipolar prosthesis is the commonly preferred method with Parkinson's disease.

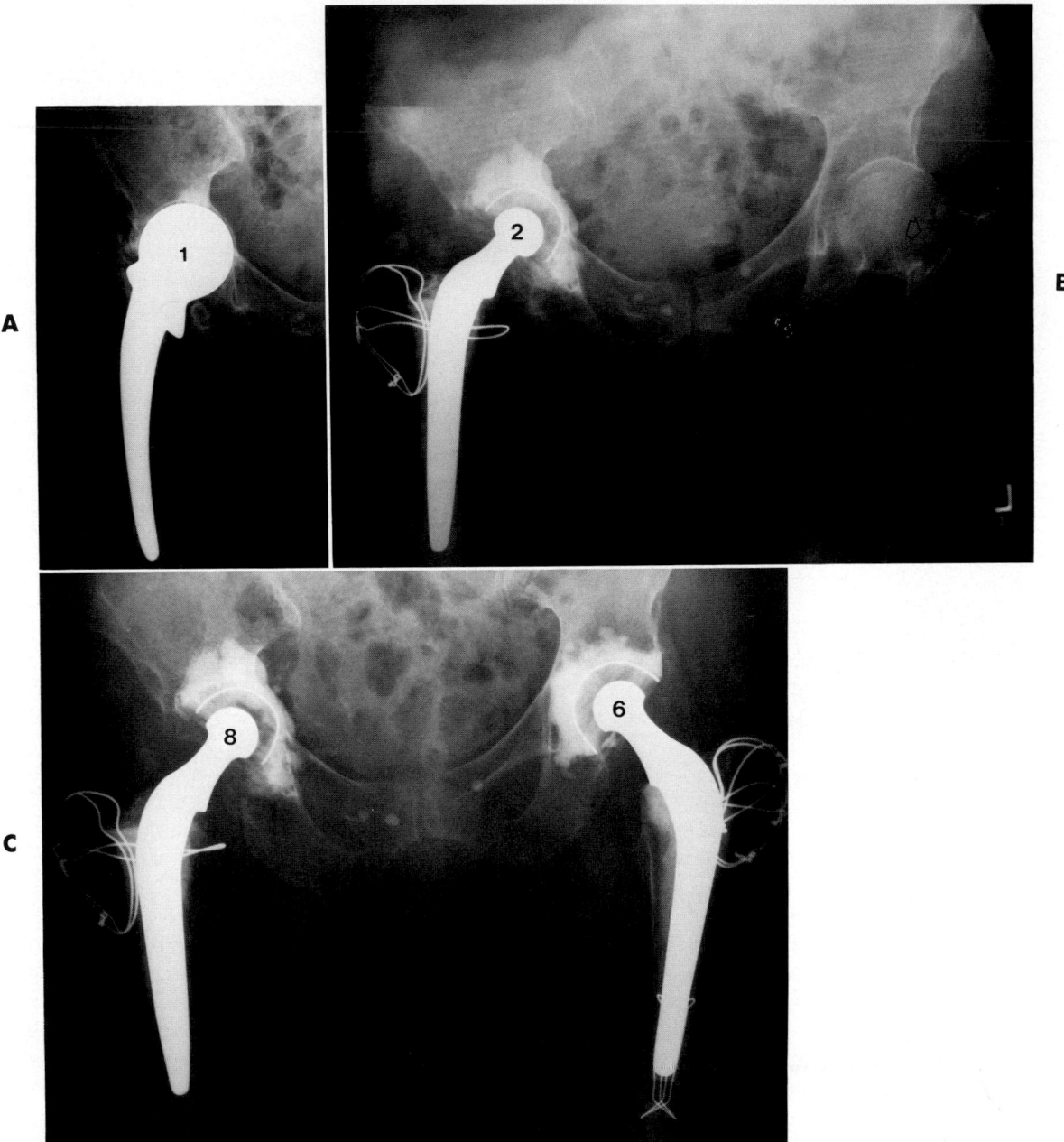

Fig. 10-34. A, A 79-year-old woman (F.G.) with severe osteoporosis experienced pain 1 year after fracture treatment with Austin-Moore prosthesis. Note migration of prosthesis. **B,** 2 years after conversion of the right hip prosthesis to a low-friction arthroplasty, patient sustained a cervical femoral fracture on the left side *(arrows)*. Patient refused to be treated by an endoprosthesis. **C,** Status 8 years after the right and 6 years after the left arthroplasties.

The dislocation rate does not appear to be higher than with patients who do not have the disease.[131]

Hip Fractures and Total Hip Arthroplasty

Relatively few small series of patients with fractured neck of the femur treated by total hip arthroplasty have been reported.[46,53,122,136] These reports indicate a high rate of local and systemic complications. For example, in one small series of 37 patients aged 70 or less, 18 (49%) had failed and required revision, and 4 more (11%) showed radiological signs of loosening. This type of surgery also has a higher rate of postoperative dislocation,[122] which in part may be caused by suboptimal operative conditions in response to an emergency, which can affect the outcome. As one might expect with the results of fractures of the hip in rheumatoid arthritis patients, total hip arthroplasty is the more acceptable treatment (Fig. 10-34). Because the bone is soft, treating osteoporotic hips of patients with rheumatoid arthritis by internal fixation or hemiarthroplasty is fraught with failure, including difficulties such as hardwear cut-outs, delayed unions, and

nonunions.[14] At present, routine use of total hip arthroplasty has a limited place in treating fresh femoral neck fractures. It should be considered for the following situations:

1. Acetabular cartilage lesion found at surgery.
2. A hip fracture in patients with rheumatoid arthritis (Fig. 10-35).
3. Osteoarthritis of the hip associated with hip fracture.
4. Pathological bone conditions associated with fracture, such as Paget's disease, sickle cell disease, etc.
5. Severe osteoporosis of the acetabulum secondary to a prolonged non-weight-bearing period (Fig. 10-36).

Hemiarthroplasty vs. Total Hip Arthroplasty

Let us now consider an interesting and provocative issue: why don't we routinely use total hip arthroplasty for hip fractures? In 95% of cases, total hip arthroplasty has a better result than femoral head replacement.

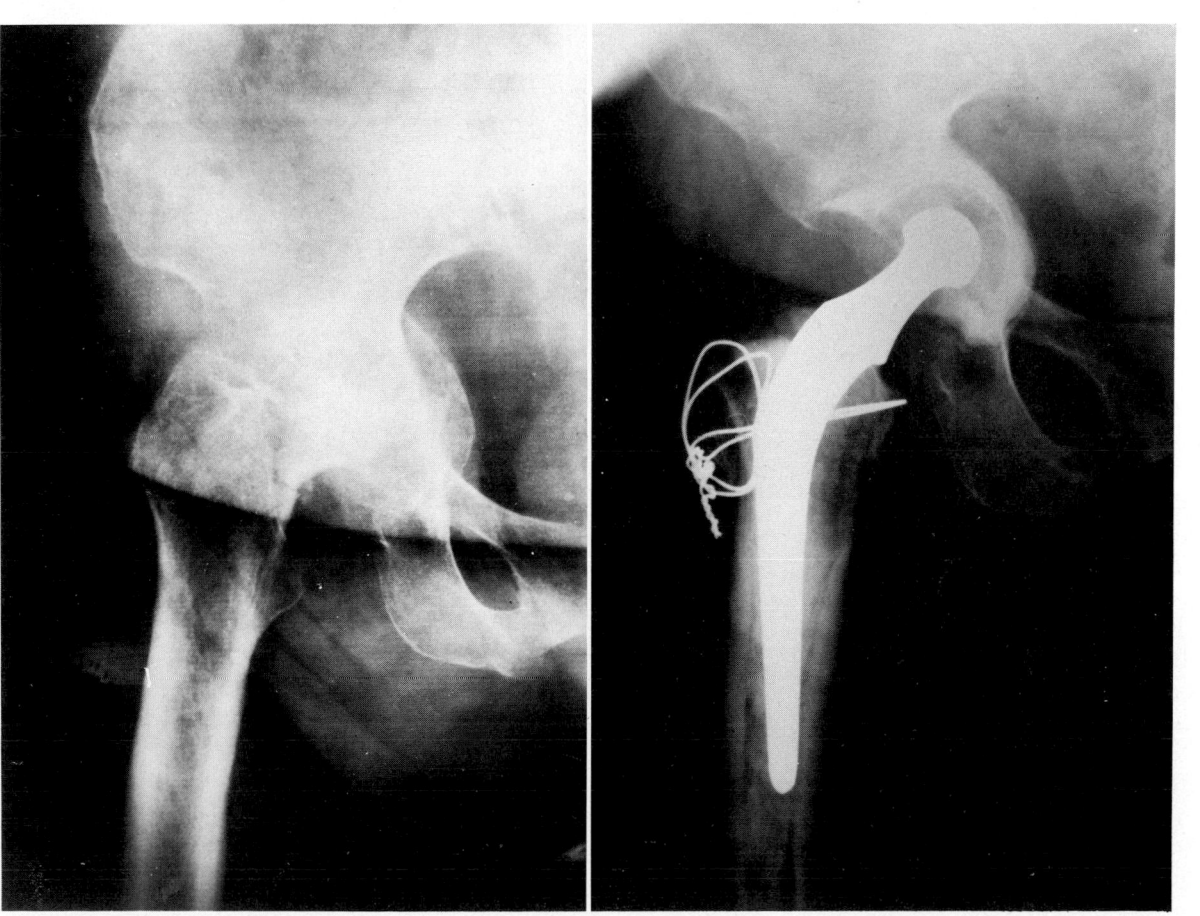

Fig. 10-35. A, Fractured neck of femur in 64-year-old woman with rheumatoid arthritis and severe protrusio acetabuli. **B,** Primary total hip arthroplasty was performed in view of preexisting arthritis in hip joint.

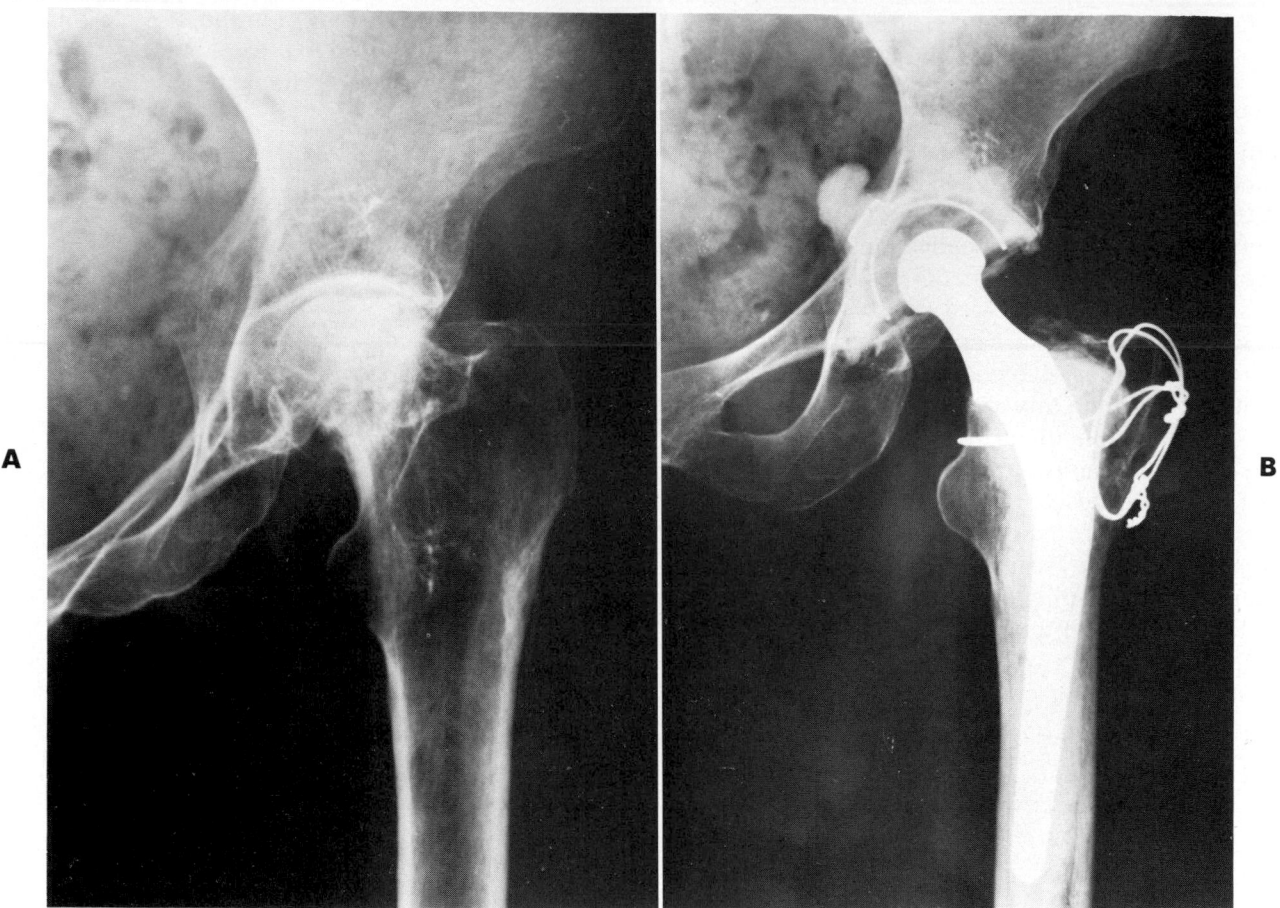

Fig. 10-36. A, Avascular necrosis of femoral head after fracture of femoral neck and internal fixation in 73-year-old female. Nail had been previously removed. **B,** Postoperative status after total hip arthroplasty. NOTE: femoral head collapse but only minor acetabular changes. Hemiarthroplasty is contraindicated in this situation. Preoperative grade was A-3,3,4; postoperative, A-6,6,6.

Further, because of the limited life expectancy of older patients with femoral neck fractures, concern about long-term complications of total hip arthroplasty may not be relevant.

Several factors argue against routine use of total hip arthroplasty in all hip fractures:

1. The high morbidity and mortality associated with total hip arthroplasty used in treating fresh femoral neck fractures.
2. The lack of available facilities and expertise to treat the large numbers of fractures involved if total hip arthroplasty is performed routinely.
3. The added burden to our already economically strained hospital system in dealing with the inherent postoperative complications and lengthy hospital stays of debilitated elderly patients.
4. The need for considerably smaller-sized implants, because the normal-sized acetabulum in women

is considerably smaller than one in an osteoarthritic hip.

5. No prosthetic replacement procedure of any kind—whether hemiarthroplasty or total arthroplasty—can substitute completely for the natural femoral head; if it can be reduced and fixed, the result is a normal or near-normal hip in most instances.

Treatment of Complications of Fracture Fixation

Because of the common occurrence of fractures of the neck of the femur in the elderly population, a relatively large number of total hip arthroplasties are being performed to correct the complications of fracture treatments. The most common initial procedure is fixation of the fracture by pins or screws, with or without side plates. Fractures are also treated by endoprostheses (unipolar or bipolar).

These procedures can become painful because of

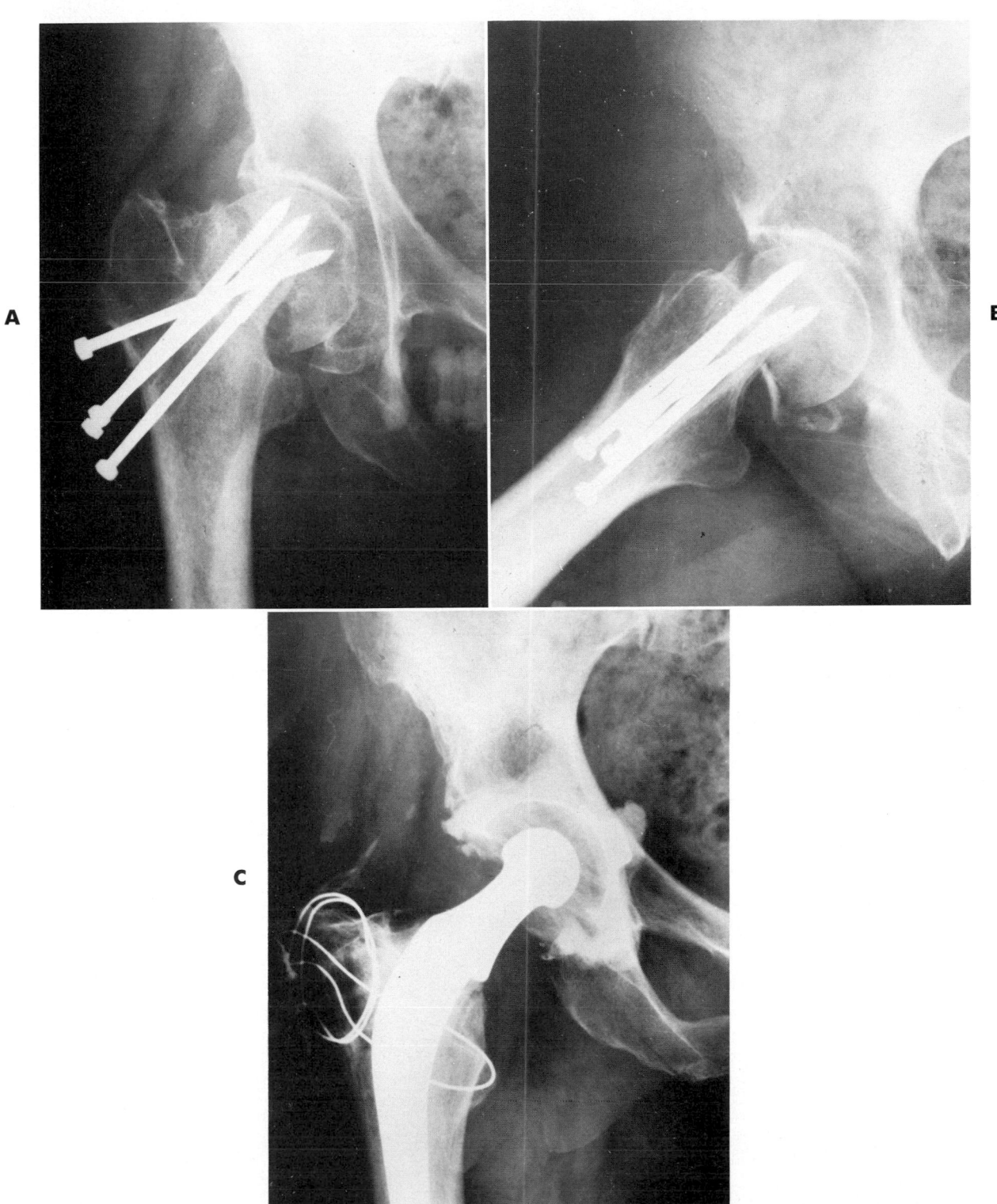

Fig. 10-37. A, Anteroposterior view. **B,** Lateral view of 63-year-old female 15 months after fracture fixation. NOTE: good joint space but severe osteoporosis. **C,** 6 years after total hip arthroplasty for nonunion of neck of femur.

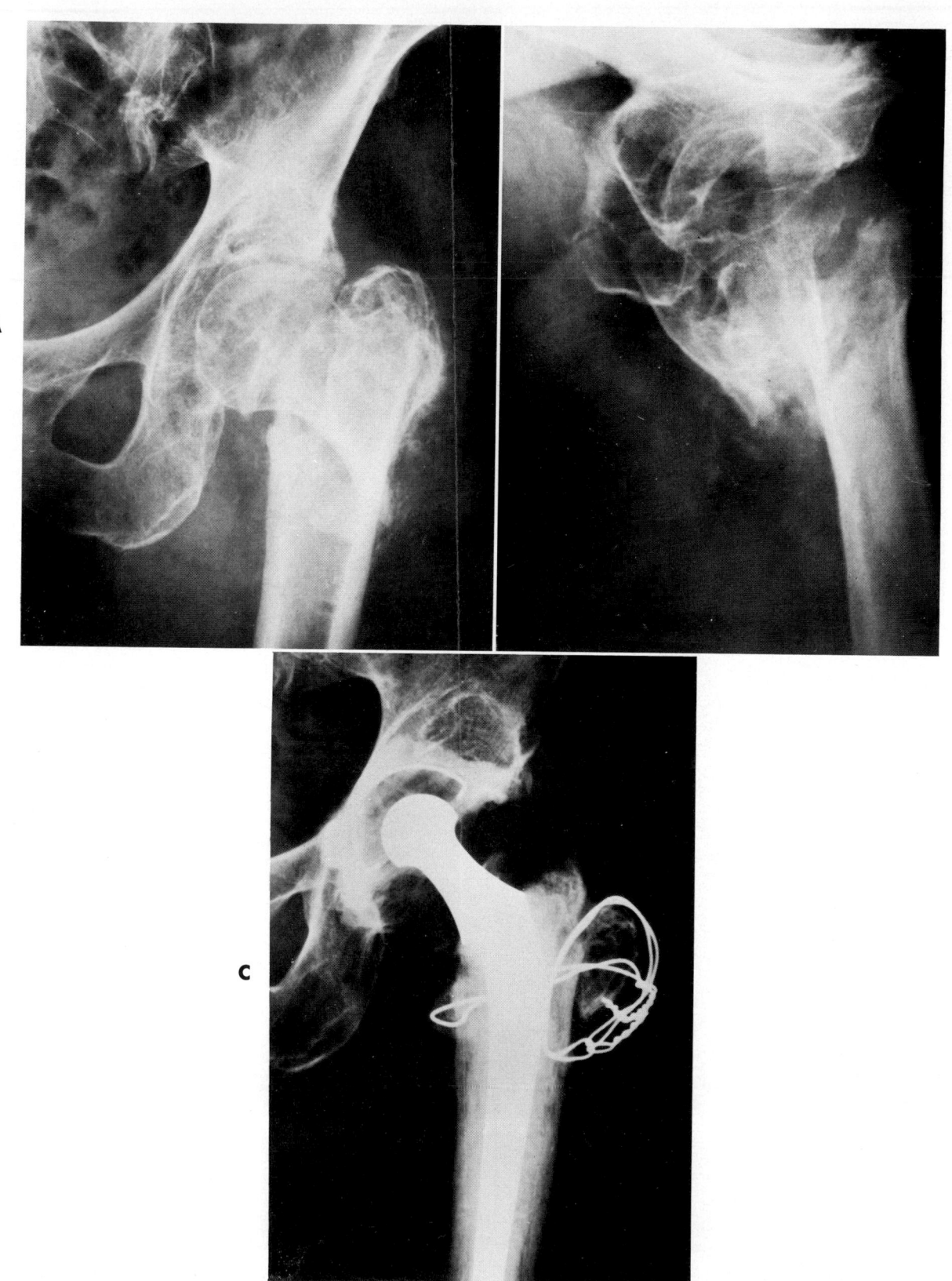

Fig. 10-38. A, Intertrochanteric fracture of neck of femur extending to shaft has been treated elsewhere by internal fixation and its subsequent removal. Patient had been kept nonweight bearing for approximately 6 months after removal of plate. **B,** Amount of displacement of fracture but no evidence of union at fracture site. Hemiarthroplasty is contraindicated because of severe osteoporosis and lack of articular cartilage nourishment during nonweight-bearing period. **C,** Postoperative total hip arthroplasty.

infection, nonunion, malunion, avascular necrosis, or migration of the prosthesis, for which conversion surgery is indicated (Figs. 10-37 and 10-38) (see Chapter 24).

The results of salvage procedures after fracture fixation are excellent but have a higher rate of complications than primary surgery.[117,143] The higher complication rate is caused by the patients' advanced age and by increased postoperative infection. A higher incidence of positive cultures from wounds of patients with previous operations has been observed.[57,60–62] The surgeon must identify the bacteria and use a prophylactic antibiotic both in the cement and systemically (see Chapters 5, 8, and 26).

Hip Fusion and Ankylosis Without Pain

Occasionally we are confronted with indications for total hip arthroplasty where there is no pain but advanced stiffness is present (Fig. 10-39). To achieve an adequate range of mobility in hips that have been completely ankylosed for many years, a bilateral operation is often needed. This is especially true when the lumbar spine is painful or the patient has another distal joint disability, such as a knee problem. It may also be a problem in young females whose hip joint arthritis have progressed to a stage where they have produced sexual difficulties. There is no guarantee that surgery will result in increased mobility, particularly if the patient has a very stiff hip preoperatively or has a tendency to form bone (as the result of previous surgery). Total hip arthroplasty complicated by heterotopic bone may be treated by revision surgery, especially if bilateral ankylosis is present or the stiff hip is in an unacceptable position (see Chapters 25 and 35).

Paget's Disease

Total hip arthroplasty is indicated in Paget's disease; hemiarthroplasty is contraindicated. Some surgeons have said that because of the pathological condition of the bone itself in Paget's disease, total hip arthroplasty may only partially relieve the pain. In this author's experience, however, total hip arthroplasty has been highly successful in relieving pain in hips with Paget's pelvis, femur, or both (Fig. 10-40). In fact, our experiences indicate that surgical results can be as good as in other conditions such as osteoarthritis of the hip joint. Because of the gradual process of bone deformity and the rapid rate of bone absorption and formation in this disease, it remains to be seen whether these results will be maintained; the ultimate rate of long-term "loosening" is unknown. Fractures of the femoral neck are notorious for their slow rate of healing. Furthermore, because of changes in the bone with Paget's disease of the upper femur, prosthetic replacement of the femoral head is not indicated, even

where the acetabulum appears normal. Prosthetic fixation without cement may not be successful; this author prefers to use cement for cup fixation.

Other results of total hip arthroplasty conform with our observations of high success after total hip arthroplasty in Paget's disease.[81,132] Medical treatment by diphosphonates, calcitonin-salmon, or other drugs is entirely independent of mechanical treatment of the diseased hip joint. Spontaneous and severe "rest pain" unrelated to activity must raise suspicions of sarcomatous changes of Paget's disease. It has recently been suggested that a high alkaline phosphate level, indicating rapid bone turnover, may cause excess bleeding intraoperatively. Such patients must be medically treated first to reduce blood loss.

ALTERNATIVES TO TOTAL HIP ARTHROPLASTY

In young and active individuals whose total hip arthroplasty has been effective only for a limited period, the surgeon must seek long-term alternatives. One of the most obvious yet neglected methods is avoidance or postponement of surgery by such methods as weight reduction, limitation of certain physical activities, and walking support (see Chapter 6). The other alternative is to improve the function of the hip joint by altering its biomechanics by performing an osteotomy before severe osteoarthritis develops. Naturally, these operative procedures must be considered early to prevent advanced arthrosis, which would require hip arthroplasty surgery too early in life.

These biological temporizing procedures must remove the pain significantly and improve quality of life until later in the patient's life, when total hip arthroplasty can more safely be performed. The surgeon should be sure that the alternative procedure will not severely alter the anatomy of the hip, thus jeopardizing the possibility of later total hip arthroplasty. Surgeons often find it difficult to justify procedures other than total hip arthroplasty: the results are often unpredictable and the procedures involve some morbidity and require long rehabilitation as compared with total hip arthroplasty.

In treating disabled patients between 20 and 40 years of age, I have stressed the nonoperative methods first but have also discussed surgical alternatives to total hip arthroplasty. Although most patients consider arthrodesis unacceptable, most young patients will agree to osteotomies as alternatives to total hip arthroplasty. Educating young patients about the potential advantages of biological procedures is essential before the patient and surgeon come to a mutual decision concerning treatment. These advantages should be weighed against the potential long-term risks of total hip arthroplasty and future revision procedures.

It has been estimated that the majority of early

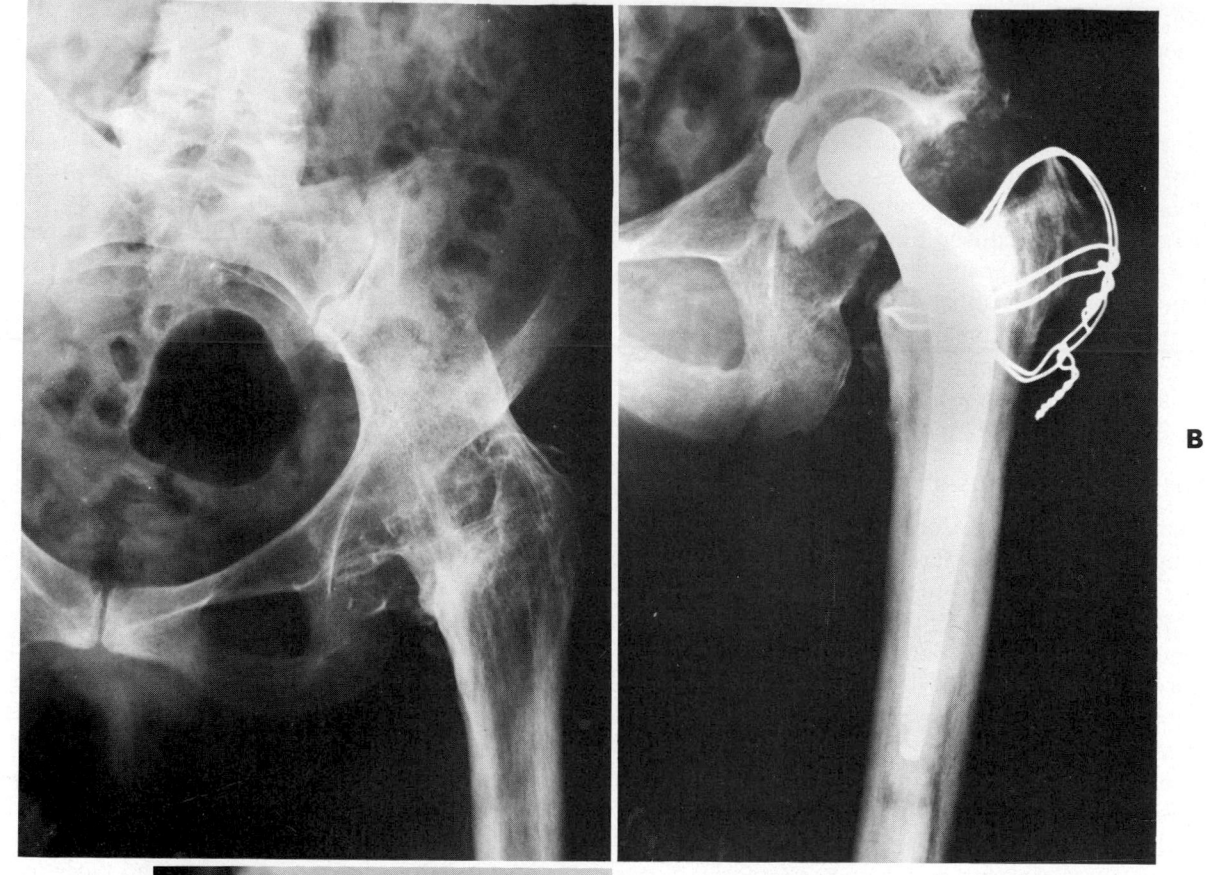

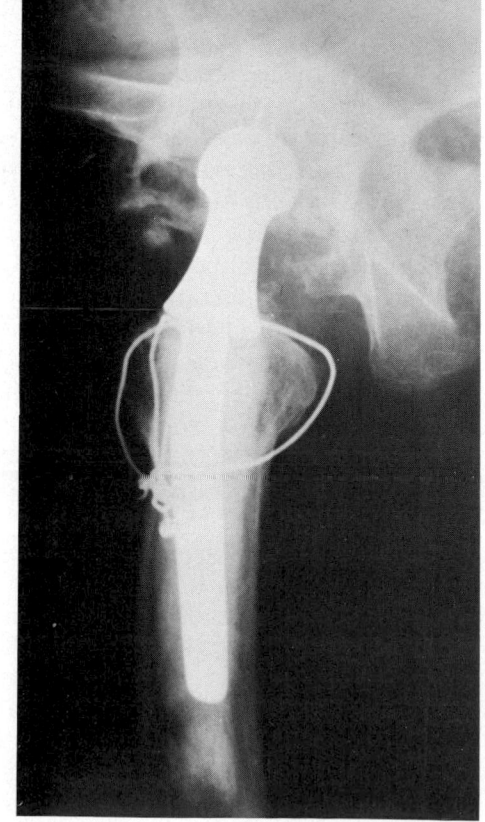

Fig. 10-39. Seventy-three-year-old woman (M.D.) with history of long-standing low back pain and left hip pain. Hip had been fused at age 30 for tuberculosis. Because of severe intractable back and ipsilateral knee pain, surgical intervention was necessary. **A,** Hip grade C-6,3,1. **B** and **C,** Postoperative grade C-6,5,5.

degenerative osteoarthritis of the hips can be attributed to some degrees of dysplasia.[98,133] It has been suggested that congenital dislocation of the hip, slipped capital femoral epiphyses, and Legg-Calvé-Perthes disease as developmental conditions, contribute considerably to early-onset osteoarthritis of the hips.[5] Aronson estimated that approximately 9000 new osteoarthritic hips in the United States are directly attributable to a preexisting congenital dysplasia of the hip, slipped capital femoral epiphyses, or Legg-Calvé-Perthes disease.[5] On the basis of these data, one can argue that a corrective osteotomy performed as early as possible after diagnosis might be indicated for most patients, with the hope of preventing early development of osteoarthritis of the hip. With certain provisions, the following procedures, based on this author's experience, have been used as alternatives to total hip arthroplasty in young-adult hip pathology:

1. Upper femoral osteotomy.
2. Pelvic osteotomy.
3. Shelf procedures.
4. Endoprostheses (bipolar).
5. Cup arthroplasties.
6. Resurfacing (double cup) arthroplasties.

Upper Femoral Osteotomy

Femoral osteotomies are used to achieve the following goals:

1. To improve the biomechanics of the hip by a varus, valgus, or rotation change.
2. To treat osteoarthritis of the hip.
3. To correct fixed deformities without altering the ankylosis or bony fusion by abduction, adduction, or rotation change.
4. To treat osteonecrosis.

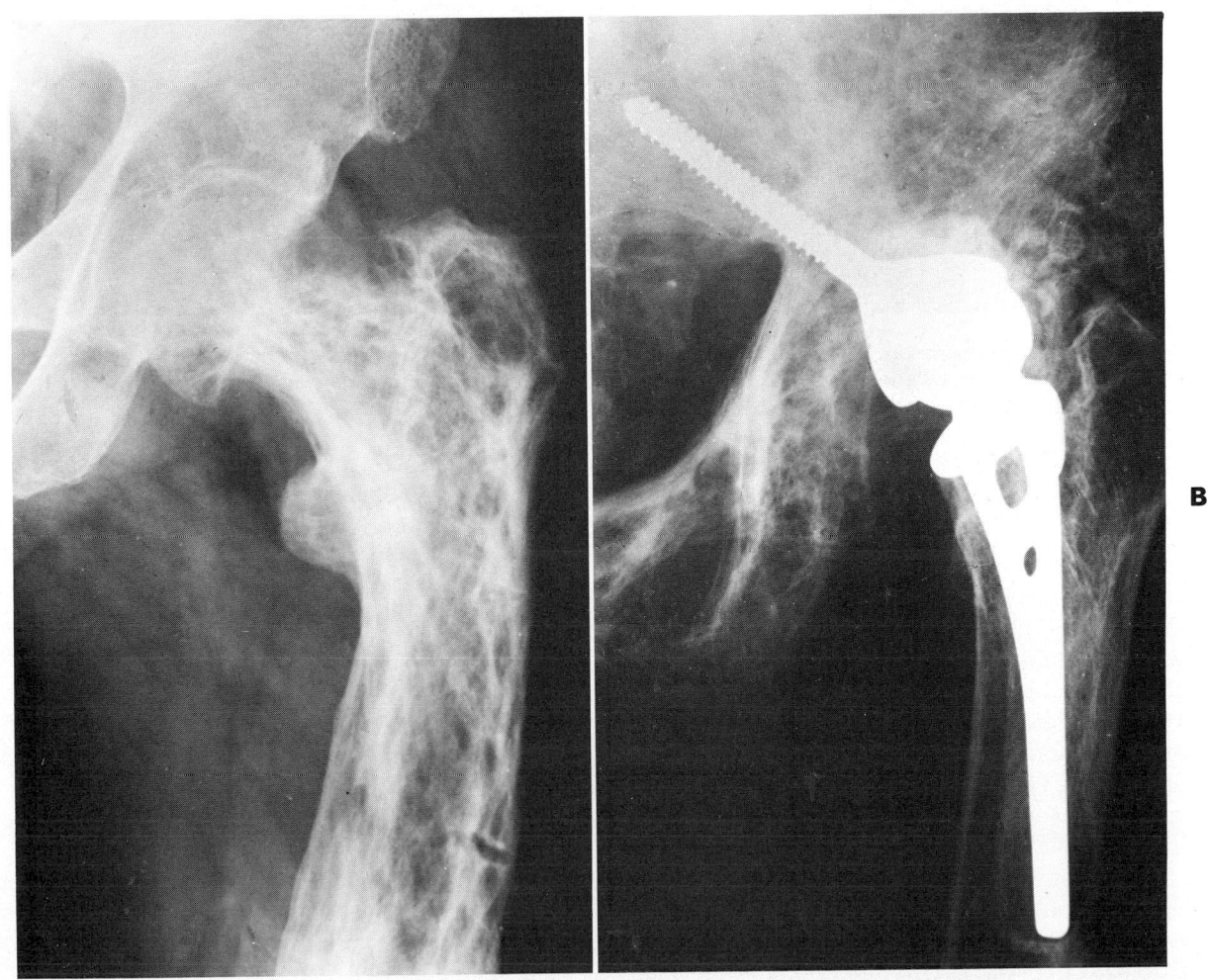

A

B

Fig. 10-40. A, Paget's disease and degenerative osteoarthrosis of left hip in 54-year-old man. **B,** 2 years after Ring total hip arthroplasty. note: marked loosening of both components and proximal migration as evidenced by sclerosis of weight-bearing portion of acetabulum.

Continued.

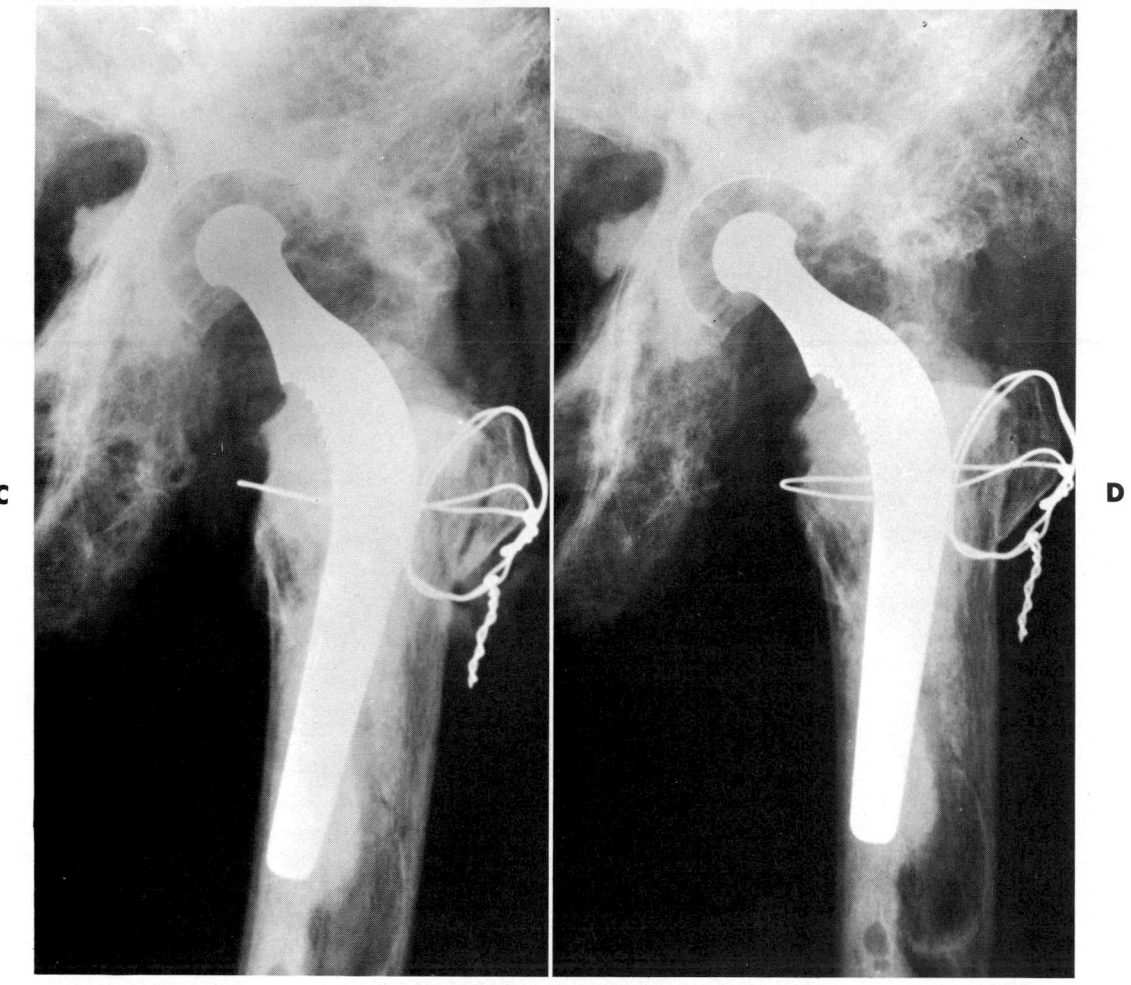

Fig. 10-40 — cont'd. C, Hip was converted to low-friction arthroplasty. **D,** Two years after arthroplasty with good functional results. Preoperative grade after Ring prosthesis (inserted elsewhere) was 2,2,2; postoperative result 2 years after surgery is 6,5,5.

Osteotomy to Improve Biomechanics of the Hip

Residual deformity of congenital dysplasia is best treated by osteotomy before osteoarthritis develops. However, symptoms of fatigue and pain and early degenerative osteoarthritis can be arrested by osteotomy. Radiological signs of dysplasia and early osteoarthritis are excellent indications for the upper femoral osteotomy.* In some instances, dysplastic acetabulum may also require correction, which must be addressed independently as a one- or two-stage operation.[120,123]

In hip dysplasia, two types of osteotomies are used, varus and valgus. Each may be combined with some degrees of derotation to accommodate excess anteversion.

VARUS OSTEOTOMY This operation is especially

indicated in patients in their late teens, twenties, or thirties to avoid a total hip arthroplasty. This type of osteotomy has been used extensively in Europe.[15,16,116]

The following principles must be observed regarding its indications:

1. Increased valgus or anteversion of the femoral neck (the coxa valga subluxant) must be present radiographically.
2. The head of the femur must be spherical by routine x-rays and CAT scan.
3. Presence of acetabular dysplasia is not a contraindication, but, when present, a pelvic osteotomy or an augmentation (shelf) procedure may be indicated as well.
4. The hip must have full or near-full range of motion.

---

* References 15, 16, 18, 105, 107.

5. Early degenerative changes and minimal arthritic pain without joint stiffness are not a contraindication.

6. Loss of abduction with or without lateral osteophyte is a contraindication for a varus osteotomy.

7. A combination of upper femoral osteotomy and pelvic osteotomy is feasible in a single stage, but it requires that the surgeon have experience and plan carefully before the operation.

Disadvantages of this osteotomy include the possibility of infection, shortening of the leg, persistent limp caused by weak abductors, and the need to remove the hardware.[15] However, pain relief and lasting results from this procedure are excellent.[17,94,116,119]

VALGUS OSTEOTOMY Bombelli and others[15,16,116] define a specific group of patients who benefit from this procedure. With the appearance of an elliptically shaped femoral head caused by flattening and the presence of an inferior medial marginal osteophyte, the neck assumes a marked valgus angulation. Several European surgeons have reported satisfactory results with this osteotomy.[15,19,94] This author has not used this type of osteotomy in congenital dysplasia of the hip. The pelvic-support osteotomy (severe valgus angulation osteotomy of the upper femur)[19,101] advocated by Lorenz and Buchelor must remain only of historical interest to the orthopedist; both cause severe disability resulting from deformity of the hips and knee and make total hip arthroplasty a complicated ordeal when necessary.

There are several indications for this procedure: conditions commonly resulting in coxa vara, such as congenital coxa vara, multiple epiphyseal dysplasia, nonunion or malunion of the neck of the femur, and slipped capital femoral epiphysis or fibrous dysplasia.

In choosing this surgery, the surgeon should observe the following principles:

1. The hip must have a normal or near-normal range of motion.

2. Minimal or no osteoarthritic changes should be visible by x-ray film.

3. Pain resulting from abduction of the hip is caused by impingement of the greater trochanter against the acetabular rim and not the arthritic joint. The source of pain can be verified by intraarticular injections of Novocain.

4. Presence of a coxa vara or coxa breva may require elongation of the trochanter and a lateral and distal transposition of the greater trochanter in addition to a valgus osteotomy.

5. Plans for a valgus osteotomy for malunion or nonunion of the femoral neck fracture must include radionucleid scintigraphy to demonstrate viability of the femoral head.

BIPLANE AND TRIPLANE OSTEOTOMIES Correction osteotomies of triplane deformity of slipped capital femoral epiphyses are best planned at the intertrochanteric level for rapid healing and stability of the osteotomy. This author has successfully corrected moderate-to-severe deformities of slipped capital femoral epiphysis (types II and III). Others have shown that excellent results (based on the long-term clinical studies) can be achieved.[31,50] Triplane osteotomies at the subtrochanteric level are slow to heal and cause severe deformities, rendering subsequent hip arthroplasty difficult (see Chapter 24).

A bipolar or total hip arthroplasty in a young patient with a unilateral hip condition and no other disabilities is not an alternative to osteotomy for this predictable short-term outcome.

The coxa plana, coxa magna, and coxa vara deformity caused by fibrous dysplasia may be helped by a valgus osteotomy. Osteotomies may also be combined with a derotational component and bone graft if indicated.

Femoral Osteotomies for Osteoarthritis

Primary or idiopathic osteoarthritis without deformity is not a candidate for osteotomies. Neither mechanical nor biological theories justify the risk of disability associated with the femoral osteotomy to be performed for osteoarthritis of the hip. As previously mentioned, good-to-excellent results may be anticipated in performing corrective osteotomies where deformity has caused symptoms and even where degenerative changes are attributable to a mismatch of the femoral head and the acetabulum. The confusion about interpreting the results of osteotomy in the past was related to the indication for this procedure being ill-defined. Accordingly the students of osteotomy schools often use the same argument for or against a given type of osteotomy. During the pre-total-hip-arthroplasty era, osteotomies were performed with the ideal of changing the biomechanics of the hip and thus reducing the load on the hip joint.[98,99,104,106] In most reports a beneficial effect was also attributed to osteotomy independent of the mechanical changes, because it relieved pain in nearly 75% of the patients.[64,65]

While Pauwels was considered a significant force in popularizing osteotomies based on biomechanical principles,[110–112] during the post-total-hip-arthroplasty era, osteotomies have become more exacting operations in their indications and techniques. These refinements owe much to our European colleagues, among whom Professor M. Muller and Renalto Bombelli must be recognized.

Corrective Osteotomies for Fixed Deformities

In patients who have a unilateral painless ankylosed hip or arthrodesis, disability can result from fixed deformity. A combination of a single- or multiple-plane deformity such as adduction/abduction/flexion and rotation deformity often leads to back or knee pain (ipsilateral or contralateral). Some of the chronic changes in the spine or knee are secondary osteoarthritic in nature, which should be evaluated. However, when the hip is fused or ankylosed with no discernible motion in young and active individuals (with or without previous history of infection), a corrective osteotomy should be performed. Because the corrective osteotomy often relieves the knee or back pain and adds to the length of the extremity, the results can be gratifying in young and active patients. When the surgeon discovers any hip motion under anesthesia, insertion of one or two pins across the joint (without a formal arthrodesis) leads to spontaneous fusion of the joints after intertrochanteric osteotomy.

Femoral Osteotomy for Avascular Necrosis

With Sujiokas's good results from rotational osteotomy,[134] there has been a resurgence of interest in osteotomy for osteonecrosis of the femoral head. Unfortunately, the operation is technically demanding, and the results in Europe and the United States have not been superior to those achieved by simple flexion osteotomy. The exact role of osteotomies for osteonecrosis has not been well defined. In Europe, where osteotomies are more frequently performed, osteotomies for avascular necrosis have a definite place in the surgeon's armamentarium. The rationale for the use of osteotomies is to place a healthy portion of the head into a new load-bearing position. The surgeon accomplishes this by performing a flexion or rotational osteotomy, moving the necrotic zone of the head further anterior and inferior, and allowing the healthy posterior portion to assume the weight-bearing position, the apical zone. When the necrotic zone is not contained as seen on the anteroposterior view, some degree of varus component, in addition to flexion, is beneficial. Preoperative x-ray films, including abduction/adduction views, should help determine the needed degrees of correction. Wagner recommended 10 to 15 degrees of valgus (to improve biomechanical efficiency) and 40 to 50 degrees flexion (in sagittal plane).[149] Ganz advocated a flexion osteotomy of 30 to 50 degrees without abduction or adduction and transfer of the greater trochanter distally and laterally.[73] The latter is performed to avoid trochanteric impingement.

In summary, we can conclude that osteotomies by flexion and valgus (Wagner) or single plane with transference of greater trochanter (Ganz) and rotation osteotomy (Sujioka) may be indicated, based on the surgeon's experience and preference. This author has combined a single sagittal plant intertrochanteric osteotomy with some degrees of varus to bring the necrotic zone within the acetabular boundary and remove it from the heavily loaded apex.

Contraindications to Osteotomy

With rare exceptions, osteotomies are contraindicated for patients over 60 years of age. In this age group, when disability is not severe, nonoperative means should be adequate until a total hip arthroplasty is indicated. The morbidity and unpredictability of the osteotomy do not justify it as an alternative to total hip arthroplasty. Osteotomy is contraindicated in the absence of anatomical deformity with anticipated correction by osteotomy.

Osteotomy is also contraindicated for patients who lack understanding, have unreasonable expectations, and are not likely to cooperate in their postoperative care. It is important that the patient understand why a total hip arthroplasty is not being performed. In such cases, more than one visit to discuss surgery is essential. The possibility of nonunion or delayed union of the osteotomy and the possible need for supportive supplemental casts must be discussed. Many hips become stiffer after surgery, despite improved pain relief.

Regardless of their age, patients with the following conditions are not good candidates for osteotomy: systemic diseases such as inflammatory or rheumatoid arthritis (including juvenile rheumatoid arthritis, lupus, and ankylosing spondylitis), infection, metabolic bone diseases, and the need to take immunosuppressive drugs. It should be emphasized that osteotomy is an exacting operation, carrying complications such as nonunion or malunion and undercorrection or overcorrection. Postoperative wound infection is the most serious complication of this procedure.

Pelvic Osteotomies

Periacetabular osteotomies are described for augmentation and head coverage in young adults with hip pain and early osteoarthritis.[43,44,66,148] Like proximal osteotomies, femoral periacetabular pelvic osteotomies should be recommended early to prevent or arrest early osteoarthrosis in young adults. Ideally (as with femoral osteotomies), pelvic osteotomies should be performed before pain or radiological signs of joint narrowing appear, although with appropriate technique, properly selected patients with mild osteoarthritis have also benefited from this operation. Chiari and others advocated this procedure for advanced degenerative osteoarthritis.[45] Most experienced surgeons consider it a useful procedure for hip dysplasia with or without signs of osteoarthritis. Additionally, it provides an improved bone stock for subsequent total hip arthroplasty. In planning a pelvic support osteotomy, the following principles must be considered:

1. The patient must have discomfort, pain, or fatigue in addition to a limp resulting from hip joint overload.
2. Acetabular dysplasia must be documented by routine radiographs and CAT scans with three-dimensional reconstruction.[33]
3. Potential mechanical improvements must be verified by examining the hip under image intensification and by placing the femoral head in various degrees of rotation and abduction to determine the femoral head coverage.
4. Three-dimensional imaging of the bone from CAT scan can be of extreme value to determine the usefulness of the planned osteotomy.[152]
5. Unlike femoral osteotomies, which can significantly alter the shape of the femur, pelvic osteotomies enhance the acetabular coverage for future arthroplasty.
6. Other osteotomies in the periacetabular region (Chiari, Salter, Dial) are equally effective in relieving pain. The anatomical morphology of the acetabulum and the surgeon's training and experience should play a role in the decision. This author prefers the Chiari osteotomy combined with a bone graft in severe acetabular dysplasia, as advocated by Simmons.[123]
7. Consider osteotomy of the upper femur if the residual deformity of the femur also contributes to the dysplasia. The femoral osteotomy can be performed as a second stage or simultaneously with the acetabular osteotomy.
8. For the combination of pelvic osteotomy and upper femoral osteotomy in adults to be safe and effective, the surgeon must be expert in performing osteotomies and take great care during preoperative planning.

Hip Arthrodesis

Hip arthrodesis in the era of total hip arthroplasty has a limited but definite place, one that the student of total hip arthroplasty must keep in mind as an alternative to total hip replacement. A hip arthrodesis in young patients (in their twenties and thirties) can eliminate pain and restore function dramatically. This procedure enables the patient to hold a job and participate in physically demanding activities, including sports, most of which are prohibited after total hip arthroplasty.[32,55]

The surgeon should offer hip fusion with confidence and a positive attitude. It is important that the patient understand that hip arthrodesis is a time-tested procedure with excellent long-term results; in fact, it can be converted to a total hip arthroplasty after many years, should it be necessary (see Chapter 24). A review of long-term studies of results of hip fusion[28,128] indicates that a high percentage of patients were satisfied with the outcome of their operations. A near-normal function and a productive lifestyle were possible with arthrodesis.[96] With a fusion rate of 91% in a series of 500 arthrodeses, Liechti also reported a high rate of success and employability.[92] Therefore arthrodesis as a surgical procedure should not be regarded as an outmoded procedure but should remain in the surgeon's armamentarium.

A successful arthrodesis of the hip results in a durable, painless joint with a functional and productive life of 20 to 30 years. On the debit side, a successful arthrodesis can be achieved only 80% to 85% of the time, 15% to 20% of the patients requiring further refusion surgery. A prolonged period of immobilization including application of hip spica cast is necessary. At best, the functional result is never as good as with arthroplasty. More significantly, only a few patients consent to a hip fusion rather than a total hip arthroplasty, which offers immediate relief of pain and a return to excellent function.

The following are this author's present indications for arthrodesis of the hip:

1. Unilateral degenerative osteoarthritis (ideally traumatic in origin) in male patients under age 30 without other joint disability. There should be no spine or knee joint involvement.
2. Hip infection in patients under 30 years of age with pain and loss of joint space.
3. Painful failed slipped capital femoral epiphyses, treated or untreated, complicated by chrondrolysis and secondary degenerative osteoarthritis.
4. Failure of multiple joint arthroplasty (unilateral) with or without infection.[86]
5. Paralytic conditions in which pain is severe and patient's muscle paralysis precludes a total hip arthroplasty.
6. Patients with mental retardation who may not be treated by total hip arthroplasty because of the lack of cooperation.
7. As an alternative to a Girdlestone pseudoarthrosis in young and active patients.[151]

Hemiarthroplasty

Primary indications for endoprosthesis since its introduction in the early 1950s by Moore and Thompson were for fresh femoral neck fractures or their complications, such as nonunion or avascular necrosis of the femoral head, in spite of a high incidence of late acetabular erosion, migration, or both, in addition to stem loosening.[102] Experimental data have clearly demonstrated that early loss of proteoglycan in carti-lage follows fibrillation and progressive loss of cartilage as a result of contact with metal. At present, a unipolar prosthesis is an accepted method of treatment for a freshly fractured neck of the femur in medically high-risk patients of advanced age and for fractures for which fixation is difficult and early ambulation is desirable.

Bipolar Endoprosthesis

Bipolar endoprosthesis, introduced by Bateman[11] and Giliberty,[75] has the following theoretical advantages:

1. Reduction of acetabular cartilage erosion by the low-friction properties of inner bearing.
2. Increased range of motion of the hip by its double-bearing design, and thus increased range of motion of the prostheses.
3. Decreased shock load and dumping effect via high-density polyethylene segment.
4. Ease of revision when necessary.
5. Decreased incidence of dislocation secondary to increased range of motion of prostheses.

Despite several theoretical advantages attributable to bipolar endoprosthesis in clinical practice, available data suggest that the results of bipolar devices are apparently only marginally better than those of the single-unit (monopolar) femoral head prosthesis. Con-sequently, some experienced surgeons have ques-tioned whether they should be indicated for routine use in the absence of well-controlled studies and have pointed out some of their distinct disadvantages[108]:

1. Bipolar prostheses are more expensive.
2. Most reports claim that operating time is longer.
3. In cases of postoperative dislocation, reduction is often impossible, requiring open reduction.
4. Failure of inner bearing (wear and creep with fractures) and dissociation of the bipolar ele-ments have been reported as a complication resulting from dislocation, requiring an open reduction, revision, or both.[100]
5. The long-term effects of wear particles of high-density polyethylene on the acetabular cartilage remain unknown.

While the basic premise that increased motion at the inner bearing reduces the stress in the acetabular cartilage, controversy exists as to the degree of motion between the inner and outer bearings. For example, Chen and associates[41] and Verberne[145] demonstrated that there was no persistent motion at the inner bearing; thus the prosthesis functioned as a monopolar device,[41,42,145] but Mess and Barmada[100] concluded that there was about equal motion between the inner and outer bearings of the bipolar prosthesis under

unloaded conditions. Other studies suggest that some movements persist between the prosthetic head and high-density polyethylene.[13,27,79,135] Others have sug-gested that lack of uniformity in the design of various types of bipolar devices and the fact that they are used to treat several different conditions may account for the disparate in vivo kinematics that have been observed; thus, reactive repair tissue and the presence or absence of cartilage in the acetabulum may play a part in these varied observations.

Bipolar Prosthesis for Treatment of Fractures

Several retrospective studies suggest that the results after insertion of bipolar prostheses show a marginal improvement compared with the unilateral prosthesis. In a large series of more than 1000 bipolar prostheses used at the Mayo Clinic, Cabanela concluded that bipolar prostheses results were only marginally better than unipolar prostheses in treating fracture of the neck of the femur in older and less active patients, however, the use of bipolar prostheses was superior in treatment of younger patients with avascular necrosis and fractured neck of the femur.[27] In their original study of bipolar prostheses, Drinker and Murray found no difference in operative complications between a bipolar and a unipolar prosthesis. They did find, however, that there were more postoperative disloca-tions requiring open reduction after 101 Bateman prostheses than after 160 cemented Thompson pros-theses.[56] Several recent studies suggest better short-term results of bipolar prostheses over fixed-head devices used for fractured neck of the femur.* Neither demographics nor technical details related to the results in these studies (some with short-term follow-up) are definitive.

Bipolar Endoprostheses and Avascular Necrosis

The concept of femoral head replacement for avascular necrosis is not new. Previous reports showed good early results but subsequent deterioration in many series thus far reported.[4] As stated elsewhere, with any degree of femoral head collapse, the corresponding weight-bearing zone of the acetabulum should be regarded as abnormal. This is so despite the absence of radiological changes (Ficat stage II). In fact, with head collapse the joint space may radiographically appear to have in-creased. This author's opinion is that endoprosthetic replacement after any degree of head collapse is contraindicated because (1) the patients are often young and not sufficiently disabled to warrant a hip replacement, and (2) regardless of the type of en-doprosthesis (unipolar or bipolar), the abnormal wear caused by preexisting cartilage fibrillation against a

---

* References 13, 87, 88, 91, 103, 135, 146, 153.

metal bearing is unavoidable, which prompts the patient to seek early corrective surgery by total hip arthroplasty.[47,52] An endoprosthesis is not a conservative operation; it violates the normal architecture of the femur and predisposes the patient to infection (see Chapter 24). According to one contemporary view, a bipolar prosthesis may obviate the acceleration in cartilage wear. This view has not yet been substantiated.

When a bipolar replacement is used for stage III or IV avascular necrosis, an acetabular migration is to be expected. Several recent reports of short-term follow-up studies substantiate that consistency is lacking in use of bipolar prostheses for treating osteoarthritis of the hip.[12,33,144] A deteriorating result clinically and radiologically may be expected because of acetabular migration, as further follow-up studies have shown.[67,72,97] Although 24 of 25 patients reported by Torisu at 2 to 6 years had no pain, acetabular migration ranging from 0 to 10 mm had been observed in many of the patients.[137] Interestingly, bipolar prostheses may be clinically acceptable for pain relief despite radiographic migration of the prosthesis. In a study by Wetherell and Hinves on 47 hips with osteoarthritis treated by bipolar prosthesis (average 5-year follow-up), only 74% had no pain or only mild discomfort.[150] Although a survival study indicated an 82% survival at 7 years in nearly half of the patients, 22 prostheses had migrated more than 2 mm.

In summary, based on personal experience and the data available in the literature, the prime indication for bipolar prosthesis is when an endoprosthesis is indicated; therefore, intercapsular and certain intertrochanteric fractures in older individuals may be reasonably treated by bipolar prosthesis. A bipolar prosthesis may also be preferred over a fixed-head endoprosthesis for early avascular necrosis. However, well-controlled studies with longer follow-up would be required to establish the true indications for bipolar prosthesis. This author prefers a fixed-socket prosthesis for stage III or IV avascular necrosis. The less common use of bipolar devices is for severe protrusio acetabuli after severe loss of acetabular bone stock when a fixed socket is not technically feasible (see Chapter 22).

Cup (Mold) Arthroplasty

This procedure is of historical significance. Cup (mold) arthroplasty as an interpositioning arthroplasty was described and popularized by Smith-Peterson as a modulation of a natural and biological repair process. This procedure includes removal of the diseased articular cartilage and bone to create a smooth surface in the acetabulum and on the femoral head. Then a highly polished cup made of Vitallium (a chromium-

cobalt alloy) is inserted as an interpositioning material. A formal fixation between the cup and the acetabulum is not intended or achieved, and this promotes formation of tissue. Under gentle range-of-motion exercises and a period of non–weight bearing, a fibrocartilage often resulted. The initial intention was for this to be a two-stage operation; the second stage included removing the interpositioning cup after the development of matured "molded" hyaline cartilage.[48] Subsequently, however, the cup was retained. In the hands of experts this procedure yielded as high as 80% to 85% good results.[6–10,124–127]

Although cup arthroplasty could be successful, pain relief after this procedure was inconsistent and loss of range of motion was often a serious problem, especially in bilateral hip disease. The length of required postoperative rehabilitation was up to 6 months, including protected weight bearing. When total hip arthroplasty was introduced, with its predictable and reproducible results, cup arthroplasty procedures were soon abandoned. This procedure was discontinued at the author's institution after the introduction of the Charnley low-friction arthroplasty technique in early 1969. Curiously, even today, extensive sections of texts refer to this procedure, yet none of the authors continue to use this technique in their practices.[48] This author can find no indication for cup arthroplasty at the present time because of the availability of the alternatives cited in this chapter.

Resurfacing ("Double-Cup") Procedures

Because of the mechanical failures of stemmed (conventional) total hip arthroplasty procedures, several European surgeons* and American surgeons[1,3,29,30] began to investigate a new procedure that eliminated the need for intramedullary stem fixation in total hip arthroplasty. Regarded as a more conservative approach, this was thought to be suitable for young and active individuals. The theoretical advantages attributed to the resurfacing procedure were preservation of the femoral head and the integrity of the upper femur by avoiding intramedullary fixation. The theoretical advantages are inadequate to compensate for the procedure's poor short-term durability, which results from the unavoidable use of a thin-walled acetabular component and thin acrylic cement mantle.[2] It is of historical interest that Charnley experimented with this procedure using Teflon as a bearing material in the 1950s. Early failures led him to abandon it.[39,40]

The failure of resurfacing procedures may be attributed to the following biomechanical failures:

1. Preserved femoral heads leave no alternative but

to use a thin high-density polyethylene cup and a thin layer of cement for socket fixation.

2. An alternative to the use of a thin high-density polyethylene cup and a thin cement layer is to expand the acetabulum, thus damaging the bony support.

3. Successful long-term results of low-friction arthroplasty have proven the soundness of the procedure, which uses a small head against a thick plastic. Such a combination also enables the prosthesis to subluxate momentarily under traumatic conditions beyond its designated range of motion, which acts as a "safety valve" to protect the socket against loosening.[34]

In clinical practice, most surgeons have now abandoned this procedure in favor of the conventional stemmed devices for all types of replacement arthroplasty. At present, this author can identify no indication for routine use of resurfacing procedures. However, this procedure may be indicated as an alternative to total hip arthroplasty when the stem of a hip prosthesis cannot be accommodated because of deformity or infection in the proximal femur. A cementless porous-coated resurfacing procedure has recently been introduced.

For indications for cemented total hip arthroplasty, cementless total hip arthroplasty, and indications for hybrid hips, see Chapter 15.

SUMMARY OF ESSENTIALS

- The extra work load imposed by total hip arthroplasty on clinics and outpatient offices poses the problem of choosing the appropriate patients for the procedure. This is particularly complicated if a nonspecialized surgeon occasionally selects a patient for total hip arthroplasty. The newer procedures should be considered only if they have been adequately tested in controlled clinical studies for comparison with more traditional procedures, some of which have been in use over 20 to 30 years.

- While awaiting the long-term results of the newer techniques, surgeons are well advised to ascertain objective signs of disability before deciding to operate. Patients will be grateful for the surgeon's decision to postpone the procedure when it is based on such logical grounds.

- Although faced with pressure from the media and patients to use the newest technology, which may have achieved spectacular results, the surgeon must resist this pressure when clinical evidence as to its efficacy is lacking.

- One of the most difficult aspects of total hip arthroplasty is selecting the patients. It is not generally realized that radiographic manifestation by itself is not an indication for hip arthroplasty. As time passes and the field evolves, indications may be altered and selection criteria for patients may be modified.

- At the time of this writing, 3 decades after the first total hip arthroplasty using acrylic cement and high-density polyethylene, it is agreed that the operation is suitable for aged patients with degenerative arthritis or rheumatoid conditions. The operation remains unchallenged because it can produce spectacular results, such as relief of pain, increased mobility, and preservation of mobility without extensive physiotherapeutic management.

- When possible, the operation must be reserved for patients with osteoarthritis over 60 years of age or those who are close to retirement; it may be considered in younger patients who are affected by systemic conditions leading to a shortened life expectancy.

- In patients with systemic disease, such as rheumatoid or ankylosing polyarthritis, surgery may be performed at almost any age when other joints remain a disabling factor.

- Osteotomy and arthrodesis are not effective in patients with bilateral hip disease. However, patients in a younger age group may be accepted despite lack of other disabling factors.

- Detailed consideration must be given to patient selection and the sequence of bilateral hip operations. Hip surgery may be particularly indicated to promote mobility when the patient has bilateral hip disease.

- When a patient has a failed total hip arthroplasty in one hip and an arthritic hip on the other side, the surgeon should perform the primary surgery first and then plan for the revision surgery. This plan gives the patient a good weight-bearing extremity, facilitating recovery from the second operation.

- In planning bilateral hip surgery, it usually is advisable to operate on the more symptomatic hip, observe the results, and project surgery of the second hip for a later date. Exceptions to this rule include patients who are in their seventies, those with severe fixed deformity, and those who have already had a failed operation on one hip with the second hip becoming symptomatic.

- Bilateral hip arthroplasty during the same anesthesia is recommended, but to minimize morbidity it should only be performed in a highly organized center for this type of operation with a first-class operating team.

- Recent experience suggests that patients with low-grade infection or those with good bone stock and bacteria sensitive to commonly used antimicrobial agents can be accepted for total hip arthroplasty provided the patient is willing to accept failure of the procedure should infection recur.

- In general, it is a good policy to advise against total hip arthroplasty in the following conditions: if the patient has unilateral hip disease, is under 60 years of age, and can continue to work without undue disability; where the pain and disability do not require pain medications or support with a cane; where the principal motivation is participation in sports activities; if the patient is overweight (over 200 pounds) and is not willing to reduce weight before surgery; and if infections caused by gram-negative organisms or active infection or osteomyelitis of the upper femur and pelvis are present.

- Obesity is a relative contraindication for surgery. Both surgeon and patient are advised to postpone a decision regarding surgery until the patient has reduced his or her weight to an optimal level.

- Pain is the cardinal sign and the major determining factor in advising total hip arthroplasty The source of pain and the patient's motivation in seeking advice should be clarified before any decision for surgery. For the next decade at least, surgeons are well advised to be certain they are operating for objective signs and symptoms. No patient should be considered for surgery if his or her present condition would be exacerbated should complications arise necessitating removal of the prosthetic device (Girdlestone pseudarthrosis test).

- Patients in their forties and fifties present a difficult problem even when severe disability is present. These patients may be cautiously selected for total hip arthroplasty if they understand that further surgery may be necessary if mechanical failure develops. In a teenager or young adult with unilateral hip disease of traumatic origin, arthrodesis is the best solution.

- While awaiting the long-term results of total hip arthroplasty, it is advisable to delay operating on active and vigorous patients who can tolerate the delay. Surgery based purely on the patient's demand should be refused, especially when objective disability is not present. This is particularly true in patients who are too young or too obese or whose subjective complaint does not correlate with objective findings.

- Although patients considering total hip arthroplasty have been examined previously by referring physicians and may be psychologically prepared to undergo total hip arthroplasty, the surgeon's decision must be completely independent of the recommendations and evaluations of the referring physician. It should be based on objective findings.

- When selecting young and active patients for total hip arthroplasty, it is best as a general rule to postpone the decision until a second interview. Preferably these patients should return with a close family member to help them fully understand the significance of the surgery. The patient must understand that total hip surgery is an irreversible procedure to be considered only when all other alternatives have been eliminated.

- An assessment of the patient's motivation is essential. Leading questions will help the surgeon assess the impact of the hip disability on the patient's life in work and recreation and whether the client is seeking correction primarily to continue hobbies and sports.

- The surgeon who selects a young patient for surgery must acknowledge a threefold responsibility: advising the patient of the potential risks involved, including further intervention if needed; accepting the responsibility of performing a technically perfect operation; and accepting the moral responsibility of an unwritten contract to provide future service should it become necessary. It is mandatory that a surgeon involved in total hip arthroplasty commit himself or herself to providing "maintenance operations" as needed.

- An important element to assess when considering a young patient for total hip arthroplasty is how cooperative the patient is likely to be in protecting the hip against dislocation, fracture, and other injuries and his or her willingness to maintain an optimal body weight and avoid athletic activities after surgery. A history of drug addiction and alcohol abuse may alert the surgeon to a possible lack of cooperation.

- A history of psychiatric disorders (including depression, hysteria, neurosis, and even Alzheimer's) is not an absolute contraindication to total hip arthroplasty. Consideration must be given, however, to the postoperative care of these patients.

- We hope it will be possible one day to replace hip joints in young people whose main concern is not so much pain but appearance. This is especially relevant to congenital dysplasia of the hip joint, which is the most difficult and challenging problem. But the young age and potential vigor of these patients would subject today's arthroplasties to enormous strain and wear; these patients should be encouraged to delay the decision for surgery as long as possible.

- The surgeon must give special consideration to hip arthroplasty associated with the following conditions: scoliosis; systemic disease; rare, congenital, and developmental conditions; bone tumors; neurovascular conditions of the limb; neurological disorders; neurotrophic joints (Charcot's); hemophilia; conditions that prevent walking; and avascular necrosis in patients with renal or cardiac transplants. An extensive medical evaluation of patients with these conditions is necessary if a total hip arthroplasty is proposed.

- Under certain circumstances a hemiarthroplasty or bipolar arthroplasty is preferred to a total hip arthroplasty. These circumstances generally involve fresh fractures of the hip. Prosthetic replacement of the femoral head must be reserved for patients whose fractures cannot be reduced, who have conditions that may limit ambulation, or who cannot be treated satisfactorily by external fixation of their fractures. Also, as a rule the use of endoprostheses and bipolar devices should be restricted to fresh femoral neck fractures with a normal acetabular cartilage. A femoral head replacement or bipolar prosthesis is commonly preferred with Parkinson's disease.

- Total hip arthroplasty after fracture of the neck of the femur is indicated if there is acetabular cartilage erosion; in rheumatoid arthritis; in preexisting osteoarthritis; in pathological conditions such as Paget's disease and sickle cell disease; and in severe osteoporosis of the acetabulum secondary to prolonged non–weight bearing resulting from nonunion of the fracture of the neck of the femur. Total hip arthroplasty is an ideal method for treating complications of fracture fixations such as nonunion and malunion.

- Several risk factors for total hip arthroplasty in fresh fractures of the neck of the femur include: a high morbidity and mortality associated with total hip arthroplasty used to treat femoral neck fractures; lack of facilities and expertise to undertake such a major procedure; the added burden to already overloaded institutions; the need for considerably smaller-sized implants because of the normal size of the acetabulum; and the extra costs of replacement by prosthesis compared with the cost of fracture fixation.

- Alternatives to total hip arthroplasty should be sought for young patients. The best alternative is to continue nonoperative means by educating the patient, limiting certain physical activities, and encouraging the use of a walking support. Another alternative is to improve the function of the hip using biological operations, including osteotomies, that alter the biomechanics of the hip. These temporizing procedures must reduce pain significantly and improve quality of life until later in the patient's life when total hip arthroplasty can be more safely performed.

- Because early degenerative osteoarthritis of the hips is attributed primarily to some degree of hip dysplasia, slipped capital femoral epiphysis, and Legg-Calvé-Perthes disease, upper femoral osteotomy, pelvic osteotomy, or shelf procedures might be indicated. These operations are designed to improve the biomechanics of the hip and generally prevent further degenerative changes rather than being therapeutic. However, under certain circumstances, these operations may be carried out therapeutically in extremely young patients.

- Hip fusion is distinctly advantageous for very young patients (in their twenties and thirties) afflicted by unilateral hip disease and no other disabling factors. A typical case for arthrodesis is a laborer in his twenties who has traumatic osteoarthritis and no back or knee disability. Arthrodesis is ideal for treatment of infection in young patients. Hip fusion may also be used in patients with unilateral chondrolysis and severe degenerative osteoarthritis, failed multiple joint replacements, paralytic conditions, and mental retardation. It may also be used as an alternative to a resection pseudarthrosis in very young individuals.

- A bipolar prosthesis should be regarded as a hemiarthroplasty because it offers no definitive advantage over total hip arthroplasty if the acetabular cartilage erosion is present at the time of its insertion. The greater durability of a bipolar prosthesis over a fixed-head prosthesis is its only theoretical advantage, and it should be used only for fresh fractures of the neck of the femur in elderly individuals. The long-term effects of wear particles of high-density polyethylene may limit its future use.

- Other procedures such as cup arthroplasty and resurfacing procedures have been abandoned by most surgeons in favor of the conventional stem total hip arthroplasty.

- The details of patient selection and contraindications are presented as guidelines rather than as a code of practice. The selection of patients is a complex matter that must be individualized while keeping all the facts in perspective.

- This author concludes that ever-increasing optimism about newer technologies in total hip technology is unfounded. In essence, the long-term results of total hip arthroplasty in young, active, and heavy individuals remain enigmatic and unresolved.

Nevertheless, the results of repeated revisionary surgery and associated problems, such as loss of bone stock, can be catastrophic. The newer technologies await many years of appraisal. Advocating and applying any new technology in total hip arthroplasty to young individuals solely on the basis of laboratory success or theoretical implications is irresponsible and must be deprecated.

REFERENCES

1. **Amstutz HC, Clarke IC, Christie J, et al:** Total hip articular replacement by internal eccentric shells: the "tharies" approach to total surface replacement arthroplasty, *Clin Orthop* 128:261, 1977.
2. **Amstutz HC, Dorey F:** The development and nine-year results of THARIES resurfacing arthroplasty. In Sevastik J, Goldie I, editors: *The young patient with degenerative hip disease*, Uppsala, 1985, Almqvist and Wiksell.
3. **Amstutz HC, Dorey F, O'Carroll PF:** THARIES resurfacing arthroplasty. Evolution and long-term results, *Clin Orthop* 213:92, 1986.
4. **Anderson LD, Hamsa WR Jr, Waring TL:** Femoral head prostheses: a review of 356 operations and their results, *J Bone Joint Surg* 46:1049, 1964.
5. **Aronson J:** Osteoarthritis of the young adult hip: Etiology and treatment, *American Academy of Orthopaedic Surgeons instructional course lectures*, vol 35, St Louis, 1986, Mosby–Year Book.
6. **Aufranc OE:** Vitallium mold arthroplasty of hip. In Crenshaw AH, editor: *Campbell's operative orthopaedics*, vol 2, St Louis, 1971, Mosby–Year Book.
7. **Aufranc OE:** The adaptability of Vitallium mold arthroplasty to difficult hip problems, *Clin Orthop* 66:31, 1969.
8. **Aufranc OE:** *Constructive surgery of the hip*, St Louis, 1962, Mosby–Year Book.
9. **Aufranc OE:** Constructive hip surgery with the Vitallium mold. A report on 1,000 cases of arthroplasty of the hip over a 15-year period, *J Bone Joint Surg* 39:237, 1957.
10. **Aufranc OE, Sweet EB:** Study of patients with hip arthroplasty at Massachusetts General Hospital, *JAMA* 170:67, 1959.
11. **Bateman JE:** Single-assembly total hip prostheses—preliminary report, *Orthop Dig* 2:15, 1974.
12. **Bateman JE, Berenji AR, Bayne O, et al:** Long-term results of bipolar arthroplasty in osteoarthritis of the hip, *Clin Orthop* 251:54, 1990.
13. **Bochner RM, Pellicci PM, Lyden JP:** Bipolar hemiarthroplasty for fracture of the femoral neck. Clinical review with special emphasis on prosthetic motion, *J Bone Joint Surg* 70:1001, 1988.
14. **Bogoch E, Ouellette G, Hastings D:** Failure of internal fixation of displaced femoral neck fractures in rheumatoid patients, *J Bone Joint Surg* [Br]73:7, 1991.
15. **Bombelli R:** *Osteoarthritis of the hip. Classification and pathogenesis: the role of osteotomy as a consequent therapy*, ed 2, New York, 1983, Springer-Verlag.
16. **Bombelli R:** *Osteoarthritis of the hip. Pathogenesis and consequent therapy*, New York, 1976, Springer-Verlag.
17. **Bombelli R, Aronson J:** Biomechanical classification of osteoarthritis of the hip with special reference to treatment techniques and results. In Schatzker J, editor: *The intertrochanteric osteotomy*, Berlin, 1984, Springer-Verlag.
18. **Bombelli R, Santore R:** Ten-year follow-up of 212 consecutive intertrochanteric femoral osteotomies for osteoarthritis of the hip. Presented at the Annual Meeting of the American Academy of Orthopaedic Surgeons, Anaheim, California, 1983.
19. **Bombelli R, Santore RF, Poss R:** Mechanics of the normal and osteoarthritic hip. A new perspective, *Clin Orthop* 182:69, 1984.
20. **Bonfiglio M:** Aseptic necrosis of femoral head in dogs; effect of drilling and bone-grafting, *Surg Gynecol Obstet* 98:591, 1954.
21. **Bonfiglio M, Bardenstein MB:** Treatment by bone-grafting of aseptic necrosis of the femoral head and non-union of the femoral neck (Phemister technique), *J Bone Joint Surg* 40:1329, 1958.
22. **Bonfiglio M, Voke EM:** Aseptic necrosis of the femoral head and non-union of the femoral neck, effect of treatment by drilling and bone-grafting (Phemister technique), *J Bone Joint Surg* 50:48, 1968.
23. **Bowman AJ Jr, Walker MW, Kilfoyle RM, et al:** Experience with the bipolar prosthesis in hip arthroplasty. A clinical study, *Orthopedics* 88:460, 1985.
24. **Boyd HB, Salvatore JE:** Acute fracture of the femoral neck: internal fixation or prosthesis? *J Bone Joint Surg* 46:1066, 1964.
25. **Bracy D, Wroblewski BM:** Bilateral Charnley arthroplasty as a single procedure. A report on 400 patients, *J Bone Joint Surg* [Br]63:354, 1981
26. **Bradford DS, Janes PC, Simmons RS, et al:** Total hip arthroplasty in renal transplant recipients, *Clin Orthop* 181:107, 1983.
27. **Cabanela ME, Van Demark RE Jr:** Bipolar endoprosthesis. In The Hip Society: *The hip: proceedings of the twelfth open scientific meeting of The Hip Society*, St Louis, 1984, Mosby–Year Book.
28. **Callaghan JJ, Brand RA, Pedersen DR:** Hip arthrodesis. A long-term follow-up, *J Bone Joint Surg* 67:1328, 1985.
29. **Capello WN, Ireland PH, Trammel TR, et al:** Conservative total hip arthroplasty: a procedure to conserve bone stock. I: analysis of sixty-six patients. II: analysis of failures, *Clin Orthop* 134:59, 1978.
30. **Capello WN, Misamore GW, Trancik TM:** Conservative total hip arthroplasty, *Orthop Clin North Am* 13:833, 1982.
31. **Carlioz H, Vogt JC, Barba L, et al:** Treatment of slipped upper femoral epiphysis: 80 cases operated on over 10 years (1968–1978), *J Pediatr Orthop* 4:153, 1984.
32. **Chandler HP, Reineck FT, Wixson RL, et al:** Total hip replacement in patients younger than thirty years old. A five-year follow-up study, *J Bone Joint Surg* 63:1426, 1981.
33. **Charnley J:** Personal communications.
34. **Charnley J:** *Low-friction arthroplasty of the hip. Theory and practice*, Berlin, 1979, Springer-Verlag.
35. **Charnley J:** *Total hip replacement following infection in the opposite hip*, Internal publication no. 48, 1974, Centre for Hip Surgery, Wrightington Hospital.
36. **Charnley J:** Present status of total hip replacement, *Ann Rheum Dis* 30:560, 1971.
37. **Charnley J:** *Total prosthetic replacement for advanced coxarthrosis*, Internal publication No. "0," 1967, Centre for Hip Surgery, Wrightington Hospital.
38. **Charnley J:** *Total prosthetic replacement of the hip joint using a socket of high-density polyethylene*, Internal publication, 1966, Centre for Hip Surgery, Wrightington Hospital.

39. **Charnley J:** Tissue reactions to polytetrafluoroethylene, *Lancet* 2:1379, 1963 (letter).

40. **Charnley JC:** Arthroplasty of the hip: a new operation, *Lancet* 1:1129, 1961.

41. **Chen SC, Badrinath K, Pell LH, et al:** The movements of the components of the Hastings bipolar prosthesis. A radiographic study in 65 patients, *J Bone Joint Surg* [Br] 71:186, 1989.

42. **Chen SC, Sarkar S, Pell LH:** A radiological study of the movements of the two components of the Monk prosthesis (hard-top 'duopleet') in patients, *Injury* 12:243, 1980.

43. **Chiari K:** Iliac osteotomy in young adults. In The Hip Society: *The hip: proceedings of the seventh open scientific meeting of The Hip Society*, St Louis, 1979, Mosby–Year Book.

44. **Chiari K:** Medial displacement osteotomy of the pelvis, *Clin Orthop* 98:55, 1974.

45. **Chiari K, Endler M, Hackel H:** Indications et résultats de l'ostéotomie du bassin selon Chiari dans l'arthrose avancée, *Acta Orthop Belg* 44:176, 1978.

46. **Coates RL, Armour P:** Treatment of subcapital femoral fractures by primary total hip replacement, *Injury* 11:132, 1980.

47. **Cook SD, Thomas KA, Kester MA:** Wear characteristics of the canine acetabulum against different femoral prostheses, *J Bone Joint Surg* [Br] 71:189, 1989.

48. **Coutts RD, Gustafson A:** Cup arthroplasty. In Steinberg ME, editor: *The hip and its disorders*, Philadelphia, 1991, WB Saunders.

49. **Coventry MB:** *Selection of patients for total hip arthroplasty. American Academy of Orthopaedic Surgeons instructional course lectures*, vol 23, St Louis, 1974, Mosby–Year Book.

50. **Crawford AH:** *Osteotomies in the treatment of slipped capital femoral epiphysis. The American Academy of Orthopaedic Surgeons instructional course lectures*, vol 33, St Louis. 1984, Mosby–Year Book.

51. **Cruess RL, Blennerhassett J, MacDonald FR, et al:** Aseptic necrosis following renal transplantation, *J Bone Joint Surg* 50:1577, 1968.

52. **Cruess RL, Kwok DC, Duc PN, et al:** The response of articular cartilage to weight-bearing against metal. A study of hemiarthroplasty of the hip in the dog, *J Bone Joint Surg* [Br] 66:592, 1984.

53. **Delamarter R, Moreland JR:** Treatment of acute femoral neck fractures with total hip arthroplasty, *Clin Orthop* 218:68, 1987.

54. **Dinley J, Duthie RB:** Hip surgery in hemophiliacs. In the Hip Society: *The hip, proceedings of the fourth open scientific meeting of The Hip Society*, St Louis, 1976, Mosby–Year Book.

55. **Dorr LD, Takei GK, Conaty P:** Total hip arthroplasties in patients less than forty-five years old, *J Bone Joint Surg* 65:474, 1983.

56. **Drinker H, Murray WR:** The universal proximal femoral endoprosthesis. A short-term comparison with conventional hemiarthroplasty, *J Bone Joint Surg* 61:1167, 1979.

57. **Dupont JA, Charnley J:** Low-friction arthroplasty of the hip for the failures of previous operations, *J Bone Joint Surg* [Br] 54:77, 1972.

58. **Eftekhar NS:** Low-friction arthroplasty: indications, contraindications, and complications, *JAMA* 218:705, 1971.

59. **Eftekhar NS:** Status of femoral head replacement in treating fracture of femoral neck. Parts I and II, *Orthop Rev* 2(6):15, 2(8):19, 1973.

60. **Eftekhar NS, Kiernan HA Jr, Stinchfield FE:** Systemic and local complications following low-friction arthroplasty of the hip joint. A study of 800 consecutive operations, *Arch Surg* 111:150, 1976.

61. **Eftekhar NS, Smith DM, Henry JH, et al:** Revision arthroplasty using Charnley low-friction technic. With reference to specifics of technic and comparison of results with primary low friction arthroplasty, *Clin Orthop* 95:48, 1973.

62. **Eftekhar NS, Stinchfield FE:** Experience with low-friction arthroplasty. A statistical review of early results and complications, *Clin Orthop* 95:60, 1973.

63. **Eftekhar NS, Tzitzikalakis GI:** Failures and reoperations following low friction arthroplasty of the hip, *Clin Orthop* 211:65, 1986.

64. **Ferguson AB Jr:** The pathological changes in degenerative arthritis of the hip and treatment by rotational osteotomy, *J Bone Joint Surg* 46:1337, 1964.

65. **Ferguson AB Jr:** High intertrochanteric osteotomy for osteoarthritis of the hip, *J Bone Joint Surg* 46:1159, 1964.

66. **Fernandez D, Isler B, Muller ME:** Chiari's osteotomy. A note on technique, *Clin Orthop* 185:53, 1984.

67. **Fischer DA, Capello WN:** *Bipolar hip prostheses in intact acetabula*. Annual Meeting of the American Academy of Orthopaedic Surgeons, Atlanta, Georgia, 1988.

68. **Freeman MAR, Bradley GW:** ICLH double cup arthroplasty, *Orthop Clin North Am* 13:799, 1982.

69. **Freeman MAR, Bradley GW:** ICLH surface replacement of the hip. An analysis of the first 10 years, *J Bone Joint Surg* [Br] 65:405, 1983.

70. **Freeman MAR, Cameron HU, Brown GC:** Cemented double cup arthroplasty of the hip: a five-year experience with the ICLH prosthesis, *Clin Orthop* 134:45, 1978.

71. **Freeman MAR, Swanson SAV, Day WH, et al:** Conservative total replacement of the hip. In Proceedings and Reports of Universities, Colleges, Councils and Associations. Great Britain, British Orthopaedic Association, *J Bone Joint Surg* [Br]57:114, 1975.

72. **Gannon JM, Kyle RF, Simonet WT, et al:** Comparison of results of bipolar and fixed acetabular components in total hip replacement using the BIAS femoral component, *Orthop Trans* 12:716, 1988.

73. **Ganz R, Jakob RP:** Partielle avaskuläre Huftkopfnekvose: Flexionsosteotonic und spongiosaplastik, *Orthopade* 9:265, 1980.

74. **Garvin KL, Pellicci PM, Windsor RE, et al:** Contralateral total hip arthroplasty or ipsilateral total knee arthroplasty in patients who have a long-standing fusion of the hip, *J Bone Joint Surg* 71:1355, 1989.

75. **Giliberty RP:** A new concept of bipolar endoprosthesis, *Orthop Rev* 3:40, 1974.

76. **Harrington KD, Murray WR, Kountz SL, et al:** Avascular necrosis of bone after renal transplantation, *J Bone Joint Surg* 53:203, 1971.

77. **Harris WH:** *Indications for major elective reconstructive surgery of the hip in the adult. American Academy of Orthopaedic Surgeons instructional course lectures*, vol 23, St Louis, 1974, Mosby–Year Book.

78. **Harris WH:** Total hip replacement for congenital dysplasia of hip: technique. In The Hip Society: *The hip: proceedings of the second open scientific meeting of The Hip Society*, St Louis, 1974, Mosby–Year Book.

79. **Hodgkinson JP, Meadows TH, Davies DR, et al:** A radiological assessment of interprosthetic movement in the Charnley-Hastings hemiarthroplasty, *Injury* 19:18, 1988.

80. **Isono SS, Woolson ST, Schurman DJ:** Total joint arthroplasty for steroid-induced osteonecrosis in cardiac transplant patients, *Clin Orthop* 217:201, 1987.
81. **Jackson CT:** *The results of low-friction arthroplasty of the hip performed in Paget's disease.* Internal publication no. 47, 1974, Centre for Hip Surgery, Wrightington Hospital.
82. **Johnston RC, Crowninshield RD:** Roentgenologic results of total hip arthroplasty. A ten-year follow-up study, *Clin Orthop* 181:92, 1983.
83. **Jaffe WL, Charnley J:** Bilateral Charnley low-friction arthroplasty as a single operative procedure. A report of fifty cases, *Bull Hosp Joint Dis* 32:198, 1971.
84. **Jayson M:** *Total hip replacement,* Philadelphia, 1972, JB Lippincott.
85. **Kenzora JE, Sledge CB:** Hip arthroplasty and the renal transplant patient. In The Hip Society: *The hip, proceedings of the third open scientific meeting of The Hip Society,* St Louis, 1975, Mosby–Year Book.
86. **Kostuik J, Alexander D:** Arthrodesis for failed arthroplasty of the hip, *Clin Orthop* 188:173, 1984.
87. **Labelle LW, Colwill JC, Swanson AB:** Bateman bipolar hip arthroplasty for femoral neck fractures. A five-to-ten-year follow-up study, *Clin Orthop* 251:20, 1990.
88. **Lausten GS, Vedel P, Nielsen PM:** Fractures of the femoral neck treated with a bipolar endoprosthesis, *Clin Orthop* 218:63, 1987.
89. **Lazansky MG:** *Total hip replacement in patients with bilateral disease. In American Academy of Orthopaedic Surgeons instructional course lectures,* vol 23, St Louis, 1974, Mosby–Year Book.
90. **Lazansky MG:** *A study of bilateral low friction arthroplasty.* Internal publication no. 3, 1967, Centre for Hip Surgery, Wrightington Hospital.
91. **Lestrange NR:** Bipolar arthroplasty for 496 hip fractures, *Clin Orthop* 251:7, 1990.
92. **Liechti R:** *Hip arthrodesis and associated problems,* New York, 1974, Springer-Verlag.
93. **Lipscomb PR:** Reconstructive surgery for bilateral hip joint disease in the adult, *J Bone Joint Surg* 47:1, 1965.
94. **Maquet P:** Charge et sollicitation de la hanche, *Rev Med Liege* 24:146, 1969.
95. **Marie P:** Acromegaly, *Brain* 12:69, 1890.
96. **McBeath AA:** Hip arthrodesis. In Steinberg ME, editor: *The hip and its disorders,* Philadelphia, 1991, WB Saunders.
97. **McConville OR, Bowman AJ Jr, Kilfoyle RM, et al:** Bipolar hemiarthroplasty in degenerative arthritis of the hip. 100 consecutive cases, *Clin Orthop* 251:67, 1990.
98. **McMurray TP:** Osteo-arthritis of the hip joint, *J Bone Joint Surg* 21:1, 1939.
99. **McMurray TP:** Osteo-arthritis of the hip joint, *Br J Surg* 22:716, 1935.
100. **Mess D, Barmada R:** Clinical and motion studies of the Bateman bipolar prosthesis in osteonecrosis of the hip, *Clin Orthop* 251:44, 1990.
101. **Milch H:** The resection-angulation operation for arthritis and ankylosis of the hip, *J Int Coll Surg* 13:750, 1950.
102. **Moore AT:** *The Moore self-locking Vitallium prosthesis in fresh femoral neck fractures. American Academy of Orthopaedic Surgeons instructional course lectures,* vol 16, St Louis, 1959, Mosby–Year Book.
103. **Moshein J, Alter AH, Elconin KB, et al:** Transcervical fractures of the hip treated with the Bateman bipolar prosthesis, *Clin Orthop* 251:48, 1990.
104. **Müller ME:** Intertrochanteric osteotomy: indications, preoperative planning, technique. In Schatzker J, editor: *The intertrochanteric osteotomy,* Berlin, 1984, Springer-Verlag.
105. **Müller ME:** Intertrochanteric osteotomies in adults: planning and operating technique. In Cruess RL, Mitchell NS, editors. *Surgical management of degenerative arthritis of the lower limbs,* Philadelphia, 1975, Lea & Febiger.
106. **Müller ME:** Intertrochanteric osteotomy in the treatment of the arthritic hip joint. In Tronzo R, editor: *Surgery of the hip joint,* Philadelphia, 1973, Lea & Febiger.
107. **Müller ME, Allgower M, Schneider R, et al:** *Manual of internal fixation. Techniques recommended by the AO Group,* ed 2, Berlin, 1979, Springer-Verlag.
108. **Murray WR:** Bipolar endoprosthesis. In The Hip Society: *The hip: proceedings of the twelfth open scientific meeting of The Hip Society,* St Louis, 1984, Mosby–Year Book.
109. **Murray WR:** Hip problems associated with organ transplants, *Clin Orthop* 90:57, 1973.
110. **Pauwels F:** *Atlas zur Biomechanik der gesunden und kranken Hufte. Prinzipien, Technik und Resuitate einer kausaien Therapie,* Berlin, 1973, Springer-Verlag.
111. **Pauwels F:** Uber eine kausale Behandlung der Coxa valga luxans, *Z Orthop* 79:305, 1950.
112. **Pauwels F:** Der Schenkelhalsbruch. Ein mechanisches Problem, *Z Orthop* 2:63, 1935.
113. **Phemister DB:** Treatment of necrotic head of femur in adults, *J Bone Joint Surg* 31:55, 1949.
114. **Ritter MA, Stringer EA:** Bilateral total hip arthroplasty: a single procedure, *Clin Orthop* 149:185, 1980.
115. **Salvati EA, Hughes P, Lachiewicz P:** Bilateral total hip-replacement arthroplasty in one stage, *J Bone Joint Surg* 60:640, 1978.
116. **Santore R, Bombelli R:** Long-term follow-up of the Bombelli experience with osteotomy for osteoarthritis: results at 11 years. In The Hip Society: *The hip, proceedings of the eleventh open scientific meeting of The Hip Society,* St Louis, 1983, Mosby–Year Book.
117. **Sarmiento A, Gerard FM:** Total hip arthroplasty for failed endoprosthesis, *Clin Orthop* 137:112, 1978.
118. **Scales JT:** Massive bone and joint replacement involving the upper femur, acetabulum and iliac bone. In The Hip Society: *The hip: the proceedings of the third open scientific meeting of The Hip Society,* St Louis, 1975, Mosby–Year Book.
119. **Schneider R:** Results of intertrochanteric osteotomies in patients with coxarthrosis 12–15 years after surgery. In Weil U, editor: *Joint-preserving procedures of the lower extremity. Progress in orthopaedic surgery,* Berlin, 1980, Springer-Verlag.
120. **Schreiber A:** Long-term results of Chiari pelvic osteotomies. In Weil U, editor: *Joint-preserving procedures of the lower extremity. Progress in orthopaedic surgery,* Berlin, 1980, Springer-Verlag.
121. **Sim FH, Chao EY, Peterson LFA:** Reconstruction following segmental resection of primary bone tumors of the hip. In The Hip Society: *The hip: proceedings of the third open scientific meeting of The Hip Society,* St Louis, 1975, Mosby–Year Book.
122. **Sim FH, Stauffer RN:** Management of hip fractures by total hip arthroplasty, *Clin Orthop* 152:192, 1980.
123. **Simmons EH:** Chiari osteotomy—a biologic alternative for the surgical management of dysplasia of the hip joint associated with arthrosis. In The Hip Society: *The hip: proceedings of the twelfth open scientific meeting of The Hip Society,* St Louis, 1984, Mosby–Year Book.

124. **Smith-Petersen MN:** Lessons learned from fourteen years experience with mould arthroplasty of the hip joint, *J Bone Joint Surg* [Br] 34:714, 1952.

125. **Smith-Petersen MN:** Evolution of mould arthroplasty of the hip joint, *J Bone Joint Surg* [Br] 30:59, 1948.

126. **Smith-Petersen MN:** Arthroplasty of the hip; a new method, *J Bone Joint Surg* 21:269, 1939.

127. **Smith-Petersen MN, Larson CB, Aufranc OE, et al:** Complications of old fractures of the neck of the femur; results of treatment by Vitallium-mold arthroplasty, *J Bone Joint Surg* 29:41, 1947.

128. **Sponseller PD, McBeath AA, Perpich M:** Hip arthrodesis in young patients. A long-term follow-up study, *J Bone Joint Surg* 66:853, 1984.

129. **Sprenger TR, Foley CJ:** Hip replacement in a Charcot joint: a case report and historical review, *Clin Orthop* 165:191, 1982.

130. **Springfield DS, Enneking WF:** Role of bone grafting in idiopathic aseptic necrosis of the femoral head. In The Hip Society: *The hip: proceedings of the third open scientific meeting of The Hip Society,* St Louis, 1975, Mosby–Year Book.

131. **Staeheli JW, Frassica FJ, Sim FH:** Prosthetic replacement of the femoral head for fracture of the femoral neck in patients who have Parkinson disease, *J Bone Joint Surg* 70:565, 1988.

132. **Stauffer RN, Sim FH:** Total hip arthroplasty in Paget's disease of the hip, *J Bone Joint Surg* 58:476, 1976.

133. **Stulberg SD, Cordell LD, Harris WH, et al:** Unrecognized childhood hip disease: a major cause of idiopathic osteoarthritis of the hip. In The Hip Society: *The hip: proceedings of the third open scientific meeting of The Hip Society,* St Louis, 1975, Mosby–Year Book.

134. **Sugioka Y:** Transtrochanteric rotational osteotomy in the treatment of idiopathic and steroid-induced femoral head necrosis. Perthes' disease, slipped capital femoral epiphysis, and osteoarthritis of the hip. Indications and results, *Clin Orthop* 184:12, 1984.

135. **Suman RK:** Prosthetic replacement of the femoral head for fractures of the neck of the femur: a comparative study, *Injury* 11:309, 1980.

136. **Taine WH, Armour PC:** Primary total hip replacement for displaced subcapital fractures of the femur, *J Bone Joint Surg* [Br] 67:214, 1985.

137. **Torisu T, Utsunomiya K, Masumi S, et al:** Bipolar hip arthroplasty in rheumatoid arthritis, *Clin Orthop* 244:188, 1989.

138. **Trentani C, Montagnani A:** Follow-up of 150 cases for more than ten years according to Paltrinieri-Trentani. In Sevastik J, Goldie I, editors: *The young patient with degenerative hip disease,* Uppsala, 1985, Almqvist & Wiksell.

139. **Trentani C, Vaccarino FP:** The Paltrinieri-Trentani hip joint resurface arthroplasty, *Orthop Clin North Am* 13:857, 1982.

140. **Trentani C, Vaccarino F:** Complications in surface replacement arthroplasty of the hip: experience with the Paltrinieri-Trentani prosthesis, *Int Orthop* 4:247, 1981.

141. **Trentani C, Vaccarino F:** The Paltrinieri-Trentani hip joint resurface arthroplasty, *Clin Orthop* 134:36, 1978.

142. **Tronzo RG, Okin EM:** Anatomic restoration of congenital hip dysplasia in adulthood by total hip displacement, *Clin Orthop* 106:94, 1975.

143. **Turner A, Wroblewski BM:** Charnley low-friction arthroplasty for the treatment of hips with late complications of femoral neck fractures, *Clin Orthop* 185:126, 1984.

144. **Vazquez-Vela G, Vazquez-Vela E, Garcia Dobarganes F:** The Bateman bipolar prosthesis in osteoarthritis and rheumatoid arthritis. A review of 400 cases, *Clin Orthop* 251:82, 1990.

145. **Verberne GH:** A femoral head prosthesis with a built-in joint. A radiological study of the movements of the two components, *J Bone Joint Surg* [Br] 65:544, 1983.

146. **Waddell JP:** The use of noncemented bipolar hip prosthesis in the management of subcapital fractures of the femur, *Orthop Trans* 11:496, 1987.

147. **Wagner H:** *Symposium on surface replacement of the hip,* American Academy of Orthopaedic Surgeons Annual Meeting, Atlanta, February 10, 1980.

148. **Wagner H:** Surface replacement arthroplasty of the hip, *Clin Orthop* 134:102, 1978.

148a. **Wagner H:** Osteotomies for congenital hip dislocation. In The Hip Society: *The hip: proceedings of the fourth open scientific meeting,* St Louis, 1976, Mosby–Year Book.

149. **Wagner H, Zeiler G:** Idiopathic necrosis of the femoral head. Results of intertrochanteric osteotomy and joint resurfacing. In Weil U, editor: *Segmental idiopathic necrosis of the femoral head,* Progress in Orthopaedic Surgery, Berlin, 1980, Springer-Verlag.

150. **Wetherell RG, Hinves BL:** The Hastings hip in osteoarthritis. A study of 47 cases with a 5-year follow-up period, *J Arthroplasty* 4:143, 1989.

151. **White RE Jr:** Arthrodesis of the hip. In Sevastic J, Goldie I, editors: *Alternatives to total hip replacement in the young adult,* Stockholm, 1985, Almqvist and Wiksell.

152. **Woolson ST, Harris WH:** Complex total hip replacement for dysplastic or hypoplastic hips using miniature or microminiature components, *J Bone Joint Surg* 65(8):1099, 1983.

153. **Yamagata M, Chao EY, Ilstrup DM, et al:** Fixed-head and bipolar hip endoprostheses. A retrospective clinical and roentgenographic study, *J Arthroplasty* 2:327, 1987.

ADDITIONAL READINGS

Amstutz HC, Christie J, Mensch JS: Treatment of osteonecrosis of the hip. In The Hip Society: *The hip: proceedings of the third open scientific meeting of The Hip Society,* St Louis, 1975, Mosby–Year Book.

Amstutz HC, Kabo M, Hermens K, et al: Porous surface replacement of the hip with chamfer cylinder design, *Clin Orthop* 222:140, 1987.

Amstutz HC, Kabo JM, Kim WC, et al: Risk factors for femoral head resurfacing. Fitzgerald RH Jr, editor: *Non-cemented total hip arthroplasty,* New York, 1988, Raven Press.

Amstutz H, Kilgus D, Kabo M, et al: Porous surface replacement of the hip with chamfered-cylinder component, *Arch Orthop Trauma Surg* 107:73, 1988.

Amstutz HC, Kilgus DJ, Thomas BJ, et al: Evaluation of bone ingrowth by technetium diphosphonate and sulfur colloid scanning in porous hip resurfacing. In *The hip,* St Louis, 1986, Mosby–Year Book.

Amstutz HC, Kim WC, O'Carroll PF, et al: Canine porous resurfacing hip arthroplasty. Long-term results, *Clin Orthop* 207:270, 1986.

Bisla RS, Ranawat CS, Inglis AE: Total hip replacement in patients with ankylosing spondylitis with involvement of the hip. *J Bone Joint Surg* 58:233, 1976.

Brewster RC, Coventry MB, Johnson EW Jr: Conversion of the arthrodesed hip to a total hip arthroplasty, *J Bone Joint Surg* 57:27, 1975.

Chandler HP, Dickson DB: Total hip replacement in the young patient, *American Academy of Orthopaedic Surgeons instructional course lectures*, vol 23, St Louis, 1974, Mosby–Year Book.

Chandler HP, Schmidt EW, Aufranc OE: Vitallium mold arthroplasty in patients under the age of 21. In Proceedings of the American Orthopaedic Association, *J Bone Joint Surg* 50:1496, 1968.

Collis DK, Johnston RC: Comparative evaluation of the results of cup arthroplasty and total hip replacement, *Clin Orthop* 86:102, 1972.

Coutts RD, Amiel D, Harwood FL, et al: Characterization of arthroplasty tissue after 14 years post-cup arthroplasty: a morphological and biochemical assessment, *J Orthop Res* 2:425, 1984.

Dunn HK, Hess WE: Total hip reconstruction in chronically dislocated hip, *J Bone Joint Surg* 58:838, 1976.

Ficat RP: Treatment of avascular necrosis of the femoral head. In The Hip Society: *The hip: proceedings of the eleventh open scientific meeting of The Hip Society*, St Louis, 1983, Mosby–Year Book.

Ghormley RK: A review of the pertinent current literature on prostheses of the hip. In *American Academy Orthopaedic Surgeons instructional course lectures*, vol 15, Ann Arbor, 1958, JW Edwards.

Hardiage K, Williams D, Etienhe A, et al: Conversion of fused hips to low friction arthroplasty, *J Bone Joint Surg* [Br] 59:385, 1977.

Harris WH: Etiology of osteoarthritis of the hip, *Clin Orthop* 213:20, 1986.

Harris WH: Power instrumentation for cup arthroplasty, *Clin Orthop* 72:219, 1970.

Harris WH: Surgical approach and technique of cup arthroplasty, *Surg Clin North Am* 49:763, 1969.

Harris WH: Traumatic arthritis of the hip after dislocation and acetabular fractures: treatment by mold arthroplasty: an end-result study using a new method of result evaluation, *J Bone Joint Surg* 51:737, 1969.

Harris WH: A new lateral approach to the hip joint, *J Bone Joint Surg* 49:891, 1967.

Harris WH, Aufranc OE: Mold arthroplasty in the treatment of hip fractures complicated by sepsis, *J Bone Joint Surg* 47:31, 1965.

Law WA: Late results in Vitallium-mold arthroplasty of the hip, *J Bone Joint Surg* 44:1497, 1962.

Law WA, Manzoni A: Smith-Petersen mould arthroplasty of the hip: results after 12–21 years, *Proc R Soc Med* 63:583, 1970.

Lorenz A, Uber die Behandlung der irreponibien angebotenen Huftluxation und der Schenkeihalspseudarthrosen mittels Gabelung (Bifurkation des oberen Femurendes), *Wien Klin Wochenschr* 32:997, 1919.

Morscher EW: Intertrochanteric osteotomy in osteoarthritis of the hip. In The Hip Society: *The hip: proceedings of the eighth open scientific meeting of The Hip Society*, St Louis, Mosby–Year Book. 1980.

Morscher E: Die intertrochantare Osteotomie bei Coxarthrose, Bern, 1971, Hans Huber, Verlag.

Reigstad A, Gronmark T: Osteoarthritis of the hip treated by intertrochanteric osteotomy. A long-term follow-up. *J Bone Joint Surg* 66:1, 1984.

Reynolds DA: Chiari innominate osteotomy in adults. Technique, indications, and contraindications, *J Bone Joint Surg* [Br] 68:45, 1986.

Santore RF: Intertrochanteric osteotomy. In Steinberg ME, editor: *The hip and its disorders,* Philadelphia, 1991, WB Saunders.

Shepherd MM: A review of 650 arthroplasty operations, *J Bone Joint Surg* [Br] 36:567, 1954.

Smith-Petersen MN: Approach to and exposure of the hip joint for mold arthroplasty, *J Bone Joint Surg* 31:40, 1949.

Steel HH: Triple osteotomy of the innominate bone, *J Bone Joint Surg* 55:343, 1973.

Stinchfield FE: Personal communication.

Stinchfield FE: Surgical treatment of the arthritic hip, *Surg Gynecol Obstet* 96:733, 1953.

Stinchfield FE, Carroll RE: Vitallium-cup arthroplasty of the hip joint; end-result study, *J Bone Joint Surg* 51:628, 1949.

Stinchfield FE, Cavallaro WU: Arthrodesis of the hip joint; a follow-up study, *J Bone Joint Surg* 32:48, 1950.

Strathy GM, Fitzgerald RH: *Conversion of the ankylosed or arthrodesed hip to total hip arthroplasty: 10-year follow-up.* Presented at the 53rd Annual Meeting of the American Academy of Orthopaedic Surgeons, New Orleans, February, 1986.

Stuck WG: The surgical treatment of degenerative arthritis of the hip, *South Med J* 42:1021, 1949.

Townley CO: Conservative total articular replacement arthroplasty (the TARA procedure) with the fixed femoral cup, *Orthop Trans* 5:463, 1981.

See Chapters 15, Principles Common to all Surgical Approaches; 20, Congenital Dysplasia and Dislocation; 21, Inflammatory, Metabolic, and Hereditary Bone Disorders; 22, Protrusio Acetabuli; 23, Tumors and Tumorous Conditions; 24, Conversion of Failed Previous Surgery; 25, Revision in Absence of Infection; 26, Revision of Infected Hip; and 32, Dislocation and Instability for additional information.

CHAPTER ELEVEN

Choice of Implants and Customization

- In the bonded configurations [cemented and porous-coated], interface stress concentrations occur on the proximal and distal sides. Stress value depends on stem rigidity. . . . [whereas] in the press-fit stem, the interface stresses are affected more by stem shape as a geometric entity and less by stem rigidity.
  R. Huiskes

Since Charnley introduced low-friction arthroplasty of the hip in the early 1960s, an explosion of innovative modifications and technologies has occurred. Efforts have focused chiefly on improving the materials and design of the prosthesis to increase durability, improve biomechanics, and consequently reduce complications and the need for revision surgery. The ultimate goal is to treat younger and more active patients by total hip arthroplasty.

Cementless vs. cemented, porous-coated vs. modular, press-fit vs. screw-in, ceramic vs. stainless steel: these are the concepts that orthopaedic surgeons must currently consider. For most patients in their sixties afflicted by osteoarthritis or rheumatoid arthritis, however, the cemented total hip arthroplasty as developed and perfected by Sir John Charnley remains the "gold standard" operation against which all newer designs must be compared. The principles Charnley incorporated into his design of the hip prosthesis were the foundation of all subsequent developments in total hip arthroplasty during the past three decades. Although recent modifications of Charnley's work have aimed largely at eliminating acrylic cement for fixation, prostheses continue to be fabricated of super-hard alloys and high-density polyethylenes.

The trend away from using cement for fixation has arisen because of fixation failures resulting from a variety of factors, some of which are attributable to the incorrect application of cement. *Since cemented fixation has demonstrated excellent long-term follow up results and reproducibility, it remains the standard for femoral component replacement for most patients.*

Early results of porous-coated cups seem promising, although long-term outcomes are not yet available.

During the past three decades, techniques, materials, and prosthetic designs for total hip arthroplasty have been improved significantly. Both cement technique and prevention of infection have improved. Consequently, follow-up studies in the literature reflect better results (see Chapter 28). Numerous hip prosthesis designs are currently on the market and others are in development. This chapter briefly outlines the author's rationale for choosing a particular prosthesis design among those he has used in the past; the discussion is not intended to be a global overview. Because of their historical and biomechanical interest, the author describes his experiences with certain types of prostheses used only briefly and abandoned when related complications surfaced. (More general biomechanical discussions of prosthesis designs appear in Chapters 4 through 6.)

THE CHOICE OF IMPLANT

The following principles are fundamental to choosing implants and improving patient care:

1. Adopt a method that is practical and has been proven successful on a long-term clinical basis.
2. Avoid modifying established techniques in the absence of adequate documentation and careful studies of the outcomes.
3. Continue surveillance of one's own results and experiences with complications to improve technique and solve problems as they arise.

4. Select patients carefully for this type of radical surgery, basing decisions on objective findings, not subjective complaints (see Chapter 10).

Certain interrelated features of prosthetic design are fundamental and must be carefully considered in total hip arthroplasty:

- Its anatomical application and surgical feasibility.
- Reduction of the forces that will act upon it.
- Mechanical optimization of wear friction and the strength of the materials from which the prosthesis is made.
- The permanent fixation of the prosthesis to the bone.

Whenever possible, arthroplasty procedures about the hip aim to change the force distribution, to reduce the total weight on the artificial joint; this goal is clearly more complicated than simply replacing the joint with a mechanical device. The principles of force reduction have been outlined in Chapter 6.

The practice of low-friction arthroplasty has included several closely related principles:

1. Use of a small-diameter femoral head.
2. Reconstruction of the hip joint through the lateral displacement of the abductor pull.
3. Medialization of the center of rotation, which can be achieved by a modest deepening of the socket. A small head, a short neck, and a valgus neck shaft angle can also medialize the center of rotation of the hip joint (see Chapter 6).
4. Allowance for subluxation (accomplished by using a small head), which provides a "safety valve" for the fixation elements, thereby reducing the forces transmitted to the cement-bone bond (Fig. 11-1).[3]

Head Size

The role of a small-diameter (22 to 26 mm) head in medializing the hip was discussed in Chapters 6 and 28. Several variables relate to head size: weight per unit area; frictional torque; distance a given point on the surface must travel when the femoral head moves against the socket; socket thickness required to absorb shock and to withstand wear; volume of wear debris (volumetric wear) generated, which influences the biological reaction; and rate of penetration of the femoral head into the thickness of the socket (linear wear). All these interrelated variables are considered in choosing a small head diameter. The small head allows the surgeon to employ a thick plastic socket and reduce volumetric wear without risking a rapid penetration into the socket, which would cause instability. On the other hand, a large femoral head (i.e., 32 to 50 mm outer diameter) requires a thin socket to fit into small acetabula. Conceivably, plastic deformation of the thin

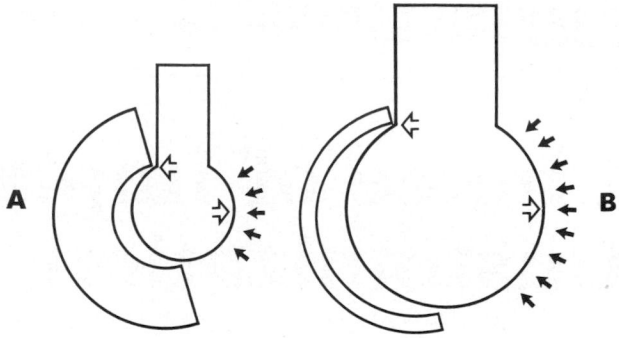

Fig. 11-1. Controlled subluxation is beneficial to survival of the hip prosthesis. **A,** In a small-diameter head, the force resisting subluxation is small, thus the force acting against (resisting) subluxation is small, so the equal opposite force reacting against socket is also small. Furthermore, with a small head a thick plastic is possible, which in turn retains the maximum external surface to resist shearing forces. **B,** In a large head the forces are increased (the opposite). (Redrawn from Charnley J: *Low-friction arthroplasty of the hip: theory and practice,* Berlin, 1979, Springer-Verlag.)

plastic under weight may be deleterious to fixation because it causes stress concentration and increased volumetric wear. In contrast, thick plastic conceivably might act as an "energy absorber," enhancing eventual fixation and favorable bone remodeling under weight bearing. The theoretical increased stability of the large head has not been supported in clinical practice (see Chapter 32). Radiographic and clinical data unequivocally support the longer survival of the smaller 22-mm femoral head prosthesis.[17]

This author considers a 22-mm or 26-mm head to be optimal. The 22-mm head is used in small acetabula and selected revision cases, while in large men whose acetabula are large enough to accommodate it, a 26-mm head is used against a thick plastic socket. In the author's own design of a total hip prosthesis, he has chosen a 26-mm outer diameter to produce a 2-to-1 ratio of the outer to the inner diameter of the socket. For smaller acetabula, he prefers a 22-mm version designed by Charnley, because it allows retention of the subchondral plate while accommodating the insertion of the cup and adequate cement (see Chapter 15).[7]

Neck Design

The prosthetic neck must have the smallest cross-sectional dimensions that will allow adequate angular motion with minimal encroachment against the socket rim (within the physiological range of hip motions). Using a kinematic simulator (Figs. 11-2 and 11-3) of the total hip, we recognize the following:

1. The smaller the diameter of the neck, the greater the range of motion it allows without impingement against the socket.

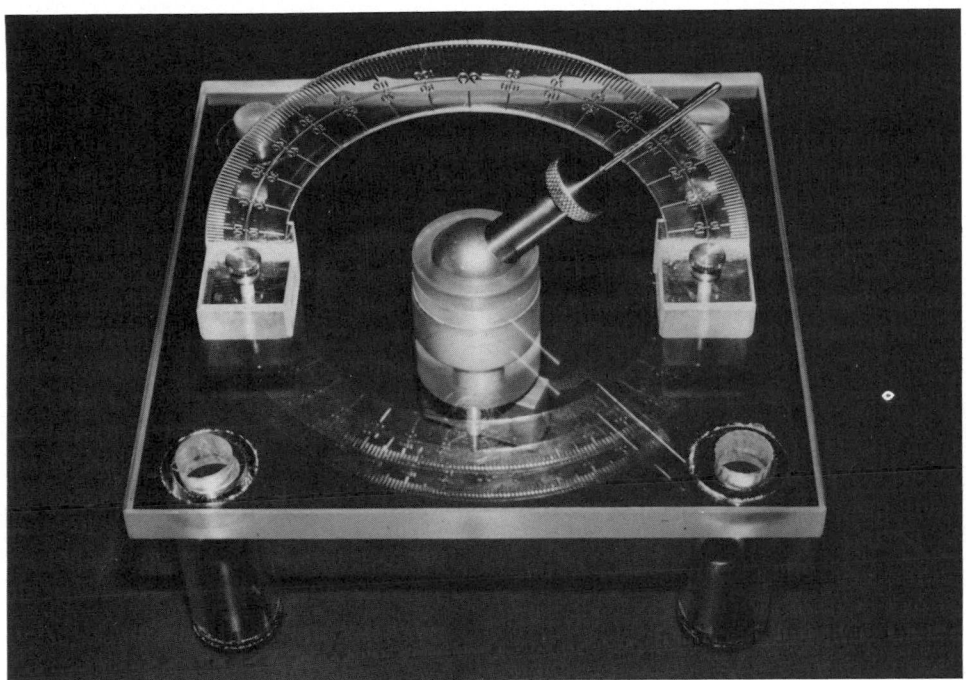

Fig. 11-2. A kinematic simulator of the total hip (designed by the author) demonstrates the role of the increased range of motion by (1) increasing the ball-neck ratio, (2) reducing the socket depth, and (3) preferentially selecting the offset of the ball on the neck. The adjusting screw mechanism changes the socket depth by lowering or raising the cup. Various necks stored in the legs of the assembly are used for simulation. The kinematic simulator may produce readings for a 22- or 26-mm-diameter head for comparison. (From Eftekhar NS: Total hip replacement using principles of low-friction arthroplasty. In Evarts CM: *Surgery of the musculoskeletal system,* New York, 1983, Churchill-Livingstone.)

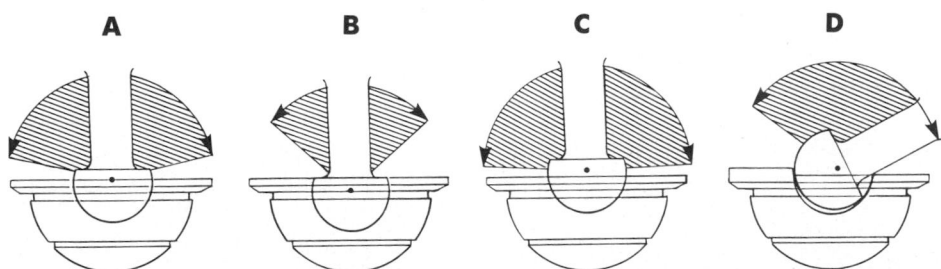

Fig. 11-3. Neck-socket-angle vs. joint stability: The neck socket impingement is demonstrated according to the depth of the socket. Range of motion (*(shaded)* is restricted proportional to the depth of penetration of the head into the socket. The head and the neck diameters remain constant in this illustration. **A,** The center of the head and the force of the cup are at the same level. **B,** The center of the head is penetrated into the acetabular cavity. **C,** The center of the head is out of the face of the cup. **D,** A long asymmetrical wall produces an asymmetrical limitation of the range-of-motion measurements in the drawing based on the kinematic simulator shown in Fig. 11-2.

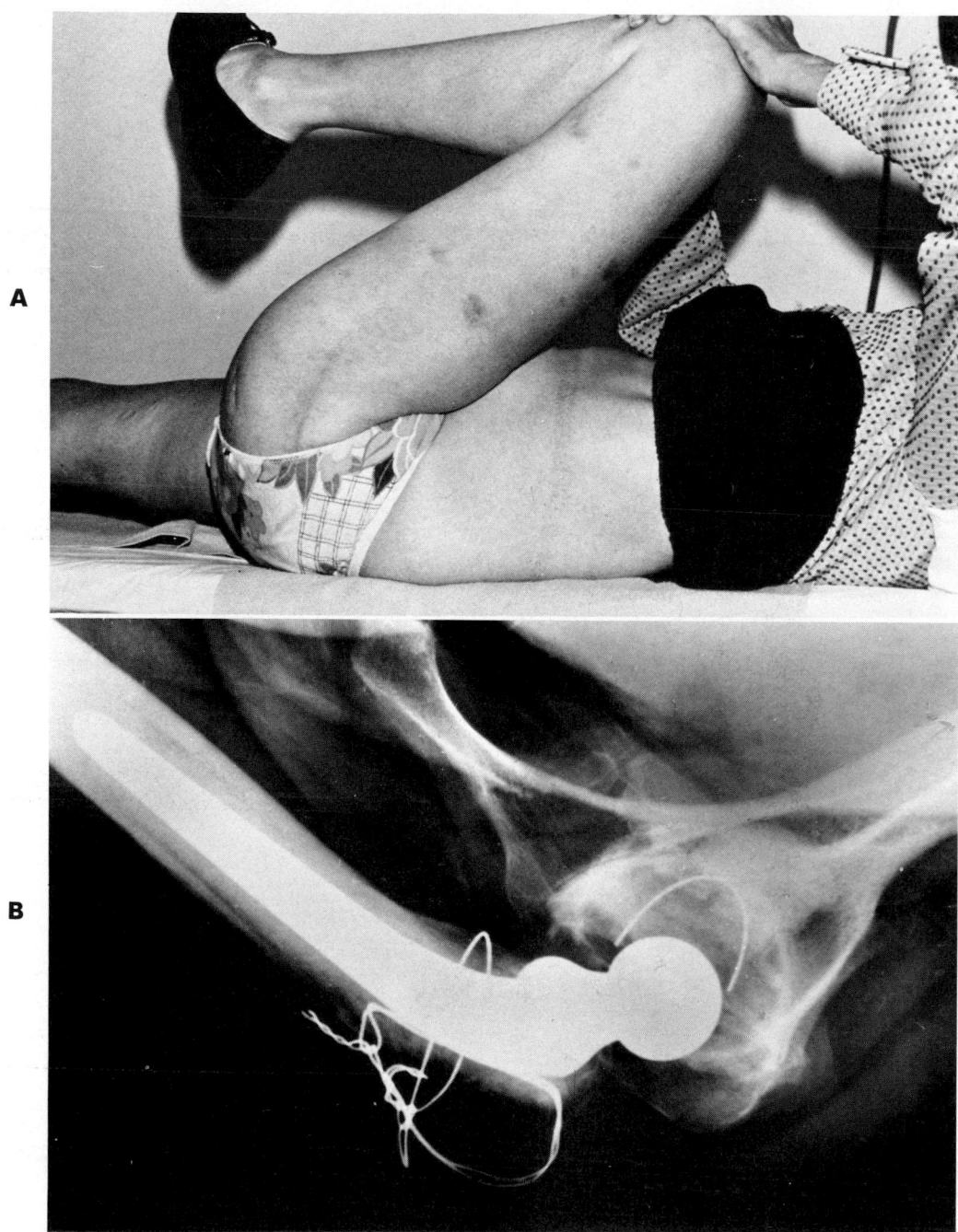

Fig. 11-4. A, Extreme range of flexion of left hip 1 year after surgery. It should be noted that once hip reaches approximately 90 degrees of flexion, it assumes slight external rotation and abduction position, which should relieve impingement of neck against socket. **B,** Shoot-through (Manfredi lateral) radiograph is attempted while hip has remained in maximum flexion as in **A**. There is a suggestion of possible migration of the head out of the depth of the socket but supported by long posterior wall of socket.

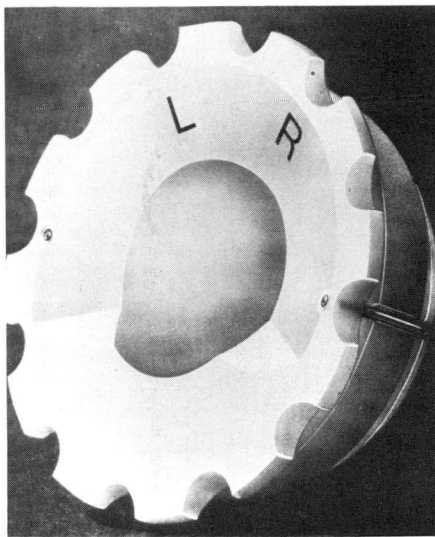

Fig. 11-5. Long posterior wall (LPW) of socket provides platform for head, preventing momentary subluxation or dislocation in extreme ranges of flexion.

2. The greater the head-neck ratio, the greater the range of motion without impingement.

3. The smaller the socket depth–ball ratio, the greater the range of motion without impingement. Obviously, increasing the depth of the socket increases resistance to dislocation; however, increased socket depth automatically reduces the "angle of impingement." For example, Charnley's original design with a 22.5-mm head produces a 90-degree range of angular movements. Reducing the neck diameter to 10 mm (the current design) will increase the angular movement to 108 degrees (see Chapters 6 and 32).

Figs. 11-4 to 11-8 illustrate an in-vivo role played by a socket with a long posterior wall (LPW). A reduced neck diameter in Charnley's design was aimed to reduce neck/socket impingement in extreme ranges of motion (Fig. 11-9).

The author has incorporated a new feature into his own design. Displacing the head inferiorly on the neck

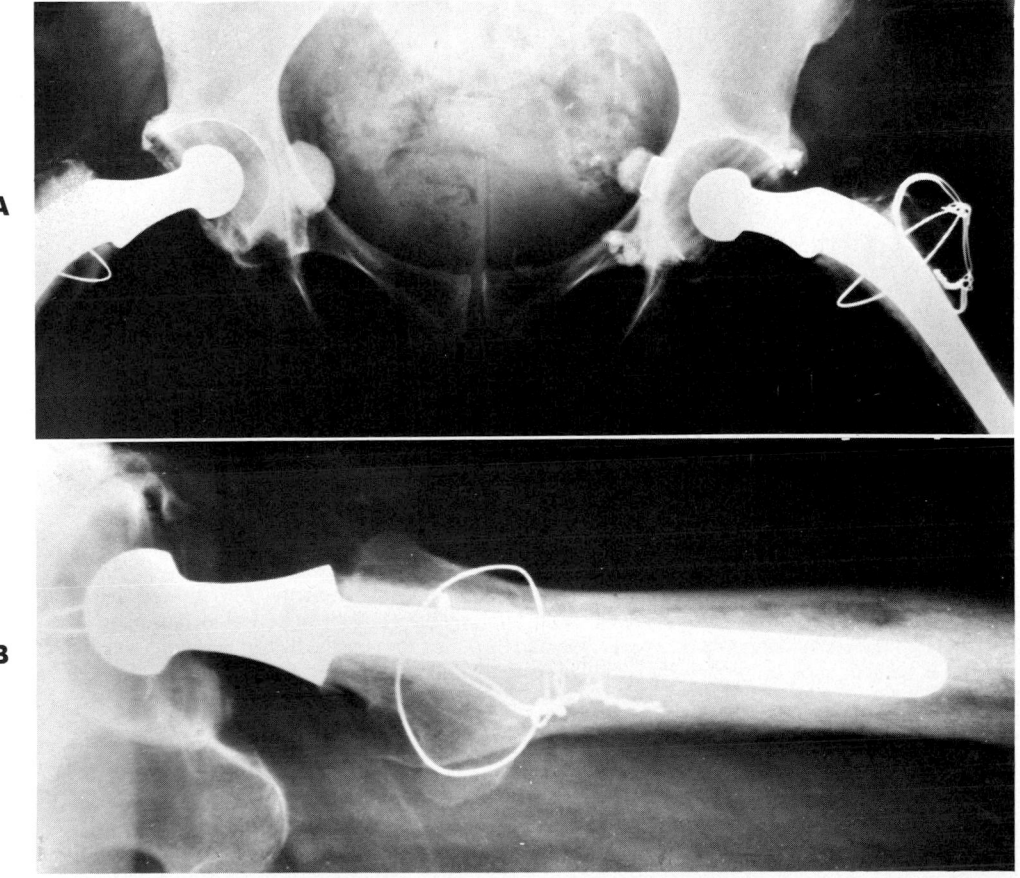

Fig. 11-6. A, Excellent range of motion is achieved in patient with rheumatoid arthritis after low-friction arthroplasty. This 36-year-old female was able to abduct to 45 degrees in each hip. **B,** Manfredi lateral radiograph of left hip illustrating position of "neutroversion" of both components.

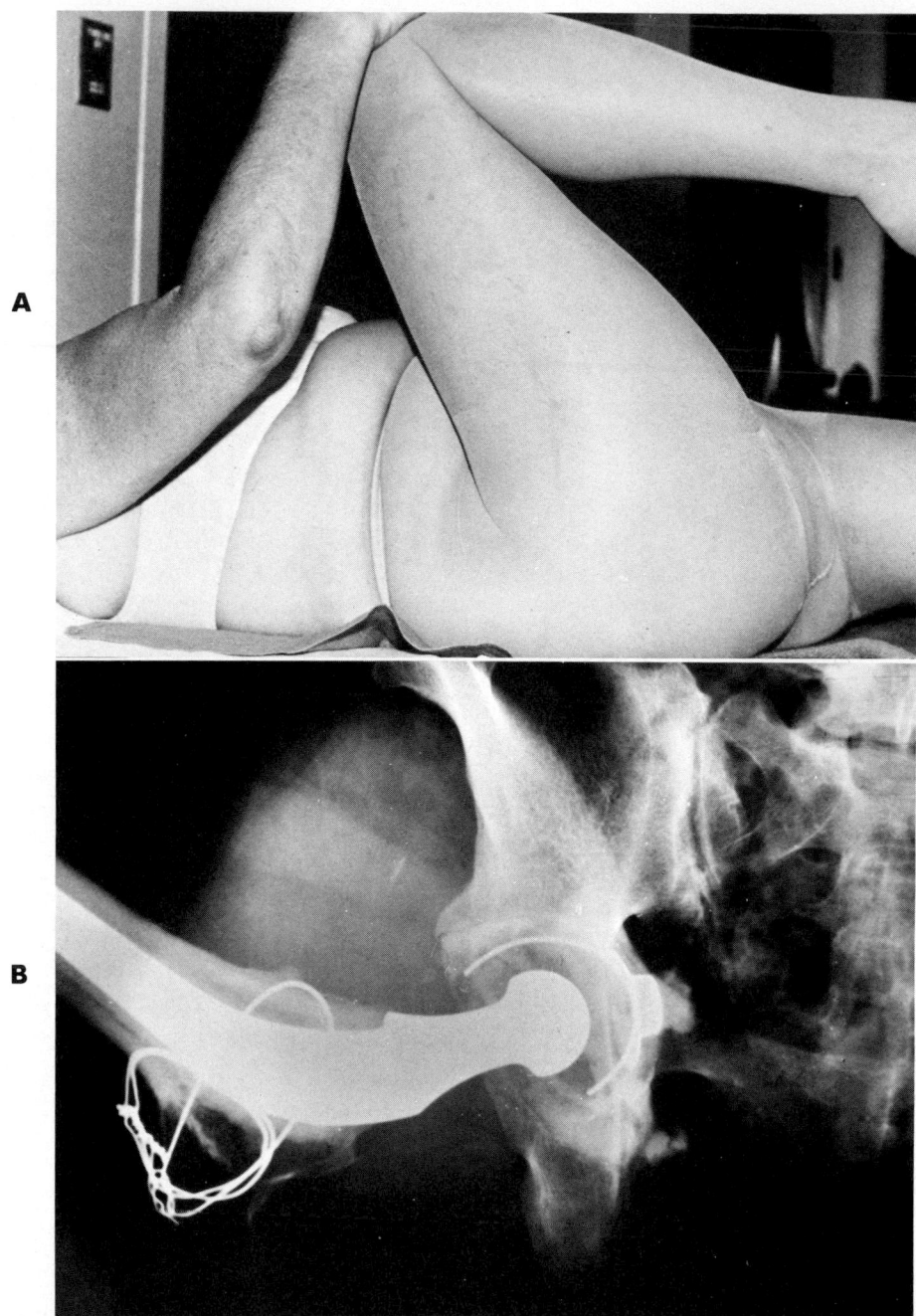

Fig. 11-7. Postoperative status of low-friction arthroplasty performed for osteoarthritis in a 58-year-old woman who has achieved good range of motion following arthroplasty. **A,** With right hip in maximum flexion, anteroposterior radiograph of pelvis and hip is obtained. NOTE: head of prosthesis has remained within depth of socket, **B,** without subluxation despite flexion beyond 90 degrees.

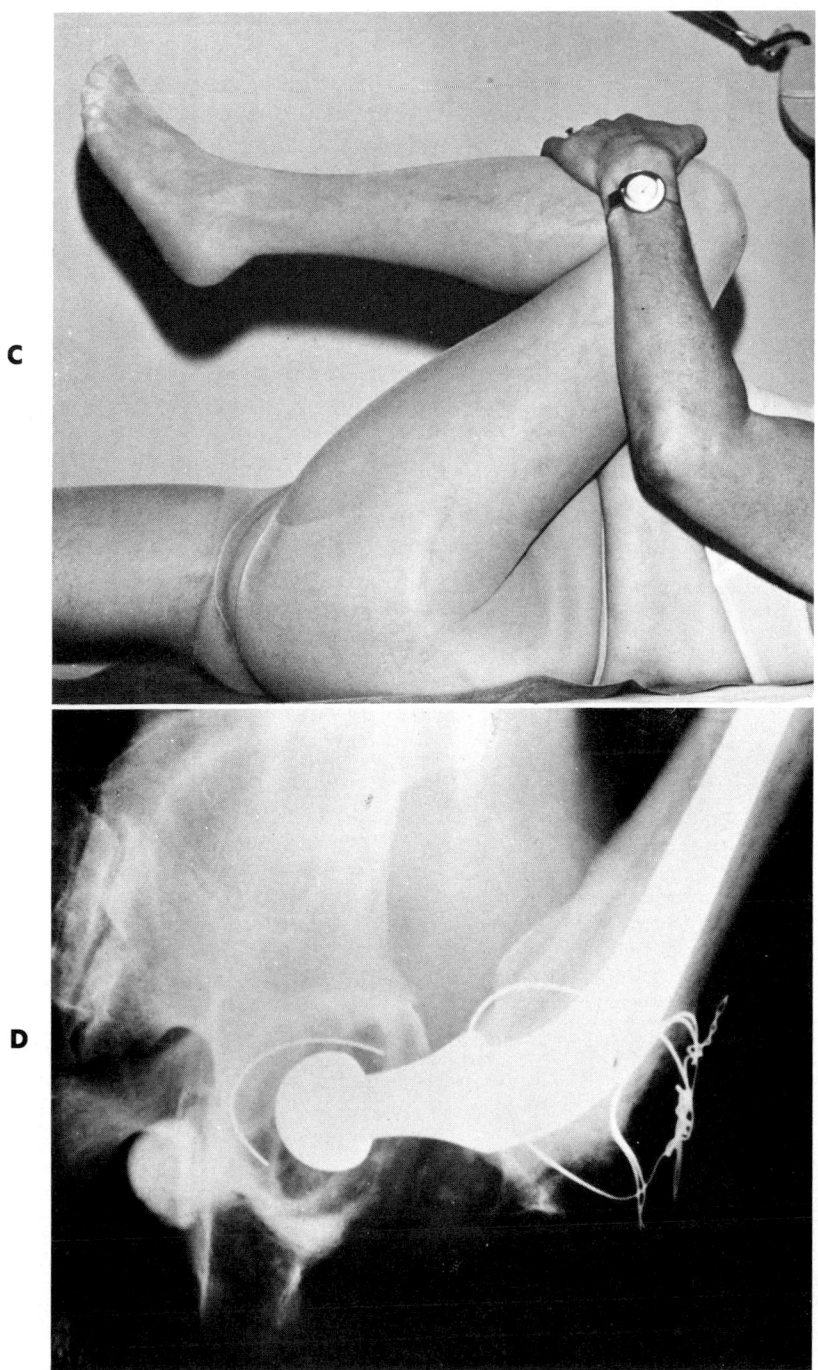

Fig. 11-7—cont'd.   C, With left hip in maximum flexion (approximately 135 degrees), x-ray film, **D,** reveals head remaining completely within depth of socket. It is possible that a few degrees of abduction and external rotation relieve neck socket impingement in addition to capsule, which tightens at extreme motions by twisting along its axis, thus retaining (stabilizing) head at depth of socket.

created an offset between the axis of the neck and the central axis of the head, thereby allowing greater range of motion in adduction and flexion and stabilizing the prosthesis in combined motions (above), or in "vulnerable positions" (Fig. 11-10).

Head-Neck Modularity

A prosthesis with a tapered neck and detachable heads has distinct advantages:

1. Modularity allows the surgeon to increase the neck length if the hip remains unstable after completing fixation of the acetabular component.
2. The surgeon can replace the head with a smaller or larger one at revision if the stem is well fixed.
3. The head is inserted as a final step following fixation of the stem, so the highly polished head is not damaged at the time of stem insertion.

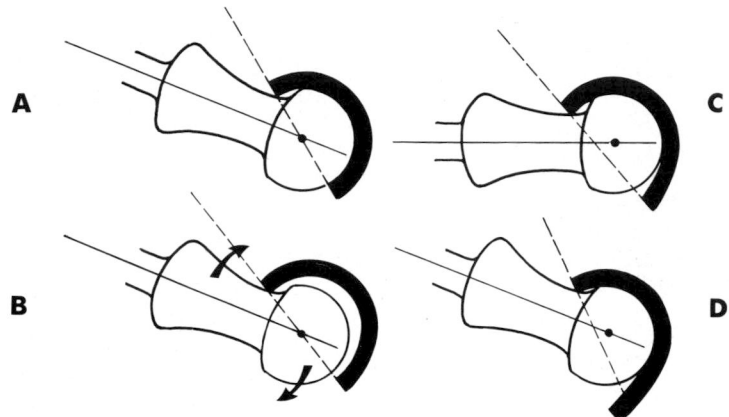

Fig. 11-8. Mechanism of dislocation by neck socket impingement. **A,** Neck socket contact (angle of dislocation) if center of ball is in same plane as mouth of cup. **B,** Greater stability of hip is achieved by placing head deep to edge of cup. **C,** Deepening of socket increases neck socket impingement but does not alter angle of dislocation (similar to angle of dislocation in **A**). **D,** Long posterior wall of prosthesis (Charnley prosthesis) allows subluxation without loss of contact between ball and socket.

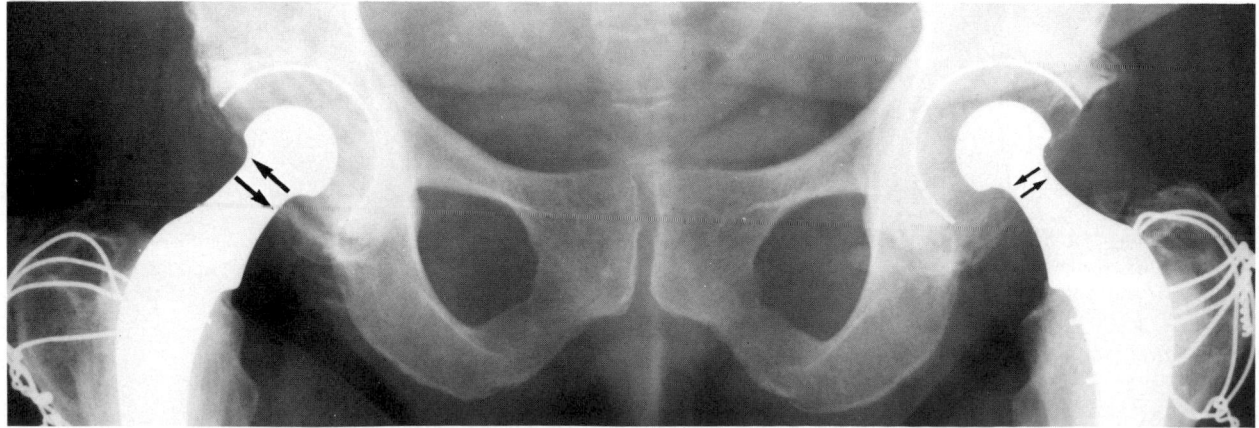

Fig. 11-9. Radiograph of bilateral hip arthroplasties in a 54-year-old woman (E.S.) whose hip arthroplasties were replaced 5 years apart. Note the difference between the neck thickness (the right hip prosthesis with a 12.5-mm neck cross-sectional diameter and the left with 10-mm diameter). Patient is unaware of the difference because the clinical range of motion is the same in both hips. However, theoretically the left hip should last longer because of a reduced neck. (See Chapters 4 and 6.)

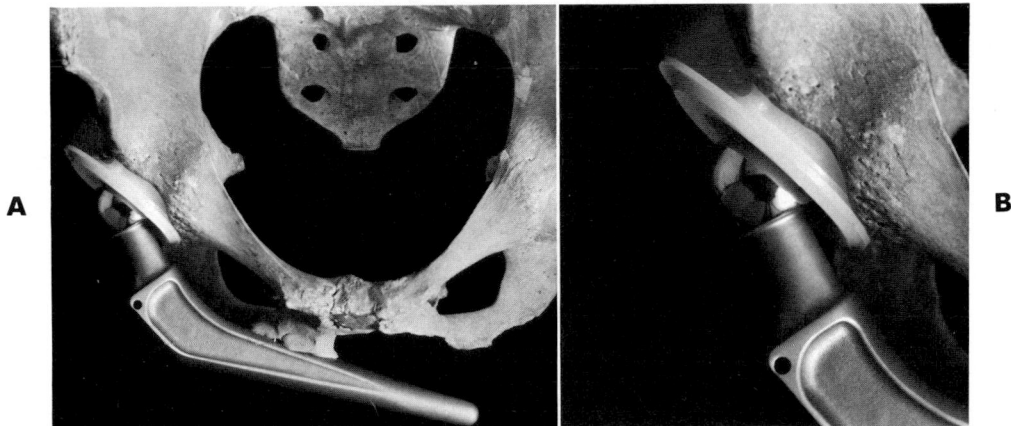

Fig. 11-10. A, Demonstration of head-neck offset; possible increase of adduction and flexion without dislocation. **B,** "Close-up" of neck-socket contact at extreme adduction without dislocation. Socket rim is demonstrated superficial to the opening of acetabulum in this rehearsal. (From Eftekhar NS: Total hip replacement using principles of low-friction arthroplasty. In Evarts CM: *Surgery of the musculoskeletal system,* New York, 1983, Churchill-Livingstone.

Modularity has drawbacks as well: it increases the manufacturing cost and the potential that the interlock between the head and the tapered neck will fail, causing disassembly and corrosion and producing particles (see Chapter 4). This author has used a modular head to accommodate a 22-mm or 26-mm head with Charnley's stem design*; Charnley never approved the large head (larger than 22.5 mm) for manufacturing.

Stem Design

The biomechanical rationale behind cemented versus cementless designs was discussed in Chapter 6. In summary, the intramedullary stem of the total hip prosthesis must have the following characteristics for use with cement:

1. A configuration and size that fit the anatomical shape of the upper femur.
2. Dimensions that do not exceed the narrowest segment of the shaft "isthmus."
3. Tapering that will facilitate cement injection.
4. A configuration that will produce maximal resistance against rotational and compressive forces at the upper third of the femur.
5. Sufficient numbers of sizes to accommodate a thick layer of acrylic cement, especially at the concave side of the prosthesis in the upper femur.
6. Sufficient strength derived through the metallurgical process to withstand cyclical long-term weight bearing without plastic deformation or fatigue failure.

7. The stem beyond the neck of the femur (at about the level of the lesser trochanter) must have a straight general configuration to allow centralization within the medullary canal of the femur.
8. The stem must be long enough to allow adequate fixation via its tapered segment, but not so long that it jeopardizes optimal orientation in the canal because of a double curve of the femur. The stem should only be long enough to prevent varus or valgus tilt.

Naturally, the design and shape of the stem influence the mechanical behavior of the prosthesis within the shaft. The stem's tensile stress is directly proportional to the bending moment but inversely related to the section modulus of the stem. Therefore, it is desirable to choose a prosthesis with the largest possible caliber (while still allowing adequate space for cement) to prevent plastic deformation of the metal and failure of the prosthesis.

While the metallurgical composition and the method of processing the metal used in the stem may generally influence the strength of the stem, the continuous bending moments generated around the stem are influenced by other factors: (1) neck-shaft angle, (2) neck length, (3) varus or valgus orientation of the stem in the shaft, and (4) offset between the center of the head and the axis of the prosthetic stem. If the stem has a double support design coupled with broadening of its calcar region, the stress is more widely distributed, thus reducing the stress on the cement. A high-modulus metal is the best material for a cemented total hip arthroplasty prosthesis. Metals such as stainless steel (such as Ortron 90 [high-nitrogen-content stain-

---

* The Elite System is supplied by DePuy U.S.A.

less steel]) and chromium-cobalt alloy have both been used with long-term success. Using titanium to make cemented stem raises concerns because of its low modulus of elasticity and its notch sensitivity; both of these factors may affect its long-term performance when used with cement (see Chapters 4 and 6).

The author's design modifies Charnley's in two ways: (1) the collar has been eliminated, and (2) double support is provided for the cement with an I-beam configuration (Fig. 11-11, *A* to *G*).

Collarless Stem

The author recommends a stem without a collar for two reasons: (1) permanent contact between the collar and the neck is not feasible, and (2) allowing controlled subsidence may keep the cement mantle under compressive load.

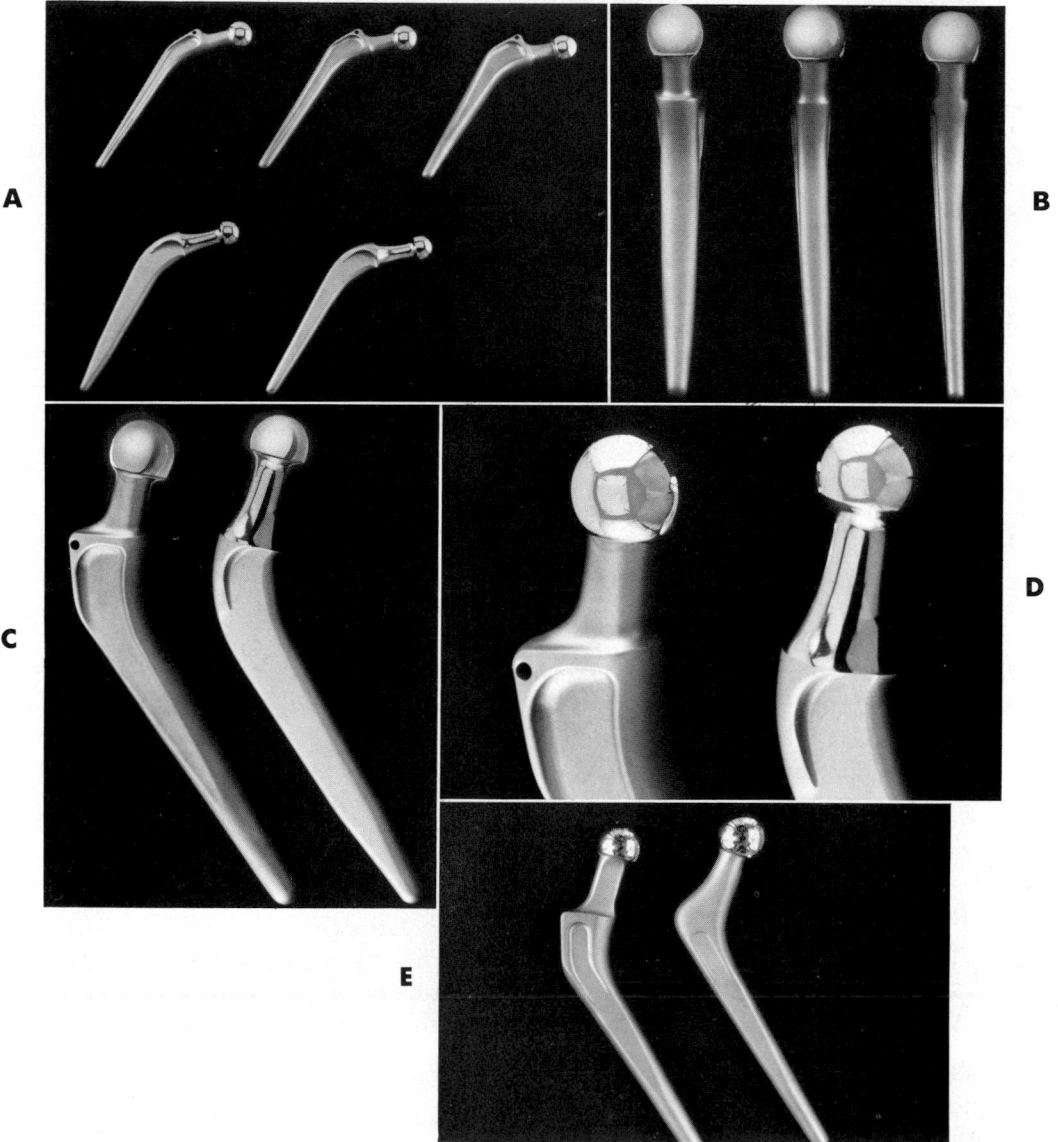

Fig. 11-11. A, The biomechanical prosthesis designed by the author, standard series: from left to right (*top*) small, medium, and heavy; compare with extra heavy (*left*) and heavy Charnley cobra design. Note comparison of 26-mm head with 22-mm Charnley. **B,** The medial aspect of the biomechanical prosthesis (examples of standard series) possesses a broad surface to reduce stress from the cement on the medial calcar. **C** and **D,** The extra-heavy cobra design of Charnley's prosthesis (*right*)) compared with the heavy author's prosthesis. Note a double support of the upper femoral component in the biomechanical design. **E,** Two examples of the author's stem designs, both in small series used in narrow canals such as congenital dysplasia.

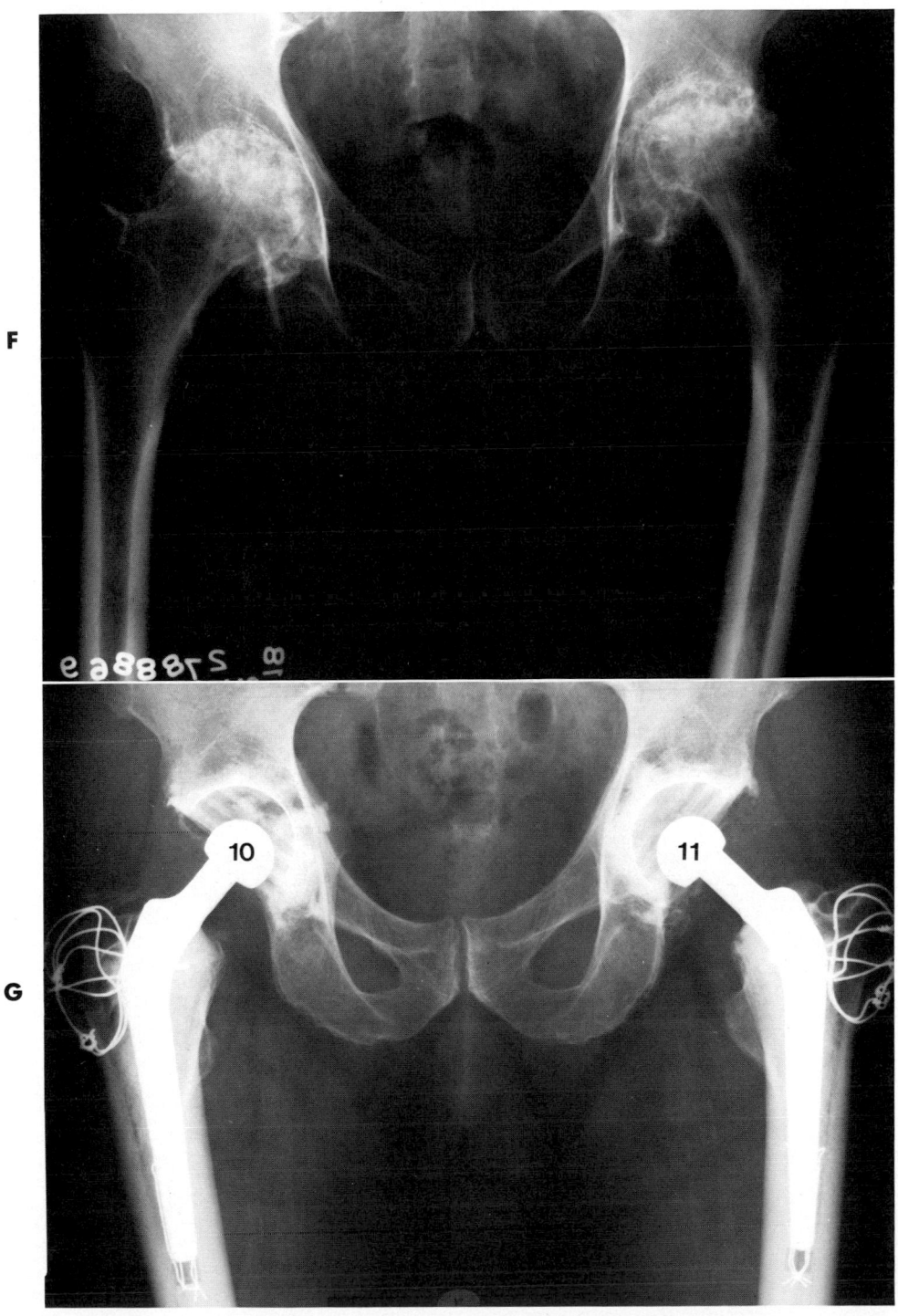

Fig. 11-11—cont'd.   F and **G,** Preoperative radiographs of a 64-year-old man (A.A.) who had bilateral total hip arthroplasty (author's prosthesis and centralization plug) 10 to 11 years after surgery. (**A** to **D** from Eftekhar NS: Total hip replacement using principles of low-friction arthroplasty. In Evarts CM: *Surgery of the musculoskeletal system,* New York, 1983, Churchill-Livingstone.)

Double Support for Cement

An I-beam cross-section configuration or a lateral flange may reduce stress from the proximal and medial cement by lateralizing the stresses.

A double-support I-beam configuration promotes load bearing via the cement in the upper femur at two areas: the outer rib and the inner rib. This feature not only reduces the compressive forces from the cement by increasing the surface area between the metal and the cement, it keeps the cement in compression.

The broad inner and outer borders of the stem strengthen the prosthesis considerably, while the "neutral axis" accommodates a thick layer of cement. The outer and inner borders fuse distally as tapering is maximized, a feature that allows the stem to pass the narrow isthmus and enter the centralization plug (see Chapter 19).

Stem Shape and Tip Design

In Charnley's design and the author's modification, the uppermost 5 cm to 7 cm at the top of the femur (the most important segment of the prosthesis) has been carefully designed to accommodate the shape of the upper femur. The straight segment of the stem (in three sizes: standard, small, and large) accommodates most canal sizes and their corresponding centralizing plugs (designed by the author; see Chapter 19). The

author's design provides an additional extra-large sized stem and Charnley provides a large stem (Magnum) for unusually large femora.

This author continues to use Charnley's total hip prosthetic design of the stem for its biomechanical superiority to other designs. At the time of this writing, he has discontinued using his own design because in his experiences with young and active patients titanium prostheses have developed early failures associated with osteolysis (see Chapter 4). The author has collaborated with biomechanical engineers to develop a modular prosthesis system based on a design derived from his own and Charnley's experience, known as the Elite Modular Charnley System. Its superiority derives from several features:

1. Its broad medial-proximal and proximal design and its even larger proximal-lateral design, including the flanged feature, which centralize the stem in the femur and keep the cement under boundary compression.
2. The stem is tapered 7 degrees in two planes.
3. The stem surface has no texture or precoating, and in the absence of a collar, subsidence may occur in the cement mantle.
4. With a stem length of 11 cm, the offset is 40 mm.
5. With a neck cross-section of 10 mm, a 22-mm or

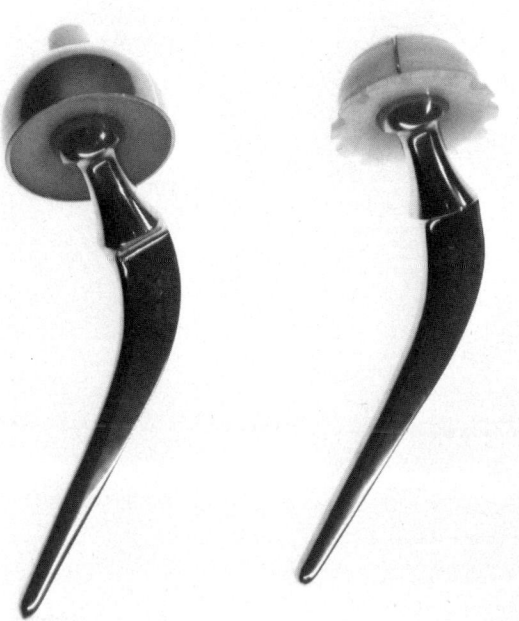

Fig. 11-12. Charnley's original designs, known as *flat-backs*, were made of annealed stainless steel; the two types of sockets, the press-fit (*left*) and cemented variety (*right*), are shown. In subsequent developments the stem was redesigned and replaced by the roundback and cobra (flanged) varieties. The stem was also made of a high-nitrogen-content stainless steel ("ORTRON90"). The flanged cups (the pressure injection and OGEE cups) replaced the original design.

Table 11–1 Specification Guide

Charnley femoral prosthesis	Dimensions							
	A	B	C	D	E	F	G	H
Roundback 45	32.00	112.66	144.75	50°	9.78	12.69	60.61	45.00
Roundback 40	32.00	112.71	141.53	50°	9.78	12.67	60.88	40.00
Flanged 45	32.00	112.98	141.75	50°	9.78	12.67	60.61	45.00
Flanged 40	32.00	112.45	141.53	50°	9.78	12.67	60.61	40.00
Flanged 35	32.00	112.23	141.31	50°	9.78	13.97	60.61	35.00
Ex H Flanged 45	32.00	112.66	141.75	50°	9.78	15.70	60.61	45.00
Ex H Flanged 40	32.00	112.45	141.53	50°	9.78	15.70	60.58	40.00
Fl. 40 Long Stem	32.00	168.06	197.14	50°	9.78	9.54	116.22	40.00
Ex H Fl 40 LS	32.00	168.06	197.14	50°	9.78	9.53	116.22	40.00
Long Neck 1	42.01	115.49	154.81	40°	9.8	11.66	63.76	38.40
Long Neck 1 Ex H	42.03	119.02	158.36	40°	9.78	14.79	67.30	38.40
Long Neck 2	51.99	115.61	165.59	32°	9.78	11.68	63.87	38.40
Long Neck 2 Ex H	51.99	115.60	165.59	32°	9.78	15.70	63.87	38.40
Long Neck 1 L S	42.00	179.15	218.48	40°	9.78	9.54	127.43	38.40
Long Neck 2 L S	51.99	186.07	236.05	32°	9.78	9.54	134.45	38.40
Roundback 40 Narrow	32.00	112.71	141.53	50°	8.18	12.67	60.88	40.00
¾ Inch Neck	25.63	92.58	117.56	50°	9.78	13.39	40.75	35.00
C D H	25.63	111.32	135.12	55°	9.78	11.61	59.97	26.00
Extra Small	20.19	119.47	140.96	50°	8.18	10.01	67.80	27.00
STS 35	32.00	112.23	141.31	50°	9.78	11.61	60.61	35.00
SNS 35	32.00	112.23	141.31	50°	8.18	11.61	60.61	35.00
C D H Ex Small	25.63	111.37	135.17	50°	8.18	10.01	60.02	26.00
Magnum 45	49.79	113.90	177.80	40°	12.22	19.60	68.90	45.00
Magnum 40	42.00	115.80	152.40	40°	10.40	17.24	64.80	40.00

Courtesy of DePuy U.S.A. These templates refer to the standard fourth generation Charnley range.

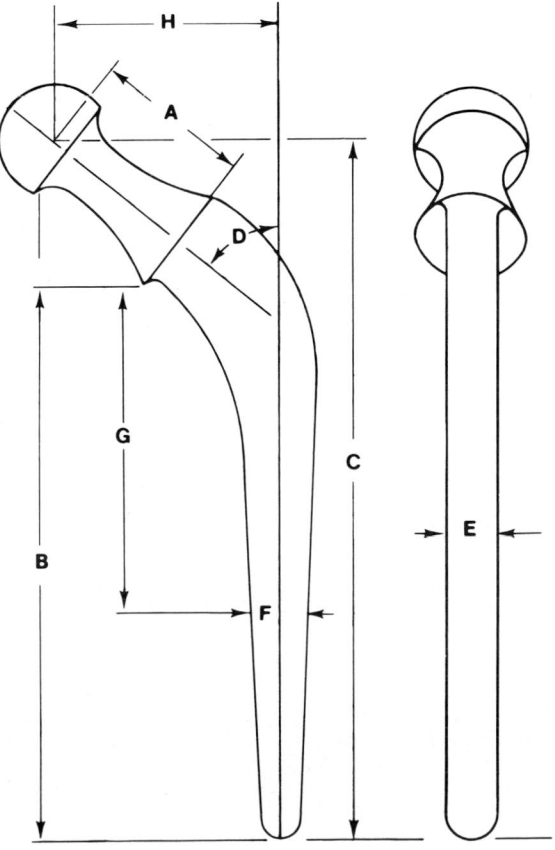

26-mm head can be incorporated to produce a range of motion of more than 120 degrees without neck socket impingement. The result is a versatile system that provides a prosthesis applicable to a variety of conditions and demands, including revision surgery; additionally, it can be used with noncemented porous-coated acetabular components currently on the market.

At the time of this writing the modular system is too new to determine its long-term advantages. A potential problem with modularity, however, is the possibility of corrosion, decoupling (dislocation), and future mechanical failures of the Morse tapered principle.

Charnley Low-Friction Arthroplasty Stem

Charnley's historical "flatback design" (in two sizes) was used with a cementless press-fit acetabular component or with a cemented socket (Fig. 11-12). Only a limited number of cementless sockets were used because they did not perform well. Charnley's design has been associated with excellent performance, despite a modest number of structural failures of the stem. Failures were caused by the sharp corners of the rectangular cross-section, the relatively narrow medial-lateral cross-section of the stem with an offset of 45 degrees, and the weak annealed stainless steel used in that design. A subsequent design improved on the "first generation" by adding metal to the flat surface of the stem, resulting in the "roundback" design. Charnley's prosthesis was further improved by adding a dorsal flange to the roundback; this is known as the *cobra design*. In addition, an extra-heavy prosthesis was designed for heavy patients (usually more than 75 kg in weight) with a larger medullary canal. Reducing the offset (from 45 mm to 40 mm), adding 3 mm of metal to the lateral border of the stem, and rounding off the flat-back effect each added approximately 10% to the strength of the stem, totaling 30%. The purposes of the dorsal flange are to keep the cement under compression while introducing the stem into the cement mantle and to increase the load-bearing capacity of the cement by keeping it under "boundary compression." The introduction of cold-coining of the stems and the use of high-strength metal (Ortron 90) have virtually eliminated stem fractures in patients.

TYPES OF CHARNLEY PROSTHESES The various types of Charnley prostheses have been developed over a period of 20 years, based on clinical experience demonstrating the need for modification (Table 11-1). The modifications were not based on mathematical calculations to produce proportionally larger or smaller prostheses relative to a standard size. They were patient-specific, based on the shape and size of the femur and biomechanical considerations. For clarity,

they are grouped into three categories:

1. Standard Series
2. Small and Short Series
3. Large and Long Series

Category I—Standard Series. This series includes heavy and extra-heavy stems. These stems are used most often and the stem and neck length remain unchanged; the only changes are in the offset and the stem thickness. They are manufactured with a flange and with different offsets (45, 40, and 35 mm). There are also two extra, extra-heavy stems and (known flanged magnum) with 45- and 40-mm offsets. This author routinely uses a 40-mm offset prosthesis. Fig. 11-13 demonstrates the use of a modular (Elite) low-friction arthroplasty prosthesis with a 26-mm head. The opposite hip is templated using a single-unit Charnley flanged 40-mm stem.

Category II—Small and Short Series. In this category, the stem thickness, stem length, neck length, or the offset may be smaller than in the Standard Series.

The flange has also been eliminated in all stems in this series. This series includes:

Roundback 45, 40

Roundback narrow 40

Roundback narrow ¾ neck

Short and narrow ¾ neck

CDH

Extra small

Straight short 35

Straight narrow 35

CDH extra small

Category III—Large and Long Series. In this category the stem length and the thickness are increased:

Flanged magnum 45, 40 (also listed with standard series)

Flanged 40 long stem

Flanged extra heavy 40 long stem

Long neck (1 cm)

Long neck (1 cm) extra heavy

Long neck (2 cm)

Long neck (2 cm) extra heavy

Long neck (1 cm) long stem

Long neck (2 cm) long stem

Flanged magnum long (1 cm)

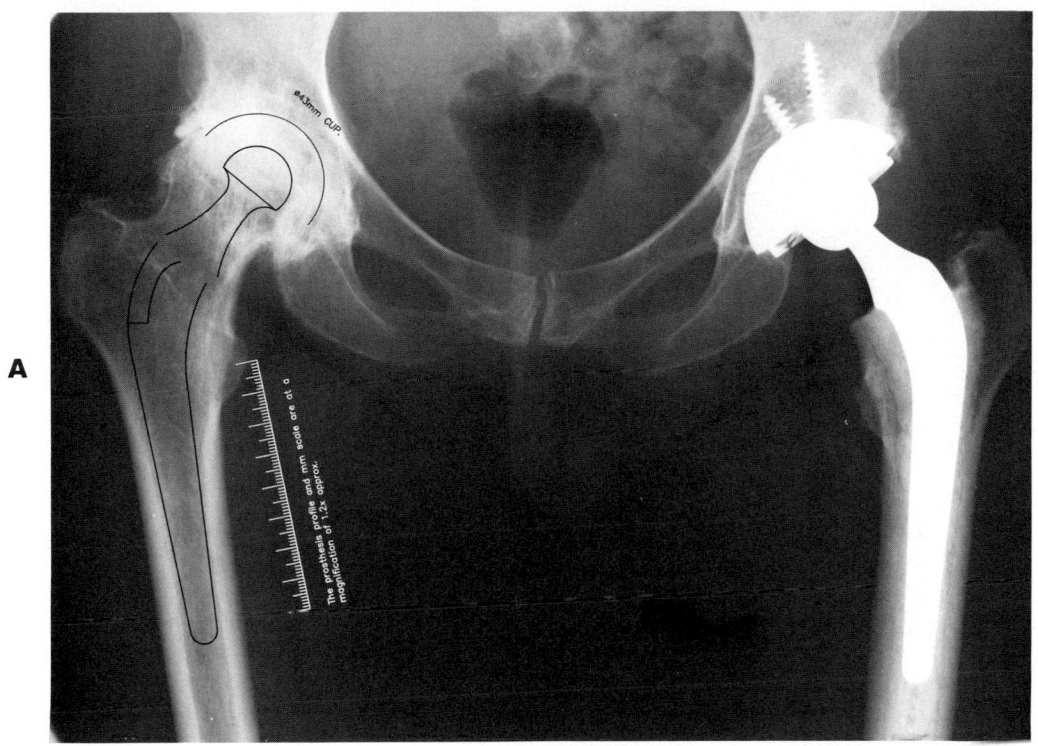

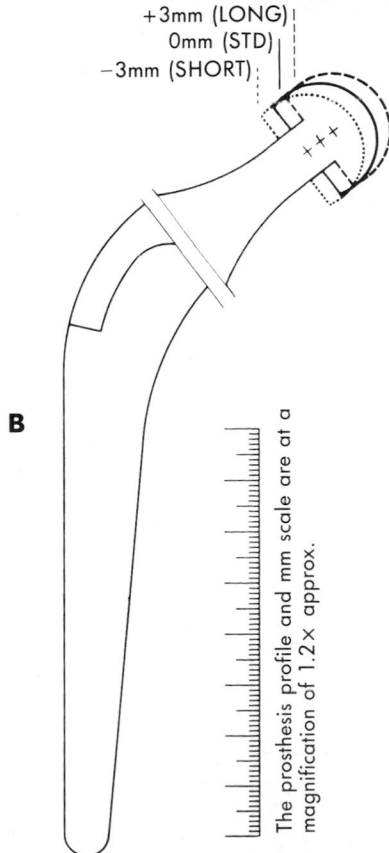

Fig. 11-13. A, Templating of osteoarthritic left hip using a standard Charnley heavy prosthesis template (40-mm offset). **B,** Right hip of 66-year-old female patient (P.L.), 3 years after low-friction arthroplasty using a modular (Elite) Charnley stem and a cementless porous-coated acetabular component. Template shows possibility of a modest shortening or elongation of the neck length after cementing of the stem.

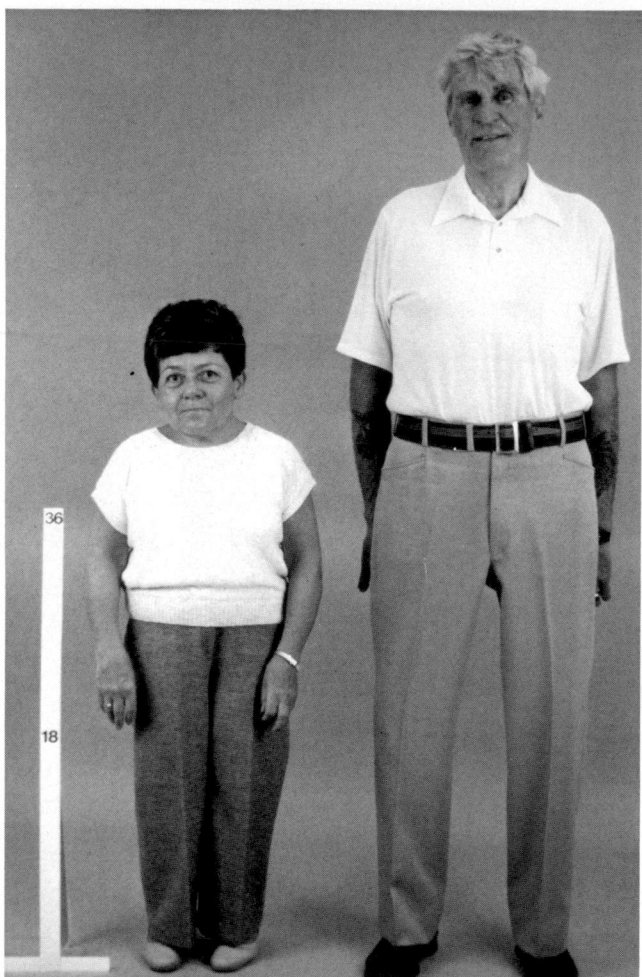

Fig. 11-14. The problem of fitting the patient with an appropriate-sized prosthesis should be anticipated even without reviewing the radiographs. Just look at the size of the patient! The patient to the right, who is 6 feet 6 inches tall, stands alongside another patient with achondroplasia. Both had hip arthroplasties (see Figs. 11-15 and 11-16).

Figs. 11-14 to 11-22 show examples of various series of Charnley and Charnley modular prostheses. The reader is encouraged to see Chapters 10, 20, 24, and 25 for examples of prosthetic selection.

Socket Design

The plastic socket must accommodate the femoral head, with clearance ranging from 0.004 to 0.010 inch. The depth of penetration of the head into the socket determines the neck-socket impingement angle.

Depth of penetration of the head in Charnley's and the author's designs is 2 mm coupled with a 2:1 head-neck ratio, which allows 108 degrees flexion in Charnley's design and 115 degrees in the author's

design without socket-neck impingement.

An extended posterior wall in the cup design augments stability, thus providing resistance against dislocation or subluxation in extreme ranges of flexion and adduction. However, this feature of the design reduces the angle of the neck-socket impingement in external rotation and extension. When using the socket with a long posterior wall (i.e., Charnley's design), allow no anteversion or retroversion at surgery. If no posterior wall has been incorporated in the design, allow 10 to 15 degrees of anteversion of the cup, a desirable feature to improve cup coverage by bone due to the commonly encountered defective anterior wall of the acetabulum and to prevent posterior dislocation (see Fig. 11-5).

Most sockets for total hip prostheses are manufactured by machine. Sockets made by injection mold techniques offer an improved surface finish and the homogeneous molecular structural density of polyethylene. Complex geometrical designs can be produced by molding techniques. However, long-term studies of the cups have not been reported. It is essential to consider the thickness of the socket in the weight-bearing zone in any given situation; therefore, from the standpoints of wear and of the "shock-absorbing property" of the plastic, it is beneficial to increase the thickness of the plastic in the weight-bearing zone (author's design), although long-term studies are needed to verify whether loosening of these cups occurs less or more than with concentric cups.

Charnley's Flanged Sockets and Pressure Injection Cup (PIJ and OGEE)

Charnley's acetabular component design is the most suitable socket to use with cemented fixation; it has the following features:

1. Hemispherical shape
2. Broad rim
3. Long posterior wall
4. No metal backing
5. No spacers

A pressure-injection cup (Charnley PIJ or OGEE, see Chapter 6)* is favored for several reasons:

1. It permits the surgeon to customize the cup (by trimming) to fit the acetabulum (Figs. 11-23 and 11-24).
2. It avoids "wobble" in the acetabulum during polymerization of the cement.

---

* DePuy, U.S.A. Use of a rimless socket is indicated only for extremely small acetabula when a rim cannot be accommodated.

3. It remains in a stable position (without bottoming) during cement polymerization.
4. It exerts an element of hydrolic pressure on the cement at insertion.
5. The semirigid flange contains cement within the acetabular cavity, allowing any excess to escape.

Fig. 11-25 shows the dimensions of the PIJ design in the standard size, along with the long posterior wall (LPW) feature.

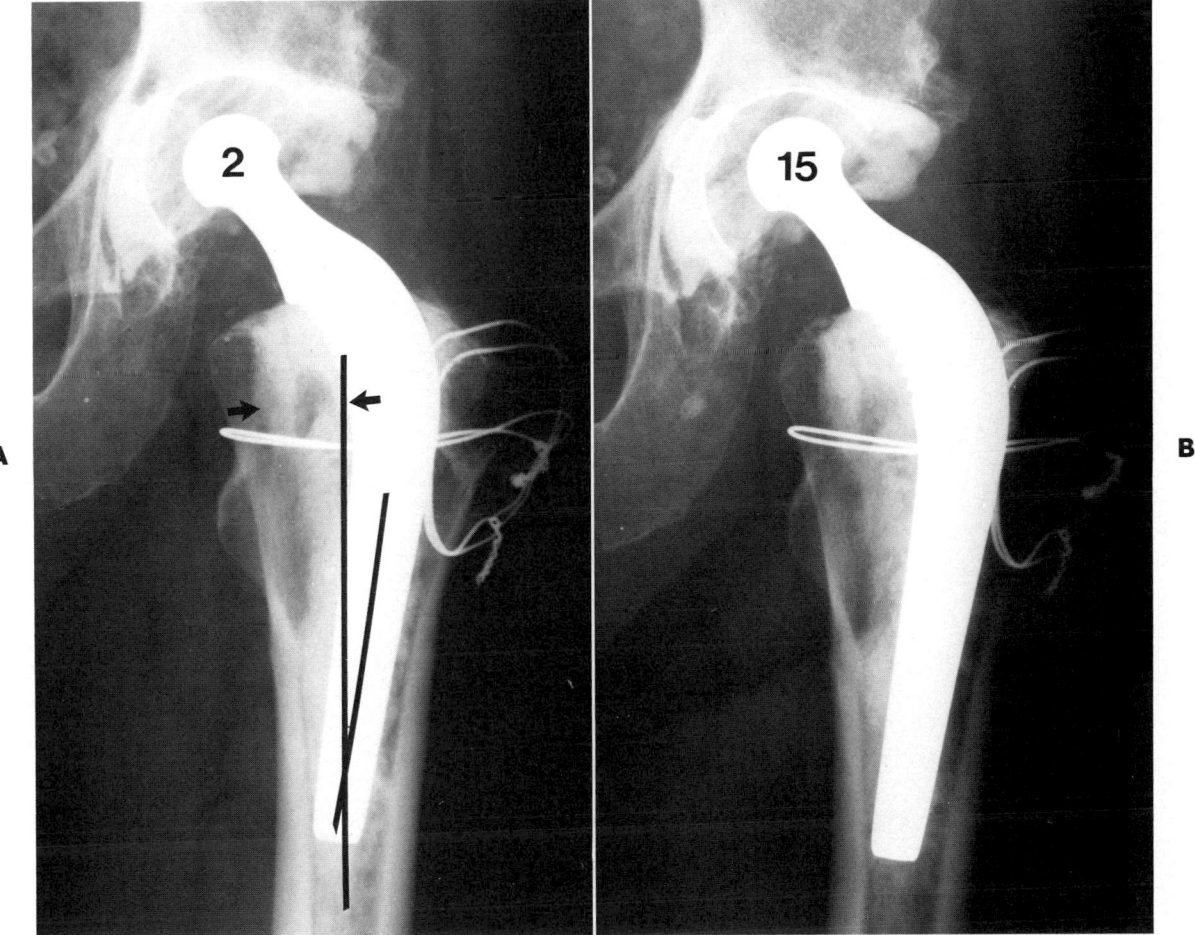

Fig. 11-15. Radiographs of same patient as in Fig. 11-14. **A,** 51-year-old male (N.E.) weighing 185 pounds 1 year after low-friction arthroplasty. NOTE: exaggerated valgus of stem measuring 12 degrees in a wide medullary canal. **B,** 15 years postoperatively, there is no loosening of either component; cup wear measures 3 mm. A well-centered position with a 26-mm femoral head would have been preferred. Note grade 3 radiolucency at cement-acetabulum interface (see Fig. 11-17).

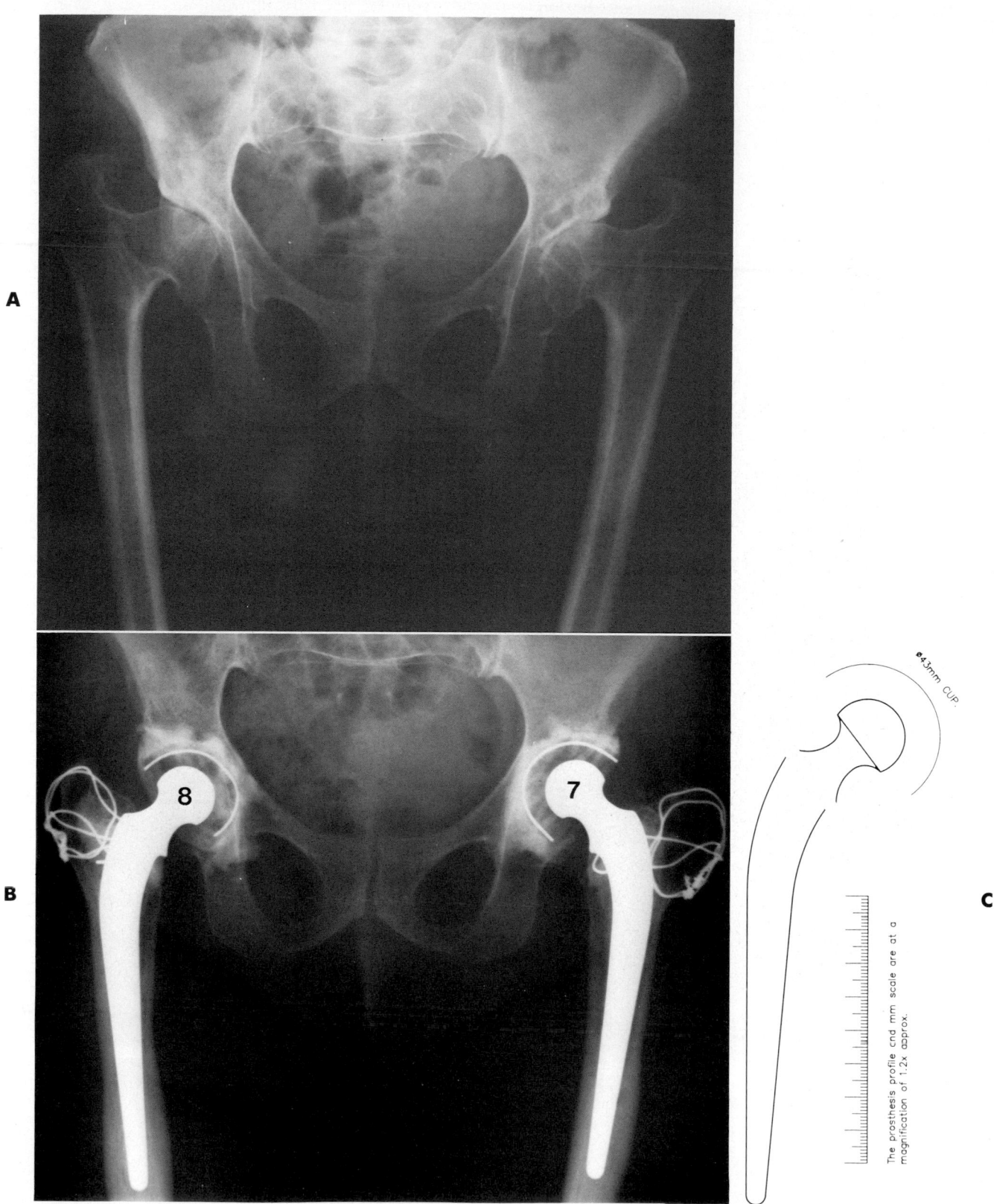

Fig. 11-16. A, Radiograph of a 50-year-old female (J.M.) with a diagnosis of achondroplasia (see Fig. 11-14). **B,** 7 and 8 years after left and right low-friction arthroplasty. NOTE: Charnley extra-small stem was inserted after modest amount of reaming of both canals. **C,** Template for prosthesis used in **B** is shown.

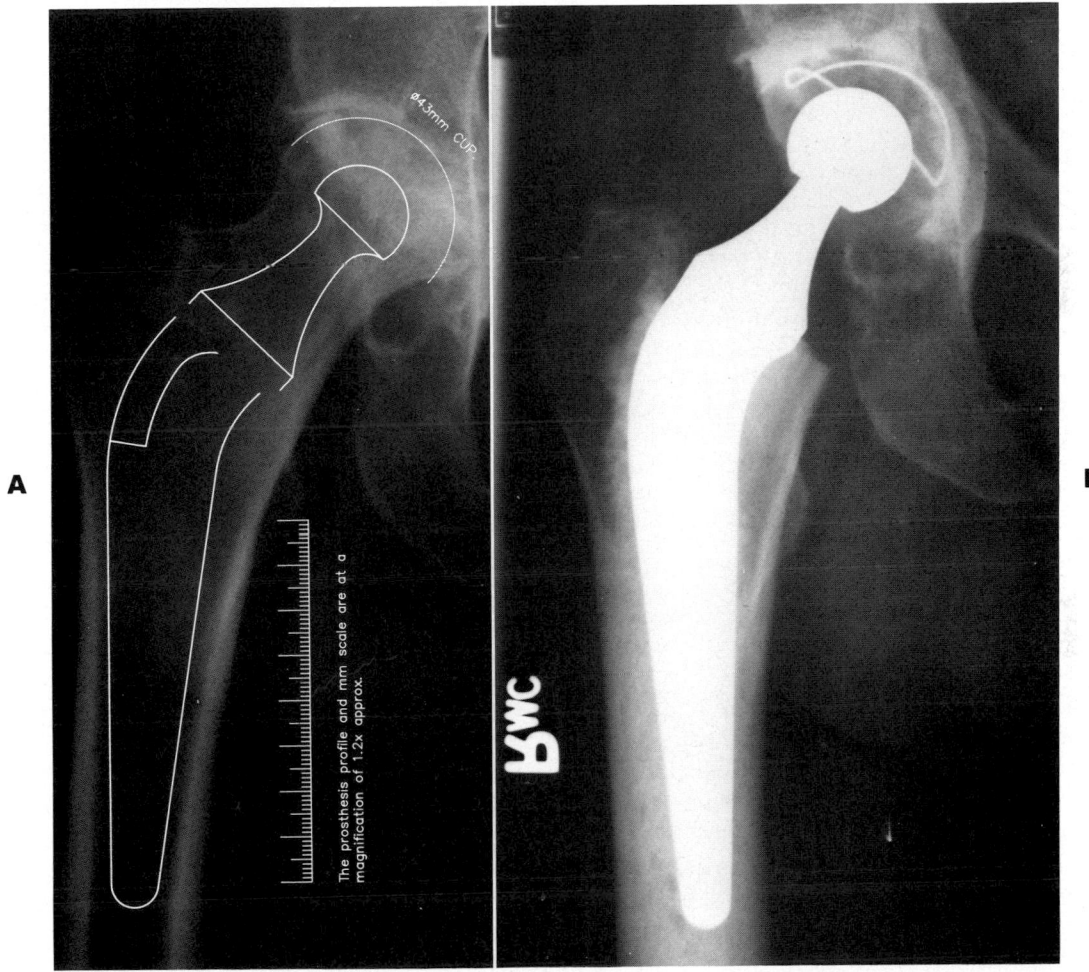

Fig. 11-17. A, A 77-year-old female (L.C.) with a large medullary canal measuring 24 mm at isthmus (stove pipe–shaped femur). **B,** Magnum stem and OGEE cup were used. NOTE: The stem could not be centered because the stem was undersized for the canal. The stem could have been larger if customization had been done.

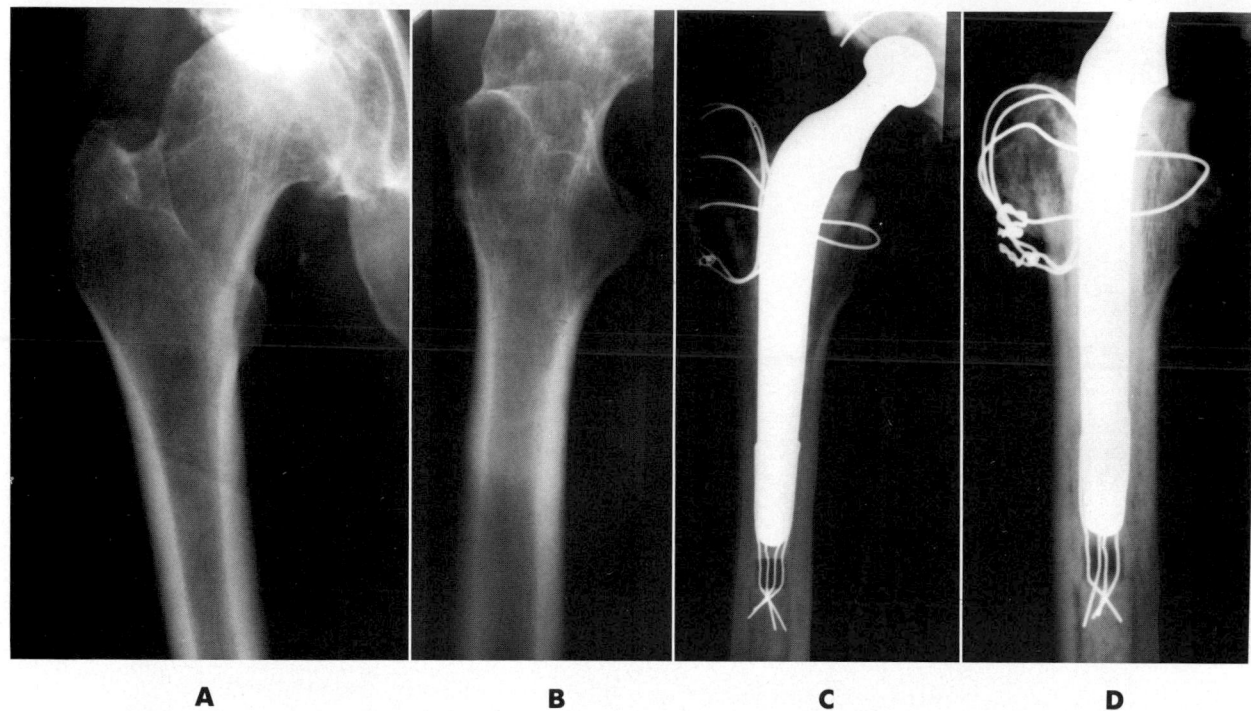

A   B   C   D

Fig. 11-18. With a large medullary canal a centralization device is necessary to center the stem in the femoral shaft (see Chapters 15 and 19). **A** and **B,** The medullary canal measures 19 to 20 mm (on anteroposterior and lateral views) at the level of isthmus. The author's centralization plug was used to center the Charnley extra-heavy stem in the canal. **C** and **D,** Anteroposterior and lateral views.

The Author's Eccentric Rimmed Cup

The author's design* originally was used in cases of protrusio acetabuli with severe medial wall defects and larger acetabuli. In cases where Charnley's original cup design (without the flange) was inadequate,[7] the author used his own modified cup (which predates Charnley's PIJ cup) in over 300 hips; it accommodates a 26-mm femoral head. As noted, the flange is in the same plane as the mouth of the cup; it was detachable after cementing of the cup (Fig. 11-26). With the introduction of the OGEE cup, it is possible to use a 26-mm- or 28-mm-diameter head, which can be helpful in revision surgery if the surgeon is revising the acetabular cup without removing the femoral component. The OGEE cups are designed for and are especially useful in dysplastic hips with anterior wall defects. The OGEE cups are now available in different cup sizes (external and internal diameter).

Other Prostheses

Since Charnley's introduction of low-friction arthroplasty, many modifications of that prosthesis have been introduced, notably, femoral heads larger than 22.5 mm, curved stems, and diamond cross-sectional stem designs, all of which have proven to be counterproductive in improving results over the original Charnley low-friction arthroplasty prosthesis.

Currently, numerous prostheses are on the market; their originators or the manufacturers make various claims for their superiority over Charnley's low-friction arthroplasty prosthesis system. Notably (with a few exceptions), long-term clinical data have not been produced with 10 to 20 years' follow up for comparison with Charnley's. While we do not intend to list all prostheses, the ones with longer history and unique features include cad hip endoprostheses, Müller straight stem and curved stem, Exeter prostheses, and HD2 prostheses. More recently, some surgeons have advocated the use of methods to encourage bonding of the prosthesis to cement proximally by precoating the proximal portion of the stem or altering the geometry of the proximal portion of the prosthesis to improve the load-bearing capacity of the stem. "Harris Precoat Prosthesis" (Zimmer U.S.A.) and "Precision Hip" (Howmedica U.S.A.) are examples of such concepts. This author prefers nontextured prostheses for use with cement. Other features of the new prostheses require careful clinical and radiographic evaluation;

---

*Zimmer U.S.A.

Text continued on p. 519.

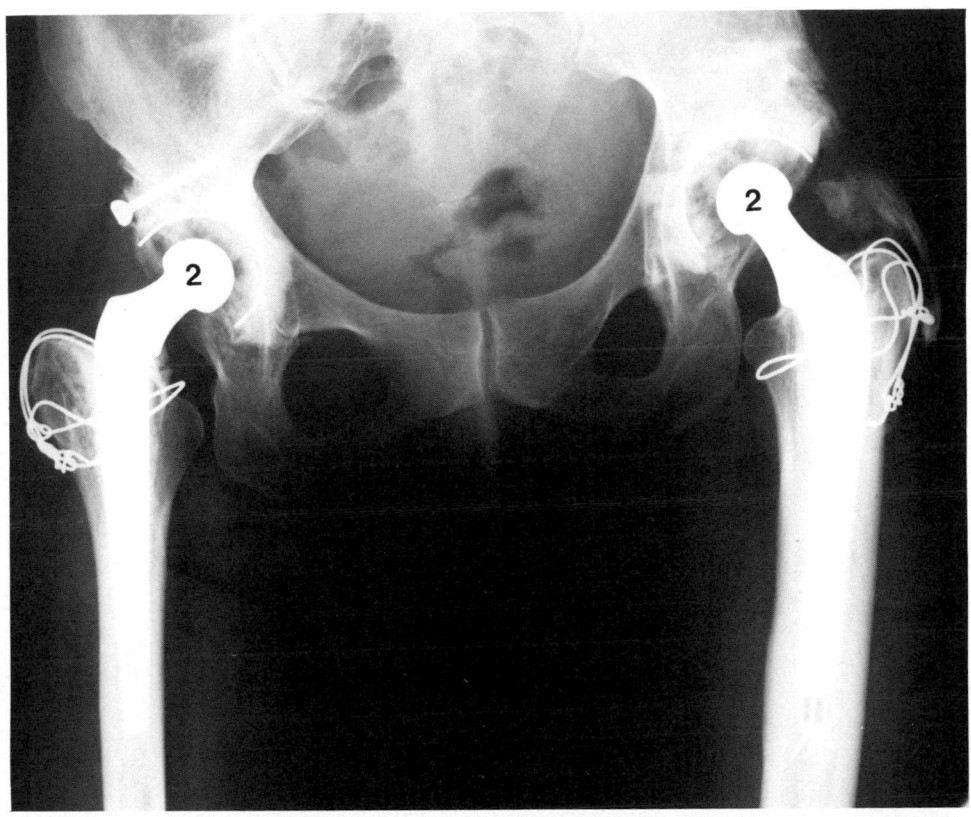

Fig. 11-19. For bilateral hip dysplasia and dislocation in the same patient, different-sized prostheses may be required. The Charnley hip system especially is suitable for dysplastic hips. Radiograph after bilateral total hip arthroplasty in 34-year-old woman (J.M.). Note that a CDH prosthesis was used on the right because the left hip accommodated a narrow roundback stem (see Chapter 20).

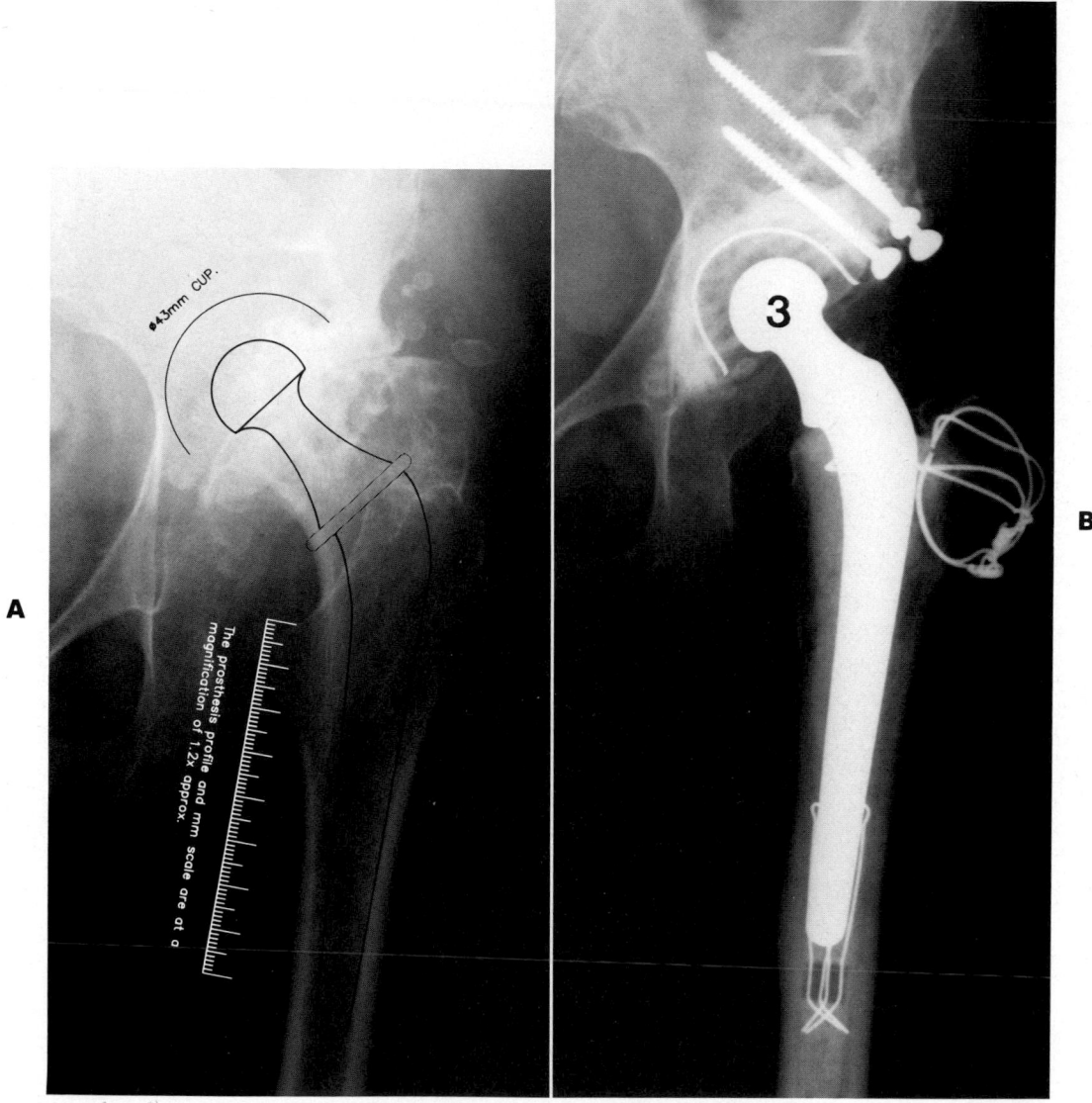

Fig. 11-20. A, Preoperative radiograph of a 46-year-old female (M.S.) with a unilateral Intermediate congenital dislocation of the hip. Femur is templated for size. Template indicates that the straight narrow stem (SNS) with 35-mm offset was not suitable. Such a prosthesis was implanted. **B,** Radiograph taken 3 years postoperatively shows bone graft has united.

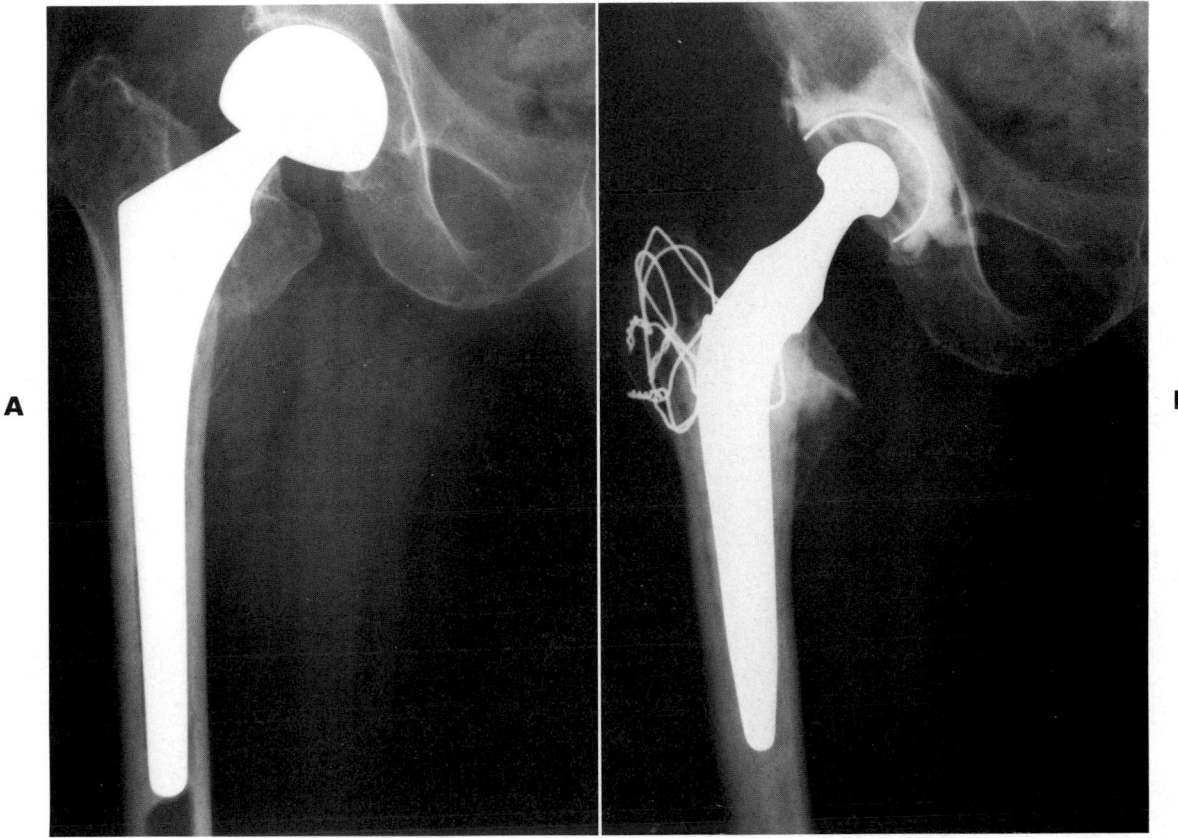

Fig. 11-21. Bone lost at neck region is best replaced by a prosthesis with an extended neck without increasing the offset. **A,** Postoperative radiograph of patient (G.M.) with failed bipolar prosthesis (loose and subsided) used for an intracapsular femoral neck fracture. **B,** After low-friction arthroplasty, a 1-cm-long-neck extra-heavy Charnley cobra prosthesis was used to correct a 5-cm leg length inequality.

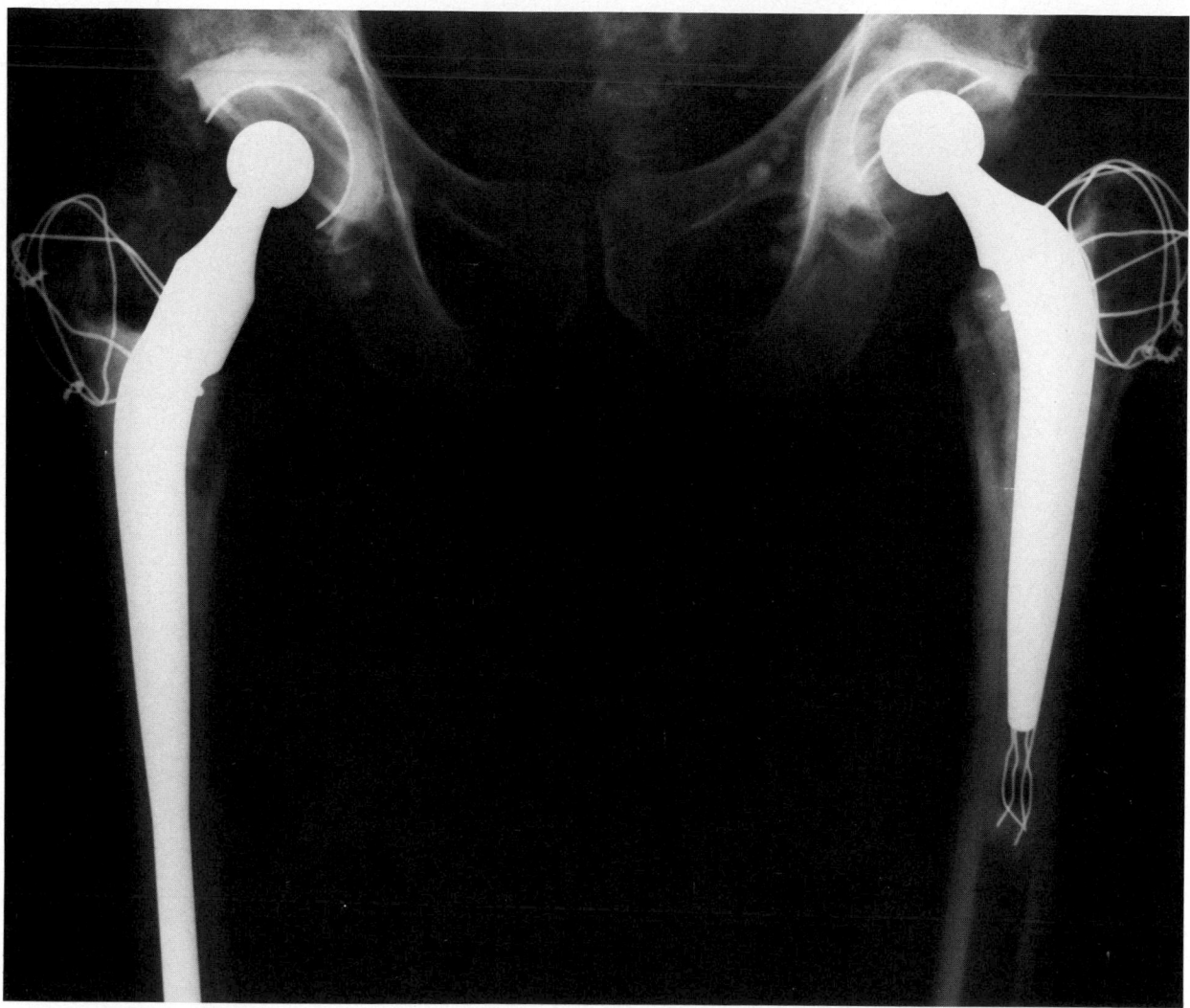

Fig. 11-22. Postoperative radiograph after bilateral low-friction arthroplasty performed in a 66-year-old man (P.L.) for primary osteoarthritis (*L*) and for revision of a failed Müller-Charnley prosthesis (*R*). NOTE: Long stem—2-cm-long-neck—was used with a 22.5-mm femoral head on the right against a pressure injection cup with 43-mm outer diameter. An extra-heavy Charnley modular stem (Elite) with a 26-mm head was used on the left. The acetabular component on the left is an OGEE cup.

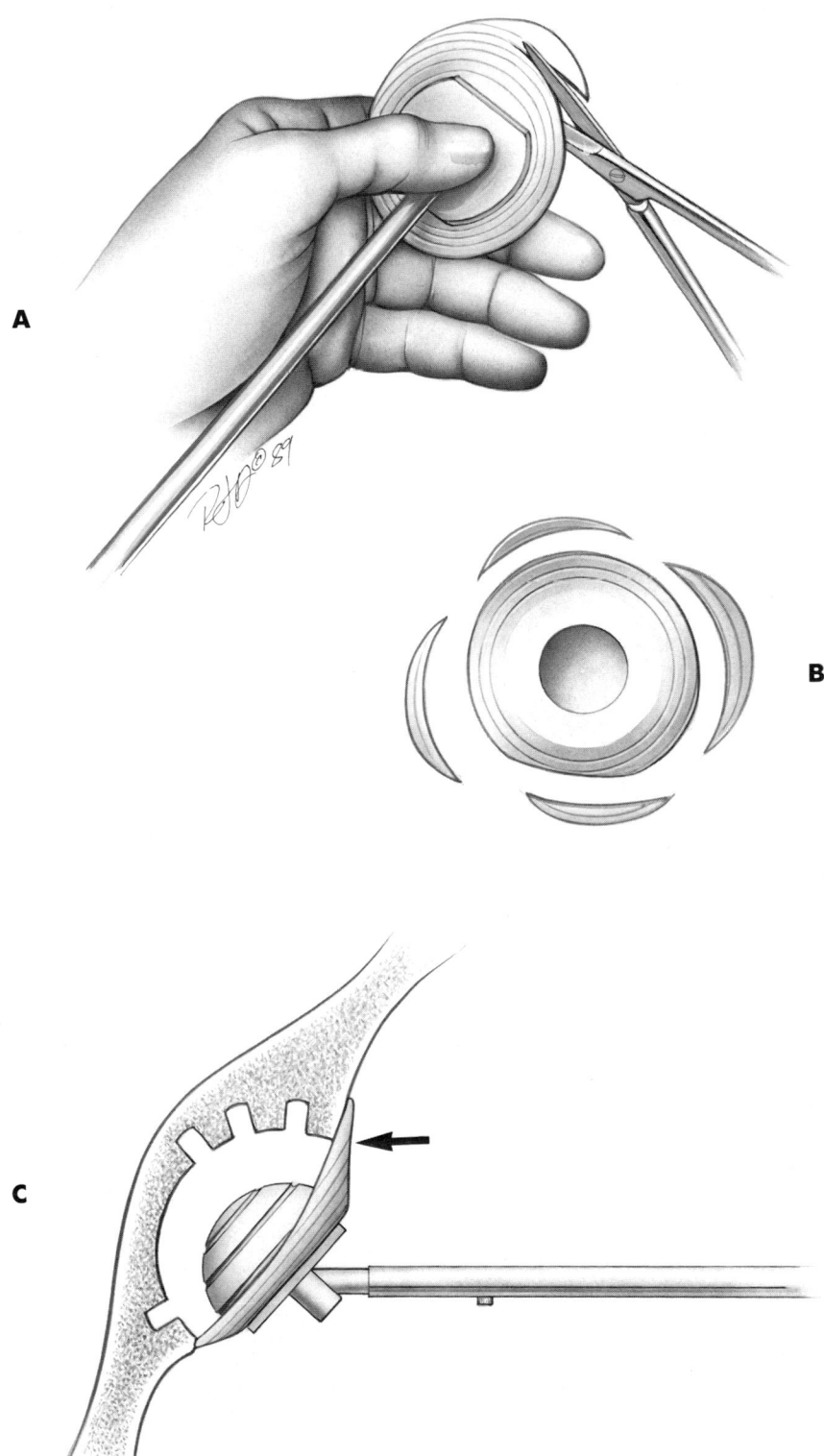

Fig. 11-23. A, Using a pair of heavy-duty scissors, trim the flange as desired. Cup is properly clipped to the holder while cutting is done along the grooves on the cup. **B,** The inferior lobe is excised first, followed by tailoring of the anterior, posterior, and finally superior lobe of the cup. **C,** After tailoring the three lobes of the flanged cup, the cup is tested for "best fit". The superior lobe is then trimmed away *(arrow)*. Ideally, the cup must be well contained and the flange must fit the inner rim of the acetabulum snugly, like a piston within a cylinder.

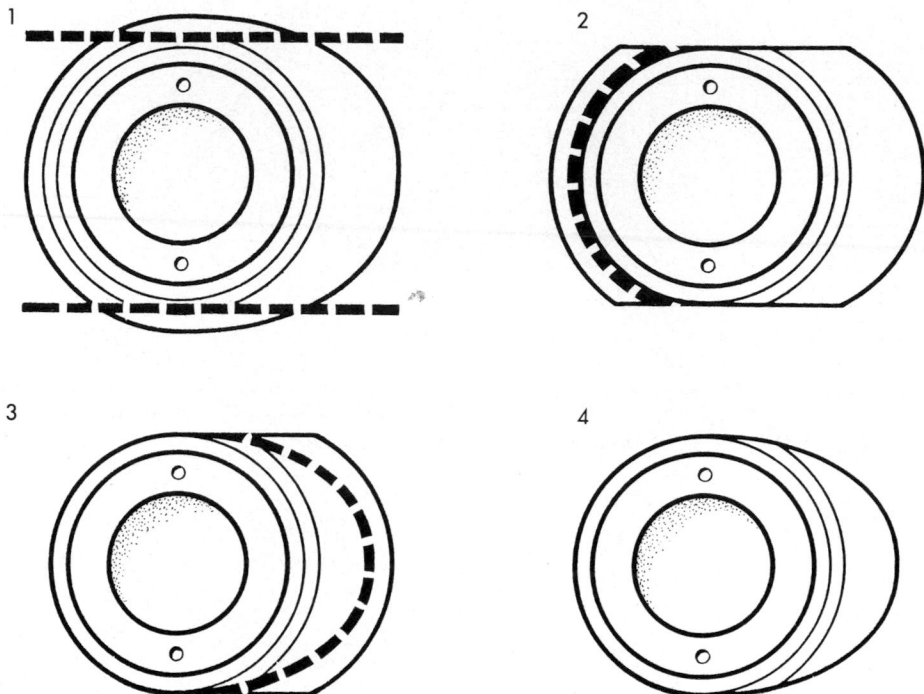

Fig. 11-24. Sequential cutting of the flanged cup (PIJ). *1,* Anterior and posterior lobe; *2,* inferior lobe; *3,* superior lobe; *4,* customized cup ready to be inserted. (Modified from Charnley J: *Low-friction arthroplasty of the hip: theory and practice,* Berlin, 1979, Springer-Verlag.

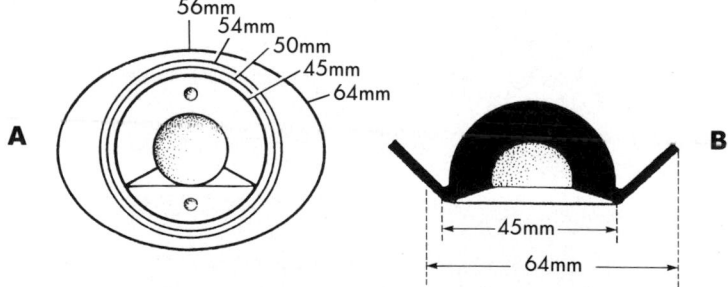

Fig. 11-25. Pressure injection cup (flanged) of Charnley's design in standard size can be customized according to the size of the acetabulum. **A,** Dimensions. **B,** Long posterior wall feature.

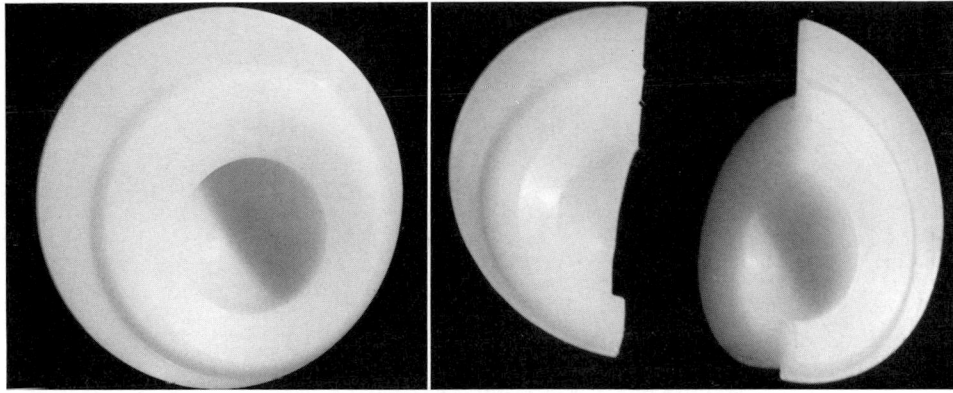

Fig. 11-26. A, The acetabular component possesses a rim to pressurize and retain the cement within the acetabular cavity. The planes of the mouth of the cup and the rim are identical; this feature is specially designed to assure cup coverage by the bony acetabulum at implantation. **B,** The vertical cross-section of the cup shows eccentric thickness of high-density polyethylene. Cups without projections, which are available, may be used. (From Eftekhar NS: Total hip replacement using principles of low-friction arthroplasty. In Evarts CM, editor: *Surgery of the musculoskeletal system*, New York, 1983, Churchill Livingstone.)

the ultimate judgment on their merits must be based on clinical experience.

Cementless Prostheses

Two original designs of cementless prostheses are (1) the anatomical medullary locking prostheses (AML*) total hip system, and (2) the porous-coated hip system (PCA†). Many subsequent designs on the market today have used some of the features of these two original designs. The newer designs include (3) Harris-Galante,‡ (4) the BIAS,‡ (5) the Omnifit,§ and (6) the S-Rom Total Hip System.‖ Indications for their use and knowledge of their advantages and disadvantages should be based on clinical performance. Unfortunately, many of these original designs have either been modified or additional sizes have been introduced, so although newer advances and innovations may have addressed some of the issues and failures of the early days, long-term studies of these designs and their modifications are still not available. In this author's experience, the short-term use of porous-coated acetabular components (Harris-Galante or AML) has been virtually trouble-free. This author only rarely uses a porous-coated femoral component due to inconsistency of the clinical results. But my own early results with Mulier intraoperative manufacturing have been encouraging, although a high percentage of clinical success has been reported

in the short-term following the use of cementless porous-coated stems. According to Galante, major problems that may predispose the patient to long-term failure of these devices can be related to component subsidence, porous surface delamination, proximal cortical atrophy, and femoral endostealysis.[12]

Figs. 11-27 to 11-31 illustrate the use of some of the contemporary cementless designs with provisions for bony ingrowth. Note that AML and Harris/Galante stems are straight but PCA, BIAS, and Intermedic stems are curved. (The inventory for curved stems must include stems for both right and left hips.)

Hybrid Hips

A combination of cementless and cemented components in total hip arthroplasty has gained popularity on the theory that this combination may increase the longevity of the procedure, especially in young and active individuals. The rationale is that long-term studies indicate excellent durability of cemented components, whereas cemented acetabular components have not performed as well (see Chapter 28). Based on the foregoing, surgeons are inclined to use a porous-coated acetabular cup with a cemented femoral component (Figs. 11-32 to 11-35). Remember, however, that in the long term (15 to 20 years), most hips fail not because of the failure of acetabular fixation, but due to wear particles of high-density polyethylene and mechanical failure of the cup itself (see Chapters 4 and 6).

CUSTOMIZATION OF IMPLANTS

The role of customization in total hip arthroplasty primarily concerns the femoral segment because of the vast variations among individuals in the shape and size

---

* DePuy Inc.
† Howmedica Inc.
‡ Zimmer Inc.
§Osteonic Inc.
‖Joint Medical Product Corporation.

Text continued on p. 524.

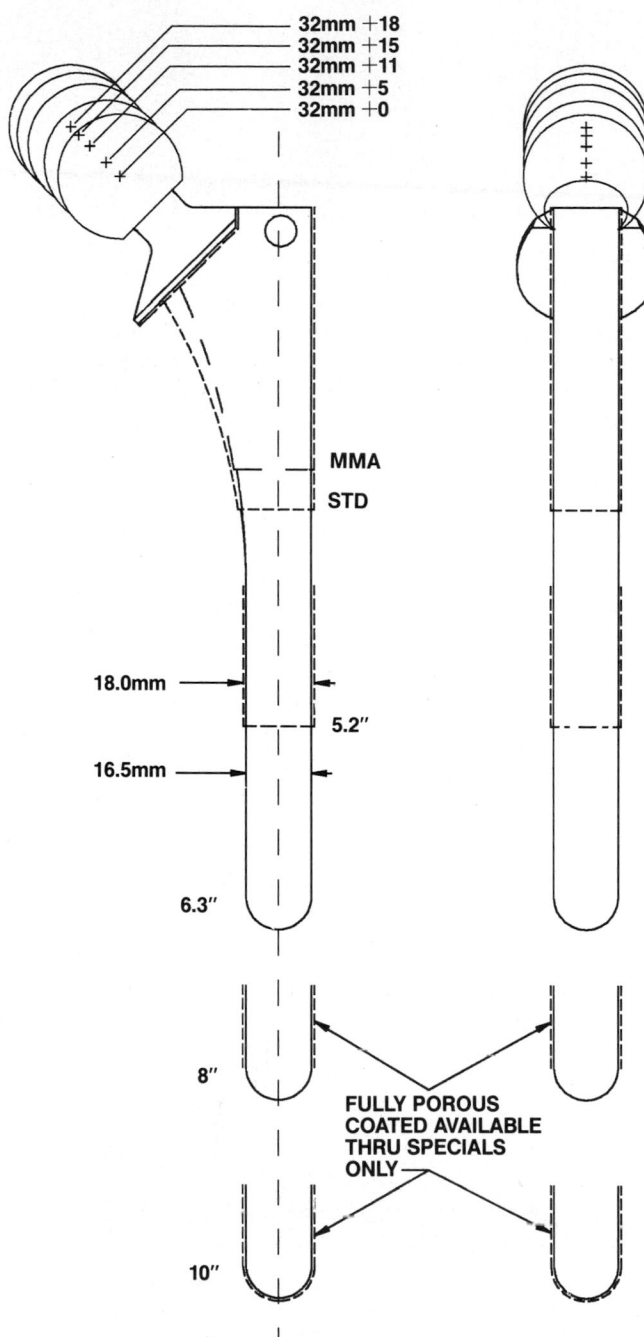

Fig. 11-27. AML "Porocoat" hip template. Note various porous-coating possibilities and neck length adjustments. The stem is straight and immediate fixation is achieved by a 3-point fixation. This is a collared prosthesis made of chromium-cobalt alloy.

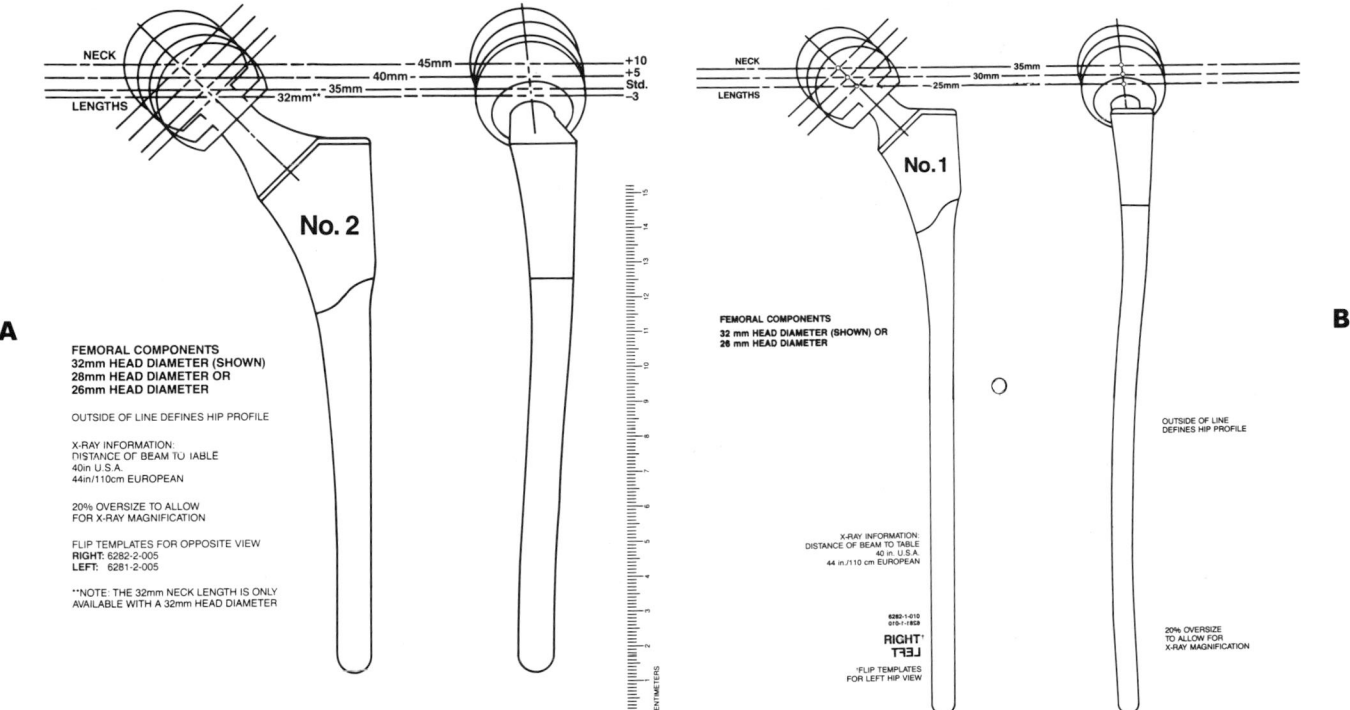

Fig. 11-28. PCA cementless porous-coated midstem total hip prosthesis (anatomical design). Note that the curve segment is designed to accommodate the anatomical bow of femur. The stem is collarless. **A,** Standard stem. **B,** Long stem.

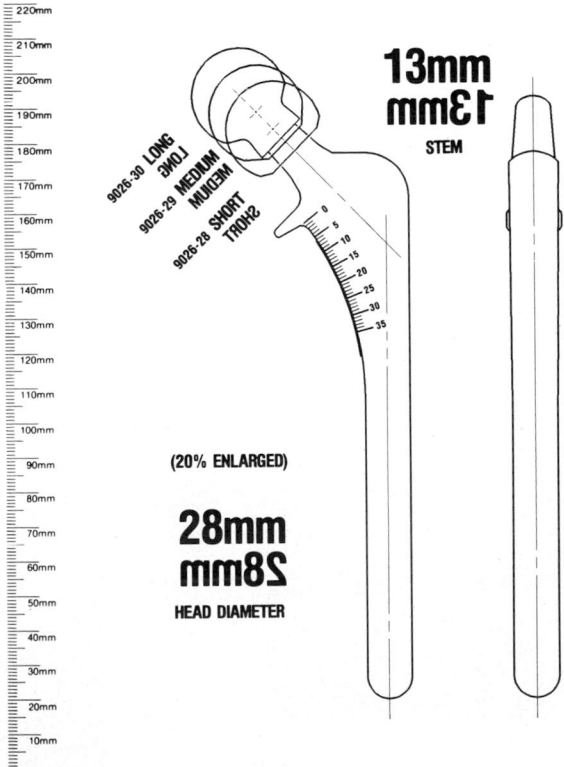

Fig. 11-29. Harris/Galante porous-coated prosthesis (with straight stem template) for 13-mm stem size. The prosthesis is collared and provides porous surface proximally by sintered titanium wire mesh. The stem is made of titanium alloy.

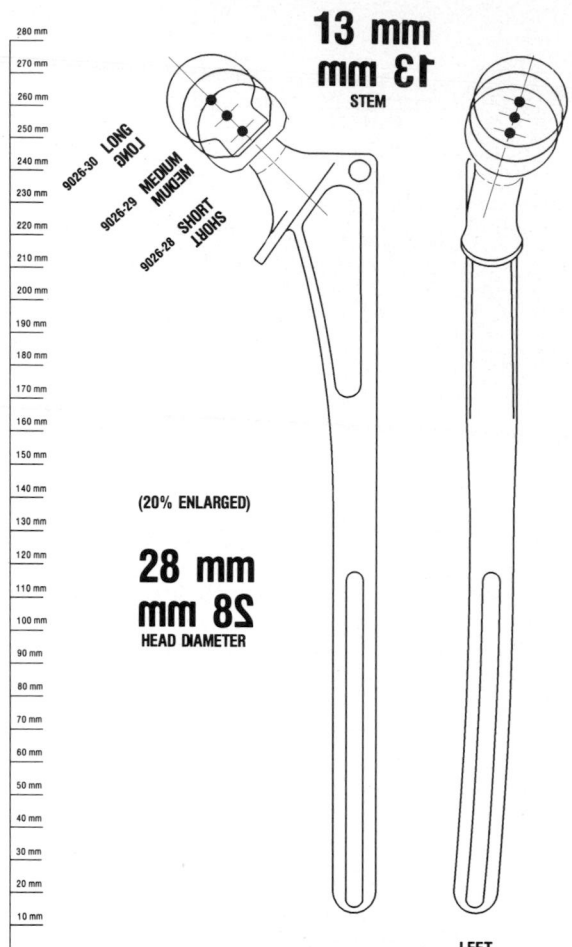

Fig. 11-30. BIAS template. This long-stem prosthesis with a curved stem (anatomical) is suitable for revision surgery when the use of cement is contraindicated (see Chapter 25). The stem is collared, and it is made of titanium alloy.

Fig. 11-31. **A,** Radiograph of a 64-year-old man (B.K.) with osteoarthritis of the hip treated by a cemented all-titanium stem (DF80) in author's institution. **B,** 2 years after revision using an APR prosthesis. **C,** Lateral of the same hip as in **B.** Note the clothespin design (*hollow arrow*), a unique feature in reducing thigh pain resulting from noncemented long-stem prostheses. Solid arrows show grafted areas of the site of osteolysis.

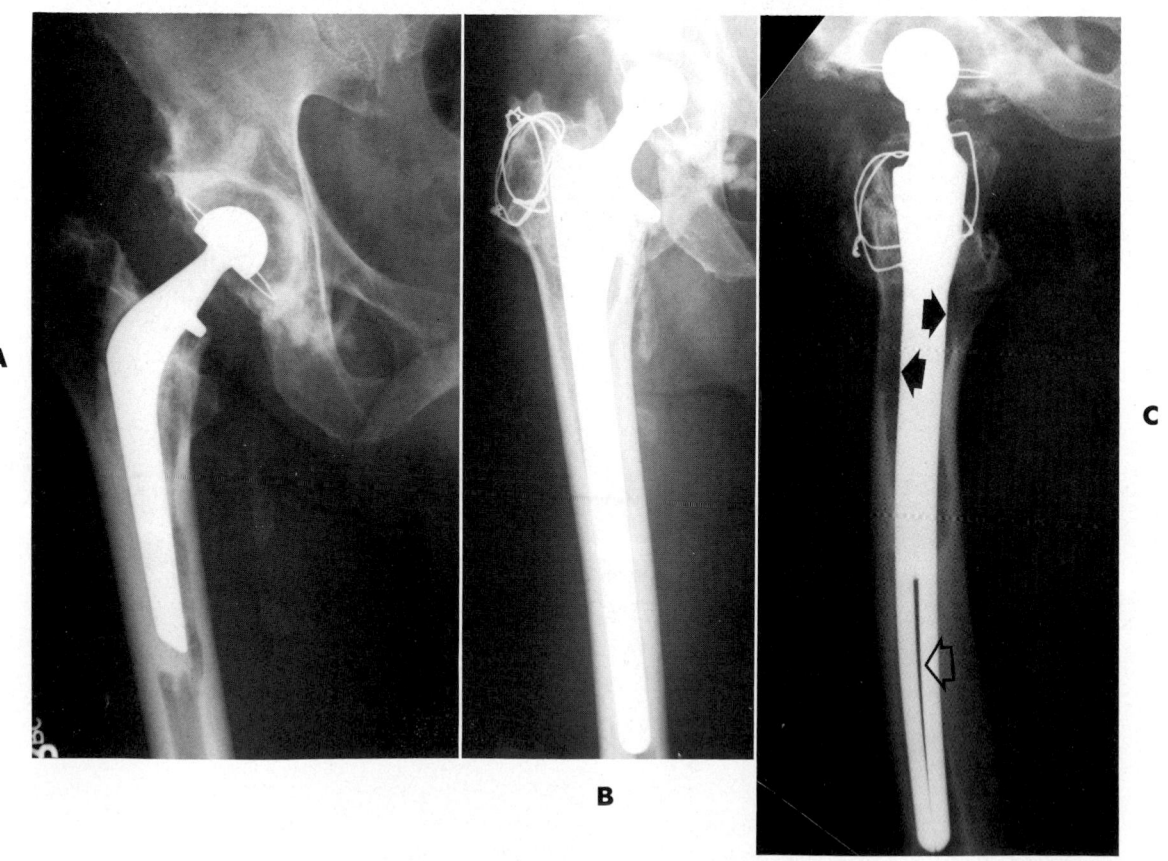

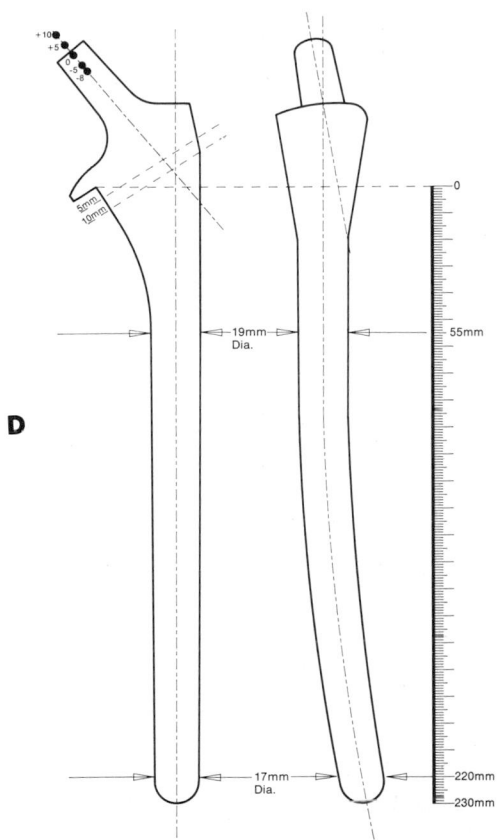

D

Fig. 11-31—cont'd. D, Template of long-stem (APR) (Intermedic) stem. This prosthesis is especially useful for revision surgery because it provides "bulk" for the proximal femur (usually associated with severe bone loss due to long-standing loosening) and a "clothespin" design (*arrow*) that collapses at insertion with the potential to reduce stress at the stem tip level (see Chapter 25).

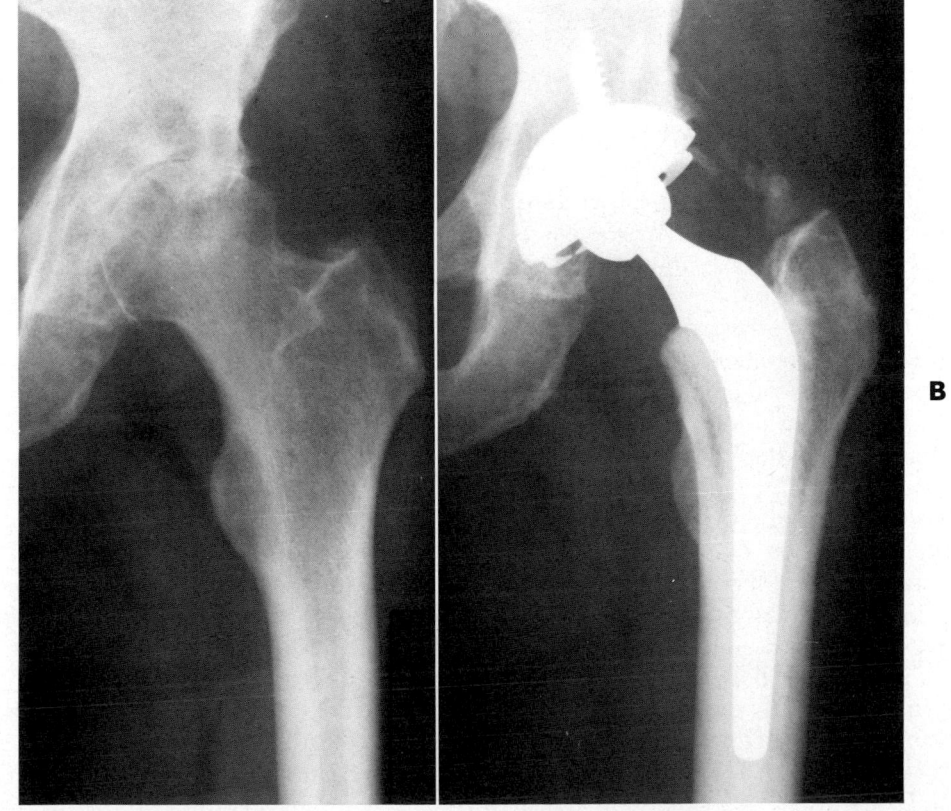

Fig. 11-32. A, Preoperative radiograph of a 66-year-old physically active man (J.D.). **B,** 1 year after a hybrid hip using a cemented Charnley (modular) heavy cobra stem, 26-mm femoral head, and a Harris/Galante porous-coated cup (hybrid hip).

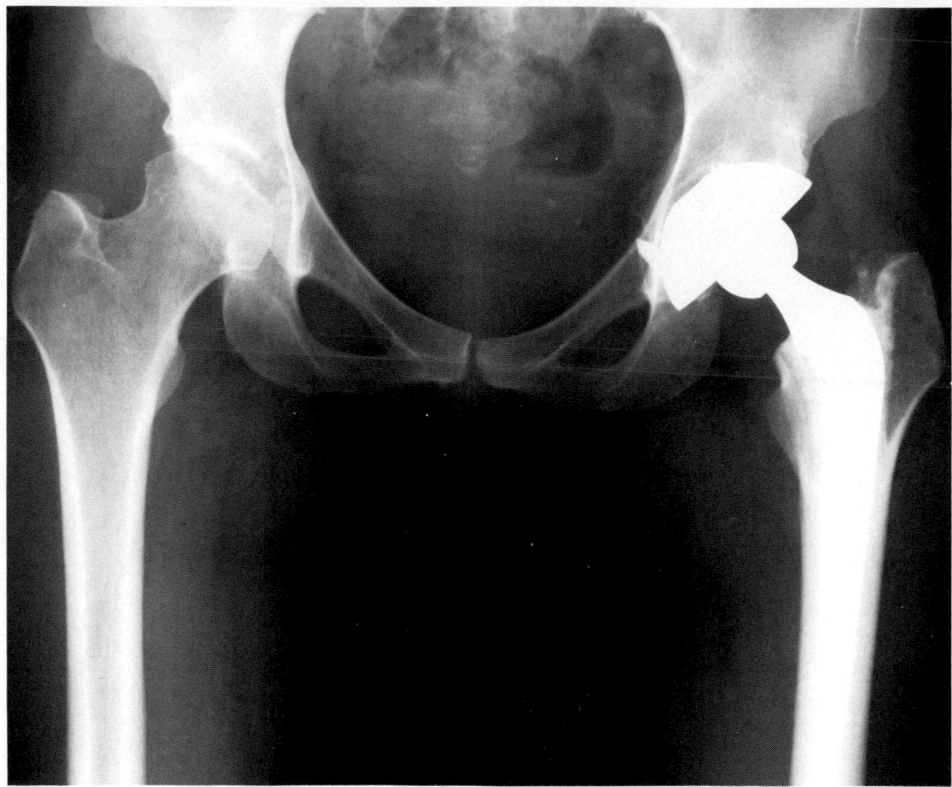

Fig. 11-33. A hybrid hip was placed in a 36-year-old female (P.R.) for degenerative osteoarthritis secondary to avascular necrosis. An AML cup and an SNS of modular Charnley (Elite) was used. Note that offset of the prosthesis (35 mm) in addition to centered stem reproduced the normal offset.

of the upper femur.[19] These variations arise because the metaphysis and diaphysis are disproportional and because the medullary canal enlarges progressively after the fourth or fifth decades of life, whereas the metaphyseal region retains its shape and size, increasing the degree of disproportion.[11,21,26,27] With the exception of certain types of revisionary surgery that are difficult because of the hemispherical geometry of the acetabulum, prefabricated acetabular components sufficiently address the requirements for the acetabular prosthesis. Therefore it is not necessary to customize the acetabular component. Customization is defined as "shaping the implant to the patient," not "shaping the patient's anatomy to fit a 'prefabricated prosthesis.'" As stated before, if we agree that the fit and fill of the prepared medullary canal are important factors in reducing micromotion and in providing optimal stress transfer to the bone, then the present success of total hip arthroplasty depends on customization of the prosthesis in one of four ways: (1) by using acrylic cement, (2) by using preoperative radiographs, (3) by using CAT scanning and computer-assisted technology, or (4) by intraoperative manufacturing of the prosthesis.

Customization by Cement

As indicated in Chapters 4, 5, 6, and 28, fixation of the stem by acrylic cement is the most practical and safest method for most patients requiring total hip arthroplasty. In this situation, the prosthetic cement composite becomes the customized device.

It is important to recognize that cemented total hip arthroplasty is the best method for custom prostheses, for several reasons:

1. It provides the best fit for the prosthetic-cement composite immediately upon insertion.
2. It produces the largest endosteal surface possible for load transfer.
3. Most of the compressive, bending, and torsional forces are resisted by PMMA bonding.
4. Painful fretting movements between the implant and bone are abolished immediately after implantation; as long as the fixation maintains its integrity, they will not recur after surgery.
5. A cemented femoral stem reduces stress and therefore strain in the proximal and/or distal femur to 9% to 35% of normal,[15,16] compared with a direct stem fit (press fit) to bone, which reduces the stresses to a much lesser extent.[31,32]

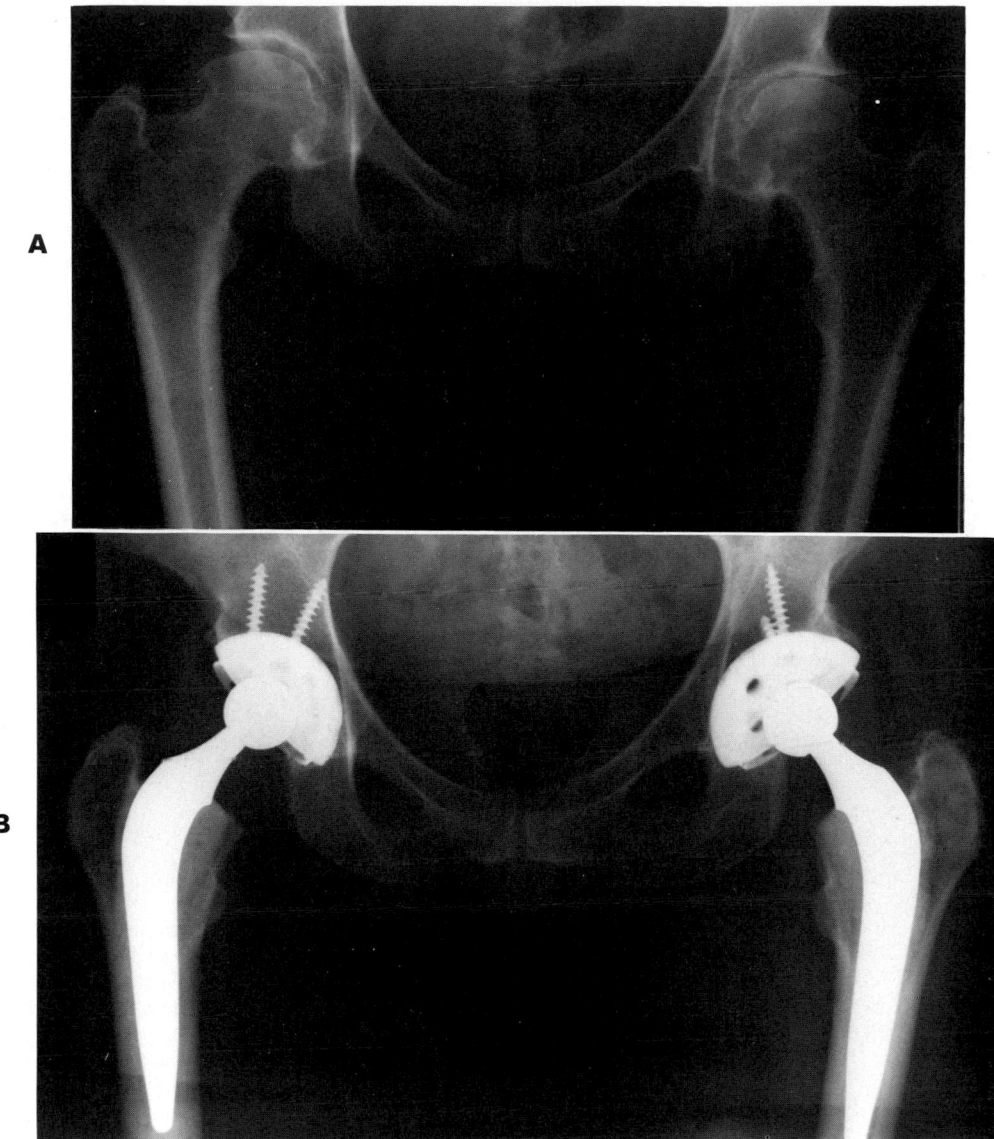

Fig. 11-34. A 62-year-old woman (A.C.) with bilateral degenerative osteoarthritis. Bilateral total hip arthroplasty (hybrid) was performed using extra-heavy modular Charnley (Elite) 1 year apart. Note normalization of the offset in both hips, despite large medullary canals.

The use of cement has been criticized for several reasons:

1. A cemented stem may loosen over time.
2. Cemented stem loosening occurs especially in young, active, and heavy patients.
3. After cement loosening, severe osteolysis occurs at the site of cement insertion.

Customizing Standard Implants

Stems using interference fit require a precision fit for optimal load transfer, both proximally and distally.

Unlike the porous-coated and cemented prostheses, which are bonded strongly, the stresses in stems using interference fit are more affected by the geometrical shape of the stem and less by its rigidity (see Chapter 6). Therefore the shape (cross-sectional dimensions) and materials used for bonded and nonbonded devices should not be the same. *Consequently, a prosthesis designed for use with cement should not be used without cement, and vice-versa.* Because the bone is not uniformly rigid, a nonbonded prosthesis (press fit) will produce a nonuniform progressive stress pattern for metaphysis to diaphysis. Although the distal load through the straight portion of the stem acts as a

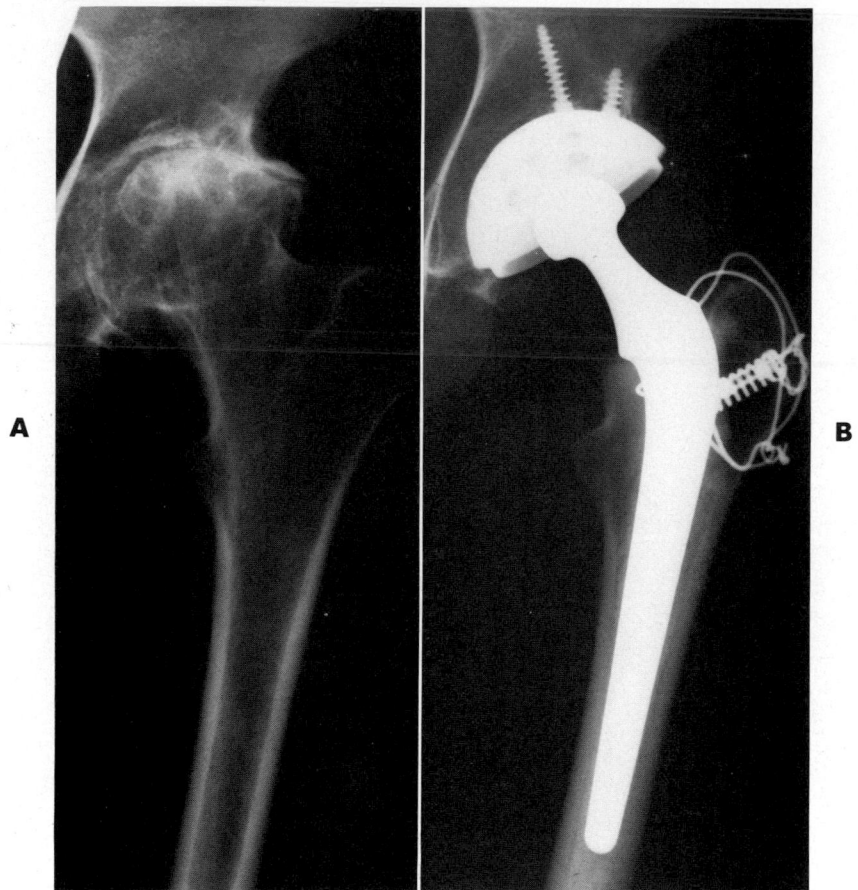

Fig. 11-35. Preoperative **A** and postoperative **B** radiographs of a 40-year-old woman (K.L.) with Legg-Calvé-Perthes disease and secondary osteoarthritis. Only a 50-mm OD cup (H/G) could be fitted in this acetabulum; a 22-mm femoral head was used. Note that wires at the stem metal (steel) and titanium alloy cup in this hybrid hip may be theoretically objectionable because they are of different metals. Mixing metals has never been a concern of the author in practice.

symmetrical cone, the proximal stem behaves differently because it is curved. Under applied compressive loads, the curved portion of the stem exerts excessive stresses medially, which can damage the bone; therefore it is desirable that a feature of the prosthetic design transfer these loads laterally and distally as much as possible (see Chapter 6).

When the load transfer is not optimal, one of the following stem conditions will lead to failure:

1. A well-fixed stem with a tight distal fit will reduce stress, causing progressive bone atrophy from stress shielding.[9,20]
2. A stem that is too loose distally will cause proximal overload. Like unloading, overloading of the proximal femur is undesirable because it leads to bone lysis and atrophy of the cortical bone, often associated with pain. Clinical failures due to mismatch resulting from micromotion of an undersized prosthesis have been document-

ed.[14,28] Therefore uncemented prostheses are more likely to exhibit micromotion than cemented components, especially in torsion. It is now abundantly clear that an oversized prosthesis is just as disadvantageous as an undersized. If the implant and bone do not fit exactly, even if poor fit does not cause fracture of the femur at surgery, poor bone remodeling will occur because of abnormal load transfer. Clinically, the result will be localized bone stress and pain.

Engh and Bobyn were among the first to observe that close-fitting femoral components yielded higher overall clinical scores than poorly matched components.[10]

It is obvious from the foregoing that to achieve optimal proximal and distal fit, a large inventory of prosthetic sizes and shapes is required.

Noble[19] recognized 45 Somatype designs that would be necessary to describe the medial-lateral endosteal contour of the femur with an accuracy of ± 1 mm. Only 17% of these designs occurred with an incidence higher than 1%. Naturally, an accuracy of ± 1 mm is not a true "press fit." Anatomical studies of the femur by Noble and others show that an actual press fit of the prosthesis to the proximal and distal femur is possible only by customization.[13,22,23,25,29]

Customizing with Preoperative Radiographs

Customizing implants in orthopaedic surgery is not new. Previously, prostheses had been customized for patients with special conditions, such as revision surgery and severe bone loss due to tumor resection. In those cases, a large segment of bone was replaced by a prosthesis and cement. These devices, known as special prostheses with either a longer neck or a longer stem with specific cross-sectional dimensions, can be conveniently manufactured to the surgeon's specifications. Magnification errors can occur, but they are not objectionable because the prosthesis is commonly made for use with cement, which can be used to fill the space between it and the bone. However, the precision of fit determined by preoperative measurements is grossly inadequate if the prosthesis is used without cement. Paradoxically, some surgeons use radiographs with unknown magnification to aid in preoperative planning for the use of cementless off-the-shelf prostheses, accepting discrepancies of 5% to 8% on the radiograph measurements and the implant as found at surgery.[2,8] Magnifications of radiographs vary from 15% to 30%, despite efforts to control this variable by using magnification markers. The variation is due to x-ray penetration and the thickness of the femoral cortex. For accurate sizing, compare the radiographs with images obtained by a CAT scan (measuring the intramedullary dimensions); they reveal that the error is due to the difference between the tube distance and the location and extent of cortical bone.[4] Another cause of the major discrepancy between the size of the medullary canal as seen on the radiograph and the actual size revealed at surgery results from failing to position the leg properly on the x-ray table; often fixed-hip flexion deformity precludes proper positioning and thus produces magnification errors. Routine radiographs fail to produce adequate information regarding the torsional deformity of the femur (anteversion of the femoral neck). Some degree of anteversion occurs commonly in osteoarthritic hips. Finally, radiographs fail to produce the cross-sectional dimensions of the femur at various levels, which is necessary in planning for sizing and prosthetic fit. Although many authors who advocate a cementless device for routine use recommend the use of templates, they also emphasize that the final selection of size must be based on the "best fit"—not on preoperative radiograph measurements.

Customization Using CAT Scanning and CAD/CAM

Customization of prosthetic joints using a computer-tomography-generated CAD-CAM was introduced because routine two-dimensional radiographs failed to produce the information needed to manufacture the prosthesis. Implants are now designed using computer-assisted-design (CAD) technology and manufactured using computer-integrated (CIN), computer-assisted manufacturing (CAM). The information used for CAD is based on the CAT scans performed on the proximal and supracondylar region of the femur according to the manufacturer's protocol.[1,29] The tapes of the scan and an anteroposterior radiograph of known magnification of the pelvis, a frog lateral, and a Manfredi lateral view (shoot-through lateral) of the involved hip are sent to the manufacturer, who makes a three-dimensional model of the femur. The drawings of the femoral component and radiographic templates are based on the design priorities prescribed by the surgeon. These drawings may be discussed and modified according to the surgeon's recommendations. The final drawing, which reflects the prescribed stem for the patient, is signed and returned to the manufacturer, and the stem is fabricated. The metal of choice is a titanium-4 aluminum-4 vanadium alloy. At present, the process takes 10 to 14 days from the final drawing to the finished product. At the surgeon's preference, porous coating (sintered beads) made of pure titanium or titanium mesh, plasma spray, or hydroxyapatite can be incorporated into the design of the implant. Early clinical results of these implants indicate that these stems achieve the most accurate fit and fill within the proximal femur.

Although this technique has been used for both primary and revision surgery, it is too imprecise to be used in planning revision surgery. The metal of the previous prosthesis in the bone causes scatter in the CAT images, making them imprecise and unreliable. Errors of from 10% to 40% have been recorded using the CAT scan.[24] Some of these errors are inevitable but are known to the experts in the field of CAT scanning and to manufacturers of the custom-made devices. Unfortunately, these errors can result in the production of prostheses that are too large or small, which is only recognized at surgery. Several commonly cited errors in CAT scanning affect the accuracy of customized devices:

1. An indication of greater bone density than is found at surgery.
2. Misinterpretation of the object's "edge definition."
3. Magnification error as the object's distance from the detector varies.
4. The need for constant monitoring of the CAT equipment to be sure it is precisely calibrated.

5. Variability in patient size and movement on the part of the patient, who must remain perfectly still for 30 to 60 minutes.

Walker and Robertson recognized the difficulty in designing a truly customized prosthesis. They suggested that inserting a stem shaped precisely to the internal anatomy of the femur is impossible, thus requiring a compromise. After incorporating the compromises made to allow insertion of the stem, the device is no longer customized.[24,30] Therefore most customization today is based on an evaluation of preoperative CAT scanning after manufacturing the stem and a broach (a replica of the stem). Unfortunately, rasping with a broach produces all the inherited potential errors of the stem. In addition to the inaccuracies cited above, the broach can produce another important inaccuracy: a mismatch between the prepared cavity of the femur and the prosthesis, caused by imprecise shaping of the femur. Because custom-made prostheses are designed for optimum fill and fit of the prosthesis in the proximal femur, they are generally bulky and stiff due to their relatively large cross-sectional dimensions. These properties may potentiate stress shielding despite the use of titanium alloy, which has a lower modulus of elasticity than other metals. Like prefabricated cementless devices, prostheses customized routinely by preoperative CAT scanning may be difficult to insert at surgery because of technical inaccuracies arising from scanning; this can lead to a mismatch between bone and implant. However, in some unique circumstances, customization using CAT designs may be helpful, particularly when intraoperative manufacturing is not available.

Intraoperative Customization
Intraoperative Manufacturing of the Stem (Identifit)*

Professor Joseph C. Mulier of Leuven, Belgium, pioneered the intraoperative manufacture of the prosthetic stem using a CAD-CAM in the late 1970s. To evaluate the feasibility and accuracy of the fit of such a prosthesis, he used a series of molds to measure the geometrical shape and size of the femur. He used this technique to prepare for a Charnley cemented total hip arthroplasty with radiographic measurements. Mulier realized that using preoperative radiographic pictures (CAT scan) and a computed digitizer could not produce a prosthesis with an identical fit because of an approximate error of +/− 1 mm; this degree of error resulted in a loose fit or an oversized prosthesis that

could potentially fracture the femur. When laser measuring of multiple points from a fixed centered line became feasible (Fig. 11-36, *A,*), a unique computer program (CAD) was introduced, which led to a practical manufacturing process still used today. Subsequently, a milling machine with sufficient versatility and speed was introduced to make it possible to build the mold expeditiously while the patient was under anesthesia. With the computer program, the surgeon could review the external geometry of the prosthesis based on such data as the area of contact, offset, anteversion, neck length, and so forth—before manufacturing the prosthesis (Fig. 11-36, *B* and *C*). Necessary alterations could be made on the existing mold or in the bone, in which case a new mold was made. These alterations were necessary only if the cavity preparation was inadequate.

Intraoperative manufacturing of the stem is quite new. The research program started in 1982 with the development of a technique to make intraoperative molds from reamed femora. The first prosthesis generated intraoperatively was inserted in Lueven, Belgium, in 1986 by Professor Mulier[18] and 2 years later in the United States in Orlando, Florida, by Dr. Louis P. Brady.

This author and colleagues at Columbia-Presbyterian Medical Center have chosen to use the intraoperative method of stem manufacturing for several reasons (they are described more fully in Chapter 6):

1. With prefabricated prostheses, it is difficult to achieve adequate medullary canal fit and fill, both proximally and distally.
2. Preoperative customization is not always satisfactory, because surgical canal preparation at surgery can result in either a loose component or one that might fracture the bone.
3. Porous-coated prostheses are fraught with such problems as stress shielding and thigh pain, which can cause prohibitive problems if extraction becomes necessary.

We used the technique of intraoperative prosthesis manufacturing for the first time in November 1990. To date, we have used only 70 such prostheses. Our standards for patient selection are extremely strict and in most cases only 2 years have passed since the procedure. This technology produces a unique opportunity to fit the pre-prepared canal to a prosthesis that has been manufactured and customized to the patient's bone. The limited longevity of cemented total hip arthroplasty in certain subgroups of patients coupled with the complexity and variability in the upper femur's shape and geometry make a good fit and fill that is impossible to achieve with an off-the-shelf

---

* The manufacturing technology was originally owned by Thackary, United Kingdom. It is now owned and manufactured by DePuy, Warsaw, Ind.

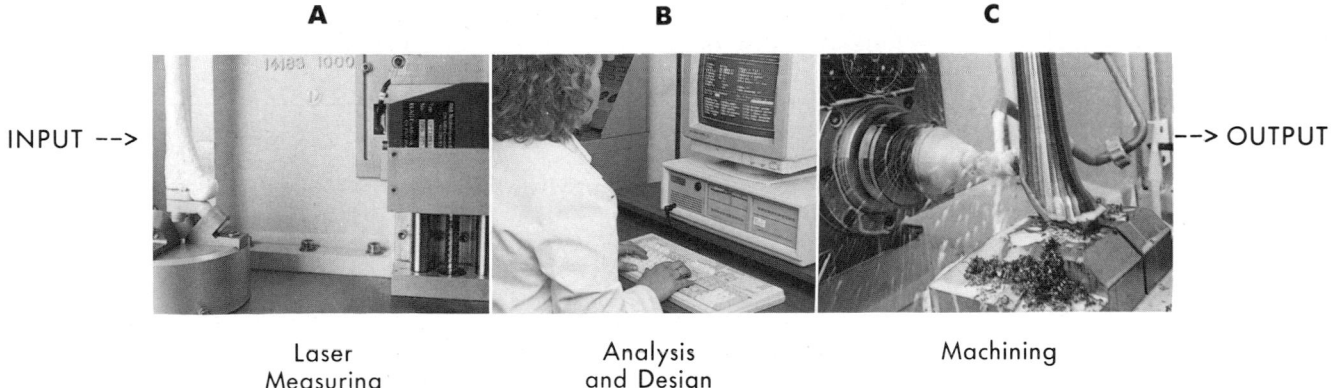

A **B** **C**

INPUT -->   --> OUTPUT

Laser
Measuring

Analysis
and Design

Machining

Fig. 11-36. **A,** Computer-assisted technology can be simply defined as a design and manufacturing system that can produce an implant in an extremely short time. Mold is being digitized for shape and size. The data may be modified as needed. **B,** Design is finalized based on the surgeon's recommendation. Certain parameters, such as anteversion offset and length, may be modified. Surface finish may be chosen at this time. **C,** The input data will be transformed to an implantable prosthesis.

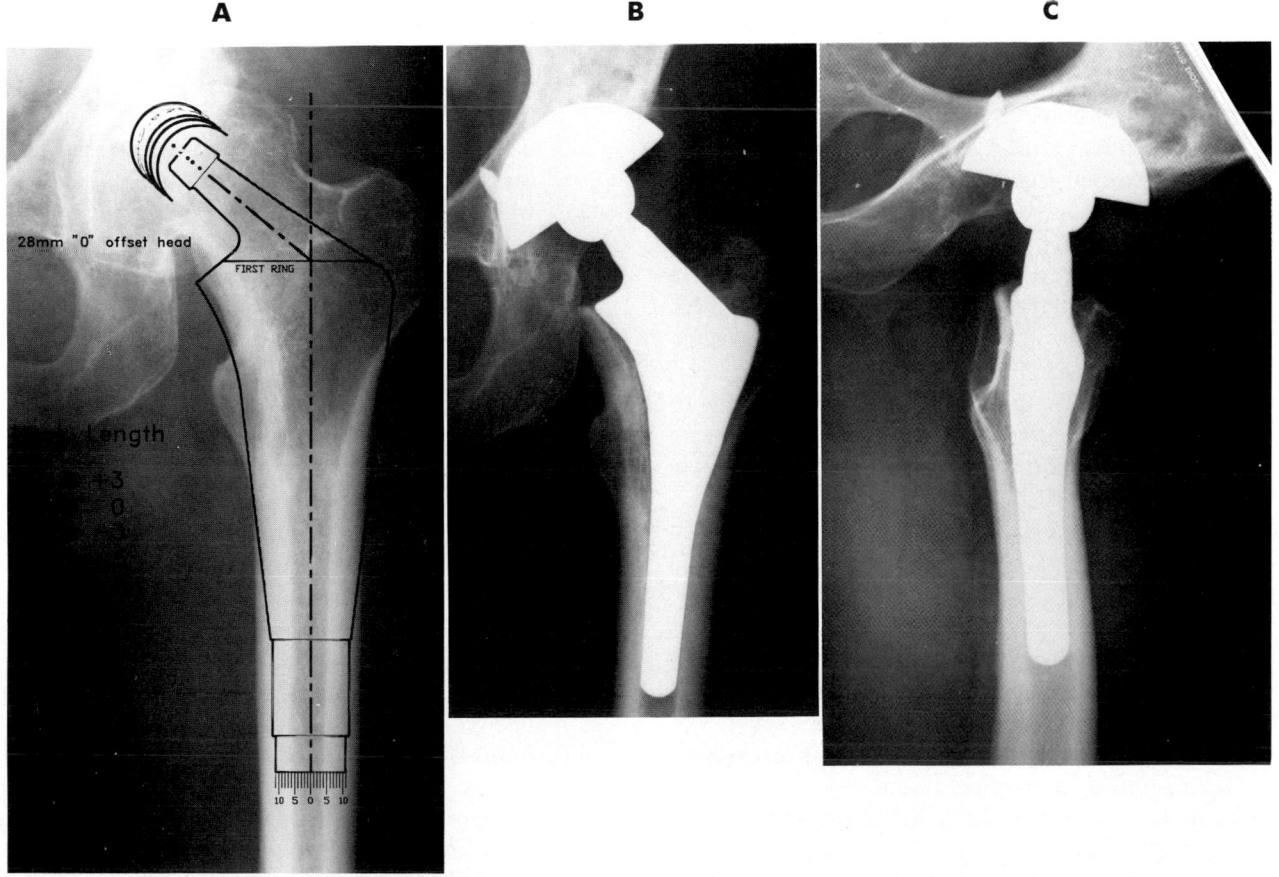

A **B** **C**

Fig. 11-37. **A,** Radiograph of 42-year-old male (M.K.) (weight 105 kg) with advanced unilateral degenerative osteoarthritis. Superimposed template determines the choice of forged titanium preform and appropriate neck length for intraoperative manufacturing of the stem (see Chapter 6). **B,** AP and **C,** lateral views showing unique shape of the prosthesis and excellent fill and fit of the stem.

prosthesis; consequently, this alternative is extremely attractive (Fig. 11-37). However, the long-term results of such radical methods are not available, and their merit can be judged only with future clinical studies.

Surgical Technique for the Identifit Prosthesis

SURGICAL APPROACH AND BONE PREPARATION
Prepare the mold with any chosen surgical approach; this author uses a posterolateral approach routinely (see Chapter 16). This step is done first; the acetabular preparation and insertion of the cup are accomplished while the prosthesis is being manufactured. Observe the following steps:

1. Position and drape the patient either supine or in the lateral decubitus position, as determined by the choice of surgical approach (see Chapter 15).
2. Expose the femoral head adequately to deliver it out of the wound (see Chapter 16).
3. Remove the femoral head to the level predetermined by templating the femur; as a rule, it should be as high as possible on the neck (see Chapter 16).
4. Remove the lateral cortical bone on the neck at the site of the digital fossa and open the medullary canal with a straight, nontapered, T-handled reamer. Progressively increase the size of the medullary reamer until the nontapered reamer engages to the femoral cortex at the isthmus.
5. Remove all the cancellous bone of the proximal femur to produce a cone shape with the widest dimension to lateralize the opening as much as possible without fracturing the thin cortex of the trochanteric region (Fig. 11-38, A).
6. Expand the medullary canal progressively to remove loose and fragile trabecular bone and strong cancellous structures and to provide cortical support for the prosthesis.
7. Use graded tapered reamers progressively in the direction and along the track of the cylindrical reamers previously used.
8. In shaping the femur, converge the metaphysis (the tapered segment) with the diaphysis (the cylindrical portion) gradually to avoid a step-cut between the two. Avoid reentrance (which will result from use of curved broaches) or careless operation of high-speed burrs.
9. Check the shape of the canal frequently, using a fiberoptic light.
10. Use long-handled curettes and high-speed burrs frequently (but with extreme caution) to maximize contact between the stem and the bone.
11. Irrigate and brush the canal, using a rotary brush and jet lavage to remove debris and bone particles.
12. Measure the isthmus of the femur and select the appropriate size injector tip.
13. Inspect the medullary canal thoroughly; pack it with a 2-inch gauze while preparing for the mold.

MAKING THE MOLD Observe the following steps:

1. Apply the latex bag to the injector. Attach the appropriate neck extension to the injector and insert the injector into the canal for rehearsal, demonstrating the location of the injector for measurements of the neck length and the offset.
2. Remove the injector and attach it to the molding gun (loaded with a cartridge containing the molding material).
3. Set the timer and begin to fill the latex bag by activating the trigger of the gun (Fig. 11-38, B).
4. Insert the injector and the partially filled latex bag (containing the molding agent) into the medullary canal and orient the injector in the proper plane of anteversion and medial/lateral displacement to produce the desirable version and offset; at the same time, place the neck-measuring device ("sugar cube") between the neck of the injector and the cut surface of the femur to maintain the rehearsed position of the injector.
5. Continue injecting the molding material until a bulge appears at the neck surface of the femur, indicating that the latex bag is completely filled. Filling the bag for a standard stem length takes approximately 2 to 2½ minutes. Release the trigger and wait 3 full minutes from the time of injection.
6. Now reactivate the trigger for a full additional 2 to 3 seconds to inject more molding material. Wait for the molding agent to solidify.
7. Extract the mold from the medullary canal after a full 5 minutes; the result should be a solid mold (Fig. 11-38, C and D).
8. Observe the mold for imperfections such as air bubbles, inadequate fillings, and other deficiencies. Also observe the mold for the proximal flare and the general shape in addition to the orientation of the neck and external parameters of the design such as anteversion, offset, etc.
9. Send the mold to the laboratory (Fig. 11-38, E) as you begin to prepare and fix the acetabular component. Repeat the procedure to make another mold if the first was unsatisfactory.
10. Review the parameters of the prosthesis based on the computer readout for the shape and proportionality of the design and the proposed contact area of the mold.
11. Approve the design or make a new mold as

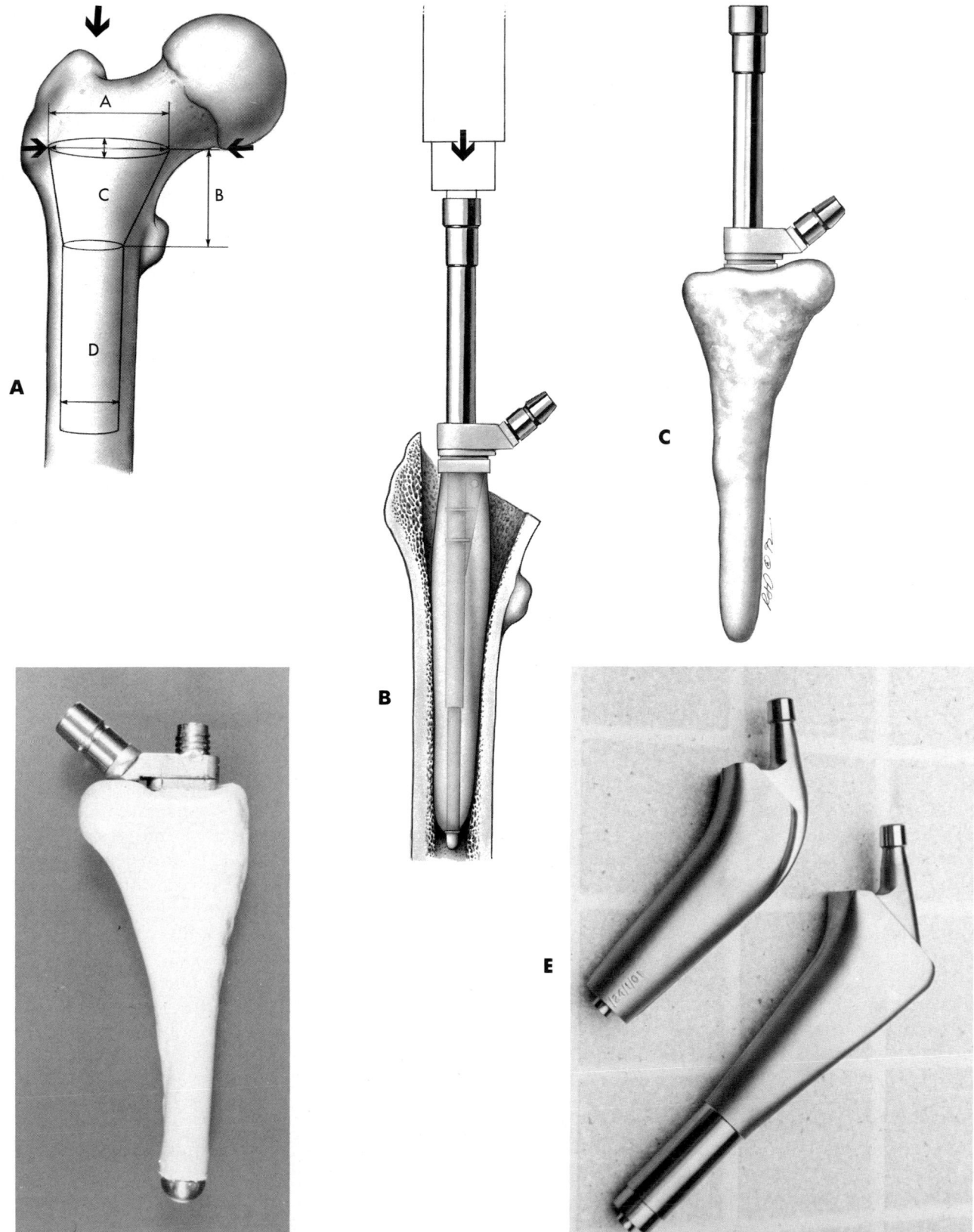

Fig. 11-38. A, The ideal cavity preparation for a press-fit prosthesis. Producing such a cavity involves preparing the metaphysis and diaphysis independently. The femoral bone must be strong to support a nonbonded prosthesis. Strong cortical or corticocancellous bone is the only bone that should remain after removing all cancellous bone. *a,* widest angles of the cone, *b,* the height of the cone, *c,* metaphysis, *d,* diaphysis. Top arrow shows the point of entry by medullary reamers to prepare the diaphysis—it must precede the metaphyseal preparation using hand broaches and high-speed burrs. Medial arrow shows a high neck section (routinely), and lateral arrow emphasizes the importance of encroaching onto the trochanteric bed to produce lateral support for the stem (see Chapter 6). **B,** Injector attached to the "air-powered gun" injecting the molding material into the latex bag after canal preparation. The depth of penetration of the injection (and latex bag) determines the length of the neck of the prosthesis (after attaching the selected neck length attached to the injector). **C,** Mold is extracted from the medullary canal at 5 minutes after injection. **D,** Actual mold after removal of the latex bag. **E,** Forged titanium preform of appropriate size is selected based on preoperative templating of the patient's radiograph from which the prosthesis is being manufactured (see Fig. 11-36).

needed by repeating the above steps.

12. Prepare and insert the acetabular component while the stem is being manufactured. Inspect the sterilized stem for any obvious defects; obtain a culture from the surface of the prosthetic stem.

13. Insert the stem by gently tapping it into the medullary cavity of the femur.

14. Fix the prefabricated chromium and cobalt modular head to the neck and reduce the prosthesis.

15. Test for range of motion and stability as discussed in Chapter 15. Reattach the greater trochanter if it was osteotomized, using a "cable grip" or wires for reattachment; prevent the prosthesis from contacting the cable* or wires. Close the wound as described in Chapter 15.

Figs. 11-39 and 11-40 illustrate examples of young, heavy, active, and physically demanding individuals for whom a cemented prosthesis might have not been satisfactory in the long term. The shape variations and variations in "flare index" in these cases would obviate the use of any single "off-the-shelf" prosthesis.

Prostheses for Uncommon Indications

As previously stated, in treating patients whose weight exceeds 85 kg and who are young and active, this author prefers a noncemented, non-porous-coated stem with a porous-coated acetabular component (AML* or Harris-Galante†). The use of a threaded acetabular cup (Mecron) by this author was associated with a high failure rate, and limited experience with porous-coated stems (primarily AML* and Harris-Galante†) has been disappointing due to a lack of consistency in the relief of pain and the appearance of abnormal bone remodeling such as "stress shielding" of the upper femur.

In addition to intraoperative customization (DePuy*), this author found three types of prostheses useful and at times indispensable for revision surgery (see Chapter 25). Those include BIAS,† APR,‡ and long-stem Osteonic.§

Three Methods of Using CAD-CAM Technology

To make customization economically feasible for a hospital, a minimum of 200 prostheses should be used annually in a given institution. The equipment and two technicians, supplied and salaried by the manufacturers, must be located in a facility within or adjacent to the hospital with no more than 1 to 2 minutes walking distance to the surgical suites. The entire system can be housed in its own self-contained unit; the only requirement is electricity and water. Operation of the unit is the responsibility of the manufacturer,* who works closely with the surgical team. The operation of the unit must also conform to the requirements of good manufacturing practice and stringent quality control standards.

An integral part of the system of CAD-CAM technology is the generation of a data base for analysis within and between patient groups, providing the surgeon with an inherent system for follow-up studies. To date, 13 in-hospital units are operational worldwide; collectively they have produced over 4000 procedures. To maximize the use of the unit, three options (Fig. 11-41 and box on p. 535) are available to the surgeon and the institution:

1. Intraoperative production of the prosthesis by making a replica of the patient's bone (most accurate fit and fill); this option is both patient- and surgeon-specific.

2. Preoperative production using information from radiographs and CAT scan. In this approach, which is *patient-specific*, the objective is to design and manufacture a prosthesis from either the patient's x-rays or CAT scans. Produced according to a strict protocol, the film is electronically transferred to the software data base. Anteroposterior and lateral images of the femur are called to the monitor screen and a shape-fitting procedure is carried out. The analysis and design software program is then used to produce the best fit prosthesis; an acetate overlay superimposed on the original film by the surgeon permits judgments to be made on the proposed implant design's acceptability.

   Up to this stage the process takes approximately 10 minutes. If the surgeon requires a model of the proposed design, it is possible to produce a plastic replica within another 10 minutes.

   Once the surgeon approves the design, an implant and matching broach can be made in about 2½ hours. If the implant requires coating and is to be supplied in a sterilized condition, the whole process will take 10 working days from approval.

3. Preoperative production based on the model-measuring concept: any geometrical or free-form shape. This approach is *surgeon-specific*. Based on preoperative templating of the x-rays and

---

*DePuy U.S.A., Warsaw, Ind.
†Zimmer U.S.A.
‡Intermedic.
§Osteonic.

---

*Orthogenesis, a division of DePuy U.S.A.

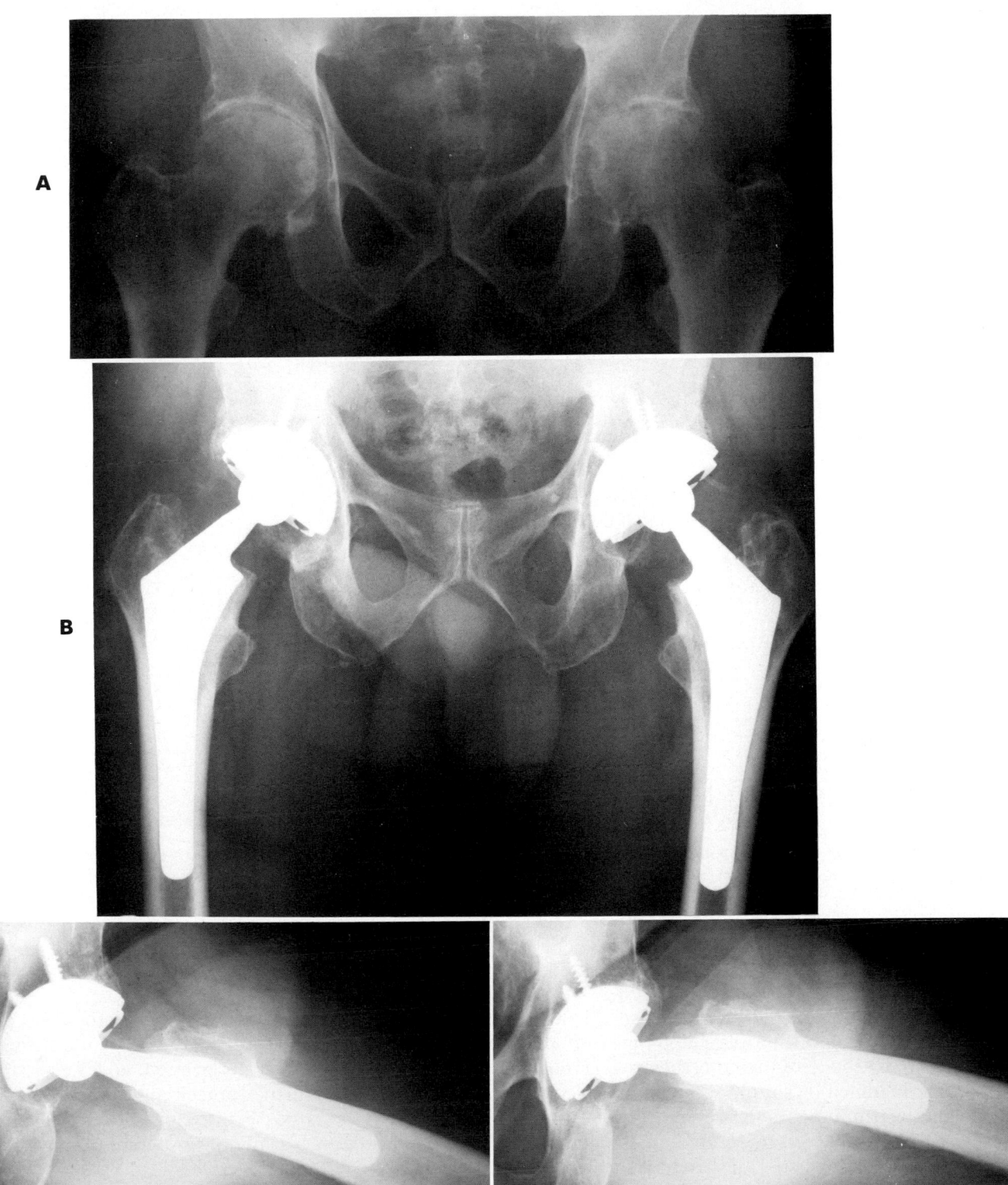

Fig. 11-39. A, Radiograph of a 59-year-old male (A.V.) with bilateral degenerative osteoarthritis, weight 100 kg, height 210 cm. **B,** Bilateral intraoperative manufacturing of the stems (Identift) was done. Note excellent canal "fill and fit." **C,** Lateral right and left same as in **B.** NOTE: Similarity of shape of the prosthesis on both sides is striking (same surgeon performed both operations).

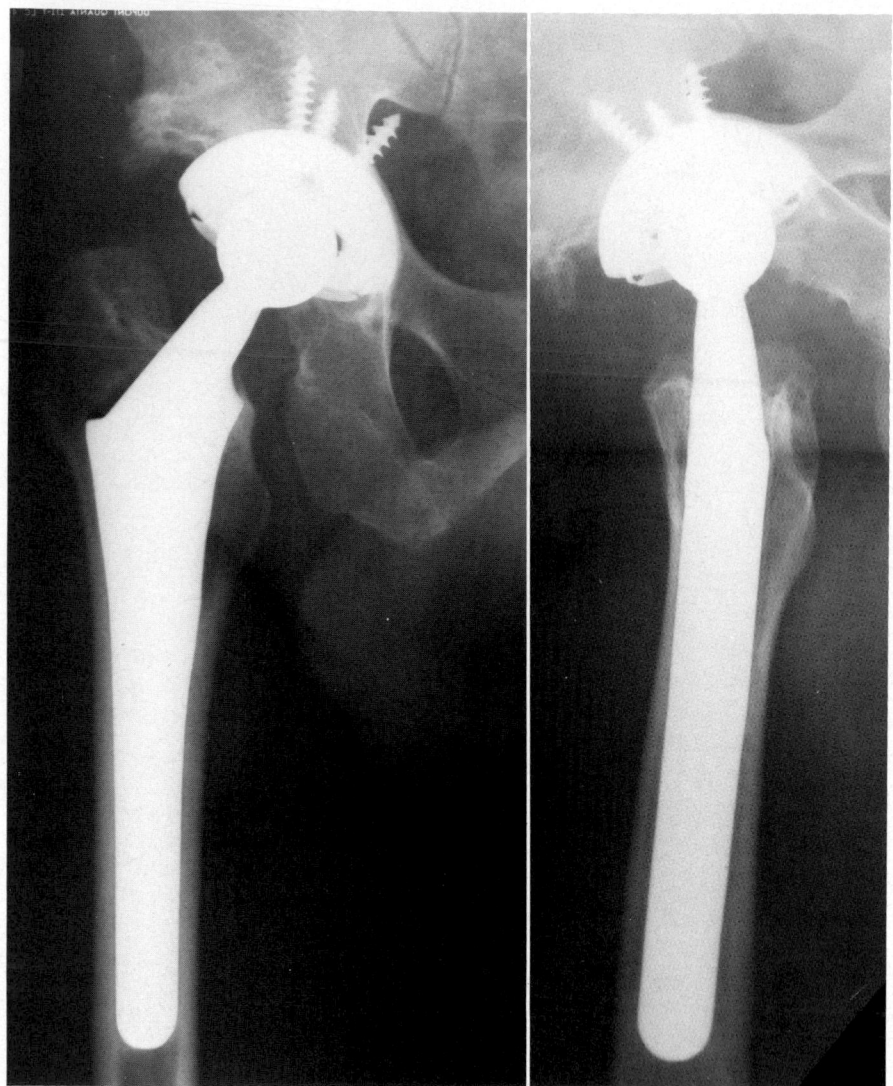

Fig. 11-40. Two years after total hip arthroplasty by intraoperative customization in a very active 51-year-old man (E.R.) with unilateral hip disease whose weight is 110 kg. Patient had an ankylosed hip from a childhood trauma. Grade: A-3,3,1. NOTE: a stovepipe-shaped femur 160 mm in length. Patient has no pain and walks without a limp. Grade: A-6,6,6.

modification (as required), a plastic model can be produced for the surgeon to preview prior to making the definitive prosthesis. The model can be modified by simply adding a suitable material or by trimming the model until the correct shape is achieved. Laser equipment is then used to measure the model and produce the final product in metal. Any number of alterations can be easily performed in this manner. The data to be used are obtained in the second stage of analysis and design. At the second stage, the software program determines the implant shape most suitable to the patient or the surgeon's specifications; it then writes the machining instructions for the equip-

ment at the third stage. The prosthesis produced in the third stage may be implanted after testing, cleaning, and sterilization; or, if necessary, it may receive further processing (e.g., surface coating) as required. The cycle time of this three-stage process is generally less than 1 hour.

A range of surgeon-specific implants can be produced in this way; they are indexed and sterilized and made available as needed for use in trauma and elective procedures. The speed of manufacturing should be commensurate with the "minimum" inventory held and with items being replaced as they are used, on a "just-in-time" basis. This system has two main

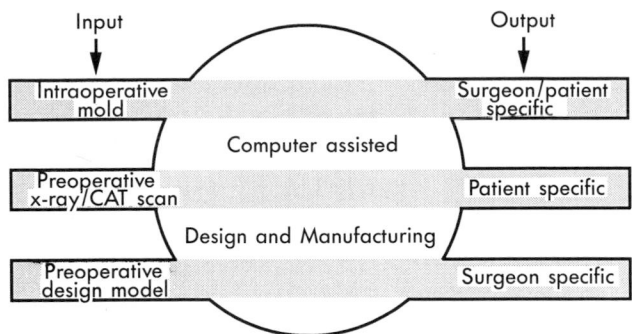

Fig. 11-41. Flow chart representation of a maximum use of a computer-assisted design and manufacturing as established within a hospital setting. The input may vary from center to center because the pattern of patient population may vary. Surgeons may use this technology for intraoperative manufacturing, preoperative manufacturing based on radiographs and CAT scanning, or design and manufacture of new models.

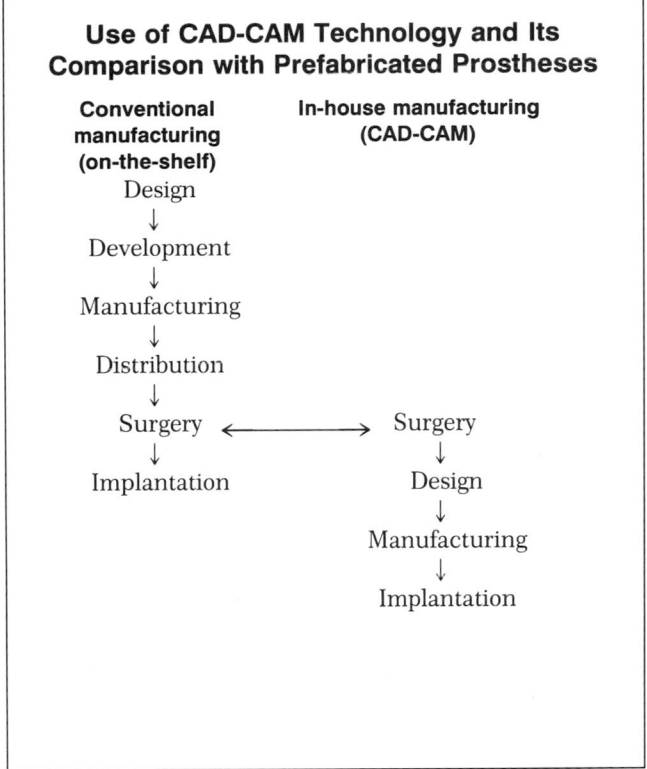

advantages: (a) several ranges of sizes can be produced from the same design and used with cement for fixation; (b) such a system minimizes the consequences of design changes, which can obviously be implemented very quickly.

It is worth reiterating that in-house customization technology is a system of design and manufacturing that can be applied generally to the production of femoral components. It is not a specific implant, but a system of customization that permits the design of an implant for each specific patient.

SUMMARY OF ESSENTIALS

- After Charnley's introduction of low-friction arthroplasty of the hip in the early 1960s, an explosion of innovative modification and technology for total hip arthroplasty resulted in a vast amount of work on both cementless and cemented devices for hip arthroplasty. Orthopaedic surgeons must consider the merits of cementless versus cemented devices, porous-coated and modular systems, press-fit versus screw-in prostheses, ceramics versus stainless steel, and titanium or chromium-cobalt, all of which may affect the future performance of hip arthroplasty in a given patient.

- Although recent modifications of Charnley's work have aimed largely at eliminating acrylic cement for fixation, cemented fixation of the stem has demonstrated excellent long-term results and reproducibility, which remain incomparable to those of subsequent developments. Early results of porous-coated acetabular components seem promising, although long-term outcomes are not yet available.

- The following principles are fundamental to choosing implants for the patient:
  1. Adopt a method that is practical and has been proven successful on a long-term clinical basis.
  2. Avoid modifying established techniques in the absence of adequate documentation and careful studies of the outcomes.
  3. Continue surveillance of one's own results and experience with complications to improve technique and solve problems as they arise.
  4. Select patients carefully for this type of radical surgery, basing decisions on objective findings, not subjective complaints.

- The surgeon must consider several interrelated features of prosthetic design, including its anatomical application and surgical feasibility, reduction of the joint force, mechanical optimization of wear, the friction and strength of the materials from which the prosthesis is made, and the permanent fixation of the prosthesis to the bone.

- The practice of low-friction arthroplasty has been successful due to several interrelated biomechanical principles: use of a small-diameter femoral head, reconstruction of the hip joint through the lateral displacement of the abductor pull, medialization of the central rotation using a small head, and allowing for subluxation as a safety valve for fixation of the components.

■ This author considers a femoral head size of 22 mm or 26 mm to be optimal. The 22-mm head is used in both small acetabula and selected revision cases. In large men whose acetabula are large enough to accommodate a 26-mm head against a thick plastic socket, a 26-mm outer diameter femoral head is used.

■ The smaller the diameter of the neck, the greater the range of motion it will allow without impinging against the socket. Therefore the greater the head-neck ratio, the greater the range of motion without impingement. The smaller the socket depth–ball ratio, the greater the range of motion without impingement. Obviously, increasing the depth of the socket increases resistance to dislocation, but increased socket depth automatically reduces the "angle of impingement."

■ The modularity of the femoral head and neck allows the surgeon to increase the neck length if the hip remains unstable after fixation of the acetabular component. The surgeon can replace the head with a smaller or larger one at revision if the stem is well fixed. The head is inserted as a final step after fixation of the stem so the highly polished head is not damaged at the time of stem insertion.

■ Modularity has drawbacks as well: it increases the manufacturing cost and the potential that the interlock between the head and the tapered neck will fail causing disassembly and corrosion and producing particles.

■ The intramedullary stem of the total hip prosthesis has different characteristics when used with and without cement. For use with cement, the stem must be of a size and shape to accommodate the anatomical shape of the femur. The dimensions should not exceed the narrowest segment of the isthmus. Tapering must facilitate cement injection. The configuration must produce maximal resistance against rotational and compressive forces. A sufficient number of sizes must be available to accommodate a thick layer of cement, especially at the concave side of the prosthesis. The strength must be adequate to withstand a lifetime of service. The stem must be straight beyond the level of the lesser trochanter, and the proximal one third of the stem should contain and pressurize the cement as it is being inserted.

■ This author prefers a stem that is collarless and provides double support for cement through a tip designed to centralize itself or through a centralizing plug within the medullary canal.

■ To facilitate access to the inventory, stems are classified into a standard series, a small and short

series, and a large and long series. The surgeon must have an adequate inventory of prostheses to be able to provide the best cement fixation for the femur according to the preoperative templating of each case.

■ An acceptable design criterion for cementless prostheses is a stem that produces the best fit in the metaphysis of the femur. A straight stem, such as AML, uses the principles of "intramedullary locking" for initial fixation, while a curved stem such as PCA depends on the anatomical shape to fill and fit the medullary cavity of the femur. A partial proximal porous coating is becoming more acceptable than a fully coated stem for ingrown prostheses. In general, in noncemented stems, the general shape (geometry) of the stem is more important than the modulus of elasticity, whereas in cemented stems the stem modulus seems to be more important in the design.

■ The acetabular components this author has found most suitable are the flanged socket and pressure injection cup, which can be customized for each case during surgery. The flanged socket is hemispherical in shape, with a broad rim, a long posterior wall, no metal backing, and no spacers for cement. The pressure injection cup permits the surgeon to customize the cup by trimming it to fit the acetabulum. It avoids wobble of the acetabular cup in the acetabular cavity and avoids bottoming during cement polymerization. It can pressurize the cement and contains the cement within the acetabular cavity at insertion.

■ The basic original porous-coated cementless designs — the anatomical modular locking prosthesis (AML) and the porous-coated hip system (PCA) — and many other modifications currently are available for use in young and active patients, although long-term results of these devices are not yet available. The amount of porous-coated segment has been modified for a larger or smaller area on these prostheses. Although excellent early results have been reported for many of the cementless devices, inconsistency regarding thigh pain and the problem of extraction (if needed) continues to be a problem. Major problems have been identified that may predispose the patient to long-term failure of these devices — component subsidence, porous surface delamination, proximal cortical atrophy, and femoral osteolysis.

■ In this author's experience (similar to others'), in the short term, the use of porous-coated acetabular components has been virtually trouble free. On the other hand, threaded acetabular cups are no longer in use, except for those with porous-coated surfaces.

- Because of excellent long-term results with cemented stems and early favorable results from porous-coated acetabular components, a combination of cementless and cemented components has gained popularity (hybrid hips). In theory, this combination may increase longevity of the procedure, especially in young and active individuals. However, the surgeon is to be reminded that in the long run, most hips may fail not because of failure of the acetabular fixation, but because of wear particles of high-density polyethylene, which could result in mechanical failure of the cup.

- Customization of prostheses is defined as shaping the implant to the patient, not shaping the patient's anatomy to fit a prefabricated prosthesis. A prosthesis can be customized by using acrylic cement, preoperative radiographs, CAT scanning and computer assisted technology, and intraoperative manufacturing of the prosthesis.

- Customization by cement is the best method because it provides the best fit for the prosthetic-cement composite immediately after insertion, it produces the largest endosteal surface possible for load transfer, it resists bending and torsional forces, and it eliminates painful fretting movements between the implant and bone. It also reduces stress and therefore strain in the proximal or distal femur as compared with a direction stem fit (press fit), which reduces the stress to a much lesser extent.

- Customization by radiographs should be regarded as inadequate because magnification errors can occur. These magnifications are related not only to the method of producing the radiographs but to actual rotational changes that can occur while taking the radiographs.

- Customization using CAT scanning is more accurate, but several commonly cited errors in CAT scanning affect the accuracy of customization via CAT scanning. CAT scans are affected by misinterpretation of the object's edge definition and by suggesting the existence of greater bone density than is actually found at surgery. Also, magnification errors as the object's distance from the detector varies, the need for constant monitoring of the CAT equipment, and variability in patient size and movement can make it extremely difficult to be accurate at all times. Therefore like prefabricated cementless devices, prostheses customized routinely by preoperative CAT scanning may be difficult to insert at surgery because of technical inaccuracies arising from scanning, leading to a mismatch between bone and implant.

- This author is currently investigating the use of intraoperative manufacturing of the prosthesis, the technique developed by Professor Mulier, with the aim at producing the replica of the prepared femur and customization during surgery. This unique technique uses advanced computer technology, laser technology, and a milling machine, controlled by the computer, that is sufficiently versatile and fast to produce the prosthesis in a short time. In this technique, the cavity is prepared first and a mold of the interior of the femur is produced. This mold is viewed by the laser and the data are transferred to the computer-assisted design–computer-assisted machine (CAD-CAM). Such a prosthesis produces excellent medullary canal fit and fill, both proximally and distally. It allows the surgeon to control variables related to contact, as well as the external geometry of the prosthesis such as anteversion, offset, neck length, etc. The same technology may use preoperative measurements of radiograph and CAT scan to produce prostheses with porous-coated designs or with application of hydroxyapatite. While it is too early to determine the long-term clinical results of this technology, its application has been limited to "high-risk" patients who are overweight, young, and active, and for whom other methods are not suitable.

- An integral part of the CAD-CAM technology is the generation of a data base for analysis within and between patient groups to provide the surgeon with a system for follow-up studies. To maximize the use of the CAD-CAM technology, three options are available to the surgeon and the institution: (1) intraoperative manufacturing of the stem; (2) preoperative production using information from radiographs and CAT scan; and (3) preoperative production based on model measuring concepts such as geometrical or free-form shapes for development of unique or experimental prostheses.

REFERENCES

1. **Bargar WL:** Shape the implant to the patient. A rationale for the use of custom-fit cementless total hip implants, *Clin Orthop* 249:73, 1989.
2. **Capello WN:** Fit the patient to the prosthesis. An argument against the routine use of custom hip implants, *Clin Orthop* 249:56, 1989.
3. **Charnley J:** *Low-friction arthroplasty of the hip: theory and practice,* Berlin, 1979, Springer-Verlag.
4. **Cherf J, Stulberg SD, Wixson RL, et al:** *Characteristics of fit in uncemented components.* Presented at the Mid-America Orthopaedic Society Meeting, Bermuda, April 19–23, 1989.
5. **Dall DM, Miles AW:** Reattachment of the greater trochanter. The use of the trochanter cable-grip system, *J Bone Joint Surg* [Br] 65:55, 1983.
6. **Davidson JA:** Characteristics of metal and the effect on longterm UHMWPE wear. Presented at the annual meeting of the Hip Society, submitted for publication to Clin Orthop 285:523, 1992.

7. **Eftekhar NS:** Total hip replacement using principles of low-friction arthroplasty. In Evarts CM: *Surgery of the musculoskeletal system*, New York, 1983, Churchill-Livingstone.

8. **Reference deleted.**

9. **Engh CA, Bobyn JD, Glassman AH:** Porous hip replacement. The factors governing bone ingrowth, stress shielding, and clinical results, *J Bone Joint Surg* 69:45, 1987.

10. **Engh CA, Bobyn JD:** *Biological fixation in total hip arthroplasty*, Thorofare, NJ, 1985, Slack.

11. **Ericksen MF:** Aging changes in the medullary cavity of the proximal femur in American blacks and whites, *Am J Phys Anthropol* 51:563, 1979.

12. **Galante JO, Jacobs J:** Clinical performances of ingrowth surfaces, *Clin Orthop* 276:41, 1992.

13. **Garg A, Deland J, Walker PS:** Design of intramedullary femoral stems using computer graphics, *Eng Med* 14:89, 1985.

14. **Harris WH:** The porous total hip replacement system: surgical technique. In Harris WH, editor: *Advanced concepts in total hip replacement*, Thorofare, NJ, 1985, Slack.

15. **Huiskes R:** Some fundamental aspects of human joint replacement. Analysis of stresses and head conduction in bone-prosthesis structures, *Acta Orthop Scand* 185 (suppl):1, 1980.

16. **Huiskes R, Boeklagen R:** Computer optimization of stem shape in THA, *Orthop Trans* 13:547, 1988.

17. **Morrey BF, Ilstrup D:** Size of the femoral head and acetabular revision in total hip arthroplasty, *J Bone Joint Surg* 71:50, 1989.

18. **Mulier JC, Mulier M, Brady LP, et al:** A new system to produce intraoperatively custom femoral prosthesis from measurements taken during surgical procedure, *Clin Orthop* 249:97, 1989.

19. **Noble PC, Alexander JW, Lindahl LJ, et al:** The anatomic basis of femoral component design, *Clin Orthop* 235:148, 1988.

20. **Page A, Jasty M, O'Connor DO, et al:** Stress shielding around proximally porous surfaced femoral components 6 months after bone ingrowth and remodeling in the canine. *Orthop Trans* [published after first edition of Eftekhar text].

21. **Poss R, Staehlin P, Larson M:** Femoral expansion in the presence of total hip arthroplasty, *J Arthroplasty* 2:259, 1987.

22. **Poss R, Walker P, Robertson DD, et al:** Anatomic stem design for press-fit and cemented total hip arthroplasty. In Fitzgerald RH Jr, editor: *Noncemented total hip arthroplasty*, Phoenix, Ariz, 1988, Raven Press.

23. **Poss R, Walker P, Spector M, et al:** Strategies for improving fixation of femoral components in total hip arthroplasty, *Clin Orthop* 235:181, 1988.

24. **Robertson DD Jr, Huang HK:** Quantitative bone measurements using x-ray computed tomography with second-order correction, *Med Phys* 13:474, 1986.

25. **Robertson DD, Walker PS, Hirano SK, et al:** Improving the fit of press-fit hip stems, *Clin Orthop* 228:134, 1988.

26. **Ruff CB, Hayes WC:** Age changes in geometry and mineral content of the lower limb bones, *Ann Biomed Eng* 12:573, 1984.

27. **Ruff CB, Hayes WC:** Subperiosteal expansion and cortical remodeling of the human femur and tibia with aging, *Science* 217:945, 1982.

28. **Saejong S, Hirano S, Granholm JW, et al:** The influence of the interface on bone strains and stem-bone micromotion in press-fit total hip stems, *Orthop Trans* 12:484, 1987.

29. **Stulberg SD, Stulberg BN, Wixson RL:** The rationale, design characteristics, and preliminary results of a primary custom total hip prosthesis, *Clin Orthop* 249:79, 1989.

30. **Walker PS, Robertson DD:** Design and fabrication of cementless hip stems, *Clin Orthop* 235:25, 1988.

31. **Walker PS, Schneeweis D, Murphy S, et al:** Strains and micromotions of press-fit femoral stem prostheses, *J Biomech* 20:693, 1987.

32. **Zhou X-M, Robertson DD, Walker PS:** Femoral strain patterns with press-fit THR — a photoelastic analysis, *Orthop Trans* 13:350, 1988.

ADDITIONAL READINGS

Eftekhar NS: *Principles of total hip arthroplasty*, St Louis, 1978, Mosby–Year Book.

Engh CA, Bobyn JD: The influence of stem size and extent of porous coating on femoral bone resorption after primary cementless hip arthroplasty, *Clin Orthop* 231:7, 1988.

Engh CA, Glassman AH, Suthers KE: The case for porous-coated hip implants. The femoral side, *Clin Orthop* 261:63, 1990.

Engh CA, Massin P: Cementless total hip arthroplasty using the anatomic medullary locking stem. Results using a survivorship analysis, *Clin Orthop* 249:141, 1989.

Hedley AK, Gruen TAW, Borden LS, et al: Two-year follow-up of the PCA noncemented total hip replacement. In The Hip Society: *The hip: proceedings of the fourteenth open scientific meeting of The Hip Society*, St Louis, 1986, Mosby–Year Book.

Kennedy W: Modes of failure of the threaded acetabular total hip replacement components, *Orthop Trans* 12:692, 1988.

Maloney WJ, Jasty M, Harris WH, et al: Endosteal erosion in association with stable uncemented femoral components, *J Bone Joint Surg* 72:1025, 1990.

Muller ME: Acetabular revision. In The Hip Society: *The hip: proceedings of the ninth open scientific meeting of The Hip Society*, St Louis, 1981, Mosby–Year Book.

Muller ME, Jaberg H: Total hip reconstruction. In Evarts CM, editor: *Surgery of the musculoskeletal system*, ed 2, New York, 1990, Churchill-Livingstone.

See Chapters 4, Biomaterials: Compatibility and Wear; 6, Biomechanics: Fixation and Loosening; 15, Principles Common to all Surgical Approaches; and 28, Results in Primary Total Hip Arthroplasty for additional information.

CHAPTER TWELVE

Clinical and Radiographic Assessment

■ An impersonal method of assessment that is comprehensive, generally applicable, and reliable is essential.
Margaret M. Shepherd

Chapter 7 discussed preoperative considerations, such as planning and surgical preparation of the patient. Plans for prophylactic measures against thromboembolism and infection were described in Chapters 8 and 9, respectively; indications for surgery based on the patient's disability were presented in Chapter 10. Chapter 11 covered the choice of prosthesis and customization.

This chapter addresses the objective clinical and radiographic assessment of the hip for prospective documentation. Such documentation is mandatory for good medical practice: the amelioration and deterioration of the patient can be assessed only if objective data document the patient's preoperative, immediate, early, and long-term progress. Comparing current data with earlier data based on the same established definitions allows the surgeon to evaluate the worth of a new surgical technique. This is especially important because modifications of procedures and devices are inevitable in medical practice.

CLINICAL METHODS OF ASSESSMENT

The importance of identical preoperative and postoperative evaluation in orthopaedic surgery has been recognized since the 1930s[19] as a necessary means of assessing outcomes. As Aufranc stated, "One should hesitate to judge the effects of a surgical procedure, even in a large series of cases, when any attempt to compare accurately the patient's condition before the operation with that after the operation was actually impossible."[13]

Establishing definitions and terminology is funda-

mental to any scientific research and reporting technique. Descriptive terms, however, are often subjective and variable from one observer to another; therefore it is essential to establish a standard system of terminology to evaluate the results of a treatment or surgical procedure. Since the mid-1940s, several numerical grading systems have been established to evaluate hip disease before and after surgery, but the criteria in each scoring system vary with the methods used for evaluation. The need for a standardized system for evaluating the results of total hip arthroplasty has been amply expressed by several investigators.[18,26,27,54]

In 1986, responding to this compelling need, the Committee on Health Care Delivery of the American Academy of Orthopaedic Surgeons asked the AAOS Task Force on Outcome Studies to define the parameters essential in evaluating total hip arthroplasty. For this purpose, the Task Force collaborated with The Hip Society and the Commission on Documentation and Evaluation of the Societé Internationale de Chirugie Orthopedique et de Traumatologie (SICOT). The Joint Commission's primary goal was to develop a system of terminology to acquire minimal data for precise scientific comparison. Their recommendations (approved in 1989 by the American Academy of Orthopaedic Surgeons) include several characteristics of the patient, the surgeon, and the institution that the Joint Commission deemed most critical to the short-term and long-term results of total hip arthroplasty (Fig. 12-1). The collaborative system of nomenclature appears in Tables 12-1 to 12-3.

The Joint Commission recommended a standard

Table 12-1 Clinical Evaluation

Pain
  Degree
    ___ None—no pain
    ___ Mild—slight and occasional pain; patient has not altered patterns of activity or work
    ___ Moderate—patient is active but has had to modify or give up some activities, or both, because of pain
    ___ Severe—major pain and serious limitations
  Occurrence
    ___ None
    ___ With first steps, then dissipates (start-up pain)
    ___ Only after long (30-minute) walks
    ___ With all walking
    ___ At all times
Work/level of activity
  Occupation (specify, including homemaker): _____
    Retired
      ___ No
      ___ Yes
    Nursing home
      ___ No
      ___ Yes (date ended: _____)
  Level of activity
    ___ Bedridden or confined to a wheelchair
    ___ Sedentary—minimum capacity for walking or other activity
    ___ Semisedentary—white-collar job, bench work, light housekeeping
    ___ Light labor—heavy house-cleaning, yard work, assembly line, light sports (e.g., walking ≤5 km)
    ___ Moderate manual labor—lifts ≤23 kg, moderate sports (e.g., walking or bicycling <5 km)
    ___ Heavy manual labor—frequently lifts 23–45 kg, vigorous sports (e.g., singles tennis or racquetball)
  Work capacity in last 3 months
    ___ 100%
    ___ 75%
    ___ 50%
    ___ 25%
    ___ 0
  Putting on shoes and socks
    ___ No difficulty
    ___ Slight difficulty
    ___ Extreme difficulty
    ___ Unable
  Ascending and descending stairs
    ___ Normal (foot over foot)
    ___ Foot over foot using banister or assistive device
    ___ 2 feet on each step
    ___ Any other method
    ___ Unable
  Sitting to standing
    ___ Can arise from chair *without* upper-extremity support
    ___ Can arise *with* upper-extremity support
    ___ Cannot arise independently

Walking capacity
  Usual support needed
    ___ None
    ___ 1 cane for long walks
    ___ 1 cane
    ___ 1 crutch
    ___ 2 canes
    ___ 2 crutches
    ___ Walker
    ___ Unable to walk
  Time walked
    Without support
      ___ Unlimited (>60 minutes)
      ___ 31–60 minutes
      ___ 11–30 minutes
      ___ 2–10 minutes
      ___ < 2 minutes or indoors only
      ___ Unable to walk
    With support
      ___ Unlimited (> 60 minutes)
      ___ 31–60 minutes
      ___ 11–30 minutes
      ___ 2–10 minutes
      ___ < 2 minutes or indoors only
      ___ Unable to walk
Satisfaction of patient
  Operation increased your function?
    ___ Yes
    ___ No
  Operation decreased your pain?
    ___ Yes
    ___ No
  Operation decreased your need for pain medication?
    ___ Yes
    ___ No
    ___ Not applicable
  Satisfied with results?
    ___ Yes
    ___ No
  Status of hip compared with your last visit?
    ___ Better
    ___ Same
    ___ Worse
Physical examination
  Limp *without* support
    ___ None   no limp
    ___ Slight—detected by trained observer
    ___ Moderate—detected by patient
    ___ Severe—markedly alters or slows gait
  Range of motion of hip
    Fixed flexion
      Left: ___ degrees
      Right: ___ degrees
    Further flexion to
      Left: ___ degrees
      Right: ___ degrees

Table 12-1 Clinical evaluation—cont'd

Abduction/adduction
  Left: __ degrees/__ degrees
  Right: __ degrees/__ degrees
External/internal rotation
  (hip in 0 degrees of flexion or maximum extension)
    Left: __ degrees/__ degrees
    Right: __ degrees/__ degrees
	Trendelenburg sign
	  Positive
	    __ Left
	    __ Right
	  Negative
	    __ Left
	    __ Right
	  Unable to test
	    __ Left
	    __ Right
	  Trendelenburg lurch (abductor lurch or Duchenne sign)
	    __ Present
	    __ Absent
	Limb lengths
	  __ Equal
	  Short left: __ cm
	  Short right: __ cm
	  Method of measurement (radiograph, blocks, other): __

From Johnston R, Fitzgerald R, Harris W, et al: *J Bone Joint Surg* 72:161, 1990.

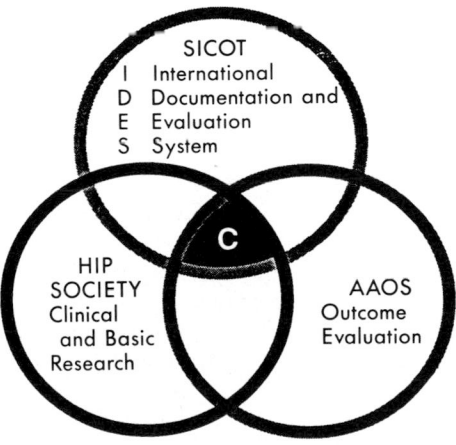

Fig. 12-1. Diagrammatic representation of the overlapping missions of the three organizations involved in the consensus (C) on evaluating total hip arthroplasty. (From Muller ME, Sledge C, Poss R, et al: Report of the SICOT presidential commission on documentation and evaluation, *Int Orthop* [SICOT] 14:221, 1990.)

system of terminology for reporting results. The Joint Commission's primary goal was to develop a system of terminology to acquire the minimum data for precise scientific comparison. This system provides a basic minimal data base to serve the needs of authors, readers, and editors when comparing the results of different studies. Recently Johnston and associates[37] published a report on the system. Remember that this basic data-acquisition format can be expanded upon when necessary, but only as long as the new parameters are objective, strictly defined, and reproducible by others.

At the New York Orthopaedic Hospital, this author developed a separate Hip Assessment Record based on the original green card used at Wrightington Hospital; it is used to assess all total hip arthroplasty candidates. Initiated preoperatively, this assessment includes a detailed history and the results of both a physical examination and a hip examination (Fig. 12-2, *A* and *B*). Roentgenographic analysis (Fig. 12-3, *A* and *B*) and details of the operative procedure are also included. Early postoperative complications (Fig. 12-4) and follow-up evaluation are also included, as well as records related to other parameters of the patient's care and management (such as anticoagulation, antibiotics, and postoperative physiotherapy).

Methods of Grading and Their Limitations

Various scales for rating hip disability have attempted to compare the preoperative and postoperative results of different types of procedures. Most hip evaluation systems record pain, walking distance, function, and the range of motion. Notably, despite all efforts to maintain objectivity, the surgeon's assessment is frequently overrated when compared with the therapist's based on the same scale system.[23]

Larson[45] suggested a scoring system based on a 100-point scale to evaluate cup arthroplasty (Table 12-4). In addition to scoring functional ability (including pain and gait), he assessed such anatomical factors as range of motion and deformity (for example, shortening of the limb). He weighed these factors,

Text continued on p. 551.

Table 12-2 Radiographic Evaluation: Cemented Prostheses

Acetabulum	Femur	
Migration of component (measurement must be related to teardrop) __ No __ Yes Superior: __ mm Medial: __ mm Location of center of rotation of hip relative to teardrop Superior: __ mm Lateral: __ mm Broken cement __ No __ Yes Zone (specify 1–3):_____ Cement-bone radiolucency (DeLee and Charnley) __ No __ Yes Maximum width Zone 1: __ mm Zone 2: __ mm Zone 3: __ mm Continuous __ No __ Yes Maximum width: __ mm Radiolucency around screws __ No __ Yes __ Not applicable Breakage of screws __ No __ Yes __ Not applicable Wear of socket: __ mm Position of component Inclination (abduction): __ degrees Version of cup Retroversion: __ degrees __ Neutral Anteversion. __ degrees	Migration of stem Varus-valgus __ No __ Yes __ Varus } qualitative only; __ Valgus } choose one Subsidence (must be related to fixed landmarks on femur: proximal tip of greater trochanter and midpoint of lesser trochanter) __ No __ Yes (__ mm) __ Within cement __ With cement Broken cement __ No __ Yes Stem __ Intact __ Bent __ Broken Radiolucency Prosthesis-cement (anteroposterior radiograph) __ No __ Yes Cement-bone Anteroposterior radiograph __ No __ Yes Maximum width Zone 1: __ mm Zone 2: __ mm Zone 3: __ mm Zone 4: __ mm Zone 5: __ mm Zone 6: __ mm Zone 7: __ mm Lateral radiograph __ No __ Yes Maximum width: Zone 8: __ mm Zone 9: __ mm Zone 10: __ mm Zone 11: __ mm Zone 12: __ mm Zone 13: __ mm Zone 14: __ mm	Resorption of medial part of neck (calcar) __ No __ Yes Loss of height (exclusive of rounding): __ mm Loss of thickness: __ mm Resorption or hypertrophy of shaft __ No Resorption (zones: _____) Hypertrophy (zones: _____) Change in density __ No Patchy loss (zones: _____) Uniform loss (zones: _____) Increased trabecular bone (zones: __) Endosteal cavitation __ No __ Yes Zones: __ Length: __ mm Width: __ mm Ectopic ossification __ Brooker I (none) __ Brooker II (mild) __ Brooker III (moderate) __ Brooker IV (severe) Position of stem __ Neutral } qualitative only; __ Valgus } choose one __ Varus Greater trochanter __ Not osteotomized __ Osteotomized __ Healed __ Not healed __ Displaced __ Nondisplaced

From Johnston R, Fitzgerald R, Harris W, et al: *J Bone Joint Surg* 72:161, 1990.

Table 12-3 Radiographic Evaluation: Uncemented Prostheses

Acetabulum	Femur	
Migration of component (measurement must be related to teardrop) — No — Yes Superior: __ mm Medial: __ mm Location of center of rotation of hip relative to teardrop Superior: __ mm Lateral: __ mm Prosthesis-bone radiolucency (DeLee and Charnley) — No — Yes Maximum width Zone 1: __ mm Zone 2: __ mm Zone 3: __ mm Continuous — No — Yes Maximum width: __ mm Radiolucency around screws — No — Yes — Not applicable Breakage of screws — No — Yes — Not applicable Porous coating — Intact — Dislodged — Progressive loss — Not applicable Wear of socket: __ mm Position of component Inclination (abduction): __degrees Version of cup Retroversion: __ degrees — Neutral Anteversion: __ degrees	Migration of stem Varus-valgus — No — Yes — Varus } qualitative only; — Valgus } choose one Subsidence (must be related to fixed landmarks on femur: proximal tip of greater trochanter and midpoint of lesser trochanter) — No — Yes (__ mm) Porous coating — Intact — Dislodged — Progressive loss — Not applicable Stem — Intact — Bent — Broken Prosthesis-bone radiolucency Anteroposterior radiograph — No — Yes Maximum width Zone 1: __ mm Zone 2: __ mm Zone 3: __ mm Zone 4: __ mm Zone 5: __ mm Zone 6: __ mm Zone 7: __ mm Lateral radiograph — No — Yes Maximum width: Zone 8: __ mm Zone 9: __ mm Zone 10: __ mm Zone 11: __ mm Zone 12: __ mm Zone 13: __ mm Zone 14: __ mm	Resorption of medial part of neck (calcar) — No — Yes Loss of height (exclusive of rounding): __ mm Loss of thickness: __ mm Resorption or hypertrophy of shaft — No Resorption (zones: ___) Hypertrophy (zones: ___) Change in density — No Patchy loss (zones: ___) Uniform loss (zones: ___) Increased trabecular bone (zones: __) Endosteal cavitation — No — Yes Zones: __ Length: __ mm Width: __ mm Ectopic ossification — Brooker I (none) — Brooker II (mild) — Brooker III (moderate) — Brooker IV (severe) Position of stem — Neutral — Valgus } qualitative only; — Varus } choose one Greater trochanter — Not osteotomized — Osteotomized — Healed — Not healed — Displaced — Nondisplaced

From Johnston R, Fitzgerald R, Harris W, et al: *J Bone Joint Surg* 72:161, 1990.

THE NEW YORK ORTHOPAEDIC HOSPITAL

IMPLANT DOCUMENTATION CENTER

PATIENT REGISTRATION

FORM **1A**

Name _____   Unit no. _____
       Last   First   MI

Birthdate ___/___/___   Height _____   Weight _____   Sex _____
        mm dd yy   Inches   Lbs.   Male/Female

Consultation date _____   Occupation _____

Address _____

City _____   State _____   Zip _____

Home telephone (___)_____   Business telephone (___)_____

Marital status   ☐ Single   ☐ Married   ☐ Widowed   ☐ Divorced   No. children _____

Mother's name _____   Father's name _____

Next of kin _____   Relationship _____   Telephone _____

Insurance _____

Referred by _____   Telephone _____

Address _____

City _____   State _____   Zip _____

Significant medical history _____

_____

Significant surgical history _____

_____

JOINT CLASSIFICATION (see codes)

HIP   KNEE

☐ A   ☐ B   ☐ C   ☐ A   ☐ B   ☐ C

A. Unilteral joint: no other functional disability   B. Bilateral joint: no other functional disability   C. Unilateral or bilateral with other joints or medical condition affecting function

CLINICAL SCORE (enter 1–6)

HIP   KNEE

Right   Left   Right   Left

___ ___ ___ ___ ___ ___   ___ ___ ___ ___ ___ ___ ___ ___
Pain Function Mobility Pain Function Mobility   Pain Stability Function Mobility Pain Stability Function Mobility

Comments _____

_____

Fig. 12-2. The New York Orthopaedic Hospital hip assessment record—patient registration form.

THE NEW YORK ORTHOPAEDIC HOSPITAL

IMPLANT DOCUMENTATION CENTER

PATIENT REGISTRATION

FORM **1B**

DIAGNOSIS (see codes below)

HIP		KNEE	
Right	Left	Right	Left

PROCEDURES (Orthopaedic Surgical History)

HIP				KNEE			
Right		Left		Right		Left	
Date	Procedure	Date	Procedure	Date	Procedure	Date	Procedure

TOTAL JOINT REPLACEMENT (CPMC and elsewhere)

HIP						KNEE					
Right			Left			Right			Left		
Date	Proc.	By	Date	Proc.	By	Date	Proc.	By	Date	Proc.	By

Date of death _____   Cause _____   Form completed by _____   Date _____

CODES

HIP

Diagnosis		Procedure-previous operations	
01. Osteoarthritis	14. Fx acetabulum	01. Cemented, fem. rep.	14. Muller (thr.)
02. Rheum. arthritis	15. Fx/dislocation	02. Non-cement fem.rep.	15. Charnley (thr.)
03. Ankyl spondylitis	16. Infection	03. Fracture fixation	16. T28 (thr.)
04. Congel. dysplasia	17. Tuberculosis	04. Acetabulum fixation	17. Other (thr.)
05. Slip. epiphysis	18. Juvenile ra.	05. Femoral osteotomy	18. Non-cemented (thr.)
06. Fx neck femur	19. Gout	06. Pelvic osteotomy	19. Bipolar
07. Traumatic arthritis	20. Gaucher's disease	07. Arthrodesis	20. Trochanteric op.
08. Non-union neck	21. Psoriatic arthritis	08. Trochanteric comp.	21. Positive preop. cult.
09. Protr. acetabulum	22. Bone tumor, benign	09. Hardware removal	22. Positive intraop.cult.
10. Perthes disease	23. Bone tumor, malig.	10. Pseudoarthrosis	23. Positive postop. cult.
11. Paget disease	24. Metastatic tumor	11. Shelf type	24. Histology (positive)
12. Avascular necrosis	25. Lupus – hem.	12. Cup arthroplasty	99. Other
13. Fx femur shaft	99. Other	13. Resurf. (D. cup)	

KNEE

Diagnosis		Procedure-previous operations	
01. Osteoarthritis	14. Fx tibia	01. Ligamentous repair	14. Fail. other (TKR)
02. Rheum. arthritis	15. Fx patella	02. Osteotomy	15.
03. Post meniscectomy	16. Infection	03. Tibial fixation	16.
04. Ligamentous injury	17.	04. Femoral fixation	17.
05. Chondromatosis	18. Juvenile ra.	05. Patellar fixation	18.
06. Rec. patella disloc.	19. Gout	06.	19.
07. Traumatic arthritis	20.	07. Arthrodesis	20.
08. Genum varus	21. Psoriatic arthritis	08.	21. Positive preop. cult.
09. Genum valgus	22. Bone tumor, benign	09. Hardware removal	22. Positive intraop.cult.
10. Genum recurvatum	23. Bone tumor, malig.	10. Fail. unicomp.(TKR)	23. Positive postop. cult.
11. Paget disease	24. Metastatic tumor	11. Fail. condylar(TKR)	24. Positive histology
12.	25. Lupus – hem.	12. Fail. cement. (TKR)	99. Other
13. Fx femur	99. Other	13. Fail. linked (TKR)	

Please return to PH 5C, Ex. 6-6220

The Presbyterian Hospital in the City of New York   Form #3: Radiological
Orthopaedic Surgery Service   A: Diagnostic
Columbia–Presbyterian Medical Center

Preoperative and Postoperative Assessment for HIP SURGERY

Name _____ Unit # _____ Hip Serial # _____ Date _____

1. Osteoarthritis (Primary)   Monoarticular (unilateral) _____ (bilateral) _____
                               Poliarticular (G O A)   _____

2. Osteoarthritis (Secondary) Perthes disease
                               Congenital subluxation
                               Congenital dislocation
                               Slipped epiphysis
                               Fracture femoral neck
                               Fracture acetabulum
                               Traumatic dislocation
                               Fracture dislocation
                               Paget disease
                               Other

3. Rheumatoid arthritis
4. Ankylosing spondylitis
5. Psoriatic arthritis
6. Protrusio acetabuli
7. Spontaneous ischemic necrosis
8. Congenital subluxation) without arthritis
9. Congenital dislocation)
10. Nonunion femoral neck without arthritis
11. Coxa vara (cervical)
12. Coxa vara (subcapital, i e, slipped epiphysis)
13. Paget disease without arthritis
14. Tuberculosis
15. Pyogenic arthritis
16. Sepsis following surgery
17. Pyogenic arthritis
18. Failure previous surgery: specify:

19. Other: specify:

_____
                          Unilateral _____ Bilateral _____

Patient's complaint

Radiological appearance

Fig. 12-3. Roentgenographic analysis form.

Findings   (side #2)

Form #3: Radiological
B: Morphology

Congruity		Nonunion		Subchondral line of cortical bone

Congruity	Nonunion		Subchondral line of cortical
none (dislocated)	Neck	Intertrochanteric area	bone

Congruity / Nonunion / Subchondral line of cortical bone

Congruity
- none (dislocated)
- minimal (marked subluxation)
- poor
- fair
- good
- normal

Joint space
- none
- very thin
- reduced
- normal

Cyst formation

Head	Acetabulum
none	none
mild	mild
moderate	moderate
severe	severe

Collapse of head
- none
- mild
- moderate
- severe

Loss of sphericity of head
- none
- minimal
- moderate
- severe

Osteophyte formation

Head	Acetabulum
none	none
mild	mild
moderate	moderate
severe	severe

Nonunion

Neck	Intertrochanteric area
present	present
absent	absent

Shenton line	Dysplasia of socket
broken	none
intact	mild
	moderate
	severe

Avascular necrosis
- none
- mild
- moderate
- severe

Protrusion	Coxa magna
none	none
mild	mild
moderate	moderate
	severe

Myositis ossificans

Volume	Restriction
none	none
mild	mild
moderate	moderate
severe	severe

Implant	Osteopenia
nail	none
nail plate	mild
pins	moderate
prosthesis	severe
cup	
total replacement	
spline	
other	
none	

Sclerosis of acetabulum
- none
- mild
- moderate
- severe

Subchondral line of cortical bone

Head	Acetabulum
normal	normal
reduced	reduced
very thin	very thin
absent	absent
irregular	irregular

Periosteal new bone along neck
- none
- minimal
- moderate
- marked

Slipped epiphysis
- none
- mild
- moderate
- severe

Head/Neck angle
- normal
- varus
- valgus
- _____ degrees
- other (specify) _____

_____

_____

Descriptive Morphology of Chronic Arthritis of the Hip (without reference to underlying pathology)

	Right	Left		Right	Left
Normal joint			Destructive head type		
Incipient arthritis (minimal changes)			Destructive acetabulum type		
Upper pole type (minimal to moderate, intact Shenton line)			Destructive tuberculous type, both acetabulum and head		
Upper pole severe (broken Shenton line)			Quadrantic head necrosis		
Medial pole type (without protrusio)			Subluxation type		
Protrusio type			Dislocation type		
Concentric type (ie, polyarthritis)			Septic type		
			Postoperative		
			Other (specify) _____		
			More than one type _____		

Fig. 12-3, cont'd.

THE NEW YORK ORTHOPAEDIC HOSPITAL

HIP SURGERY
HIP # _____

IMPLANT DOCUMENTATION CENTER

FORM **2A**

Name _____   Age _____   Unit no. _____
        Last   First   MI

Surgery date __/__/__   Site ____/____   Surgeon _____   Resident _____
             mm dd yy   L   R

DIAGNOSIS (see codes)

OPERATED SIDE

_____

_____

_____

_____

OPPOSITE SIDE

_____

_____

_____

_____

Pre-op Hip Scores

_____   _____   _____   _____   _____   _____
Pain   Function   Mobility   Pain   Function   Mobility

JOINT CLASSIFICATION (see codes)

HIP

☐ A   ☐ A'   ☐ B   ☐ B'   ☐ C

KNEE

☐ A   ☐ A'   ☐ B   ☐ B'   ☐ C

A. Unilateral joint: no other functional disability   B. Bilateral joint: no other functional disability   C. Unilateral or bilateral with other joints or medical condition affecting function
A'. Unilateral joint replaced: no other functional disability   B'. Bilateral joint replaced: no other functional disability

SURGERY

SURGERY TYPE _____

1. Primary   2. Primary bilateral simult.   3. Revision with primary
                                                             at CPMC
4. Revision with primary 5. Conversion   6. Revision of prior revisions
   elsewhere

BONE GRAFTING

☐ None   ☐ Femur   ☐ Acetabulum   ☐ Both

CONVERSION TYPE ONLY

Previous operation type _____

Reason failed _____

Comments _____

REVISION TYPE ONLY

Failed hip system _____

Reason failed _____

Operated on by (surgeon) _____

EXTENT OF REVISION

Femur _____

Acetabulum _____

Both _____

SURGICAL APPROACH _____

1. Anterior   2. Lateral   3. Posterior   4. Trans. Troch.   5. Other

ANESTHESIA TYPE _____

1. Normotensive   Hypotensive   3. Regional

PROSTHETIC SYSTEM

TYPE

Cup   Stem   Plug

_____

Prosthesis manufacturer _____

SIZE

Cup (OD-mm)   Stem (describe)   Head (OD-mm)

_____

Cement manufacturer _____

CODES: If more than one diagnosis or previous procedure, list chronologically.

HIP

Diagnosis

01. Osteoarthritis	08. Non-union neck	15. Fx/dislocation	21. Psoriatic arthritis
02. Rheum. arthritis	09. Protr. acetabulum	16. Infection	22. Bone tumor, benign
03. Ankyl spondylitis	10. Perthes disease	17. Tuberculosis	23. Bone tumor, malig.
04. Congel. dysplasia	11. Paget disease	18. Juvenile RA	24. Metastatic tumor
05. Slip. epiphysis	12. Avascular necrosis	19. Gout	25. Lupus – hem.
06. Fx neck femur	13. Fx femur shaft	20. Gaucher's disease	99. Other
07. Traumatic arthritis	14. Fx acetabulum		

Procedure-Previous operatios

01. Cemented, fem. rep.	08. Trochanteric comp.	14. Muller (thr.)	20. Trochanteric op.
02. Non-cement fem.rep.	09. Hardware removal	15. Charnley (thr.)	21. Positive preop. cult.
03. Fracture fixation	10. Pseudoarthrosis	16. T28 (thr.)	22. Positive intraop.cult.
04. Acetabulum fixation	11. Shelf type	17. Other (thr.)	23. Positive postop.cult.
05. Femoral osteotomy	12. Cup arthroplasty	18. Non-cemented (thr.)	24. Histology (positive)
06. Pelvic osteotomy	13. Resurf. (D. cup)	19. Bipolar	99. Other
07. Arthrodesis			

Please return to PH 5C, Ex. 6-6220

Fig. 12-4. The New York Orthopaedic Hospital hip assessment record—hip surgery.

THE NEW YORK ORTHOPAEDIC HOSPITAL

IMPLANT DOCUMENTATION CENTER

HIP SURGERY
HIP # _____
FORM **2B**

FIXATION SYSTEM

TYPE: Indicate: Cement, Ingrowth, Pressfit, Threaded cup,
Multiple screws, Wires, Other.

SURGEON'S OPINION AT OPERATION
Indicate: E=Excellent, G=Good, P=Poor

	Quality of bone	Surgical exposure	Quality of fixation
☐ Acetabulum _____	_____	_____	_____
☐ Femur _____	_____	_____	_____
☐ Trochanter _____	_____	_____	_____

OPERATING ROOM ENVIRONMENT

☐ Standard OR   ☐ Clean air room   ☐ Gown-hood-suction   ☐ Standard gown   ☐ Other

ANTIBIOTICS

	YES	NO	TYPE
Systemic	☐	☐	_____
Local irrigation	☐	☐	_____
In cement	☐	☐	_____

ANTICOAGULANTS

TYPE

COMMENTS

_____

_____

_____

_____

_____

_____

EARLY COMPLICATIONS IN-HOSPITAL (list all that apply)

GENERAL _____

1. None	2. Death	3. Pleurisy	4. Pneumonia	5. Cardiac failure	6. Pulm. embol.
7. Coronary occl.	8. Fat. embolism	9. Paral. ileus	10. Urinary ret.	11. Urinary inf.	12. Psychosis
99. Other					

LOCAL _____

| 1. None | 2. Hematoma | 3. Sup. w. inf. | 4. Deep wound inf. | 5. Dislocation | 6. DVT (ipsil.) |
| 7. DVT (contr.) | 8. Drop foot | 10. Skin necrosis | 99. Other | | |

TECHNICAL _____

| 1. None | 2. Fract. femur | 3. Fract. acet. | 4. Nerve palsy | 5. Arter. injury | 6. Troch. det. |
| 7. Dislocation | 8. Ectopic cement | 9. Poor tech. | 10. In-hosp. troch. prob. | 99. Other | |

SPECIAL STUDY   ☐ YES   ☐ NO

Description

Comments

_____

_____

_____

_____

_____

Form completed/updated by _____   Date _____

Please return to PH 5C, Ex. 6-6220

Fig. 12-4, cont'd.

Table 12-4 Iowa Hip Scale

Chart 1. Hip evaluation

Name _____ Date _____

Age _____

100-Point Scale for Hip Evaluation

Total points _____

A. Function (35 points)

Does most of housework or job which requires moving about...	5
Dresses unaided (included tying shoes and putting on socks)..	5
Walks enough to be independent..........................	5
Sits without difficulty at table or toilet..................	4
Picks up objects from floor by squatting...............	3
Bathes without help..	3
Negotiates stairs foot over foot...........................	3
Carries objects comparable to suitcase..................	2
Gets into car or public conveyance unaided and rides comfortably..	2
Drives a car..	1

B. Freedom from Pain (35 points) (Circle 1 only)

No pain..	35
Pain only with fatigue.......................................	30
Pain only with weight-bearing.............................	20
Pain at rest but not with weight-bearing...............	15
Pain sitting or in bed..	10
Continuous pain...	0

C. Gait (10 points) (Circle 1 only)

No limp; no support..	10
No limp using cane...	8
Abductor limp...	8
Short-leg limp...	8
Needs 2 canes...	6
Needs 2 crutches...	4
Cannot walk..	0

D. Absence of Deformity (10 points)

No fixed flexion over 30 degrees..........................	3
No fixed adduction over 10 degrees......................	3
No fixed rotation over 10 degrees........................	2
Not over 1 inch shortening (ASIS-MM)..................	2

E. Range of Motion (10 points)

Flexion extension (normal 140 degrees)................._____°

Abduction-adduction (normal 80 degrees)............._____°

External-internal rotation (normal 80 degrees)........_____°

Total degrees............................_____°

Points (1 point/30 degrees)..........._____

Muscle Strength (no points)

Straight leg-raising:

Less than gravity _____ Gravity _____

Gravity + resistance _____

Abduction:

Less than gravity _____ Gravity _____

Gravity + resistance _____

Extension:

Less than gravity _____ Gravity _____

Gravity + resistance _____

Chart 2. Hip evaluation

Name _____ Diagnosis _____

Age ___ Sex ___ Date of operation_____

Date of follow-up _____

Previous surgery: Date _____ Type _____

Subsequent surgery: Date _____ Type _____

I. Pain — 40%

None..	40
Pain with fatigue...	35
Pain with weight-bearing:	
Mild..	30
Moderate...	20
Severe...	10
Persistence with non-weight bearing............. (less than above)	10
Continuous pain..	0

II. Functional Ability — 30%

Work and household duties	
Full day—usual occupation...........................	10
Modified work or duties................................	6
Severe restriction of former...........................	2
Walking tolerances:	
Long distances...	10
Shorter distances...	6
2 blocks or less..	1
Self-reliance:	
Dresses self unaided.....................................	3
Help with shoes and socks.............................	2
Sits at table and toilet..................................	3
Stairs:	
Normal...	2
One at a time..	1
Gets into car or public conveyance without difficulty...	2

III. Gait — 15%

No limp—No support..	15
No limp—with cane...	12
Limp—mild—without cane..................................	12
Limp—mild—with cane......................................	9
Limp—moderate—without cane or crutch.............	9
Limp—moderate—with cane or crutch..................	6
Limp—severe—without cane or crutch..................	3
Limp—severe—with cane or crutch......................	2
Two canes or crutches......................................	1

IV. Anatomical Assessment — 15%

A. Motion:	
Flexion—Up to 80 degrees in range 0 degrees– 100 degrees × 0.1..	8
Abduction—Up to 20 degrees in range 0 degrees–30 degrees × 0.1..............................	2
B. Shortening:	
None—½ inch...	3
½–1 inch..	2
1–2 inches..	1
C. Trendelenburg—absent..................................	2

100%

From Larson CB: Rating scale for hip disabilities, *Clin Orthop* 31:85, 1963.

allowing 35 points for pain, 25 for function, 10 for gait, 10 for the absence of deformity, and 10 for motion. Alternatively, Harris's[35] 100-point scale (Table 12-5) gives 44 points for pain, 47 for function, 5 for range of motion, and 4 for the absence of deformity. Obviously, both systems involve an arbitrary loading, which defeats the advantage of assessing the patient using one numerical scale. Shepherd[63] further modified the Larson method to improve its effectiveness in evaluating hip disability. She suggested incorporating the variables to make them equally applicable to different problems and treatment methods. However, her system does not integrate function with motion and lacks a single overall value for all ratings.

In attempting to compare the results of cup arthroplasty with osteotomy or arthrodesis, Shepherd uses the Gade[25] index, granting fewer points to a flexion of more than 45 degrees than to a flexion of less than 45 degrees. Her purpose is to evaluate the benefit derived from an operation, the results of which cannot be compared to a normal hip joint. Although somewhat more comprehensive, this approach is rather complicated and subject to the same criticism for loading as the other systems. This inadequacy is especially important because the results of total hip arthroplasty should approximate a normal hip condition, and mobility should merit equally weighted points with function and pain.

In 1954, Merle d'Aubigne and Postel[53] (Table 12-6) suggested the first objective scoring system, using three units: one for pain, one for function, and one for mobility. Each unit ranges from 1 to 6; 1 represents complete disability and 6 represents normalcy. Judet and Judet later added one digit to describe the patient's "amelioration factors."[38]

Lazansky[46] adopted 26 separate items of clinical information (the "green card" used at the Wrightington Centre for Hip Surgery) to develop an objective system representing the patient by a single digit. His method was largely derived from the methods of Shepherd, the Judets, d'Aubigne, and Postel. Although Lazansky's grading system expresses the condition of the entire patient rather than just the hip (whether unilateral or bilateral), like the other systems it applies "loading" in scoring, and therefore the total score is weighted to emphasize mobility.

Charnley[18] modified the Merle d'Aubigne and Postel numerical classification (Table 12-7). This author[24] adopted this modified 6-6-6 grading system (popular in Great Britain and continental Europe) at the New York Orthopaedic Hospital at Columbia-Presbyterian Medical Center when the total hip arthroplasty program began there in 1969. The advantage of this method is its simplicity; the reviewer can quickly and separately evaluate the three parameters of hip disability: pain,

function, and mobility. In addition, he or she can compare the results directly with those of a larger series, such as Charnley's. By assigning the patient to one of three groups (A, B, and C) it is possible to describe the patient as a whole, not merely as a hip. Group A includes patients with unilateral hip disease; group B consists of patients with bilateral hip disease without other restraining factors; and group C comprises patients with either unilateral or bilateral hip disease who also have systemic or other conditions restricting their function. For example, a rheumatoid arthritis patient with multiple joint involvement and another with excessive obesity would both be placed in group C if these conditions limited their function overall. This division is extremely valuable when assessing the results of hip arthroplasty as a surgical procedure and also in terms of the overall performance of the patient's functions. Fig. 12-5 shows the hip evaluation form used by the author at the New York Orthopaedic Hospital; it evaluates the patient's preoperative status on the basis of 54 factors. A similar postoperative evaluation sheet is completed at each subsequent hospital or office visit.

Other systems of evaluation have been developed and used at the Hospital for Special Surgery in New York (Table 12-8) and at the Mayo Clinic in Rochester, Minnesota. Modifications of old systems have also been introduced.[5,56] As complications of total hip arthroplasty surfaced, it became increasingly obvious that a system of radiographic evaluation was highly desirable to evaluate the zonal failure of the interface and such parameters as wear and the status of fixation. The earliest radiographic evaluation for the acetabulum was proposed by Delee and Charnley[20]; Gruen and associates[34] introduced the first for the femur. A newer rating system incorporates the radiographic score into the evaluation, resulting in a single value scale for both.[40]

Evaluating Pain by Numerical Grades

As can be seen from Form 1 (Fig. 12-5), assessment of the pain before and after total hip arthroplasty is largely a subjective matter; it requires not only an in-depth interview with the patient, but also close observation of his or her function. A definition of the degrees of pain varies from one evaluation system to another. In evaluating the pain, it is necessary to concentrate on its intensity and whether it is provoked by activity. Assess "night pain" only when the patient volunteers the subject; do not emphasize the subject by asking a leading question because such a question may elicit mention of night pain or rest pain in most patients who want a total hip arthroplasty.

Most patients with osteoarthritis of the hip fall into

Text continued on p. 557.

Table 12-5 Hip Evaluation System (Harris Hip Score)

I. Pain (44 possible)

A. None or ignores it.. 44

B. Slight, occasional, no compromise in activities... 40

C. Mild pain, no effect on average activities, rarely moderate pain with unusual activity, may take aspirin............... 30

D. Moderate pain, tolerable but makes concessions to pain. Some limitation of ordinary activity or work. May require occasional pain medicine stronger than aspirin.. 20

E. Marked pain, serious limitation of activities.. 10

F. Totally disabled, crippled, pain in bed, bedridden... 0

II. Function (47 possible)

A. Gait (33 possible)

   1. Limp

      a. None... 11

      b. Slight.. 8

      c. Moderate.. 5

      d. Severe... 0

   2. Support

      a. None... 11

      b. Cane for long walks.. 7

      c. Cane most of the time.. 5

      d. One crutch.. 3

      e. Two canes... 2

      f. Two crutches.. 0

      g. Not able to walk (specify reason).. 0

B. Activities (14 possible)

   1. Stairs

      a. Normally without using a railing... 4

      b. Normally using a railing... 2

      c. In any manner.. 1

      d. Unable to do stairs.. 0

   2. Shoes and socks

      a. With ease.. 4

      b. With difficulty.. 2

      c. Unable.. 0

   3. Sitting

      a. Comfortably in ordinary chair one hour... 5

      b. On a high chair for one-half hour... 3

      c. Unable to sit comfortably in any chair... 0

   4. Enter public transportation... 1

III. Absence of deformity points (4) are given if the patient demonstrates:

A. Less than 30 degrees fixed flexion contracture

B. Less than 10 degrees fixed adduction

C. Less than 10 degrees fixed internal rotation in extension

D. Limb-length discrepancy less than 3.2 cm

IV. Range of motion (index values are determined by multiplying the degrees of motion possible in each arc by the appropriate index)

A. Flexion 0–45 degrees × 1.0
     45–90 degrees × 0.6
     90–110 degrees × 0.3

B. Abduction 0–15 degrees × 0.8
     15–20 degrees × 0.3
     over 20 degrees × 0

C. External rotation in extension 0–15 × 0.4
     over 15 degrees   × 10

D. Internal rotation in extension any × 0

E. Adduction 0–15 degrees × 0.2

To determine the overall rating for range of motion, multiply the sum of the index values × 0.05. Record Trendelenburg test as positive, level, or neutral.

From Harris WH: Traumatic arthritis of the hip after dislocation and acetabular fractures: treatment by mold arthroplasty. An end-result study using a new method of result evaluation, *J Bone Joint Surg* 51:737, 1969.

Table 12-6 Method of Grading Functional Value of Hip—Merle d'Aubigne and Postel

Grade	Pain	Mobility	Ability to walk
0	Pain is intense and permanent.	Ankylosis with bad position of hip.	None.
1	Pain is severe even at night.	No movement; pain or slight deformity.	Only with crutches.
2	Pain is severe when walking; prevents any activity.	Flexion under 40 degrees.	Only with canes.
3	Pain is tolerable with limited activity.	Flexion between 40 and 60 degrees.	With one cane, less than 1 hour; very difficult without cane.
4	Pain is mild when walking; disappears with rest.	Flexion between 60 and 80 degrees; patient can reach his foot.	A long time with a cane; short time without cane and with limp.
5	Pain is mild and inconstant; normal activity.	Flexion between 80 and 90 degrees; abduction of at least 15 degrees.	Without cane but with slight limp.
6	No pain.	Flexion of more than 90 degrees; abduction to 30 degrees.	Normal.

From Merle d'Aubigne R, Postel M: Functional results of hip arthroplasty with acrylic prosthesis, *J Bone Joint Surg* 36:451, 1954.

Table 12-7 Charnley's Modification of Merle d'Aubigne and Postel's Numeric Classification

Grade	Pain	Grade	Movement	Grade	Walking (Function)
1	Severe and spontaneous.	1	0–30 degrees	1	Few yards or bedridden. Two sticks or crutches.
2	Severe on attempting to walk.	2	60 degrees	2	Time and distance very limited without sticks.
3	Tolerable, permitting limited activity.	3	100 degrees	3	Limited with one stick. Difficult without a stick. Able to stand long periods.
4	Only after some activity.	4	160 degrees	4	Long distances with one stick. Limited without a stick.
5	Slight or intermittent. Pain on starting to walk but less with normal activity.	5	210 degrees	5	No stick but a limp.
6	No pain.	6	260 degrees	6	Normal.

From Charnley J: *J Bone Joint Surg* 54[Br]:61, 1972.

THE PRESBYTERIAN HOSPITAL
in the City of New York
Department of Orthopaedic Surgery
Columbia–Presbyterian Medical Center

Form #2 Assessment

Hosp. No.

Preoperative and Postoperative Assessment for Hip Surgery

Type operation: _____

Date operation: _____

Work: _____

Last Name	First Name	M.I.	Age	Weight

Type and Number of Pain Tablets/day

Spontaneous Pain at Night   YES ☐   NO ☐

A①

PAIN

	BEDRIDDEN OR CHAIR LIFE	TWO CRUTCHES	TWO STICKS	ONE STICK ALWAYS	ONE STICK OUTSIDE	NO STICKS
	1 Severe Spontaneous	**2** Severe on attempting to walk Prevents all activity	**3** Pain tolerable permitting limited activity	**4** Pain only after some activity; disappears quickly with rest	**5** Slight or intermittent. Pain on starting to walk but getting less with normal activity	**6** No pain
	R L	R L	R L	R L	R L	R L

FUNCTION

	1 Bedridden or few yards; two sticks or crutches	**2** Time and distance very limited with or without sticks	**3** Limited with one stick (less than one hour) Diffi-without stick. Able to stand long periods	**4** Long distances with one stick; limited without a stick	**5** No stick but a limp	**6** Normal
	R L	R L	R L	R L	R L	R L
GAIT WITHOUT STICKS	Cannot walk	Just able to walk	Walks but with gross limp	Walks with moderate limp	Slight limp	Normal gait

Gait (Describe)

Limp   Short leg limp   YES ☐   NO ☐   Hip limp   YES ☐   NO ☐

Trendelenburg: Positive   R: L   ;   Negative   R: L

Length of stride: (estimated by sight)

Dresses self	With Difficulty	YES ☐ NO ☐	Can climb stairs	With Difficulty	YES ☐ NO ☐
Puts on stockings	With Difficulty	YES ☐ NO ☐	— with banister	With Difficulty	YES ☐ NO ☐
Ties shoes	With Difficulty	YES ☐ NO ☐	— one at time	With Difficulty	YES ☐ NO ☐
Walks outside	With Difficulty	YES ☐ NO ☐	Cuts toenails	With Difficulty	YES ☐ NO ☐
Bathing self	With Difficulty	YES ☐ NO ☐	Drives car	With Difficulty	YES ☐ NO ☐
Regular toilet	With Difficulty	YES ☐ NO ☐	Sits comfortably	With Difficulty	YES ☐ NO ☐
Public transportation	With Difficulty	YES ☐ NO ☐	— only high chair ½ Hr.	With Difficulty	YES ☐ NO ☐

CATEGORICAL CLASSIFICATION FOR FUNCTION

A) Unilateral hip: no other functional disability
B) Bilateral hip; no other functional disability
C) Unilateral or bilateral WITH other joints or medical condition affecting function

Category 'C' Cases

☐ CVS
☐ RS
☐ CNS
☐ Senility
☐ Obesity
☐ Psychiatric
☐ Other

☐ orthopaedics

COMMENTS:

Fig. 12-5. A, Preoperative and postoperative assessment for pain, function, and mobility— form used at Columbia-Presbyterian Hospital.

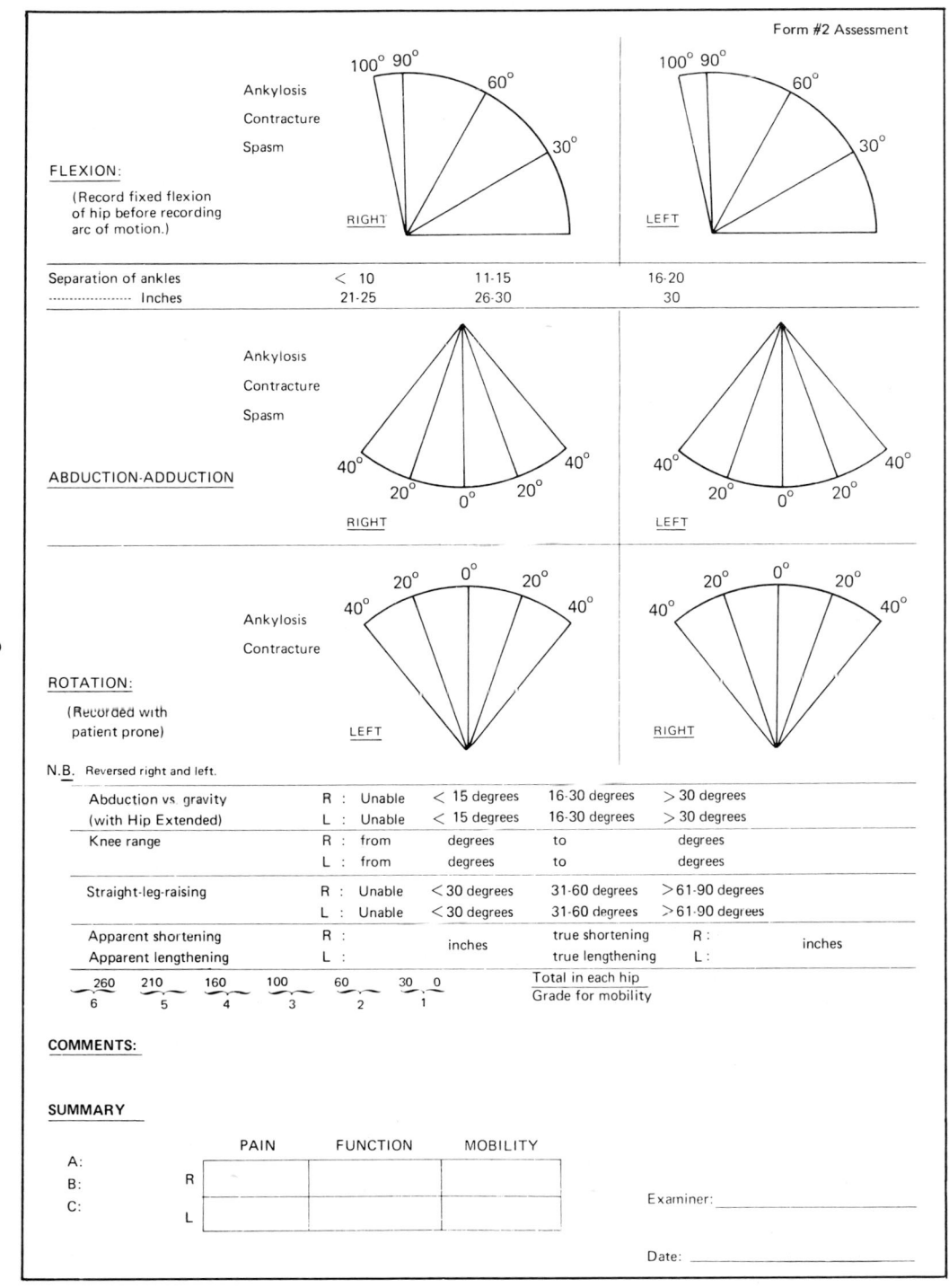

A②

Form #2 Assessment

FLEXION:

(Record fixed flexion of hip before recording arc of motion.)

Ankylosis
Contracture
Spasm

RIGHT   LEFT

Separation of ankles .... Inches

| < 10 | 11-15 | 16-20 |
| 21-25 | 26-30 | 30 |

ABDUCTION-ADDUCTION

Ankylosis
Contracture
Spasm

RIGHT   LEFT

ROTATION:

(Recorded with patient prone)

Ankylosis
Contracture

LEFT   RIGHT

N.B. Reversed right and left.

Abduction vs. gravity (with Hip Extended)	R : Unable	< 15 degrees	16-30 degrees	> 30 degrees
	L : Unable	< 15 degrees	16-30 degrees	> 30 degrees
Knee range	R : from	degrees	to	degrees
	L : from	degrees	to	degrees
Straight-leg-raising	R : Unable	< 30 degrees	31-60 degrees	> 61-90 degrees
	L : Unable	< 30 degrees	31-60 degrees	> 61-90 degrees
Apparent shortening	R :	inches	true shortening	R : inches
Apparent lengthening	L :		true lengthening	L :

| 260 | 210 | 160 | 100 | 60 | 30 0 |
| 6 | 5 | 4 | 3 | 2 | 1 |

Total in each hip
Grade for mobility

COMMENTS:

SUMMARY

A:
B:
C:

	PAIN	FUNCTION	MOBILITY
R			
L			

Examiner: _____

Date: _____

Fig. 12-5, cont'd.

Continued.

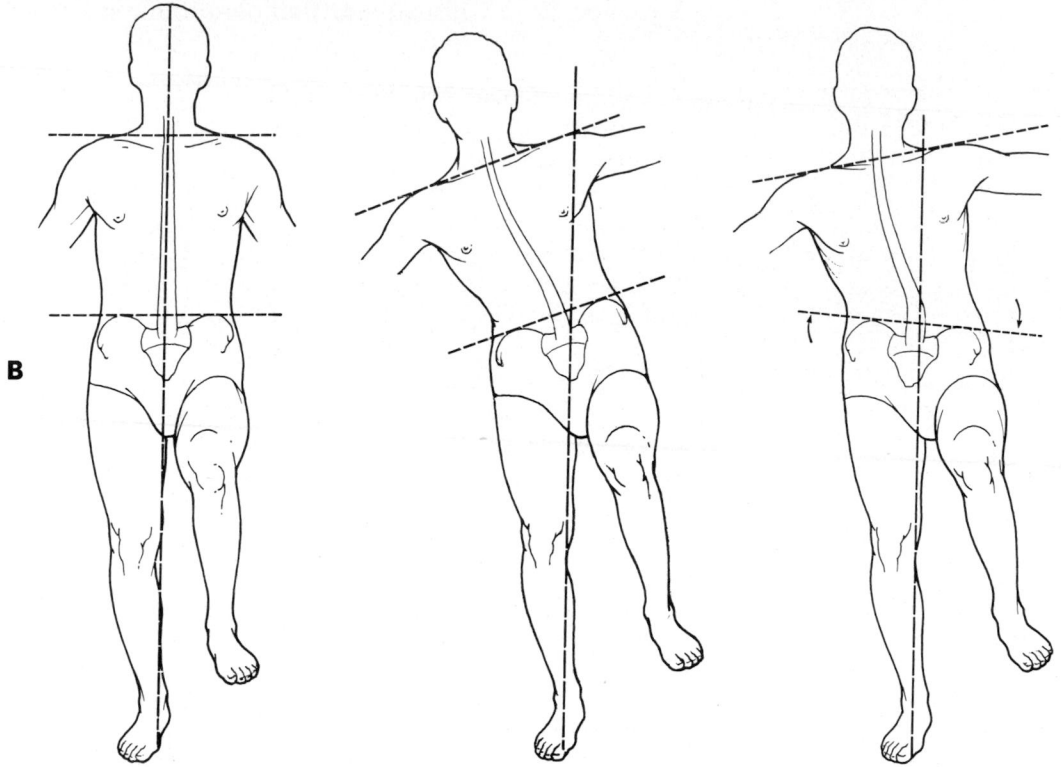

Fig. 12-5—cont'd. **B,** Demonstration of Trendelenburg sign and Trendelenburg lurch (Duchenne's sign). Left, negative Trendelenburg sign and lurch. Center, negative Trendelenburg sign and positive Trendelenburg lurch. Right, positive Trendelenburg sign and lurch. (**B** redrawn from Johnston RC, Fitzgerald RH Jr, Harris WH, et al: Clinical and radiographic evaluation of total hip replacement: a standard system of terminology for reporting results, *J Bone Joint Surg* 72:161, 1990.)

Table 12-8 Hospital for Special Surgery—Hip Rating System

Pain

0. All the time. Unbearable. Strong medication frequently.
2. All the time but bearable. Strong medication occasionally. Salicylates frequently.
4. None or little at rest. With activities. Salicylates frequently.
6. When starting, then better, or after a certain activity. Salicylates occasional.
8. Occasional and slight.
10. No pain.

Muscle Power and Motion*

0. Ankylosis with deformity.
2. Ankylosis with good functional position.
4. MP—Poor to fair. Arc of flexion less than 60 degrees. Restricted lateral and rotary movement.
6. MP—Fair to good. Arc of flexion up to 90 degrees. Fair† lateral and rotary movement.
8. MP—Good or normal. Arc of flexion over 90 degrees. Good‡ lateral and rotary movement.
10. MP—Normal. Motion—Normal or almost normal.

Walking

0. Bedridden.
2. Wheel chair. Transfer activities with walker.
4. No support—housebound or
   One support—less than one block } Markedly
   Bilateral support—less than three blocks } restricted
6. No support—less than one block
   One support—up to five blocks } Moderately
   Bilateral support—unrestricted } restricted
8. No support—limp } Mildly
   One support—no limp } restricted
10. No support or appreciable limp—unrestricted

Function

0. Completely dependent and confined.
2. Partially dependent.
4. Independent. Limited housework, shops limitedly.
6. Most housework, shops freely, desk-type work.
8. Very little restriction. Can work on feet.
10. Normal activities.

From Wilson PD Jr, et al: *J Bone Joint Surg* 54:226, 1972.
*Precedence in rating was given to active movement, but usually both active and passive movement were the same.
†Fair lateral movement: 10 degrees abduction, 10 degrees adduction. Fair rotary movement: internal rotation 10 degrees, external rotation 20 degrees.
‡Good lateral movement: 20 degrees abduction, 20 degrees adduction. Good rotary movement: internal rotation 20 degrees, external rotation 40 degrees.

grade 2 or 3 based on the Merle d'Aubigne and Postel grading system. In grade 3, the patient's activities are severely limited because of pain; any attempt to move the hip causes pain or spasm. Although grade 2 pain is rather uncommon in osteoarthritis, it is often present in the acute stage of rheumatoid arthritis.

Grade 1 pain is found in infections, tumors, and fresh fractures of the neck of the femur. Pain at the level of grade 4 is the minimum to qualify the patient for a total hip arthroplasty. Grade 4 is often tolerable in unilateral hip disease without surgery, providing the patient uses a cane and can tolerate nonsteroidal antiinflammatory drugs. Grade 5 pain is not enough to recommend surgery; even with a limp grade 5 patients can function well without surgery.

Evaluating Pain by a Scoring System

Pain is often the major component of arthritis; it requires special evaluation before and after treatment by total hip arthroplasty. Although subjective, pain can be measured by a variety of techniques[9,42]; use simple numerical scales in a standardized format.

Because pain is one of the most critical issues for patients seeking total hip arthroplasty (see Chapter 10) and because the success or failure of total hip arthroplasty depends on eliminating pain, it should be evaluated without introducing a "loading" factor. Because a cemented arthroplasty should offer total pain relief, a successful arthroplasty should be compared with a normal joint. The results of other methods of arthroplasty should be compared in a similar manner. For this purpose a numerical scale that quantifies the severity of pain is needed.[43] Because operations such as osteotomy and cup arthroplasty do not relieve pain completely or restore mobility, a number of scores were developed by giving an arbitrary "loading" value to the grade for pain.[35,45] Any numerical grading system that does not arbitrarily load the grade offers the distinct advantages of simplicity and clarity. For example, Merle d'Aubigne and Postel's grading system expresses the two extremes of the pain spectrum in a 1 to 6 grading system: 1 denotes extreme pain, and 6 represents no pain. With this system, any arthroplasty graded less than 6 is considered defective.

In an attempt to determine the effectiveness of the hip score to judge the success or failure of a total hip arthroplasty procedure, Ritter applied both Harris and Charnley hip evaluation forms[59] to 191 ingrowth total hip arthroplasties. The Harris hip evaluation form demonstrated a significantly lower score than the Charnley hip score; it consequently failed patients more often because of pain. It is of interest that 32% of the hips that failed on the basis of pain with Harris's hip score did not fail in terms of the total score. Clearly, it can be misleading to judge the success of a hip

operation based on one average hip score; despite a high average score, the patient may experience significant pain.

The sensitivity of the hip score for pain can be further reduced when the scoring includes other parameters, such as radiography. Kavanaugh and Fitzgerald introduced a hip score to represent the patient's status.[40] To assess the patient's status before and after surgery on a 100-point numerical scale, they combined 80 points of clinical assessment with 20 points of radiographic assessments. Although with their system the patient with signs of radiological failure would have a reduced total score, their assessment also shifts the emphasis from the pain score, which should be regarded as the most important parameter in assessing the results of arthroplasty. In conclusion, in evaluating the results (outcome) of a new surgical technique or prosthesis, the overall score may indeed not really reflect whether the procedure has achieved its main goal: the relief of pain.

In his own 100-point score, Larson (Iowa Hip Rating, 1963) designated 35 points for pain (see Table 12-4); Harris allows 44 points in his modified scoring system (see Table 12-5). In treating an arthritic hip joint, always compare the pain in the operated hip with that of a healthy joint (no pain). Remember that the level of pain in the musculoskeletal system can be greatly modified by using analgesics, antiinflammatory agents, or assistive devices (such as a cane or crutches), or simply by limiting the patient's functional activities. Therefore also consider the level of pain in the context of the patient's activity; when this is done it may be more reliable to evaluate the function than the pain. Adopt a simple numerical scale that can be administered easily.

Evaluating Function

In evaluating function by the simple numerical grades (Merle d'Aubigne and Postel's or Charnley's modification, see Tables 12-6 and 12-7), grades 1, 2, or 3 designate patients whose disability is severe enough to indicate the need for a total hip arthroplasty. Grade 3 most commonly designates patients with osteoarthritis demanding total hip arthroplasty. Grades 1 or 2 represent patients with systemic arthritis, such as rheumatoid disease.

Grade 4 is a borderline category; it often includes young patients (under age 50) who have a unilateral hip that is stiff and deformed, some shortening of the leg, and possibly some flexion and adduction deformity. These patients demand surgery to relieve their limp (which also may be associated with back pain) and to be able to walk without the cane. Grade 5 patients should never be considered for a total hip arthroplasty; this grade may reflect a "less than perfect" outcome of total hip arthroplasty. Charnley recognized that evaluation of a unilateral operation may be confused by the patient's remaining disabilities in the opposite hip (the unoperated side) or other disabling diseases (such as polyarthritis in the knees or ankles) or systemic diseases, such as heart failure. He considered the "acid test" for the success of arthroplasty to be determined in patients with unilateral hip disease and with no other factors restricting their function.

The use of the prefixes A, B, and C in describing the patient's condition has been extremely valuable. Category A represents unilateral hip disease without other conditions that interfere with function: the patient is fit in all respects relating to function, with allowance for age, and has no other defect than the arthritic hip. Category B indicates bilateral hip disease with no other condition that might interfere with walking. The patient is fit for his or her age, and no other factors impede a normal function. Category C incorporates patients suffering from a unilateral or bilateral hip disease who also suffer from a generalized systemic factor (such as senility, a neuromuscular disorder, or widespread arthritis of one or more joints) that affects the patient's function (see Figs. 12-2 and 12-4).

Annual follow ups of the patient after total hip arthroplasty may reveal progressive changes if factors emerge that affect the patient's function. An A patient whose hip function deteriorates 5 years after surgery (because of the development of osteoarthritis of the opposite hip) may be downgraded from A to B; if at 15 years after surgery the patient is homebound (because of a cerebrovascular accident), he or she will be further downgraded to C. It should be emphasized that category C must be reserved only for patients whose walking ability is affected by a supervening condition. If the patient's desire to walk more has been impeded by factors unrelated to the hip, the patient may not fit in category C.

To evaluate the outcome of surgery, the surgeon may examine the range of motion of the hips (checking for Trendelenburg's sign or a lurch) and take a specific history related to each function of daily living activities. Record the patient's walking (gait) objectively, asking whether he or she uses assistive walking devices (such as one cane, two canes, crutches, or a walker). Specifics of daily functional activities (such as cutting toenails, reaching the foot to put on shoes, bathing, dressing, stair climbing, sexual intercourse, using a toilet seat, driving a car, and so on) are interdependent parameters; they are affected not only by the level of pain, but by the mobility of the other joints (in some cases the joints of the upper extremities may also affect the patient's pain level).

Reemployment alone cannot be used as a criterion to measure the success or failure of total hip arthroplasty, because many complicating factors enter into the decision to resume work. Gaining employment after total hip arthroplasty can reflect improved function, but it can also reflect a personal need to be productive or a need for increased income. Consider the patient's age and work status before total hip arthroplasty; your records should show whether the patient is retired and if so whether retirement was caused by the hip disease.

Evaluating Hip Motion

The range of motion of the hips (affected and unaffected) is examined according to the standard criteria[4] for flexion, extension, and internal and external rotation. To evaluate the hip objectively, the most effective measure is a simple scale (1 to 3, 6, 10, or 100) that incorporates all the important parameters. While various numerical scales have been developed to provide an objective comparison, many of them incorporate arbitrarily designated loading numbers; they are not objective because they may distort the evaluation, representing it overly optimistically or pessimistically. For example, using the Iowa or Harris hip scores, a unilateral arthrodesed hip in an otherwise healthy patient scores extremely high because of the patient's freedom from pain and good function. The Iowa score allocates 70 points for the absence of pain and a normal function; such patients may receive another 20 points if they do not limp or need to use crutches or a cane. Iowa scoring may give up to 90 points for a well-positioned, pain-free arthrodesis. Nevertheless, the results of such an operation are very displeasing to the patient compared to those of a total hip arthroplasty with an equal score. Such patients might also have good-to-excellent outcomes using Harris's hip score, on which they will score 95 or more. Although Merle d'Aubigne and Postel's grading system only scores flexion and abduction (see Table 12-6), Charnley's modification of that system assesses movement on the basis of flexion/extension, abduction/adduction, and internal/external rotation. This modification evaluates movement without giving any special significance to one plane of motion versus the other. Patients with advanced arthritis may preserve a good range of flexion (even in protusio acetabuli) but lose abduction or rotation. Charnley also modified Merle d'Aubigne and Postel's system to include one numerical representation of the range of motion by adding the scores of motion in various planes (see Table 12-7). Some of the hip score systems use the range of motion (sitting, ability to reach the foot, etc.) to measure functional results. However, Levac[47] found that the range of motion as measured by the patient's ability to reach his or her foot is a poor indicator of function. In other words, it is pointless to assess certain functional activities (reaching one's foot to put on shoes or cutting one's toenails) on the basis of range of motion of the hip alone. These functional activities can be evaluated and recorded independent of the hip score.

Designating a specific number (loading factor) for the range of motion reduces the importance attributed to range of motion in daily functional activities. For example, the zero points given in the Iowa hip score and the 5 of 100 points given in Harris's hip score reflect the era of osteotomy and cup arthroplasty, when loss of motion was common after those operations. The results of total hip arthroplasty must be compared with the "normal" hip, as a normal or near-normal range of motion is achievable; Grade 5 or 6 condition before surgery (Grade 5 or 6 on Charnley's modification of the Merle d'Aubigne and Postel hip score).

Comparison of Various Scales

The Joint Commission's primary goal was to develop a system of terminology to acquire minimal data for precise scientific comparison; they did not recommend a method for presenting the data (i.e., a "system of score"). Their goal was to allow individual investigators sufficient latitude to present their data as they desire. If the primary data acquisition is exact and uniform, a uniform language results (see Tables 12-1 to 12-3); each investigator may add facts, observations, or comments as deemed necessary. At this time, however, there is no system of evaluation that is without limitations, even though most systems provide viewers with information that enables them to compare different operations, prostheses, and patient populations preoperatively and at various times postoperatively. This author believes that the best method of evaluation presents the results without subjectively emphasizing the importance of one parameter over another. With a system like Charnley's modification of Merle d'Abugine and Postel's, the surgeon can evaluate the patient's condition preoperatively and postoperatively as a whole by averaging three scores: pain, function, and mobility. By adding a prefix for function (A, B, or C), it can also illustrate whether the patient's poor function results from causes other than the hip disability or the hip arthroplasty.

However, adding the score of radiographic parameters to the clinical score (for ease of interpreting the patient's clinical and radiographic data in a single digit[40]) creates significant discrepancies between the clinical and radiographic features of arthroplasty. In one study,[41] nearly one third of the patients with radiographic component loosening exhibited pain at the time of evaluation. This technique is flawed, for several reasons:

1. The natural history of early radiographic changes is not well established, so indexing and incorpo-

rating nonprogressive radiolucencies produces inferior results.
2. The patient with marked radiological loosening and migration may score well clinically and so receive a high overall score.
3. The radiographic criteria for cementless arthroplasties have not been established; therefore a well-performed hip arthroplasty may be regarded as a failure and vice versa.

In comparing nine different methods of hip assessments in 1954, Andersson concluded that the results varied significantly and emphasized the importance of achieving a standard evaluation system.[7] In 1985, Galante[27] pleaded for a standardized system; he found it difficult to compare the results of two series of arthroplasties when one used a modified Harris hip score system and the other used the Mayo hip score system (a 20-point system to measure the radiographic hip score).[40] To compare the results of various hip scoring systems, Callaghan and associates[16] used five different rating systems to evaluate 100 total hip arthroplasties: the Merle d'Aubigne and Postel (1954) system, Larson's system (Iowa hip score, 1963), the Harris hip score (1969), the Hospital for Special Surgery hip score (1972), and the Mayo Clinic (modified) hip score (Kavanagh and Fitzgerald, 1985). Each of these ratings (as well as the patient's own assessment) produced different results (Fig. 12-6, Table 12-9). The Hospital for Special Surgery's rating system produced the most optimistic results; the most pessimistic were obtained using Merle d'Aubigne and Postel's rating scale. Callaghan and associates[16] also concluded that it was important to include Charnley's A, B, and C functional classes in the evaluation (Fig. 12-7).

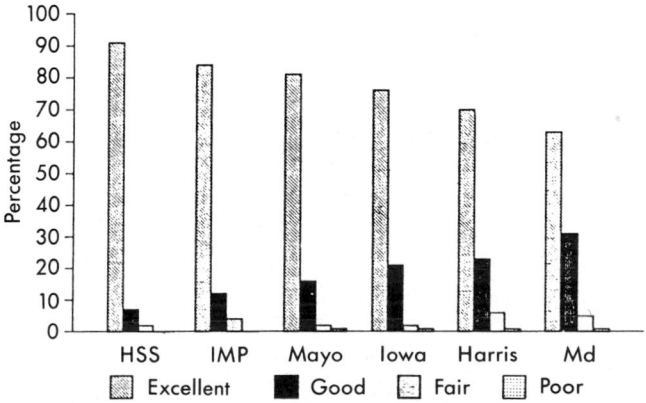

Fig. 12-6. Overall results of 100 hips. *HSS,* Hospital for Special Surgery; *IMP,* Patient's own impressions; *Md,* Merle d'Aubigne. (From Callaghan JJ, Dysart SH, Savory CF, et al: Assessing the results of hip replacement. A comparison of five different rating systems, *J Bone Joint Surg* 72[Br]:1008, 1990.)

Table 12-9 Comparison of the Patient's Own Assessment with the Ratings of the Five Systems (*percentage*)

Patient's own assessments	Result by hip scoring	Percentage in each category				
		HSS	Mayo	Iowa	Harris	Merle d'Aubigné
Excellent (n = 84)	Excellent	95.3	87.0	84.5	76.4	71.4
	Good	4.7	13.0	15.5	20.0	27.4
	Fair				3.6	1.2
Good (n = 12)	Excellent	83.3	58.3	33.3	41.7	25
	Good	8.3	33.3	58.3	41.7	50
	Fair	8.4	8.4	8.4	16.6	25
Fair (n = 4)	Excellent	25	25	25	25	0
	Good	50	25	25	25	50
	Fair	25	25	25	25	25
	Poor		25	25	25	25

From Callaghan JJ, Dysart SH, Savory CF, et al: Assessing the results of hip replacement. A comparison of five different rating systems, *J Bone Joint Surg* 72[Br]:1008, 1990.

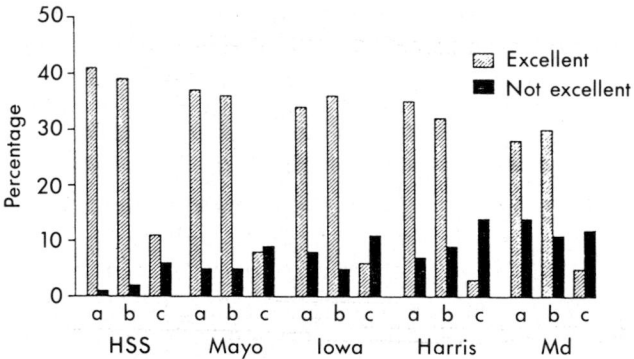

Fig. 12-7. The ratings of each system in each of Charnley's functional classes. (From Callaghan JJ, Dysart SH, Savory CF, et al: Assessing the results of hip replacement. A comparison of five different rating systems, *J Bone Joint Surg* 72[Br]:1008, 1990.)

RADIOGRAPHIC ASSESSMENT

Radiographic imaging for total hip arthroplasty is required preoperatively and postoperatively; occasionally it is also necessary for intraoperative evaluation. The relevant image studies include plain radiography, tomography (laminograms), arthrography, computerized axial tomography (CAT), nuclear imaging, single-photon emission computerized tomography (SPECT), ultrasonography, and magnetic resonance imaging (MRI). Special studies such as selected and enhanced angiography (angiography and CAT scanning) may also be required.

Plain Radiographs

In evaluating the hip joint before and after total hip arthroplasty, the single most helpful and frequently

used diagnostic tool is high-quality radiographs. They are important in establishing the diagnosis and in planning surgical treatment. Even more important than their role in the clinical course is that they allow the surgeon to establish a means of follow-up evaluation.

A careful review of preoperative radiographs and recording of the radiological morphology are essential to appreciate the diagnostic and technical aspects of total hip arthroplasty. In this context the study of radiographs is as essential to the surgeon as analysis of blueprints is to the engineer and builder.

1. Generally, a distinction between osteoarthritis, rheumatoid arthritis, and a septic hip can be made. Although diagnosis is not always possible by radiographs alone, radiological study may establish telltale signs and clinical symptoms.
2. Conditions such as suppurative arthritis or tuberculosis may be screened out.
3. Difficult anatomical situations may be verified and technical problems anticipated so that appropriate measures can be taken during surgery. An outstanding example is equalization of leg length after replacement of one or both hips. Conditions such as fusion of the hip, ectopic bone, protrusio acetabuli, and severe osteoporosis are all indications for special technical requirements.
4. Types of hardware inserted in previous surgery may be identified so that its removal at surgery can be anticipated and special instruments or prostheses made available when necessary.
5. Mechanical failure often can be distinguished from infection only by examination of serial radiographs.

Text continued on p. 579.

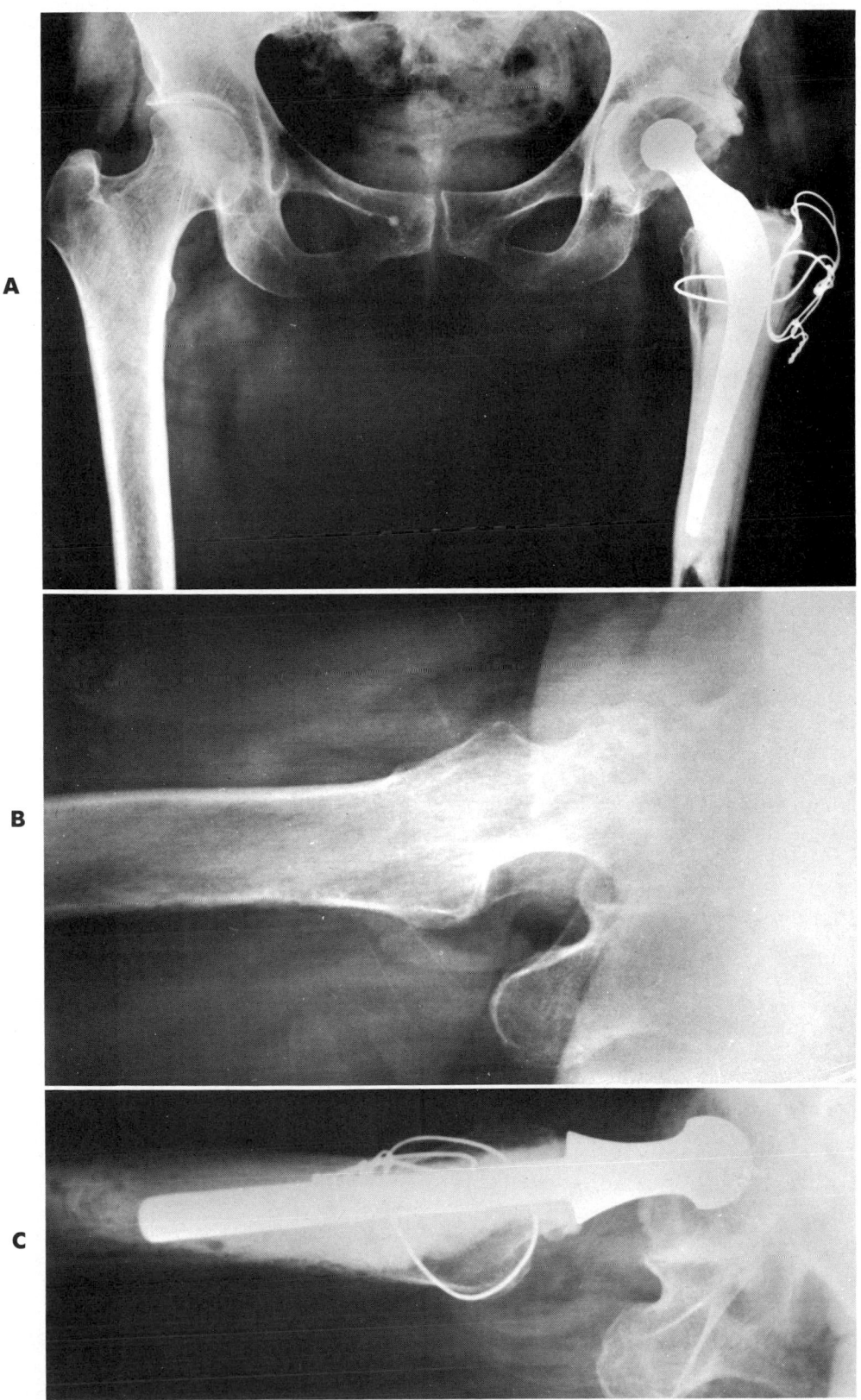

Fig. 12-8. Good-quality radiographs that include upper third of femurs and the isthmus of femur are essential. Anteroposterior view must include both hips and upper third of femurs. **A,** Manfredi lateral. **B** and **C,** Shoot-through is preferable since frog-lateral position is not usually possible because of stiffness of hip in arthritic conditions.

Continued.

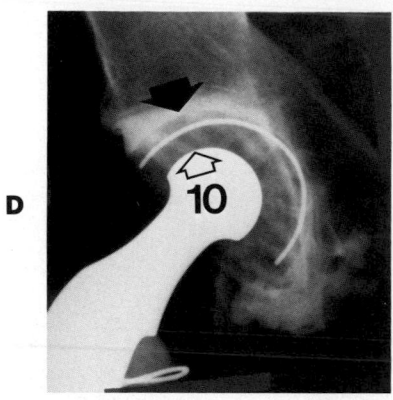

Fig. 12-8—cont'd. D, The wear of the socket is measured between the femoral head and the radiographic marker. This distance is "true" linear wear resulting from penetration of the head into the socket provided that the wire marker remains in a frontal plane of the pelvis (without anteversion or retroversion). NOTE: the "true wear" of the socket in 51-year-old woman (D.P.) 10 years after low-friction arthroplasty measures less than 1 mm (the distance between the two arrows), whereas the "apparent wear" (the distance between the femoral head and the radiographic marker) is only 5 mm, indicating a false assumption of 5-mm wear. In this case the cup has been inserted with some degrees of anteversion.

An aware and interested radiologist familiar with specific problems of total hip arthroplasty is invaluable in performing certain diagnostic procedures or establishing a correct diagnosis.

Generally, an anteroposterior view of both hips and the upper third of both femurs is obtained on a single film. Although radiographs cannot be centered on both hip joints on one film, such a film provides details adequate for diagnostic purposes.

A standard x-ray table with a Potter-Bucky diaphragm is used. For a standard image, the distance of tube to film is 42 inches, which usually produces a 1.2× magnification of the bone and prosthesis.

A lateral view of the hip is helpful to compare cortical changes of the bone with postoperative films, that is, to verify the possibility of infection or loosening. A Manfredi lateral (shoot-through) view of both hips is preferable, since a "frogleg" lateral position is not suitable. External rotation on abduction often is painful or impossible in patients with arthritis (Fig. 12-8). Good-quality radiographs that include the upper third of the femur and the isthmus of the femur are essential. X-ray films that do not adequately show the upper femur may result in unrecognized pathology. Fig. 12-9 is an example of a case where the stem of a previous prosthesis extends from the femoral shaft and is not recognized in the anteroposterior view.

Documentation of the details of x-ray films in the evaluation record is an effective teaching tool and insurance against loss of the radiographs, since the descriptive details become a permanent record on the patient's chart. Fig. 12-3 represents the form used for recording the radiological morphology of the hip.

Figs. 12-10 to 12-22 illustrate examples of various radiographic morphologies of the hip commonly observed and documented during assessment of the hip for arthroplasty.

Clinical Course Examination

Radiographs not only help the surgeon to evaluate the performance of the artificial joint, they also indicate the presence of tissue reactions to the artificial joint (such as those caused by particulate materials, plastic, or metals) before symptoms develop. Serial radiographs also reflect the status of bone remodeling, revealing a gross measure of bone atrophy or hypertrophy. To establish a standard nomenclature, several zones of the interface between and around the implant and bone have been established (Fig. 12-23). Other radiographic landmarks are used for reference (Figs. 12-24 and 12-25).

To be of value for follow up, radiographic studies must have several characteristics:

1. They must be of high quality and resolution.
2. Their magnification, x-ray penetration, and orientation must conform with previous studies of the same patient.
3. They must provide views of the upper third of the

Text continued on p. 579.

Fig. 12-9. To find actual location of stem within shaft, two perpendicular plane films are essential. On anteroposterior view, hip must be in neutral rotation; shoot-through lateral view to include upper third of femur must also be obtained. **A,** Postoperative x-ray film of low-friction arthroplasty in 61-year-old man, suggestive of femoral stem penetration through medial cortex. **B,** With internal rotation, stem looks as if it has penetrated through lateral cortex. **C,** Hip in neutral position; stem is within shaft of femur. **D,** Situation was not well appraised until lateral view was obtained (Manfredi lateral) where actual penetration was discovered to be posterior.

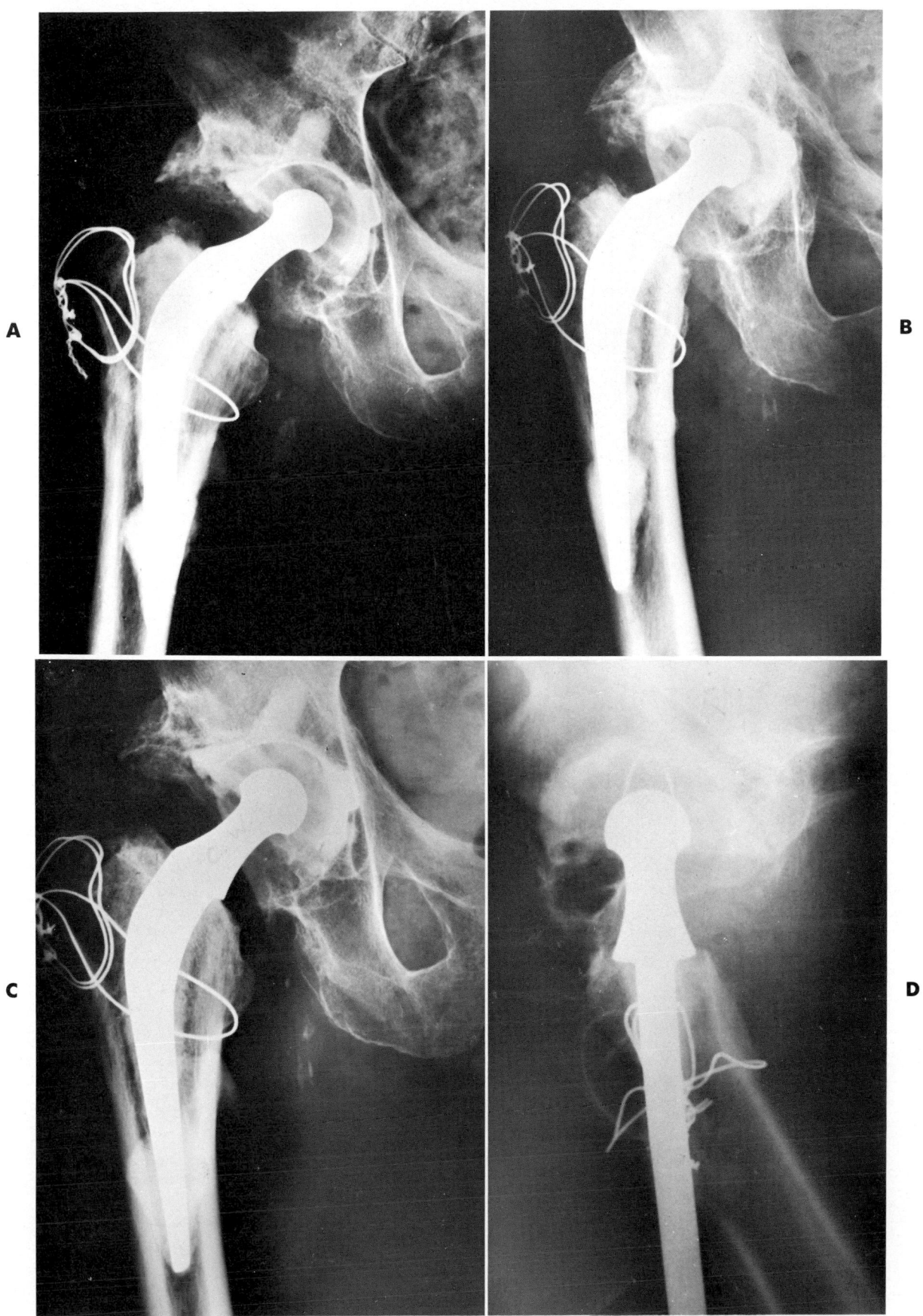

Fig. 12-9. See legend on opposite page.

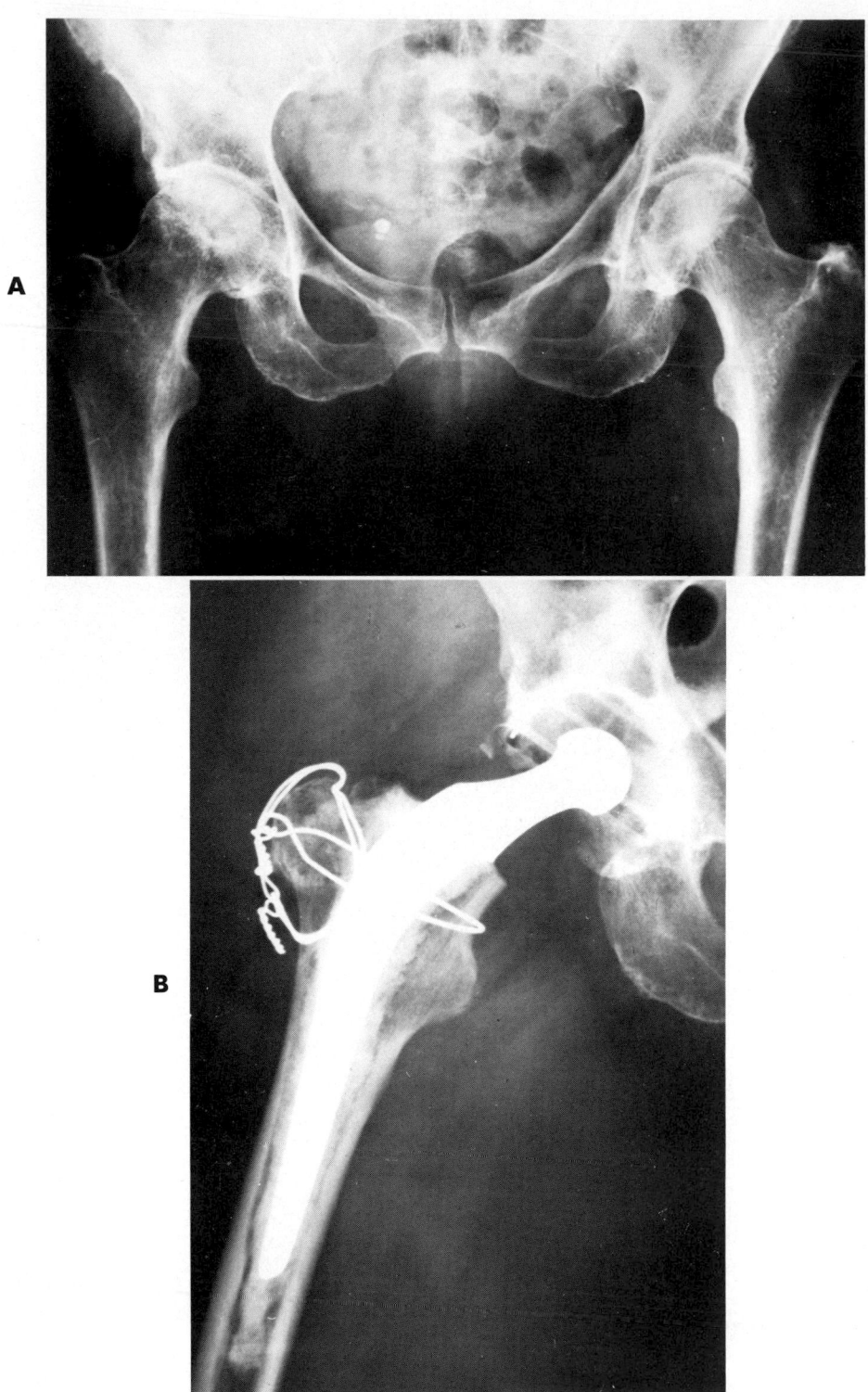

Fig. 12-10. A, Early phase of osteoarthritis is usually characterized by slight osteophytic formation and slight narrowing of joint space *(left hip).* This is regarded as an "incipient form" of arthritis. Osteoarthritis at times may show only minimum joint space narrowing, but the main feature may resemble that of "quadrantic head necrosis" without collapse *(right hip).* **B,** Postoperative low-friction arthroplasty performed on right side.

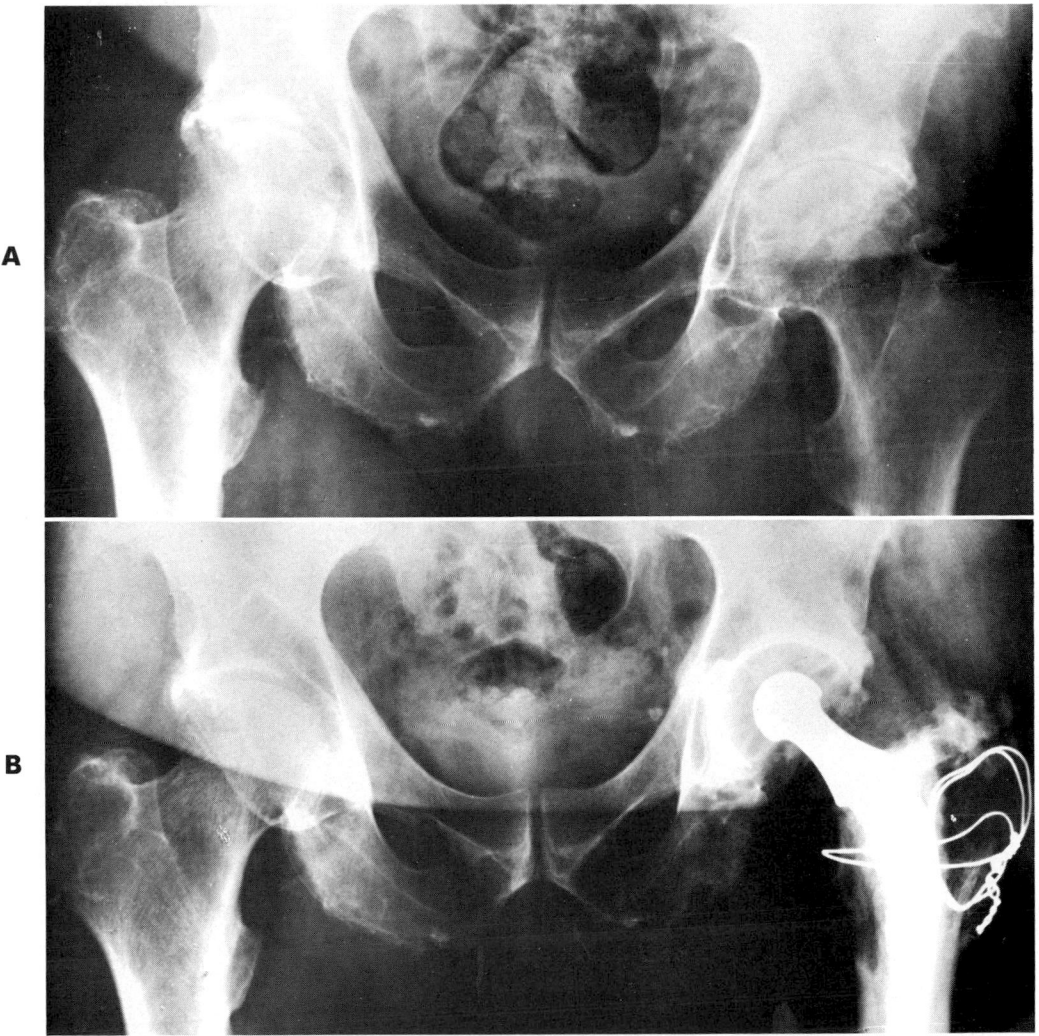

Fig. 12-11. A, Another example of nonmigratory-type osteoarthritis known as *concentric type.* Left hip: narrowing of joint space is uniform but secondary sclerosis may be seen. Right hip: evidence of similar changes but predominantly at this stage over medial pole. **B,** Postoperative low-friction arthroplasty performed for same.

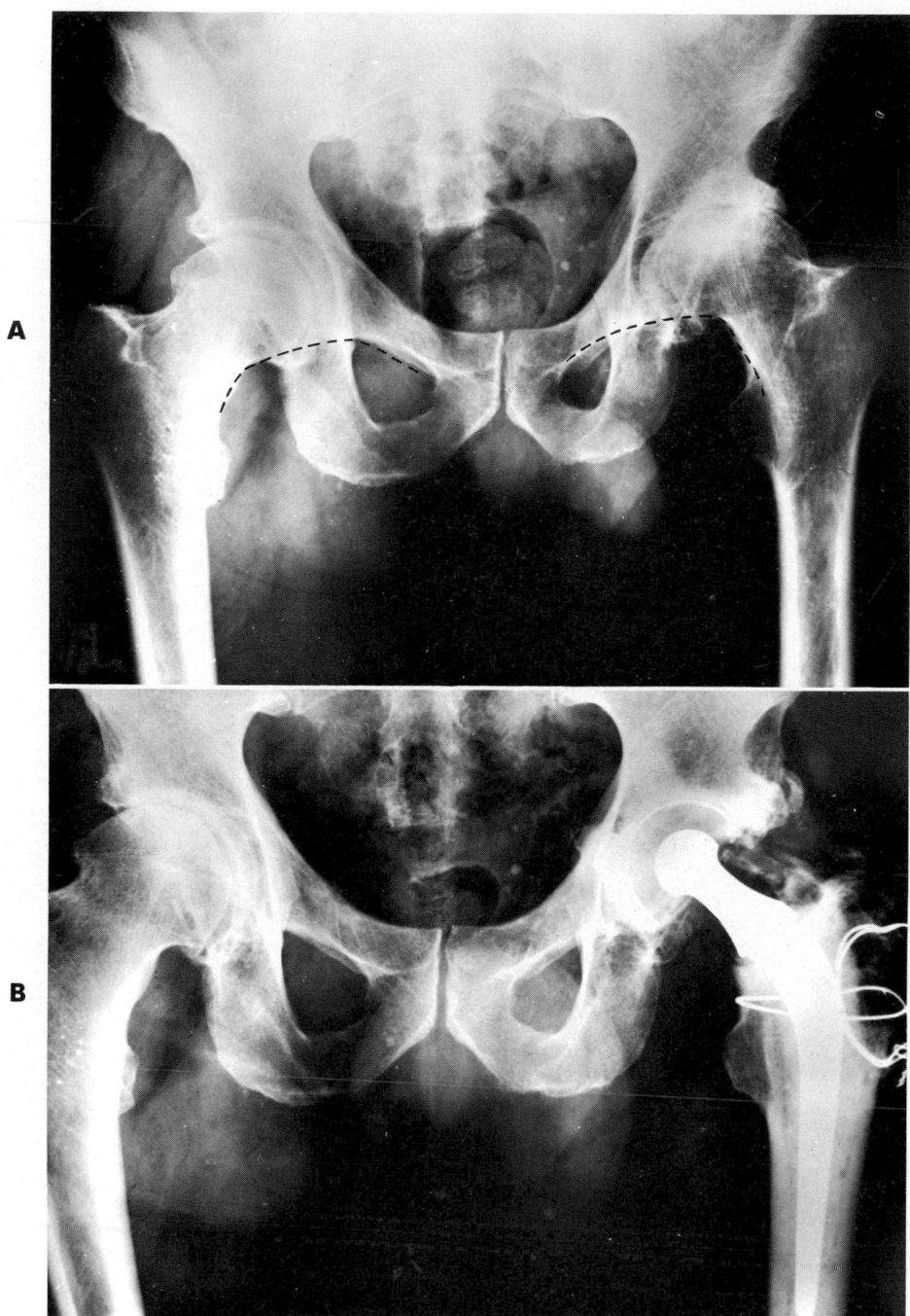

Fig. 12-12. A, Right hip depicts upper pole grade 1, in which joint space is narrowed at level of upper pole of femoral head. Here femoral head remains more or less spherical. Small osteophyte is present, but there is no evidence of proximal migration of head. Left hip depicts grade 2 upper pole; head is flattened on top, and moderate-sized inferior acetabular osteophyte is present, although head is slightly subluxated out of socket. Shenton's line is still intact. **B,** Postoperative low-friction arthroplasty performed on left.

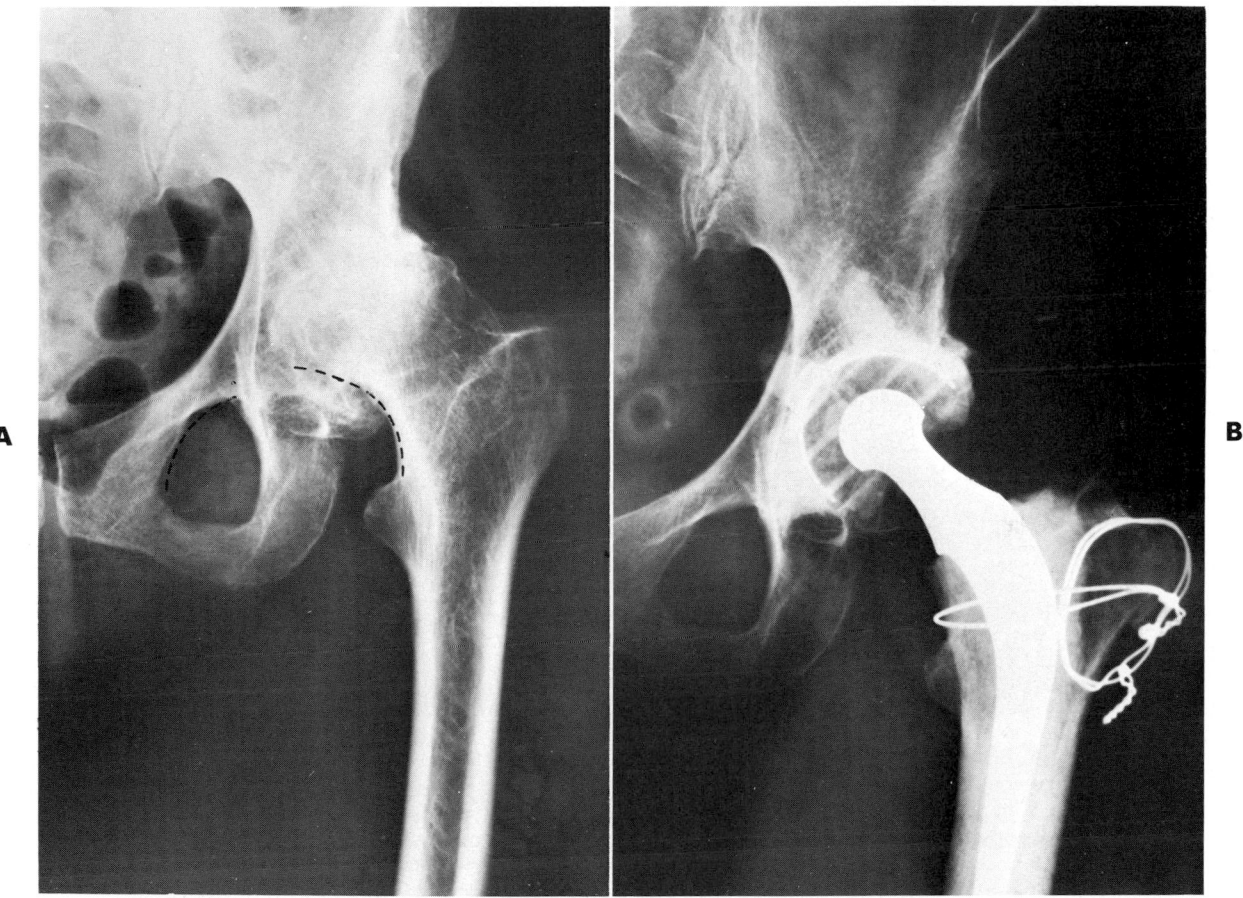

Fig. 12-13. A, Upper pole grade 3, disease is advanced. NOTE: loss of head substance and flattening of acetabular roof. Head is subluxated proximally. Large inferior osteophyte is also present. Shenton's line is broken. **B,** Postoperative low-friction arthroplasty for same.

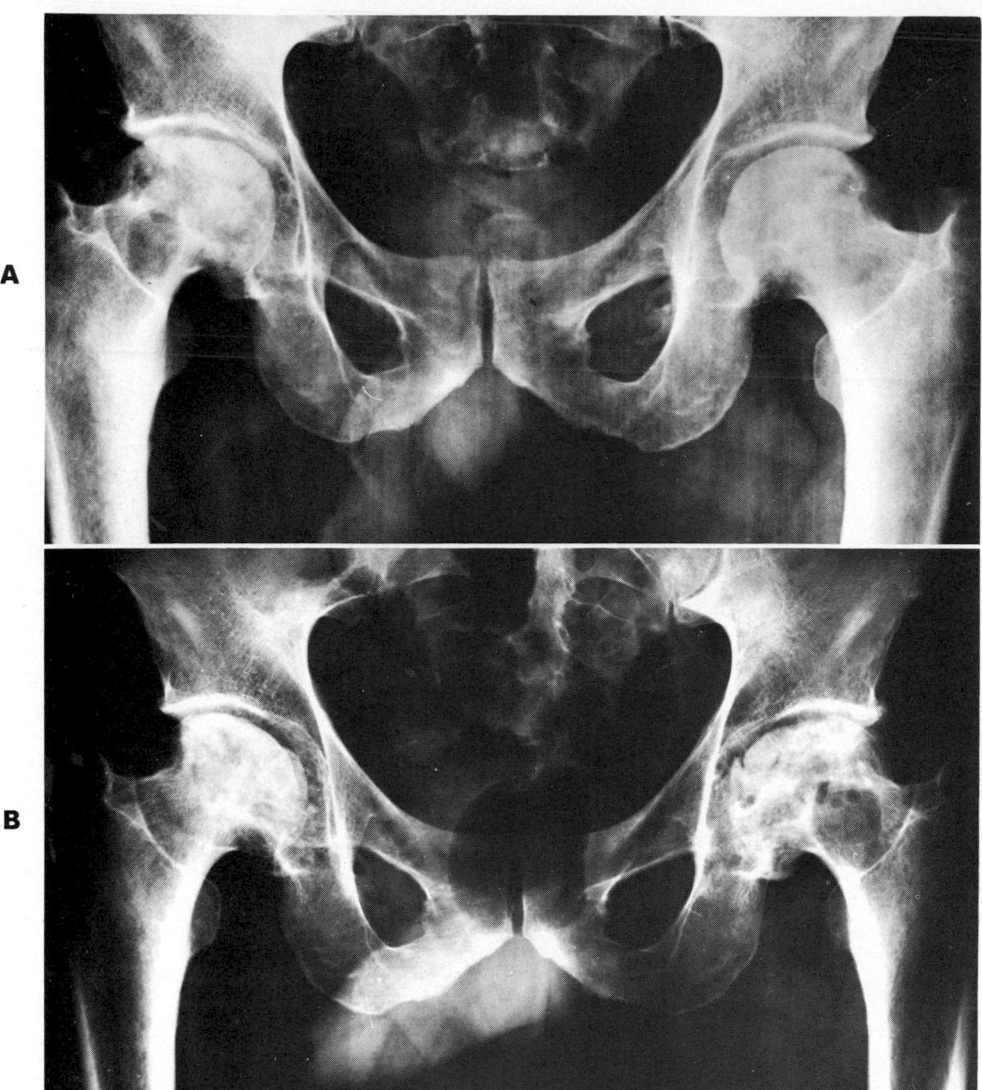

Fig. 12-14. Bilateral avascular necrosis of femoral heads initiating degenerative osteoarthritis in otherwise healthy person. There was no history of alcoholism or systemic condition to explain presence of avascular necrosis. With proximal migration of head and disruption of Shenton's line, condition becomes obvious. **A,** Bilateral changes more severe on right with some flattening of head as result of collapse. Although acetabulum appears normal, even at this stage acetabular cartilage involvement is inevitable. **B,** Within 6-month interval, further collapse of head on left and right is observed. **C,** Postoperative insertion of cemented endoprosthesis, 2 years after surgery, shows evidence of proximal migration of prosthesis and clinical evidence of failure because of acetabular cartilage wear. Absence of acetabular changes by radiograph does not necessarily indicate healthy acetabular cartilage; therefore hemiarthroplasty is not indicated.

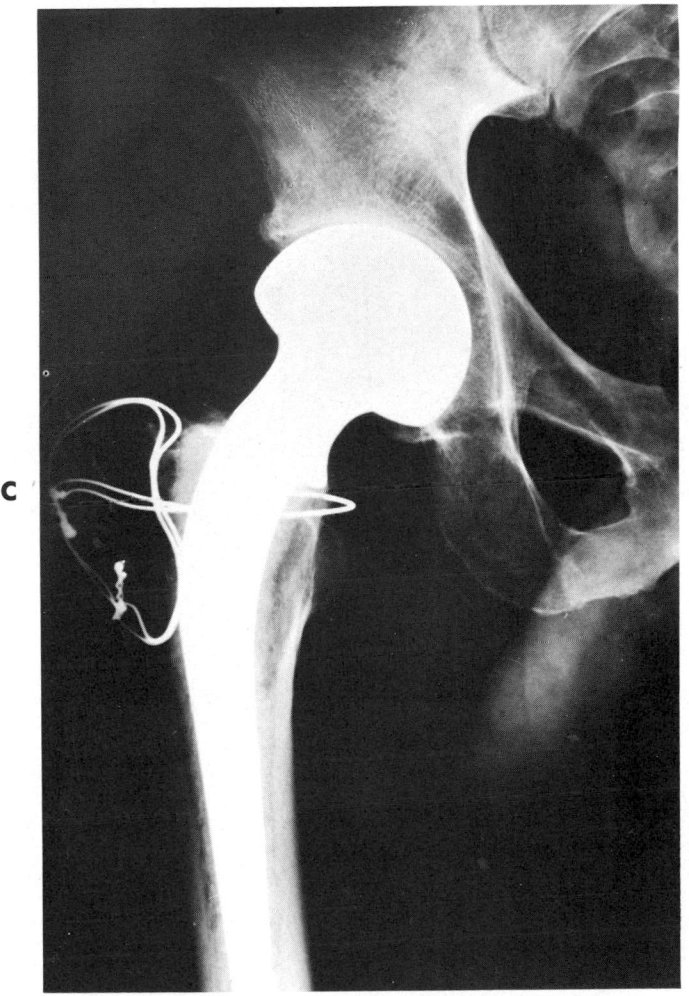

Fig. 12-14, cont'd. See legend on opposite page.

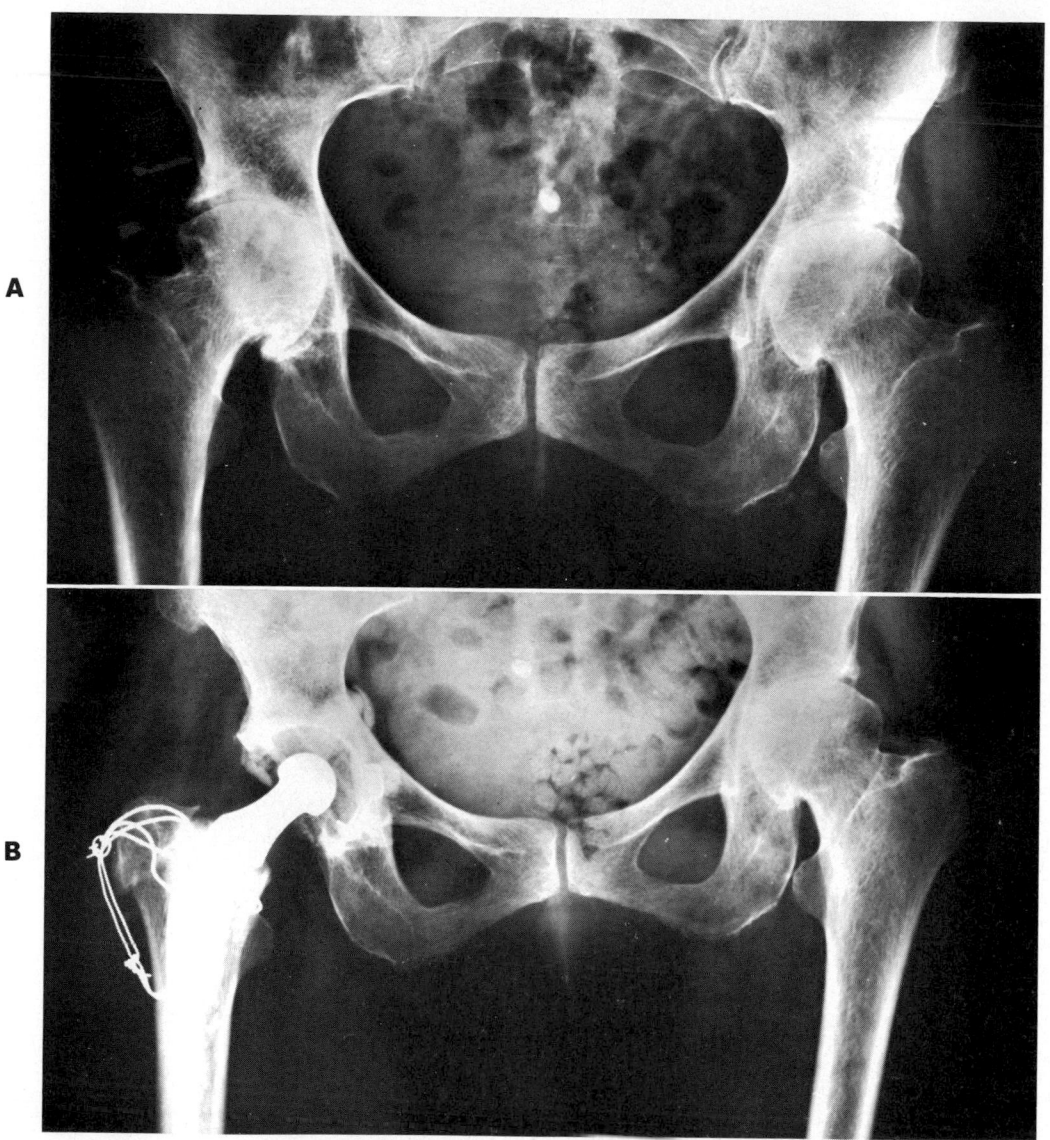

Fig. 12-15. A, Bilateral medial pole arthritis in 65-year-old female. **B,** Postoperative replacement of same on right hip.

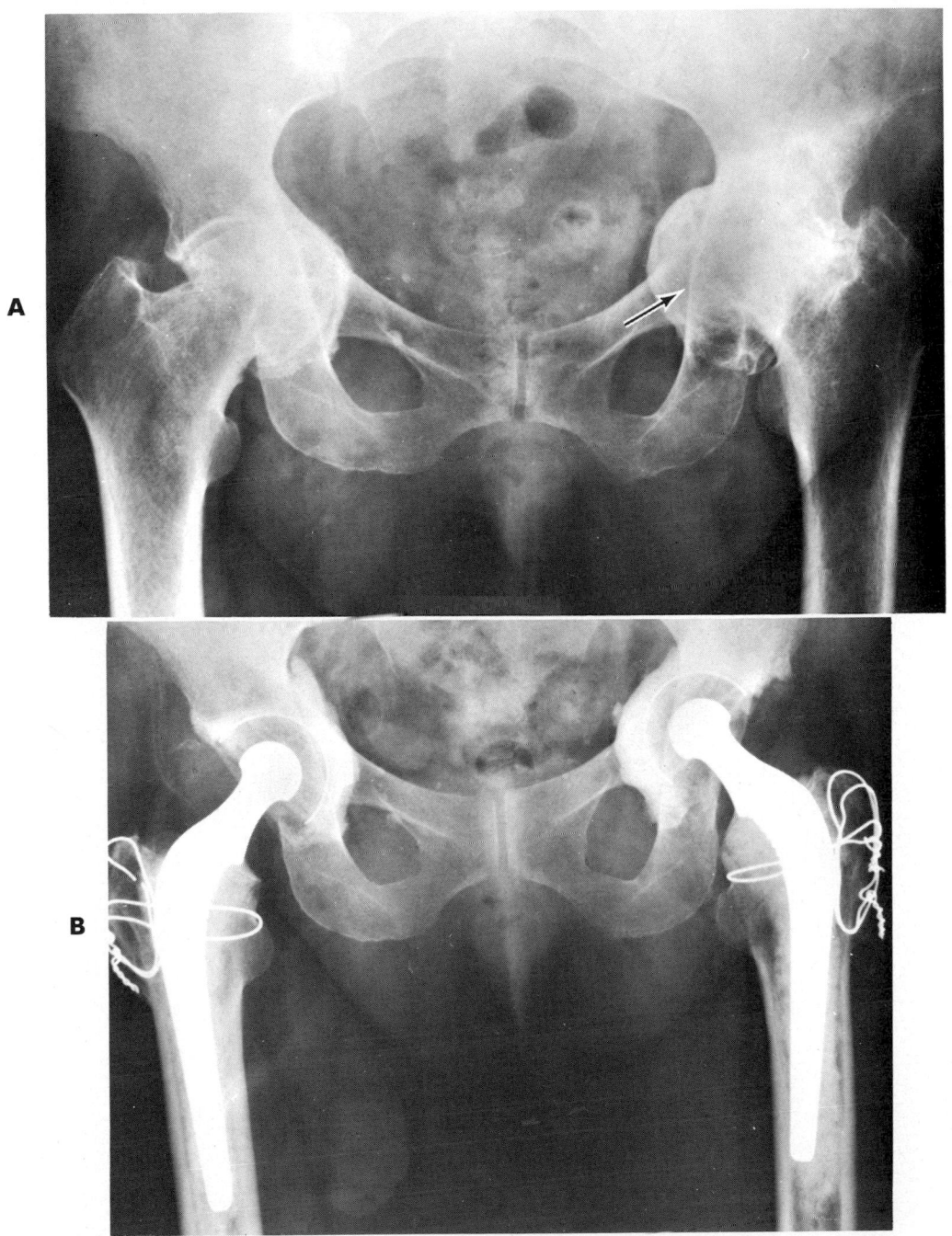

Fig. 12-16. A, Bilateral protrusion of acetabulum in 58-year-old female, more severe on left than right. NOTE: so-called teardrop formed laterally by acetabular floor and medially by pelvic wall can be taken as point of reference to determine degree of medial protrusion. **B,** Postoperative radiographs of same after bilateral low-friction arthroplasty procedure.

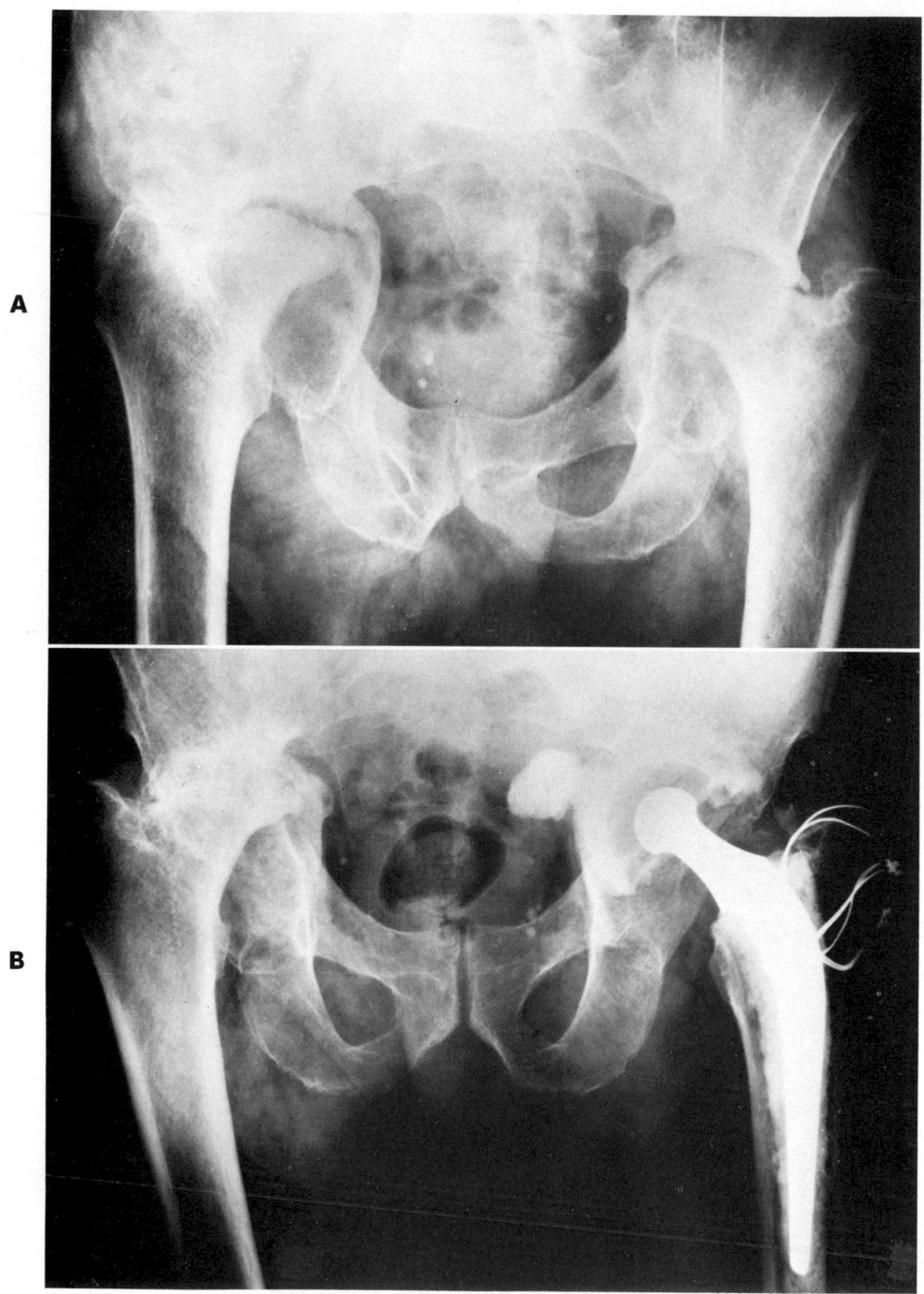

Fig. 12-17. A, Bilateral protrusio acetabuli in 68-year-old man with clinical diagnosis of osteoarthrosis. NOTE: head collapse and "wandering acetabulum." Protrusion is not only medial but proximal. **B,** Postoperative radiograph of replacement of left hip 6 years after surgery. This patient became active, and symptoms of right hip did not require surgical intervention.

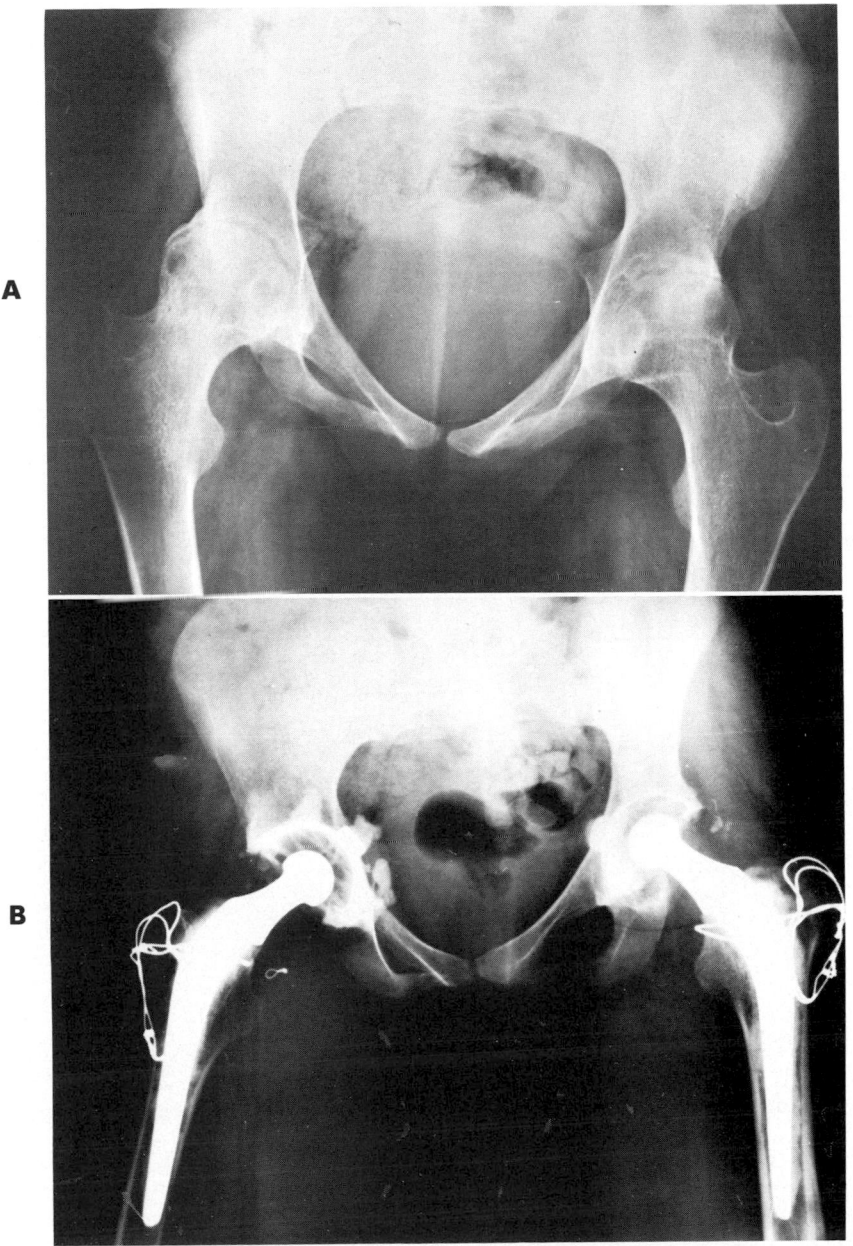

Fig. 12-18. Severe osteoporosis, microcystic changes, and symmetrical involvement of hips is common in rheumatoid arthritis. **A,** 22-year-old female affected by rheumatoid arthritis at age 18 with rapid progression. NOTE: symmetrical hip involvement. **B,** Postoperative radiograph after bilateral low-friction arthroplasty 4 years after surgery.

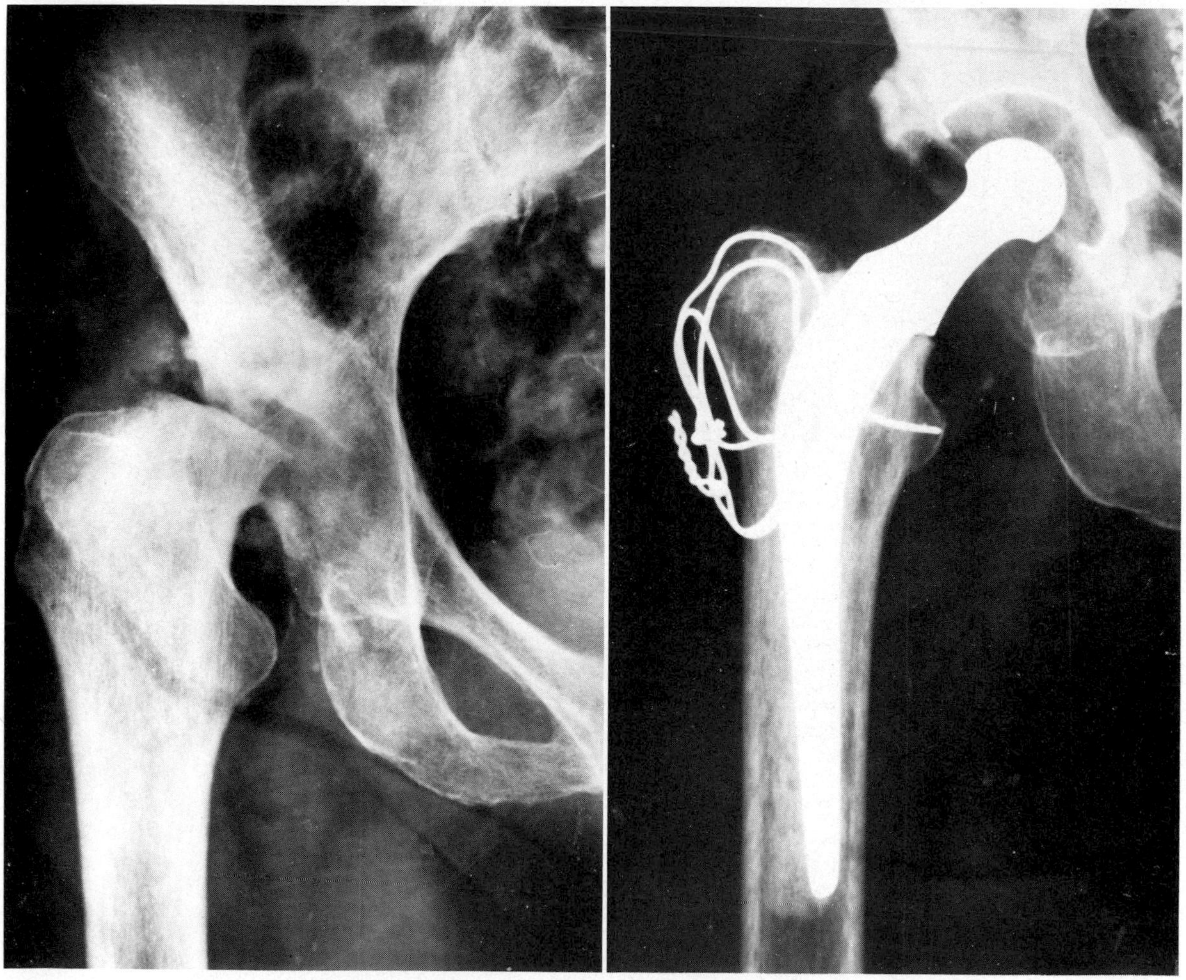

Fig. 12-19. A, Upward subluxation and collapse in hip of 52-year-old female gives impression of "Charcot type" of infection. Patient also has received steroids for many years. **B,** Postoperative radiograph of **A** 8 years after replacement. Cultures were negative for aspirate and biopsy material.

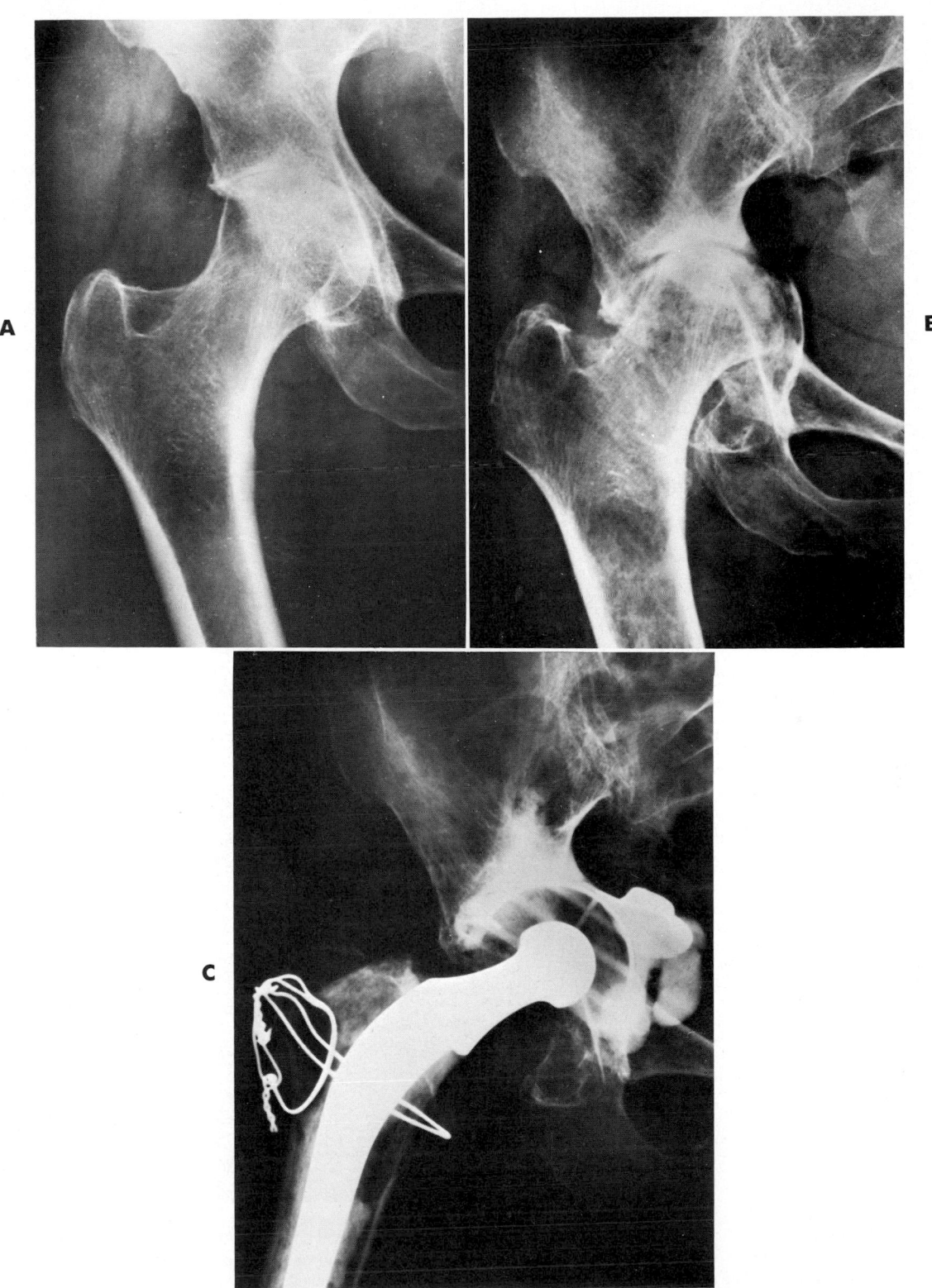

Fig. 12-20. A, Classic appearance of early involvement of rheumatoid hip. **B,** Rapid and progressive protrusion of femoral head into pelvis and defective floor created within only 2 years from onset of disease in hip. **C,** After arthroplasty, note defective floor has led to escape of cement restrictor into pelvis.

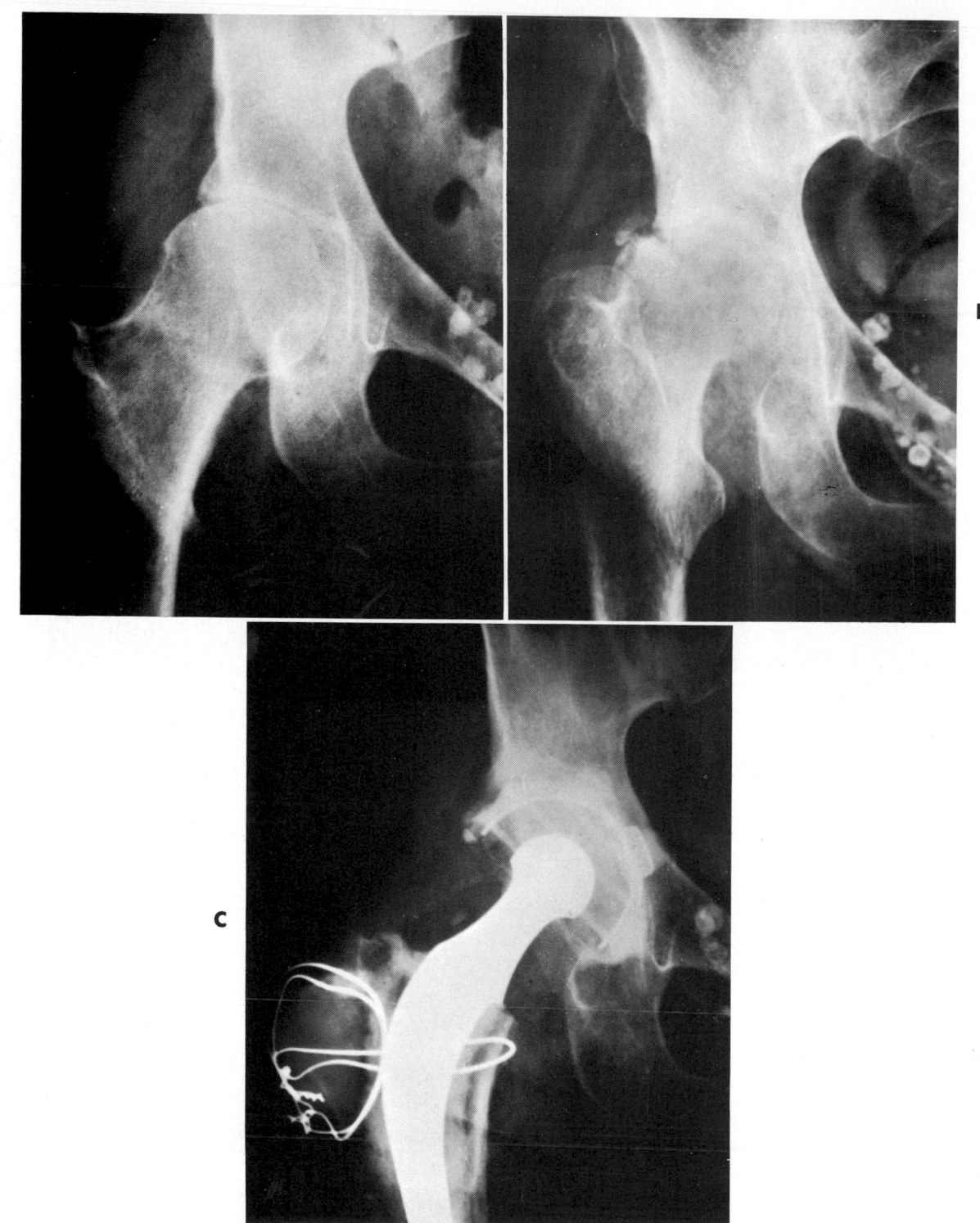

Fig. 12-21. Avascular necrosis of femoral head may only be recognized after development of osteoarthritis in hip. Collapse of femoral head subsequently may clarify diagnosis. **A,** Preoperative radiograph of right hip in 54-year-old female suffering from Cushing's disease treated by corticosteroids. NOTE: joint narrowing but no evidence of avascular necrosis of head at this stage. **B,** One year after onset of hip pain, femoral head collapse is obvious. **C,** Postoperative radiograph after hip arthroplasty.

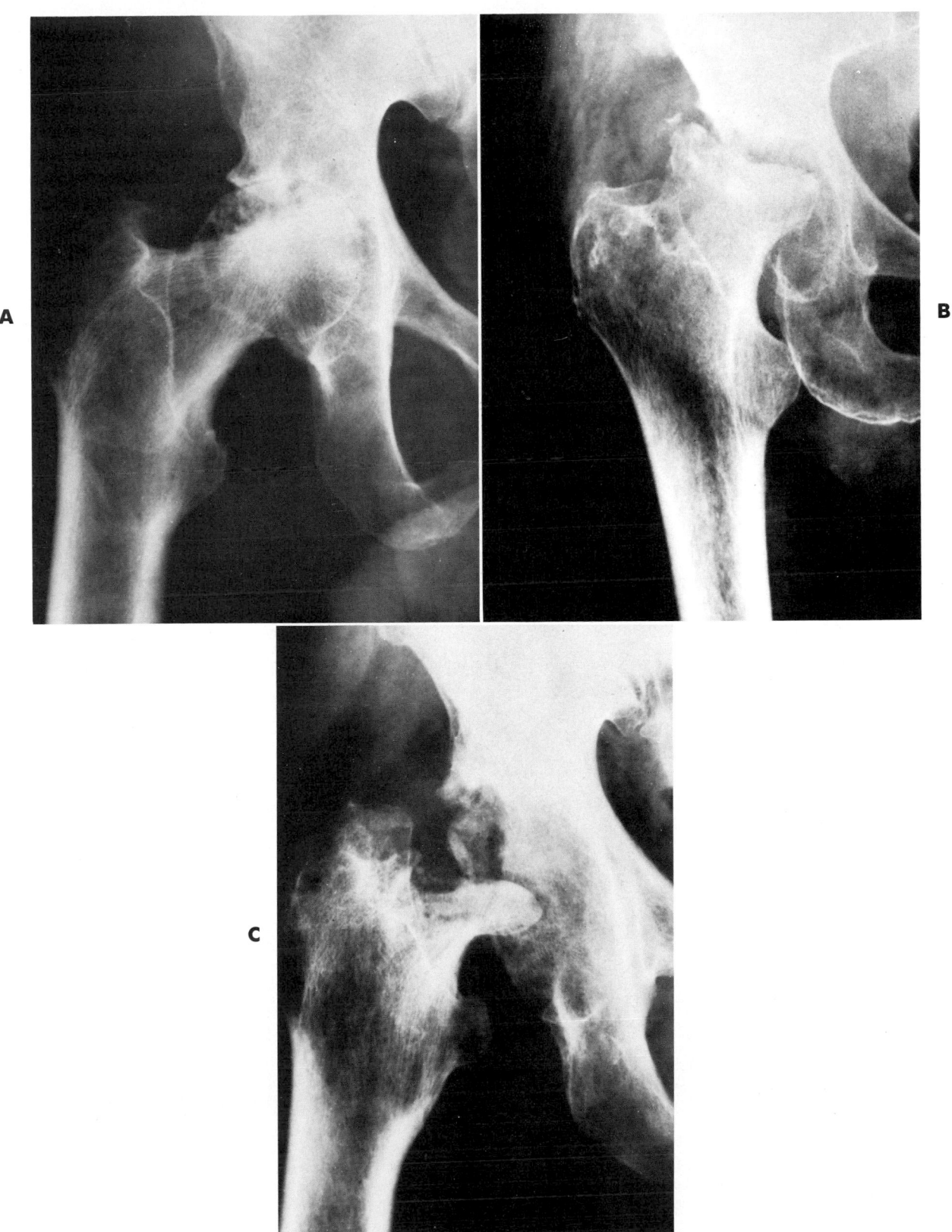

Fig. 12-22. A, Avascular necrosis of femoral head in 44-year-old male; rheumatoid arthritis is shown. Concentric involvement of hip and microcystic changes with secondary sclerosis are main features. **B,** Six months later, head collapse and upward migration of femoral head can be seen. **C,** Further dissolution of femoral head giving radiological pattern similar to Charcot-like joint.

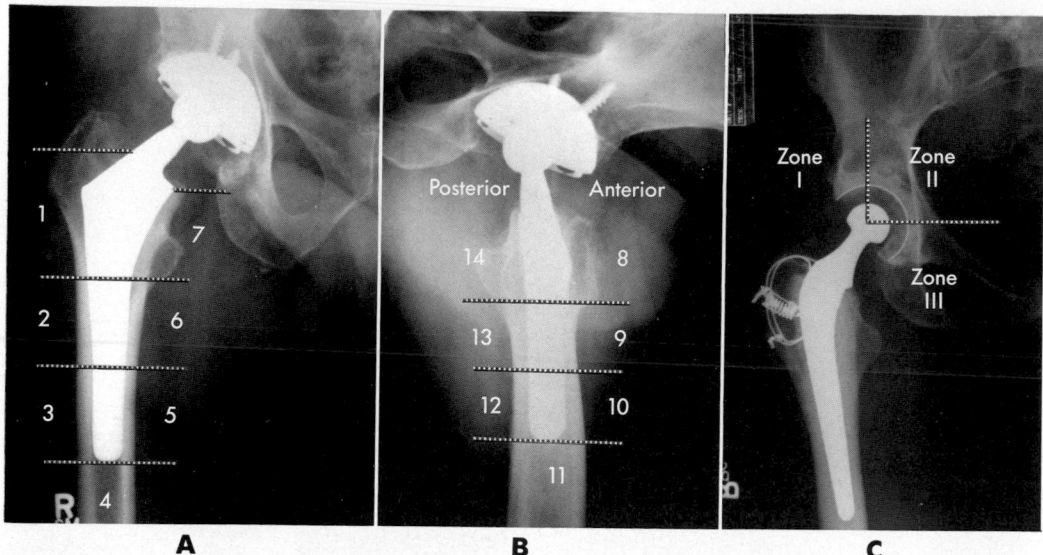

Fig. 12-23. Radiographic interpretation of interface between prosthesis and bone. **A,** Anteroposterior radiographic zones (1 to 7). **B,** Lateral view radiographic zones (8 to 14). **C,** Acetabular zones (1 to 3).

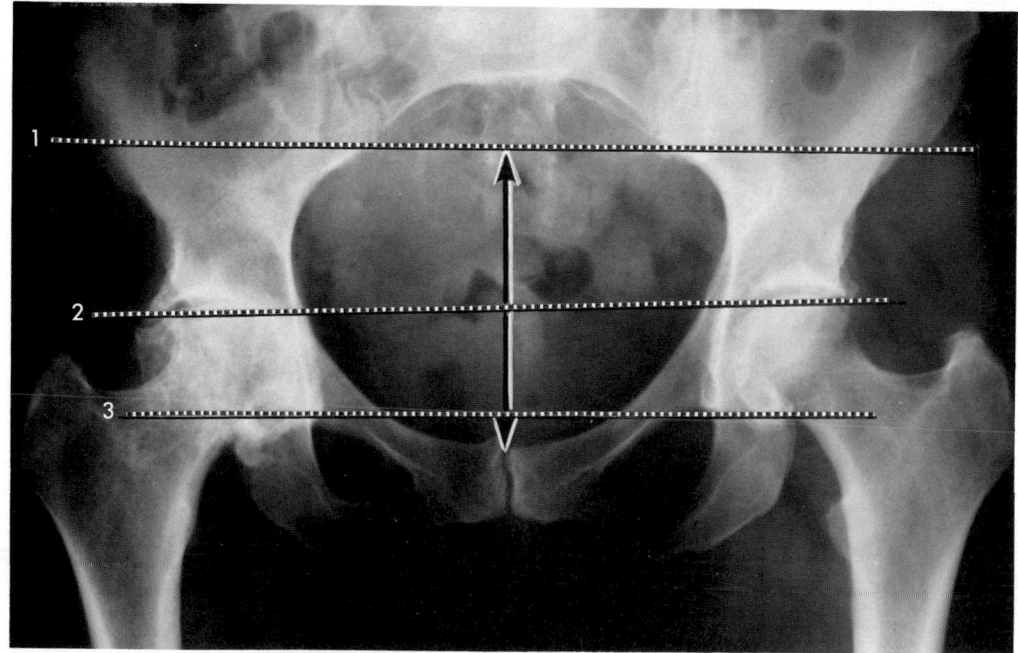

Fig. 12-24. Three horizontal lines for vertical migration of the acetabulum or the femoral head include: (1) sacroiliac line *(SI)*, (2) acetabular line *(A)*, and (3) teardrop line *(T)*. Note that two other horizontal lines (not shown) may be drawn along the upper margins of iliac crests or ischial tuberosities. These lines are less defined than the ones shown in this figure. Sacroiliac-symphysis distance *(arrows)* is shown.

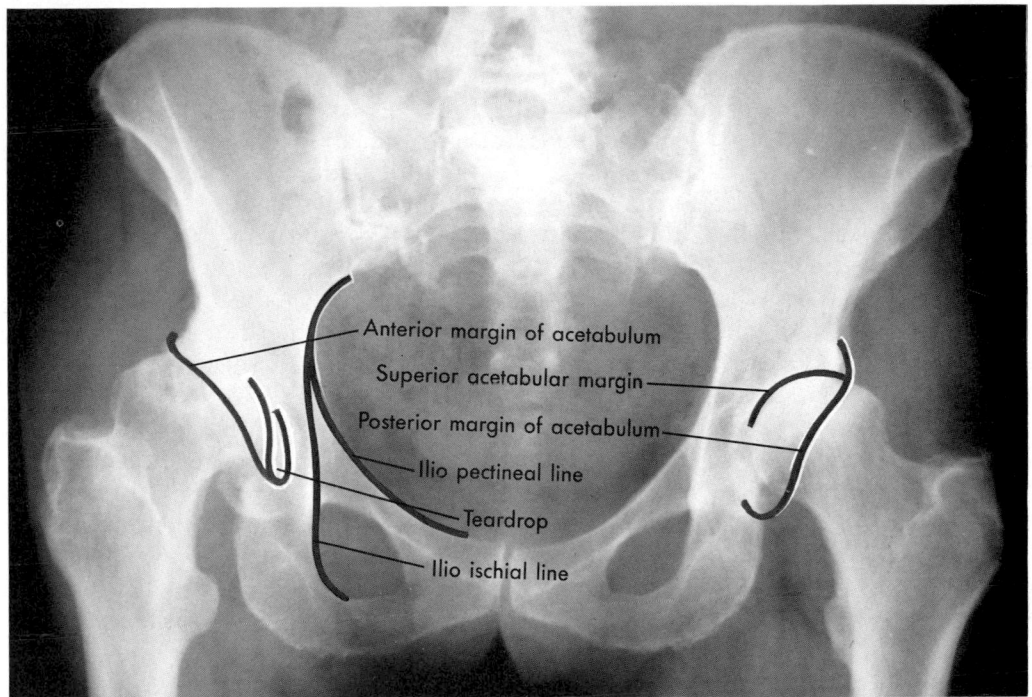

Fig. 12-25. Six important acetabular lines include: (1) arcuate (iliopectineal line), (2) illioischial line, (3) anterior margin of the acetabulum, (4) teardrop, (5) posterior acetabular margin, and (6) superior acetabular margin.

femur in two perpendicular planes (AP and lateral views), as well as a standard anteroposterior view of the pelvis, including both hips.

4. Serial radiographs (AP and lateral views) of the patients with total hip arthroplasty should be regarded as a "blueprint" of the reconstructed joint. In some institutions (including this author's institution) all radiographs of inactive patients (those who were not seen for 5 consecutive years) are burned because of a shortage of space without being copied on microfilms or electronically digitized. Such documents must be kept separate from the patient's main x-ray folder (in a general hospital setting) to provide better protection against accidental damage, loss, or misfiling.

5. When preparing for a cementless device, the magnification scales must be appropriate for preoperative planning and sizing of the prosthesis. Radiographs of good quality must show all of the anatomical landmarks on the pelvis; the landmarks provide intraoperative guidance for placing the acetabular cup and also give a good impression of the size and shape of the medullary canal.

6. The bone quality (the degree of osteopenia) can be judged qualitatively from x-ray films of the hip as a correlation is made with Singh's index.[64]

Note, however, that plain radiographs are unreliable for diagnosing osteoporosis because they depend on technical factors, including positioning, body habitus, and overlying soft tissues.[60,61,65] In his study of bone histology and radiographic indices, Stulberg found no correlation between the two.[65]

7. Good-quality films show the compressive and tensile trabeculae and the poorly defined trabeculae in the trochanter; these factors can form the basis for judging the severity (or lack) of osteoporosis.

8. Radiographs must be taken in the same way at every follow-up visit for comparison.[6,44] The main advantage of reproducible serial radiographs is to allow the surgeon to track changes in component positions, such as migration; these factors can be spotted by superimposing one radiograph over another. Reproducibility requires the use of special devices.[6,44] On supine anteroposterior radiographs, a relatively small (15 degrees or less) rotation can cause significant changes in the proximal femoral dimensions. According to Bell and Brand,[13] 15 degrees of rotation can increase or decrease the width of the medullary canal by 3 mm. These changes are comparable to the amount of medullary canal expansion in a normal adult femur over a 5- to 10-year period.

In addition to the potential errors that can result from altering the position of the femur, errors are also inherent in the quantitative densitometric analysis of orthopaedic radiographs. West and associates[69] concluded that despite efforts to normalize variables (such as the film and developing process, exposure, target distance magnification, field differences, orientation of the bone, soft tissue, skin folds, and so on), their nature and number made it impossible to evaluate the growth and resorptive changes in bone retrospectively by densitometric analysis, even with radiographs made under controlled conditions. However, West and co-workers[69] concluded that the quantitative information obtained can be reliable if the following parameters are kept uniform in serial radiographs on the same subject under study:

1. The type of film
2. The exposure
3. The development
4. The x-ray apparatus
5. The size of the window
6. The target distance
7. The orientation

Stereophotogrammetry

Baldursson and associates[11] were the first to use stereophotogrammetry to assess the position of the acetabular component and thus to detect any changes caused by migration. This elaborate method produces better-defined radiographs with reference points marked by small metallic beads inserted at surgery or percutaneously after surgery. One set of stereoscopic films of the hip is made with the patient supine; to determine the degree of displacement resulting from weight bearing, a set with weight bearing is also made. A software program enables the investigator to locate the implant in relation to the skeleton. A comparison of such films with weight-bearing films or radiographs taken previously allows the surgeon to determine whether the position of the implant has changed. This method has been estimated to measure differences between serial films with an accuracy of up to 0.8 mm in linear measurement at 95% confidence. The use of this method is currently limited to research because it is too costly and time-consuming for routine clinical use. Amstutz described using a radiographic grid-coordinate method to achieve consistently high resolution of the hip image.[6] This method has several advantages over stereophotogrammetry: not only is it less complicated, it facilitates better positioning of the patient and the x-ray beam, eliminates inconsistencies in magnification, and provides better visualization of the metal-cement and bone interfaces.[6,44]

To determine leg length during preoperative planning, it is possible to superimpose grid lines over a radiograph that presents an AP view of the pelvis. A frog-lateral position is adequate for routine preoperative evaluation; however, a shoot-through lateral (Manfredi-lateral) is preferred to determine the anterior bow of the femur.

X-ray magnification can be minimized by placing the femur as close as possible to the x-ray film cassette; the distance between the tube and the top of the table is 40 inches. With the grid cassette placed between the patient's thighs on the top of the table, magnification is less than 5% to 10%, whereas with the x-ray film placed in a Bucky tray 2 inches below the table top, the magnification is 15% to 20%. Significant magnification errors can occur if the patient has hip or kee contractures that raise the femur and move it away from the table. In that event, prop the patient on the table in a manner that will flatten the femur on it; the patient will be in a semiseated position with the knee flexed at 90 degrees over the end of the table. For templating, obtain a lateral view of the femur; place the ipsilateral knee (flexed at 90 degrees) as close as possible to the table top, ensuring a view perpendicular to that of the previous film (anteroposterior with the patient at the end of the table). A cross-table view (shoot-through) is not suitable for templating: the x-ray beam for this view is usually 30 to 40 degrees off the perpendicular, and most templates of the prostheses produced by manufacturers use a frog-lateral view of the femur.

Surgeons who template the femur based on radiographs should be alerted that despite diligent care, errors of magnification can occur because of the patient's size, the deformity of his or her hip, and the radiographic technique. To overcome magnification errors, templates supplied by manufacturers typically have known magnifications ranging from 12% to 25% (as marked on the templates). In practice, place a magnification ruler of 100 mm length parallel to the femur and on top of the cassette. Compare the length of the image of the ruler to the ruler's actual length (100 mm) to determine the degree of magnification: the increase in length of the image is the percentage of magnification. For example, if the image of the 100 mm ruler measures 120 mm, the magnification is 20%. After determining the magnification error, template the femur for size by selecting a comparably magnified template.

Radiographic Evaluation of the Acetabulum

A normal or pathological acetabulum without distortion can be measured with the standard radiographic templates. Judge the site of insertion and the amount of bone to be removed by orienting the template relative to the radiographic "teardrop sign" in two coordinates; the teardrop is located inferomedially in the acetabulum, just superior to the obturator foramen. The lateral lip is the exterior acetabular wall; the medial lip is the interior wall (see Chapter 2).[31]

The vertical and horizontal migration of the acetabular component of total hip arthroplasty can be determined by comparing two radiographs with an accuracy of 3 mm. However, statistically valid comparisons between two groups of radiographs can still be made when they differ (collectively) by only a fraction of a millimeter.[55] Wetherell and Heatly[70] studied the effect of pelvic rotation on commonly described landmarks. In an experimental radiography of a dried pelvis, the pelvis was tilted and rotated, various lines were evaluated, and the accuracy of each was compared with new landmark lines: the "acetabular line" and the "obturator/brim line" were found to be most accurate in measuring acetabular erosion caused by disease or prosthetic migration (see Chapter 22).

Cup Orientation

The angle of cup orientation can be measured easily on the anteroposterior view as the angle between two lines, one drawn along the plane of the opening of the acetabular cup and the other drawn on the sagittal plane with the pelvis in the anatomical position. The alignment angle can also be determined by measuring the angle between the transverse plane of the pelvis and the opening of the acetabular cup; the alignment is known as the *abduction angle* of the cup, or the angle of vertical tilt. Define the transverse plane of the pelvis by drawing a line through both ischial tuberosities, the anterior/superior iliac spines, or the lower margin of teardrops.

The orientation of the acetabular component seen from the frog-lateral view is similar to that of the anteroposterior view. They are similar because the position of the pelvis does not change when the hip is rotated externally to obtain the frog-lateral view of the hip (providing that the hip is fully mobile).

The Manfredi lateral view (shoot-through) provides a profile of the cup that may represent the amount of anteversion; however, it is not accurate because centering the x-ray beams through the hip joint makes them variable. Random tests on skeletons reveal considerable variation by different technicians.[62] Furthermore, the angle of anteversion (as viewed by shoot-through lateral films of the hip) can change according to the amount of flexion or extension of the pelvis. Thus the actual angle of anteversion relative to the body axes varies with several factors: the mobility of the lumbar spine; the presence of a fixed deformity of the spine or a fixed-flexion deformity of the hip; and changes that occur when the patient moves from a

standing to a supine position.[50]

The angle formed between the opening of the acetabular cup (face) and the sagittal plane of the pelvis is known as the *angle of anteversion*. Ackland and associates[2] improved definition of this angle. They recognized two planes about which the acetabular cup rotation can take place, one true transverse plane of the body (termed *true anteversion*) and the anatomical plane of the normal acetabulum (termed *planar anteversion*). Therefore the actual amount of the cup anteversion in relation to the pelvis can be based on true anteversion, planar anteversion, or both. The two planes of anteversion are related to one another geometrically. Their effect in positioning the cup in relation to the pelvis may be additive. The combination can be calculated with a computation table.[2]

Because excess anteversion or retroversion of the cup has been proven to cause postoperative dislocation,[3] the surgeon must remember that a combination of excessive true and planar anteversion may have an additive effect, leading to serious malpositioning of the cup (see Chapter 32). Because the degrees of anteversion of the cup on the holder vary in different designs, the surgeon must also be familiar with the cup positioners. For example, the plane of anteversion in the Aufranc-Turner and the Harris-Galante cup positioners is in the true anatomical plane; in the Charnley-Müller, the positioner is planar; in the Charnley cup positioner, the cup is positioned without anteversion or retroversion.

A method for determining the exact amount of anteversion of the cup is highly desirable, especially when dislocation of the hip prosthesis is recurrent and revisionary surgery is planned.

Several ways to determine the amount of anteversion have been described:

1. Fluoroscopic methods and biplanar methods as described by Ghelman[28,29]
2. Lateral standing radiographs as described by McCollum and Gray[50]
3. Mathematical methods of Visser[68] and Ackland[2]
4. CAT
5. Stereophotogrammetry

The fluoroscopy method has drawbacks: poor screen resolution and exposure to irradiation.

To prevent postoperative dislocation, McCollum and Gray observed that the safe range for acetabular cup positioning is 30 to 50 degrees of abduction and 20 to 40 degrees of flexion from the horizontal (anteversion). They used a true lateral radiographic projection that was reproducible within 10 degrees of accuracy.[50]

Visser developed a mathematical method for measuring the acetabular cup orientation and abduction. The femoral anteversion and the valgus of the femoral component could also be measured by calculations based on an anteroposterior radiograph of the hip, when the length of the neck of the femoral component and the diameter of the acetabular cup were known.[68] This method may be difficult for surgeons who are not well acquainted with mathematics and when the x-ray film cannot fully show the details of the component.

Ackland and associates used a simpler and more practical mathematical method.[2] They described the radiographic measurement of anteversion and distinguished between true and planar anteversion. Using mathematical calculations, they proposed a method of measuring the angle of the acetabular cup. Their method exploits the fact that some acetabular cup designs (nonmetal-backed) use a metal wire (ring) in the periphery; when seen at an angle on routine standard AP radiographs, this ring projects as an ellipse. The amount of anteversion or retroversion can be calculated mathematically using a general formula for all ellipses. This method requires a conversion table and a second radiograph (taken with a tube angled 10 degrees caudally) to distinguish between anteversion and retroversion. No other special views are necessary.

CAT may yield images of sufficient clarity to determine the amount of the cup anteversion; the amount of scatter with the titanium alloy prosthesis is significantly less than with prostheses made of chromium and cobalt.

Stereophotogrammetry is based on shifting the source of illumination to produce pairs of radiographs; the radiographs are then measured by stereophotogrammetric techniques.

Other Imaging Techniques
Aspiration Arthrography

Aspiration of the hip joint under image intensification is useful, but it has limited value in distinguishing a loose or infected implant (see Chapter 32). Observe the following disciplines:

1. Perform the test fluoroscopy in extremely aseptic conditions (either in the operating room or in a dedicated radiological suite).
2. Inject x-ray dye through the same needle used for aspiration; the dye must verify the intraarticular location of the needle.
3. Do not use bacteriostatic solutions as a local anesthetic agent; the x-ray dye is not bacteriostatic.[51]
4. Perform multiple aspirations of the periosteum if indicated.
5. Place the aspiration fluid immediately in the culture medium, and send it to the bacteriology laboratory.
6. If the joint space extends into muscle planes, demonstrate the extent of the abscess by injecting more dye.

Arthrography is not helpful in diagnosing loosening of the total hip arthroplasty, for the following reasons:

1. Only occasionally and only when a gross loosening is present will contrast media trace along the adjacent cement or metal.
2. A small amount of dye may not be visible if it is adjacent to the radiopaque metal or cement.
3. Radiographic dye is rather viscous and may not penetrate the thick membranes or the viscous synovial-like fluid present at the interface.[30,32,33]
4. Enhanced arthrography (by using a subtraction arthrography technique) may detect small amounts of radiopaque dye adjacent to radiopaque cement or metal, but again this technique is demanding and prone to diagnostic errors; the patient must remain motionless during the test.[8,32,66] Arthrography can be of value in establishing the presence or absence of extension of infection from the joint to soft tissue (Fig. 12-26).

Radionucleid Imaging

As discussed in Chapter 31, bone scanning using technetium 99m methylene phosphate (99m Tc-MDP) has limited diagnostic value unless it is used in combination with other studies (such as gallium/indium and aspiration of the joint) and correlated with a detailed history, a physical examination, and other laboratory data as well as plain radiographs. Gallium-67 citrate (^{76} Ga) and indium 111 oxine (^{111} In WBG) are now commonly preferred and used to diagnose infection (see Chapter 31).

Several observations are noteworthy:

1. Indium WBC studies have shown 83% to 100% sensitivity, 73% to 89.9% specificity, and 50% to 93.3% accuracy in diagnosing infection.[49,52,57]
2. Reports indicate that indium-labeled WBC is more sensitive and accurate than a combination of technetium and gallium scan[5] in diagnosing infection in total hip arthroplasty.
3. Indium-labeled WBC seems to be more sensitive than hip aspiration in diagnosing infection in total hip arthroplasty.[17,49]
4. Sequential indium-labeled WBC and 99m Tc-MDP scans may increase specificity for diagnosing infection; a combination of 67 gallium and technetium phosphate to increase diagnostic specificity for infection is sometimes recommended.[17]
5. Radioisotope arthrography is accomplished by injecting technetium 99m sulfur colloid (99m Tc-SC) into the joint under fluoroscopic image.[1,58,67] This method can be of value if arthrography is absolutely indicated in patients who are sensitive to radiographic dye. The diagnostic value of this method for routine use cannot be

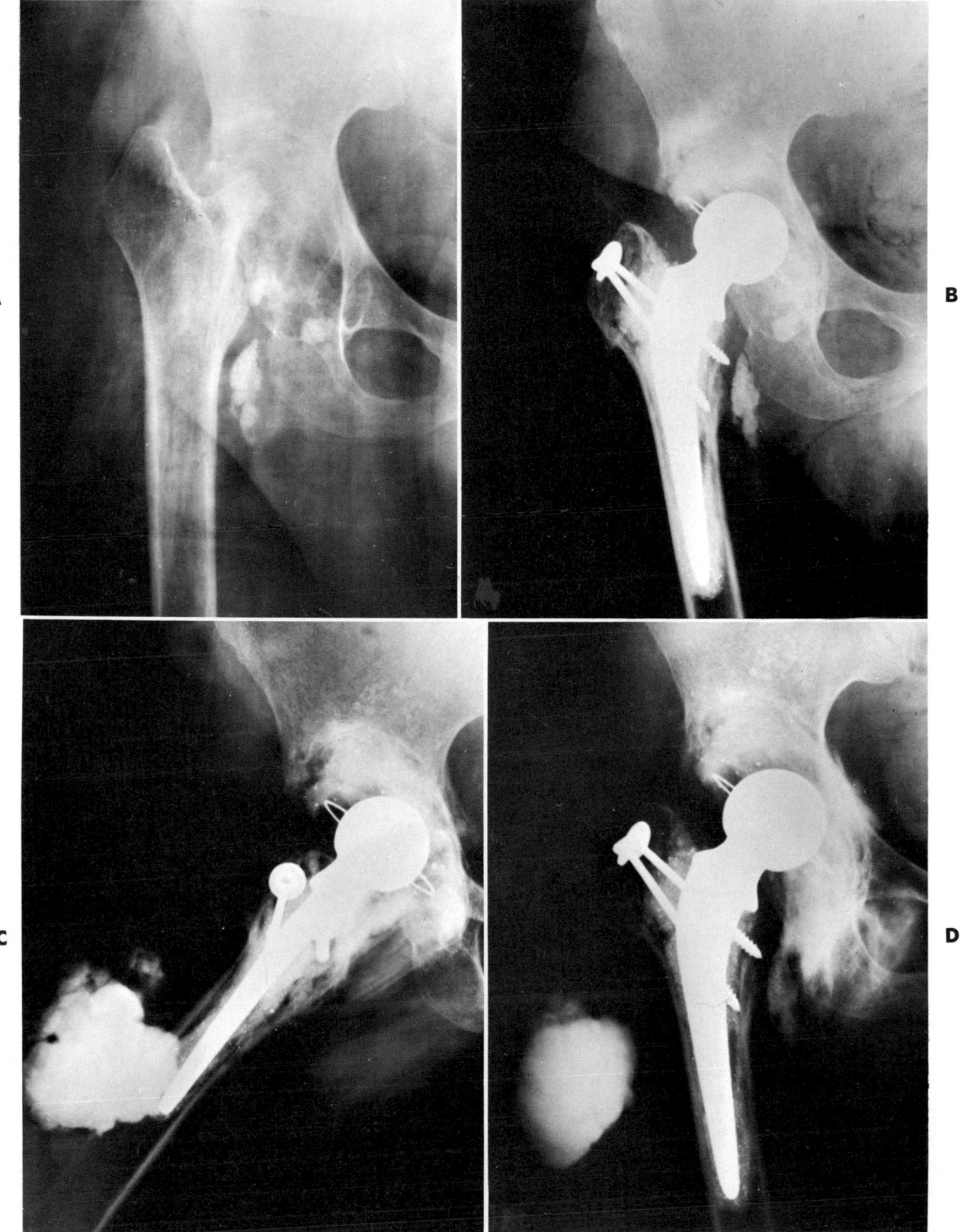

Fig. 12-26. Special studies using contrast media may be useful in elaborating certain conditions of the hip. Arthrograms may reveal soft tissue collection of pus or infective cavities about the hip joint. **A,** Preoperative radiograph of 56-year-old accountant without history of tuberculosis but with radiological appearance of hip tuberculosis and calcific area within vicinity of hip joint. **B,** Postoperative x-ray film of hip arthroplasty performed in another institution with early successful results. **C,** One year after surgery, hip was painful, and swelling appeared in lateral aspect of thigh. **D,** Contrast medium, 20 ml, was injected into soft tissue located at level of tip of prosthesis. No communication was observed between soft tissue abscess and bone.

Continued.

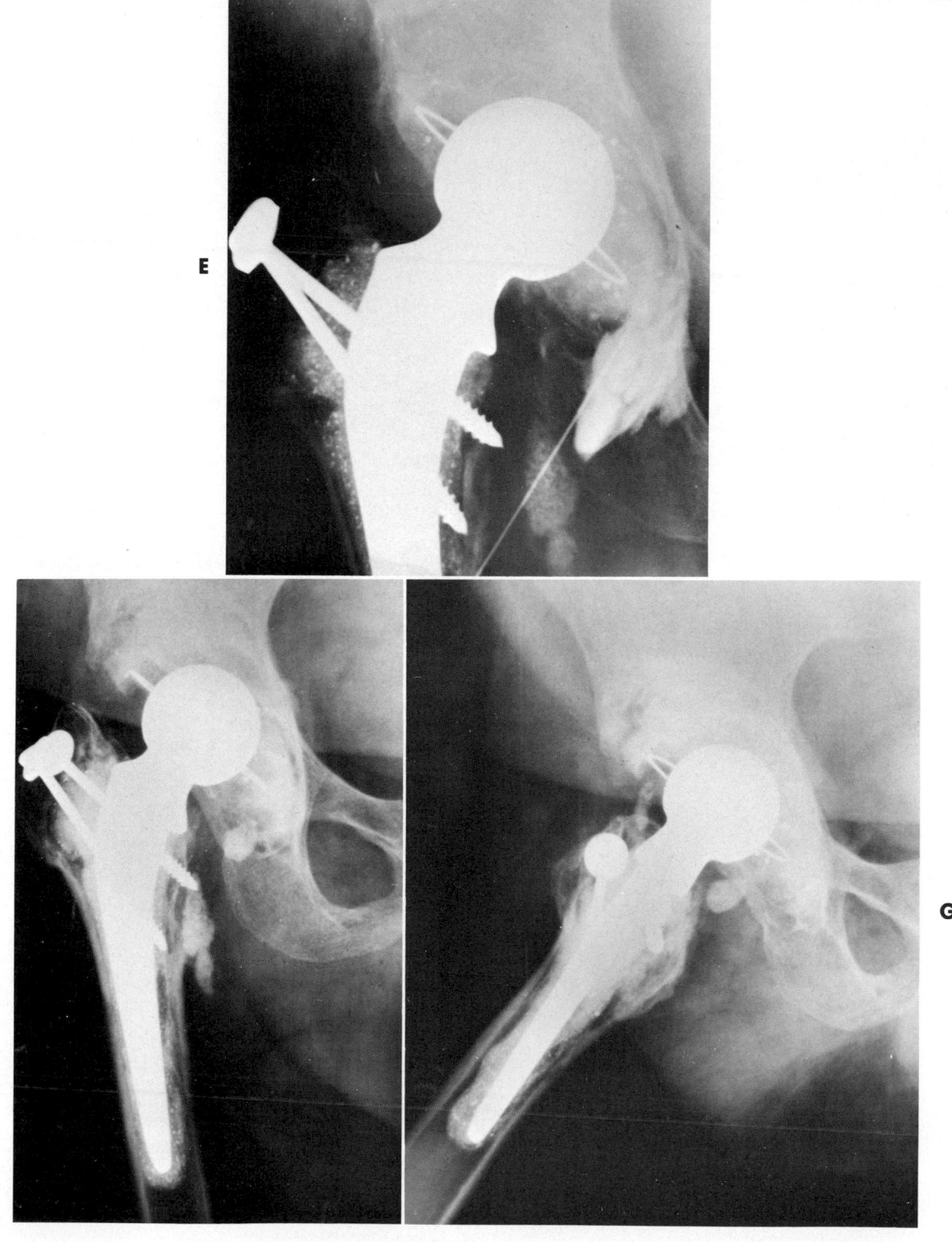

Fig. 12-26—cont'd.   E, Subsequently, needle was also inserted into hip joint to obtain arthrogram in addition to injection of contrast media at interface between cement and bone. No communication was detected between soft tissue abscess and hip joint. **F and G,** Three years after removal of soft tissue abscess and exploration of joint, which confirmed original impression of diagnosis of tuberculous abscess and extension of hip joint. Artificial hip joint was not disturbed because of good mechanical fixation; patient, who had not originally received chemoprophylaxis for tuberculosis, was placed on antituberculous drugs for 2 years.

determined at this time because its use has been very limited.

Computerized Axial Tomography (CAT)

CAT scanning can be of value preoperatively and postoperatively in the following ways:

1. To assess the availability of bone stock in the pelvis (especially the periacetabular region) and in the femur.
2. To assess bone abnormality resulting from invasive tumors, infection, or previous surgery.
3. To assess the topographic anatomy of the bone (based on software that generates reformatted images in the sagittal or coronal planes).
4. To assist the surgical procedure by producing three-dimensional images displayed in an interactive format.
5. To create three-dimensional images to produce models and customize prostheses (see Chapter 11).
6. To evaluate bone details (especially occult bone defects, hypertrophy, or severe atrophy) that might not be picked up by routine x-ray films.
7. To detect intraarticular bone or cement fragments.

The presence of implants in or near the joints to be scanned will produce artifacts; this may result in a less precise image. X-ray attenuation and the production of artifacts occur with all implants, but to varying degrees; chromium and cobalt prostheses are the most severely affected, plastic components the least. The imprecision, however, is not great enough to make this technique entirely useless.[12,15]

MRI and Ultrasound

MRI has limited diagnostic value in total hip arthroplasty. Its usefulness as a diagnostic tool in the early (preradiographic stage) diagnosis of avascular necrosis of the femoral head has been established. Occasionally MRI may also be helpful in diagnosing a mass (tumor or abscess) near the joint that is not revealed by aspiration or arthrogram.

The risk from heating or motion caused by MRI in the presence of orthopaedic implants is only theoretical, although it is essential to screen for any contraindications for its use: the presence of cardiac pacemakers, ferromagnetic clips used in intracranial surgery, certain vena cava embolism filters, spinal cord simulators, and cochlear implants. However, other metal prostheses can be imaged safely: total joint prostheses, dental devices, intrauterine devices, and some surgical clips (other than intracranial aneurysm clips, coronary bypass clips, cardiac valves, and cerebral ventricular shunts).[36]

Ultrasound is occasionally indicated as a diagnostic tool. The ultrasound beam does not penetrate metallic devices; it stops abruptly when it reaches the level of metallic implants. However, because MRI and CAT scans are difficult to interpret, ultrasound may be used to visualize a soft tissue mass or abscess near a metallic implant. It has no diagnostic value in total hip arthroplasty failure (such as infection or loosening).

For further radiographic and other imaging diagnostics on specific topics, see Chapters 10 and 20 through 25.

ASSESSMENT BY SURVIVORSHIP METHODS

Because of progressive loss of patients to follow up, evaluating the clinical and radiographic results becomes increasingly difficult. Obviously, the number of patients available for follow up varies with time lapsed from the index operation. The number of patients available at each follow-up year must be known (Fig. 12-27). The number of patients in a given study may be reduced by death, lack of follow up, or revision because of failure. Therefore the study of all available patients at any given point does not provide an accurate estimate of failure or success. If all patients having a given type of operation underwent surgery on a designated date and the end point of study occurred on a designated date, an "all-inclusive" method would determine the percentage of success or failure of that operation. However, because the beginning and the end results of any procedure vary and because some patients die, are lost to follow up, or their operation fails, the statistical problem must be handled by actuarial methods based on life table methods. In this method, survival time is lumped into annual time intervals. Berkson in 1950[14] used this method for cancer patients. Dobbs in 1980[21] and Dorey and Amstutz[22] in 1986 adopted this method of survivorship to analyze orthopaedic implants. Many investigators have adopted the actuarial analysis method described by Kaplan and Meier[39] to estimate survivorship of the total hip arthroplasty. The greatest advantage of survivorship methods is that they include all available information on all patients and do not eliminate data from patients who were not followed for more than a minimum follow-up time. In other words, all patients contribute information to data until they are eliminated by failure, inadequate follow up, or death. In this method, one assumes that patients lost to follow up and those who died by natural causes are recorded as failures. This method does not distinguish between patients whose operations remain successful and did not return for follow up and those whose revision operations were performed elsewhere and who did not attend the follow-up study. Dorey and Amstutz concluded that estimates are less accurate when fewer patients remain

THE NEW YORK ORTHOPAEDIC HOSPITAL
HIP SURVIVORSHIP FOLLOW-UP

HIP # _____

FORM **3A**

Name _____ Age _____ Unit no. _____
　　　Last　　　　　　　　　　　First　　　　　　　　　　MI

Attending (private pt.) _____ Resident (clinic) _____

Surgery date _____/_____/_____　　Side _____/_____
　　　　　　　mm　　dd　　yy　　　　　　　　L　　R

	F/U date	Hip scores P F M	Jt. class	Wound infect.	Femoral comp	Acetab. comp	Cement	Troch.	Other compl.	Operat. status	Pt. f/up status	X-rays (y/n)	Wt.
1													
2													
3													
4													
5													
6													
7													
8													
9													
10													
11													
12													
13													
14													

CODES

WOUND INFECT

1. None　　　2. Deep w. infect.　　　3. Infect. (elsewhere)

FEMORAL COMP.

1. None　　　　　　　2. Thigh pain fem.　　3. Radiolucency　　　4. Subsidence　　　5. Gross loosening　　　6. Gross lysis
7. Bend/fract. stem　　99. Other

ACETAB. COMP.

1. None　　　2. Gross pain acetab.　　3. Radiolucency　　　4. Migration　　　5. Gross loosening　　　6. Gross lysis
7. Wear　　　8. Fracture　　　　　　99. Other

CEMENT

1. None　　　2. Fracture　　　3. Fragment　　　4. Inadequate　　　5. Poor technique　　　6. Ectopic cement
99. Other

TROCHANTER

1. None　　　2. Pain-tender　　　3. Wire breakage　　　4. Non-union　　　5. Migration　　　6. Ectopic bone
99. Other

OTHER COMP.

1. None　　　　　　2. Subluxation　　　3. Dislocation　　　4. Ectopic bone　　　5. Fracture femur　　　6. Fract. acetab.
7. Leg lgth. discrep.　99. Other

OPERAT. STATUS

1. Satisfactory　　　2. Pend. fail. no reop.　　3. Reop. not removed　　4. Rev. cup　　　5. Rev. stem　　　6. Exc. not replaced
7. Rev. both comp.　99. Other　　　　　　　9. Death (unrelated)

PAT. F/U STATUS

1. Active　　　2. Deceased　　　3. X-rays sent　　　4. Not fit to f/up　　　5. Lost to F/up

Please return to PH 5C, Ex. 6-6220

Fig. 12-27. The New York Orthopaedic Hospital Hip Survivorship form.

THE NEW YORK ORTHOPAEDIC HOSPITAL
HIP SURVIVORSHIP FOLLOW-UP

HIP # _____

FORM **3B**

Surgery date _____/_____/_____   Side _____/_____
mm   dd   yy   L   R

	F/U date	Hip scores P F M	Jt. class	Wound infect.	Femoral comp	Acetab. comp	Cement	Troch.	Other compl.	Operat. status	Pt. f/up status	X-rays (y/n)	Wt.
15													
16													
17													
18													
19													
20													
21													
22													
23													
24													
25													
26													
27													
28													
29													
30													
31													
32													
33													
34													
35													
36													
37													
38													
39													
40													

VISIT DATE   COMMENTS

_____   _____

_____   _____

_____   _____

_____   _____

_____   _____

_____   _____

_____   _____

Please return to PH 5C, Ex. 6-6220

Fig. 12-27, cont'd.

THE TOTAL HIP ARTHROPLASTY OUTCOME EVALUATION FORM
FACTORS AFFECTING THE RESULTS OF TOTAL HIP ARTHROPLASTY

Characteristics of the patient
  Age
  Sex
  Race
  Height
  Weight
  Educational attainment
  Socioeconomic status (income and health-
    insurance coverage)
  Social supports
  Marital status
  Primary diagnosis (check those that apply)
    Osteoarthrosis
      Primary
      Secondary (e.g., slipped capital femoral
        epiphysis, Legg-Perthes disease, con-
        genital dysplasia, or dislocation of the hip)
    Inflammatory arthritis (e.g., rheumatoid arthritis
      or juvenile rheumatoid arthritis)
    Fracture
      Acute (e.g., femoral head with or without dis-
        location, femoral neck, or femoral shaft)
      Remote
    Osteonecrosis (e.g., idiopathic, posttraumatic,
      or steroid-associated)
    Deposition or metabolic disease or bone disease
      (e.g., gout, chrondro-
      calcinosis or pseudogout, Gaucher
      disease, ochronosis, or Paget disease)

	Left	Right
Previous operation on the hip		
None	_____	_____
Internal fixation	_____	_____
Cup arthroplasty	_____	_____
Osteotomy	_____	_____
Arthrodesis	_____	_____
Girdlestone procedure	_____	_____
Femoral head prosthesis (hemiarthroplasty)	_____	_____
Double cup arthroplasty (surface replacement)	_____	_____
Number of previous total hip replacements	_____	_____
Number of femoral revisions	_____	_____
Number of acetabular revisions	_____	_____

Medications
  During the last month, has the patient taken any
  of the following medications on a regular basis?
  Yes   No
  _____ _____ Antiinflammatory drugs (e.g., aspirin com-
              pounds, ibuprofen, or naprosyn [naproxen])
  _____ _____ Oral steroids (prednisone or dexamethasone)
  _____ _____ Hydroxychloroquine
  _____ _____ Disease-modiffying antirheumatic drugs
              (methotrexate, cyclophosphamide, arathio-
              prine, etc.)
  _____ _____ Oral gold
  _____ _____ Minor analgesics (acetaminophen)
  _____ _____ Narcotic analgesics (codeine, propoxyphene,
              or oxycodone)

Indications for operation
  Progression of disease
    Clinical _____ Yes _____ No
    Radiographic _____ Yes _____ No
  Failure of previous operations other than total hip arthroplasty
    _____ Yes _____ No
  Complication of previous total hip arthroplasty
    _____ Yes _____ No
    (If yes, specify)
    _____ Loosening
    _____ Dislocation
    _____ Fracture
    _____ Infection
    _____ Other
Sources of infection present
  _____ Chronic respiratory infection
  _____ Urinary tract infection
  _____ Poor dental hygiene (gingivitis or abscess)
  _____ Breakdown of skin
Patient's reason for operation

Medical conddition
  Co-morbidity and severity of disease
  Potential sources of infection
  Nutritional status
    Hemotocrit level
    Albumin level
  Previous nonoperative management
    of the hip and disability

Operative factors
  Surgeon
    Number of primary total hip replacements each year
    Type of first assistant in the performance of the total hip arthroplasty
      Orthopaedic resident
      General surgery resident
      Other orthopaedic surgeon
      Other physician
      Physician's assistant
      Nurse
      Other (identify)
    How many different total hip systems are stocked by the hospital
      on a regular basis?
      Porous systems
      Cemented systems
      Revision systems
    Experience of the operative support staff (nurses, anesthesiologists,
      and therapists of various types [physical, respiratory, etc.])
      Highly experienced
      Average experience
      Less-than-average experience
      Minimum experience
    Percentage of patients for whom at least one nurse or equivalent
      person was assigned to orthopaedic service full time
      Has person received special training in the technique and
        instrumentation of total hip arthroplasty
    Orthopaedic surgeon
      Years in practice
      Duration and date of orthopaedic residency
      Date of Board certification
      Duration and date of hip fellowship
      Duration and date of other fellowship
      Practice profile (estimated percentage ratio of volume of
        operations on the hip to total volume of operations)
  Operative technique
    Type of prothesis
      Cemented or cementless
    Operative or technical approach
    Use of prophylactic antibiotics
    Use of anticoagulants
    Use of Foley catheter (during or after operation)
    Length of the operation
    Type of anesthesia
    Amount of blood lost
    Concomitant operations

Institutional characteristics
  Total of primary total hip arthroplasties performed in
    the institution each year
    Number performed each year for osteoarthrosis
  Type of air-sterilization system used in operating rooms
    in which hip arthroplasties are performed
    Standard operating-room construction
    Ultraviolet light
    Unidirectional airflow system
    Unidirectional airflow system and body-exhaust apparatus
    Name of airflow system
    Other
  Payer mix
  Orthopaedic residency program
  Written protocol for rehabilitation
  Preoperative and postoperative education program for patients
  Type of institution
    Academic medical center (medical school and hospitals)
    Medical school-affiliated hospital
    Community hospital
    County hospital
    City hospital
    Veterans Administration hospital
  Bed-capacity of hospital

Fig. 12-28. The total hip arthroplasty outcome evaluation form. (From Liang MH, Katz JN, Phillips C, et al: The total hip arthroplasty outcome evaluation form of the American Academy of Orthopaedic Surgeons. Results of a nominal group process, *J Bone Joint Surg* 73:641, 1991.)

and more accurate when a higher percentage of patients remain in the study.[22] For further details on survivorship see Chapters 28 and 29.

DATA ACQUISITION FOR OUTCOME STUDIES

The Task Force on Outcome Studies of the American Academy of Orthopaedic Surgeons incorporated into its model the following criteria considered essential for outcome studies in total hip arthroplasty[48]: history, clinical and radiological evaluation (see Tables 12-1 to 12-3); work activity; activities of daily living; gait; complications; and the patient's satisfaction and expectations. Other important patient-related characteristics are age, race, socioeconomic status, social support, primary diagnosis, indications, operative factors, operative technique, the type of implant, and characteristics of the institution. Important medical factors include co-morbidity, patient's health status and quality of life, risk of infection, and current use of medications. For further details, see the Total Hip Arthroplasty Outcome Evaluation Form of the American Academy of Orthopaedic Surgeons, Results of Nominal Group Process (Fig. 12-28).[48]

SUMMARY OF ESSENTIALS

- An objective clinical and radiographic assessment of the hip for prospective documentation is mandatory for good medical practice. The amelioration and deterioration of the patient can be assessed only if objective data document preoperative, immediate, early, and long-term progress. Comparing current data with earlier data based on the same established definitions allows the surgeon to evaluate the worth of a new surgical technique and modify treatment and technique accordingly.

- A standardized system to evaluate the results of total hip arthroplasty is needed. One should hesitate to judge the effects of a surgical procedure even in a large series of cases when the patient's condition before and after operation cannot be compared.

- A system has been developed to provide a basic minimal data base to serve the needs of authors, readers, editors, and practitioners alike, which could help in comparing the results of different studies. The parameters included must be objective, strictly defined, and reproducible by others.

- To compare the preoperative and postoperative status of the patient, most hip evaluation systems record pain, walking distance, function, and range of motion. It is notable that despite all efforts to maintain objectivity, surgeons frequently give higher ratings than therapists using the same scale system.

- Merle d'Aubigne and Postel suggested the first objective scoring system using three units, one for pain, one for function, and one for mobility. Each unit ranges from 1 to 6; 1 represents complete disability, and 6 represents normalcy.

- Charnley modified Merle d'Aubigne and Postel's model by placing each patient in one of the three categories: A, B, and C. In this way it was possible to describe the patient as a whole, not merely as a hip. Group A includes patients with unilateral hip disease; group B consists of patients with bilateral hip disease without other restraining factors; group C comprises patients with either unilateral or bilateral hip disease who also have systemic or other conditions restricting their function. This division is extremely valuable when assessing the results of hip arthroplasty as a surgical procedure and also the overall performance of the patient.

- In evaluating pain, it is necessary to concentrate on its intensity and whether it is provoked by activity. Assess "night pain" only when the patient volunteers the subject; do not emphasize the subject by raising a leading question because such a question may elicit mention of night pain or rest pain in most patients who want a total hip arthroplasty.

- Any numerical grading system that does not arbitrarily load the grade offers the distinct advantages of simplicity and clarity. For example, in 6-number grading, 1 denotes extreme pain, and 6 represents no pain. When a 100-point numerical scale system is used, a patient may have a high average score and still experience significant pain.

- The sensitivity of hip score to pain can be reduced when the scoring includes other parameters, such as radiography. In evaluating the results (outcome) of a new surgical technique or prosthesis, the overall score may not reflect the main concern of arthroplasty—the relief of pain.

- In comparing various hip assessment systems, the Hospital for Special Surgeries rating system produced the most optimistic results; the most pessimistic were obtained using Merle d'Aubigne and Postel's rating scale.

- Regarding data acquisition for outcome studies, a minimum data base of information is required. The factors affecting the results of total hip arthroplasty may be assessed by prospective evaluation forms that cover clinical and operative factors, as well as information related to institutional characteristics.

- Serial radiographs are most commonly used to evaluate total hip arthroplasty for success and failure. To be of value, radiographs must be of high quality and resolution. Their magnification, x-ray penetration, and orientation must conform with those used in previous studies of the same patient. They must provide views of the upper third of the femur in two perpendicular planes, as well as a standard anteroposterior view of the pelvis including both hips. Such documents must be kept separate from the patient's main x-ray folder to better protect them against accidental damage, loss, or misfiling. When they are used for preoperative planning for a cementless device, magnification scale must also be known.

- Despite efforts to normalize variables affecting the quality of the x-ray films, certain quantitative information can be obtained reliably if the following parameters are kept uniform in serial radiographs: the type of film, the exposure, the development, the x-ray apparatus, the size of the window, the target distance, and the orientation.

- Other radiographic studies, including stereophotogrammetry, scanograms, special views of the femur and pelvis for orientation, and fluoroscopic methods, are helpful. CAT scanning and aspiration arthrography are adjunctive methods of evaluating the hip preoperatively.

- Radionucleid imaging techniques are particularly helpful in differentiating loosening of the implant and infection. Indium and gallium bone scans are commonly used for this purpose. Sequential indium-labeled WBC and 99m Tc-MPD scans may increase the specificity for diagnosing infection.

- CAT scanning is extremely helpful to evaluate the bone stock in the pelvis in the periacetabular region and the femur. It shows abnormality of bone resulting from invasive tumors or infection, as well as from previous surgery.

- A three-dimensional image produced by CAT scanning in an interactive format may be useful in the surgical procedure and to produce models and customize the prosthesis. Additional information may also be obtained by the use of MRI and ultrasound in evaluating a painful total hip arthroplasty.

- Because of progressive loss of patients to follow up, evaluating clinical and radiographic results over time becomes increasingly difficult. Because the beginning and end results of any procedure vary and some patients die, are not followed up, or their operation fails over a span of time, it becomes necessary to handle the statistical problem by actuarial methods based on life table methods. In this method, survival time is lumped into annual time intervals. The greatest advantage of survivorship methods is that they include all available information on all patients and do not estimate data

from patients who were not followed more than a minimum follow-up time. As such, all patients contribute to data until they are eliminated for the reasons of failure, inadequate follow up, or death. It may be concluded that despite the advantages of survivalship analysis, the estimates are less accurate when fewer patients remain in the study and more accurate when a higher percentage of patients remain in the study.

REFERENCES

1. **Abdel-Dayem HM, Bardowala YM, Papademitro T, et al:** Loose hip prosthesis. An appearance in radionuclide arthrography, *Clin Nucl Med* 11:713, 1986.
2. **Ackland MK, Bourne WB, Uhthoff HK:** Anteversion of the acetabular cup. Measurement of angle after total hip replacement, *J Bone Joint Surg* 68[Br]:409, 1986.
3. **Ali Kahn MA, Brakenbury PH, Reynolds ISR:** Dislocation following total hip replacement, *J Bone Joint Surg* 63[Br]:214, 1981.
4. **American Academy of Orthopaedic Surgeons:** *Joint motion. Method of measuring and recording,* rev ed, Chicago, 1965, The American Academy of Orthopaedic Surgeons.
5. **Amstutz HC, Ma SM, Jinnah RH, et al:** Revision of aseptic loose total hip arthroplasties, *Clin Orthop* 170:21, 1982.
6. **Amstutz HC, Ouzouian T, Grauer D, et al:** The grid radiograph. A simple technique for consistent high-resolution visualization of the hip, *J Bone Joint Surg* 68:1052, 1986.
7. **Andersson G:** Hip assessment: a comparison of nine different methods, *J Bone Joint Surg* 54[Br]:621, 1972.
8. **Apple JS, Roberts L Jr, Gamba J, et al:** Digital subtraction arthrography of the prosthetic hip, *South Med J* 79:808, 1986.
9. **ARA Glossary Committee:** *Dictionary of the rheumatic diseases,* vol III: *Health status measurement.* Bayport, NY, 1988, Contact Associates International.
10. **Aufranc OE:** Preoperative and postoperative treatment of patients with reconstructive surgery of the hip, *Clin Orthop* 38:40, 1965.
11. **Baldursson H, Hansson LI, Olsson TH, et al:** Migration of the acetabular socket after total hip replacement determined by roentgen stereophotogrammetry, *Acta Orthop Scand* 51:535, 1980.
12. **Barmeir E, Dubowitz B, Roffman M:** Computed tomography in the assessment and planning of complicated total hip replacement, *Acta Orthop Scand* 53:597, 1982.
13. **Bell AL, Brand RA:** Roentgenographic changes in proximal femoral dimensions due to hip rotation, *Clin Orthop* 240:194, 1989.
14. **Berkson J, Gage RP:** Calculation of survival rates for cancer, *Proc Staff Meet Mayo Clin* 25:270, 1950.
15. **Berman AT, McGovern KM, Paret RS, et al:** The use of preoperative computed tomography scanning in total hip arthroplasty, *Clin Orthop* 222:190, 1987.
16. **Callaghan JJ, Dysart SH, Savory CF, et al:** Assessing the results of hip replacement. A comparison of five different rating systems, *J Bone Joint Surg* 72[Br]:1008, 1990.
17. **Chafetz N, Hattner RS, Ruarke WC, et al:** Multinuclide digital subtraction imaging in symptomatic prosthetic joints, *Am J Radiol* 144:1255, 1985.
18. **Charnley J:** *Low-friction arthroplasty of the hip. Theory and*

practice, Berlin, 1979, Springer-Verlag.

19. **Codman EA:** *The shoulder,* Boston, 1934, privately printed.

20. **DeLee JG, Charnley J:** Radiological demarcation of cemented sockets in total hip replacement, *Clin Orthop* 121:20, 1976.

21. **Dobbs HS:** Survivorship of total hip replacement, *J Bone Joint Surg* 62[Br]:168, 1980.

22. **Dorey F, Amstutz H:** Survivorship analysis in the evaluation of joint replacement, *J Arthroplasty* 1:63, 1986.

23. **Ehrlich GE,** editor: *Total management of the arthritic patient,* Philadelphia, 1973, JB Lippincott.

24. **Eftekhar NS, Stinchfield FE:** Experience with low-friction arthroplasty. A statistical review of early results and complications, *Clin Orthop* 95:60, 1973.

25. **Gade HG:** A contribution to the surgical treatment of osteoarthritis of the hip-joint. A clinical study. Comments on the follow-up examination and the evaluation of the therapeutic results, *Acta Chir Scand* 95(suppl):1, 1947.

26. **Galante J:** Evaluation of results of total hip replacement, *J Bone Joint Surg* 72:159, 1990 (editorial).

27. **Galante J:** The need for a standardized system for evaluating results of total hip surgery, *J Bone Joint Surg* 67:511, 1985 (editorial).

28. **Ghelman B:** Radiographic localization of the acetabular component of a hip prosthesis, *Radiology* 130:540, 1979.

29. **Ghelman B:** Three methods for determining anteversion and retroversion of a total hip prosthesis, *AJR* 133:1127, 1979.

30. **Goldring SR, Schiller A, Roelke M, et al:** The synovial-like membrane at the bone-cement interface in loose total hip replacements and its proposed role in bone lysis, *J Bone Joint Surg* 65:575, 1983.

31. **Goodman SB, Adler SJ, Fyhrie DP, et al:** The acetabular teardrop and its relevance to acetabular migration, *Clin Orthop* 236:199, 1988.

32. **Griffiths HJ, Burke J, Bonfiglio TA:** Granulomatous pseudotumors in total joint replacement, *Skeletal Radiol* 16:146, 1987.

33. **Griffiths HJ, Lovelock JE, Evarts CM, et al:** The radiology of total hip replacement, *Skeletal Radiol* 12:1, 1984.

34. **Gruen TA, McNeice GM, Amstutz HC:** "Modes of failure" of cemented stem-type femoral components. A radiographic analysis of loosening, *Clin Orthop* 141:17, 1979.

35. **Harris WH:** Traumatic arthritis of the hip after dislocation and acetabular fractures: treatment by mold arthroplasty. An end-result study using a new method of result evaluation, *J Bone Joint Surg* 51:737, 1969.

36. **Hear MM, Montgomery WJ:** *Imaging of total joint replacement in total joint replacement.* In Petty W, editor: Philadelphia, 1991, WB Saunders.

37. **Johnston RC, Fitzgerald RH Jr, Harris WH, et al:** Clinical and radiographic evaluation of total hip replacement: a standard system of terminology for reporting results, *J Bone Joint Surg* 72:161, 1990.

38. **Judet R, Judet J:** Technique and results with the acrylic femoral head prosthesis, *J Bone Joint Surg* 34[Br]:173, 1952.

39. **Kaplan EL, Meier P:** Nonparametric estimation from incomplete observations, *J Am Stat Assoc* 53:457, 1958.

40. **Kavanagh BF, Fitzgerald RH Jr:** Clinical and roentgenographic assessment of total hip arthroplasty. A new hip score, *Clin Orthop* 193:133, 1985.

41. **Kavanagh BF, Ilstrup DM, Fitzgerald RH Jr:** Revision total hip arthroplasty, *J Bone Joint Surg* 67:517, 1985.

42. **Kazis LE, Meenan RF, Anderson JJ:** Pain in the rheumatic diseases. Investigation of a key health status component, *Arthritis Rheum* 26:1017, 1983.

43. **Keele KD:** The pain chart, *Lancet* 2:6, 1948.

44. **Kirkpatrick JS, Clarke IC, Amstutz HC, et al:** Radiographic techniques for consistent visualization of total hip arthroplasties, *Clin Orthop* 174:158, 1983.

45. **Larson CB:** Rating scale for hip disabilities, *Clin Orthop* 31:85, 1963.

46. **Lazansky MG:** A method for grading hips, *J Bone Joint Surg* 49[Br]:644, 1967.

47. **Levack B, Rassmussen GL, Day S, et al:** Range of movement poor index of hip function, *Acta Orthop Scand* 59:14, 1988.

48. **Liang MH, Katz JN, Phillips C, et al:** The total hip arthroplasty outcome evaluation form of the American Academy of Orthopaedic Surgeons. Results of a nominal group process, *J Bone Joint Surg* 73:639, 1991.

49. **Magnuson JE, Brown ML, Hauser HF, et al:** In-111-labeled leukocyte scintigraphy in suspected orthopedic prosthesis infection: comparison with other imaging modalities, *Radiology* 168:235, 1988.

50. **McCollum DE, Gray WJ:** Dislocation after total hip arthroplasty. Causes and prevention, *Clin Orthop* 261:159, 1990.

51. **Melson GL, McDaniel RC, Southern PM, et al:** *In vitro* effects of iodinated arthrographic contrast media on bacterial growth, *Radiology* 112:593, 1974.

52. **Merkel KD, Brown ML, Dewanjee MK, et al:** Comparison of indium-labeled-leukocyte imaging with sequential technetium-gallium scanning in the diagnosis of low-grade musculoskeletal sepsis. A prospective study, *J Bone Joint Surg* 67:465, 1985.

53. **Merle d'Aubigne R, Postel M:** Functional results of hip arthroplasty with acrylic prosthesis, *J Bone Joint Surg* 36:451, 1954.

54. **Müller ME, Sledge C, Poss R, et al:** Report of the SICOT presidential commission on documentation and evaluation, *Int Orthop* 14:221, 1990.

55. **Nunn D, Freeman MAR, Hill PF, et al:** The measurement of migration of the acetabular component of hip prostheses, *J Bone Joint Surg* 71[Br]:629, 1989.

56. **Pellicci PM, Wilson PD Jr, Sledge CB, et al:** Long-term results of revision total hip replacement. A follow-up report, *J Bone Joint Surg* 67:513, 1985.

57. **Pring DJ, Henderson RG, Keshavarzian A, et al:** Indium-granulocyte scanning in the painful prosthetic joint, *Am J Radiol* 147:167, 1986.

58. **Resnik CS, Fratkin MJ, Cardea JA:** Arthroscintigraphic evaluation of the painful total hip prosthesis, *Clin Nucl Med* 11:242, 1986.

59. **Ritter MA, Fechtman RW, Keating EM, et al:** The use of a hip score for evaluation of the results of total hip arthroplasty, *J Arthroplasty* 5:187, 1990.

60. **Schneider R:** Radiologic methods of evaluating generalized osteopenia, *Orthop Clin North Am* 15:631, 1984.

61. **Schneider R, Freiberger RH, Ghelman B, et al:** Radiologic evaluation of painful joint prostheses, *Clin Orthop* 170:156, 1982.

62. **Seradge H, Nagle KR, Miller RJ:** Analysis of version in the acetabular cup, *Clin Orthop* 166:152, 1982.

63. **Shepherd MM:** Assessment of function after arthroplasty of the hip, *J Bone Joint Surg* 36[Br]:354, 1954.

64. **Singh M, Nagrath AR, Maini PS:** Changes in trabecular pattern of the upper end of the femur as an index of osteoporosis, *J Bone Joint Surg* 52:457, 1970.

65. **Stulberg BN, Bauer TW, Watson JT, et al:** Bone quality. Roentgenographic versus histologic assessment of hip bone structure, *Clin Orthop* 240:200, 1989.
66. **Tehranzadeh J, Schneider R, Freiberger RH:** Radiological evaluation of painful total hip replacement, *Radiology* 141:355, 1981.
67. **Uri G, Wellman H, Capello W, et al:** Scintigraphic and x-ray arthrographic diagnosis of femoral prosthesis loosening: concise communication, *J Nucl Med* 25:661, 1984.
68. **Visser JD, Konings JG:** A new method for measuring angles after total hip arthroplasty. A study of the acetabular cup and femoral component, *J Bone Joint Surg* 63[Br]:556, 1981.
69. **West JD, Mayor MB, Collier JP:** Potential errors inherent in quantitative densitometric analysis of orthopaedic radiographs. A study after total hip arthroplasty, *J Bone Joint Surg* 69:58, 1987.
70. **Wetherell RG, Amis AA, Heatley FW:** Measurement of acetabular erosion. The effect of pelvic rotation on common landmarks, *J Bone Joint Surg* 71[Br]:447, 1989.

ADDITIONAL READINGS

Beabout JW: Radiology of total hip arthroplasty, *Radiol Clin North Am* 13:3, 1975.
Brand RA, Yoder SA, Pedersen DR: Interobserver variability in interpreting radiographic lucencies about total hip reconstructions, *Clin Orthop* 192:237, 1985.
Buchli R, Boesiger P, Meier D: Heating effects of metallic implants by MRI examinations, *Magn Reason Med* 7:255, 1988.
Burk DL Jr, Karasick D, Kratz AB, et al: Rotator cuff tears: prospective comparison of MR imaging with arthrography, sonography, and surgery, *Am J Radiol* 153:87, 1989.
Christensen RA, Van Sonnenberg E, Casola G, et al: Interventional ultrasound in the musculoskeletal system, *Radiol Clin North Am* 26:145, 1988.
Clarke IC, Gruen T, Matos M, et al: Improved methods for quantitative radiographic evaluation with particular reference to total-hip arthroplasty, *Clin Orthop* 121:83, 1976.
Datz FL, Thorne DA: Effect of antibiotic therapy on the sensitivity of indium-111-labeled leukocyte scans, *J Nucl Med* 27:1849, 1986.
Datz FL, Thorne DA: Effect of chronicity of infection on the sensitivity of the In-111-labeled leukocyte scan, *Am J Radiol* 147:809, 1986.
Eftekhar NS, et al: Perioperative management of total hip replacement, *Orthop Rev* 3:17, 1974.
Fishman EK, et al: Metallic hip implants: CT with multiplanar reconstruction, *Radiology* 160:675, 1986.
Harcke HT, Grissom LE, Finkelstein MS: Evaluation of the musculoskeletal system with sonography, *Am J Radiol* 150:1253, 1988.
Hendrix RW, Wixson RL, Rana NA, et al: Arthrography after total hip arthroplasty: a modified technique used in the diagnosis of pain, *Radiology* 148:647, 1983.
Hunter JC, Baumrind S, Genant HK, et al: The detection of loosening in total hip arthroplasty: description of a stereophotogrammetric computer assisted method, *Invest Radiol* 14:323, 1979.
Iida H, Tamamuro T, Okumura H, et al: Socket location in total hip replacement. Preoperative computed tomography and computer simulation, *Acta Orthop Scand* 59:1, 1988.
Johnson JA, Christie MJ, Sandler MP, et al: Detection of occult infection following total joint arthroplasty using sequential technetium-99m HDP bone scintigraphy and indium-111 WBC imaging, *J Nucl Med* 29:1347, 1988.
Lewinnek GE, Lewis JL, Tarr R, et al: Dislocations after total hip-replacement arthroplasties, *J Bone Joint Surg* 60:217, 1978.
Mjöberg B, Hansson LI, Selvik G: Instability, migration and laxity of total hip prostheses. A roentgen stereophotogrammetric study, *Acta Orthop Scand* 55:141, 1984.
Newberg AH, Wetzner SM: Digital subtraction arthrography, *Radiology* 154:238, 1985.
O'Neill DA, Harris WH: Failed total hip replacement: assessment by plain radiographs, arthrograms, and aspiration of the hip joint, *J Bone Joint Surg* 66:540, 1984.
Phillips WC, Kattapuram SV: Prosthetic hip replacements. Plain films and arthrography for component loosening, *Am J Radiol* 138:677, 1982.
Post M: Constrained arthroplasty of shoulder, *Orthop Clin North Am* 18:455, 1987.
Reckling FW, Asher MA, Dillon WL: A longitudinal study of the radiolucent line at the bone-cement interface following total joint-replacement procedures, *J Bone Joint Surg* 59:355, 1977.
Resnick D, Derr R, Andre M, et al: Digital arthrography in the evaluation of painful joint prostheses, *Invest Radiol* 19:432, 1984.
Roberson DD, Weiss PJ, Fishman EK, et al: Evaluation of CT techniques for reducing artifacts in the presence of metallic orthopedic implants, *J Comput Assist Tomogr* 12:236, 1988.
Rosenthall L, Lisbona R, Hernandez M, et al: 99mTC-PP and 67Ga imaging following insertion of orthopedic devices, *Radiology* 133:717, 1979.
Schneider R, Hood RW, Ranawat CS: Radiologic evaluation of knee arthroplasty, *Orthop Clin North Am* 13:225, 1982.
Schneider R, Soudry M: Radiographic and scintigraphic evaluation of total knee arthroplasty, *Clin Orthop* 205:108, 1986.
Shepherd MM: A further review of the results of operations on the hip joint, *J Bone Joint Surg* 42[Br]:177, 1960.
Shepherd MM: A review of 650 hip arthroplasty operations, *J Bone Joint Surg* 36[Br]:567, 1954.
Wientroub S, Boyde A, Chrispin AR, et al: The use of stereophotogrammetry to measure acetabular and femoral anteversion, *J Bone Joint Surg* 63[Br]:209, 1981.
Weisman BN: The radiology of total joint replacement, *Orthop Clin North Am* 14:171, 1983.
Weisman BN, Sledge CB: *Orthopedic radiology*, Philadelphia, 1986, WB Saunders.
Woo RYG, Morrey BF: Dislocations after total hip arthroplasty, *J Bone Joint Surg* 64:1295, 1982.
Yoder SA, Brand RA, Pedersen DR, et al: Total hip acetabular component position affects component loosening rates, *Clin Orthop* 228:79, 1988.
Zlatkin MB, Iannotti JP, Roberts MC, et al: Diagnostic performance of MR imaging, *Radiology* 172:223, 1989.
Zwas ST, Elkanovitch R, Frank G: Interpretation and classification of bone scintigraphic findings in stress fractures, *J Nucl Med* 28:452, 1987.

See Chapters 28, Results in Primary Total Hip Arthroplasty; 29, Results in Revision Total Hip Arthroplasty; 31, Postoperative Wound Infection; and 32, Dislocation and Instability for additional information.

CHAPTER THIRTEEN

Postoperative Management

- This is the greatest error in the treatment of human sickness, that there are physicians for the body and physicians for the soul, yet the two are one indivisible.
  Plato

Postoperative care is provided using a team approach that combines orthopaedic, medical, and physical therapy care. Patients should be prepared for the postoperative period by being informed of what will be expected of them after surgery. Specific problems should be discussed with them in detail preoperatively. Patients also should receive written instructions describing the procedure and postoperative steps. This chapter discusses routine postoperative procedures in the hospital, ambulation and preparation for discharge, and rehabilitation. The postoperative details of anticoagulation and antibiotics are covered in Chapters 8 and 9.

ABDUCTION SPLINTING

Immediately after applying the dressing, apply the antiembolic stocking or elastic bandages to both extremities, and place the patient in the abduction splint (Fig. 13-1). Routinely use a specially designed abduction splint, shown in Fig. 13-1, C,* in all cases at the end of surgery. This splint has the advantage of ease of application and removal. It is well padded to prevent pressure necrosis, and the foam padding is replaceable for maintenance purposes.[8,10]

Wedge-shaped pillows made from blocks of foam are useful because of their low cost and disposable nature. To properly place such pillows, hold the blocks in place to avoid overtightening, which can cause peroneal nerve palsy at the level of the fibular neck or skin maceration. Both complications have occurred at my institution.

---

* Abduction splint designed by the author.

Place the abduction splint proximal to the malleoli. Keep in mind that the amount of abduction achieved is governed by the mobility of the hips, the width of the pelvis, and the height of the patient. Two sizes of abduction splints, small and large, have been found to be adequate for all patients. The size used depends on the degree of bimalleolar separation. Using an abduction splint too large for a patient with bilateral hip disease causes undue discomfort in the unoperated hip. Too small an abduction splint in a tall patient with unilateral hip disease and good range of motion may not provide adequate abduction.

PATIENT TRANSFER PROCEDURE

The surgeon must supervise the transfer procedure. Never use only a draw sheet under the hip and buttocks to lift the patient because of the danger of dislocating the head out of the socket. Additionally, removal of the draw sheet by an inexperienced individual may cause skin injuries similar to first- and second-degree burns. Transfer the patient directly from the operating table to the bed, obviating the need for further transfer, as is common in conventional operations. Transfer the patient by lifting the lower lumbar spine while one helper holds the legs and another holds the shoulders. The anesthetist should support the head and neck during transfer. Protect the wound drain and urinary bladder catheter against inadvertent pull, which may accidentally remove them.

RECOVERY ROOM PROCEDURES

In the recovery room the Hemovac tubes must be immediately connected to the wall suction. To mea-

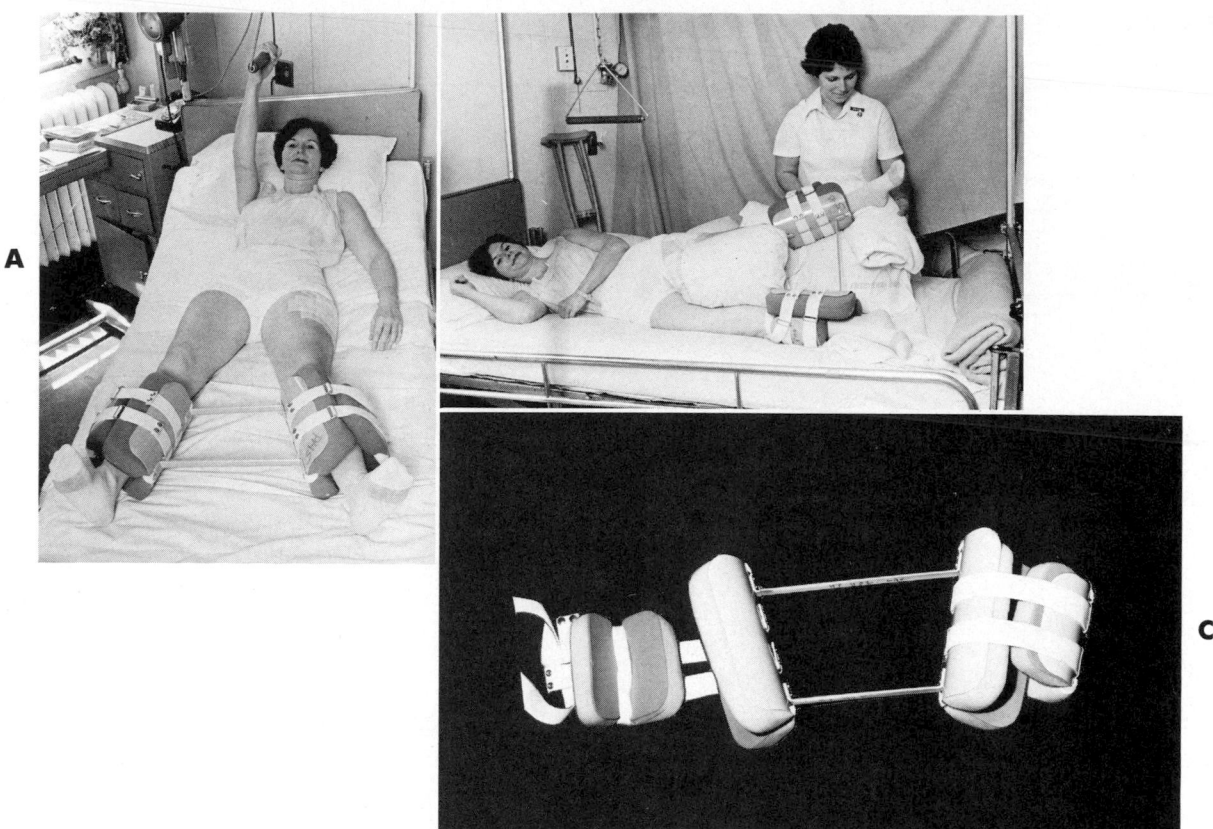

Fig. 13-1. A, Patient in bed wearing abduction splint. **B,** Position of legs in abduction splint with patient on side. Patient is propped on pillows to maintain lateral position. Splint allows frequent turning of patient with minimal risk of accidental adduction. Lateral positioning of patient requires support by two or three regular pillows placed along patient's back and legs to maintain this position. **C,** Abduction splint.

sure the amount of blood in the Hemovac bottle, it is best to mark the bottle periodically. Repeated evacuation of these bottles is unnecessary and may increase the chance of contamination.

A hematocrit level is obtained when the patient arrives in the recovery room and is repeated daily for 5 days. Frequently a postoperative transfusion is needed. The practice at my institution is to keep the hematocrit level above 30% in all patients and above 35% in high-risk patients with a history of coronary or cerebrovascular disease. However, younger and healthy patients can tolerate a hematocrit level of between 25% and 35% (see Chapter 7).

Most patients who have deposited their own blood in the blood bank for autologous transfusion (which is now our routine) have a relatively low hemoglobin/hematocrit level, and it is prudent that most, if not all, of the patient's own blood be transfused. Any blood collected during surgery by a Cell Saver that was not used during surgery should be transfused only after the patient's own banked blood is used up.

Supportive measures, including blood and fluid replacement and close monitoring of the patient, are

conducted by the anesthesia team in the recovery room, and the patient remains there until his or her condition completely stabilizes and he or she regains consciousness.

Postoperative x-ray evaluation is discussed elsewhere. Confirm by radiograph taken before the patient leaves the recovery room that the components are properly placed; the prosthesis may have been dislocated during the patient's transfer from the operating table to the bed.

OTHER POSTOPERATIVE PROCEDURES

Obtain an electrocardiogram on the first postoperative day to evaluate unrecognized surgical ischemia and to provide a baseline should further complications arise. Obtain laboratory studies relative to anticoagulation as indicated. Repeat an SMA 12/60 before discharge.

The initial dressing applied in the operating room remains undisturbed during the first 5 postoperative days; thus it is essential to check the fullness of the thigh daily. If the patient complains of undue pain or sudden onset of pain, especially while taking anticoagulants, the dressing may be removed to search for a hematoma. This complaint of pain is common and should be diagnosed and anticoagulation therapy reversed if necessary. As previously stated (see Chapter 9), our policy is not to drain or aspirate hematomas at the bedside. For the most part they resolve spontaneously. If evacuation is necessary, we carry it out under sterile conditions in the operating room.

If for any other reason the dressing is changed within the first 5 days, the patient is taken to a treatment room so that the procedure can be performed under sterile conditions. Serous or old clots accompanied by dehiscence of the wound are significant and must be reported to the operating surgeon. Repeated dressing changes without investigation of the wound for possible infection are to be deprecated. If infection occurs, the patient should not receive antibiotics until adequate cultures are obtained (see Chapter 31).

The surgeon usually inspects the wound by the fifth postoperative day when a fresh dressing is applied. The retention sutures (foam pads) should remain contained in the dressing to protect them from being damaged.

AMBULATION

Early ambulation is essential. Timing depends on the patient's recovery from surgery. Many patients are very ill from surgical trauma and uninterested in early ambulation because of postoperative pain and a low-grade postoperative temperature elevation. Premature ambulation, when the patient is not physiologically or psychologically ready, can be very discouraging. Patients usually have considerable incisional pain during the first 2 to 3 days after surgery, but normally by the third day they are ready to stand up and take a few steps. Ambulation starts with the patient attempting to stand, aided by the physical therapist.

The out-of-bed period the first day may be limited to two 10- to 15-minute sessions. These periods are increased to a longer time as tolerated by the patient. Usually during the second week, when the patient masters the technique of transfer from the bed to standing and walking, he or she attempts further ambulation without the therapist but with the assistance or presence of a nurse or nurse's aid.

Before attempting to ambulate the patient receives

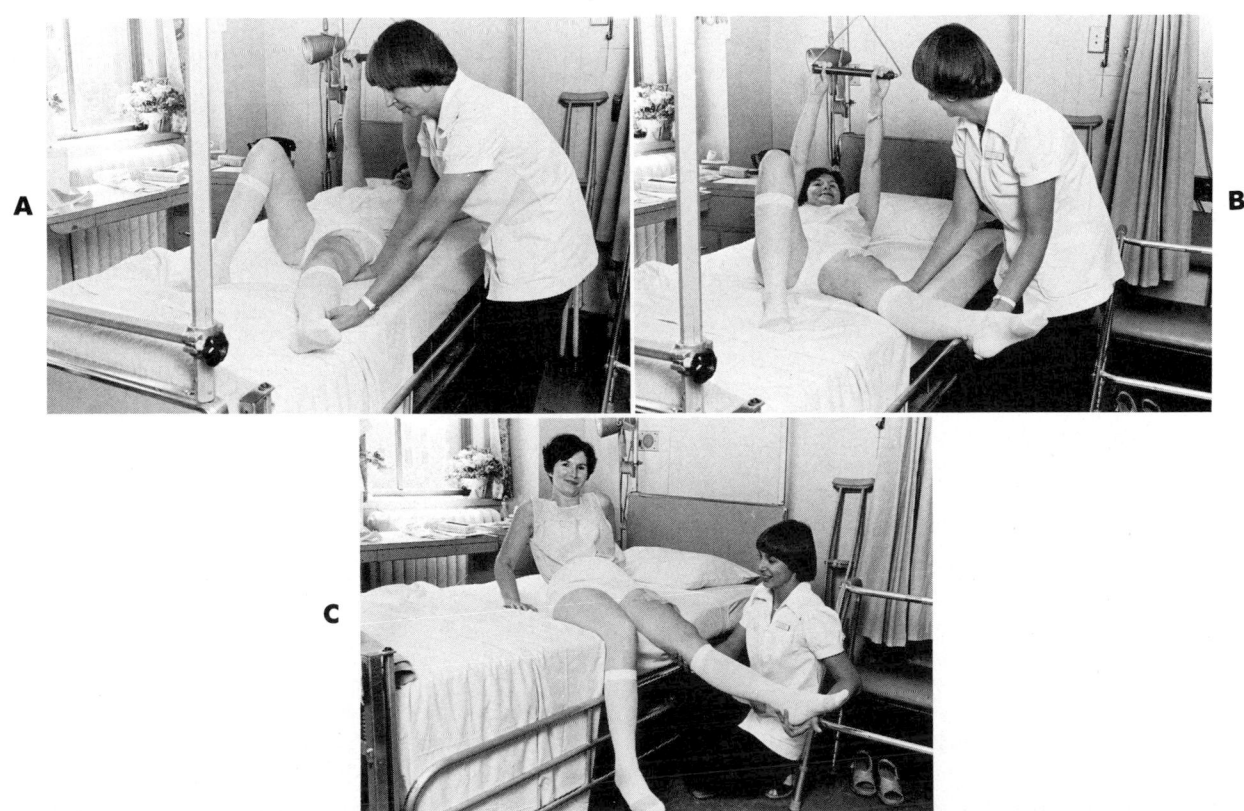

Fig. 13-2. A, Ambulation is initiated with removal of abduction splint. Patient uses trapeze and is assisted by therapist to maintain operated hip in abduction, while unoperated extremity of patient is flexed to raise buttocks and move toward edge of bed. **B,** Same as **A** in a more advanced stage. NOTE: therapist supporting operated extremity while patient turns in bed; in horizontal plane hip is maintained in extended position. **C,** Patient has assumed semi-sitting position with hip in only slight flexion and stabilized by upper extremities; position is maintained by therapist.

Continued.

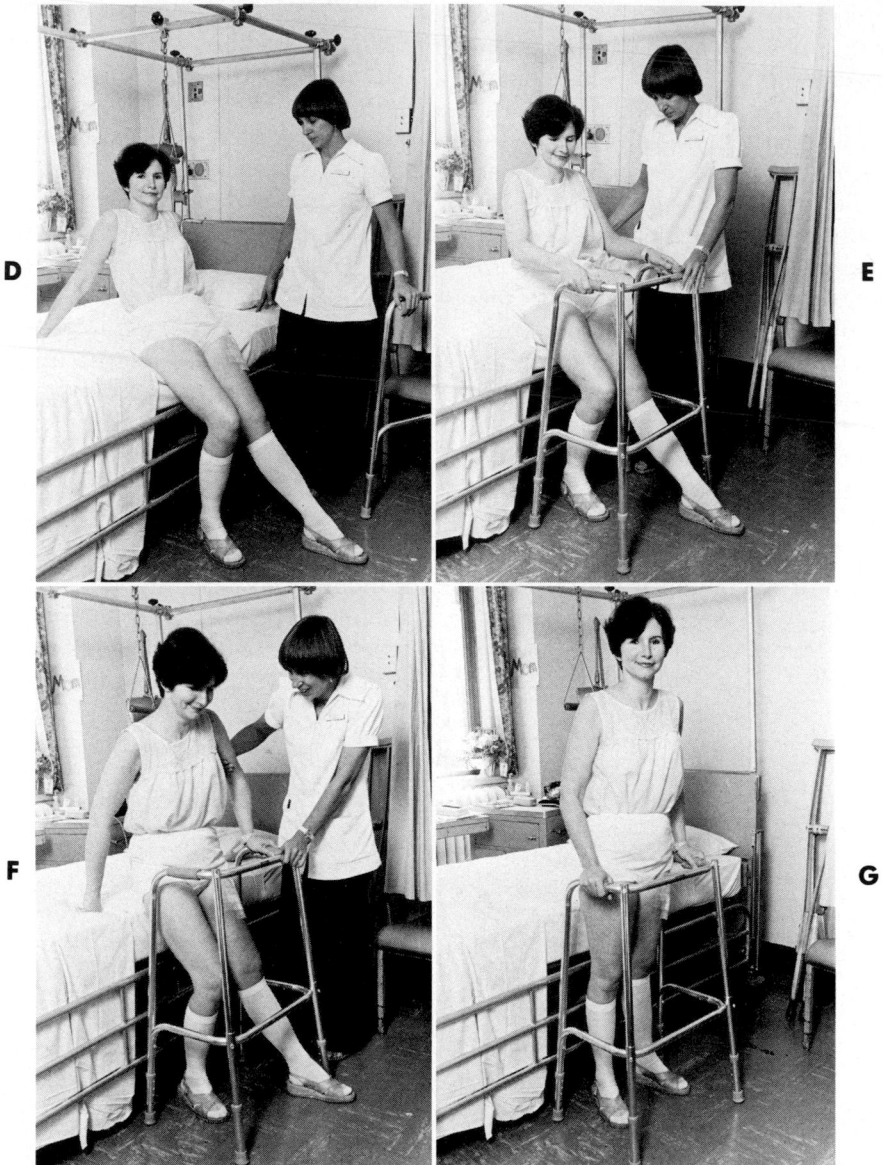

Fig. 13-2 — cont'd. **D,** Patient's main weight is supported by unoperated hip *(right)* and two arms leaning back onto bed. In this position patient momentarily rests and overcomes dizziness or apprehension during first day out of bed. **E,** Walker may be used for start of ambulation. It is appropriately adjusted to patient's height and placed properly in relation to position of standing. NOTE: operated hip *(left)* is still in extension. Main weight is to be transferred onto unoperated side *(right hip)*. **F,** Standing. Maximum support is obtained by pushing on bed while standing; unoperated leg *(right leg)* lifts patient off bed. **G,** Standing. Standing is encouraged with weight equally distributed on both hips.

instruction in methods of transfer from bed to the standing position. The patient keeps the hip in maximum extension while getting out of bed, with the knees apart to maintain abduction at the hip. The patient uses a trapeze for turning toward the edge of the bed (Fig. 13-2, *A and B*). This maneuver can be done in two stages: (1) flexing the knee of the unoperated side and using the trapeze to turn 90 degrees to the edge of the bed and then (2) assuming a semi-sitting posture at the edge of the bed (Fig. 13-2, *C and D*). For a tall person, the bed is raised from the floor. Slippers are adequate for the first day of ambulation, but shoes are preferable for walking. A slippery floor or unsuitable bed may cause insecurity or falls and should be avoided. The first one or two ambulatory attempts may be limited to standing, especially when there is lightheadedness caused by orthostatic hypotension, which is common in these patients. The physical therapist may initiate ambulation with a walker or crutches at his or her discretion (Fig. 13-2, *E to G*). Patients initially are encouraged to avoid weight bearing on the operated extremity but to use flat foot contact for balance, using crutches or walker and both upper extremities for support from the first day of ambulation. This pattern of weight bearing is suggested when cementless devices are used, but more weight bearing may be recommended based on the surgical approach used and the surgeon's preference. Patients tend to keep the operated hip in abduction during walking, which need not be discouraged at first, but a more normal gait should be expected after a week of ambulation (Fig. 13-3).

Ambulation with crutches is encouraged in all patients. The continuing use of a walker may be limited to a very old and debilitated patient. Crutch walking is basically a two-point gait, with the crutch on the operated side synchronized with the unoperated extremity. With the next step the crutch on the unoperated side supports the operated hip, and so on.

SITTING OUT OF BED

Contrary to the patient's expectations, ambulation does not begin with sitting. In fact, the patient should be walking about a week before being allowed to sit in a chair. The abduction splint, replaced while the patient is in bed, may be removed after the first week, and the head of the bed may be raised 45 degrees for reading, eating, and so on. At no time should the patient sit straight up in bed or on the edge of the bed. This should be discouraged if attempted. While the patient sits in bed, even at a 45-degree angle, the knees should be

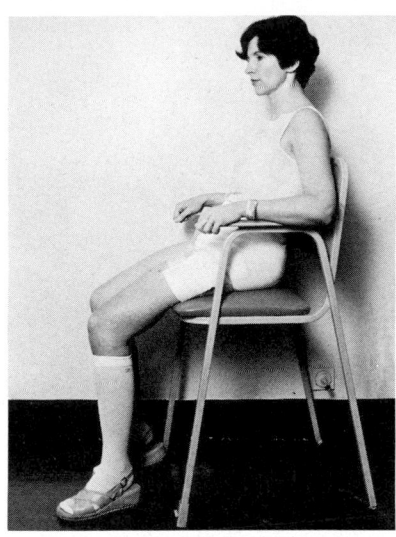

Fig. 13-4. After ambulation has begun and patient has achieved approximately 50 to 60 degrees of range in flexion, patient may be allowed to sit on high, raised chair.

extended to stabilize the hip. The abduction splint may be discarded during the resting period after 1 week. However, it should be replaced if the patient is lying on his side. After the patient begins ambulation and achieves approximately 50 to 60 degrees range of motion, the patient may be allowed to sit on a high, raised chair (Fig. 13-4), a chair with two pillows, or preferably a high-seated chair to avoid excessive flexion at the hip. A high armchair with a firm seat is very helpful for all patients. While the patient is sitting on the chair, the knee remains extended. Patients prefer high-seated chairs and also enjoy using them at home for the first 6 weeks postoperatively. I also recommend a raised toilet seat, which may be used as soon as the patient is allowed to sit out of bed. Before the use of the raised toilet seat and ambulation, the patient uses a flat orthopaedic bedpan. The use of the trapeze is essential in raising the pelvis onto the bedpan. The unoperated hip and knee are flexed to assist placement of the bedpan. The operated hip and leg need not be removed from the splint (Fig. 13-5).

PREPARATION FOR HOME DISCHARGE

At the end of the second week or just before discharge, a second radiograph verifies the details of arthroplasty and trochanteric fixation. A good anteroposterior film includes both hips and the upper third of the femurs. This radiograph must be of good quality, since it is the only documentation before the patient's discharge from the hospital.

Home transfer can be facilitated by a large car, with the patient preferably seated in the front seat with the hip elevated on one pillow. A sport or compact car

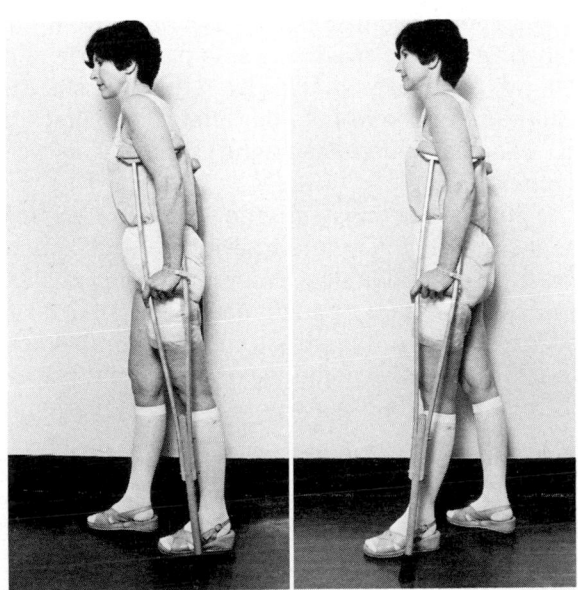

Fig. 13-3. Initiation of walking with crutches is by forward placement of unoperated extremity and support by crutch from operated side.

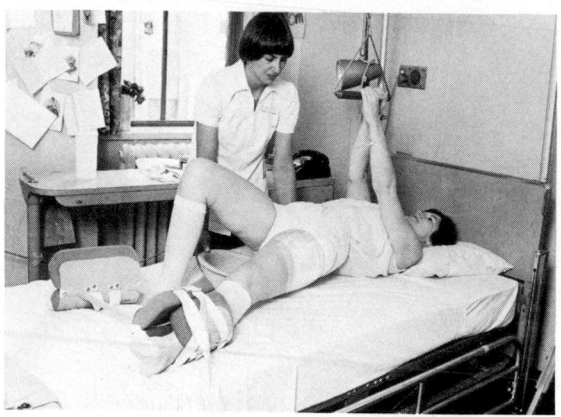

Fig. 13-5. To use a bedpan, patient uses trapeze to elevate buttocks. Operated hip may remain in brace while patient flexes unoperated hip and bends knee to 90 degrees. By using arms and applying pressure on unoperated extremity, patient raises buttocks, thus allowing placement of bedpan.

forces the hip into excess flexion, making the trip home unpleasant and possibly even causing hip dislocation. For patients who live in an upstairs apartment without an elevator, transportation by ambulance should be encouraged. The height of the bed at home should be raised 6 to 12 inches, either by placing blocks under the bed or by adding a second mattress.

Patients are reminded to avoid extreme flexion such as sitting on a low chair or trying to put on their own stockings. They also should avoid adduction by crossing the legs.

Encourage the patient to use crutches for 6 weeks after the operation. Thereafter, the patient may progress to one cane. At this point, the patient may ride in a car but should postpone driving until at least 3 weeks after the first postoperative outpatient visit (9 weeks after surgery).

REHABILITATION
Preoperative Instruction

Ideally, every patient admitted to the hospital for total hip arthroplasty should be referred to the physical therapy department at least 1 day before the scheduled surgery. The preoperative treatment program includes the following:

1. Instruction and practice in deep breathing and coughing.
2. Active ankle exercises, especially plantar flexion and dorsiflexion.
3. Instruction in postoperative bed-to-standing transfer, avoiding hip flexion and adduction of the operated hip.
4. Instruction on crutch walking.
5. Explanation of the physical therapy program to be used during the recovery period.

The preoperative outpatient visit enables the physical therapist to establish a good working relationship at a time when the patient is best able to comprehend instructions. It also allows the therapist to clarify any questions the patient may have regarding the role of physical therapy.

The nursing staff also gives the patient preoperative instruction. The nurses cover postoperative bed positioning and motion and use of the bedpan. They also reinforce the physical therapist's instructions on deep breathing and coughing.

A video production of perioperative patient care, including physical therapy management, is a luxury that can be helpful to the patient before or at the time of admission.

Postoperative Physical Therapy Management

Some patients are overly anxious about returning to normal activities. They should be encouraged to proceed slowly. In the postoperative period the psychological aspects of rehabilitation are probably as important as the physical. Physical therapists usually have more time than other medical staff to spend with the patient, and their sensitivity to psychological and physical handicaps could be instrumental in the patient's overall assessment and management.

The physical therapist must be fully acquainted with the patient's rate of progression. The therapist's role is to guide the patient in a relaxed manner through activities that are now possible because of the new pain-free hip joint. However, the patient should be reminded that the muscles require time to be reeducated and strengthened. At the same time the physical therapist must reinforce that no set timetable exists and that each patient is expected to progress at his or her own rate. This reassurance is particularly necessary if two patients recovering from this type of surgery are in the same room, and one is not able to do certain active exercises, such as straight leg raising, as well as the other.

The physical therapist must be willing to adapt to the patient's temperament and individual needs concerning restrictions, additional encouragement, and exercises. For example, if a patient does not wish to do stair climbing (because there is no need to climb stairs at home), it should be eliminated from that patient's individual program.

First Postoperative Week

After surgery, the physical therapist sees the patient immediately on return to the recovery room. For the first 2 postoperative days, the physical therapy program consists of deep breathing and coughing and bilateral active ankle exercises. Isometric contraction of the quadriceps muscles is initiated after removal of the wound drains, usually on the second or third postoperative day. Active assisted hip and knee flexion and straight leg raising, with the abduction splint removed only during the exercise period, commence on the fourth postoperative day. For most patients this is the first experience of pain-free motion after several years of hip disability. The hip feels mobile ("lubricated"), and there is only incisional discomfort at the site of the wound. Passive hip flexion is to be avoided, so elevation of the head of the bed should be limited to no more than 45 degrees. During this period the nursing staff turns the patient on the unoperated side, with the abduction splint in place and with the side-lying position maintained with several regular bed pillows. The "bed-to-standing" transfer is executed by the patient without sitting on the edge of the bed and with the therapist helping to maintain the hip in abduction position. Full weight bearing as tolerated is encouraged on ambulation with a walker or crutches (see Figs. 13-2 and 13-3) for techniques without trochanteric osteotomy and for totally cemented hips. For patients with noncemented, porous-coated devices and those with a transtrochanteric approach, a period of 6 to 8 weeks without weight bearing is advisable. This method of rehabilitation is designed to minimize the possibility of nonunion of the trochanter and postoperative subluxation.

Second Postoperative Week

During the second postoperative week, physical therapy continues with active assisted hip and knee flexion, straight leg raising exercises, and the gait-training program. In most instances the patient is now able to walk with crutches in a three-point gait. Should the patient have pain and limitation in the unoperated hip, he or she is instructed in a four-point gait. The patient avoids sitting until the end of the second postoperative week or until at least 55 degrees of hip flexion has been achieved (see Fig. 13-4).

When the physical therapist is sure that the patient is able to transfer from the bed to the standing position and walk independently, the patient is allowed out of bed as desired. When sitting is permitted, the patient uses an armchair with a pillow on the seat to avoid extreme flexion of the hip. The patient receives instruction in stair climbing toward the end of the second week or earlier if the patient is to be discharged at 10 to 12 days postoperatively.

Third Postoperative Week

Abduction on a powder board may be added to the exercise program during the third postoperative week. Instruction in stair climbing with crutches also begins at this time. If necessary, the patient is referred to the occupational therapist for instruction in dressing techniques involving the lower extremities. Many patients are discharged from the hospital during this period, usually the first or second day of the third postoperative week. Thus this portion of the program is aborted in patients who can walk independently and climb stairs.

Specific Place and Means of Physical Therapy

Routine management requires little or no specific training; with attention to the details of postoperative routine, personnel could be trained to assist the therapist or to take the place of the therapist after the first week. Personnel instructed to assist the patient out of bed and walk with the patient could alleviate demands on the nursing staff. They could serve in the capacity of technicians, assistant nursing staff, or nurses' aides. These trainees would also be available to the patient over the weekend, when other trained staff is normally not available. These patients must continue their activities during the weekend so that daily ambulation is not disrupted.

On the other hand, for patients with polyarticular involvement, as in rheumatoid arthritis, an expert physical therapist is invaluable. The therapist is instrumental in rectifying postoperative rehabilitation problems, including splinting of the lower or upper extremities, and in making modifications to walking aids and lifts when required. The physical therapist discusses the problems of these patients with the surgeon in charge, plotting a sensible and individualized rehabilitation approach. Often, whirlpool or other hydrotherapy is beneficial in polyarticular rheumatoid conditions.

Because of slow healing and fragility and muscle wasting, the rheumatoid patient may progress more slowly than patients with osteoarthritis. Chair- and bed-bound patients need continuous appraisal before surgery for the potential of becoming ambulatory. However, because of extreme osteoporosis of these individuals, they may be susceptible to stress fractures. Pain can also be promoted in the bones and joints of their lower extremities.

Because psychological and physical aspects of rehabilitation are equally important, a therapist who is able to answer questions with intelligence and concern conveys cheerful confidence to the patient and is indispensable during the rehabilitation course.

Speed of Rehabilitation and Therapy

Many surgeons and therapists claim successful results in patients who achieve early and spectacular ranges of motion within the first 2 weeks during recovery. I consider this effort ineffective, however, because most patients gain the same range of motion without jeopardy to the hip joint within 3 to 6 months. Extreme ranges of motion may damage the artificial hip joint and should not be encouraged at any time. With an ambitious therapist and the extroverted (usually male) patient, the surgeon must request dampening the enthusiasm for exercise (see Chapters 32 and 37). Nature is the greatest guide in attempting and achieving range of motion in most instances. Passive forceful range of motion directed by a therapist must be avoided; it is for this reason that no physiotherapeutic modality should be prescribed for the patient when he or she leaves the hospital.

In contrast to range of flexion, gain in abduction postoperatively is essential and fundamental to a successful total hip arthroplasty. If an adduction deformity is not corrected during surgery or if patients develop adduction contractures, a therapist must specifically attend to these problems (to overcome such a fixed deformity with consequential pelvic obliquity). Fixed adduction deformities must be corrected by powdered board exercises coupled with pelvic-shrugging exercises.[1,4,10]

Gain in Range of Motion and Management of Fixed Deformity

If a patient suffers considerable restriction of the range of motion before surgery, some postoperative restriction should be expected. Usually about 75% to 80% of the total range to be gained is achieved within the first 3 weeks after arthroplasty. A patient's mobility occasionally improves up to a year or more. When accompanied by a few degrees of abduction, patients may flex as much as 100 to 120 degrees. In a patient with a good preoperative range of motion, active and passive flexion of about 90 to 100 degrees will probably take place without any physiotherapeutic effort. This has been seen even in patients who were put in plaster after total hip surgery and achieved similar ranges of motion. It seems that the soft tissue about the hip largely determines the range of motion, and other factors not yet fully understood may also contribute to this phenomenon. A 90-degree flexion range is quite adequate for most daily functional activities, and forceful passive manipulation beyond that may jeopardize the hip joint. Gain in mobility does not seem to be related to degrees of exercises to promote mobility.[9]

Recovering the range of motion from a fixed adduction deformity is really a matter of surgical correction. A flexion deformity corrected at surgery is usually eliminated postoperatively provided that (1) the patient remains flat on his back during recovery, and (2) the opposite hip does not have a severe flexion deformity leading to lumbar lordosis, and thus resumption of the flexion deformity of the operated hip. If severe flexion deformity exists in both hips and both operations are planned within 2 to 3 weeks, it is advantageous to keep

the operated hip in extension by supporting the opposite hip in a flexion position, that is, propped over several pillows. This position keeps the lumbar spine flat and avoids recurrence of flexion deformity. As an alternative method, if the patient has had release of flexion contracture deformity, he or she may be placed prone during recovery as opposed to the supine position.

The problem of fixed adduction deformity is serious and commonly found in combination with a short lower extremity. After adductor tenotomy surgery and complete mobilization of the medial aspect of the hip joint augmented by transfer of the abductor muscles to a new position, the therapist must take care to maintain abduction postoperatively, especially by passive and active development of abduction power. Special emphasis on pelvic tilt exercises is necessary to overcome recurrence of this deformity.

To achieve abduction the patient is taught to shrug the pelvis, hiking it by alternately lengthening and shortening the limbs. The patient, in effect, abducts the previously adducted hip to a more favorable position. The opposite hip must be normal for this exercise (Fig. 13-6). A program of active abduction exercises, instituted early during the postoperative course, is especially necessary in patients with a tendency to develop adduction deformity (Fig. 13-7).

Fixed external rotation deformity is also a serious problem that, like the flexion deformity, must be completely corrected during surgery. Occasionally the lower extremity resumes external rotation despite correction. Recurrence of external rotation deformity after surgery creates the hazards of postoperative peroneal nerve palsy and consequently of foot drop, a disturbing complication to patient and surgeon alike. While postoperative testing for foot function is routine, recording of dorsiflexion of the ipsilateral foot is essential. When, because of lateral pressure near the head of the fibula as a result of deformity, the patient has a radiation of pain to the lateral aspect of the dorsum of the foot, the pressure must be elucidated at once, and preferably a small, soft-foam pillow or a bean bag should be placed under the knee to relax the nerve. When palsy is manifested, an L-shaped orthotic device may be worn in the shoe during the postoperative course. Fortunately, most palsies, if they are detected early and the pressure is relieved, resolve within 6 months postoperatively. Insertion of a tibial pin postoperatively may correct severe external rotation deformities (more than 30 to 40 degrees).[5,7] The therapist can keep the hip in internal rotation during exercise, and with effort the patient can learn to practice active internal rotation during walking to overcome resistant external rotation deformity during the postoperative course.

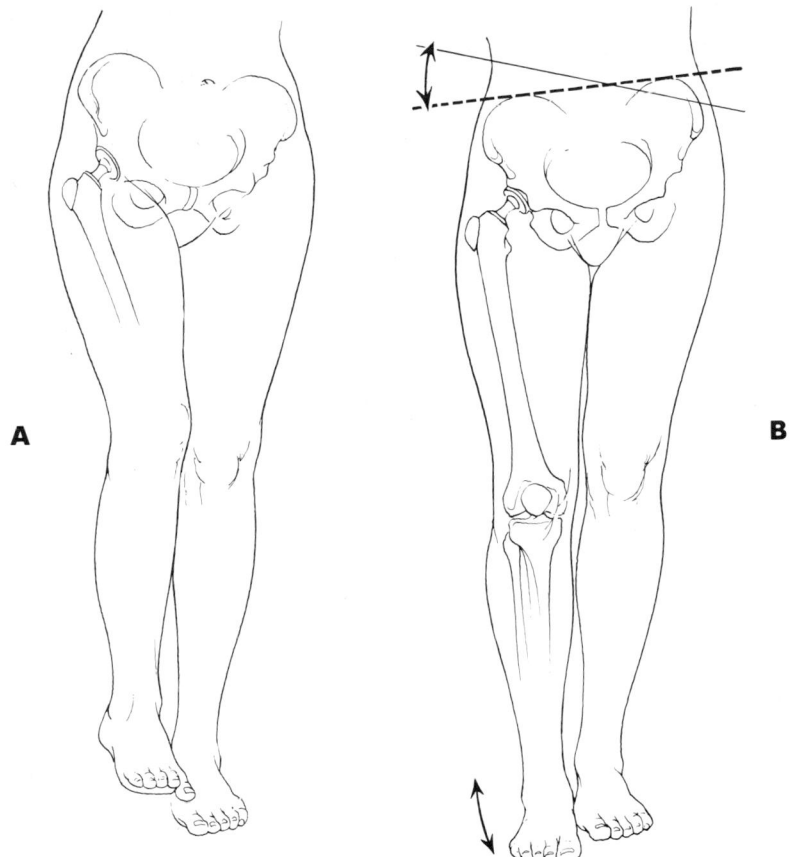

Fig. 13-6. "Pelvic shrug" exercise in which patient is taught to hike pelvis alternatively by lengthening, **B,** and shortening, **A,** limb while in supine position. Opposite hip must be normal to perform this exercise. NOTE: effect of lengthening and shortening is producing abduction of "adducted hip."

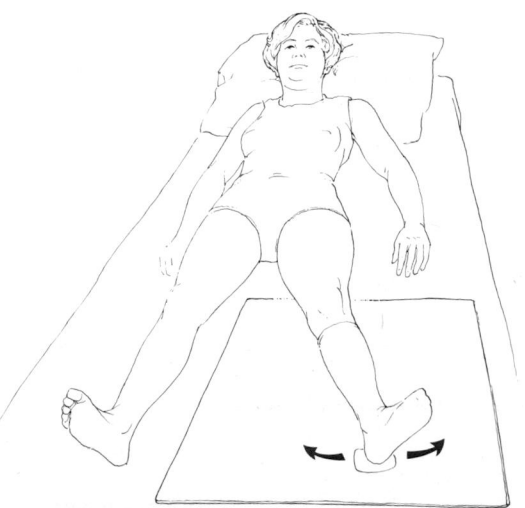

Fig. 13-7. An active program of abduction exercises is especially needed in patients with a tendency to develop adduction deformity. Powdered board and rolled stockinette (or a roller skate) may be used to provide low-friction apparatus and prevent heel irritation while doing this exercise.

Postoperative Knee Pain

Not infrequently, patients complain of knee pain postoperatively while the operated extremity is held in extension in the abduction splint. I find no objection to placing a rolled towel, a small pillow, or similar device made of foam under the knee for comfort. Such a procedure may also protect the lateral division (superficial) of the peroneal nerve by flexion of the knee and elimination of contact with the mattress if the limb has a tendency to externally rotate.

Use of a Knee Immobilizer

Routine use of a knee immobilizer, in addition to an abduction splint for protection against accidental excess flexion, to avoid dislocation is not indicated and is overkill. It is true, however, that if the knee (ipsilateral) is held in extension, it is more difficult for the patient to dislocate the hip. I find the temporary use of a knee immobilizer with an abduction splint attractive if the patient is agitated or mentally confused, and thus uncooperative.

Ace Bandages and Heel Pads

This author finds Ace bandages potentially dangerous if improperly applied. Too much tension during application causes severe problems in patients with poor venous circulation and sensitive skin; as such they cause pressure sores proximal to the heel, along the Achilles tendon, or along the dorsum of the foot along the line of the extensor tendons. To avoid these complications, Ace bandages must be applied gently in the operating room without too much tension and must be replaced by compressive stretch stockings (thromboembolic disease, or TED, stockings) upon the patient's arrival to the floor.

Heels are also especially vulnerable if they are not protected and routinely inspected by the nursing staff. The use of heel pads or an IV-solution plastic bag placed proximal to the calcaneal tuberosity along the Achilles tendon is a useful detail.

Fig. 13-8 summarizes the timetable for different activities after total hip arthroplasty.

Patient Instructions on Discharge

Patients should receive written instructions on discharge. This author has produced a handout that contains information such as a description of the total hip arthroplasty and preoperative and postoperative steps including nursing, physiotherapy, and postdischarge instructions. If a handout is not available the therapist or the surgeon must provide the patient with an outline of "dos" and "don'ts." These instructions should be simple and include all the activities that the patient has been doing while in the hospital.

The patient should be encouraged to walk a lot, since this improves the hip more than any other specific exercise. On discharge the patient may be instructed to avoid bathing in a tub but should be encouraged to shower, if possible. The patient may start swimming after the 6-week postoperative visit. Sexual intercourse can be commenced about 2 to 3 months after surgery. It must be frankly discussed, with specific instructions regarding positioning. The patient must avoid excessive flexion or adduction at sexual engagement. The patient may drive a car after the 3-week postoperative visit. Normal activities may be resumed as the patient feels able.

The patient instructions should include a list of dos and don'ts, such as the following lists, which the patient can use as a reminder at home.

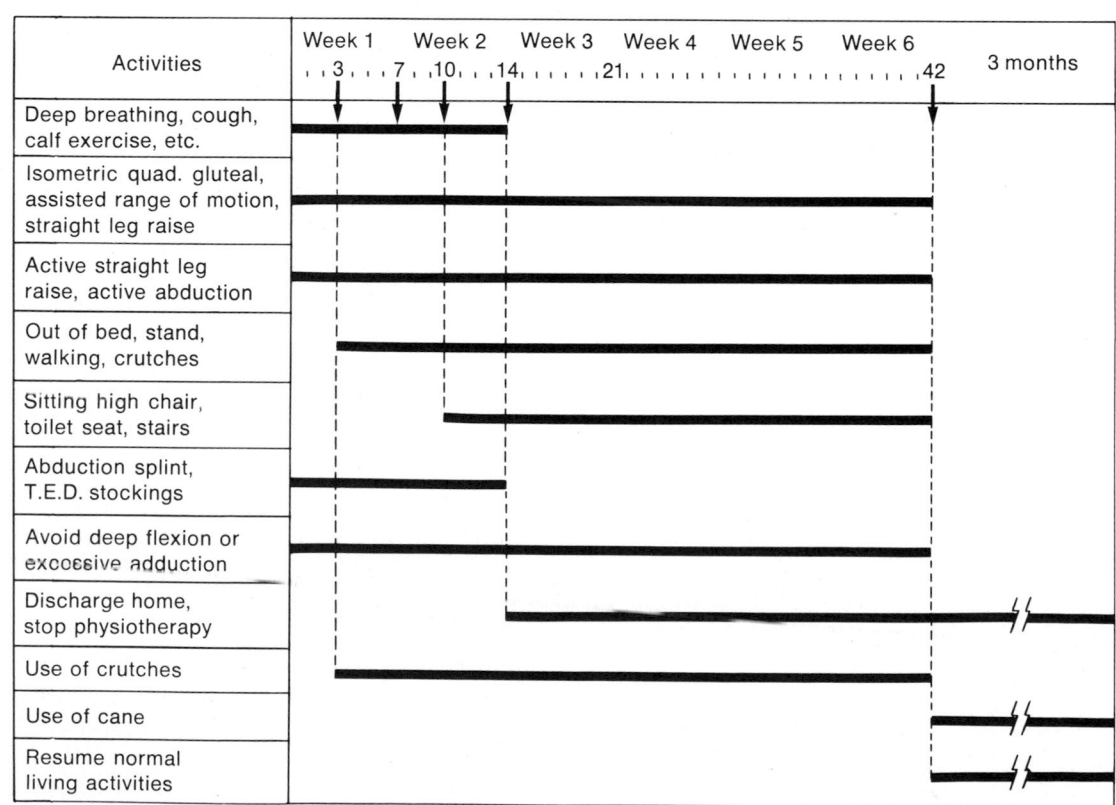

Fig. 13-8. Summary of beginning and end of exercises during postoperative course. NOTE: most restrictions and therapeutic modalities are stopped at end of 6 weeks after surgery. In routine cases, by 3 months the patient may resume all routine daily living activities but is discouraged from engaging in strenous sports such as skiing or tennis.

Dos

- Take your Ace bandages or TED stockings with you and wear them during walking; you may remove them while resting and at bedtime.
- Have someone assist you with tying your shoelaces and cutting your toenails until you obtain adequate mobility in the hip.
- Take an occasional aspirin, Bufferin, or other mild analgesic, if necessary, for mild aches or muscle spasm. You are not expected to have much pain upon departure from the hospital. The incisional discomfort should disappear gradually. Strong medications are not needed.
- Follow the instructions regarding your anticoagulation regimen, and contact your physician as instructed.
- Call your surgeon if you have severe pain in the hip area or undue swelling of the ankle and leg.
- Continue the postoperative activities you were engaging in while in the hospital, particularly walking within your tolerance. This is your principal exercise. No physical therapy is needed. Walk as long and as far as you want using two crutches. Use two crutches for 6 weeks and then a cane for another 4 to 6 weeks.
- Use a straight, high chair with arms to facilitate getting out of the chair. Avoid using a sofa.
- Women may wear a soft girdle when home, if desired.
- Shower and wash hair as necessary.

Don'ts

- Don't cross your legs for 6 weeks.
- Don't lie on your operated side; when lying on the other side, don't permit the operated leg to cross over. Place a pillow between your knees as a precaution.
- Don't sit on a low sofa or chair for 6 weeks.
- Don't bend down to pick up objects, bending your hips in excess.
- Don't worry about range of motion of your hips. This usually improves within 1 year after the operation. Remember that the hip gets better with passage of time; gradual increases in walking (time and distance) will progressively strengthen your hip during the first 6 weeks postoperatively.
- Don't adduct your hips excessively.
- Never engage in activities that involve:
  1. Placing heavy loading forces on the hip joint, that is, running, jumping, or carrying heavy loads (more than 25 kg).
  2. Placing excessive bending and twisting stresses on the hip joint, that is, lifting, shoveling, or forceful turning.

Discontinuation of Walking Aids

As I stated elsewhere, I consider crutch walking (6 weeks) and use of a cane (6 weeks) for a total of 3 months after surgery advisable. On the other hand, if after 3 months after surgery a pronounced limp exists and the gluteal muscles have not recovered fully, I then encourage a continuance of walking with a cane for a total of 6 to 12 months. I encourage elderly patients who are unsteady to use a cane permanently if they wish. It is essential to transmit cheerful confidence during the patient's recovery period, emphasizing nature as a guideline rather than comparing the patient's performance with that of other patients who have undergone the same procedure.[10]

Modification of Routine

Pathological Conditions and Special Conditions Encountered at Surgery

The surgeon may prescribe a specific modification of the postoperative regimen according to the special conditions encountered at the time of surgery; similarly, certain pathological conditions may necessitate modification of basic routine in postoperative management. The following situations indicate the need to modify routine management:

1. Extreme osteoporosis with fragmentation of the trochanter at surgery or an inability to achieve any perfect fixation of the trochanter at the time of surgery. A slow rehabilitation is recommended to prevent further separation of the trochanter or the possibility of postoperative dislocation.
2. Instability at surgery, especially in revision operations where extensive soft tissue releases are necessary and the tension of the tissue across the hip is inadequate to produce stable reduction.
3. Revision for recurrent dislocation of total hip arthroplasty. Because of possible recurrence of dislocation with a revision performed for instability caused by hypermobility, it is advisable to limit the patient postoperatively by use of a short hip spica cast made of light fiberglass for a period of 6 weeks, followed by an abduction brace for a period of 3 to 6 months. The brace is only a limited restriction and assists as a reminder rather than as an immobilizer (see Chapters 32 and 35).
4. Fracture of the shaft or acetabulum during preparation or cementing technique. When traumatic or pathological fracture of the femur is encountered during total hip arthroplasty, it is prudent for both the patient and the therapist to participate closely in managing the patient. In such a case the rehabilitation and status of weight bearing are determined largely by the strength of fixation of the fracture at surgery and the process

of healing of the fracture. With this condition, fracture healing should take precedence over recovery of the arthroplasty (see Chapter 36).

In addition, the patient should be guarded against excess mobility where extreme ranges of motion of the hip were present preoperatively or if the patient is overly enthusiastic and initiates a lot of range-of-motion exercises within the first week despite the therapist's instructions. Caution is necessary to guard against possible dislocation and subluxation of the hip joint. If dislocation or trochanteric problems exist at surgery, the modification may involve applying a hip spica cast or treating the patient in a balanced suspension apparatus. The total immobilization period may be increased up to 8 to 12 weeks when the failure to achieve good fixation of the trochanter is noted intraoperatively or postoperatively. Another situation that requires drastic modification of postoperative management is when the shaft of the femur fractures during operation. The best response is to fix these fractures immediately at surgery (see Chapter 36) and then to place the patient in a balanced suspension apparatus for comfort. Depending on the severity of the fracture or the method of fixation at surgery, a hip spica cast may be applied within 2 weeks after surgery upon removal of the sutures. The patient may resume walking (with the cast) if the fracture has been securely fixed, and partial weight bearing may be resumed within 2 to 3 months after surgery. The combination of a fracture of the shaft of the femur and total hip arthroplasty requires diligent observation concerning the status of the fracture healing before the surgeon authorizes weight bearing and independent walking (see Chapter 36).

Other modifications of the program may include the number and duration of the patient's exercises. For example, patients with borderline cardiac problems are advised to be out of bed once a day only, as opposed to twice daily in routine cases. Postoperative standing in younger patients may be modified to the second or third day postoperatively, as opposed to the routine fourth day. The earlier the patient can stand and walk, the better the chance of preventing thromboembolic disease.

Postoperative Management for Rheumatoid Arthritis

Charnley emphasized a new method of rehabilitation after low-friction arthroplasty, with a less cautious attitude that included discarding the wedge pillow between the third and seventh postoperative day, lying freely in bed, not restricting movement in any direction, and encouraging flexion.[6] He also encouraged the patient to sleep on the unoperated side with pillows

between the legs after the first week. These changes in Charnley's postoperative recommendations reflected changes in his operative technique by two measures: (1) improved tissue tension by use of a neck-length jig, and (2) the cruciate wiring technique and the use of a staple clamp for reattachment of the greater trochanter. The change in policy emphasized that with the above improved techniques in preventing postoperative dislocation, rehabilitating the patient early and vigorously was possible without fear of dislocation after detachment of the greater trochanter. My policy has been somewhat more conservative (as outlined in this chapter) despite a good trochanteric reattachment and the use of provisions against postoperative instability of the joint. I believe that overactivity has no benefit during the first 6 weeks after surgery. On the other hand, excessive exercise, especially flexion and extension exercises, may cause many problems. These potential problems include (1) preventing loose capsule formation with subsequent instability, (2) immediate instability and dislocation in an overzealous or uncooperative patient, (3) detachment of the greater trochanter, which can manifest itself by early wire breakage while the patient is still in the hospital, (4) formation of hematoma, and (5) muscle spasm and pain, which can damage the patient's confidence about normal progressive gain in range of motion and muscle strength. I strongly encourage patients to use only partial weight bearing, to avoid flexion beyond 70 degrees, to avoid any adduction, and to spare weight bearing on the operated leg when sitting in a high chair or in getting to a standing position during the first 6 weeks postoperatively.

A modified program for total hip arthroplasty is also required for patients with rheumatoid arthritis and multiple joint involvement. In rheumatoid conditions the patient is affected not only by the hip, but also by the knees, the ankles, and the joints of the upper extremities. Consequently, these patients need individually modified crutches and assistive devices. They also need more assistive support during the first few days of rehabilitation; it may be necessary to schedule a modified program of early sitting for these individuals rather than extensive walking before allowing them out of bed. They will require longer postoperative recuperation and rehabilitation periods. Specific therapies, including hydrotherapy, are essential for many severely handicapped patients with rheumatoid arthritis. Additionally, it may be necessary to splint their lower extremities during their ambulation period.

The routine postoperative course calls for weight bearing using crutches for support as soon as the patient can tolerate it on the operated extremity, but partial weight bearing may be required in patients with additional bone graft procedures, the transtrochanteric approach, or precarious anatomical defects based on observation at surgery. Patients showing signs of overactivity (reaching a range of motion of 80 to 90 degrees within the first 10 days after surgery) should be restricted and reminded of the consequences of possible dislocations and trochanteric problems. It is essential to inhibit the patient from further exercises and from sitting in bed with knees flexed or on a low chair leaning forward. If recovery of postoperative range is slow and the patient is not gaining range of motion by the second week, the patient should be instructed to sit at more of a right angle (against conventional advice), and range of motion, including flexion, should be encouraged.

While the straight leg-raising exercise is routinely encouraged after cemented hip arthroplasty, patients who fail to perform it must be psychologically supported, and the surgeon must insist on their continuing to attempt the exercise. The degree of rehabilitation is not related to the ability to do straight leg raising before ambulation. Straight leg-raise exercise is a good method to strengthen the quadriceps and hip muscles to prepare the patient for independent walking. However, patients whose hips were replaced by a porous-coated stem or cup should avoid attempts to do straight leg raising because this maneuver increases the joint "reaction force" by twice the body weight (see Chapter 6).

Postoperative Weight Bearing for Bilateral Arthroplasty

When bilateral arthroplasties are performed sequentially during the same hospitalization or during the same anesthesia, the patient's rehabilitation is modified. Weight bearing is resumed using 50% weight bearing on each hip with a four-point gait starting 3 to 4 days postoperatively and carried out for 6 to 8 weeks postoperatively. At that time the rehabilitation must be individualized for the use of a single cane or crutch as an alternative to using both crutches a bit longer. When the patient's operations are 7 to 10 days apart, protection is first eliminated for the first hip; that is, the crutch or cane from the hand opposite the first hip operation is discarded.

Postoperative Care After Revision Surgery

As one might expect, postoperative rehabilitation after revision surgery must be modified because of problems related to trochanteric reattachment and porotic bone. I routinely use a short hip spica (see Chapters 24 and 25) or a hip abduction brace after revision surgery. Most patients are prepared for a slow postoperative rehabilitation, including weight bearing. When bone graft or a cementless porous-coated implant is used, recommended weight-bearing status may be deferred

up to 3 months. The decision regarding resumption of weight bearing must be highly individualized based on the extent of bone damage found at surgery and on the surgical methods used, including the extent of bone grafts. Additionally, because of the potential for soft tissue impairment and muscle atrophy, the gain in postoperative range of motion and strength must be slow and supervised to avoid postoperative dislocation or muscular pain. Patients at risk for recurrence of postoperative heterotopic ossification (HTO) may receive the currently used regimen of radiation postoperatively before application of a light fiberglass cast (see Chapters 24 and 25).

Postoperative Management for Cementless Implants

There is common agreement among the proponents of cementless implants, those with porous-coated surfaces (femoral or acetabular component), that a period without weight bearing after surgery is essential in promoting bone ingrowth. Engh believes that postoperative weight bearing in primary or revision surgery must be individualized based on factors such as "sensation" of tightness of friction fit of the implant during impaction at surgery, the patient's bone quality, and, in particular, the bone density adjacent to the implant, as well as the immediate postoperative x-ray films demonstrating the amount of bone contact.[12] Six weeks of nonweight-bearing toe touch is followed by the use of one crutch for 4 weeks, and an additional 4 weeks using a cane has been recommended. It is natural that standard protocol after the use of cementless devices has not been established, and currently some surgeons believe that postoperative rehabilitation of cementless devices should be similar to that of cemented prostheses. The occurrence of thigh pain in some patients after use of cementless devices remains an unsolved problem that requires postoperative rehabilitation modifications; usually the patients improve when they resume partial weight bearing and the use of crutches.

POSTOPERATIVE LEG LENGTH DISCREPANCY AND SHOE LIFT

Recommendations regarding leg length discrepancies — often a source of complaint from the patient — must be addressed earlier than 3 months after surgery. This lapse of time between surgery and a complete evaluation of leg length discrepancy is necessary to allow the spine to adjust to the new position of the hip joint (thus allowing correction of pelvic tilt resulting from an arthritic condition). In general, the lengthening of an extremity as the result of surgery (an unfortunate complication) is quite disturbing to the patient, but, again, it is possible to rectify this situation if time is allowed for pelvic level adjustment. We have found a small insole lift (¼ inch) and a small heel lift (¼ inch) to be adequate for minor adjustments, but this is rarely necessary if 3 to 6 months are allowed for the lumbar spine to adjust to the leg length after arthroplasty. Patients who have been told before surgery of the possibility that they will need a shoe lift accept this recommendation postoperatively without disappointment.

POSTOPERATIVE ANKLE EDEMA AND SWOLLEN LEG

Patients who sit in a chair with the operated leg down and extended may experience some ankle edema. This often occurs after discharge from the hospital toward the end of the second or third week and results from added periods of sitting out of bed, despite wearing their support stockings. This is usually interpreted as a benign form of postoperative venous compromise caused by blockage of veins and does not require any studies by sonography or other means or special treatment such as anticoagulation therapy. Patients are encouraged to continue walking and other activities, limiting sitting to no more than 10 to 15 minutes at a time. They should be instructed not only to avoid sitting for long periods but to keep the leg elevated while in bed. They should support the foot on a stool while sitting and intermittently extend the knee (every ½ to 1 hour) and flex. In addition they should get into bed frequently with the operated leg elevated on pillows during the first 3 to 4 weeks at home. The ankle should be higher than the knee, the knee higher than the hip, and so on (see Chapter 9).

REMOTE INFECTION AND ANTIBIOTIC COVERAGE

Instructions are necessary regarding the use of prophylactic antibiotic coverage for patients who may develop a source of infection elsewhere. Because of the importance of the possibility of infection of the total hip secondary to a remote source, patients should be advised to remain in touch with their surgeon any time they may risk bacterial infection or surgical manipulation. They are advised to suggest to their family physician (or other medical professionals) that if any infectious lesions (dental, skin, genitourinary, and so on) develop, they should receive prophylactic antibiotics; depending on the source of infection and the type of organism, specific prophylactic antibiotics covering a broad spectrum for both gram-positive and gram-negative organisms have been recommended. During surgery and for genitourinary infections or dental manipulations, patients must receive the appropriate antibiotics in large doses to combat possible bacteremia and the risk that these organisms will seed into the artificial hip joint (see Chapter 8).

SUMMARY OF ESSENTIALS

- The overall postoperative management of the patient uses a team approach headed by the surgeon; equally important are the roles of the medical consultants, physical therapists, and nursing staff. An informed patient (who is instructed properly preoperatively) facilitates the postoperative rehabilitation and recovery program, thereby minimizing complications.

- The initial dressing applied at surgery should remain undisturbed for the first 4 to 5 days. Wounds are not repeatedly examined, and hematomas are not drained at the bedside. Postoperative x-ray evaluation is essential in the recovery room and at the time of the patient's discharge from the hospital. The role of early ambulation in preventing thromboembolic disease and other complications cannot be overemphasized.

- Supportive measures such as blood transfusions, anticoagulation regimens, and handling of medical complications should be coordinated with the surgeon and not left to the discretion of the most junior members of the staff. A standard policy for managing most complications will evolve only in an organized center handling a large number of operations of this type.

- While early ambulation is essential, many patients are too ill from surgical trauma to ambulate the first or second day after surgery. However, on the third or fourth day postoperatively, most patients can begin ambulation. The details of nursing and therapeutic management are vital in preventing postoperative complications. The rehabilitation program must be coordinated by a physical therapist in accordance with the patient's performance and ability rather than a standard formula applied to all patients.

- It is essential that crutch walking, bed-chair transfer, and walking be rehearsed with the patient before surgery to facilitate postoperative recovery. Contrary to the patient's expectations, ambulation does not begin with sitting out of bed. Walking precedes sitting out of bed by at least 1 week.

- The use of a high, raised chair, avoidance of sitting in bed, and avoidance of passive flexion at the hip are necessary to develop a capsule around the artificial joint and further stabilize the hip joint. Excessive early motion within the first 2 weeks is discouraged, but patients who are too slow in gaining motion are to be encouraged to gain mobility.

- Specific physiotherapeutic management includes instruction in deep breathing and coughing, active ankle exercises, instructions regarding bed-to-standing transfer, crutch walking, and abductor-strengthening exercises. During the first postoperative week, isometric exercises, including quadriceps exercises and attempts at straight leg raising, are encouraged. Most patients' ambulation begins with crutches on the third or fourth postoperative day, but an older patient may ambulate with a walker. Weight bearing is resumed as soon as it can be tolerated.

- During the second postoperative week, further muscle strengthening exercises (isometric) in addition to a gait-training program are encouraged. During the second week, the patient is able to sit out of bed using an elevated seat (to avoid extreme flexion of the hip). Stair climbing may begin toward the end of the second week.

- Hospitalization for the third postoperative week is required only of patients who have not achieved complete independence in their rehabilitation and have not demonstrated a total independent transfer from the bed to a standing position and a satisfactory gait. During this period, besides additional gait training, stair climbing, and the like, an exercise program that includes powdered board abduction exercises is incorporated.

- At discharge, a list of dos and don'ts is given to the patient, and the importance of obeying it is emphasized. Basically, the patient is discharged with a program of activities similar to those engaged in during the second and third week of the hospital stay.

- The role of physical therapy in total hip arthroplasty is as much one of psychological as of physical support. (The therapist should express cheerful confidence to the patient and provide reinforcement.) A knowledgeable physical therapist is indispensable in supervising the patient's activities and answering the questions that often worry the patient.

- One area in which the physical therapist is involved concerns managing rheumatoid arthritic patients who have multiple joint involvement requiring physical modalities for joint disabilities other than the hip. Patients with fixed deformities usually need attention similar to that of patients with severe upper extremity involvement.

- One of the most difficult aspects of handling total hip arthroplasty is the psychological outlook of the therapist and the patient regarding improved range of flexion after total hip arthroplasty. Contrary to most conventional arthroplasties—that is, cup arthroplasty and Moore self-locking prosthesis—patients with total hip arthroplasty gain range of motion that is generally related to the preoperative

range of motion. Most patients achieve a 90-degree flexion, which is quite adequate for most daily functional activities, regardless of a regimented exercise program. Early gain in range of flexion to this degree (within the first week) must be avoided because it invites complications such as detachment of the greater trochanter or dislocation. Fixed adduction and external rotation deformity require special attention (specific exercises and management).

- With technical surgical complications (fragmentation of the greater trochanter, instability noted at surgery, etc.) the surgeon should consider modifying the routine postoperative course. The method of rehabilitation must be adjusted to the patient's physiological needs.

REFERENCES

1. **Aufranc OE:** *Constructive surgery of the hip,* St Louis, 1962, Mosby–Year Book.
2. **Aufranc OE:** Preoperative and postoperative treatment of the patient with reconstructive surgery of the hip, *Clin Orthop* 38:40, 1965.
3. **Blume R:** Personal communication.
4. **Charnley J:** Total prosthetic replacement of the hip in relation to physiotherapy. The Founder's Lecture. Annual Congress, Chartered Society of Physiotherapy, Sheffield, England, 1968.
5. **Charnley J:** *Postoperative management of total hip reconstruction by low friction method,* Internal Publication No. 27, England, 1970, Centre for Hip Surgery, Wrightington Hospital.
6. **Charnley J:** *Low-friction arthroplasty of the hip. Theory and practices,* New York, 1979, Springer-Verlag.
7. **Charnley J:** Personal communication.
8. **Eftekhar NS:** Abduction splint for hip surgery, *Orthop Rev* 3:51, 1974.
9. **Eftekhar NS, Stinchfield FE:** Experience with low friction arthroplasty, a statistical review of early results and complications, *Clin Orthop* 95:60, 1973.
10. **Eftekhar NS, Bush DC, Freeman AR, et al:** Perioperative management of total hip replacement, *Orthop Rev* 3:17, 1974.
11. **Ehrlich GE, editor:** *Total management of the arthritic patient,* Philadelphia, 1973, JB Lippincott.
12. **Engh CA, Bobyn JD:** *Biological fixation in total hip arthroplasty,* Thorofare, NJ, 1985, Slack.
13. **Janecki CJ, DeHaven KE, Benton JW:** Preoperative and postoperative management in total hip reconstruction, *Orthop Clin North Am* 4:523, 1973.
14. **Thomas WH:** Postoperative program for patients having cup arthroplasty, *Surg Clin North Am* 49:779, 1969.

See Chapters 8, Prevention of Infection; 9, Prevention of Thromboembolic Complications; 24, Conversion of Failed Previous Surgery; 25, Revision in Absence of Infection; 31, Postoperative Wound Infection; and 32, Dislocation and Instability for additional information.

CHAPTER FOURTEEN

Bone Grafts and Bone Banking

■ It is important to recognize that incorporation is a partnership between recipient's site and the bone graft, each providing unique and indispensable contributions.

Gary E. Friedlander

Bone grafts have been used in surgery for many years after bone loss caused by trauma or disease. Their value in restoring the structural integrity of the host through osteogenic potential, substitution, and incorporation has been recognized for over a century.*

The use of bone grafts in reconstructive hip surgery is designed to serve two functions: (1) to provide a source of osteogenesis; and (2) to serve as a mechanical support. The clinical demand for the use of bone grafts in reconstructive orthopedics is caused by increases in limb salvage procedures, severe trauma, and number of failed total joint arthroplasties. Because biological and mechanical responses between autogenous and allogenic grafts and between cortical and cancellous grafts are vastly different, a full understanding of the biological processes related to these grafts is necessary.

Bone grafts that have been used in reconstructive surgery include autogenous grafts (autografts) – the patient's own tissue, allografts, homografts, xenografts, and heterografts. Because of the availability of allografts and autografts, xenografts are rarely used in practice.

Bovine bone (processed) used in the 1960s and 1970s as a xenograft now is considered unacceptable for clinical use as bone grafts or bone substitutes. Rejection of these grafts (similar to other xenogenic grafts) is marked by severe inflammation, resorption, and sequestration. However, some reports of their clinical use with mixed results have been published.[87,104] Bovine bone no longer is used in the United States.

Although systematic use of bone transplants dates to the early 1800s, many successful results were reported at the turn of the century. Axhausen was the first to report on extensive basic research on histology and incorporation of the bone grafts. He coined the phrase "creeping substitution for mechanism of bone repair."[15] Albee and Lexer are among the early pioneers in the field with extensive experience and documentation of the fate of bone transplants.[1,72] While early work substantiated that bone could successfully be transplanted, the failure rate remained high because of mechanical instability, rejection, and infection. A major breakthrough began in the 1950s as more information regarding the immunogenicity of bone allografts became available.[21,57,59,121] Although autologous bone grafts are commonly used as fresh grafts, the allogenic bone grafts are procured and stored frozen, lyophilized (freeze dried), or chemically sterilized. The storage procedures significantly decrease the immunogenicity of allografts.

The vast amount of research on osteogenic potential repair and remodeling of the bone grafts suggests that the process of incorporation of bone grafts is a predictable sequence of events that is not only unique to the bone graft but also to the recipient bone bed. As such, in the process of incorporation, factors such as mechanical properties of the graft, mechanical stability of the graft, and certain systemic factors may determine the fate of the graft incorporation. All of these factors are poorly understood at this time.[35]

Two aspects of bone graft and repair must be emphasized.

1. A distinction must be made between autologous

---

* References 1, 5, 72, 77, 98, 103.

and allogenic grafts.

2. Cortical-cancellous bones (autogenous grafts or allografts) behave somewhat differently than cancellous bone in revascularization and have different structural strengths.

INCORPORATION OF BONE GRAFTS

Bone remodeling results from an initial phase of activation, which is followed by bone absorption (osteoclastic) and bone formation (osteoblastic) phases.* The biological environment (that is, related immunological factors, humoral controls, and various physical factors such as mechanical stress and electromagnetic fields) may determine the initiation and the rate of incorporation of the grafts.[26,110] See Table 14-1.

To survive, a bone graft must become vascularized. Invariably, bone grafts undergo necrosis, which causes a local inflammatory reaction. After surgery, a hematoma forms (in a process similar to fracture repair), which initiates the subsequent stages for the bone graft to be incorporated to the host bone. The process of graft incorporation involves two additional phases of osteoconduction and osteoinduction, both of which are as necessary as the initial phase of incorporation.[128] Invasion of the bone graft by vascular buds seems essential for both osteoclasis and osteoblastic activities, leading to viability and incorporation of the graft. Although the incorporation is often incomplete, good function is often compatible with partial vascularization of the graft. Delayed or incomplete incorporation of the allograft can result from genetic disparity between the donor and recipient. In practical terms, such biologically incompatible grafts may succeed by their altered immunological state resulting from preparation of the graft.† It is now well recognized that unlike fresh allografts, which are immunologically active and produce severe inflammatory response and absorption, frozen allografts (at $-80°C$) have a markedly decreased immune response.[39,40,49,83] Clearly, deep-freeze and freeze-dried allografts are capable of incorporating to the host bone in a manner similar to that of autogenous bone graft, but at a slower rate, and perhaps less completely.[15,39,57,101]

There are three basic differences in vascularization and repair of cancellous and cortical bone grafts.[15]

1. Cancellous grafts are vascularized more rapidly and completely than cortical grafts.
2. In cancellous bone, creeping substitution includes appositional bone formation followed by a resorptive phase, whereas cortical bone undergoes a reverse process.

---

* References 20, 26, 98, 105, 110.
† References 21, 39, 40, 83, 106.

3. Significantly, cancellous bone grafts tend to repair completely. Cortical grafts do not and the grafted site remains an admixture of dead and living bone.

The various forms of allograft preparation must be weighed against their intended use because each method alters the mechanical properties of the grafts. For example, different forms of preparation produce different degrees of loss of mechanical properties of support and weight bearing for the graft in the acetabulum or femur. Consequently, most grafts used in the acetabulum are simply used as a filler, while in the femur grafts are mostly segmental replacements of the cortical bone.

The immunogenicity of bone is markedly reduced by irradiation or sterilization by ethylene oxide. Demineralization in combination with lyophilization and even autoclaving of bone have been attempted to reduce the immunogenicity of bone allografts.[21,55,102,106]

Factors Influencing Bone Graft Incorporation

Physiological, skeletal, and metabolic factors influence the rate and completeness of bone graft incorporation. Factors that can influence the vascularity or availability of progenitor cells, that is, osteoblastic and osteoclastic cells, may affect the incorporation process. These factors may be local and systemic. Examples of local factors include loss of tissue viability surrounding the recipient site; presence of debris and foreign material; extensive tissue scarring (loss of blood supply); active infection; and osteoporosis. Other local factors, such as poor quality of recipient bone caused by rheumatoid and other conditions, fibrous relacement of bone tissue, or neoplastic bone with accompanying poor blood supply, are deleterious to incorporation of the bone graft to the host bone. Other important local factors are the size, shape, and degree of stability of the graft at the implanted site, which may affect its survival or incorporation. Finally, optimal stress is necessary during revascularization when the mechanical strength of the bone is suboptimal.

Systemic factors include the use of immunosuppressive drugs, a history of radiation to the site of the implantation, and use of myelodepressive drugs or antimetabolic drugs, all of which may affect bone remodeling and incorporation.[41] Antiinflammatory drugs (steroidal and nonsteroidal), diphosphonates, indomethacin, and even certain hormones also adversely affect the outcome of the process of bone formation and incorporation (see Table 14-1).[26]

CELLULAR MORPHOLOGY

As early as 1893, Barth concluded that bone grafts die after removal from the body and that to survive they must be revascularized in the host's bed.[5] Numerous

Table 14-1 Factors Influencing Graft Incorporation

Positive influence	Negative influence
Graft type:	Graft type:
Vascularized	Allografts
Autogenous	Fresh allograft
Graft preparation and	Graft preparation and
preservation:	preservation:
Fresh	Preservatives
Deep freeze	Autoclave
Lyophilization	Small size/large size
Irradiation	
Sterilization	
Optimal size	
Graft vascularization:	Graft vascularization:
Vascular bed	Sclerotic-nonvascular
	bed
Systemic factors:	Systemic factors:
Good health, young age	Poor health, immuno-
	suppression,
	steroids, rheumatoid
	disease, hormones,
	medications
Local factors:	Local factors:
Rigid fixation	Infection, debris,
	necrosis, loose
	fixation
Stress:	Stress:
Optimum stress	Too much
Absence of motion	Too little
	Motion

histological studies of many types of bone grafts have proven this principle to be accurate. Therefore as Friedlander stated, "It is important to recognize that incorporation is a partnership between recipient's site and the bone graft, each providing unique and indispensable contributions."

Extensive histological studies in man and animal indicate that they have similar patterns of bone-graft biology.[57,58] The pattern of cellular events during incorporation of nonvascularized autogenous bone grafts can be summarized in three phases.

Phase I

After initial necrosis of the bone graft (at the site of hematoma), cell death stimulates a localized inflammatory response, leading to formation of a fibrovascular stroma. The newly formed fibrovascular medium provides new vascularity and thus new precursor cells to the graft. This phase lasts about 3 weeks in a dog.

Phase II

In phase II both osteoblastic and osteoclastic activities are present, as are osteoconduction and osteoinduction. The graft provides a scaffolding onto which the bone is deposited (osteoconduction), while graft-derived factors stimulate the recipient to invade the structure with osteogenic activity (osteoinduction).[26] This phase lasts 3 to 12 weeks. It has been suggested that the source of stimulation may be in part cells of the graft or, most certainly, the matrix in the form of bone morphogenic protein.[26,127] During this phase cortical bone absorption is via expansion of preexisting Haversian and Volkmann's canals, by invasion by capillaries.

Phase III

During phase III, remodeling takes place whereby reinforcement of trabeculae leads to a more normal cellular pattern depending on the quantity and pattern of bone strain. This phase of repair in a dog may be complete by 1 year.

AUTOLOGOUS CANCELLOUS AND CORTICAL BONE GRAFTS

There is little controversy that autogenous cancellous bone is the best material for bone grafting because of its potential for healing, the rapidity with which it incorporates, and its reduced immunogenicity. During the first 2 weeks, some of the cells on the graft surface may survive by diffusion.[15,33] The process of revascularization is rapid while the graft is gradually replaced by living bone. Autologous cortical bone exhibits a similar inflammatory response, as does cancellous bone, but the process of revascularization in cortical bone is slow and incomplete. Revascularization begins in the periphery because absorption occurs primarily in the Volkmann and Haversian canals, thus leading to increased bone porosity.[33,57] Although the new Haversian canals are formed, the porosities of the cortical bone may never be completely replaced because the dead bone remains bonded by the new bone. The histology of cortical grafts therefore is a mosaic of the new bone and the old graft bone.

Burchardt[15] and Enneking[33] demonstrated that several major differences exist in incorporation of cancellous and cortical bone grafts. In cortical bone graft, the process of revascularization is slower. The osteoclastic resorption must occur before osteoblastic bone formation, and the cortical bone grafts are not, as a rule, completely substituted by living bone. It is imperative that cortical bone grafts be fixed rigidly and that fixation be maintained for a long time to promote osteosynthesis because of the slow incorporation to the recipient host bone.

ALLOGENIC CANCELLOUS AND CORTICAL BONE GRAFTS

It is well established that both cancellous and cortical allografts show slower vascularization and incorporation to the host bone than autogenous bone grafts. There is a similarity between allografts and autografts, however, in the cellular response process. There is first an inflammatory response (which is very severe for fresh allografts) that is followed by revascularization. It has been observed that new blood vessels penetrate 2 to 3 mm into allografts, although reinforcement occurs from the periphery and the surface of the allograft. The interior of the bone grafts, for the most part, remains avascular. The allografts, which are qualitatively similar to autogenous bone grafts, undergo replacement by creeping substitution but over a much longer period than autogenous bone grafts. A greater portion of the bone remains necrotic than in autogenous bone grafts.

Several studies on the quality of incorporation of allografts are based on radiographs. Radiographs are notoriously inaccurate for determining the incorporation of bone graft.[123] However, an improved technique combining radioisotopes and CAT scanning techniques is now available to study revascularization of the bone grafts.[47] These studies have shown that allograft bone fragments (morcellized bone) and combined cortical-cancellous allografts incorporate between 1 and 2 years. However, some large bulk allografts and failed osteochondral segmental (cortical) allografts may never be incorporated. Kandel and co-workers[65] showed inadequate bone remodeling and incorporation 7 years after implantation in their failed specimens. Approximately 5% of allografts undergo massive osteoclasis, which is thought to be an immunological response leading to rejection of allografts.

Immune Response

It has been estimated[60] that over 200,000 allograft procedures are performed annually in the United States, and this number is rapidly growing. Most of these graft implantations are done without the use of tissue typing and immunosuppressive drugs and evidently, in short and intermediate follow up, are not rejected clinically. Although several animal experiments have demonstrated the value of antigen profile matching, its clinical application in humans has not yet been defined.[9,10] Therefore the most crucial aspect to be elucidated is whether the recipient's immune system recognizes the graft as foreign or self. Substantial evidence indicates that bone allografts induce a different immune response than autogenous grafts.[15,21,39] Although the nature of immune response is not fully understood, bone allografts appear to be influenced by the same immunological factors as other tissues. Burchardt, Enneking, Friedlander, and others have demonstrated that frozen bone is immunogenic by demonstrating cytotoxin antibodies and cell-mediated immunity in allografts.[38,70] According to Friedlander, the tissue antigens recognized

by the recipient are on the surface of the bone marrow cells. The bone matrix itself is less antigenic, although matrix macromolecules are additional antigenic elements in the grafts. Therefore the rejection of bone allografts seems to be cellular in origin rather than humeral, although a humeral component also may play a part. The antigenic cells are all derivatives of mesenchymal precursors, including osteogenic, chondrogenic, fibrogenic, and hemopoietic cells. As stated, fresh allografts are extremely antigenic. This has been thought to be related not entirely to the bone itself, but to plasma, blood cells, and so on. Several types of treatment of allografts have been shown to significantly reduce their antigenicity. These include boiling of the graft, freezing, lyophilization, sterilization, irradiation, and antigen extraction.

Reduction of Antigenicity of the Grafts
Boiling, Deproteinization, and Decalcification

Clinical reports indicate isolated instances of excellent results after the use of boiled allografts and xenografts.[44,74] Generally these grafts have poor ability to incorporate, since boiling has destroyed the induction repair capacity.[15] Boiling also denatures the bone collagen and coagulates the Haversian canals, thus impeding revascularization and the normal repair process.[15,31]

Deproteinization of the bone by chemical agents has resulted in various divergent conclusions regarding its antigenicity, but often agreeable conclusions on considerable mechanical weakening of the grafts.[4,58,61]

Several investigators, who used decalcified bone under different conditions, agreed that organic decalcified bone grafts healed bone defects better than inorganic grafts.[13,58,126] Bone grafts treated by merthiolate in both laboratory and clinical settings have been associated with a higher failure rate and poor healing because of inferior osteogenesis.[7]

Irradiation

Irradiating the grafts has two purposes: to sterilize the bone and to destroy the antigens. Irradiation is highly desirable because of its potential to eradicate all viruses and bacteria. However, the high megarads required for sterilization destroy the inductive and mechanical properties of the bone graft[12] because they affect the collagen solubility and damage the bone matrix.[31,127] The required level of radiation for sterilization is 2 to 3 megarads.[127]

Freezing

Since frozen allografts (also known as *fresh frozen*) have been shown to reduce antigenicity, they have been used extensively in orthopaedic reconstructive procedures and fracture repair. However these grafts (both clinically and in laboratory studies) have been shown to retain some antigenicity.[15] The intensity of cellular reaction after freezing is much less than with fresh allografts. In clinical practice, varying degrees of success with large frozen allografts have been cited, ranging from 20% by Imamaliev[63] to just over 50%.[82,84,96,99] Mankin and co-workers, in a study of 76 patients with 79 allografts, concluded that 76% had excellent or good results and 24% had failed. In the long term, failures were caused by fractures, nonunions, and graft absorptions. The rate of infection in their experience was 14%. The main advantage of freezing allografts is long-term preservation for bone banking and sufficient time to allow for donor screening for bacterial and viral contaminations.

Freeze-Drying (Lyophilization)

Freezing allografts in liquid nitrogen at $-170°$ C eliminates all molecular motion, thus allowing indefinite storage time. Freeze-drying, like freezing of allografts, decreases antigenicity.[78,80,81] However, lyophilization alters the biomechanical strength of the graft, and it is also expensive. Only a few bone banks can afford to produce and lyophilize bone for general use. The antigenicity of the graft after lyophilization is reduced despite the presence of plasma and blood cells, which remain chemically and electrophoretically stable after lyophilization for many years. Despite clinical success with lyophilized allografts, recipients developed donor graft–specific anti–human leukocyte antigen (HLA) antibodies.[37] Long-term results of lyophilized allografts suggest that the complications, such as fatigue fracture, nonunion or delayed host-graft union, and occasional complete resorption of the graft, may be similar to those found in frozen bone allografts.[15–19]

Chemical Treatment

Because of potential autolysis resulting from storage of bone grafts and allergic and toxic side effects, the use of chemicals for sterilization and antigenic suppression has been limited.[119]

Tissue Typing

If the assumption is correct that late failure of large grafts (especially allografts) is caused by tissue incompatibility, it would be logical that tissue typing might enhance the long-range results of massive allografts and osteochondral grafts.

The degree of histocompatibility and the value of practical application of HLA-matching in bone transplantations is a subject for future basic research. At present, several studies indicate that a gross mismatching between the host and the donor may increase the incidence of graft failure.[9,10,46,91]

As mentioned earlier, at present neither antigen

screening nor precise tissue-typing techniques are used in allograft transplantation. A prospective study by Friedlander and associates[40] did not demonstrate any deleterious affects caused by host sensitivity to the graft antigen. Studies involving larger samples with longer follow up are needed to better define the HLA-matching concerning the rate of union, incorporation of the graft, absorption, and other parameters in bone grafts.

Immunosuppression

An interesting aspect of the antigen-antibody response to bone grafts has been the attempt to administer immunosuppressive drugs to reduce immune response. The beneficial effects of immunosuppression have been investigated. According to Burchardt and co-workers,[17,18] the mechanism of incorporation of the cortical bone may call for an immunosuppressed host. In addition to having immunosuppression effects, the repair process of allografts resembles that of autografts in experiments. The long-term side effects of immunosuppressive durgs and the lack of clinical experience do not warrant their use in conjunction with the use of allografts at the present time.

BONE BANKING

The first practice of bone banking for subsequent use has been attributed to MacEwen,[77] who saved the bones removed from the osteotomy sites of children with tibial deformities and used them to replace a missing portion of a humerus of a child in 1881. With more demand for reconstruction of skeletal tissue, bone and cartilage banking expanded rapidly throughout the world.*

Regional tissue banking was established in the United States as early as the 1950s.[117] Throughout the world, the use of banked bone for major limb-saving procedures and other complex segmental bone reconstructions was introduced.†

Currently 600 tissue banks have been established in the United States. With increasing need for donor tissues and enactment of routine donor inquiry legislation by most states, the banks are better supplied and the bone-banking industry has become better defined. Despite the expansion of bone banking, the demand for certain types of tissue is greater than the supply. Since the formation of the American Association of Tissue Banks in 1975, a set of quality and safety standards has been enforced and donor screening criteria have been established. Tissue donation and banking are beyond the scope of this book, but it should be emphasized that the surgeon's familiarity with the "source of bone"—

* References 22, 62, 64, 68, 133.

† References 10, 36, 67, 84, 97, 99.

where the bone has been sterilized, stored, and processed—is of fundamental importance.

Until recently, most hospitals operated a small bone bank with a simple registry. Limited information was gathered on bone donors. The retrieved bones were mainly femoral heads removed during primary total hip arthroplasty. However, because of fear of human immunodeficiency virus (HIV) transmission, most hospitals now acquire the bone from major commercial or voluntary suppliers.

A good bone bank should expeditiously supply any size or shape graft. Quality control based on the guidelines set by the American Association of Tissue Banks must be strictly followed. The donor's medical history and circumstances related to the death must be reviewed. Any systemic infection or contamination of tissue should eliminate the use of the graft.

Retrieved specimens must be cultured appropriately. Blood and body fluids should be cultured for aerobic and anaerobic organisms. Serological tests for syphilis, hepatitis, and HIV should be routine. Repeated testing of living donors such as in the case of femoral head or ribs 90 to 180 days after donation is also indicated to identify those with latency window[118,124] or HIV.[3,108] Patients with neoplasms or those who use steroids or toxic substances are also excluded.

Graft sterility must be guaranteed. Retrieved nonsterile grafts must be sterilized by irradiation or gas. Because of their longer shelf life, lyophilized allografts are advantageous compared to frozen allografts. From a mechanical properties standpoint, however, they are inferior to the frozen grafts. Retrieved bone is either from deceased or from living donors. The requirements regarding acquisition of history and donor screening tests are basically the same for living and deceased donors. Tests for infection are included as outlined previously. Retrieval of specimens from donated bodies is ideally carried out under sterile conditions similar to a surgical procedure. However, it is permissible to retrieve specimens cleanly but not under operating conditions and to subsequently sterilize the specimens by use of chemicals such as ethylenoxide, strong acids, alcohol, or thimorsal.[35,40] When radiation is chosen for sterilization, a dose of 1 to 2.5 megarads is effective against most bacteria and some viruses. However, as stated previously, the mechanical properties of the graft are adversely affected by the use of more than 3 megarads. Further, because methods of sterilization may fail to ultimately eliminate all pathogens, it is essential that the donor-selection process remain fundamentally sound. The same vigorous methods for donor selection and the procedures regarding sterility must be adhered to during procurement of samples such as femoral heads and ribs during the surgical procedures.

Grafts kept at -70 to $-80°$ C can be safely stored for months and even years because of the absence of enzyme activities.[34] On the other hand, lyophilized grafts can be stored at room temperature for an indefinite period, providing the residual moisture of lyophilized bone is within 3% to 5% and the bone is stored in an evacuated sealed container.[78] For further details on tissue banking, see a recent publication of the American Academy of Orthopaedic Surgeons.[36]

Procurement and Storage of Femoral Heads

With the increasing number of revisions and the expense and scarcity of the femoral bone allografts, surgeons doing revision surgery frequently are well advised to consider banking femoral heads during primary total hip arthroplasty. Procurement storage is done under sterile conditions during the surgical procedure, does not require any elaborate equipment or personnel,[120] and is economically feasible.[32] A large number of these grafts can be stored because primary total hip arthroplasty is frequently performed. The age of the patient should not be a factor, but the diagnosis is. For example, osteoarthritic patients and patients with a fractured neck of the femur are good donors unless extremely osteoporotic. Inflammatory arthritis and AVN heads are excluded for their poor quality. Patients should be carefully screened for a history of venereal disease, HIV, or other infectious processes. Patients are asked for permission to donate their femoral heads.

At surgery, the retrieved femoral head is cultured by the surgeon and placed in a sterile jar labeled with the donor's name and unit number, surgeon's name, and date. The specimen is then placed in a freezer where the temperature is maintained at $-80°$ C. A freezer of 7 cubic feet (0.2 cubic meter) is recommended to be equipped with an alarm that sounds if the temperature rises or falls 10° C from $-80°$ C. If the result of culture is negative, the specimen is registered in the femoral head bone bank inventory along with the size of the head, the surgeon's name (who provided the graft), laboratory reports of cultures, and the patient's blood type. If the culture report is positive, the specimen is discarded. When using a banked head, the head is again cultured and soaked in an antibiotic solution of 500,000 units bacitracin and 500,000 units polymyxin B in Ringer's solution until it is used. The donor's name and a charge slip (submitted to the Accounting Department of the hospital) must be included in the recipient's records. During the past 20 years, at our hospital, our nursing staff has managed our small bone bank, which also has contributed not only to the hip surgeons for revision surgery but also to the other surgeons in the hospital. Because of the HIV epidemic

Steps in Procurement of Bone Grafts and Storage

Before Surgery

- Obtain written consent from patient to donate bone.
- Obtain health histories from patients (Fig. 14-1).
- Draw blood samples for required tests including HIV and hepatitis.
- Inform bone bank personnel that bone will be ready to be picked up.

At Surgery

- Open the surgical bone-collect kit. Fill the blood tubes with the donor's blood before administering any blood products.
- Open the second nonpermeable wrapping on the sterile field, making sure that the sterility of the kit has been maintained (the strip has not changed color).

The Surgeon

- Obtain a small bone chip containing marrow, and place it in a thioglycolate tube held by the circulating nurse.
- Obtain culture swabs from the entire bone surface.
- Place the donor bone in the small inner jar, and screw on the lid. Place the small jar in the larger outer jar, and screw the lid tightly.
- The scrub nurse hands the bone jars to the circulating nurse.
- The circulating nurse checks and identifies the bone jar and blood tube labels for accuracy.
- Send the specimen to the Red Cross at the earliest possible time for storage, or store it in the hospital bone bank refrigerator.

and the need for more stringent bookkeeping, our bone bank now operates in collaboration with the Red Cross using the established protocol (see box).

The American Red Cross will store the bone grafts and supply them to the physician on request after a "window period" of approximately 6 months after a history and a blood test for HIV are repeated.

The shape and approximate size of bone grafts supplied by the American Red Cross transplant service are shown in Fig. 14-2, A. Clinical examples of bone graft used in hip surgery are shown in Fig. 14-2, B.

BIOMECHANICAL BEHAVIOR OF BONE GRAFTS

Bone grafts, regardless of the origin or type, have diminished biomechanical properties compared to similar viable bone. The biomechanical properties of bone are adversely affected by sterilization, preservation, deep freezing, lyophilization, and irradiation.*

---
* References 15, 66, 101, 102, 125.

The mechanical strength of cancellous and cortical grafts depends on the reparative process because the cancellous grafts tend to strengthen first whereas cortical grafts weaken.[15] Although deep freezing does not alter the mechanical strength of allografts, lyophilization reduces the torsional and flexural strengths of the graft without affecting the compressive or tensile strengths. A combination of lyophilization and irradiation significantly reduces both the compressive and the torsional strength of allografts.[66,134]

CLINICAL APPLICATION AND RESULTS

Bone grafts are used to reconstruct the femur or acetabulum in both primary and revision surgery. Bone grafts serve a dual function, providing mechanical support for the prosthesis and promoting osteogenesis. The following clinical situations often require bone augmentation:

- Acetabular reconstruction using a fixed socket (cemented or cementless).
- Acetabular reconstruction using bipolar prosthesis.
- Acetabular reconstruction in revision surgery.
- Two-stage acetabular reconstruction.
- En-bloc acetabular allograft replacement.
- Bone graft femoral deficiencies.
- Femoral allograft prosthetic composites.

Acetabular Bone Grafts

Acetabular bone grafts are commonly used for primary protrusio acetabuli or protrusio acetabuli prosthetica (see Chapters 22 and 25). As noted, autogenous bone grafts are readily available and ideal for reconstruction of protrusio acetabuli. The femoral head (bone in osteoarthritis and rheumatoid arthritis) can be shaped and used as a solid or made into the bone chips.

In most revision surgery, bone chips are adequate for cavitary defects, but for extensive defects a combination of slabs and chips is used. Femoral head allografts are most suitable for this procedure. One or two femoral head allografts may be needed in most revisions. I prefer to use autogenous iliac bone grafts mixed with allografts whenever available.

In severely bone-deficient acetabula, segmental defects are best handled by using appropriately shaped and sized solid bone autografts or allografts, which may or may not be fixed to the host bone (see Chapters 24 and 25). The choice of cement or porous-coated noncemented devices is based primarily on the patient's age, gender, availability of host bone for contact with porous-coated surfaces, and the ability of the cup to achieve a good initial fixation. In general, one attempts to avoid using cement in a failed cemented device in young and active male patients whose bone stock shows contact of at least 50% of the porous surface with the cup.

American Red Cross

Bone Bank Use Only		Place Bar-Coded Label Here
Donor No.	**SURGICAL BONE COLLECTION PROGRAM**	

Patient Name	Date of Health History
Patient Address	Social Security Number
Hospital	Patient Hospital Number
Admitting Diagnosis/Physician	Date of Birth
Date/Time of Bone Collection_____	Sex_____M_____F
Type of Tissue Collected_____	Surgical Procedure_____

I have read and I understand the brochure *Give a Little Something of Yourself.*

I have deferred myself from donating my bone if I feel I fall into any of the high-risk categories specified in the brochure *Give a Little Something of Yourself.*

I understand the procedure that will be used to collect the bone removed during the scheduled surgical procedure, and I understand that there are **NO** additional risks for me because of this collection, outside the risks involved in the scheduled surgery itself.

I understand that a blood sample will be drawn prior to my scheduled surgery to test for hepatitis B, syphilis, and HIV antibodies (an indicator of past exposure to the AIDS virus).

I understand that my attending physician and I will be notified directly and confidentially by the American Red Cross if any of the blood tests are positive.

I have been asked questions concerning my present and past health to detect diseases that could be transmitted through donated bone, and I have answered each question accurately.

I understand that my bone may be used for transplantation purposes. If my bone is not used for transplantation, it may be used for research or discarded.

I voluntarily donate my bone to the American Red Cross for any of these purposes.

Signature of Patient	Signature of Witness	Date

HEALTH HISTORY QUESTIONS

	YES	NO		YES	NO
1. Have you ever...			6. Have you been to Haiti or Central Africa since 1977?	___	___
(a) had yellow jaundice/liver disease?	___	___	7. Have you ever ...		
(b) had hepatitis or a positive test for hepatitis?	___	___	(a) had a blood disease or cancer?	___	___
(c) been exposed to anyone with AIDS or a positive HTLVIII antibody test?	___	___	(b) had a slow virus such as rabies or Creutzfeldt-Jacob disease?	___	___
(d) had a biopsy?	___	___	(c) had an autoimmune disease such as rheumatoid arthritis, systemic lupus erythematosus, sarcoidosis, polyarteritis nodosa, or multiple sclerosis?	___	___
2. Have you ever taken self-injected drugs?	___	___	(d) had an infectious disease such as meningitis, encephalitis, syphilis, or TB?	___	___
3. In the past six months, have you ...			(e) had radiotherapy, such as cobalt?	___	___
(a) received any blood transfusions, blood injections, or tattoos?	___	___	(f) been exposed to toxic substances, such as gold, lead, fluoride, mercury, or dioxin?	___	___
(b) been exposed to anyone with yellow jaundice or hepatitis or to someone on a kidney machine?	___	___	8. Have you ever had night sweats; unexplained fever or weight loss; lumps in the neck, armpits, or groin; discolored areas of the skin or the mouth (bluish-purple or white); persistent cough or shortness of breath; persistent diarrhea?	___	___
(c) been hospitalized?	___	___			
(d) taken any medications, such as antibiotics or steroids?	___	___			
(e) had surgery?	___	___			
4. Have you ever had malaria?	___	___			
5. In the past three years, have you traveled outside the United States?	___	___			

REMARKS: _____

_____

_____

_____

_____

ACCEPTED_____   DEFERRED_____

Signature of Health Historian_____Date_____

Fig. 14-1. American Red Cross bone donor health history form for Surgical Bone Collection Program. (From the American Red Cross.)

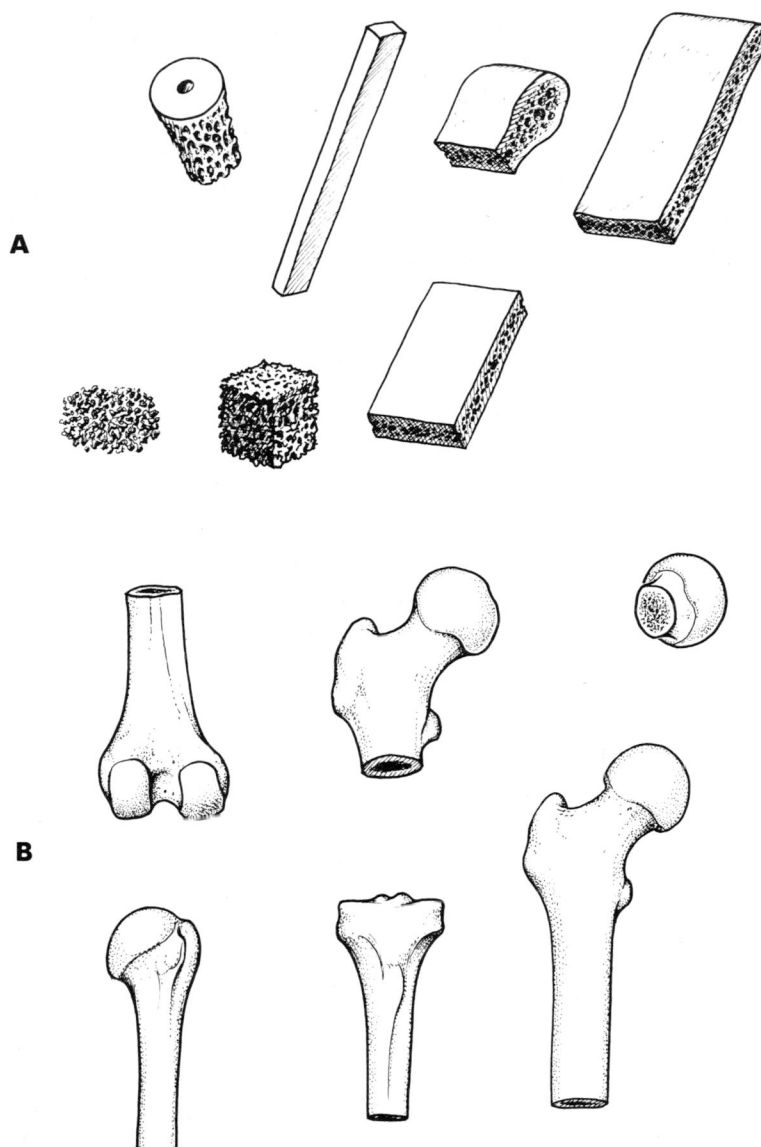

Fig. 14-2. Bone grafts of various sizes and shapes are available commercially. **A,** These grafts are used to fill bony defects and are best used when mixed with autogenous bone grafts. **B,** Denuded segments of bone can be obtained from a central bone bank. Femoral head allografts are the most commonly used and available. An order for allografts should include a radiograph with known magnification.

Augmentation of Acetabular Deficiencies (Autografts)

Harris and associates described the use of autogenous femoral heads for reconstruction of severely dysplastic hips.[52,54] A 5- to 7-year follow-up study of the experience was reported by Gerber and Harris[45]; all grafts united but five hips failed (approximately 10%) and required reoperation (four for aseptic loosening and one for infection). Six additional sockets (15%) were also radiographically loose, with an additional 10% dislocated. Despite a high rate of complication, patients considered the procedure justifiable and rewarding 5 years later.[45] Mulroy and Harris[89] reported on the same series with an average follow up of 11.8 years.

Nine hips (20%) had failed, requiring a second operation, two had resection arthroplasties, seven needed complex revision arthroplasties, and an additional infected hip required resection operation. Definite acetabular loosening was observed in the remaining 12 of 36 hips. Thus, definite acetabular loosening was observed in 20 (46%) of 44 hips. This study may be significant since the authors used large cortical/cancellous autografts. The failure may have been time-dependent; the first sign of a definite loosening was noted 6.4 years after the index operation.[89] It should be emphasized, however, that the operations in this series studied by Mulroy were done for severe acetabular deformities for which no alternative procedure had been available except resection pseudarthrosis. The bone graft reconstruction remains today the only solution for this difficult problem of severely dysplastic hips (see Chapter 20).[45,53,54]

Acetabular Augmentation by Allograft

Superolateral acetabular bone grafts for minor acetabular deficiencies of up to one third are commonly used, and the results of such bone grafts, autografts, or allografts are good in the short-to-intermediate range.[23,79,113] Generally, these grafts do not significantly contribute to load transfer, and they are small in size; both factors may contribute to their survival and their clinical success.

Acetabular reconstruction using allografts is relatively recent. During revision surgery, segmental defects often require reconstruction. The cortical/cancellous bone grafts (usually femoral heads) are used for their geometric adaptability and availability (Figs. 14-3 to 14-5).

The early results of their use are satisfactory. In a study of 13 hips with augmented acetabular deficiency resulting from failed previous surgery, Harris found no failure at an average follow up at 17 months (range 6 to 36 months).[51] Again, at follow up of 3.9 years in 29 hips, Harris and associates reported 10% failures requiring further corrective surgery. It was thought that the union of the previous grafts was beneficial for support during reoperation. In another study, Trancik and associates reported on the fate of 17 hips receiving allografts at revision surgery[123] and followed for 2 to 5 years (with an average follow up of 3.5 years). Two had progressive radiolucency and one remodeling by stress shielding, with evidence of definite loosening in one. Good short-term results with allografts of various sizes and combinations have been reported by Gross,[48] Borja and Mnaymneh,[8] Cameron,[23] and Samuelson.[115] Protrusio and other cavitary and segmental acetabular defects are treated by filling the defects with chips (obtained from the femoral head) using the reamers for impaction (Fig. 14-6).

Solid bone grafts of suitable sizes may be shaped conveniently from femoral head grafts (Figs. 14-7 and 14-8) and used in acetabular medial wall defects with or without protrusion.

Bone Grafts with Bipolar Prosthesis

In the 1960s, bone grafts were used in conjunction with an Austin-Moore prosthesis to augment acetabular defects associated with protrusio acetabuli. Although early reports were encouraging, late failures were common and were attributed to the graft absorption and secondary acetabular wear and pain with migration. With the recent popularity of the bipolar prosthesis[6] for fracture fixation, it has been suggested (at least theoretically) that the procedure may reduce acetabular stress and friction and thereby diminish acetabular cartilage wear. Murray[90] reported on the use of bipolar prosthesis for salvage of acetabular insufficiency in conjunction with bone grafts. The prime indication was massive loss of bone stock that precluded the possibility of a fixed socket. The large

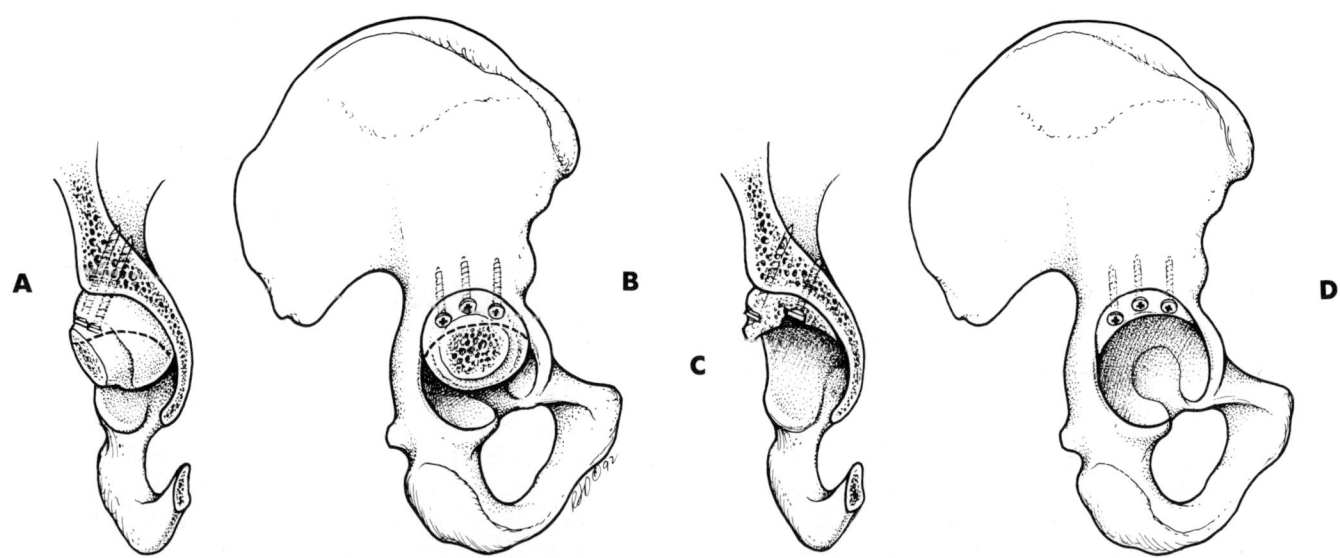

Fig. 14-3. A, Femoral head can be fitted and fixed onto defect for superior acetabular bone deficiency. **B,** Excess bone (allograft or autograft) is excised. **C** and **D,** Intraarticular bone grafts *(solid)* can be fixed to the defects. NOTE: countersinking of the screw is necessary.

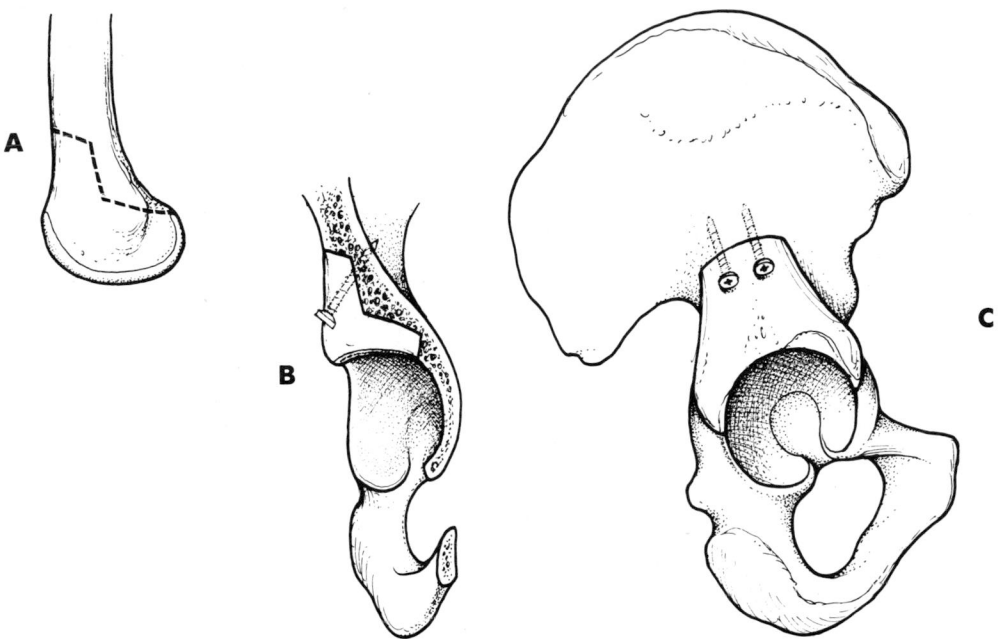

Fig. 14-4. A, Distal femoral allograft may be used to replace a large acetabular bone defect. **B** and **C,** Allograft provides a rim and superior segmental replacement.

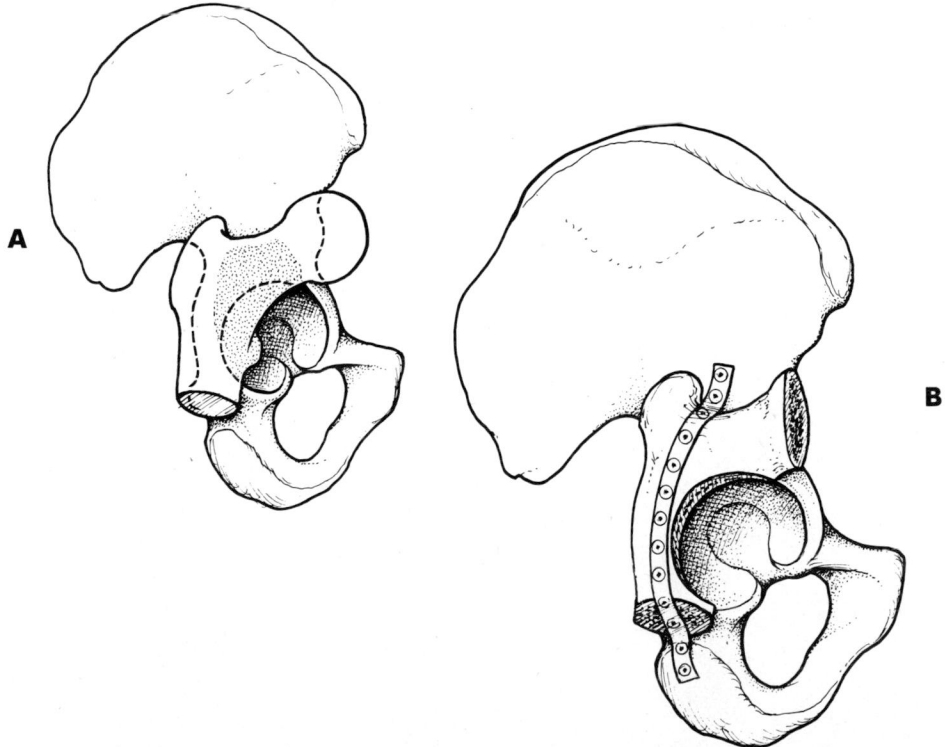

Fig. 14-5. A, Proximal femoral allograft must be firmly fixed to pelvis for a more severe acetabular deficiency. **B,** Long, malleable plate fixes the allograft to the patient's pelvis. Excess bone is removed (this method is technically demanding).

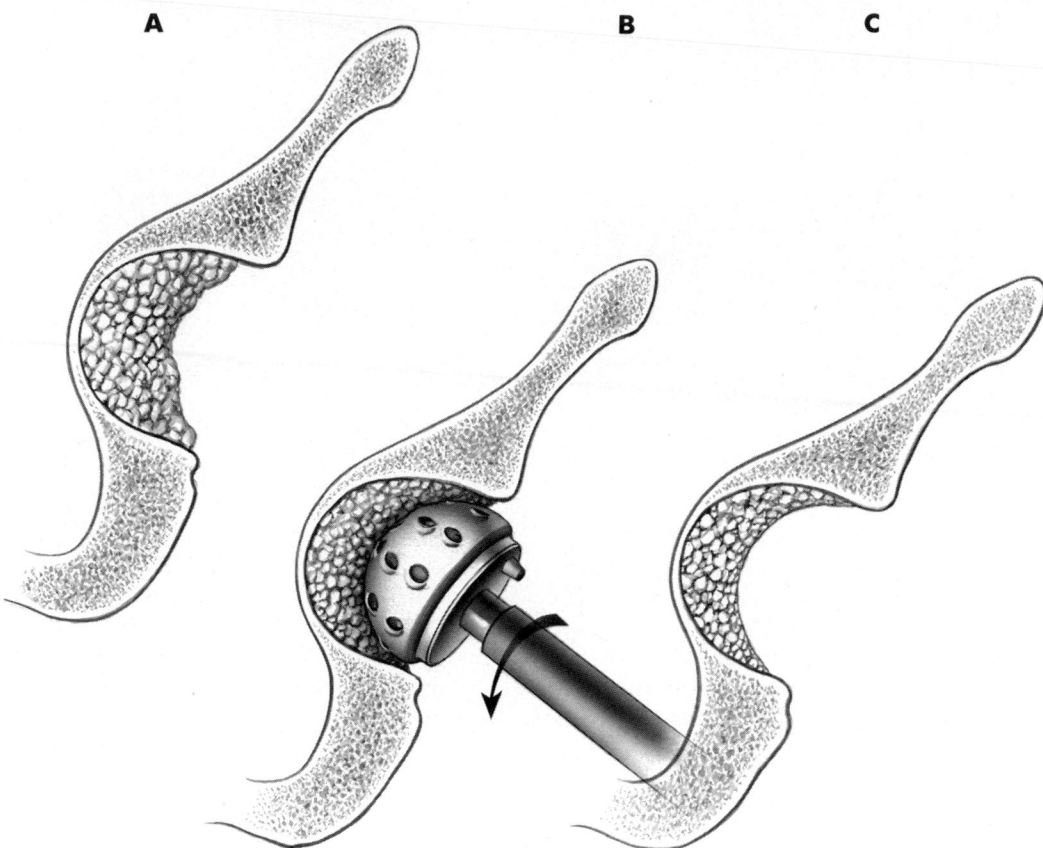

Fig. 14-6. Cavitary and segmental defects in the acetabulum may be treated by bone chips produced from femoral heads (allografts or autografts). **A,** Bone chips packed manually into acetabular cavity. **B,** Debris-retaining reamer is placed onto the graft and turned only briefly (five to six turns) in a reverse mode to impact the bone graft into the cavities. **C,** Prepared bed before insertion of acetabular component.

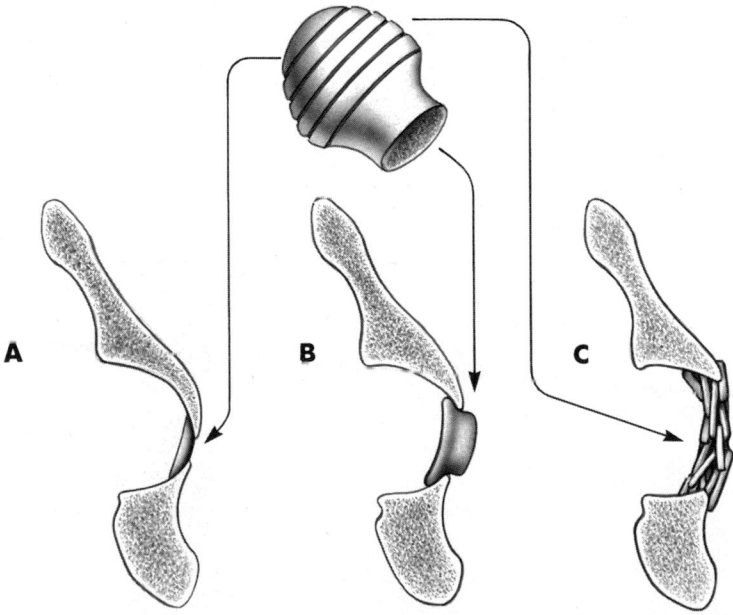

Fig. 14-7. Without a severe protrusio acetabuli, bony defects of medial wall may be treated by different shapes and sizes of bone grafts obtained from a femoral head. **A,** Slice of femoral head. **B,** Champagne-cork shape. **C,** Multiple slices and struts.

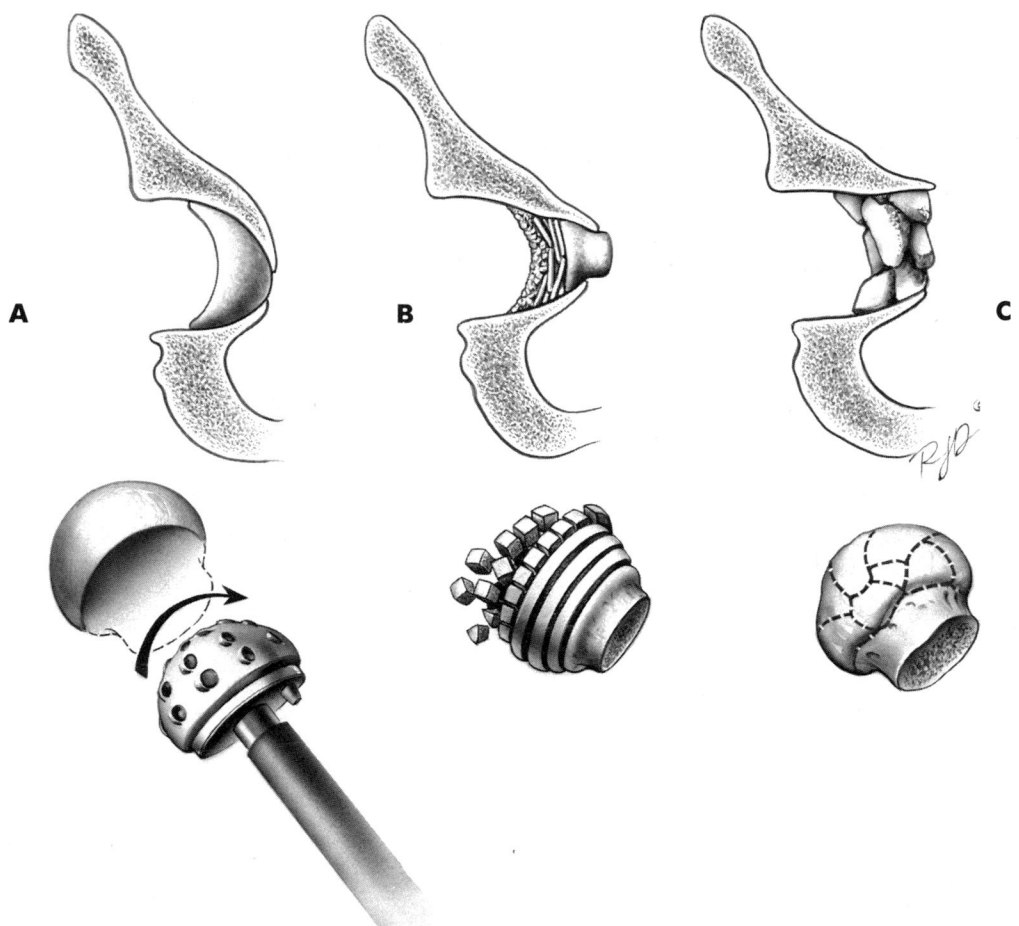

Fig. 14-8. With severe protrusio acetabuli, grafts may be used in greater bulk and in combinations of various forms. The following graft preparations are illustrated: **A,** Slice of head is being prepared; **B,** Combination of grafts; and **C,** Packing of bone grafts for a two-stage replacement (see Chapter 25).

acctabular cavity was filled with crushed bone, and a large bipolar prosthesis was used. In this technique, morcellized frozen femoral allograft bone fills the cavity as the reamers, in reverse mode, mold and impact the allograft into a hemispherical shape. An intact acetabular rim is considered essential in transferring the load to the acetabulum, which in turn will reduce excess stress transfer to the graft. A tight rim fit is regarded as the key to success. Therefore preoperative templating is recommended, although the final selection of the cup size must be determined at surgery. It must be emphasized that the surgeon must avoid over-zealous packing of too much bone so that the cup is lateralized excessively. The cup must be contained and tightly fit inside the acetabular rim with maximum stability.

The patient should be kept nonweight bearing for 3 to 6 months until radiographs show evidence of graft incorporation. The early results of this procedure have met with mixed reviews. Reasonably good early function and pain relief have been reported, but as one might expect, a superior and medial migration of the prosthesis occurs in most instances after 2 years.[93] In a study of 19 hips, Scott and associates[116] observed eight hips with no progressive migration but eleven had some detectable early migration. Two additional cases also showed evidence of progressive migration, which was attributed to poor contact and medial wall defects. Other studies provide grounds for cautious early optimism.[24,114,122,132]

Wilson and co-workers recently reviewed radiographs of 32 hips of 31 patients to establish the fate of acetabular bone grafts used in conjunction with bipolar prosthesis after failed total hip arthroplasty. The grafts used were solid and crushed bone. The acetabular defects were categorized as periacetabular or rim defects and their severity as contained or noncontained (depending on the integrity of the medial acetabular wall). In their study, central contained solid grafts had less resorption than comparable crushed bone grafts and less socket migration. The grafts that were not contained (medial or peripheral) showed the highest absorption and acetabular socket migration.[132] In a study by Allan[2] there was also a definite progressive bone loss in the proximal and medial direction with the use of bipolar components.

From the bulk of the literature and the author's experience, the author concludes the following:

1. A "floating cup" that is a bipolar prosthesis has limited use on conjunction with bone grafts in severely migrated failed prostheses.
2. A fixed cup and bone grafts produce the best results. A bipolar prosthesis should not be used as an alternative to a fixed cup.
3. Some degree of migration with a bipolar prosthesis and bone grafts is to be expected (in a majority of cases). Recurrence of symptoms requires revision surgery. The best results are achieved when the acetabular rim is intact and a large prosthesis is used (Fig. 14-9).
4. The combination of a bipolar prosthesis and bone grafts should be limited to acetabuli that demon-

strate such a severe bone loss that a fixed cup (with or without cement) is not feasible.
5. A bipolar prosthesis and bone grafts should be regarded as an alternative to resection pseudoarthrosis for a failed total hip arthroplasty in the absence of infection.
6. Further clinical studies are needed to redefine the indications for the use of bipolar prostheses and bone grafts.

Massive Solid Bone Grafts to the Acetabulum

Severe acetabular destruction after trauma, severe injuries, repeated surgery, and failed total hip arthroplasty has been treated in the past by hemipelvectomy. Such an operation is devastating to the patient; physiologically and physically the functional results are unacceptable. It should be recommended only as a life-saving measure.[88] Resection of pelvic tumors has resulted in severe disability but if feasible is superior to hemipelvectomy.[25,92] Isolated reports pertaining to arthrodesis of the femur to the remaining pelvis after

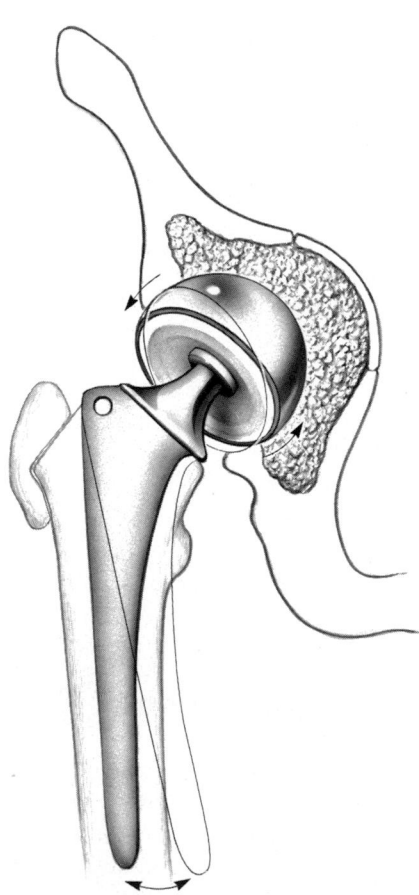

Fig. 14-9. Fixation of the acetabular component may not be possible with severely damaged acetabulum (combined cavitary and segmental defect); thus, a bipolar prosthesis may be used. The bipolar prosthesis may be placed directly onto the bone grafts, filling the acetabular cavity. The prosthesis must be large enough to transfer the load to the rim of the acetabulum.

major pelvic resection or failed total hip arthroplasty are fraught with failure, poor clinical function, and lengthy rehabilitation. Reconstruction by allograft-prosthesis has been suggested as a good alternative to hemipelvectomy and other salvage procedures.[50] CAT scanning and MRI have made the resection of tumors more effective and easier. Guest and associates reported that in a series of ten patients with periacetabular sarcomas treated by an allograft composite, three had recurrence of tumor, one of which was salvaged with repeated surgery. Hip dislocation occurred immediately postoperatively in four of ten patients; one required reoperation. Six of nine hips had a satisfactory outcome with a follow up of 7 to 85 months (median = 18 months). Two patients died as a result of their disease at 8 and 12 months follow up.

Langlais reported satisfactory results with allograft-prosthetic reconstruction in four patients with malignancy with a mean follow up of 19 months.[71] Allen and associates[2] reported on a large series of allografts used in revision total hip arthroplasty between 1978 and 1989. They used 263 solid fragments and 110 morcellized allografts in 176 revision operations. Twenty-two procedures used minor column allografts (shelf), and 28 procedures required major column acetabular allografts. The results of both major and minor allografts were generally acceptable. For example, with follow up of 36 months (range: 24 to 71 months), the overall success of major column allografts was 71% (20 of 28 procedures).

Fig. 14-10 demonstrates a properly shaped massive acetabular allograft fixed to the host bone before and after implantation of the acetabular component. Figs. 14-11 to 14-15 are examples of various bone grafts used in clinical practice. For an example of a solid acetabular bone graft, see Fig. 14-20.

Femoral Allograft-Prosthetic Composites

Massive bone loss of the proximal femur caused by benign or malignant tumors and failed revision surgery associated with severe bone loss require replacement that can be done by either an all-metal proximal femoral replacement or an allograft-prosthetic composite (Fig. 14-16). Allen,[2] Mankin,[85] Head,[56] and others have reported good early results with proximal femoral-prosthetic composites in a relatively small number of cases with relatively short-term follow up. Of more than 500 allografts used to manage bone tumors at the Massachusetts General Hospital between 1971 and 1989,[85] 38 included proximal femoral allografts. Mankin believes that results of bone grafts based on survivorship are encouraging in that patients appear to do well if infection and fracture can be avoided; more than 80% of patients did well by any standard of analysis.

Text continued on p. 627.

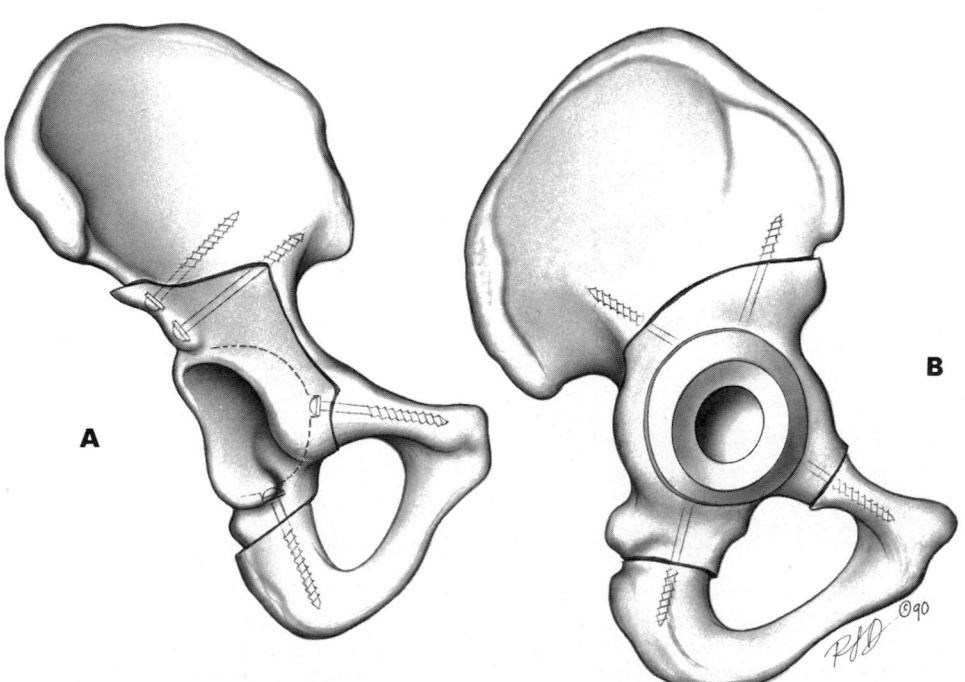

Fig. 14-10. A, Properly shaped and sized bulk acetabular allograft fixed to host bone with partially threaded screws. **B,** After implantation of the prosthesis.

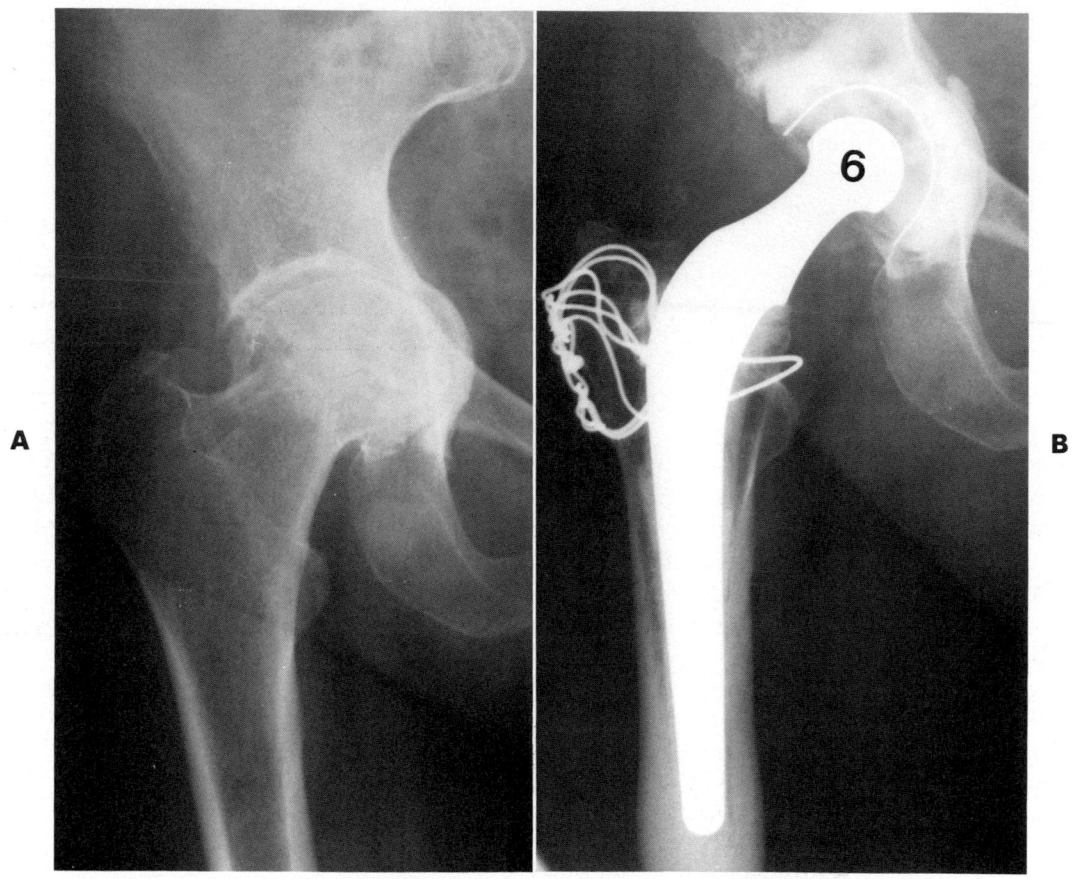

Fig. 14-11. An example of a contained bone graft in primary surgery is shown. **A,** Radiograph of 59-year-old female (M.B.) with unilateral protrusio acetabuli. **B,** Radiograph 6 years after use of autologous bone graft (femoral head) to lateralize socket. Preoperative grade 2,3,1. Postoperative grade 6,6,6.

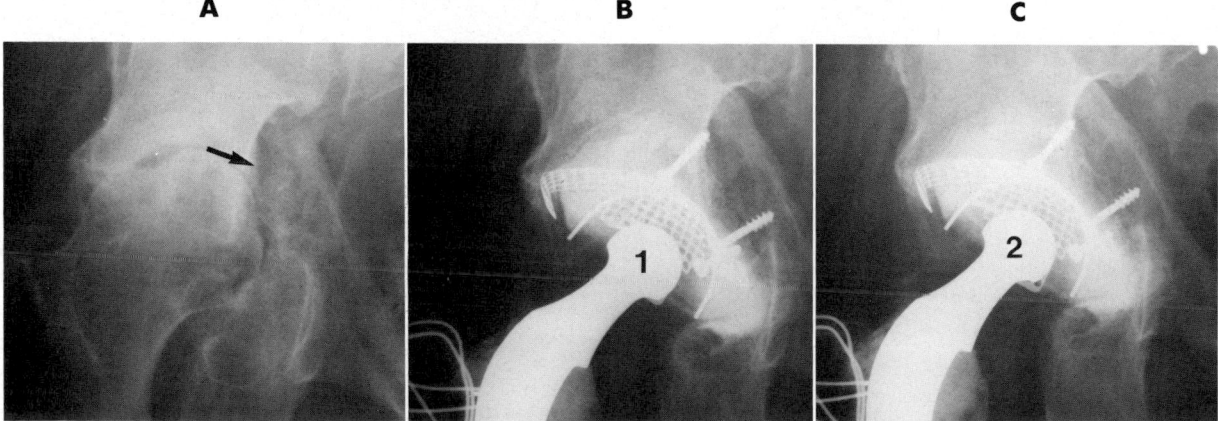

Fig. 14-12. A, 60-year-old man (A.P.) developed double-column pelvic fracture with subsequent nonunion and osteoarthritis. **B,** 1 year after arthroplasty and use of autologous bone graft to repair nonunion. The grafts were fixed to the pelvis from within the acetabulum using partially threaded screws. NOTE: union has occurred at 1 year. **C,** 2 years after surgery, excellent remodeling of bone in periacetabular region is established. Grade: A-6,6,6.

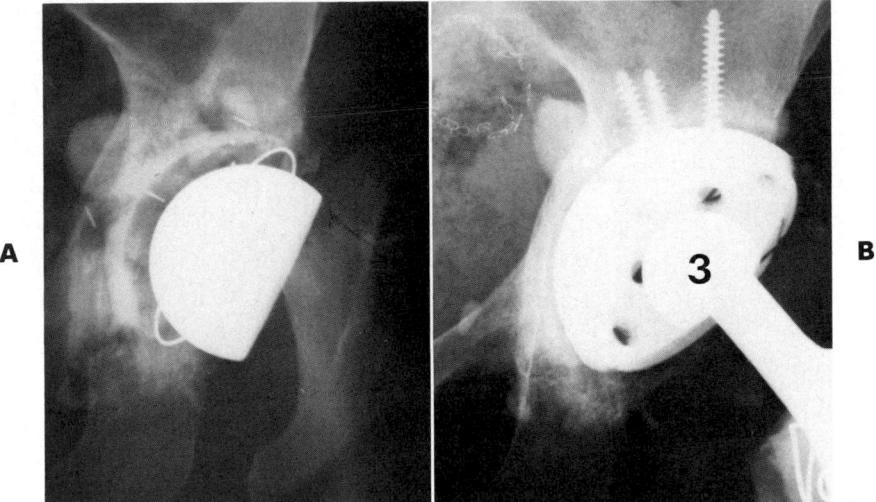

Fig. 14-13. One-stage acetabular revision using femoral head bone allograft. **A,** 69-year-old woman (I.G.) with a failed resurfacing and severe acetabular damage. Grade: B-3,3,5. **B,** 3 years after revision using 2 femoral head allografts and a porous-coated acetabular cup. Grade: B-6,6,6.

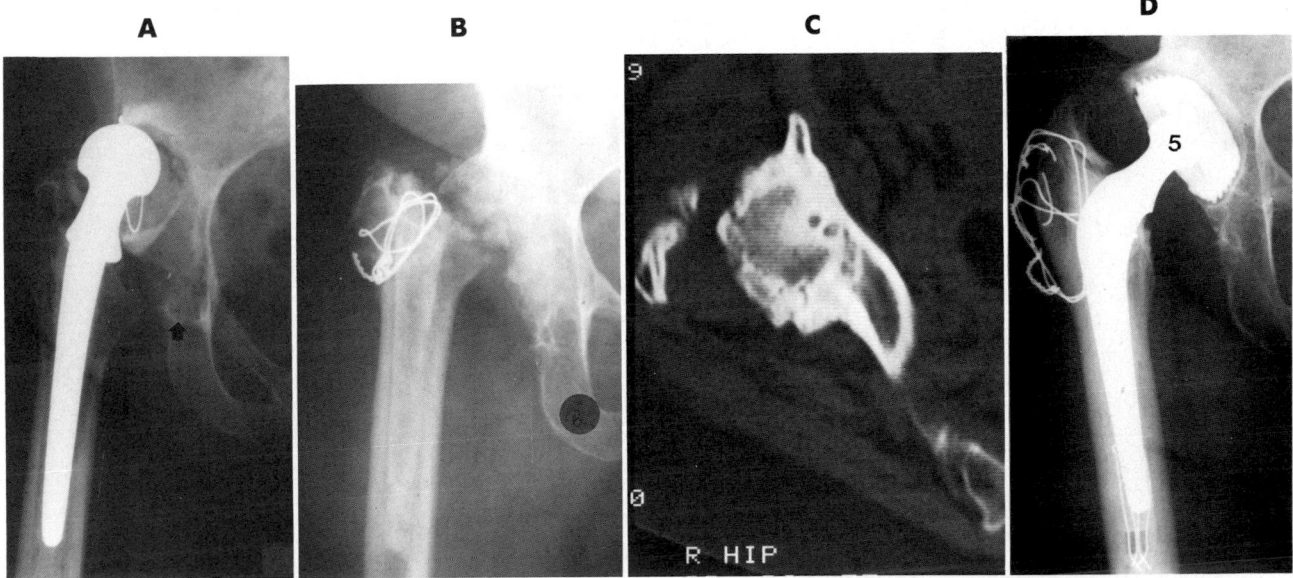

Fig. 14-14. A, Radiograph of severely migrated total hip arthroplasty in 64-year-old woman (P.L.). NOTE: severe bone loss in periacetabular region. Arrow indicates the site of originally implanted socket (operation was performed at another institution). A two-stage revision was planned. **B,** The first stage of planned two-stage reconstruction; removal of prosthesis and fixation of three femoral head allografts to the site of the defects in the acetabulum. **C,** CAT scan at the acetabular region 1 year after bone grafting indicates excellent incorporation of the allograft (incorporation was confirmed at revision surgery). **D,** 5 years after revision arthroplasty (second stage). NOTE: excellent support has been provided for the threaded acetabular cup. Grade: 6,6,6. Radiolucency between cup and bone has remained unchanged for the past 4 years.

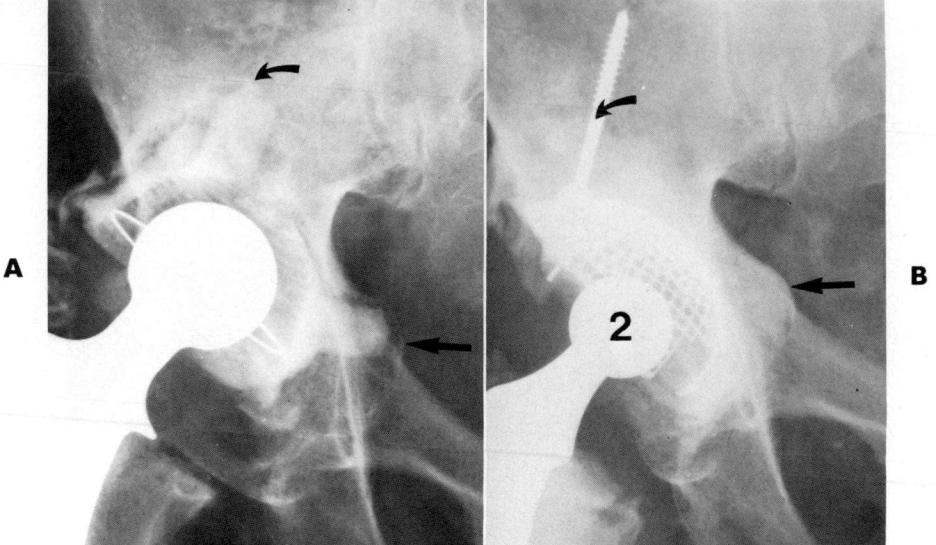

Fig. 14-15. Superior and medial bone allograft in revision surgery. **A,** Radiograph of 76-year-old man (K.H.) 3 years after total hip arthroplasty shows migration and loosening *(arrows).* Operation was performed at another institution. **B,** Two years postrevision. NOTE: the solid piece of femoral head allograft is fixed onto the ilium intraarticularly. NOTE: bone incorporation at the medial acetabular wall and lateralization of the socket using acrylic cement for fixation.

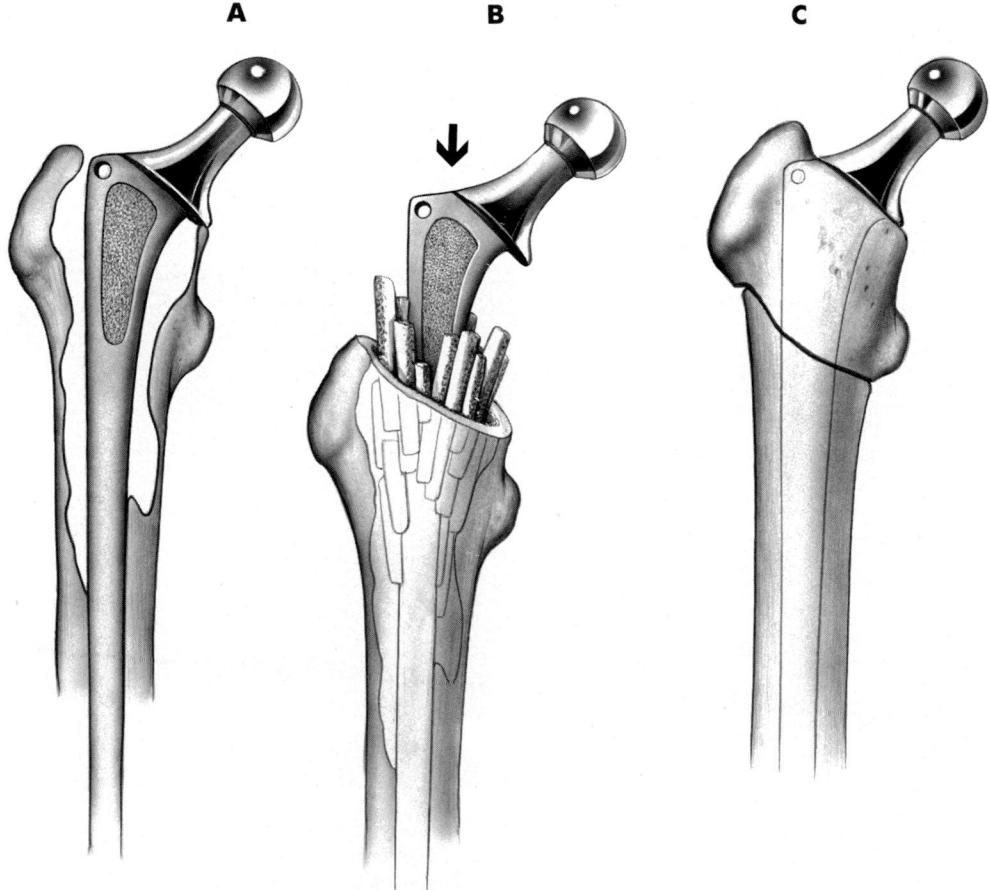

Fig. 14-16. Massive osteolysis (medullary cavity corticocancellous loss) caused by cement fragmentation in young patients is an indication for the use of allografts mixed with autogenous bone grafts. **A,** The extent of bone loss after cement removal. **B,** "Strips and sticks" of bone are packed around the stem as it is inserted into the canal of the femur. **C,** A small, segmental replacement without cement fixation.

Head and associates[56] reported that in using lyophilized proximal femur allografts in the revision of 14 hips, all patients had a complete union and encouraging results between 16 and 30 months. Other significant series of allograft-prosthesis combinations have been reported by Gross[48,49] and subsequently by Allen.[2] The overall performance of the allograft appears to be satisfactory. The host-allograft junction uniformly healed and did not appear to be a problem. Functional results were good without infection and recurrence of dislocations. With this type of allograft-prosthesis composite, a good early result may be anticipated. The small calcar grafts, however, are not as good as large fragment allografts to reconstruct substantial bone loss.[2] The available literature suggests that bulk allografts seem to maintain their structural integrity even though some absorption and slow revascularization take place over time. Allograft osseous union and structural stability are satisfactory in the short and medium range. Because revascularization is extremely slow, the biological changes resulting from immunological incompatibility do not seem to affect the graft in the short term. The process of healing of the allograft is by creeping substitution. Nonunion and fractures can be readily repaired using supplemental fixation and autogenous bone grafts.

Mankin,[85] who has extensive experience with allografts, attributes several advantages to allografts over other methods used to compensate for bone loss. These include (1) their availability in appropriate sizes and shapes; (2) joint replacement can be readily performed without customized devices; (3) biological attachment of the functioning graft tissue is possible; (4) without donor site morbidity, the allograft will predictably convert to host tissue; and (5) with complications such as infection or fractures, more options are available for reconstruction. Mankin[85] also notes some disadvantages, including (1) at best, the success rate is approximately 80% to 85%; (2) infection and nonunions occur at high rates; (3) inadequate remodeling; (4) inadequate availability of large quantities of allografts (even in large tissue banks); and (5) difficulty in restoring ligaments and tendinous reattachments. Examples of partial (cortical and corticocancellous) and proximal femoral allografts and femoral allograft-prosthesis composites are illustrated in Figs. 14-17 to 14-20.

COMPLICATIONS
Infection in Allografts

Hepatitis of various types, HIV, syphilis, Creutzfeldt-Jakob disease, and other diseases are known to have been transmitted via blood or bone. A fundamental question is whether the infection after allograft is caused by contamination of allografts or other sources.

Since the introduction of allografts, reports have periodically indicated a high incidence of postoperative

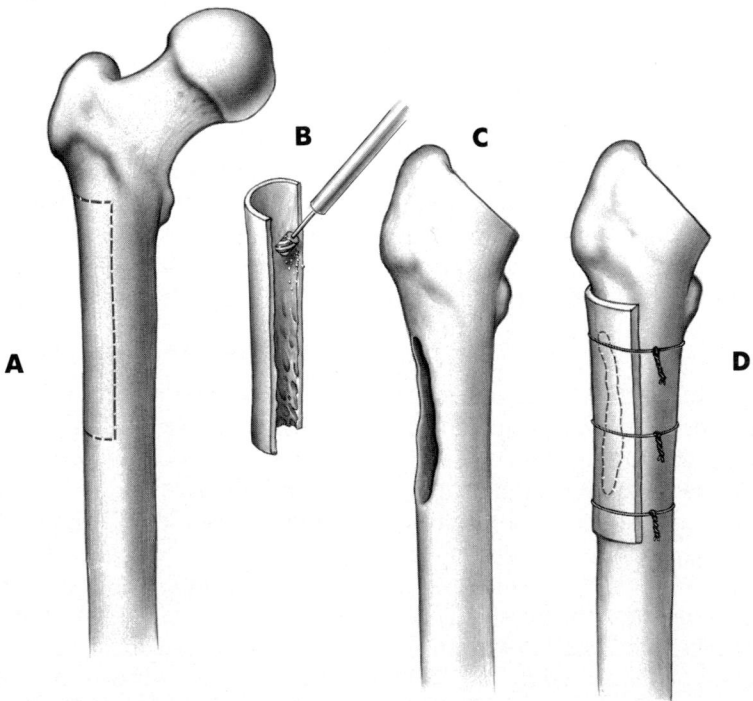

Fig. 14-17. Proximal femoral allograft is especially suitable for repair of various defects found in revision surgery. **A,** Desired segment is mapped on the allograft. **B,** Graft is being shaped. **C,** Defect is treated. **D,** Bone defect is repaired by onlay cortical allograft.

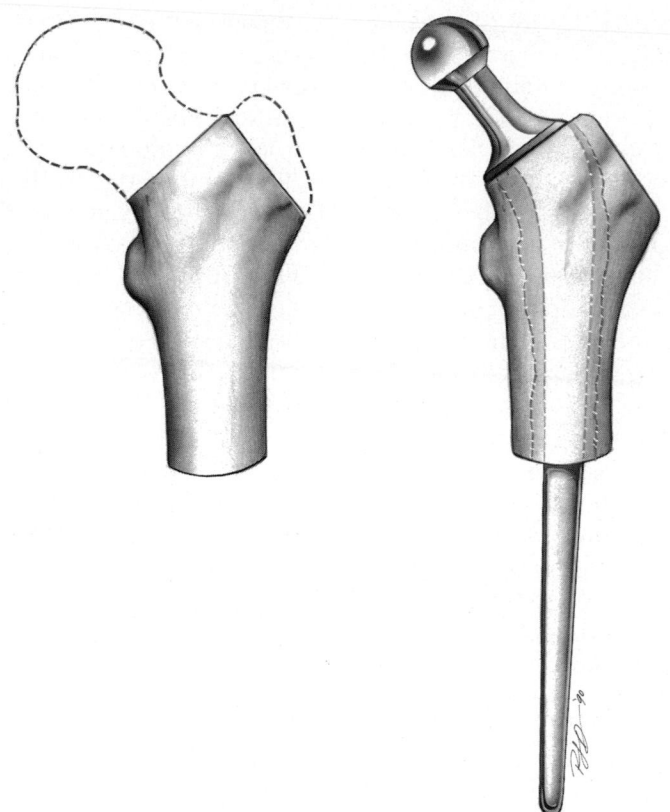

Fig. 14-18. Proximal femoral allograft of appropriate size is prepared and fixed to the remaining host bone by a long-stem prosthesis. **A,** Head and neck and trochanter are amputated. **B,** Long-stem prosthesis is fixed to allograft by acrylic cement.

infections (as high as 14%) after the use of massive allografts.[40,75,83] In some series, the single most significant complication has been infection. Mankin reported an overall infection rate of 13% along with other significant complications, such as a 17% rate of allograft fracture and an 11% nonunion rate. Immunological factors related to patients (who often receive immunosuppressive drugs) and other immunological factors such as graft rejection may compromise the host response, thus making them susceptible to infection. However, prophylactic measures such as systemic antibiotics and improved operating room environment have reduced the rate of these infections (see Chapter 26).

The only study that largely disputes the possibility of infection transmission by processed bone-bank bone is that by Tomford.[121] In a follow-up study of 333 lyophilized allograft transplants, 21 patients showed signs of infection, 11 of whom had positive cultures as proof of their infection. This relatively low rate of infection was considered for orthopaedic procedures using autogenous bone grafts. For management of infected allografts, see Chapter 26. Two examples of bone graft absorptions (failures) and fracture of a massive femoral allograft are shown in Figs. 14-21 to 14-23.

Complications of the Iliac Donor Site

Complications at the donor site after removal of the bone graft for spinal fusion or other elective procedures are uncommon.[28] Nevertheless, complications such as "meralgia paresthetica" (lateral femoral cutaneous nerve damage),[86,130] fracture of the anterior superior iliac spine,[69,113] iliac crest fractures,[109] hematomas, and infections have been frequently reported. An uncommon yet significant complication of bone grafts is a hernia through the donor's site for iliac-bone grafts.[43,73,76,111] This complication was first reported by Oldfield in 1945.[94] Cowley reviewed 11 cases in the literature and added 4 cases of his own.[29] The signs and symptoms of bowel herniation (small or large) can be insidious and manifested only by mild discomfort in the

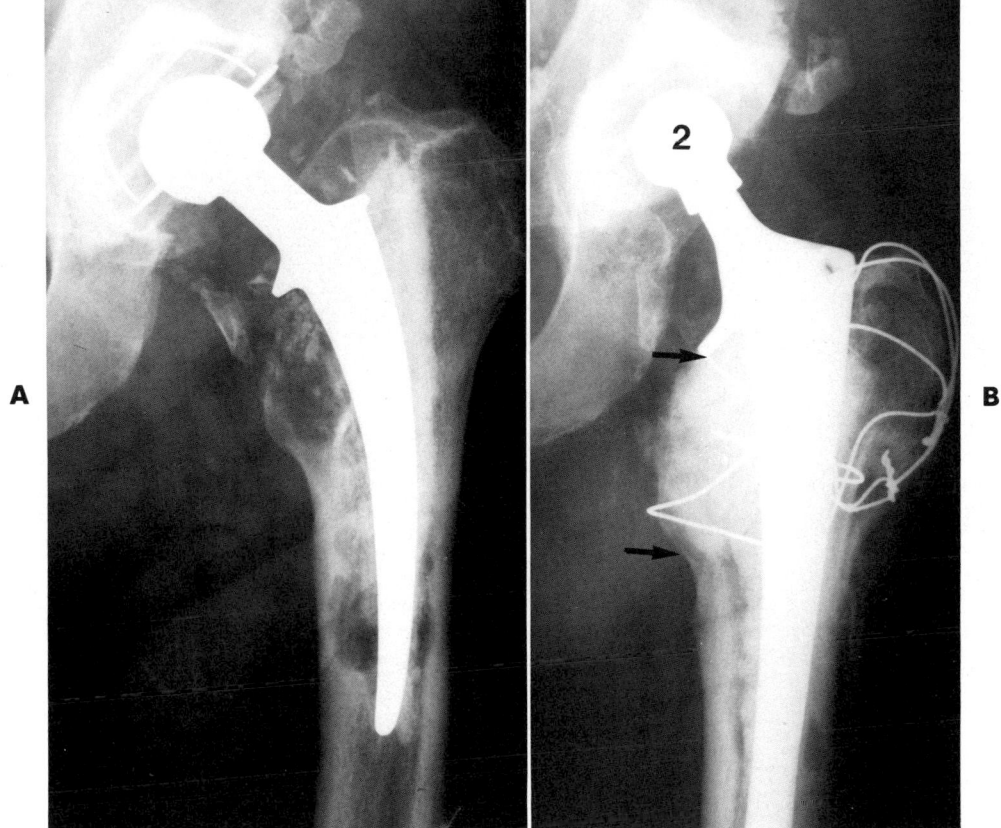

Fig. 14-19. Calcar replacement bone graft and intramedullary bone graft with cement. **A,** Severe proximal, medial, and diaphysial bone loss caused by long-standing loosening of total hip arthroplasty performed in 71-year-old physician (H.S.) at another institution. Segmental replacement with corticocancellous bone allograft was used and bone defects were packed with cancellous bone chips before insertion of cement. **B,** 2 years after surgery, no demarcation is present. Grade: A-6,6,6.

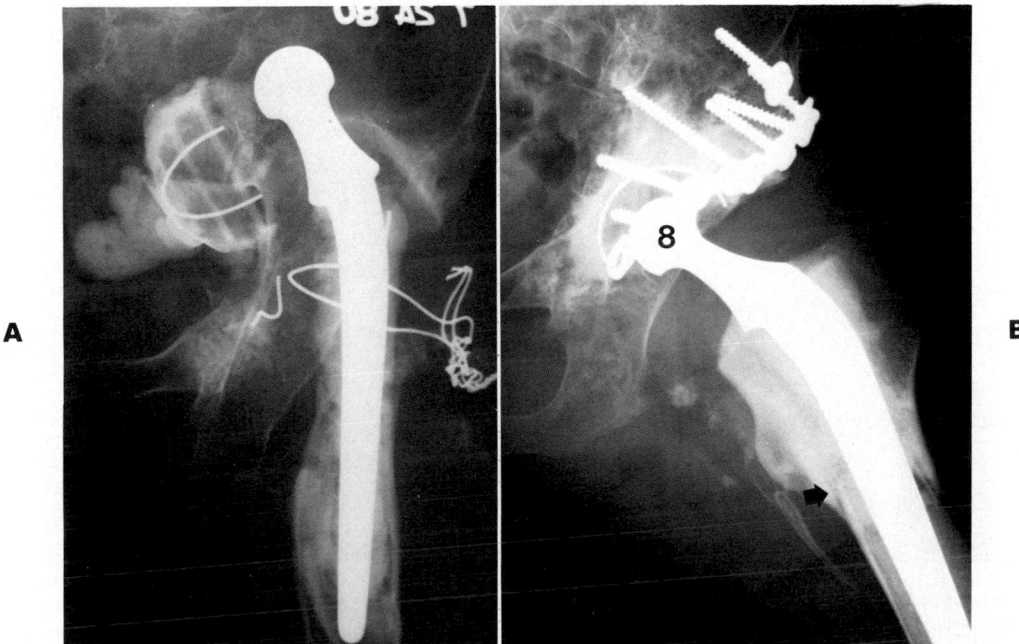

Fig. 14-20. Massive pelvic and femoral allograft. **A,** Severe intrapelvic migration of LFA in 33-year-old woman (D.M.) after multiple previous surgeries. **B,** 8 years after reconstruction procedure including a massive acetabular and segmental femoral allograft prosthesis composite. NOTE: distal femoral allograft was inserted into the host bone femoral canal to maximize contact; union was achieved at 6 months *(arrow)*. Patient has no pain but walks with a cane. Grade: A-5,5,5.

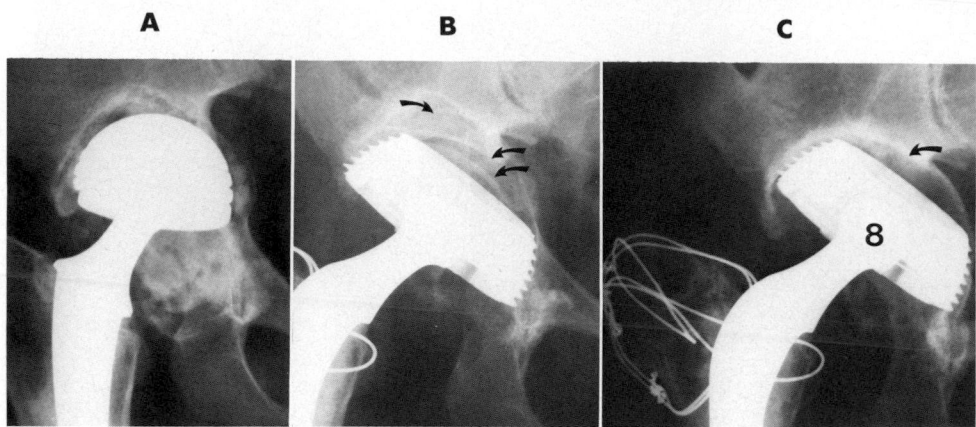

Fig. 14-21. Bone graft absorption, perhaps caused by lack of stress. **A,** Radiograph of 26-year-old male (J.V.) after three previous hip arthroplasties performed in other institutions. **B,** Radiograph taken 2 months after surgery shows corticocancellous bone used at surgery. The grafts were well packed before the acetabular Mecring was used *(arrows)*. **C,** 2 years after surgery the bone allograft has been absorbed.

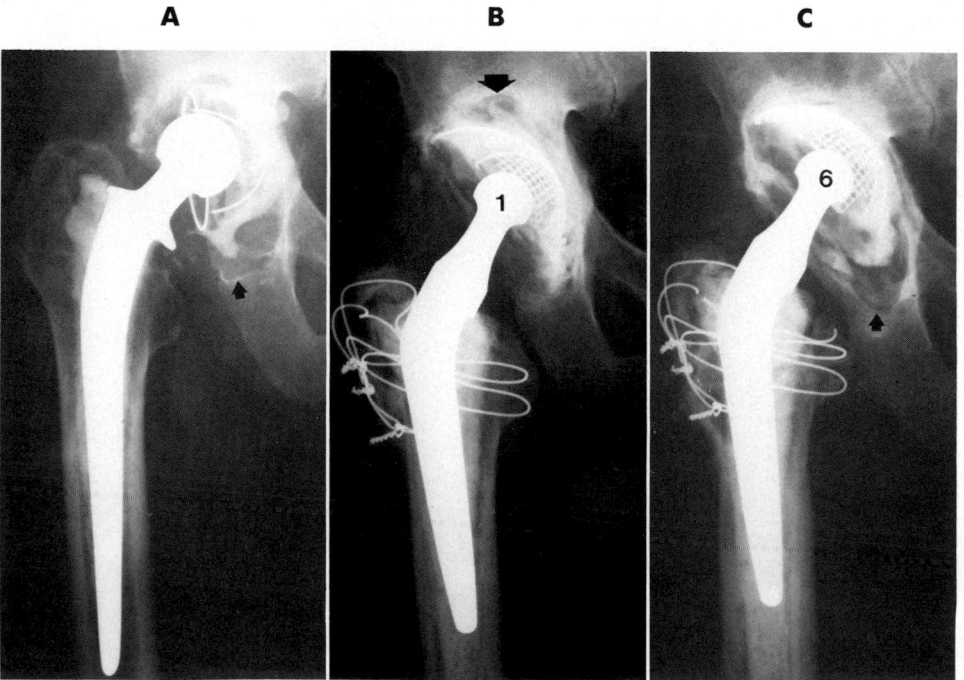

Fig. 14-22. Failed allograft fixation in the acetabulum. **A,** Radiograph of 66-year-old male (P.A.) with a failed long-stem Müller total hip arthroplasty caused by loosening of both components. (Operation was performed in another institution.) Arrow shows site of original fixation. **B,** 1 year after LFA including femoral bone allograft. NOTE: a radiolucent zone has appeared superiorly *(arrow)*. **C,** At 6 years postoperatively, note loosening of socket with proximal migration *(arrow)*. The femur remains intact. Grade: A-5,5,5.

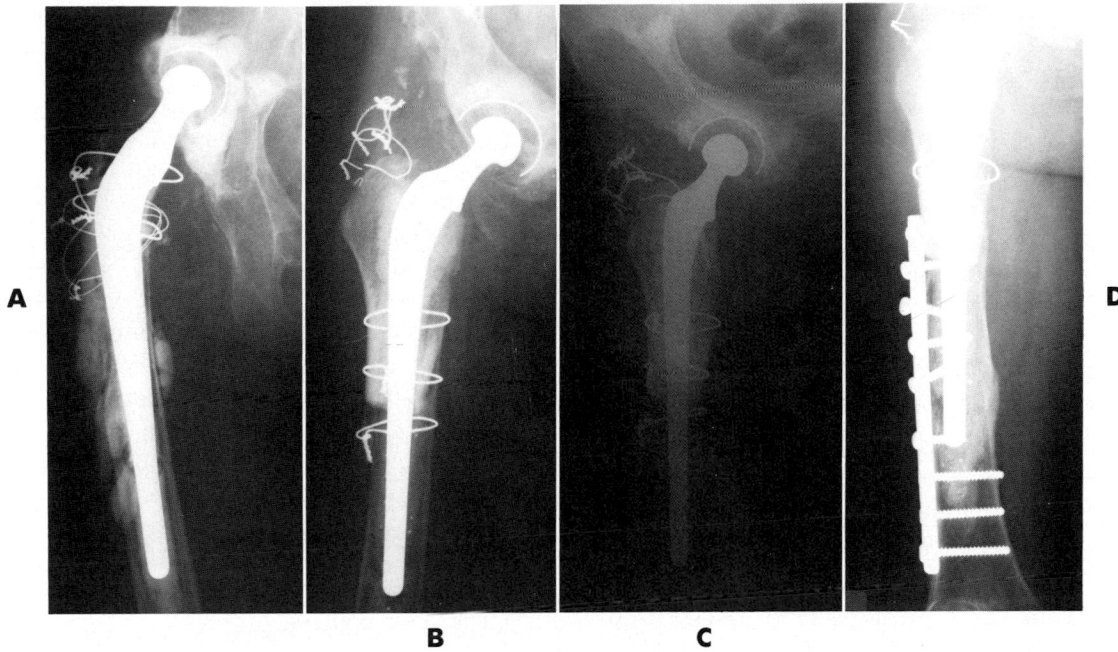

Fig. 14-23. A, Radiograph of 63-year-old female (O.L.) with multiple surgical procedures (performed at another institution) including three total hip arthroplasties. Because of severe bone loss, an allograft replacement was necessary. NOTE: the acetabular site was dysplastic, and cup had been placed in the false acetabulum. **B,** 1 year after reconstruction procedure, allograft is united, and patient has no pain. Grade B-6,6,6. **C,** Radiograph taken after patient sustained femoral fracture at level of tip of stem extending to allograft. **D,** 3 years after fixation of allograft prosthesis and the patient's femur by a plate and screws with a rapid union of femoral fracture (at 6 months).

donor's side as early as 24 hours after surgery to as late as 15 years.[27] The condition, however, can become significant and life threatening if the hernia becomes irreducible or is accompanied by strangulation.[27,107] However, the mass is usually reducible and diagnosis is relatively easy by auscultation, x-ray films, and CAT scans of the pelvis. In the past, various repairs, including the use of Marlex mesh, have been advocated. However, according to Cowley, the most effective method of repair is the technique described by Bosworth.[11] In Bosworth's technique, the iliac crest defect is enlarged by removing enough bone from the crest of the ilium to allow mobilization of the abdominal fascia (including insertion of transversalis and oblique muscles) so that it can be directly attached to the remaining crest of ilium.[11]

BONE ALLOGRAFTS AND HIV

An epidemic of HIV has caused concern among patients and surgeons regarding the safety of banked homologous allografts.[42] Obviously, this real concern has placed an additional responsibility on the agencies who prepare and supply the grafts to hospitals and surgeons. The main safeguards (standards set by the Centers for Disease Control) are rigorous donor selection and repeat screening for HIV antibodies and

antigens and detailed morphologic tissue studies.

Buck and associates[14] concluded that with rigorous selection and exclusion criteria followed by screening for HIV and antigen antibodies and histological studies of donor tissues, the chances of transmitting disease via bone graft were one in well over one million.

The American Association of Tissue Banks has established guidelines that must be followed by the bone banks and local hospital bone banks. These guidelines must be strictly followed to eliminate the risks of bacterial and viral infections. Regarding HIV transmission, the current recommendation for bone banking is that the donors be tested for HIV and that the test be repeated at 3 months to rule out the false negative results. Freezing bone ($-70°$ to $-80°$ C) does not inactivate HIV.

SUMMARY OF ESSENTIALS

- Bone grafts are used in reconstructive hip surgery to provide a source of osteogenesis and to serve as a mechanical support and substitution for lost bone.

- Although autogenous bone grafts are biologically best, allografts are in great demand because of the inadequate supply of autogenous bone grafts. Xenographs are rarely used today.

- Although autogenous bone grafts are commonly used as fresh grafts, allogenic bone grafts are procured and stored frozen, lyophilized, or chemically sterilized and are available in large quantities. The storage procedures decrease the immunogenicity of allografts significantly.

- Bone grafts incorporate into the host bone in a predictable and sequential manner, a process that is unique not only to the bone grafts but to the recipient bone bed as well. Many factors may affect the incorporation process, including mechanical properties of the bone grafts, the mechanical stability of the bone grafts, and certain systemic factors.

- The remodeling process occurs as the result of an initial phase of activation followed by bone absorption and bone formation.

- All bone grafts are dead at the time of transplantation (with the exception of vascularized grafts). To survive, a bone graft must become vascularized. Invariably, bone grafts undergo necrosis. This causes a local inflammatory process that initiates the subsequent stages for bone grafts to be incorporated to the host bone; the process of incorporation involves two additional phases of osteoconduction and osteoinduction. Although the incorporation is often incomplete, good function is often compatible with partial vascularization of the graft.

- Unlike fresh allografts, which are immunologically active, procured bone grafts (frozen allografts at $-80°$ C or lyophilized allografts) are capable of incorporation and are less immunogenic.

- Graft incorporation is more likely when grafts are vascularized or autogenous, irradiated, sterilized, and of optimal size. The bed of the recipient bone must also be vascularized. Patient youth and good health also promote healing of the bone grafts, as does rigid fixation of the bone graft with optimum stress and absence of motion.

- Allografts that are fresh, have been autoclaved, are extremely small or large, and that are applied to a nonvascular bed are less likely to incorporate. Poor health, immunosuppression, use of steroids, rheumatoid disease, hormonal imbalance, medications, and local factors such as infection, debris, necrosis, and loss of fixation also adversely affect bone graft incorporation. Finally, too much or too little stress and increased motion adversely affect incorporation.

- Physiological studies of humans and animals show a similar pattern of biology of bone grafts. After initial necrosis, the bone graft site has localized inflammatory response followed by formation of a fibrovascular medium that provides a new source of precursor cells to the graft. During the second phase, which lasts 3 to 12 weeks, both osteoblastic and osteoclastic activities occur. During this phase, cortical bone absorption is via expansion of preexisting Haversian and Volkmann's canals by invasion of capillaries. The last phase of bone graft healing includes remodeling, which takes place by reinforcement of trabeculae, leading to a more normal pattern depending on the quality, quantity, and pattern of bone strain. In dogs, this phase of repair may be complete by 1 year. Because of their potential for healing and the rate of incorporation, autologous, cancellous, and cortical bone grafts are the best.

- Autologous, cortical bone exhibits an inflammatory response similar to cancellous bone, but the process of revascularization is slow and incomplete in cortical bone. It must be recognized that although new Haversian canals are formed, the porosity of the cortical bone may never be completely replaced because the dead bone remains bonded by the new bone. The histology of cortical grafts therefore is a mosaic of new and old graft bone.

- Both cancellous and cortical allografts show a slower vascularization and incorporation to the host bone than autogenous bone grafts. Both show similar processes of cellular response. They first exhibit an inflammatory response, which is followed by revascularization. New blood vessels penetrate 2 to 3 mm into the allografts, but reinforcement occurs from the periphery and the surface of the allograft. The interior of the bone grafts remains avascular for the most part. Although qualitatively similar to autogenous bone grafts, allografts undergo replacement by creeping substitution over a much longer time period and much less completely than autogenous bone grafts.

- Radiographs are notoriously inaccurate to determine incorporation of the bone grafts, but improved techniques using radioisotopes are now available to study revascularization.

- Several types of treatments of allografts have been shown to significantly reduce their antigenicity. These include boiling the graft, freezing, lyophilization, sterilization, irradiation, and antigen extraction. The purpose of radiating the bone grafts is to sterilize the bone and destroy the antigens. Frozen allografts (also known as *fresh frozen*) have been used extensively in orthopaedic reconstruction procedures because of their availability and ease of application. Freezing in liquid nitrogen at $-170°$ C eliminates all molecular motion, thus allowing indefinite storage time. Lyophilization alters the biomechanical strength of the grafts and is also expensive. The long-term results suggest that complications such as fatigue fracture, nonunion, and delayed host-graft union may be similar to those found in frozen bone allografts. While further studies involving larger samples and longer follow up are needed to define the role of HLA matching in rate of union, incorporation of the graft, absorption, and other parameters of the bone grafts, immuno-suppressive drugs do not at present seem warranted in conjunction with the use of allografts.

■ A good bone bank should expeditiously supply various sizes and shapes of bone grafts. Bone banks at the national and local levels should strictly adhere to the guidelines set by the American Association of Tissue Banks. Retrieved specimens must be cultured appropriately; blood and body fluids are cultured for aerobic and anaerobic organisms. Serological tests for syphilis, hepatitis, and HIV should be performed routinely. Repeated testing 90 to 180 days after donation of the bone by living subjects is indicated to identify those with a "latency window" of transmission of HIV. Patients with neoplasm and those who have used steroids and other toxic substances are strictly excluded. The sterility of the bone graft must be guaranteed. Freeze-dried allografts are advantageous because of their longer shelf life than frozen allografts, but they are inferior to frozen grafts from a mechanical property standpoint. Grafts kept at −70° to −80° C can be safely stored for months and even years because of the absence of enzyme activities.

■ The clinical application of bone grafts in total hip arthroplasty includes acetabular reconstruction associated with fixed sockets (cemented or cementless), acetabular reconstruction using bipolar prosthesis, acetabular reconstruction in revision surgery, two-stage acetabular reconstruction, en-bloc acetabular allograft replacement, bone graft femoral deficiencies, and femoral allograft prosthetic composites.

■ Weight-bearing bone grafts demand that the patient remain nonweight bearing for 3 to 6 months or longer, if necessary, until the bone graft has incorporated adequately.

■ From the available literature, it seems that bulk allografts maintain their structural integrity even though some absorption and slow revascularization take place over time. Allograft-osseous union and structural stability are satisfactory in the short and medium range. Because the process of revascularization is extremely slow, the biological changes resulting from immunological incompatibility do not seem to affect the graft in the short term. Since the process of healing is by creeping substitution, nonunion and fractures can be readily repaired using supplemental fixation and autogenous bone grafts.

■ The advantages of the allograft-composite prosthesis include the availability of different sizes and shapes of bone grafts, the ability to customize the prosthesis at surgery, biological acceptance by the host, and biological attachment and functioning of the graft tissue with the possibility of repair in the face of failure. The disadvantages are infection or fracture of the graft and difficulty in restoring the ligaments and tendinous attachments.

■ Available data suggest that with proper procurement of the grafts under extremely aseptic conditions, including the use of antibiotics, an acceptable infection rate can be achieved.

REFERENCES

1. **Albee FH:** Fundamentals in bone transplantation. Experience in three thousand bone graft operations, *JAMA* 81:1429, 1923.
2. **Allan GD, Lavoie GJ, Rudan JF, et al:** The use of allograft bone in revision total hip arthroplasty. In Friedlaender GE, Goldberg VM, editors: *Bone and cartilage allografts*, Park Ridge, Ill, 1991, AAOS Workshop.
3. **American Association of Tissue Banks:** 180-day quarantine for HCV and HIV for living donors effective April 1, 1991, *ATTB Newsletter* 3:1, 1990.
4. **Anderson KJ, Schmidt J, Clawson DK:** The vascularization and cellular response induced by homogenous deproteinized bone transplants in the anterior chamber of the rat eye, *Transplant Bull* 6:97, 1959.
5. **Barth A:** Zur frage der vitalität replantier knochenstucke, *Berhmet Klm Wochenschr* 31:340, 1894.
6. **Bateman J:** Salvage of failed hip arthroplasties using a multiple bearing implant, *Orthop Trans* 5:357, 1981.
7. **Bonfiglio M:** Repair of bone-transplant fractures, *J Bone Joint Surg* 40:446, 1958.
8. **Borja FJ, Mnaymneh W:** Bone allografts in salvage of difficult hip arthroplasties, *Clin Orthop* 197:123, 1985.
9. **Bos GD, Goldberg VM, Powell AE, et al:** The effect of histocompatibility matching on canine frozen bone allografts, *J Bone Joint Surg* 65:89, 1983.
10. **Bos GD, Goldberg VM, Zika JM, et al:** Immune responses of rats to frozen bone allografts, *J Bone Joint Surg* 65:239, 1983.
11. **Bosworth DM:** Repair of herniae through iliac-crest defects, *J Bone Joint Surg* 37:106, 1955.
12. **Bright RW, Burchardt H:** The biomechanical properties of preserved bone grafts. In Friedlaender G, editor: *Osteochondral allografts. Biology, banking and clinical applications*, Boston, 1983, Little Brown.
13. **Brooks DB, Heiple KG, Herndon CH, et al:** Immunological factors in homogeneous bone transplantation. IV. The effects of various methods of preparation and irradiation on antigenicity, *J Bone Joint Surg* 45:1617, 1963.
14. **Buck BE, Malinin TI, Brown MD:** Bone transplantation and human immunodeficiency virus. An estimate of risk of acquired immunodeficiency syndrome (AIDS), *Clin Orthop* 240:129, 1988.
15. **Burchardt H:** The biology of bone graft repair, *Clin Orthop* 174:28, 1983.

16. **Burchardt H, Busbee GA 3rd, Enneking WF:** Repair of experimental autologous grafts of cortical bone, *J Bone Joint Surg* 57:814, 1975.

17. **Burchardt H, Enneking WF:** Transplantation of bone, *Surg Clin North Am* 58:403, 1978.

18. **Burchardt H, Glowczewskie FP, Enneking WF:** Allogeneic segmental fibular transplants in azathioprine-immunosuppressed dogs, *J Bone Joint Surg* 59:881, 1977.

19. **Burchardt J, Jones H, Glowczewskie FP, et al:** Freeze-dried allogeneic segmental cortical-bone grafts in dogs, *J Bone Joint Surg* 60:1082, 1978.

20. **Burger EH, van der Meer JWM, Nisweide PJ:** Osteo-clast formation from mononuclear phagocytes: role of bone-forming cells, *J Cell Biol* 99:1901, 1984.

21. **Burwell RG:** The fate of bone grafts. In Apley AG, editor: *Recent advances in orthopaedics*, London, 1969, Churchill Livingstone.

22. **Bush LF:** The use of homogenous bone grafts: a preliminary report on the bone bank, *J Bone Joint Surg* 29:620, 1947.

23. **Cameron HU, MacDiarmid A:** Major acetabulum reconstruction using autograft bone in cemented hip arthroplasty, *Orth Rev* 16:845, 1987.

24. **Cameron HU, Jung YB:** Acetabular revision with a bipolar prosthesis, *Clin Orthop* 251:100, 1990.

25. **Campanacci M, Salzer M, Pritchard D, et al:** Functional results of reconstruction of peri-acetabular pelvic resection requiring sacrifice of the hip joint. In Enneking WF, editor: *Limb salvage in musculoskeletal oncology*, Edinburgh, 1987, Churchill Livingstone.

26. **Canalis E:** Effects of growth factors of bone cell replication and differentiation, *Clin Orthop* 193:246, 1985.

27. **Challis JH, Lyttle JA, Stuart AE:** Strangulated lumbar hernia and volvulus following removal of iliac crest bone graft, *Acta Orthop Scand* 46:230, 1975.

28. **Cockin J:** Autologous bone grafting-complications at the donor site, *J Bone Joint Surg* 53[Br]:153, 1971.

29. **Cowley SP, Anderson LD:** Hernias through donor sites for iliac-bone grafts, *J Bone Joint Surg* 65:1023, 1983.

30. **Conway B, Tomford WW, Hirsch MS, et al:** Effects of gamma irradiation on HIV-1 in a bone allograft model, *Trans Orthop Res Soc* 15:225, 1990.

31. **Devries PH, Badgley CE, Hartmann JT:** Radiation sterilization of homogenous bone transplants utilizing radioactive cobalt, *J Bone Joint Surg* 40:187, 1958.

32. **Doppelt SH:** Operational and financial aspects of a hospital bone bank, *J Bone Joint Surg* 63:1472, 1981.

33. **Enneking WF, Burchardt H, Puhl JJ, et al:** Physical and biological aspects of repair in dog cortical-bone transplants, *J Bone Joint Surg* 57:237, 1975.

34. **Ehrlich MG, Lorenz J, Tomford WW, et al:** Collagenase activity in banked bone, *Trans Orthop Res Soc* 8:166, 1983.

35. **Friedlaender GE:** Current concepts review bone grafts. The basic science rationale for clinical applications, *J Bone Joint Surg* 69:786, 1987.

36. **Friedlaender GE, Goldbert VM, editors:** *Bone and cartilage allografts: biology and clinical applications* (workshop Aivie House, Warrenton, Va, 1989 Publication) American Association of Orthopaedic Surgeons, 1990.

37. **Friedlaender GE, Strong DM, Sell KW:** Donor graft specific anti-HLA antibodies following freeze-dried bone allografts, *Trans Orthop Res Soc* 2:87, 1977.

38. **Friedlaender GE, Strong DM, Sell KW:** Studies on the antigenicity of bone. I. Freeze-dried and deep-frozen bone allografts in rabbits, *J Bone Joint Surg* 58:854, 1976.

39. **Friedlaender GE:** Immune responses to osteochondral allografts. Current knowledge and future directions, *Clin Orthop* 174:58, 1983.

40. **Friedlaender GE, Mankin HJ, Sell KW:** *Osteochondral allografts. Biology, banking and clinical applications*, Boston, 1983, Little Brown.

41. **Friedlaender GE, Tross RB, Doganis AC, et al:** Effects of chemotherapeutic agents on bone. 1. Short-term methotrexate and doxorubicin (Adriamycin) treatment in a rat model, *J Bone Joint Surg* 66:602, 1984.

42. **Friedland GH, Klein RS:** Transmission of the human immunodeficiency virus, *N Engl J Med* 317:1125, 1987.

43. **Froimson AI, Cummings AG Jr:** Iliac hernia following hip arthrodesis, *Clin Orthop* 80:89, 1971.

44. **Gallie WE:** The use of boiled bone in operative surgery, *Am J Orthop Surg* 16:373, 1918.

45. **Gerber SD, Harris WH:** Femoral head autografting to augment acetabular deficiency in patients requiring total hip replacement. A minimum five-year study and an average seven-year follow-up study, *J Bone Joint Surg* 68:1241, 1986.

46. **Goldberg VM, Bos GD, Heiple KG, et al:** Improved acceptance of frozen bone allografts in genetically mismatched dogs by immunosuppression, *J Bone Joint Surg* 66:937, 1984.

47. **Gordon SL, Binkert BL, Rashkoff ES, et al:** Assessment of bone grafts used for acetabular augmentation in total hip arthroplasty. A study using roentgenograms and bone scintigraphy, *Clin Orthop* 201:18, 1985.

48. **Gross AE, Lavoie MV, McDermott P, et al:** The use of allograft bone in revision of total hip arthroplasty, *Clin Orthop* 197:115, 1985.

49. **Gross AE, McKee NH, Pritzker KPH, et al:** Reconstruction of skeletal deficits at the knee. A comprehensive osteochondral transplant program, *Clin Orthop* 174:96, 1983.

50. **Guest CB, et al:** Allograft-implant composite reconstruction following periacetabular sarcoma resection, *J Arthroplasty* 5 (suppl):525, 1990.

51. **Harris WH:** Allografting in total hip arthroplasty: in adults with severe acetabular deficiency including a surgical technique for bolting the graft to the ilium, *Clin Orthop* 162:150, 1982.

52. **Harris WH:** Total hip replacement for congenital dysplasia of hip: technique. In The Hip Society: *the hip: proceedings of the second open scientific meeting of The Hip Society*, St Louis, 1974, Mosby–Year Book.

53. **Harris WH, Crothers OD:** Autogenous bone grafting using the femoral head to correct severe acetabular deficiency for total hip replacement. In The Hip Society: *the hip: proceedings of the fourth open scientific meeting of The Hip Society*, St Louis, 1976, Mosby–Year Book.

54. **Harris WH, Crothers O, Oh I:** Total hip replacement and femoral-head bone-grafting for severe acetabular deficiency in adults, *J Bone Joint Surg* 59:752, 1977.

55. **Harrington KD, Johnston JO, Kaufer HN, et al:** Limb salvage and prosthetic joint reconstruction for low-grade and selected high-grade sarcomas of the bone after wide resection and replacement by autoclaved autogeneic grafts, *Clin Orthop* 211:180, 1986.

56. **Head WC, Malinin TI, Berklacich F:** Freeze-dried proximal femur allografts in revision total hip arthroplasty. A preliminary report, *Clin Orthop* 215:109, 1987.

57. **Heiple KG, Chase SW, Hernidon CH:** A comparative

study of the healing process following different types of bone transplantation, *J Bone Joint Surg* 45:1593, 1963.

58. **Heiple KG, Goldberg VM, Powell AE:** The biology of cancellous bone graft repair. In Friedlaender GE, Mankin HJ, Sell KW, editors: *Osteochondral allografts,* Boston, 1983, Little Brown.

59. **Herndon CH, Chase SW:** The fate of massive autogenous and homogenous bone grafts including articular surfaces, *Surg Gynecol Obstet* 98:273, 1954.

60. **Horowitz MC, Friedlaender GE:** The immune response to bone grafts. In Friedlaender GE, Goldberg VM, editors: Bone and cartilage allografts—biology and clinical applications, *Am Acad Orthop Surg* 85, 1990.

61. **Hurley LA, Zeier FG, Stinchfield FE:** Anorganic bone grafting. Clinical experiences with heterografts processed by ethylenediamine extraction, *Am J Surg* 100:12, 1960.

62. **Hyatt GW, Butler MC:** Bone grafting: Bone grafting—the procurement, storage and clinical use of bone homografts. *American Academy of Orthopaedic Surgeons instructional course lectures,* vol XIV, Ann Arbor, 1957, JW Edwards.

63. **Imamaliev AS:** The preparation, preservation, and transplantation of articular bone ends. In Apley AG, editor: *Recent advances in orthopaedics,* Baltimore, 1970, Williams & Wilkins.

64. **Inclan A:** Use of preserved bone graft in orthopaedic surgery, *J Bone Joint Surg* 24:81, 1942.

65. **Kandel RA, Gross AE, Ganel A, et al:** Histopathology of failed osteoarticular shell allografts, *Clin Orthop* 197:103, 1985.

66. **Komender A:** Influence of preservation on some mechanical properties of human haversian bone, *Mater Med Pol* 8:13, 1976.

67. **Koskinen EV:** Wide resection of primary tumors of bone and replacement with massive bone grafts: an improved technique for transplanting allogenic bone grafts, *Clin Orthop* 134:302, 1978.

68. **Kreuz FP, Hyatt GW, Turner TC, et al:** The preservation and clinical use of freeze-dried bone, *J Bone Joint Surg* 33:863, 1951.

69. **Kuhn DA, Moreland MS:** Complications following iliac crest bone grafting, *Clin Orthop* 186:224, 1986.

70. **Langer F, Czitrom A, Pritzker KP, et al:** The immunogenicity of fresh and frozen allogeneic bone, *J Bone Joint Surg* 57:216, 1975.

71. **Langlais F, Vielpeau C:** Allografts of the hemipelvis after tumour resection. Technical aspects of four cases, *J Bone Joint Surg* 71[Br]:58, 1989.

72. **Lexer E:** Joint transplantation and arthroplasty, *Surg Gynecol Obstet* 40:782, 1925.

73. **Lewin ML, Bradley ET:** Traumatic iliac hernia with extensive soft tissue loss, *Surgery* 26:601, 1949.

74. **Lloyd-Roberts GC:** Experiences with boiled cadaveric bone, *J Bone Joint Surg* 34[Br]:428, 1952.

75. **Lord CF, Gebhardt MC, Tomford WW, et al:** Infection in bone allografts, *J Bone Joint Surg* 70:369, 1988.

76. **Lotem M, et al:** Lumbar hernia at an iliac bone graft donor site. A case report, *Clin Orthop* 80:130, 1971.

77. **MacEwen W:** Observations concerning transplantation of bone. Illustrated by a case of inter-human osseous transplantation, whereby over two-thirds of the shaft of the humerus was restored, *Proc Roy Soc London* 32:232, 1881.

78. **Malinin TI, Wu NM, Flores A:** Freeze-drying of bone for allotransplantation. In Friedlaender GE, Mankin HJ, Sell KW, editors: *Osteochondral allografts: biology, banking, and clinical applications,* Boston, 1983, Little Brown.

79. **Malkin C, Tauber C:** Total hip arthroplasty and acetabular bone grafting for unreduced fracture-dislocation of the hip, *Clin Orthop* 201:57, 1985.

80. **Malinin TI, Martinez OV, Brown MD:** Banking of massive osteoarticular and intercalary bone allografts—12 years experience, *Clin Orthop* 197:44, 1985.

81. **Malinin TI, Wagner JL, Pita JC, et al:** Hypothermic storage and cryopreservation of cartilage. An experimental study, *Clin Orthop* 197:15, 1985.

82. **Mankin HJ, Gebhardt MC, Springfield DS:** Osteoarticular and intercalary allograft transplantation in the management of malignant tumors of bone, *Cancer* 50:613, 1982.

83. **Mankin HJ, Doppelt S, Tomford W:** Clinical experience with allograft implantation. The first ten years, *Clin Orthop* 174:69, 1983.

84. **Mankin HJ, Fogelson FS, Trasher AZ, et al:** Massive resection and allograft transplantation in the treatment of malignant bone tumors, *N Engl J Med* 294:1247, 1976.

85. **Mankin HJ, Gebhardt MC, Springfield DS:** The clinical use of frozen cadaveric allografts in management of bone tumors. In Friedlaender GE, Goldberg VM, editors: *Bone and cartilage allografts,* Park Ridge, Ill, 1991, AAOS Workshop.

86. **Massey EW:** Meralgia paresthetica secondary to trauma of bone graft, *J Trauma* 4:342, 1980.

87. **McMurray GN:** The evaluation of Kiel bone in spinal fusions, *J Bone Joint Surg* 64[Br]:101, 1982.

88. **Michaut E, Rabeux B, Lefèvre MY, et al:** Désarticulations de hanche et amputations enter-ilio-abdominales: appareilage et résultat fonctionel, *Rev Chir Orthop* 61:547, 1975.

89. **Mulroy RD, Harris WH:** Failure of acetabular autogenous grafts in total hip arthroplasty: Increasing incidence, a follow-up note, *J Bone Joint Surg* 72:1536, 1990.

90. **Murray WR:** Salvage of acetabular insufficiency with bipolar prosthesis. In The Hip Society: *the hip, proceedings of the twelfth open scientific meeting of The Hip Society,* St Louis, 1984, Mosby–Year Book.

91. **Muscolo DL, Caletti E, Schajowicz F, et al:** Tissue-typing in human massive allografts of frozen bone, *J Bone Joint Surg* 69:583, 1987.

92. **Nilsonne U, Kreicbergs A, Olsson E, et al:** Function after pelvic tumour resection involving the acetabular ring, *Int Orthop* 6:27, 1982.

93. **Ochsner JG Jr, Perenberg BL, Dorr LD, et al:** *Results of bipolar endoprosthesis and bone graft for acetabular component revision.* Paper published at the 55th annual meeting of AAOS, Atlanta, 1988.

94. **Oldfield MC:** Iliac hernia after bone-grafting, *Lancet* 1:810, 1945.

95. **Ollier LXE:** *Traité expérimental et clinique de la régénération des os et de la production artificielle du tissu osseux,* Paris, 1867, Masson.

96. **Ottolenghi CE:** Massive osteo and osteo-articular bone grafts. Technic and results of 62 cases, *Clin Orthop* 87:156, 1972.

97. **Ottolenghi CE:** Massive osteoarticular bone grafts. Transplant of the whole femur, *J Bone Joint Surg* 48[Br]:646, 1966.

98. **Owen M:** Cell population kinetics of an osteogenic tissue, *Int J Cell Biol* 19:19, 1963.

99. **Parrish FF:** Allograft replacement of all or part of the end

of a long bone following excision of a tumor: report of twenty-one cases, *J Bone Joint Surg* 55:1, 1973.

100. **Parrish FF:** Treatment of bone tumors by total excision and replacement with massive autologous and homologous grafts, *J Bone Joint Surg* 48:968, 1966.

101. **Pelker RR, Friedlaender GE, Markham TC, et al:** Effects of freezing and freeze-drying on the biomechanical properties of the rat bone, *J Orthop Res* 1:405, 1984.

102. **Pelker RR, Friedlaender GE, Panjabi MM, et al:** Radiation-induced alterations of fracture healing biomechanics, *J Orthop Res* 2:90, 1984.

103. **Phemister DB:** The fate of transplanted bones and regenerative power of its various constituents, *Surg Gynecol Obstet* 19:303, 1914.

104. **Pieron AP, Bigelow D, Hamonic M:** Bone grafting with Boplant. Results in thirty-three cases, *J Bone Joint Surg* 50[Br]:364, 1968.

105. **Pritchard JJ:** The osteoblast. In Bourne GH, editor: *The biochemistry and physiology of bone*, ed 2, vol 1, New York, 1972, Academic Press.

106. **Prolo DJ, Rodrigo JJ:** Contemporary bone graft physiology and surgery, *Clin Orthop* 200:322, 1985.

107. **Prytek LJ, Kelly CC:** Management of herniation through large iliac bone defects, *Ann Surg* 152:998, 1960.

108. **Ranki A, Valle SL, Krohn M, et al:** Long latency precedes overt seroconversion in sexually transmitted human-immunodeficiency-virus infection, *Lancet* 2:589, 1987.

109. **Reale F, Gambacorta D, Mencattini G:** Iliac crest fracture after removal of two bone plugs for anterior cervical fusion. Case report, *J Neurosurg* 51:560, 1979.

110. **Reddi AH, Wientroub S, Muthukumaran N:** Biologic principles of bone induction, *Orthop Clin North Am* 18:207, 1987.

111. **Reid RL:** Hernia through an iliac bone-graft donor site. A case report, *J Bone Joint Surg* 50:757, 1968.

112. **Reynolds AF Jr, Turner PT, Loeser JD:** Fracture of the anterior superior iliac spine following anterior cervical fusion using iliac crest. Case report, *J Neurosurg* 48:809, 1978.

113. **Ritter MA, Trancik TM:** Lateral acetabular bone graft in total hip arthroplasty. A three- to eight-year follow-up study without internal fixation, *Clin Orthop* 193:156, 1985.

114. **Roberson JR, Cohen D:** Bipolar components for severe periacetabular bone loss around the failed total hip arthroplasty, *Clin Orthop* 251:113, 1990.

115. **Samuelson KM, Freeman MAR, Levack B, et al:** Homograft bone in revision acetabular arthroplasty. A clinical and radiographic study, *J Bone Joint Surg* 70[Br]:367, 1988.

116. **Scott RD, Pomeroy DL, Oser E, et al:** *Two- to four-year follow-up of bipolar revision hip arthroplasty using morcellized acetabular bone graft.* Paper presented at the 54th annual meeting, AAOS, San Francisco, 1987.

117. **Sell KW, Friedlaender GE, editors:** *1975: tissue banking for transplantation; a transplantation proceedings report*, New York, 1976, Grune & Stratton.

118. **Shutkin NM:** Monologous-serum hepatitis following use of refrigerated bone-bank bone; report of a case, *J Bone Joint Surg* 36:160, 1954.

119. **Tomford WW, Doppelt SH, Mankin HJ, et al:** 1983 bone bank procedures, *Clin Orthop* 174:15, 1983.

120. **Tomford WW, Ploetz JE, Mankin HJ:** Bone allografts of femoral heads: procurement and storage, *J Bone Joint Surg* 68A:534, 1986.

121. **Tomford WW, Starkweather RJ, Goldman MH:** A study of the clinical incidence of infection in the use of banked allograft bone, *J Bone Joint Surg* 63:244, 1981.

122. **Torisu T, Utsunomiya K, Maekawa M, et al:** Use of bipolar hip arthroplasty in states of acetabular deficiency, *Clin Orthop* 251:119, 1990.

123. **Trancik TM, Stulberg BN, Wilde AH, et al:** Allograft reconstruction of the acetabulum during revision total hip arthroplasty. Clinical, radiographic, and scintigraphic assessment of the results, *J Bone Joint Surg* 68:527, 1986.

124. **Transmission of HIV through bone transplantation**: Case report of public health recommendations, *MMVR* 37:597, 1988.

125. **Triantafyllow N, SotibropoulosE, Traintafyllou JN:** The mechanical properties of lyophilized and irradiated bone grafts, *Acta Orthop Belg* 41(suppl):35, 1975.

126. **Urist MR:** Surface-decalcified allogenic bone (SDAB) implants. A preliminary report of 10 cases and 25 comparable operations with undecalcified lyophilized bone implants, *Clin Orthop* 56:37, 1968.

127. **Urist MR:** Practical applications of basic research on bone graft physiology. *American Academy of Orthopaedic Surgeons instructional course lectures,* vol 25, St Louis, 1976, Mosby–Year Book.

128. **Urist MR, Silverman BF, Büring K, et al:** The bone induction principle, *Clin Orthop* 53:243, 1967.

129. **Volkov M:** Allotransplantation of joints, *J Bone Joint Surg* 52[Br]:49, 1970.

130. **Weikel AM, Habal MB:** Meralgia paresthetica: a complication of iliac bone procurement, *Plast Reconstr Surg* 60:572, 1977.

131. **Williams G:** Experiences with boiled cadaveric cancellous bone for fractures of long bones, *J Bone Joint Surg* 46[Br]:398, 1964.

132. **Wilson MG, Scott RD:** Reconstruction of the deficient acetabulum using the bipolar socket, *Clin Orthop* 251:126, 1990.

133. **Wilson PD:** Experiences with a bone bank, *Ann Surg* 126:932, 1947.

134. **Withrow SJ, Oulton SA, Suto TL, et al:** Evaluation of the antiretroviral effect of various methods of sterilizing/preserving corticocancellous bone, *Trans Orthop Res Soc* 15:226, 1990.

ADDITIONAL READINGS

Blakemore ME: Fractures at cancellous bone graft donor sites, *Injury* 14:519, 1983.

Dooley BJ, Clifford MJ, Hjorth DP: Total hip replacement combined with bone grafting for acetabular dysplasia causing severe osteoarthritis of the hip joint, *Aust NZ J Surg* 55:195, 1985.

Harris WH: Traumatic arthritis of the hip after dislocation and acetabular fractures: treatment by mold arthroplasty. An end-result study using a new method of result evaluation, *J Bone Joint Surg* 51:737, 1969.

Harris WH: Bone grafting for acetabular deficiency in association with total hip replacement. In The Hip Society: *the Hip: proceedings of the fourteenth open scientific meeting* of The Hip Society, St Louis, 1986, Mosby–Year Book.

Harris WH, Penenberg BL: Further follow-up on socket fixation using a metal-backed acetabular component for total hip replacement. A minimum ten-year follow-up study, *J Bone Joint Surg* 69:1140, 1983.

McCollum DE, Nunley JA, Harrelson JM: Bone-grafting in total hip replacement for acetabular protrusion, *J Bone Joint Surg* 62:1065, 1980.

Mendes DG, Roffman M, Silberman M: Reconstruction of the acetabular wall with bone graft in arthroplasty of the hip, *Clin Orthop* 186:29, 1984.

Murray WR: Acetabular salvage in revision total hip arthroplasty using the bipolar prosthesis, *Clin Orthop* 251:92, 1990.

Pelker RR, Friedlaender GE, Markham TC: Biomechanical properties of bone allografts, *Clin Orthop* 174:54, 1983.

Urist MR: Osteoinduction in undemineralized bone implants modified by chemical inhibitors of endogenous matrix enzymes. A preliminary report, *Clin Orthop* 87:132, 1972.

See Chapters 20, Congenital Dysplasia and Dislocation; 22, Protrusio Acetabuli; 25, Revision in Absence of Infection; and 26, Revision of Infected Hip for additional information.

PART FIVE

SURGICAL TECHNIQUES FOR PRIMARY SURGERY

■ If it could be guaranteed that the greater trochanter would unite within 3 weeks when reattached, and without imposing restrictions which would impede rehabilitation, few surgeons would fail to avail themselves of the easy and beautiful access to the hip provided by the lateral approach.
Sir John Charnley

INTRODUCTION

Choice of a surgical approach in performing total hip arthroplasty depends largely on circumstances such as the anatomical pathology of the hip, surgeon's training, the choice of positioning of the patient, and so on. *Certain steps are common to all total hip arthroplasties regardless of the surgical approach or prosthesis used. These procedures are presented in Chapter 15 to avoid duplication in the succeeding surgical chapters, and therefore it is essential that this chapter be read first.*

The reader should review the detailed discussion of the advantages and disadvantages of each surgical approach for total hip arthroplasty in Chapter 3. The surgeon must choose an approach that is most reproducible and provides the patient with a long-term satisfactory result. When the surgeon uses one surgical approach routinely, his or her skills are refined and better serve the patient. This author prefers a posterolateral approach (Chapter 16) without trochanteric osteotomy for a routine and uncomplicated total hip arthroplasty. However, I prefer a transtrochanteric approach when performing anatomically difficult and revision surgery.

The surgical exposure must cause no undue injury (other than what might be occasioned by dissection of the tissue) to the soft tissues, including abductor muscles. It should produce a circumferential view of the acetabulum and unimpeded surgical access to the top of the femur and medullary canal so that the stem can be inserted. The transtrochanteric approach meets all these requirements (Chapters 18 and 19). However, this approach has been criticized on the basis of troublesome complications, described in Chapter 37.

Because the major gluteal muscle fiber mass is located anterior to the greater trochanter, acetabulum, and femur, use of a transgluteal or anterolateral approach (see Chapter 3) renders the gluteal muscles and their nerve supply more prone to injury than use of the posterolateral approach (Fig. 1).

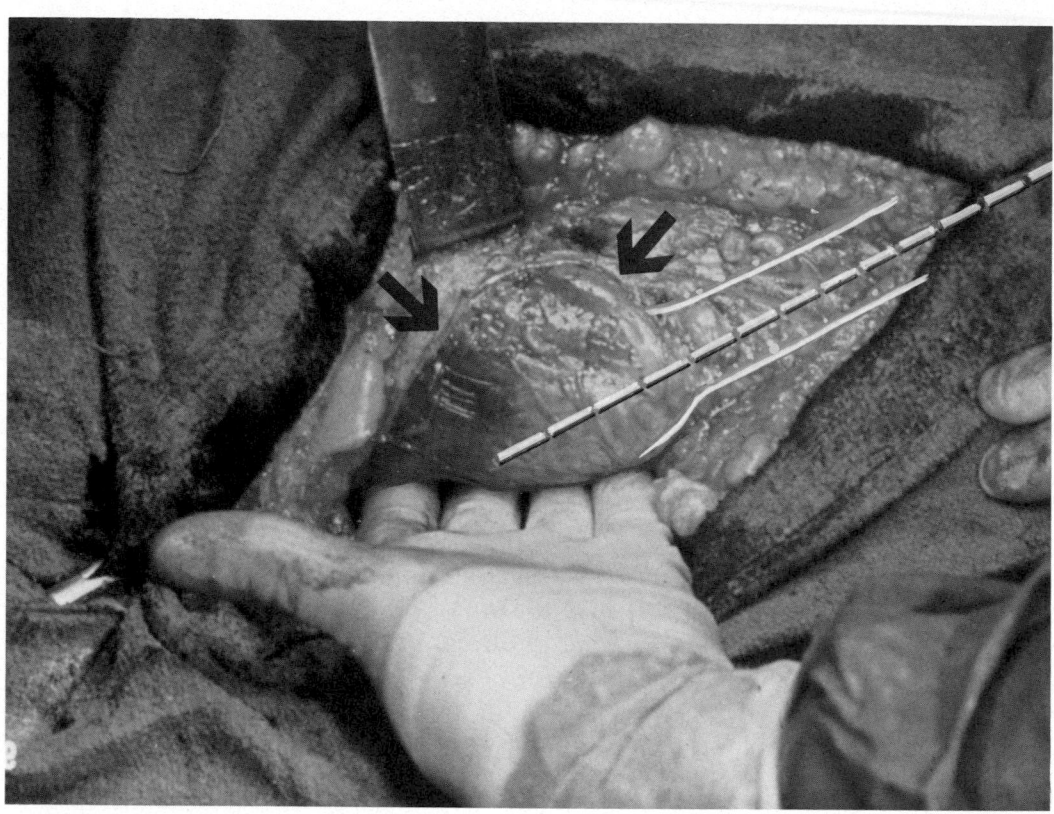

A major portion of the gluteus medius and the tendon of gluteus minimus lies anterior to the trochanter and femoral axis. Intraoperative photograph illustrates the surgeon's hand inserted behind the trochanter demonstrating the teninous portion of the gluteus medius and the trochanteric crest. Note the extent of the abductor mass located anterior to the trochanter and femur *(arrows)*, which is prone to injury during retraction using an anterolateral approach. Similarly a transgluteal approach (along the interrupted line) renders the gluteal muscles and branches of the superior gluteal nerve more prone to injury.

CHAPTER FIFTEEN

Principles Common to All Surgical Approaches

■ . . . Many surgeons thought that it was an adhesive, and many subconsciously still do, as indicated by the fact that it is still frequently called a "glue".
Sir John Charnley

This chapter presents some technical details related to all total hip arthroplasty procedures that have been demonstrated clinically to be effective. They apply to all surgical approaches and all prostheses and instrumentation. The chapter is organized to avoid repetition of the common steps shared by all techniques, regardless of the surgical approach, the patient's position, or the instrumentation used. It is hoped that the student of hip arthroplasty will be neither discouraged by the details outlined here nor dissuaded from improving or improvising on his or her method according to his or her training. Modifications are justifiable if they are based on objective data supporting the logic behind the modifications. In Chapters 4, 5, and 6 the basic principles related to biomaterials and biomechanics have been detailed. Chapter 11 discusses the fundamentals of prosthetic choice and customization. Because acrylic cement currently is the material of choice for bonding the prosthesis, a section on the practical aspects of its use is presented at the end of this chapter.

Chapters 16 through 19 and others on technique will frequently refer the reader back to this chapter because many steps discussed here are common to all techniques.

The most common causes of failure in total hip arthroplasty requiring revision are loosening, recurrent dislocation, and infection. Although these complications are not entirely preventable, they can be minimized by improved technique and by attention to the surgical details described in this and subsequent technique chapters.

A very high rate of success can be achieved in most patients with hip disease when cement is used with modern prostheses, providing the surgeon attends to the essential details of technique. Cementless devices are still largely in the developmental stage, with less than a 10-year follow up; consequently, they should be considered with caution and only for those patients for whom a cemented hip is contraindicated (see Chapter 10).

The principle in improved cement fixation is to achieve microinterlock resulting from (1) exposure of firm trabecular bone free of debris and clots, (2) improved intrusion of the cement into the trabecular bone, (3) pressurization of the cement after containment, and (4) checking of the "bleeding pressure" by sustained pressurization of cement while it is being polymerized.

The principle in improved cementless fixation of the prosthesis (including those with porous-coated surfaces or press-fit devices) is (1) to create a bony cavity that conforms to the shape of the prosthesis, (2) to produce a maximum surface area conforming to the shape of the prosthesis, and (3) to maintain initial rigid fixation long enough to achieve bony ingrowth (or ongrowth).

Theoretically, bone ingrowth in patients with adequate bone stock can occur and is seemingly the ideal fixation method for young and active patients, but in practice these devices have not gained universal popularity. Because of the lack of long-term evaluation, the routine use of these devices is not warranted. Several problems have been associated with the use of these cementless devices including abnormal bone remodeling, stress shielding (particularly in the femur and when the surgeon uses large-caliber stems), persistent thigh pain, and problems associated with their removal.

The use of hemispherical, porous-coated cups in patients with good bone quality is producing a more consistent and reproducible result than do porous-coated femoral components; the latter undergo continual changes with respect to the geometric shape, the porous coating, and so on. For most patients age 60 or younger, except those with inflammatory disease and bone-deficient hips, this author favors a combined cementless, porous-coated acetabular component and a cemented femoral design (see Chapter 10). For older patients, who comprise most patients undergoing total hip arthroplasty, a completely cemented hip is advisable in view of excellent early and long-term results.

Total hip arthroplasty demands a more extensive exposure of the acetabulum and femur than most other surgical procedures about the hip (such as hip fracture, osteotomy, etc.). Regardless of the surgical approach, time spent developing a good view of the acetabulum and delivering the upper femur (thus providing a straight entry to the femur), ensures the safety and accuracy of bone preparation and component placement while avoiding damage to the hip. With proper surgical training and appropriate instrumentation, most total hip arthroplasty procedures may be performed without osteotomy of the trochanter.

The surgeon must be familiar with and should perform a trochanteric osteotomy when exposure is difficult and when complex reconstruction such as in revision surgery is necessary. Careful planning and execution are necessary to avoid complications related to trochanteric osteotomy. On the other hand, the surgeon should remember that serious complications, such as neurovascular or bone damage, can result from inadequate exposure without trochanteric osteotomy. These can be more serious than the complications resulting from trochanteric nonunion. This risk is especially present in revision surgery, in which reconstruction of the hip demands reorganization of the muscles and leg-length equalization in the presence of abnormal bone and accompanying deformities (see Chapter 25). For a discussion on indications for and the controversy regarding trochanteric osteotomy see Chapter 3; for details on detachment and reattachment of the trochanter see Chapters 18 and 19; and for complications of trochanteric osteotomy see Chapter 37.

OPERATING SUITE, POSITIONING, AND PREPARATION*
Operating Suite Requirements

The operation should be performed in a clean air operating room (OR). The OR should preferably be enclosed and equipped with ultrafiltration equipment. If it is not enclosed, the colony count must be low and traffic kept to a minimum (see Chapter 8). When available the surgeon and team should wear a body exhaust system, preferably with a communication system. I prefer a vertical flow-type enclosure ("greenhouse"), but a horizontal clean air room is equally satisfactory (see Chapter 8).

An induction room for anesthetization and wash-up adjacent to the OR is essential. Body exhaust systems are available for both laundered ventile cloth materials (almost completely impervious) and synthetic materials (totally impervious). Wide-bore exhaust tubes must provide good air circulation, since an inadequate circulation makes the gown intolerably hot. The design of the body exhaust gown should not include belts that would impede a free flow of air within the gown. Although a one-piece suit is advantageous for an effective air flow, a two-piece suit (with head and neck piece and the body piece) is easier to wear.

A standard operating table with an x-ray cassette holder and special "arm-holder" for positioning the upper extremities is used. A good adjustable light is of paramount importance to allow complete

---

* This description of OR requirements, draping, and preparation is designed to assist those performing surgery outside specialized centers and without the assistance of regular personnel who are fully familiar with the surgical procedure. Impervious laundered drapes are illustrated (similar to Wrightington Hospital).

illumination both horizontally and vertically; it should also have a focal length that will provide the deepest view of the wound and the acetabulum.

Induction Room

A trained technician or nurse and the most junior member of the team prepare the patient in the induction room under the supervision of the surgeon. The patient is anesthetized and placed on the operating table with the ipsilateral arm (or both arms if the frame is so designed) directly over his shoulder; the arm is held with the shoulder at 90 degrees flexion (Fig. 15-1).

The endotracheal tube must be secured before the arm is placed in the holder. This same arm usually carries the blood pressure cuff and the pulse stethoscope. The elbow is flexed to 90 degrees and well-padded to avoid pressure over the ulnar nerve. Stretching the brachial plexus by shoulder hyperabduction must be avoided. If this positioning of the arm is not possible because of rheumatoid arthritis or other conditions, improvisation is necessary. The surgeon is responsible for proper positioning and must remain aware that excess forward flexion or hyperabduction of the shoulder during surgery (poor positioning of the arm) can result in partial brachial and ulnar nerve palsy.

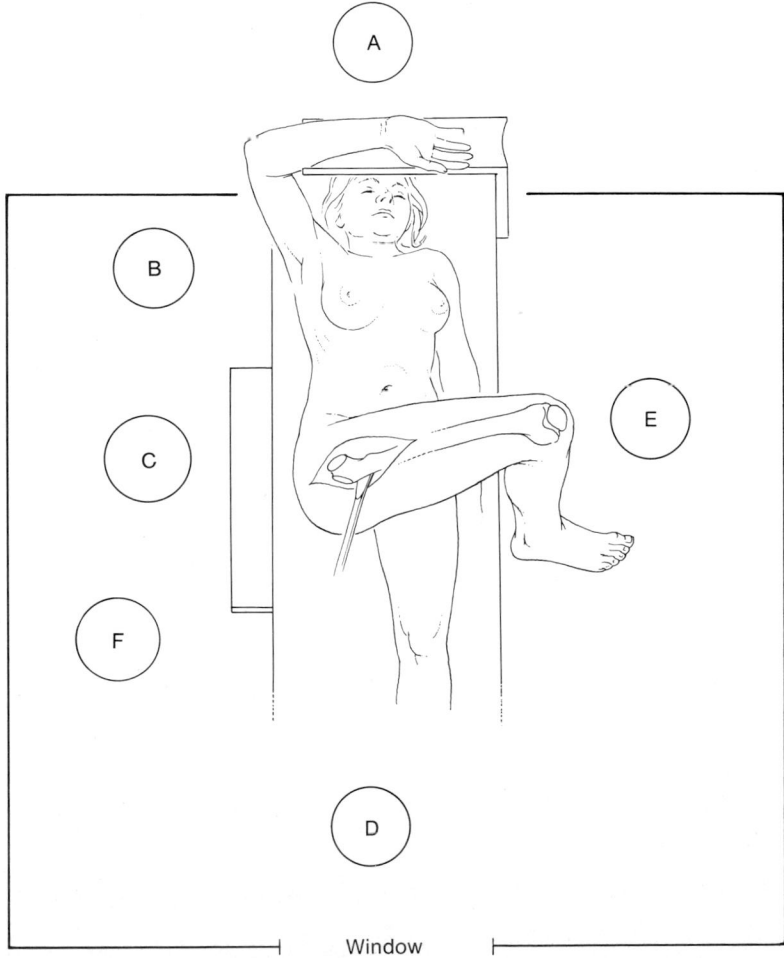

Fig. 15-1. The patient is positioned and anesthetized, and the skin is prepared in the induction room adjacent to the operating room proper. General view of the operating room enclosure. Positions of patient, operating table, and personnel and their relationship to the operating and instrument tables. *A*, Anesthetist; *B*, first assistant; *C*, surgeon; *D*, nurse; *E*, second assistant at the beginning of the operation; *F*, second assistant may move to this position after application of the octomerous retractor to observe the operation. Rectangular-shaped space attached to the operating table in front of the surgeon *(C)* is the surgeon's instrument table. This table is used to place the instruments as they arrive in the enclosure.

When a supine position is used a side table is attached to the operating table. The instrument side table is attached to the OR table so that the greater trochanter is located equidistant from either end (all subsequent draping will cover it). An 8 × 16 inch design is quite adequate; a larger table would prohibit free access to the field, as would placement excessively distal from the center of the wound (see Fig. 15-1).

In both male and female patients with arthritic hips and limited range of motion a complete preparation of the perineum may be difficult; it is therefore advisable to isolate the perineum from the surgical field before skin preparation. Assisted by a technician, the surgeon positions an adhesive sterile sheet at the periphery of the perineum (Fig. 15-2). The perineum adhesive sterile sheet must be applied so that it will remain fixed to the skin throughout the operation and isolate the perineum from the surgical field. The indwelling catheter is inserted before the adhesive sheet is applied. Apply tincture of benzoin solution to the skin before using the adhesive sterile sheet.

Positioning

Preoperative preparation is generally based on the individual surgeon's customary choice and training, as well as the facilities offered by the particular hospital. The suggested positioning, preparation, draping, and surgical exposure are this author's personal preference and can be modified as required according to the operating circumstances.

This author prefers a posterolateral approach with the patient in lateral decubitus position for all noncomplicated primary arthroplasties (see Chapter 16). However, I use a transtrochanteric approach in all revision operations and in cases with difficult anatomical deformities requiring extensive exposure. For the latter I use a supine position, although a lateral decubitus might be equally satisfactory (see Chapters 18 and 19).

LATERAL DECUBITUS POSITION After the anesthetist administers the anesthesia and secures the endotracheal tube, turn the patient to the side with the hip in a perfect lateral decubitus position, and follow the steps described:

1. Insert an in-dwelling Foley catheter before turning the patient. Place the electric cautery Bovie pad over the ipsilateral shoulder or lateral aspect of the contralateral thigh. Apply an occlusive perineal adhesive sheet (Steri-drape) in the same manner as used for supine position (see Fig. 15-2). Have the technician abduct the ipsilateral hip proximally. Apply tincture of

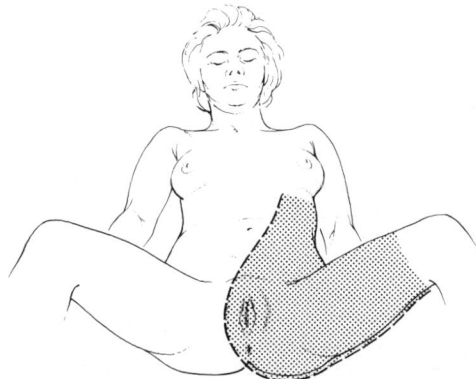

Fig. 15-2. Adhesive sheet is applied to isolate perineum. Both legs are abducted maximally and flexed to about 45 degrees to expose perineum. Sheet is then applied starting from abdomen to genitalia to perineum; avoid adductor region on medial side of ipsilateral thigh, extending to buttock at level of gluteal fold (at this point adhering to inner side of gluteal fold of ipsilateral side). It should then extend to buttock of other side. Site of insertion of adductor longus to pubis must not be covered in case adductor tenotomy becomes necessary during surgery. In this way no preparation or washup of contralateral medial thigh is necessary (in this case left medial thigh). Genitalia and anus are isolated from surgical field.

benzoin from the chest to the back extending from the umbilicus to the adductor region onto the ipsilateral of the buttock, thereby insulating the genitalia and the anal region from the surgical field. The insertion site of the adductor longus must not be covered in case an adductor tenotomy is necessary during surgery.

2. Bring the patient to the edge of the table in the direction of the operative hip and then turn him or her onto the opposite side. Adjust the two support clamps while supporting the ipsilateral arm with an armrest (Fig. 15-3).

3. Support the upper thorax with an axillary roll thus avoiding compression of the brachial plexus by the weight of the patient's chest and the ipsilateral upper limb.

4. Flex the contralateral knee from 45 to 60 degrees, and support the bony prominences (lateral malleolus, fibular head, lateral femoral condyle) on soft pads.

5. Secure the flexed knee (contralateral) to the operating room table with a cross-table Velcro strap placed over 2 to 3 cm thick foam pillow.

Observe the following details:

1. Ensure the safety of the "down leg" (contralateral), and obviate any venous or arterial occlusion that may result from the pubic support device. This omission may result in catastrophe as a result of either arterial or venous damage to the opposite limb. Heavy and obese patients are particularly prone to this complication (see Chapter 16). As a safeguard, check the color and pulse of the down leg after positioning and just before draping. Adjust the position of the pubic support as necessary.

2. Ensure the safety of the brachial plexus, and locate the axillary roll in an appropriate position. Such an axillary roll can be made from firmly rolled soft pads or towels to contour, approximately 2 to 4 inches in diameter. Place it just distal to the axilla to elevate the contralateral chest wall, which relieves pressure from the trunk on the brachial plexus. You should be able to feel with your hand the space between the dome of the axilla and the roll. The exact location of the roll is shown in Fig. 15-3.

3. Conduct any final examination regarding leg length discrepancy (clinically) before positioning the patient in the lateral decubitus position.

4. Make certain that the patient is in true lateral decubitus position before draping; any change in the patient's position after draping may risk malpositioning, which cannot be conveniently corrected.

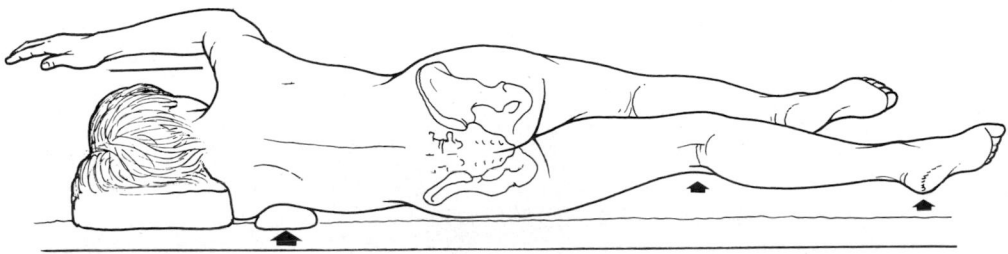

Fig. 15-3. The surgeon and assistants must ensure the safety of brachial plexus and the neurovascular structures of the down leg in the lateral decubitus position. *1,* Be sure the patient is in a true lateral position relative to the table. *2,* Protect the down arm (brachial plexus) with firmly rolled towels placed 7 to 10 cm distal to the dome of axilla to elevate the chest *(arrow). 3,* Protect the upper arm by placing it in forward flexion (shoulder), and place the flexed elbow over a well-padded support. *4,* Stabilize the patient by using sacral and pubic pads (clamps) as shown in Fig. 15-4. *5,* Place soft pads under the bony prominences of the fibular head and the malleolus of the down leg to protect them. *6,* Finally check the vascular supply (venous and arterial) of the down leg before starting preparation and draping.

5. Make sure that hip flexion and adduction (during surgery) are not impeded by the pubic pad and clamp that have been used to secure the patient (Fig. 15-4). Rehearse the ranges of motion of the hip before draping.

SUPINE POSITION The patient is placed on the operating table in the supine position with the pelvis flat and the trochanter located beyond the edge of the table on the surgeon's side. This is done in the following manner:

1. The feet are brought to the end of the table, and the hip is brought to the edge of the table (on the side of the operator) so that the level of the greater trochanter and the table edge is the same.
2. An electric cautery (Bovie) pad is placed under the patient's opposite shoulder.
3. An in-dwelling Foley catheter is inserted.
4. Apply the occlusive perineal adhesive sheet (Steri-drape). Both legs are abducted maximally and flexed to about 45 degrees, exposing the perineum. The sheet is then applied, running from the abdomen to the perineum, avoiding the adductor region on the medial ipsilateral thigh and extending onto the medial ipsilateral buttock, thereby walling off the genitalia and the anal region (see Fig. 15-2). The insertion site of the adductor longus tendon to the pubic ramus must not be covered in case adductor tenotomy is necessary during surgery. In this way no preparation or wash-up of the contralateral thigh is necessary, and the genitalia and anus are isolated from the surgical field.

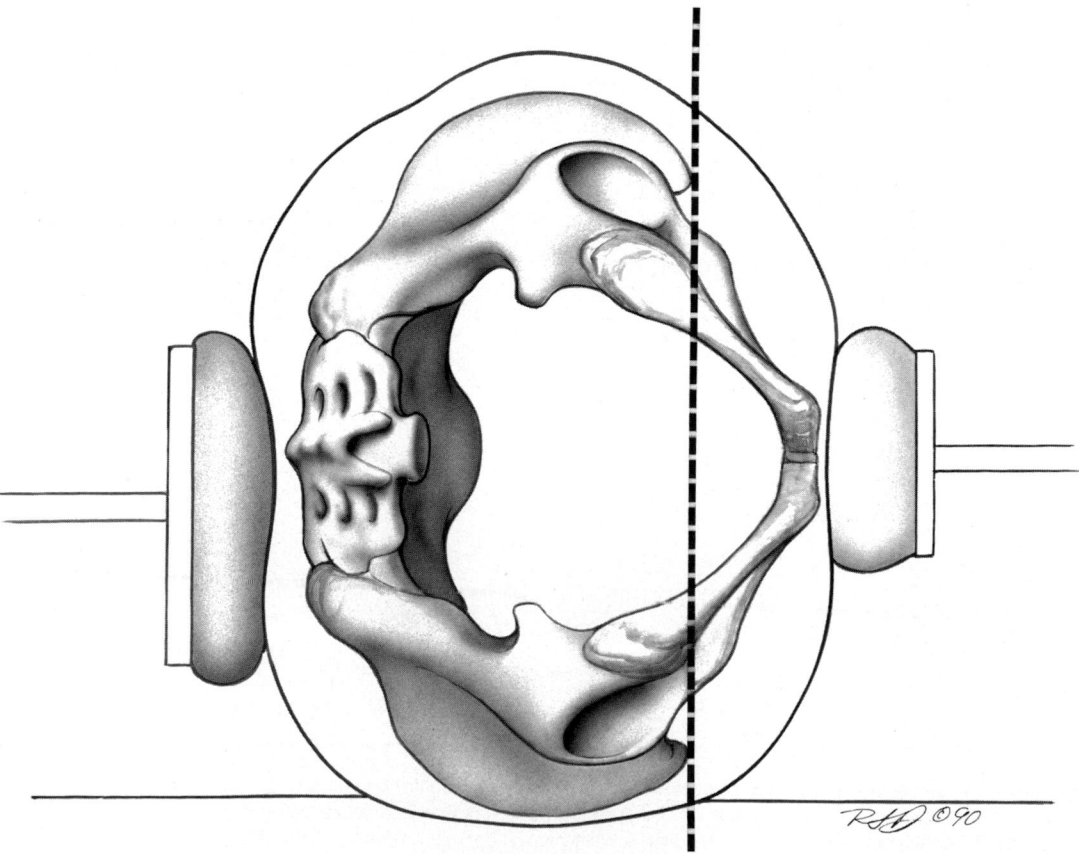

Fig. 15-4. Pelvis is secured in a "true" lateral position. A forward or backward tilt results in malpositioning of the acetabular component. Illustration shows the exact location of the small *(round)* anterior pubic pad and the large *(square)* posterior pad with the transaxis line of the pelvis at right angle to the table and operating room floor.

An alternative method for positioning the arms in those patients with restricted upper extremity joint motion should also be available (see Chapter 21). If an intraoperative radiogram is needed, a cassette holder is centered under the hip. A pelvic support is placed on the contralateral side of the operating table and adjusted to prevent any displacement of the pelvis away from the surgeon during surgery. Sand bags should not be used to elevate the operated side. The surgeon may sit while operating with the instruments prewrapped and placed on the instrument table attached to the operating table (see Fig. 15-1). A general view of the operating room enclosure and designated areas for the surgeons, assistant, and scrub nurse is shown in Fig. 15-1.

Wash-up and Skin Prep

Any remaining hair is clipped or shaved before wash-up, then a gloved but not gowned second assistant or trained technician prepares the surgical site with a 5-minute wash-up using surgical soap—povidone-iodine (Betadine) or hexachlorophene (pHisoHex). If a surgical prep team is available in the hospital, the practice of induction room wash-up is unnecessary. The surgical field can be prepared before patient arrival and the entire lower extremity is wrapped in sterile towels, so that the patient can be brought to the OR after anesthetic induction, positioning, and removal of the wrapping. The wash is from the nipple line to the toes on the affected side and from the anterior to the posterior midline. Using two bath sponges and soap, the wash first extends down to the ankle while the technician holds the patient's foot and flexes the hip to about 45 degrees; the technician then holds the calf with a folded sterile towel while the assistant finishes the wash by scrubbing the foot. The patient is finally moved into the surgical area in this position for the final preparation.* Use a degreasing agent such as Freon before applying a 2% tincture of iodine in 70% alcohol or Betadine solution.

Solutions and Towel Clips

- Solutions: surgical alcohol, Freon or ether, tincture of iodine (2%) in 70% alcohol
- 18 Moynihan clamps, 2 Turkish towels (24 inch × 18 inch), 8 standard towel clips

---

* If a prep room is not available adjacent to the clean air OR, wash-up and skin prep are carried out within the clean air room.

Reusable (Laundered) Drapes

1 Impermeable sterile sheet (70 inch × 40 inch)
1 Double-thickness sheet (for covering the end of the table) (52 inch × 47 inch)
1 Special double-thickness lateral sheet (72 inch × 45 inch)
1 Special double-thickness medial sheet (72 inch × 45 inch)
1 Double-thickness bottom sheet (104 inch × 94 inch)
1 Double-thickness top sheet
2 Side sheets (104 inch × 94 inch)
1 Double-thickness bag (for covering surgeon's sitting stool)
1 Large fenestrated sheet (98 inch × 180 inch) (18 inch long fenestration)
2 Rolled stockinettes (6 inch and 8 inch wide)

Disposable Drapes*

1 Disposable sterile plastic sheet (70 inch × 40 inch)
1 Disposable sheet for covering the end of the table (52 inch × 47 inch)
1 Special disposable lateral sheet (72 inch × 45 inch)
1 Special disposable double-thickness medial cloth* (72 inch × 45 inch) sheet
1 Bottom sheet (104 inch × 94 inch)
1 Top sheet
1 Double-thickness bag (for covering surgeon's sitting stool)
1 Large fenestrated sheet (98 inch × 180 inch) (18 inch 45 cm long)
1 Plastic bag for the leg
1 Rolled stockinette (8 inch wide)
1 Small adhesive plastic drape
1 Large adhesive plastic drape
1 Ioband (Steri-drape)

---

*Disposable impervious drapes are considered state of the art. The only laundered sheet is a double-thickness sheet.

Draping

Although rewashable textiles and sterilization are becoming obsolete in Western industrialized nations because of excess cost and manpower required to perform these tasks, it will be a long time before disposable textiles are universally available. The draping technique in this chapter can be adapted to reusable drapes, as well as disposable ones.

The entrance to the enclosure is sealed off by special curtains, and the window (instrument hatch) and instrument table are draped with special sterile sheets by the scrub nurse. Gowns are prewrapped and handed to personnel as they arrive in the OR. We currently use a two-piece paper gown consisting of the helmet aspirator section and a standard paper gown. A one-piece, single hood and gown are preferred. The two-piece suits used in a teaching hospital environment are easier to don (see Chapter 8).

The scrub nurse stays behind or at the side of the instrument table organizing the trays, handing out the sheets as needed during draping, cutting suture material, and so on, although no instrument table is required if prewrapped instruments are used because they are passed through the window of the enclosure during the operation. The double-glove technique is used for all personnel.

Upon arrival of the operating table in the OR, a double-thickness sheet is placed over the foot of the table as an added precaution against contamination. The table is not fully inserted into the enclosure at this point, so the nurse may continue setting up the instrument table and draping the instrument window (when an enclosure is used). The surgeon and the first assistant prepare the foot and ankle by removing the soap with alcohol, defatting the skin with a defatting agent, and finally painting the area with 2% tincture of iodine. The foot is then held by the second assistant with a plastic leg cover and rolled-up stockinette, while the surgeon and the first assistant finish applying the solutions to the hip and the entire extremity as described (Fig. 15-5).

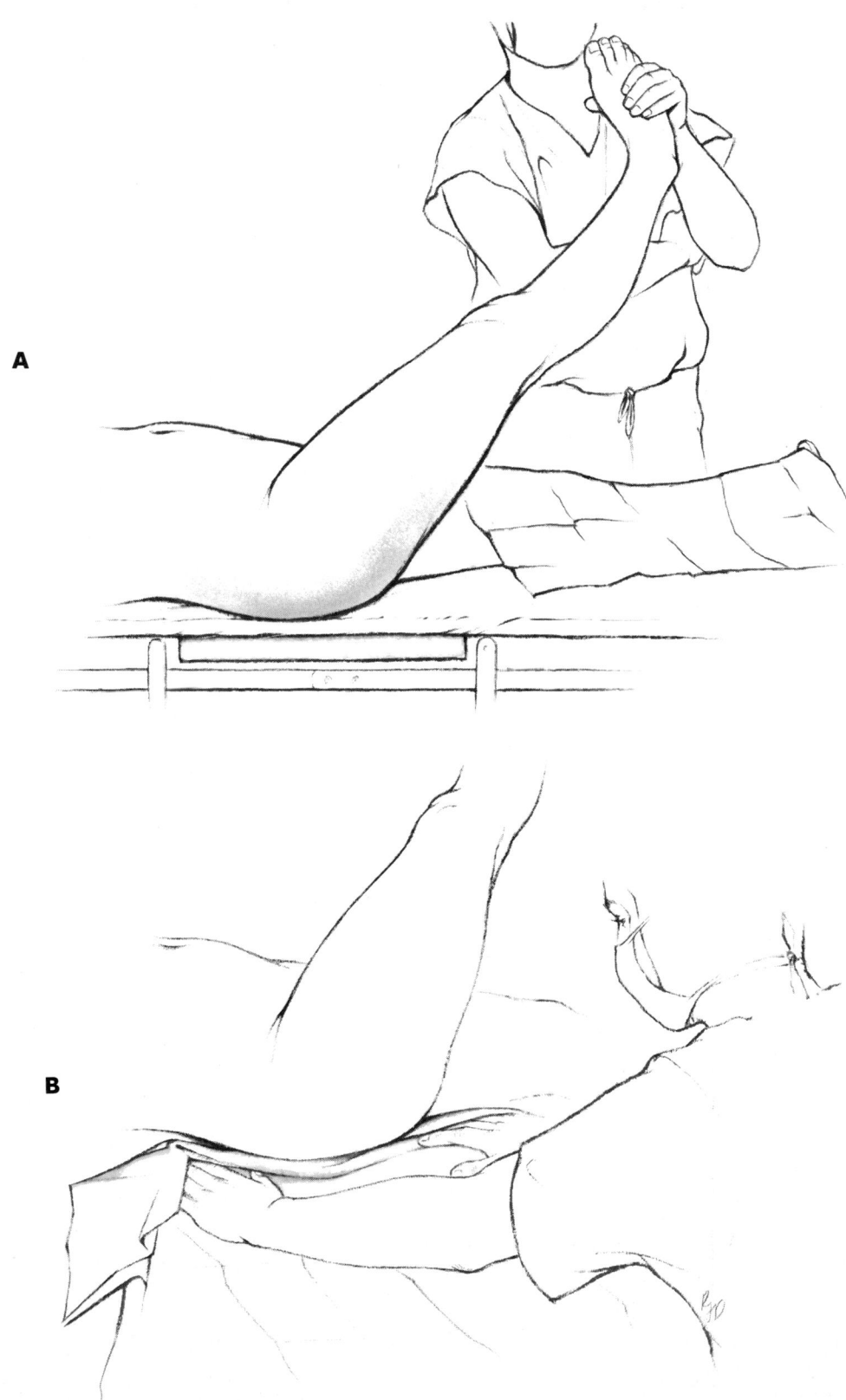

Fig. 15-5. A, The patient is positioned on the operating table in a supine position. An x-ray cassette holder is positioned and centered under the hip with the instrument table centered on that position. The pelvis is flat on the operating table; no sandbags are used. **B,** The orderly places the hip in flexion and maximum adduction, elevating the buttock so that the second assistant can put the impermeable sterile sheet in place. The orderly need not wear sterile garments or gloves.

Continued.

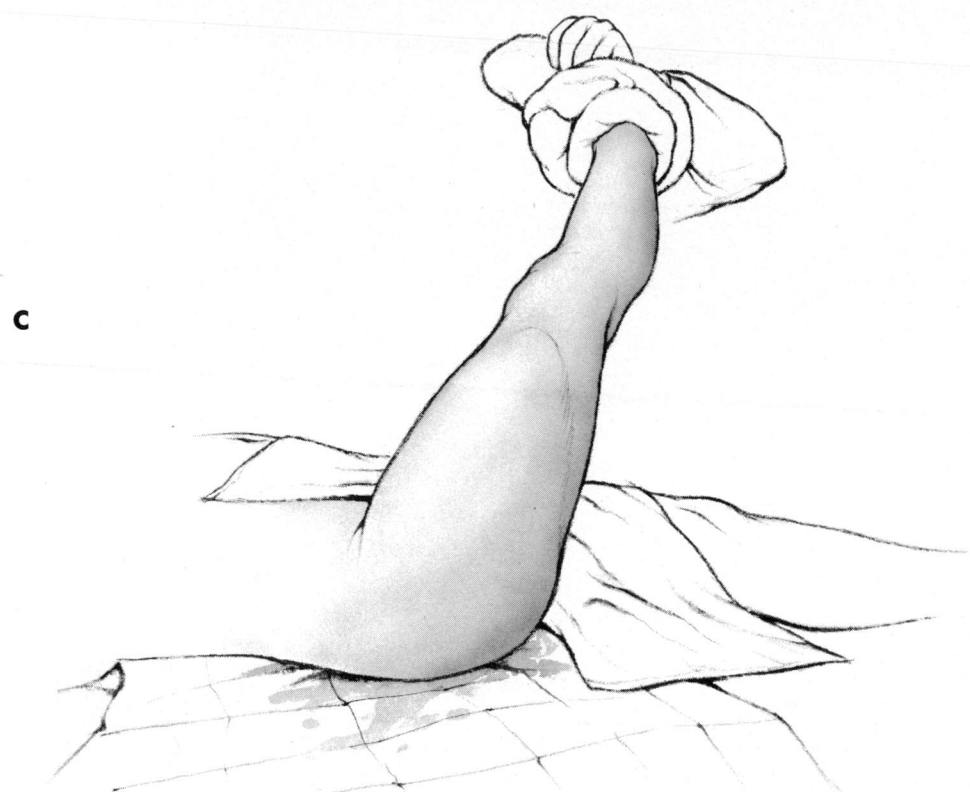

Fig. 15-5—cont'd. C, After the lower extremity is washed, the second assistant, holding the foot covered by a double stockinette, flexes and maximally adducts the hip. The surgeon and first assistant apply the prep solution. A sterile towel is placed over the medial aspect of the opposite thigh to prevent contamination by maximal adduction of ipsilateral thigh. NOTE: the original sterile sheet applied in induction room is still in place.

The following steps detail the draping technique for the patient in supine position (Figs. 15-6 to 15-10). A similar method can be adapted for draping the patient in the lateral decubitus position.

1. The first impermeable posterior sheet is exchanged for a new one and it, in turn, is covered by double-thickness sheet number 1 (Fig. 15-6). Particular care must be taken so that the initial posterior impermeable sheet used for wash-up does not come in contact with the surgical site as it is removed. The bottom of the table is now covered with double-thickness sheet number 2, which is placed across the table only to the level of the perineum (Fig. 15-7).

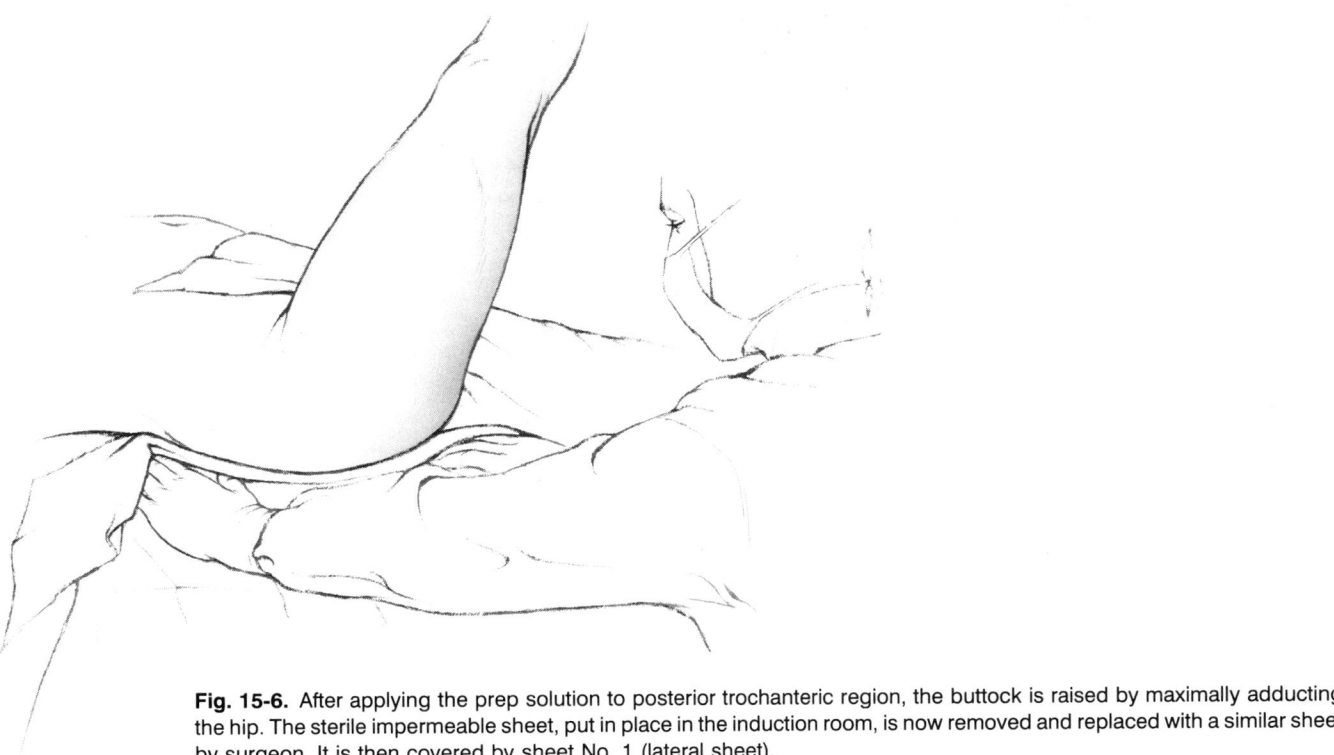

Fig. 15-6. After applying the prep solution to posterior trochanteric region, the buttock is raised by maximally adducting the hip. The sterile impermeable sheet, put in place in the induction room, is now removed and replaced with a similar sheet by surgeon. It is then covered by sheet No. 1 (lateral sheet).

Fig. 15-7. Sheet No. 2 (bottom sheet) is applied. It is placed across end of table under lower extremity while the second assistant holds hip in flexed position. This sheet is brought to level of perineum covering small towel (medial thigh towel) and lower portion of lateral sheet (sheet No. 1). NOTE: stockinettes are unrolled toward hip region.

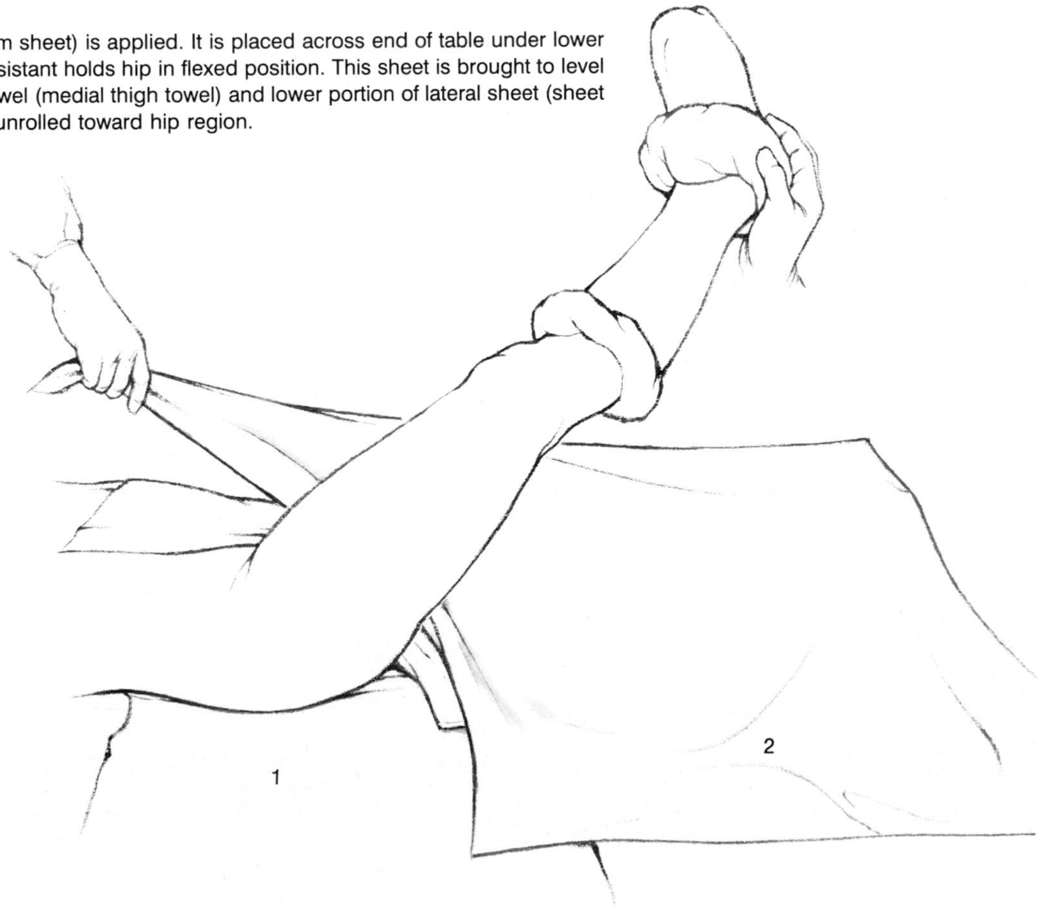

2. The stockinettes are then unrolled toward the hip, the impermeable (plastic) stockinette to above the knee level only. Unrolling the large stockinette requires some adduction of the limb so that it can be applied to the buttock area and held firmly against the rib cage. It is stretched taut over the crest of the ilium (Fig. 15-8, *A*) while the third sheet (special medial sheet number 3) is applied. The top (upper) sheet (number 4) is now lowered and fastened along with the third sheet and the unrolled top to the stockinette over the patient's abdominal wall (Fig. 15-8, *B*).

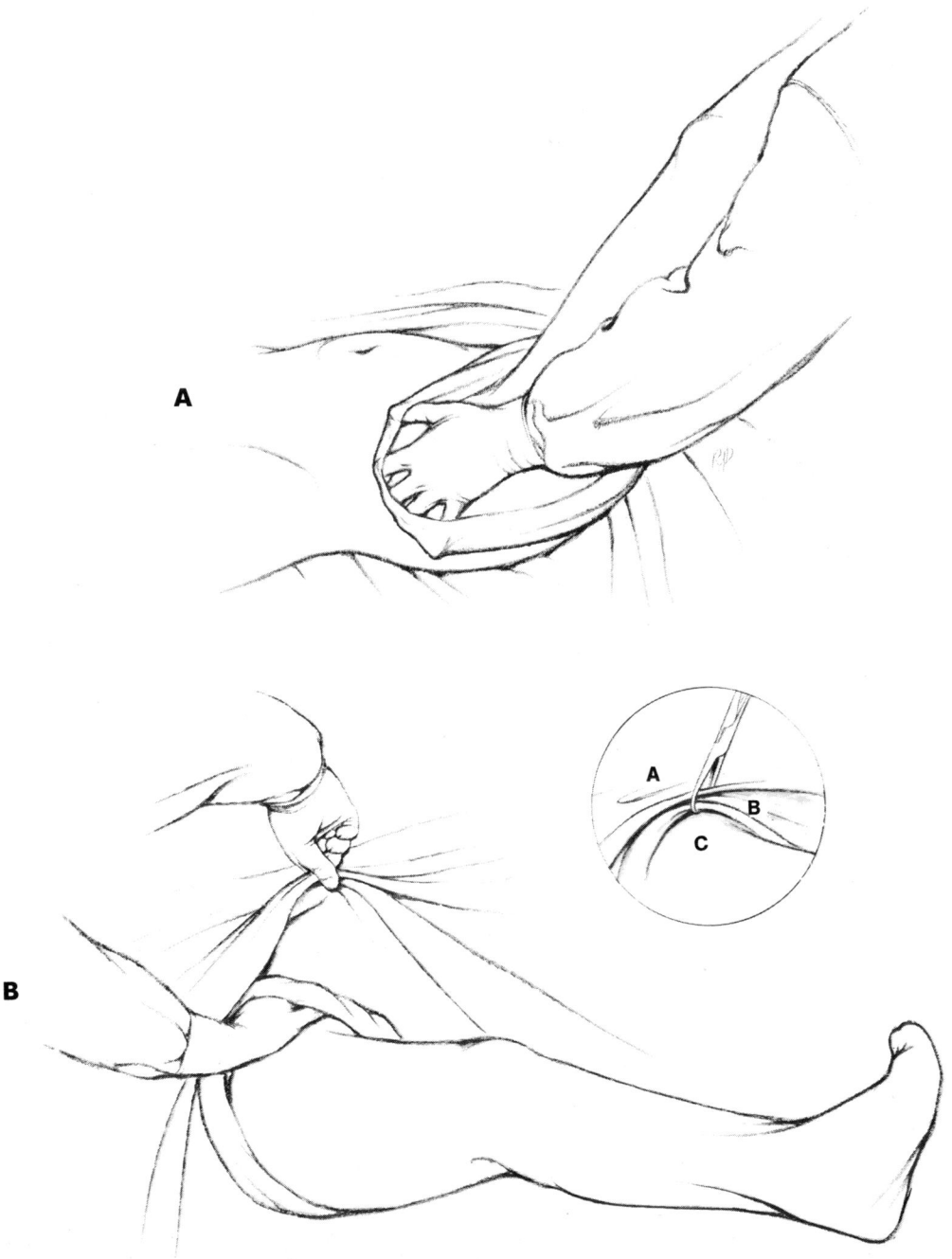

Fig. 15-8. A, Supine position: Stockinette is unrolled by surgeon and held against hip proximal to crest of ilium. **B,** Supine position: Medial and top sheets (Nos. 3 and 4) are placed on opening of stockinette while it is being unrolled toward patient's abdomen. Inset 1, Illustrates application of first towel clip to include medial sheet, *B,* top sheet, *A,* and unrolled stockinette, *C,* clipped together onto patient's abdominal wall. First towel clip should be applied approximately 2 inches proximal and 2 inches medial to anterosuperior spine. Inset shows stockinette, medial sheet, and top sheet, held and fastened to the abdominal wall.

3. Four standard towel clips are used to anchor the draping. The first is placed approximately 2 inches medial to the anterosuperior spine and fastens sheets 3 and 4 and the unrolled stockinette together over the abdominal wall as described. With the hip flexed to 90 degrees, sheet 3 is brought tightly across the medial thigh over the stockinette and fastened onto the midbuttock region with the second clip (Fig. 15-9, *A*). The assistant then adducts the hip, rolling the patient to the opposite side so that the buttock is slightly raised off the table and the surgeon is able to anchor sheet 4, the stockinette, and sheet 3 to the skin 3 or 4 inches from the level of the greater trochanter (Fig. 15-9, *B*). It is essential to provide the maximum amount of space proximal to the level of the greater trochanter to allow adequate operative exposure and prevent cramping of the wound. The third clip must anchor sheets 3 and 4 tautly, encompassing the unrolled stockinette. The sheets are applied counterclockwise for the right hip and clockwise for the left hip.

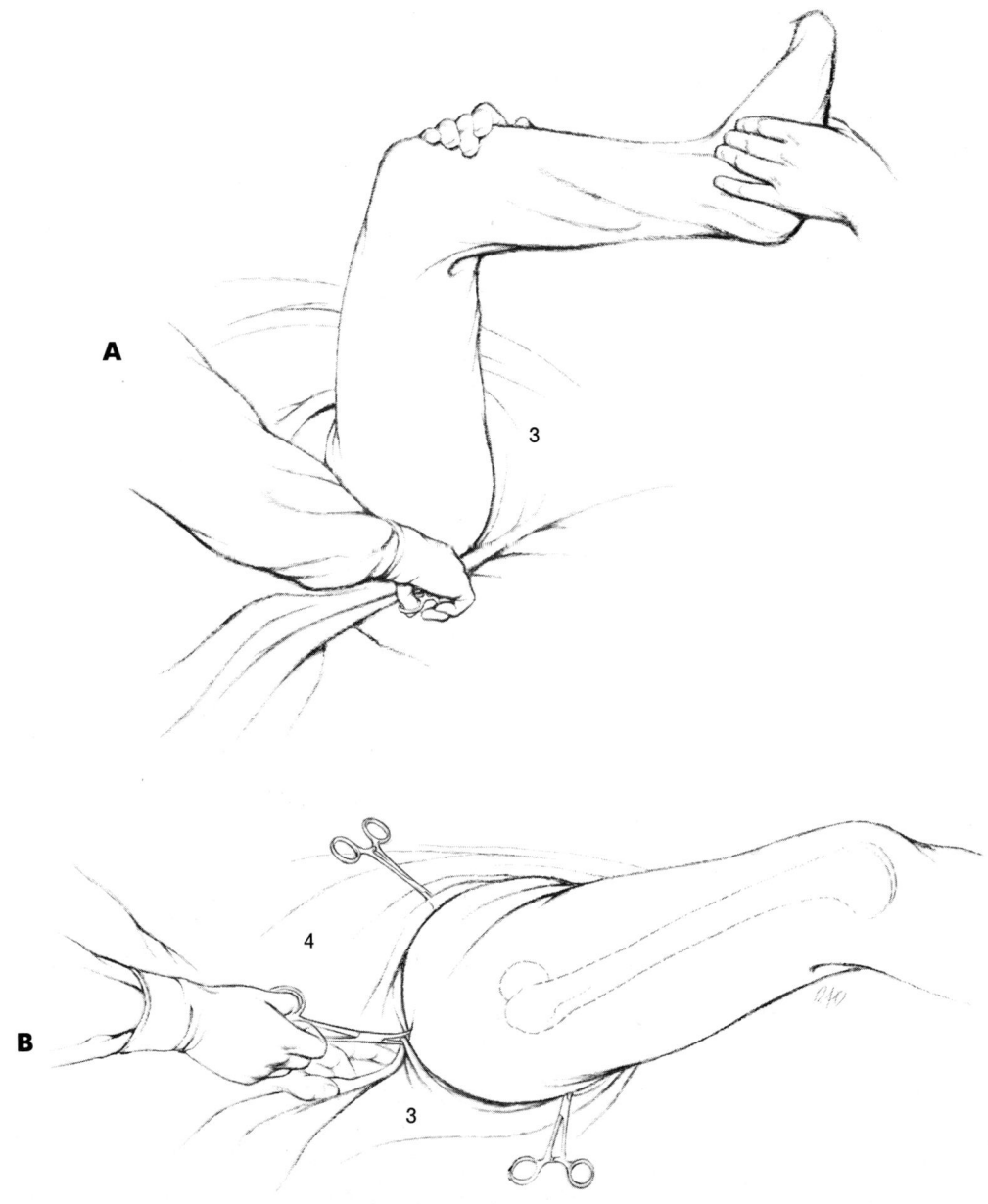

Fig. 15-9. A, Medial sheet (No. 3) is brought to medial thigh and gluteal fold of buttock and fastened to midbuttock region with second towel clip. **B,** By adducting hip and rolling patient to opposite side, buttock is slightly raised off table, while surgeon anchors top sheet (No. 4) and medial sheet (No. 3) onto skin 3 or 4 inches proximal to level of greater trochanter.

4. A large, fenestrated sheet is now applied, stretched toward the head of the table and anchored proximally with the fourth towel clip to eliminate slack in the aperture (Fig. 15-10) while taking care, however, not to limit the exposure. An opening is cut in the stockinette over the greater trochanter and extended 3 inches proximally and 6 inches distally; the rolled sheet of adhesive plastic Steri-drape is then applied to the skin (Fig. 15-11).

This is best done with the hip flexed about 30 degrees and adducted about 20 degrees by the second assistant. The first assistant opens a slit in the stockinette without touching the "painted skin." The corners of the Steri-drape are held by the first and second assistants (one each) and the backing is peeled from the adhesive surface by the surgeon. This drape further isolates the operative field from its surroundings. An alternative technique involves the application of an adhesive solution (that is, acrylic base spray) to the skin, causing the stockinette to adhere; in this way the stockinette is incised together with the skin, and the need for the adhesive plastic drape is eliminated.

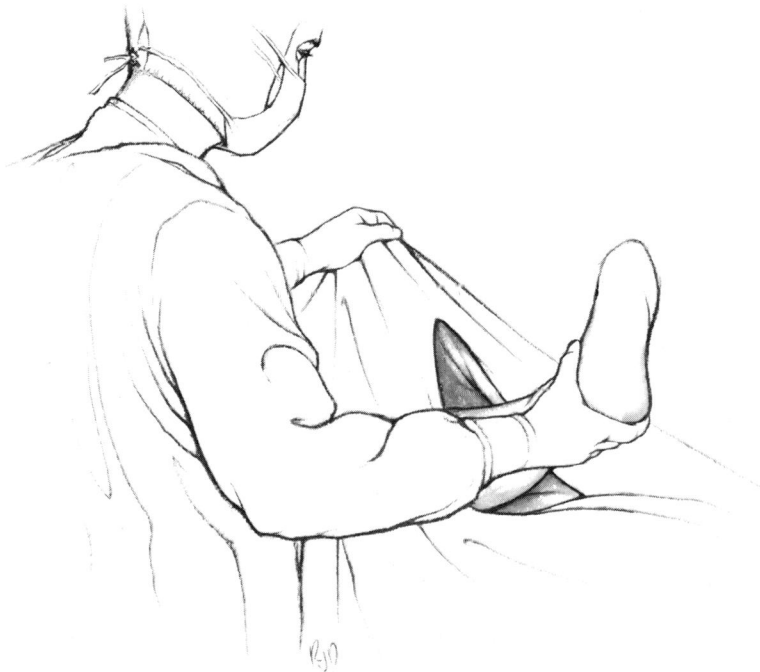

Fig. 15-10. Supine position: Large fenestrated sheet completes draping. Drape stretches toward head of table. Fenestration is anchored to remainder of drapes with fourth towel clip to eliminate slack in aperture.

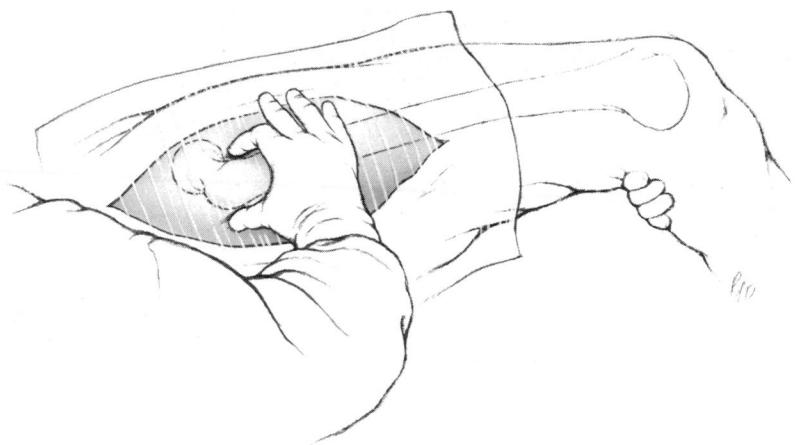

Fig. 15-11. Supine position: Opening is scissored in stockinette centered over greater trochanter. Adhesive plastic drape (Steri-drape) is then applied to skin.

5. The surgical team, now gowned and gloved,* guides the table into position well inside the enclosure. The sterile cover for the stool and the two side sheets are used to encompass the side of the operating table and the instrument table. The light is adjusted so that illumination is optional. Range of motion of the hip may be measured and recorded in the operating notes.

   The electric cautery, cutting apparatus, and suction tubing are now clipped to the drapes. The stool height is adjusted for the surgeon's comfort. The surgical team is now positioned for surgery (see Fig. 15-1), and the entire team exchanges its outer gloves for new ones. The basic steps for draping the patient in the lateral decubitus position are similar to those for the supine position. The only added step is to place four towels in the surgical field (anteriorly/posteriorly, superiorly/inferiorly). These towels are fastened to the skin with four towel clips before the stockinette is placed over the hip region.

SURGICAL EXPOSURE OF THE HIP JOINT
Skin Incision

The importance of a properly placed incision of adequate length cannot be overly emphasized. Undue trauma to soft tissue and bone resulting in complications certainly can be more damaging than a longer skin incision. Complications related to limited exposure are hematomas, infection, nerve and artery damage, malposition of components, and so on. The surgeon's pride in the brevity of the exterior scar is rarely acknowledged by the patient after surgery.

Plan for incision carefully using available landmarks and according to the anatomical planes used in each specific surgical exposure. Use a longer incision in obese, large muscled men, and in those

---

* The surgeon may use hexochlorophene (pHisoHex) or povidone-iodine soap, which will leave a protective film of disinfectant on the skin while gloves are worn.)

with severe anatomical deficiency that requires extra dissection and exposure and more complex reconstruction. Provide adequate space proximal to the level of the greater trochanter. Carefully drape the anterosuperior spine so it can be palpated during the procedure. Ensure that the patient is properly positioned since he or she may have moved during the preparation.

Observe any pelvic obliquity resulting from a fixed deformity. An unnoticed fixed pelvic obliquity may result in malposition of the cup in relation to the pelvis. Misplacement of the incision may occur as a result of fixed flexion deformity of the hip, excessive internal rotation, fixed external rotation, or faulty draping, so the surgeon must be fully cognizant of the position of the hip when the incision is made.

Three major points of reference should be kept in mind: the anterosuperior spine, the vastus lateralis ridge, and the shaft of the femur. The configuration of the muscle planes of the thigh (the hollow area of the iliotibial tract) is also visible and can be better seen by slight flexion and adduction of the hip (see Chapter 2).

Insulating the Skin Edges

This author recommends routinely applying a Steri-drape to the skin before making the incision. I also protect the skin by applying two towels clipped or sewn to the skin to isolate the wound and prevent trauma to the skin edges during surgery.

To protect the skin edge from trauma, as well as the hair follicles and sweat glands opened by the skin incision, the skin edge is walled off with two Turkish towels, each secured by nine Moynihan clamps (complete hemostasis is attained before their application). The anterior skin edge towel is applied first. After centering it over the wound, the distal and proximal towel clips are applied to stretch the towel to its full length. The remainder of the towel is secured by seven more clamps equally spaced along the edge of the wound, after which the second towel is applied to the posterior skin edge in the same manner. Four standard sharp-ended Mayo towel clips, two applied to either end of the incision, secure the towels together and complete the procedure. Forceful compression of the skin edge by the clamps results in skin necrosis and should be avoided. The towels should not be clipped to the drapes nor should they be pulled by the second assistant, since they are adequately held in place by the chain and weight of the initial incision retractor. Because of the tendency for Moynihan clamps to unspring, they are held together in groups of three, using rubber bands. As the final step, the surgeon applies 2% tincture of iodine to the skin edges pinched by the Moynihan towel clips.

Incision of Fat

The subcutaneous tissue is generally partially incised with the original skin incision before application of the towels; approximately 1 cm of fat should be cut with the skin knife. A change of outer gloves by the surgeon at this point may be a good practice. In a thin person, the incision should not be made boldly, to prevent opening the fascia inadvertently; undercutting the skin should also be avoided. Ideally, the incision of the skin, fat, and fascia is done in the same plane. Any deviation from the line of incision should be adjusted, keeping the trochanter as a point of reference, continually palpating it as the incision is made through the fat, and adjusting it before opening the fascia. Incision of the fat should be completed without changing the position of the limb, except in an obese patient, in whom it is helpful to elevate the buttock by increasing hip adduction. This will keep the subcutaneous tissue from falling across the wound and interfering with exposure (a common problem in obesity). The first assistant can improve the exposure by retracting the anterior flap of skin and subcutaneous tissue.

Veins and small arteries often cover the outer surface of the deep fascia and should be cauterized before incising the innermost layer of fat covering the fascia. Temptation to undermine the fat and detach it from the fascia must be avoided; this is done only if the incision has deviated from its original direction. Finally, the fat incision must use the full length of the skin incision to maximize exposure.

Fascial Incision

The effective use of self-retaining retractors (Charnley's initial incision retractor or Eftekhar's Octomerous retractor) (see Chapters 18 and 19) will expedite the proper placement of the fascial incision. Inadequate exposure of the acetabulum often is the result of too distal placement of the fascial incision.

From the point of the greater trochanter ridge, carefully incise the gluteal fascia for approximately 7.5 to 10 cm. Gently separate the underlying fibers of the gluteus maximus along the line of the incision. This important technical detail prevents damage to the gluteus maximus and allows wide opening of the fascia along with the deep muscle fibers of the gluteus maximus. Opening the fascia distal to the vastus lateralis ridge requires little effort since the fibers are parallel, and separation can take place with ease.

Maximum mobilization of the fascia is necessary before applying the self-retaining retractors. If the incision has been made excessively anterior, the iliotibial tract obstructs access to the back of the joint (this can be rectified by T-ing the fascia posteriorly). On the other hand, if the incision is placed excessively posterior (near the shaft of the femur), there is insufficient posterior fascial edge for anchoring the retractor.

Additional mobilization of the fascial edge may be obtained by running one's thumb beneath the edge anteriorly and posteriorly. This technique breaks up adhesions and intermuscular septa between the tensor fascia femoris and gluteus medius anteriorly by placing the hip in maximum external rotation and approximately 30 degrees flexion, and posteriorly by placing the hip in maximum internal rotation and 30 degrees flexion. Therefore the posterior aspect of the trochanter can be reached to detach the areolar connective tissue from the fascia at the level of the gluteus maximus tendon, the gluteus medius bursa, and the trochanteric bursa.

Since the initial incision retractor can facilitate exposure throughout the operation, it must be carefully placed. When applied properly at the trochanter level, the wound will be diamond-shaped with equal exposure proximally and distally to the trochanter. Ideally, approximately 5 to 7.5 cm of abductor muscle with its tendinous insertion and about 5 to 7 cm of vastus lateralis musculature should appear in the wound.

In an obese person the retractor may be difficult to apply. The posterior jaw is applied first (detached from the frame); the tensor fascia femoris may be T'd; then the frame is inserted in situ onto the lower jaw, with the limb abducted to relax the fascia and facilitate placement. The chain and hook carrying the weight are then attached to the upper jaw to provide a somewhat horizontal plane for the retractor. The higher the level of the chain and hook, the more horizontal the position of this retractor. The tilt of the retractor provides better access to the neck of the femur.

Unplanned Trochanteric Osteotomy

The role of trochanteric osteotomy for improving exposure and for the safety of abductors and neurovascular structures was discussed in Chapter 3. When the surgeon anticipates difficulty in exposing the hip adequately (because of deformity or stiffness), trochanteric osteotomy should be planned in advance (see Chapters 18 and 19).

However, if the exposure proves inadequate, the surgeon faces intraoperative difficulties in dislocating the hip, there is severe intraoperative instability, or the femur fractures, a trochanteric osteotomy should be performed. Trochanteric osteotomy is by far superior to detaching the abductors from the trochanter. For details of detachment and reattachment of the trochanter see Chapters 18 and 19.

Leg Length Equalization

A careful measurement of "actual" and "relative" leg length is essential to reproduce the preoperative leg length, although shortening of the limb is present. As such, leg length must be restored to the preoperative status if the patient did not wear a lift preoperatively.

In complex hip reconstruction, revision, and conversion surgery, the patient must understand that despite attempts to equalize the length at surgery, occasionally a slightly longer or shorter leg is inevitable, which may be caused by the stability of the hip at surgery (see Chapters 24, 25, and 32). Thus a shoe-lift may be prescribed.

To evaluate leg length equality, several methods are available to the surgeon that must be used in combination to assist in equalizing the leg lengths during surgery:

1. Preoperative clinical leg length measurements of the distance between the anterosuperior spine and medial malleolus.
2. Preoperative templating of the radiographs with known magnification.
3. Intraoperative measurements through drapes of the leg length from bony landmarks, that is, anterosuperior spine and medial mallelus.
4. Intraoperative measurements between two fixed points on the pelvis and femur.

Preoperative Measurement Between Bony Landmarks

The distance between the anterosuperior iliac spine and medial malleolus (for "actual" leg lengths) and measurements for "relative" leg lengths when pelvis obliquity is present (between a fixed central point on the midline of the body and medial malleolus,) should be carefully recorded and kept available to the surgeon during surgery. However, these clinical measurements should be matched with measurements on radiographic templates of x-rays with known magnification and recorded. Knowledge of the patient's height and the condition of the opposite hip or fixed pelvic obliquity is important in equalizing leg length. Minor degrees of overlengthening (in short persons) and shortening (in tall persons) may lead to severe pelvic tilt in the former and hip instability or dislocation of the hip in the latter.

PREOPERATIVE TEMPLATING The vendors of most prostheses currently on the market provide the surgeon with a transparent sheet depicting the outline of the stem and the cup with 15 to 20 degrees magnification, which can determine the exact level of the cut on the femur and the exact site for placement of the new socket.

By American standards, a 40-inch distance between the tube and the cassette holder and 2 inches between the table top and cassette results in a magnification between 17% and 24%. Errors of magnification can occur under the following circumstances:

1. Smaller and thinner patients have less while larger and fatter patients have greater magnification because of the changes in the distance between the patient's bone and the cassette. Routine measurement by radioopaque marker should be done to reflect the true magnification for accuracy.
2. A fixed hip contracture may lead to fixed "pelvic flexion" and changes in magnification because of a shorter distance between the femur and the tube. In this case it is necessary to position the femur flat on the table by propping the patient's back on pillows. Using radiographs with known magnification, the surgeon should be able to equalize the leg length within 0.5 to 1.0 cm. Despite careful x-ray measurements the surgeon may be forced to use a longer prosthetic neck length if the hip is unstable or a prosthesis with a shorter neck if the hip cannot be reduced after fixation of the socket.

Intraoperative Measurement Between Bony Landmarks

The classic measurement of leg length (anterosuperior spine to medial malleolus) can be used for the intraoperative measurement only if (1) the patient is in the supine position on the operating table and (2) both the anterosuperior spine and medial malleolus are available for palpation through the drapes during surgery (see Fig. 15-1).

MEASUREMENT BETWEEN PELVIS AND FEMUR In this method the leg length is measured intraoperatively by selecting two fixed points, one on the pelvis and the other on the femur. Insert two screws or Steinmann nails perpendicular to respective bones before hip dislocation. The same distance is measured after inserting the femoral component. The surgeon compares the recorded distance before dislocation and that after replacement, thus determining the degree of lengthening or shortening of the limb.

The length of the operated leg can be affected by the location of the socket on the pelvis, the location of the femoral component (varus/valgus) in the shaft, the neck length, and the offset of the prosthesis. The surgeon must record the intended lengthening or shortening of the limb based on his or her preoperative templating and also be guided by the leg length measurement (as indicated by the changes in the space between the pelvis and the femur).

Perform the intraoperative measurements as follows:

1. Insert the acetabular pin retractor or staple (see Chapters 16 and 19) 2 cm proximal to the lip of the acetabulum before dislocating the hip and removing the femoral head.
2. Mark a fixed point on the femur using cautery so that the bone is marked at the mid trochanteric ridge (vastus tubercle). Tag this site with a stitch.
3. Measure the distance between the tag and the acetabular pin with a ruler, and record it on the drape.
4. Repeat the measurements between the two points after inserting the components at test rehearsal.
5. Repeat the measurements after the actual prosthesis is inserted.
6. Make sure that the position of the leg on the operating table remains unchanged as measurements are being made. To prevent this error, which may affect the outcome, trace the operated leg on the drape and place the leg on the same tracing at each measurement.

This predictable and reproducible technique is applicable to all arthroplasty methods.

Finally, the surgeon should combine all of the methods (clinical, radiographic, and accurate intraoperative measurement) in every case for the best results in equalizing the leg length.

Leg length equality after total hip arthroplasty is desired by the patient and surgeon alike. Equalization helps restore the mechanics of the hip. It is desirable not only to equalize the lengths of the extremities during the total hip arthroplasty but also to avoid overlengthening the operated extremity. Overlengthening of the limb after surgery can cause back pain and an unhappy patient despite an excellent arthroplasty; rarely is a slight shortening of the extremity a concern to the patient.

When performing total hip arthroplasty for the following conditions, the surgeon must avoid leg length changes.

1. Unilateral arthroplasty with a normal opposite hip offers a singular opportunity to equalize the leg length. Careful intraoperative measurement and preoperative templating are required to equalize the leg lengths at surgery. In bilateral sequential replacement, further adjustments of the leg length equality may be possible at the second hip operation. Clearly, the patient must be reminded that the operated leg may be longer than the nonoperated leg because of the hip pathology in the latter, which may be corrected by lengthening during the second operation.
2. Patients with severe shortening caused by congenital dislocation of the hip must be informed that their operated leg will be lengthened but perhaps not to its normal length because of restrictions imposed by the myofascial length of the thigh (see Chapter 20).
3. Patients with fixed pelvic obliquity resulting from long-standing adduction contracture of the hip or suprapelvic obliquity and spinal arthrosis are especially prone to back pain if the operated leg becomes longer or shorter after total hip arthroplasty.

Capsulectomy and Capsulotomy

To facilitate dislocation of the hip, capsulectomy may be indicated, especially for anterolateral and transgluteal approaches (see Chapter 3). Capsulotomy is accomplished by using a diathermy knife. It should be performed at three sites: (1) anteriorly at 10 to 11 o'clock for the right hip and 1 to 2 o'clock for the left hip. Division of the acetabular labrum is also included; (2) posteriorly at 7 to 8 o'clock for the right hip and 4 to 5 o'clock for the left hip. Division of acetabular labrum is also included; and (3) a circumferential cut between 1 and 2. Similarly, a radial capsular release permits insertion of the inferior retractor and thus a better visualization and definition of the inferior margin of the acetabulum (3 o'clock for the right and 9 o'clock for the left hip).

In patients with protrusio acetabuli, excise the marginal osteophytes posteriorly, laterally, and anteriorly as needed when dislocation of the hip is not possible despite capsulotomy or capsulectomy. During capsulectomy or capsulotomy the surgeon must be aware of the location of the sciatic nerve posteriorly and the femoral artery, vein, and nerve anteriorly.

Dislocating the Hip

Although conventionally an anterior dislocation of the hip can be achieved by flexion abduction and external rotation (FABER) and a posterior dislocation by flexion adduction and internal rotation (FADIR), these maneuvers are contraindicated since they may cause intraoperative femoral fractures (see Chapter 37). Dislocation must be accomplished with adduction without rotation. Resistance to dislocation occurs as the result of one or more of the following:

1. The vacuum created as the head is moved from the depth of the socket.
2. Persistent posterosuperior or anterior capsular attachments and intact acetabular labrum.
3. A peripheral osteophyte or an excessively deep acetabulum, that is, protrusio acetabuli.
4. A coxa magna senilis larger than the opening of the acetabulum restricted by capsule and labrum.
5. Residual ligamentum teres.
6. A hypertrophied labrum.

Complete dislocation and delivery of the head into the wound may be facilitated by:

1. Placing the Watson-Jones bone gouge between the head and the acetabulum and levering the head out as the hip is adducted (Fig. 15-12).
2. Successively flexing and extending the hip to break the vacuum.
3. Further release of residual capsular and ligamentous structures.
4. Removing the overhanging acetabular osteophytes if present.
5. Incising the labrum along the superior acetabular rim.
6. Most important, maximal posterior capsular release.

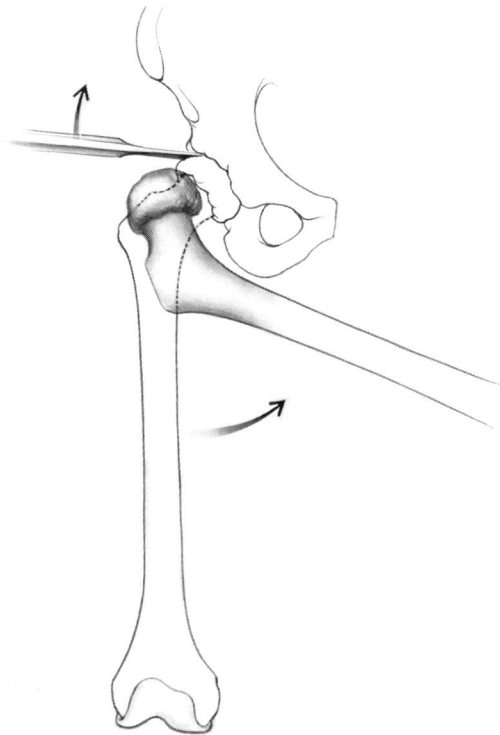

Fig. 15-12. Dislocation may be facilitated by inserting a Watson-Jones gouge between head and roof of acetabulum to pry head out of socket, while adduction force is applied to hip.

An excessively flexed hip in an adducted posture is more difficult to dislocate. An experienced second assistant is valuable at this stage of the operation; however, the surgeon is fully responsible for the act of dislocation.

In summary, dislocation is achieved by maximum adduction without external or internal rotation or flexion. Forceful external or internal rotation can cause a spiral fracture of the femur if the head is still engaged in the acetabulum. When dislocation is not possible the surgeon must decide to perform a trochanteric osteotomy or to perform an in-situ osteotomy of the neck of the femur and remove the head in a retrograde fashion.

AMPUTATING THE FEMORAL HEAD

This author prefers using a power saw to amputate the head of the femur. The level of the amputation must have already been estimated by a radiographic template (see Chapter 12). Using the radiographic template, direct the line of amputation toward the proximal edge of the greater trochanter osteotomy site. While amputating the head, the second assistant keeps the knee flexed and the tibial shaft perpendicular (90 degrees) to the floor. The plane of section of the neck is judged in relation to the vertical position of the tibia (Fig. 15-13, *A*). Ignore any anteversion or retroversion that may be present in the femoral neck. Fig. 15-13, *B*, illustrates various optional levels for sectioning the neck.

Observe the following:

- Adduct the femur strongly to facilitate passage of the Gigli saw.
- Protect adjacent soft tissue with narrow Hohmann retractors.
- Use a reciprocating saw to amputate the head.
- Use a cholecystectomy clamp to facilitate the passage of the saw.
- Avoid excess shortening of the neck. If the neck is too long, it can be shortened as needed at a later stage.
- Never use an osteotome, since it may fracture (split) the neck.
- Do not drop the femoral head out of the sterile surgical field, since it will be unusable as a bone graft or for bone banking.

PREPARATION OF THE ACETABULUM AND FIXATION OF THE SOCKET
Maximizing the Peripheral Exposure (Rim)

A complete exposure of the acetabular rim is essential to determine the acetabular depth and deficiencies. Observe the following:

- Remove cartilaginous labrum.
- Incise the capsule anterosuperiorly, posterosuperiorly, and inferiorly, and retract the superior and posterior capsule using Hohmann-type acetabular retractors.
- A routine excision of the capsule is unnecessary although it may be needed to achieve exposure or correct a fixed deformity and in certain approaches (see Chapter 17).
- Divide short external rotators and the posterior capsule to improve exposure where fixed external rotation deformity exists.
- Use one or two pin retractors (to retract the superior, posterior, and anterosuperior capsule) thus exposing the bony rim of the acetabulum. These pins are inserted parallel to the transaxis of the pelvis and should be fully engaged into both cortices of the pelvic bone.
- Avoid doing a complete capsulectomy (routinely) to obtain exposure since it adds to bleeding, causes loss of time, and removes "protection barrier" between it and the neurovascular structures.
- Use Hohmann-type retractors to produce the best results in exposing the acetabular rim and in excising the labrum or capsule.

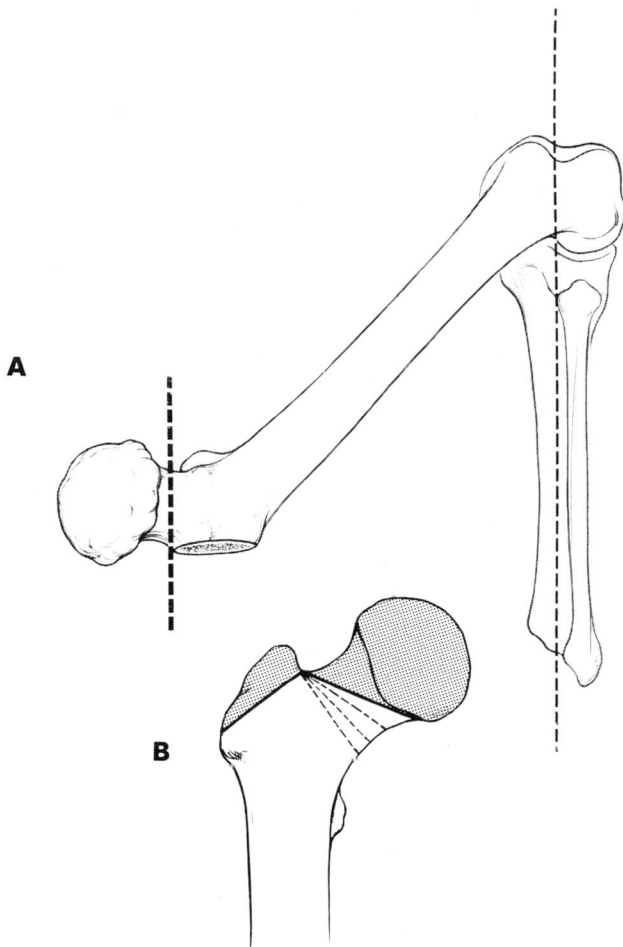

Fig. 15-13. A, Plane of section of neck is judged in relation to vertical position of tibia. This plane of section of neck ignores any anteversion or retroversion that may be present in neck of femur. **B,** Femoral head is divided at "meeting point" of cut surface of greater trochanter with femoral head. In this drawing several optimal lines *(dashed lines)* show meeting points. These optional lines indicate further shortening of neck of femur when it becomes necessary.

Maximizing the Exposure of the "Fossa" (Pulvinar)

The "fossa," or nonarticulating portion of the acetabulum, is the most important "landmark" because its direct visualization enables the surgeon to determine the limit to which the acetabulum can be safely deepened (Figs. 15-14 and 15-15). This zone of acetabulum can easily be visualized in a normal acetabulum by removing the ligamentum teres and synovial fold and fat (collectively termed the Haversian gland), and in some arthritic hips without severe changes caused by osteophytes or medial migration (Fig. 15-16, *A*). However, occasionally the nonarticulating segment may be partially or totally covered by hypertrophic marginal acetabular osteophytes. This phenomenon can usually be recognized on x-ray film and requires special attention when preparing the acetabulum (Fig. 15-17).

Text continued on p. 670.

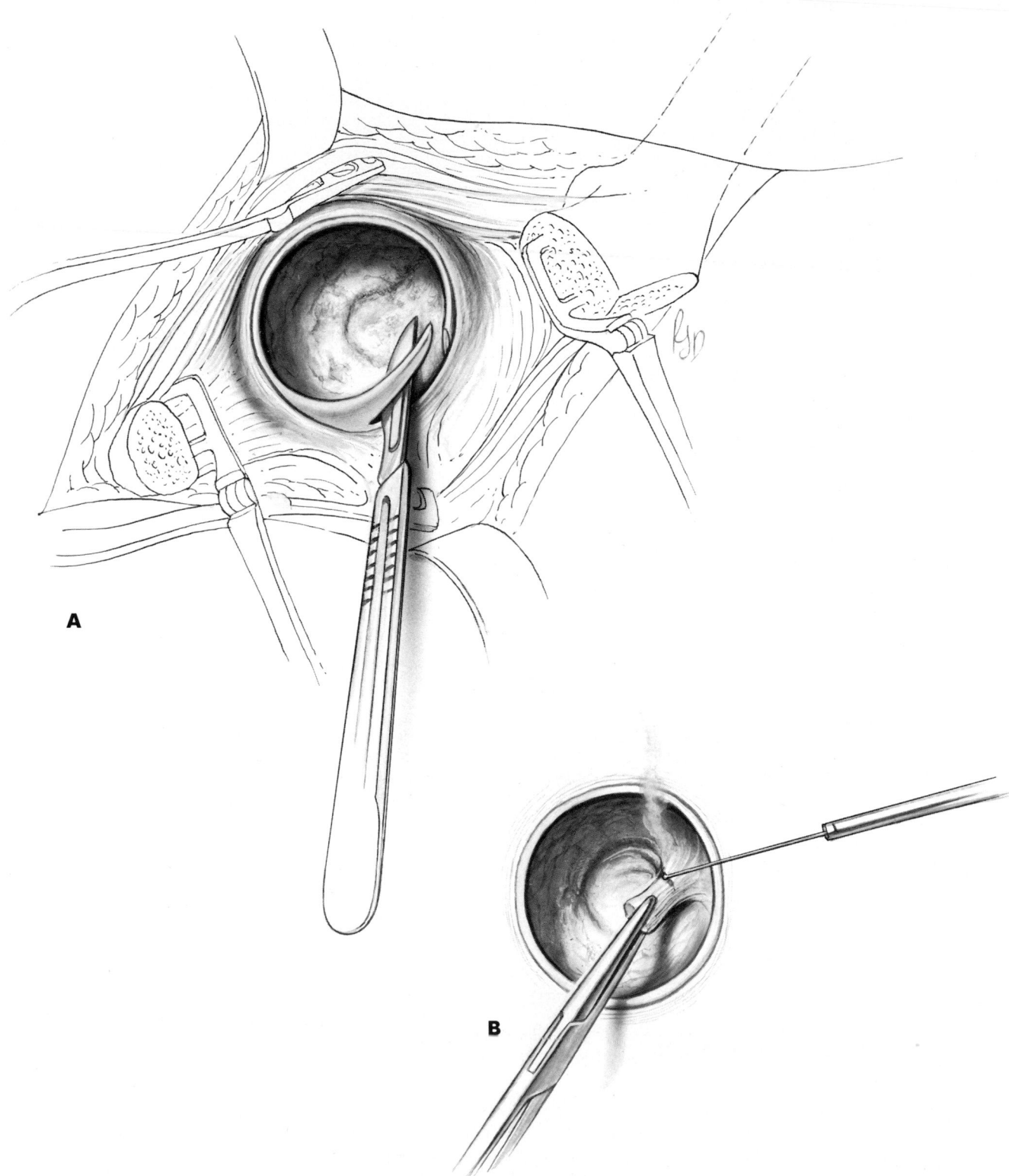

Fig. 15-14. A, North-south retractor should be replaced by Hohmann retractor to visualize anterior lip of acetabulum. Similar retractor may be placed additionally inferior to acetabulum at level of intercotyloid notch if necessary. **B,** Complete excision of labrum (intracapsularly) is necessary to expose bony rim.

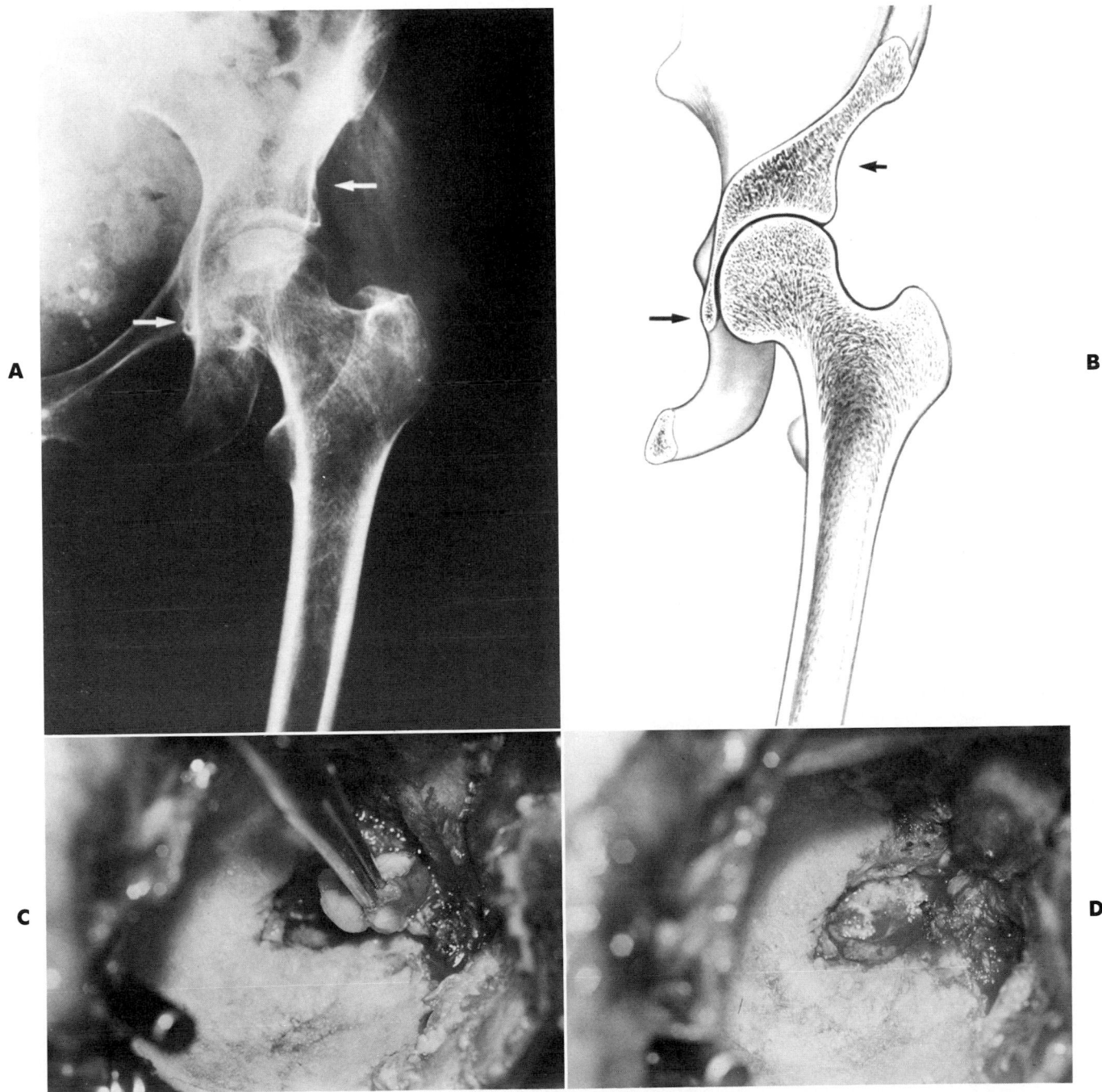

Fig. 15-15. A and **B,** Radiograph and artist's rendering of the medial and superior walls of the acetabulum (the limits of cephalad and medial walls of the acetabulum). Note lower arrows correspond to radiographical teardrop sign while upper arrows indicate the cancellous structure of the ilium that progressively becomes thinner in a cephalad direction. **C,** The content of the nonarticulating segment of the acetabulum is being removed. **D,** The outer margin of the floor (corresponding to the outer margin of the teardrop sign) has been visualized.

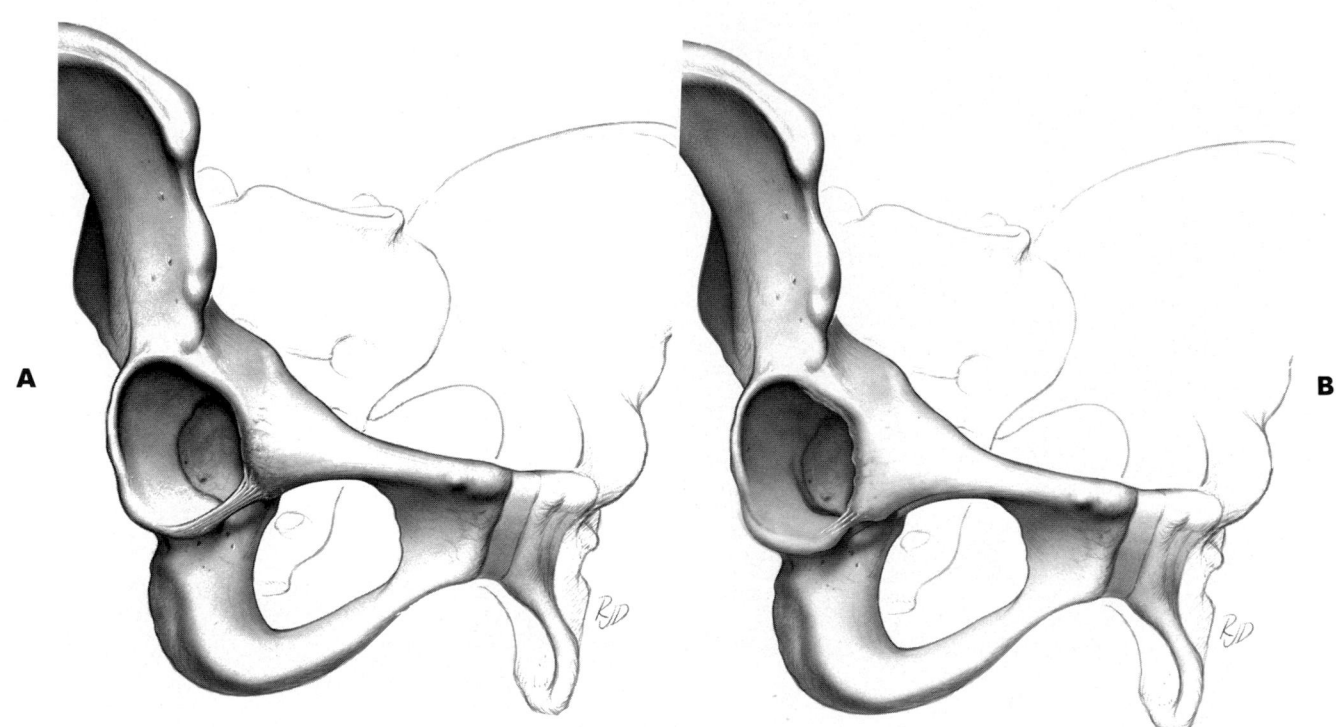

Fig. 15-16. A, In a less deformed acetabulum the transverse ligament is readily visible while it leads to the lower margin of the acetabulum. **B,** Inferior margin of the acetabulum may be covered by osteophytes requiring excision to visualize this margin.

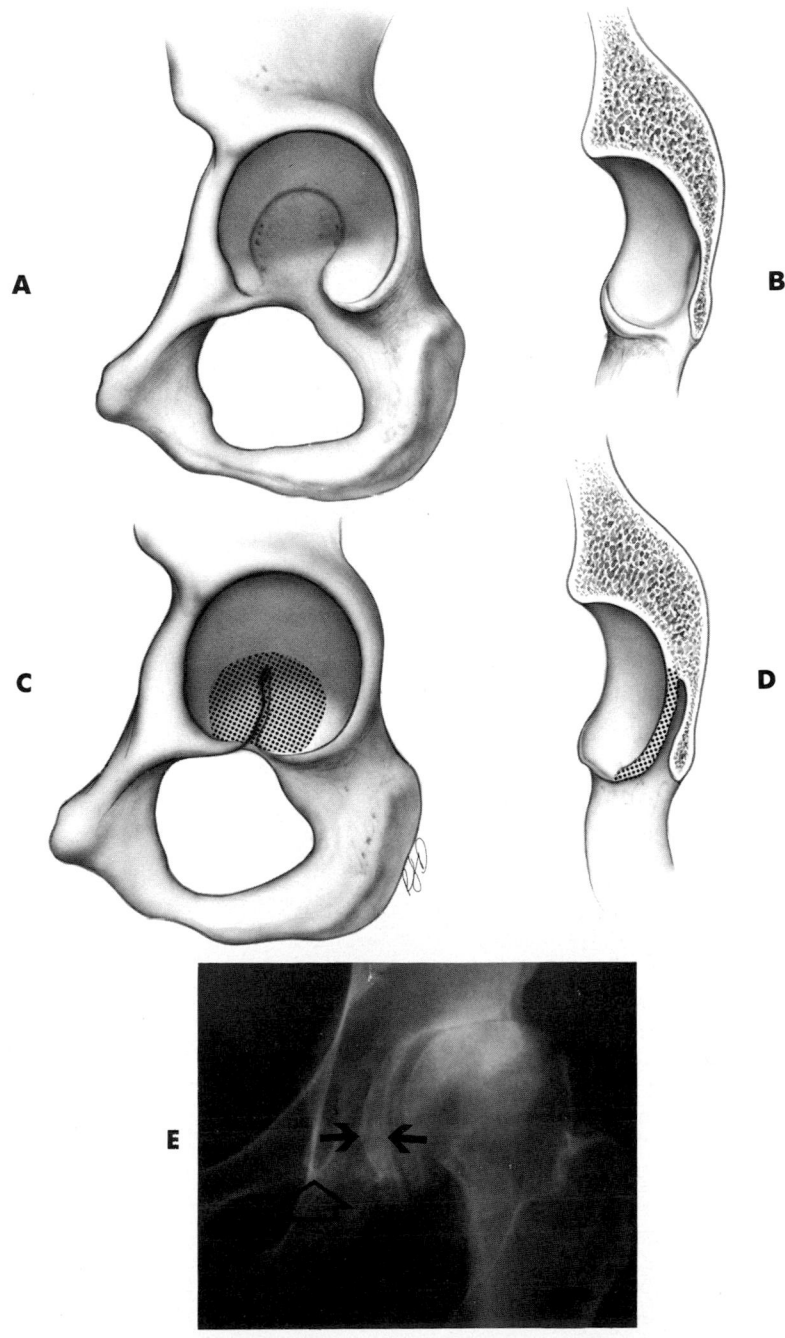

Fig. 15-17. A and **B,** Drawing of pelvis (front and profile) at acetabular zone shows the articulating and nonarticulating (pulvinar) portion of the normal acetabulum. **C** and **D,** The same views as shown in **A** and **B** illustrating the presence of significant inferior and medial marginal osteophytes covering the nonarticulating portion of the acetabulum. Shaded areas must be removed to expose the true medial wall of the acetabulum. **E,** Radiographic representation of medial osteophyte covering the nonarticulating portion of the acetabulum (*solid arrows*). The hollow arrow points to the teardrop.

Socket Preparation Vis-a-Vis Acetabular Pathology

Most acetabula lend themselves to one of the following four morphological types: normal acetabular configuration, medial pole migration, upper pole arthritis, and mild acetabular dysplasia. Using graded debris-retaining reamers appropriately directed to remove cartilage and bone, socket preparation can be accomplished with consideration to the morphological changes in the acetabulum.

Type I: Normal Acetabular Configuration

Normal acetabular configuration demonstrates a normal hemispherical shape and intact subchondral bone, with only loss of cartilage. The nonarticulating portion is revealed after removal of the ligamentum teres and synovial fold. This type is exemplified by early osteoarthritis after avascular necrosis of the femoral head with minimal acetabular deformity. The teardrop remains normal on the AP x-ray film, and the acetabular roof is at the same level as the opposite side. In this case the reamers are directed to the anatomical plane of the acetabulum, that is, 45 degrees to the AP transaxis of the pelvis and 15 to 20 degrees anteverted to accommodate the anteversion of the normal acetabulum. Fig. 15-18 shows preoperative and postoperative x-ray films that illustrate the specifics of the technique.

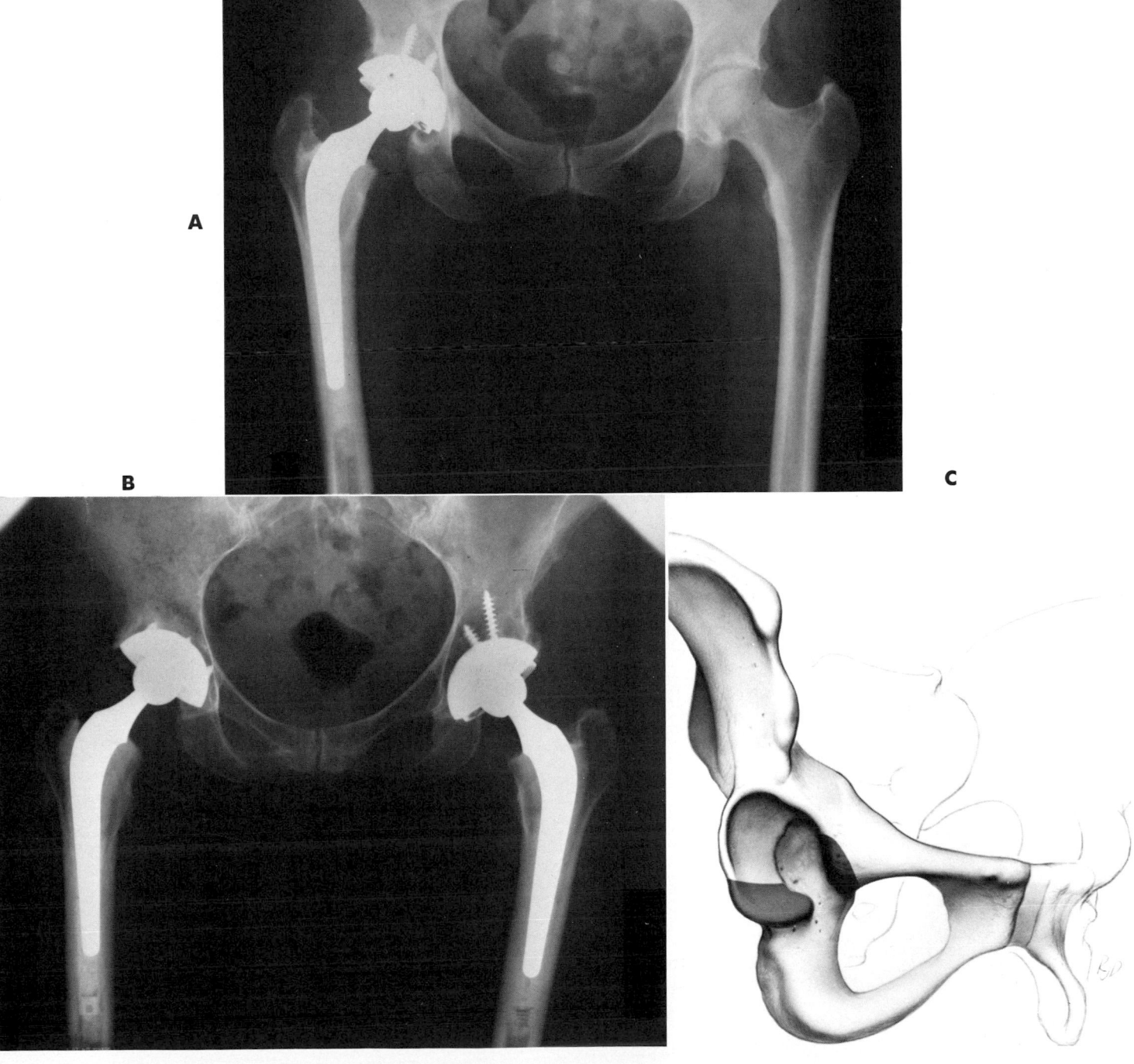

Fig. 15-18. A, A unilateral degenerative osteoarthritic hip, with only minimal acetabular deformity, was replaced with a porous-coated cup and a cemented stem using a 22-mm femoral head. Note the center of rotation was kept at the level of the opposite side (normal) by a universal expansion—the leg length remained equal. **B,** Bilateral "hybrid" hips with symmetrically positioned cups from different vendors (AML cup and H/G cup). The stem used in **A** and **B** is standard modular (Elite) Charnley prosthesis. **C,** Shaded area illustrates where maximum reaming in a nondeformed acetabulum must be carried out to retain the subchondral bone of the roof of the acetabulum.

Type II: Medial Pole Migration*

In medial pole migration cases, the head has migrated medially, causing thinning of the floor. The superior joint space is still present, and the teardrop sign is thin or slightly curved on x-ray film. Severe actual migration (protrusio acetabuli) has not occurred, but the floor is thin and may bulge inward slightly (medial to Kohler's line). Preparation of this type of acetabulum is carried out in a manner similar to that of type I; however, the surgeon must be careful not to medialize the socket (by transverse reaming), which has already been medialized by the disease. Only fibro-fatty material or remaining cartilage can be scraped away from the depth of the acetabulum toward the medial wall. Any further deepening may perforate the medial wall. Fig. 15-19, *A* and *B*, shows a case radiographically preoperatively and postoperatively. The best method to prepare the acetabulum is to use a reamer with a caliber 2 to 3 mm larger in diameter to enlarge the narrow opening of the acetabulum. The reamer must not penetrate fully to avoid damaging the thin acetabular floor (Fig. 15-19, *C* and *D*).

---

* For protrusio acetabuli, see Chapter 22.

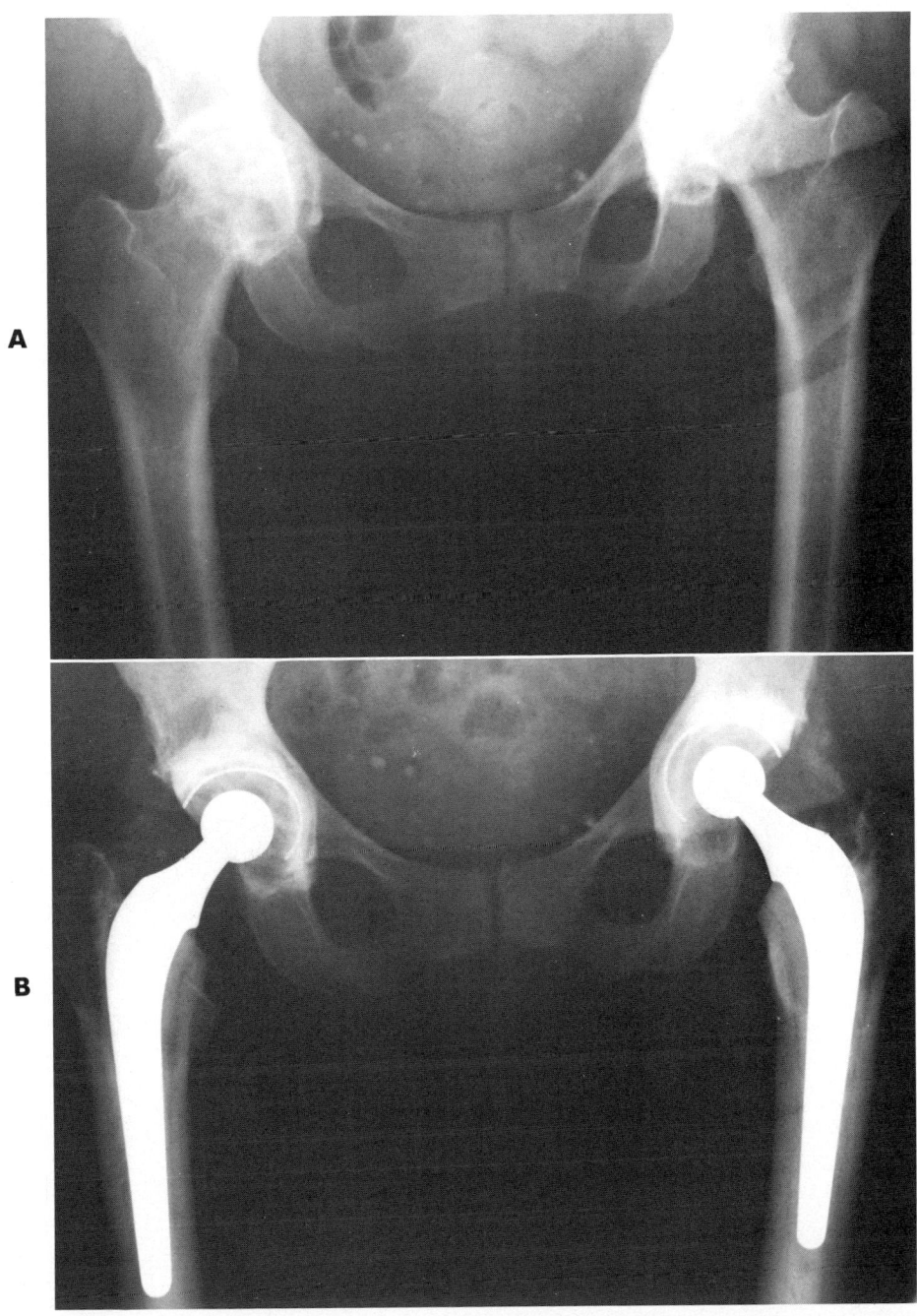

Fig. 15-19. A, Radiograph of bilateral "medial pole" arthritis with only mild bilateral protrusion (protrusio acetabuli). **B,** Status after bilateral low-friction arthroplasty using a modular Elite Charnley (Large Ogee Cup) and 26-mm femoral head. Only minor expansion of the bony acetabulum was required to accommodate the cup.

Continued.

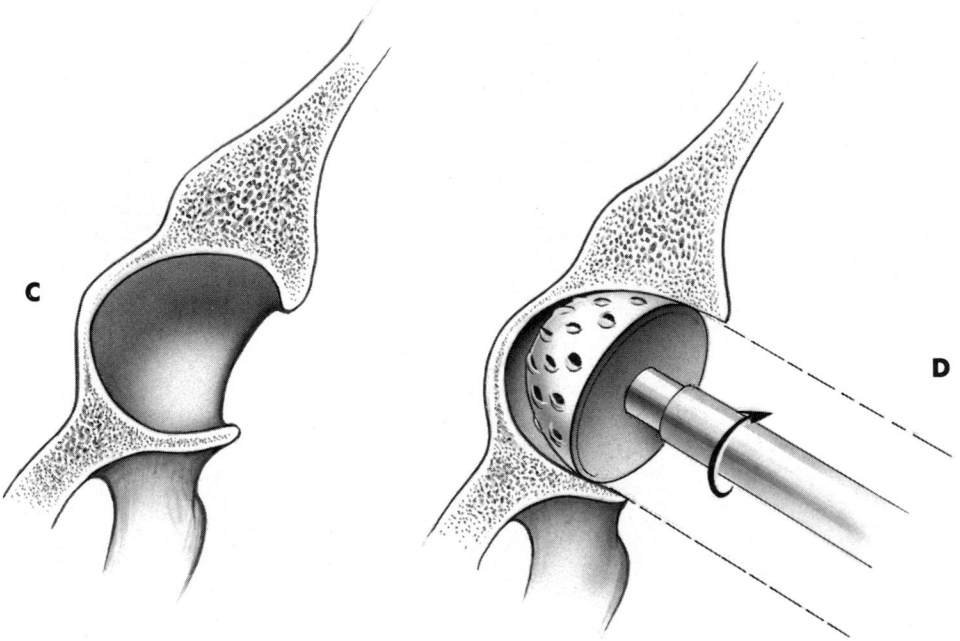

Fig. 15-19—cont'd. C and **D,** Shaded area on the pelvis indicates the necessary "expansion zone" to be created by reamers.

Type III: Upper Pole Arthritis

Upper pole arthritis is often present in hyperproductive osteoarthritis (hypertrophic) in male patients and accompanied by (1) a large inferior acetabular osteophyte (Fig. 15-20), (2) cephalad migration of the head accompanied by shortening of the limb with apparent dysplasia (Fig. 15-21), and (3) occasionally severe cystic or destructive changes of the roof. In this type the acetabulum must be prepared low at its original site. The cup can be contained by deepening the acetabulum in a low position, since there is no real dysplasia. Cysts may require bone grafting. The main concern here is to lower the cup and locate the center of rotation of the hip at its original site. Fig. 15-20 shows a case radiographically.

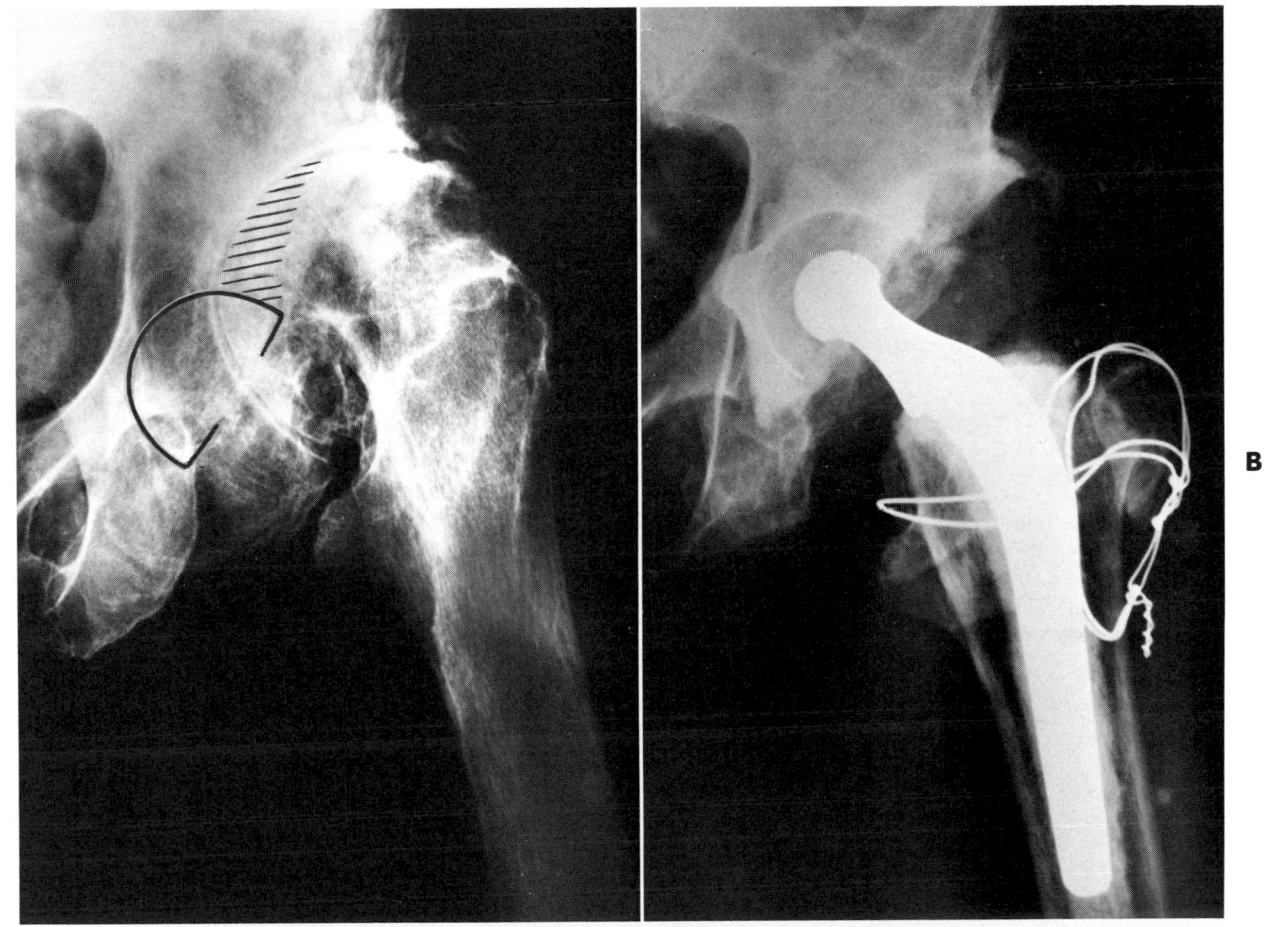

A   B

Fig. 15-20. Two essential features of surgery in patient with productive osteoarthrosis and large bony skeleton are demonstrated in this case. **A,** Site of preparation of acetabulum and its relationship to teardrop and obturator foramen. NOTE: large marginal osteophyte present in this individual. Marked external rotation of femur and lateral subluxation in addition to proximal migration of head should be observed. **B,** Replacement after lowering of socket. NOTE: lateral portion of acetabulum is supported by cement, which in turn is supported by outer segment of old acetabulum (shaded area in **A**).

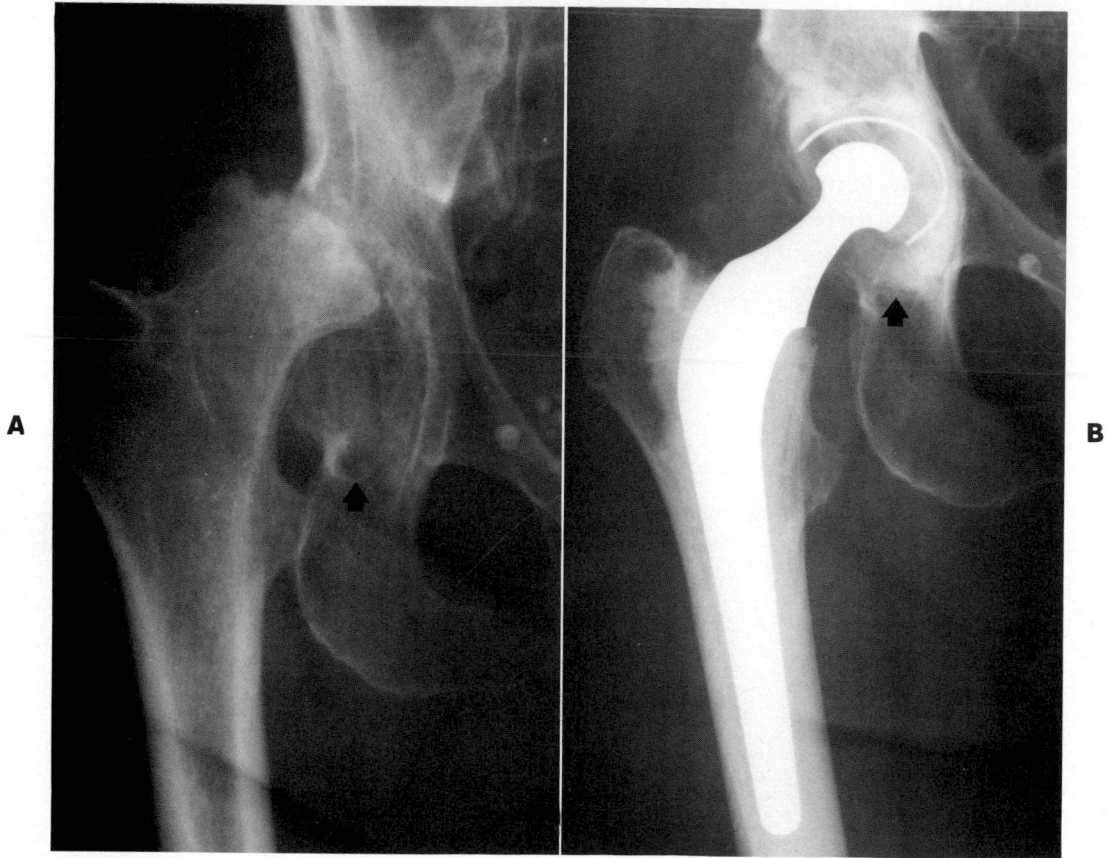

Fig. 15-21. A, Radiograph of a 55-year-old (G.D.) woman with a "wandering acetabulum" and avascular necrosis of the femoral head. **B,** The center of hip rotation has been lowered to the anatomical site (note the relationship of the cup to the teardrop).

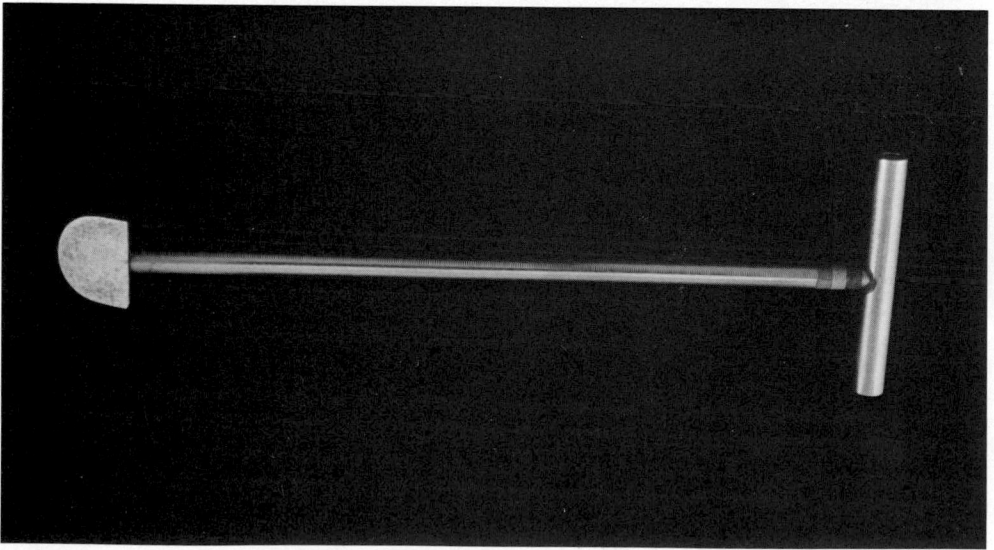

Fig. 15-22. Acetabular scraper (designed by the author) with a T handle and a half-moon-shaped cutting edge facilitates scraping the cartilage and soft bone from the acetabulum.

Type IV: Mild Acetabular Dysplasia

Mild acetabular dysplasia is commonly accompanied by a medial wall that manifests a widened teardrop sign, anterior deficiency, and lateralization of the center of hip rotation. Such sockets require medialization by medial reaming and replacing the center of rotation to its original site while preserving the subchondral bone (see Chapter 20) and the roof of the acetabulum. In most cases with a modest amount of deepening, bone grafting is unnecessary.

Acetabular Preparation

In preparing the acetabulum, aim to do the following:

1. Produce a cavity large enough to accommodate the acetabular component and cement.
2. Protect the integrity of the acetabulum by preserving the subchondral bone of the roof of the acetabulum.
3. Provide a bony cavity after reaming that can contain the cup and cement with full bony support from the ilium, ischium, and pubis.
4. Locate the center of rotation (acetabular cavity) at the original site of the normal acetabulum (comparable to normal).
5. Provide a precise hemispherical cavity to accommodate the cup when a cementless cup is to be used.

These goals may be reached by using one of the following two methods of acetabular preparation based on altered morphology of the normal acetabulum resulting from arthritis. The four types of changes that have just been described can be identified from the preoperative x-ray films. Removal of fatty tissue and remnants of ligamentum teres must precede the socket preparation. Marginal inferior osteophytes covering the acetabular fossa are removed with a sharp Volkmann's spoon.

Method A: Preparation In Situ for Types I and II Acetabula

Direct an appropriately sized (best fit for the size of acetabulum) reamer, remove cartilage, and deepen the socket concentrically. Observe the following: (1) do not deepen beyond the level of the nonarticulating portion of the "pulvinar" that corresponds to the outer table of the acetabular floor; (2) select larger reamers, using judicious control to avoid damaging the least developed wall of the acetabulum; (3) repeatedly check for adequate depth and thickness of the walls; (4) do not allow the reamers to drift in a cephalad direction; (5) use the sharp Volkmann's spoon and acetabular scraper (Fig. 15-22) frequently to assess the progress and need for localized scraping; (6) changing the direction of the reamers (Fig. 15-23) can be helpful in the selective removal of cartilage to the subchondral bone, thus creating space in a selected direction.

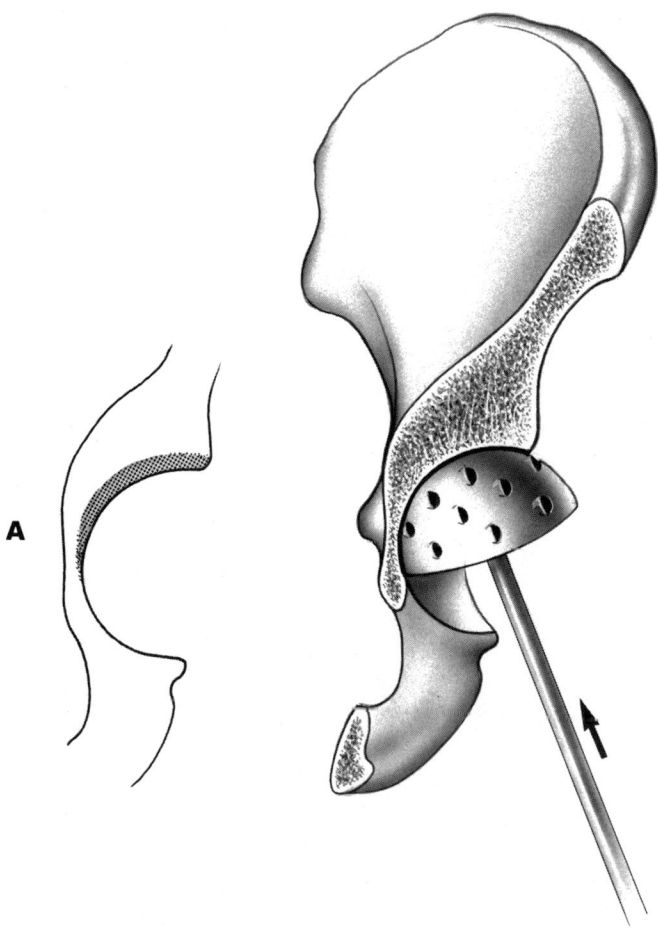

Fig. 15-23. Priority reaming is illustrated: **A,** Debris retaining reamer is directed toward the superior (roof) segment of the acetabulum. **B,** While the reamer shaft is kept parallel to the transaxis of the pelvis, a medial reaming is carried out. **C,** Demonstration of removal of inferior marginal osteophytes by directing the reamer in a caudal direction.

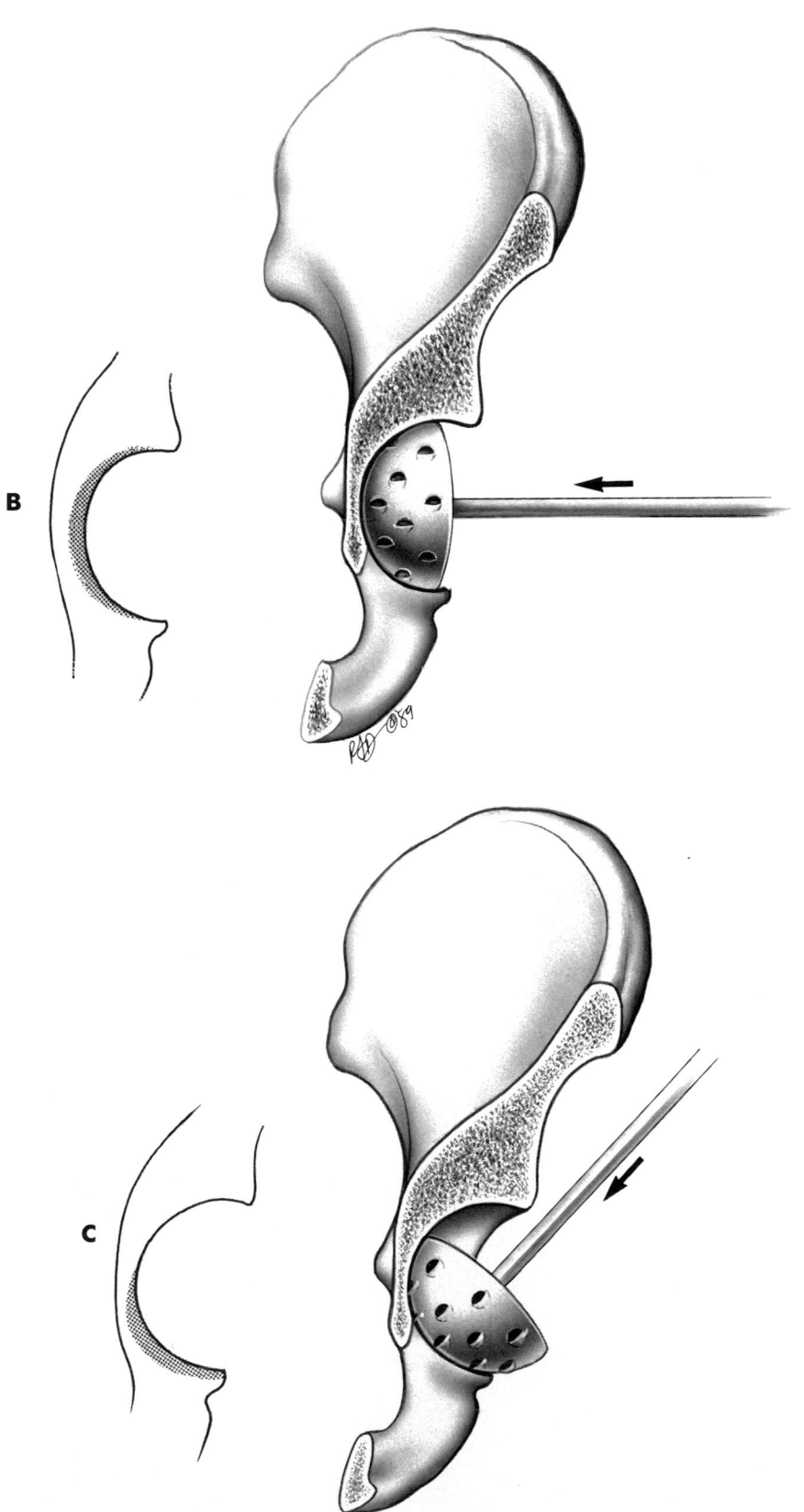

Fig. 15-23—cont'd. For legend see opposite page.

Method B: Preparation in Lower Position (Types III and IV Acetabula)

In method B the acetabular site (center of rotation of the hip) is lowered to its original position by locating the site of the reamers low (distal) in relation to the pelvis. This is accomplished best by a spigotted acetabular reamer and according to the technique described by the author.

Preparation of the socket at a lower position, such as the original site of the acetabulum (site of triradiate cartilage), requires the following steps:

1. Use a small (40 mm) diameter or large (45 mm) outer diameter acetabular gauge-drill guide, depending on the size of the acetabulum. Drill to locate the site of a spigot hole for spigotted reamer. The drill should be parallel to the transaxis of the pelvis.
2. Use corresponding debris-retaining reamers with a spigot that is 2 mm larger than the acetabular gauge (42 or 46 mm outer diameter) for small and large acetabula, respectively.
3. Check frequently for adequacy of depth; the reamer is always used in the exact direction of the drill, that is, parallel to the transaxis of the pelvis (Fig. 15-24).
4. Repeat step 1 if the spigot hole is shallow and does not permit full penetration of the reamer.
5. Do not change reaming direction until full cup depth is created.
6. The offset between the site of the reamer and margin of unprepared bone becomes greater as further reaming proceeds.

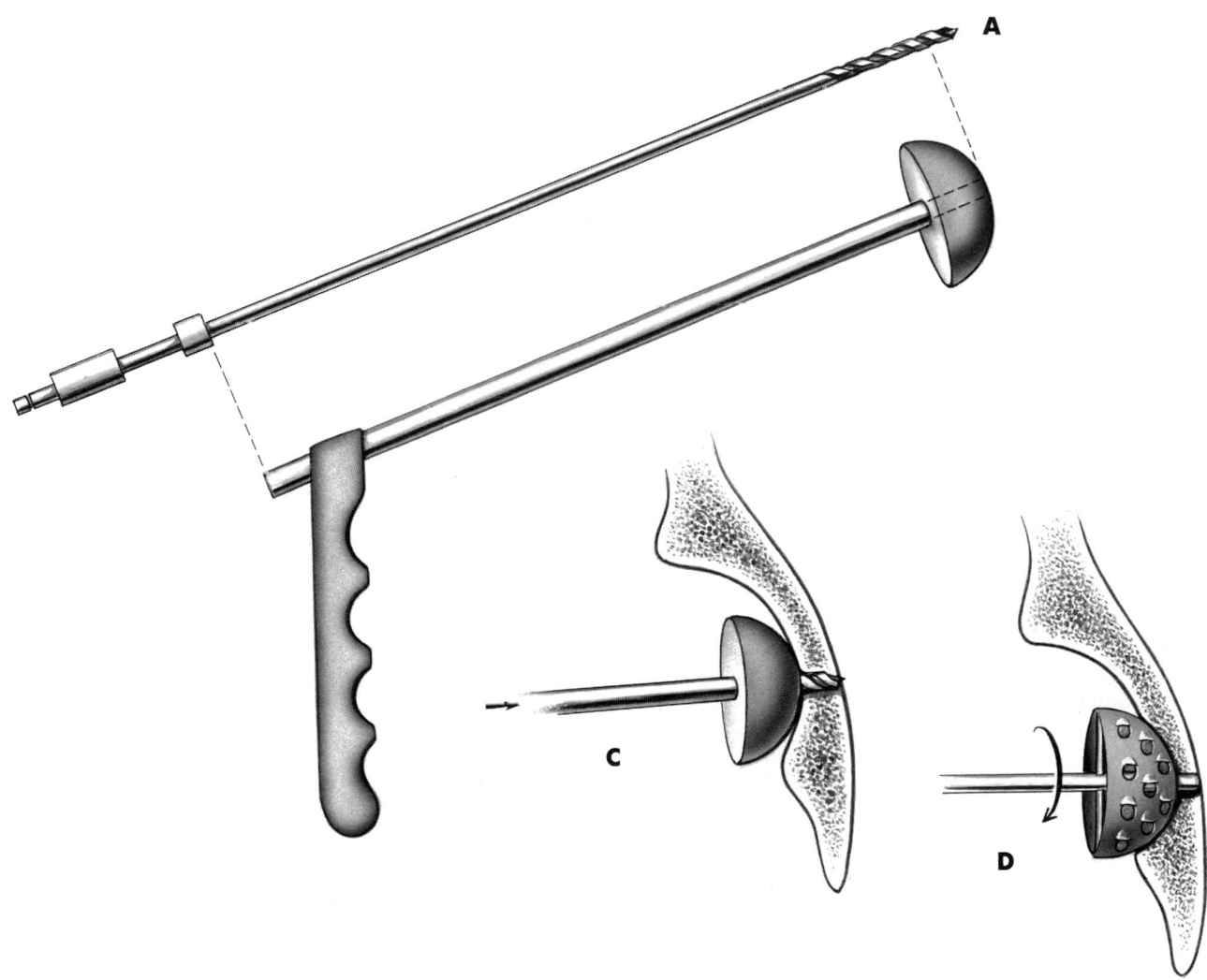

Fig. 15-24. Technique for lowering socket to the level of true acetabulum. **A,** Drill. **B,** Acetabular gauge–drill guide. **C,** Spigot drill hole is drilled in a low position. **D,** Note deepening of the socket at the site of original acetabulum where most bone stock is available. (From Eftekhar NS: Total hip replacement: low-friction arthroplasty. In Evarts CM: *Surgery of the musculoskeletal system,* New York, 1983, Churchill Livingstone.)

Preparation Vis-a-Vis Socket Fixation Type

As noted, two distinctly different types of acetabular preparations are required: (1) preparation for cementless fixation and (2) preparation for cement fixation.

PREPARATION FOR CEMENTLESS CUPS WITH OR WITHOUT POROUS COATING Preparation for cementless cups demands precision in cavity preparation in a predetermined direction. While the subchondral bone is preferably retained, it should be reamed sufficiently to provide a bleeding surface to ensure bony ingrowth. There should be maximum contact with the porous coating of the cup. Socket preparation must be concentric to maximize contact with the cup. Increased deepening in a headward direction may jeopardize good contact. This cannot be corrected by further enlarging the cavity, since adequate bone stock may not be available anteriorly or posteriorly. In this case a high socket position for the cup is desirable. Brushing the acetabular cavity is not indicated, since it can remove good cancellous bone needed for fixation of the ingrowth prosthesis. A cup trial must indicate good bony coverage superiorly, posteriorly, and anteriorly with proper orientation of the cup before its insertion. Cysts, when exposed during reaming, should be packed with cancellous bone obtained from the femoral neck or head.

PREPARATION FOR CEMENTED CUPS Socket fixation by cement requires sizing and trimming the cup rim. The following principles should be observed:

1. Prepare the cavity of the acetabulum larger than the cup size to accommodate a minimum thickness of 2 to 3 mm of cement.
2. Ensure that at final rehearsal the flange seals the acetabular cavity, thus pressurizing and containing the cement while the cup is fully covered by the acetabular margins.
3. Use multiple (6 mm diameter) drill holes in addition to one to three large ones (12.5 mm diameter) to increase the surface area of the cement and provide anchorage for PMMA (Figs. 15-25 and 15-26).
4. Irrigate and brush to facilitate removal of debris and search for any unremoved soft tissue within the acetabular cavity (Fig. 15-27). Pack the acetabulum tightly with a sponge soaked in hydrogen peroxide (Fig. 15-28, *A*).
5. Identify any penetration of the medial wall, and seal it with bone. If penetration occurs and goes unnoticed, pressurization is completely ineffective, and a large bolus of cement will escape into the pelvic cavity.
6. Note that large defects may require bone grafting and the use of a separate mix of cement that should be allowed to polymerize before it is pressurized. Pressurization of cement in the acetabulum by a mechanical device and independent of the use of a flanged cup should be encouraged when (1) the acetabular cavity is intact and the cement can be contained, (2) the pressurization device seals the bony rim, and (3) cement is adequately viscous to allow penetration. Pressurization devices introduced by Ling,[15] Oh,[25] and others are satisfactory for this purpose (Fig. 15-29). Pressurization of the cement can also be achieved by a closed-cavity technique described by Ling and others.[15] In this two-step technique, low-viscosity cement is first introduced and pressurized into bony trabeculae, and then the cup is inserted into a newly added bolus of high-viscosity cement that allows accurate positioning of the implant.[15]
7. Steadily maintain cup position until the cement is polymerized (see Chapter 19).
8. Completely remove excess cement from around the acetabular area (Fig. 15-30).

Text continued on p. 688.

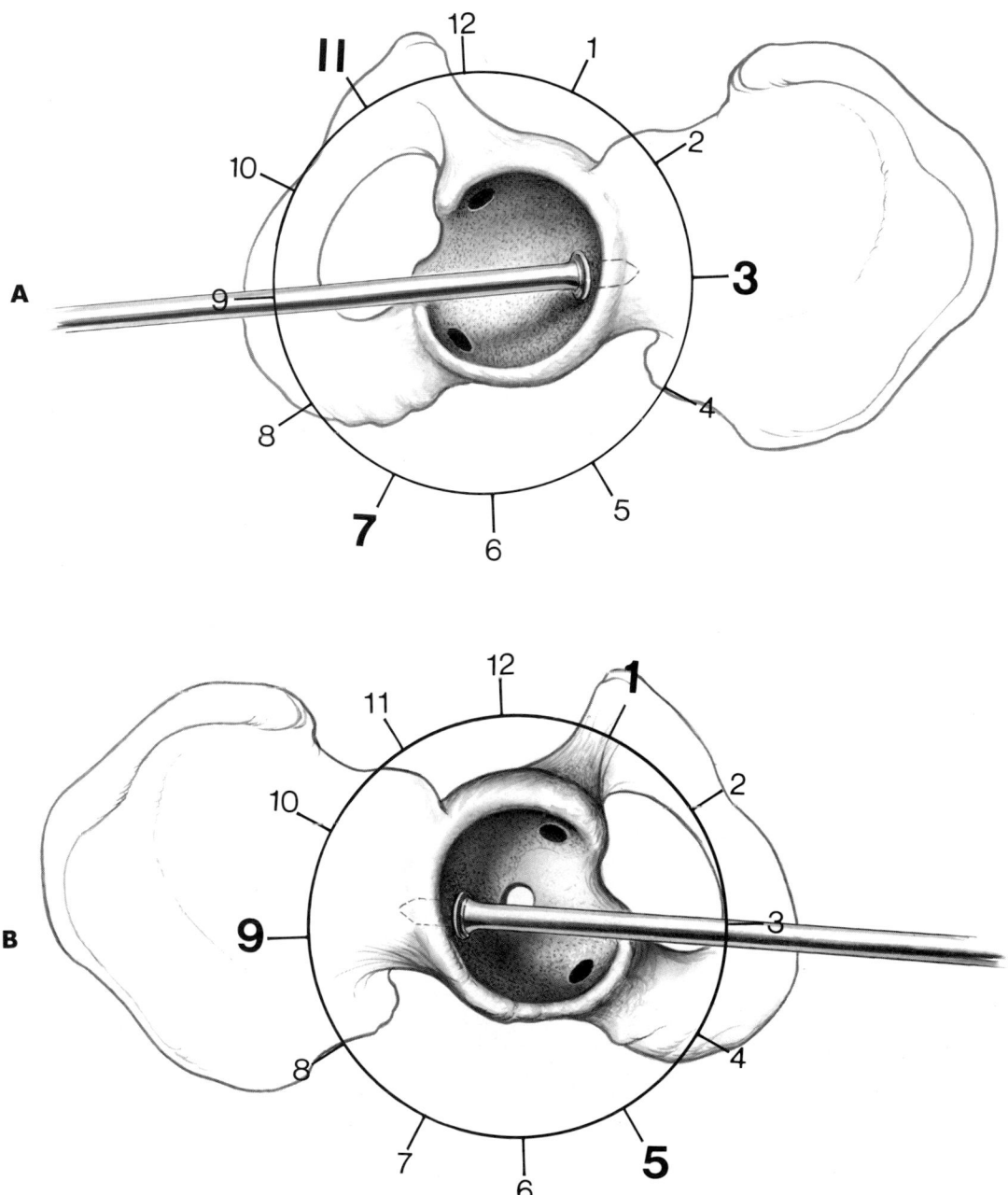

Fig. 15-25. With the patient in supine position; 12.5-mm outer diameter drill holes must be centered in each bone contributing to the acetabulum formation. **A,** The sites of anchor holes for the left hip correspond to 3, 7, and 11 o'clock. **B,** The sites of anchor holes for the right hip correspond to 1, 5, and 9 o'clock. Two 12.5 mm anchor holes for cement, one in direction of ilium and one in direction of ischium usually suffice. Anchor hole toward pubis is used only in large, bony individuals.

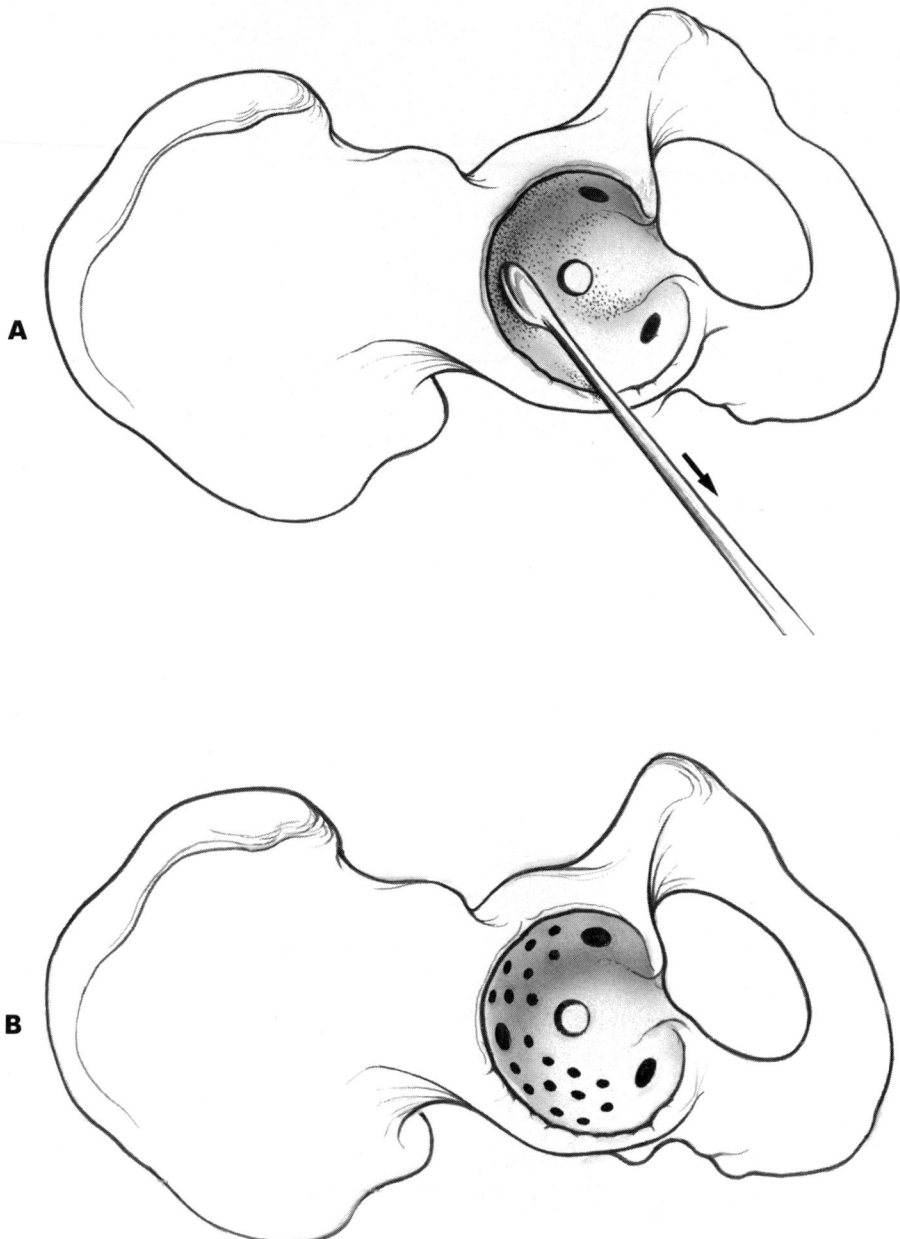

Fig. 15-26. A, All cartilage and loose fragments of bone are scraped away using a sharp Volkmann's spoon. **B,** Additional 15 to 25, 6-mm outer diameter drill holes (depending on the acetabular size) are evenly distributed throughout the weight-bearing zones of the acetabulum.

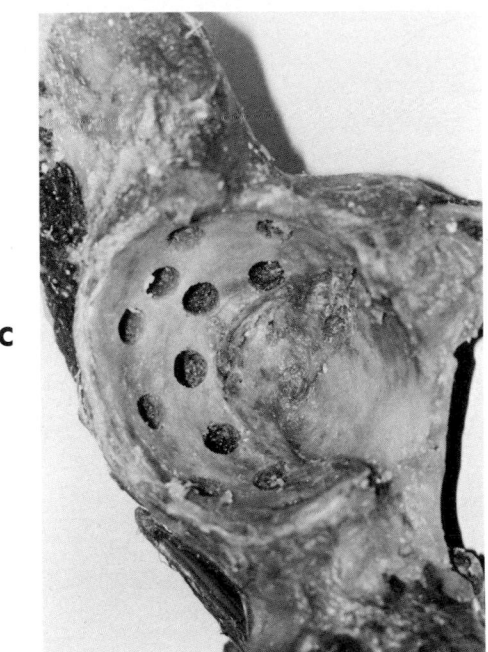

Fig. 15-26—cont'd. C, Final preparation of the acetabulum on an anatomical specimen.

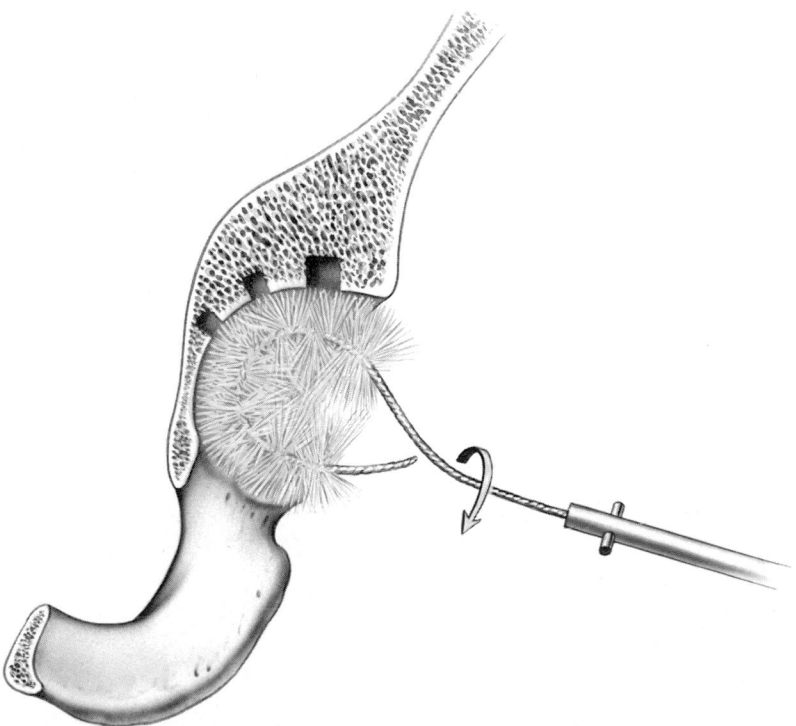

Fig. 15-27. A firm brush attached to a power drill (using drilling speed), accompanied by jet lavage (using Ringer's solution) removes bone and soft tissue debris.

A

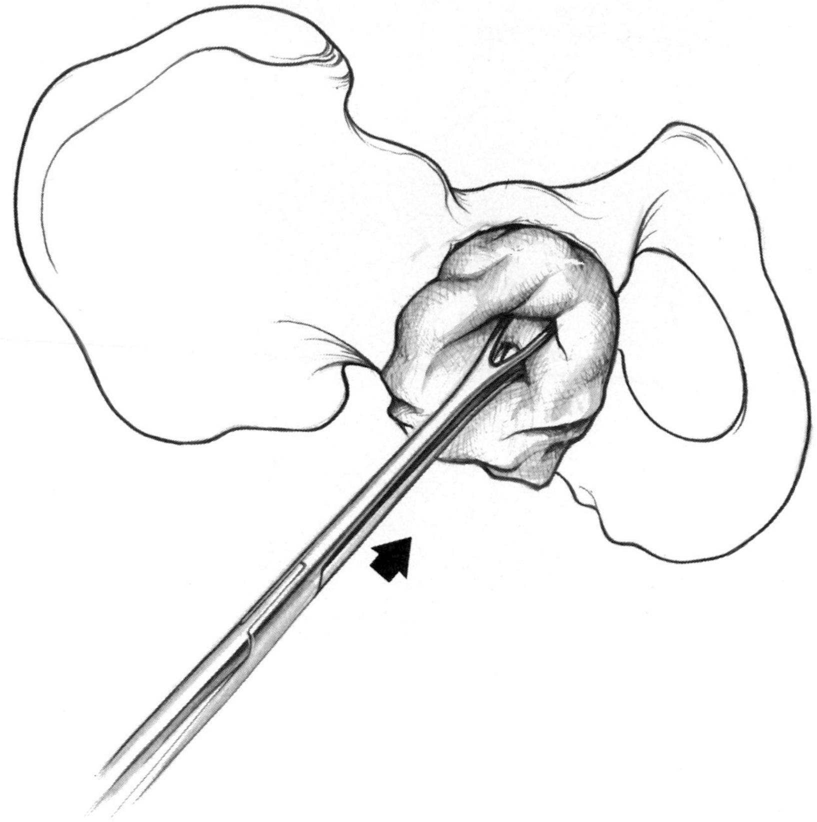

B

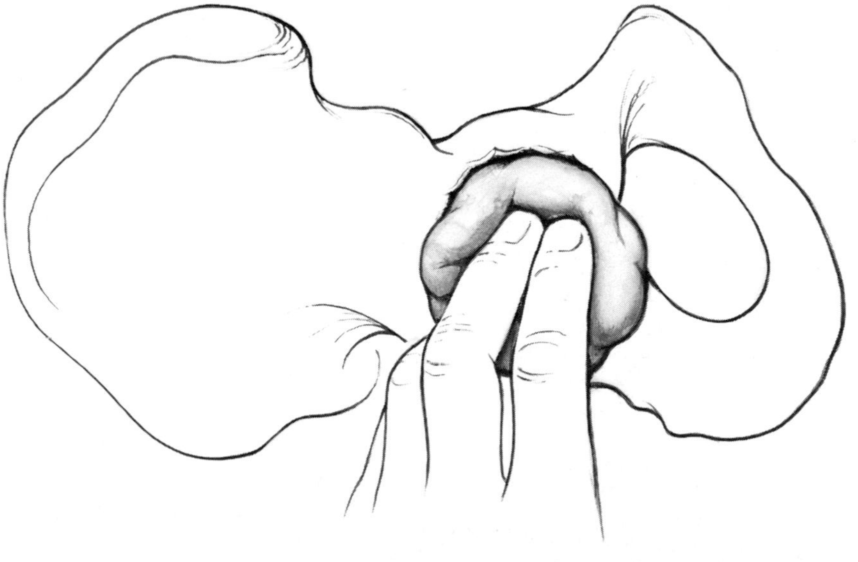

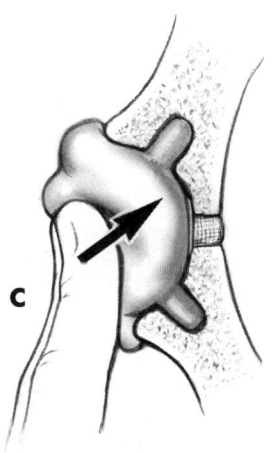

C

Fig. 15-28. A, Sponge soaked with hydrogen peroxide is packed tightly into the acetabulum while cement is mixed by the sterile nurse. **B** and **C,** Bolus of cement is inserted immediately after removal of the sponge using two or three fingertips to push cement toward depth of acetabulum. Cement is pressurized especially in areas of anchor holes using a pressurization device.

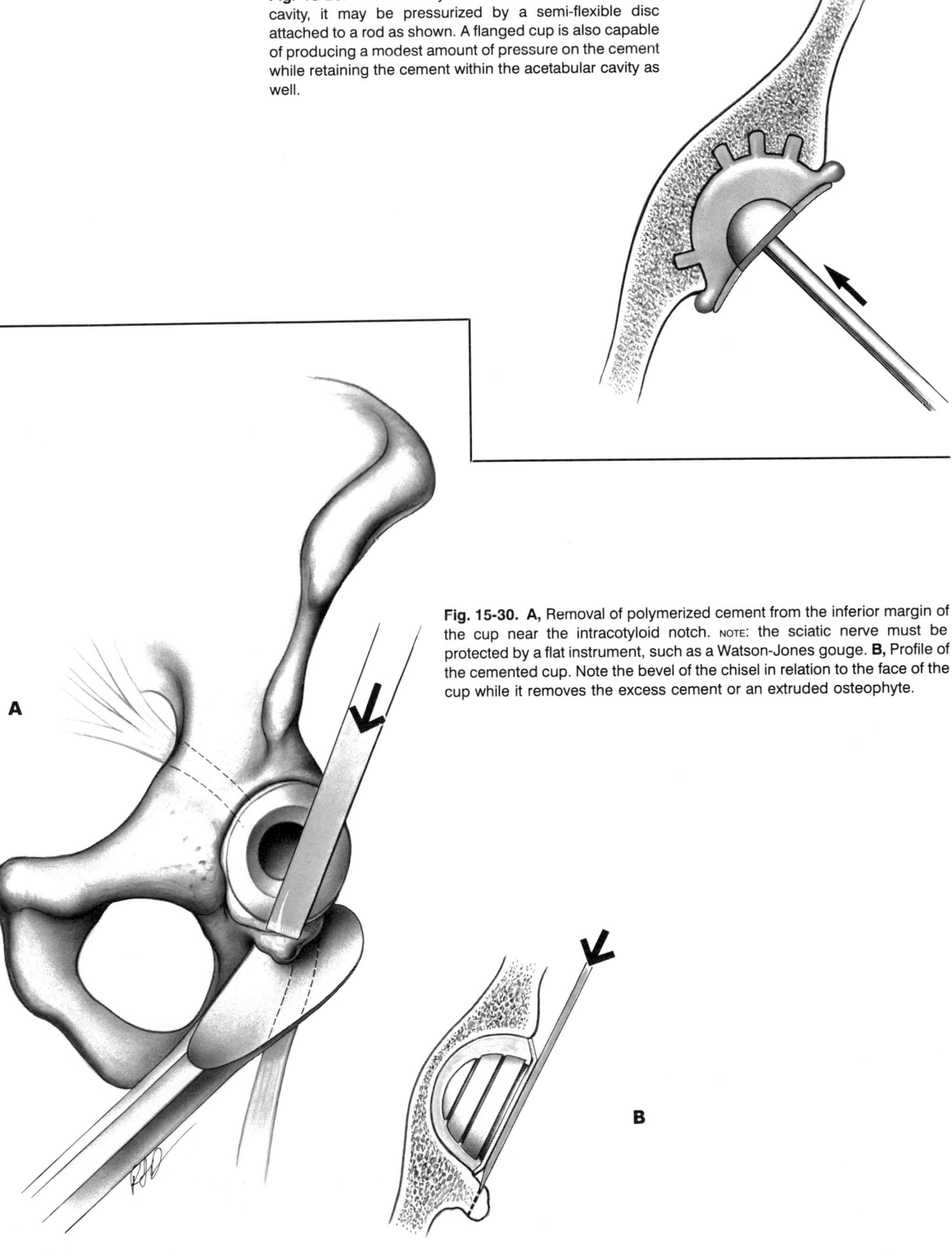

Fig. 15-29. After delivery of cement into the acetabular cavity, it may be pressurized by a semi-flexible disc attached to a rod as shown. A flanged cup is also capable of producing a modest amount of pressure on the cement while retaining the cement within the acetabular cavity as well.

Fig. 15-30. A, Removal of polymerized cement from the inferior margin of the cup near the intracotyloid notch. NOTE: the sciatic nerve must be protected by a flat instrument, such as a Watson-Jones gouge. **B,** Profile of the cemented cup. Note the bevel of the chisel in relation to the face of the cup while it removes the excess cement or an extruded osteophyte.

A

B

Gauging for Socket Size

An acetabular gauge is used to select the appropriate acetabular size (Fig. 15-31, *A*). Fig. 15-31, *B*, shows the actual prosthesis clipped to the holder to show orientation for final position. The acetabular gauge is oriented on the handle at 45 degrees. Therefore at insertion (with the aligning rods in appropriate alignment with the pelvis): (1) fully insert the selected cup gauge inside the bony acetabulum; (2) allow at least 3 to 4 mm of space for cement; (3) make a visual assessment of the width of the rim to be trimmed from the acetabular cup. While the acetabular gauge is in place, assess the amount of anteversion. With the long posterior wall socket, no more than 5 degrees of anteversion is allowed. This applies to both the 26 mm and 22 mm inner diameter acetabular cups.

Socket Selection and Trimming

Socket selection should be based on the size of the acetabular component to be used and the coverage needed by bone and the shape of the existing reamed acetabulum. This author has used a 26 mm outer diameter head for large-boned individuals and patients whose acetabuli are deep enough to accommodate a thicker acetabular wall. For most hips a 22 mm outer diameter head is preferred. If dysplasia of the anterior rim of the acetabulum is present, the design of an OGEE cup is preferred to the pressure injection cup, which has a asymmetrical pressure injection rim (see Chapter 11).

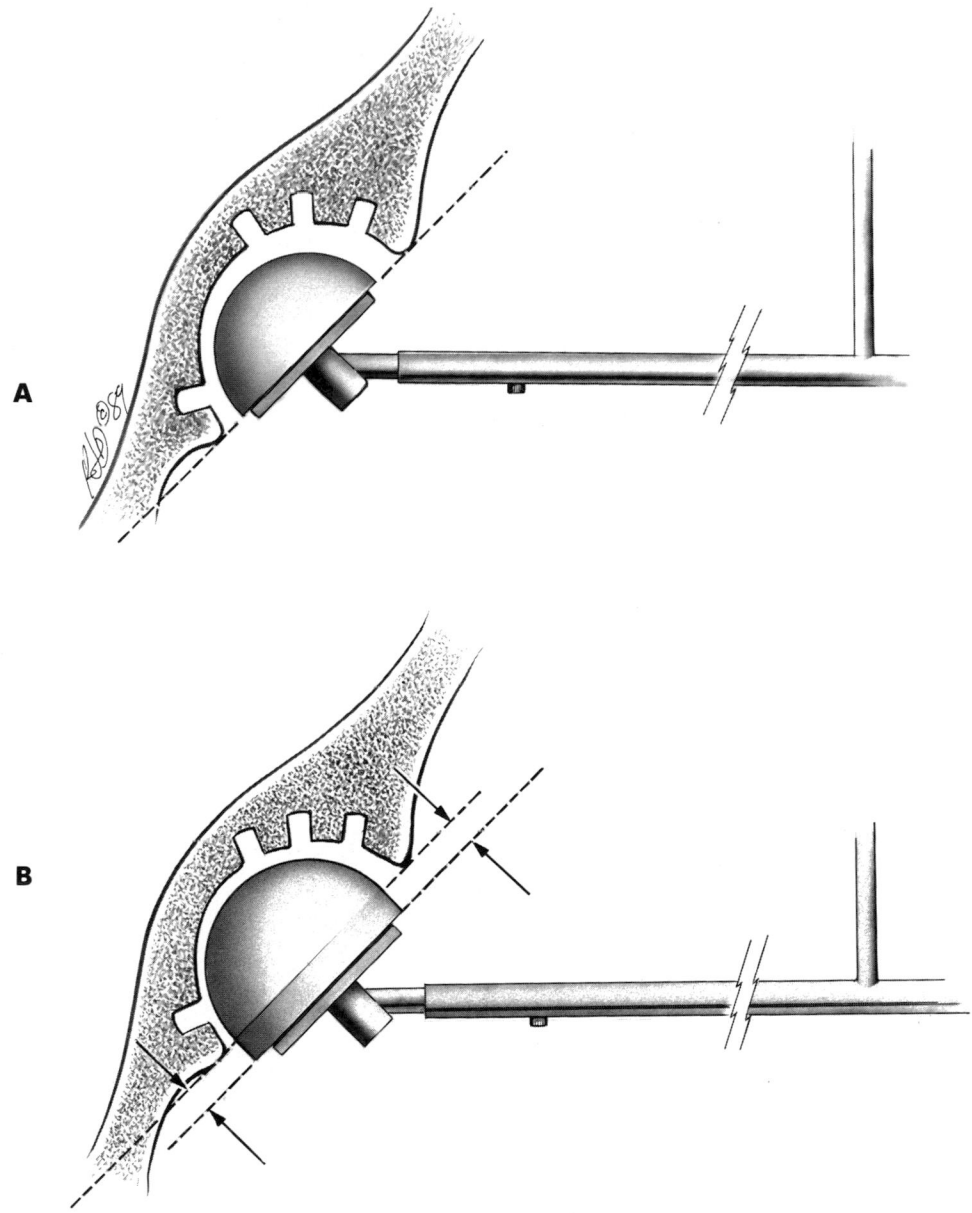

Fig. 15-31. Gauging the acetabulum for socket size selection is demonstrated. **A,** Small size cup (40 mm outer diameter) is well contained by the prepared acetabulum. The cup is positioned at a 45-degree angle to the transaxis line of pelvis. **B,** Large size acetabular cup (44 mm outer diameter) is tried. NOTE: for the same size acetabulum as in **A;** the cup is not covered by the bony acetabulum; the acetabular depth and circumferential size determine the appropriate size of the cup to be used.

Containment and Orientation

Trim the flange of the pressure injection cup or an Ogee cup shown in Figs. 15-32 to 15-34. Ideally, the socket must be fully supported by bone. Most prosthetic hip systems provide a series of cup gauges that enable the surgeon to determine the relationship of the cup to the acetabulum for size and orientation. One cup gauge designed by the author is shown in Fig. 15-31. Containment of the cup within the acetabulum is a fundamental principle in all designs. The surgeon must accept only minor imperfections regarding bone coverage; however, the limits regarding the absence of bone support compatible with a satisfactory result have not been scientifically verified. In terms of the risk of loosening, this author believes that deficiency in the anterior wall (iliopubic ramus) is more acceptable than any lack of coverage superiorly or posteriorly. Cement and bone graft must be contained if they are to transmit load to pelvis. It is therefore necessary that the cup be placed as medial as possible in dysplastic hips and that a smaller outer diameter cup be used to obtain coverage (see Fig. 15-31). Osteophytes may be used for coverage as needed in the shallow acetabula.

Orientation of the cup must always be determined at rehearsal before inserting the actual prosthesis. All hip systems provide a cup holder that is fixed to the cup for orientation, and this can provide a reference for the plane of the cup in two or three directions (planes). Such a device must be used to verify the actual acetabular orientation before its permanent insertion. In the case of a cup with a pressure injection rim, it is essential that the trimmed cup be attached to the holder and tested for fit and orientation before inserting the cement into the acetabulum (see Fig. 15-34).

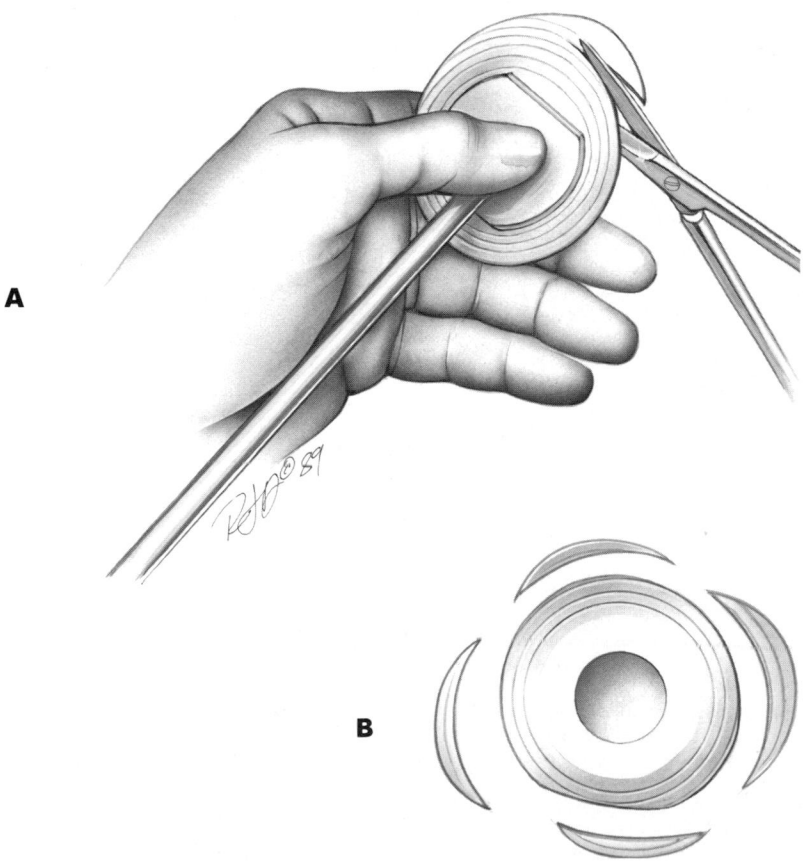

Fig. 15-32. Trimming a flanged cup is demonstrated. **A,** Using a pair of heavy duty scissors, trim the flange as desired. Cup is properly clipped to the holder while cutting is done along the grooves of the cup. **B,** The inferior lobe is excised first, followed by tailoring of the anterior, posterior, and finally superior lobe of the cup.

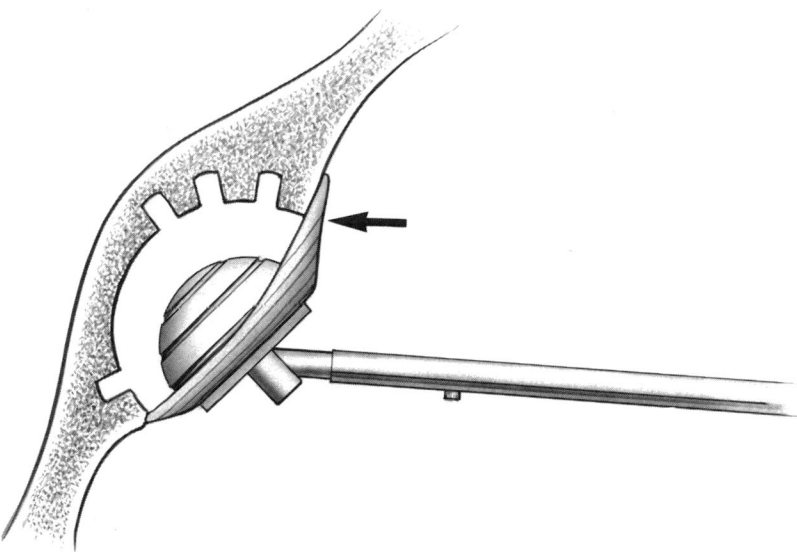

Fig. 15-33. After tailoring the three lobes of the flanged cup, the cup is tested for "best fit." The superior and the final remaining lobe is then trimmed away *(arrow)*. Ideally, the cup must be well contained and the flange must fit the inner rim of the acetabulum snugly like a piston within a cylinder.

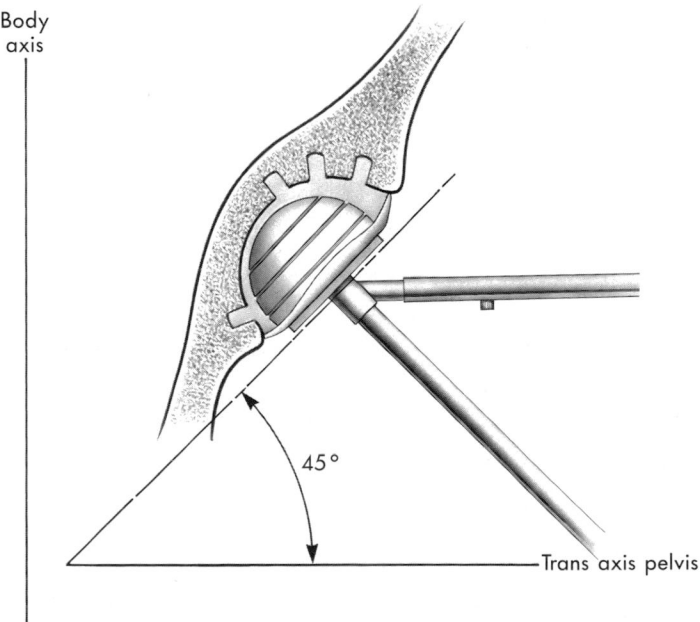

Fig. 15-34. Well-fitted (trimmed) pressure injection cup is demonstrated. NOTE: with proper alignment (45 degrees to the body axis) the cup is well covered by bone.

Acetabular Cement Thickness

As Blacker and Charnley have pointed out, a thin layer of PMMA may fragment under heavy load, leading to mechanical and biological failure of the implant.[2] Although the ideal thickness of the cement between the acetabular cup and bone has not been established, Kwak and colleagues have recommended a 3 to 4 mm thickness of cement for retention between the prosthesis and bone, based on their experimental work.[14]

One of the technical difficulties in controlling cement thickness as the cup is pushed into the dough cement is that the acetabular cup may "bottom in," thus eliminating the appropriate thickness of cement from critical load-bearing zones. The following two methods are available for maintaining a 2 to 3 mm minimum cement thickness.

Method I: Use of Spacers Between Cup and Bone

Spacers are composed of PMMA and comprised of short cylinders 5 mm in diameter. They are driven into the bone at desired positions via their stainless steel 0.75 mm diameter inserting pins.[19] The cup is pushed deep against the PMMA spacers by standard cementing techniques. The bolus of PMMA bonds satisfactorily with the precured PMMA spacers, since the space between the cup and the bone is maintained by the spacers. Although this technique is a novel idea, this author is not aware of any long-term clinical results or comparative studies in support of the advantages of this method over the conventional methods in clinical practice. Cement also is not contained and pressurized as the cement is being polymerized.

Method II: Use of a Flanged Cup

The use of a flanged cup provides a space between the cup and the bone, thus controlling the cement thickness and containment. With final positioning of the cup after trimming, the rim prevents the cup from bottoming into the acetabulum (unless it is overtrimmed as its flange contacts the bone) (see Fig. 15-34). This author's experience with spacers and flanged cups indicates that the latter is a most useful method of retaining and controlling the thickness of cement in the acetabulum. By trimming the flange, five parameters related to cup fixation can be met.

1. The flange allows retention of the cement within the acetabulum.
2. The flange allows pressurization at insertion.
3. The flange locates the center of the cup at the desired level, that is, at the original anatomical site.
4. The flange renders the use of any "stand-offs," that is, spacers, on the cup or the bone unnecessary.
5. Cup orientation can be reproduced after insertion of cement (similar to the test performed without cement) as a result of the contact between the cup rim and the acetabulum.

Inserting a Rimless Cup

Rimless cups are more difficult to insert with precision than pressure injection cups. The correct placement of the cup on the socket holder is verified. Insertion of the cup may be divided into the following six steps (Figs. 15-35 and 15-36):

Fig. 15-35. Plastic socket fixed on socket holder is pressed into cement with face of socket directed toward patient's feet. When socket has reached full depth of acetabulum, surgeon presses cement with finger into gap between socket and superior lip of acetabulum. Socket holder is maintained in position by pusher that allows socket to remain steady at depth of acetabulum. (Pusher has been removed here.) Final position of socket is obtained by moving socket holder to its final transverse position (inset).

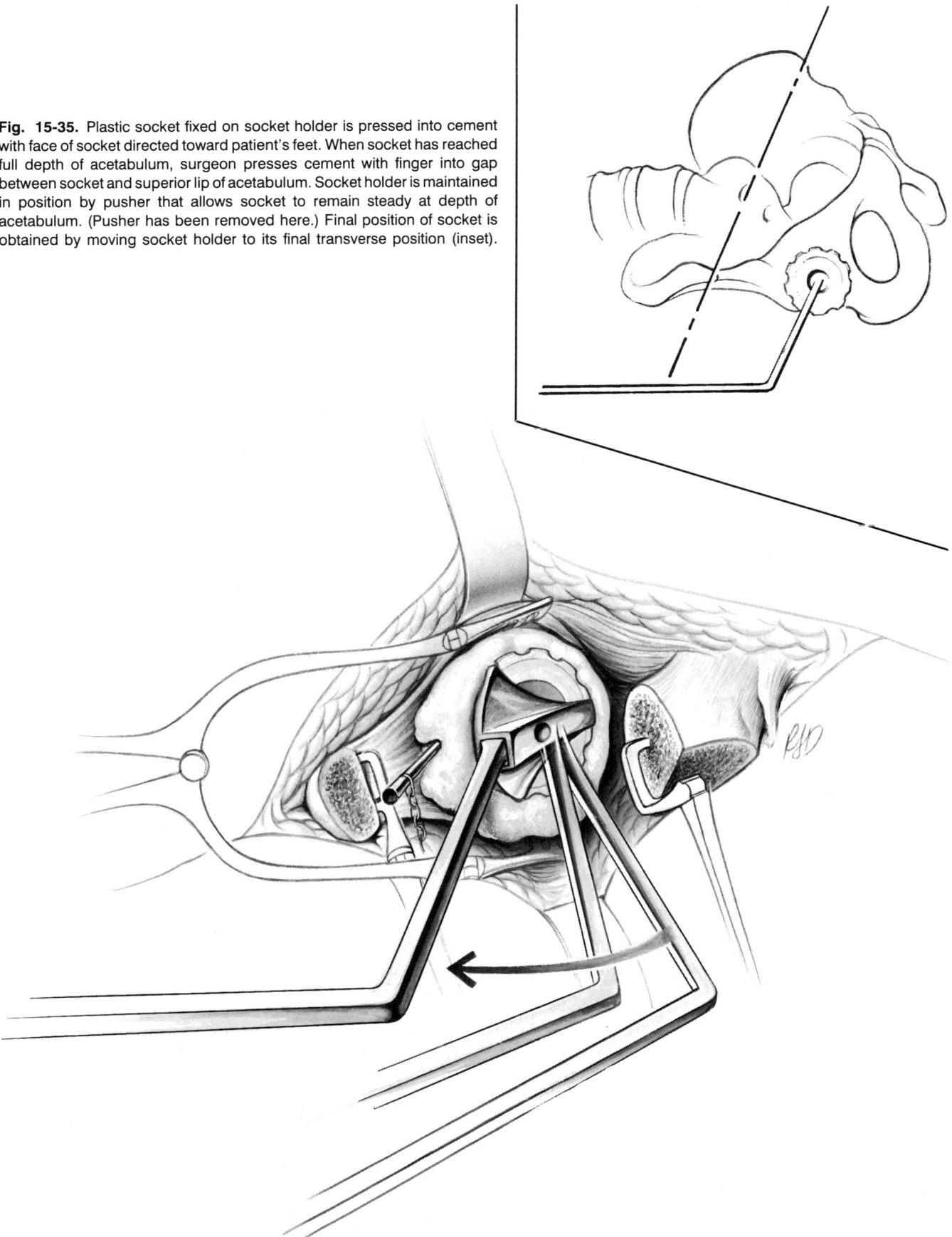

1. Insert the socket into the depth of the acetabulum (Fig. 15-36, *A*). While pressing on the socket holder, push the socket into the inferior aspect of the acetabulum (the guide handle is maximally tilted toward the patient's foot). Oscillate the socket holder back and forth a few degrees to sink the cup in deeply. The handle is not yet brought up to the final position.

2. Place the "socket pusher" in the depression in the socket holder (Fig. 15-36, *B*); bring the handle of the holder gradually up toward the patient's head without oscillation. This causes the space between the superior aspect of the cup and the acetabulum to become filled with cement as it extrudes over the top edge of the cup. The cement must be pushed back into the space with the tip of a finger or the tip of a Kocher clamp to completely fill the superior portion of the acetabulum. If the broad-rim pressure injection cup (tailored at surgery to the size of the socket) is used this is not necessary, since the rim of the cup will inject the cement into the acetabulum as the final position is reached.

3. Bring the handle of the cup holder up to the final desired position (Fig. 15-36, *C*). The handle should be lined up with the transverse axis of the pelvis. In this way the cup assumes a 45-degree orientation to the axis of the body. No more than 5 degrees of anteversion should be allowed. Once the socket and socket holder are in the optimal position, the assembly is held steady. Under no circumstances should the holder be readjusted. Do not move the socket back to a more horizontal position.

4. The first assistant must immobilize the holder while the surgeon maintains steady pressure with the "pusher" through the depressed area of the cup holder. Maintain the 45-degree orientation with minimum anteversion. This is the final fixation position, and no further changes should be made. Remove excess cement from the anterior and posterior portions of the socket with a small Volkmann's spoon. Take care not to pull the cement away from underneath the cup or change the orientation of the socket. The first assistant should not attempt to help remove cement, since his or her movements may change the socket's position. Instead, the assistant should hold the socket holder until it is removed by the surgeon. Avoid excessive pressure on the pusher because too much cement will be squeezed out of the acetabular cavity. If this occurs (most often in a large acetabulum), there will be no cement between the socket and the contact point of the acetabulum.

5. The surgeon should test the degree of polymerization using the leftover sample. When the cement is in the rubbery stage, one or two light taps of the hammer against the pusher will "coin" the socket into the cement and the cement into the bony trabeculae of the acetabulum. Do not leave coining until the cement reaches the final stage of stiffening, since it may not inject the stiff cement into the bone and might even be harmful and cause loosening of the cup.

6. Disengage the socket holder from the cup by pressing its release mechanism (Fig. 15-36, *D*). Place the tip of the pusher concentrically within the depth of the cup. Maintain pressure at a 45-degree angle. The surgeon should observe the true orientation of the cup. While the cement is still soft, "stuff" and "butter" it into the periphery of the cup between the cup and the bone, and remove any excess with a curette. Irrigate the area thoroughly and remove the retractors.

Remember the following:

1. A steady pair of hands is mandatory. Clumsy disengagement of the socket holder from the face of the cup causes cement to pull away from the bone, creating an imperfect fit. Likewise, if the first assistant moves the holder excessively, spaces are created between the cement and bone.

2. Early excessive pressure on the cup squeezes cement from the interface, causing direct contact between bone and cup that results in defective fixation.

3. Early removal of cement with a curette from the periphery of the acetabulum may pull cement away from the interface and must be avoided.

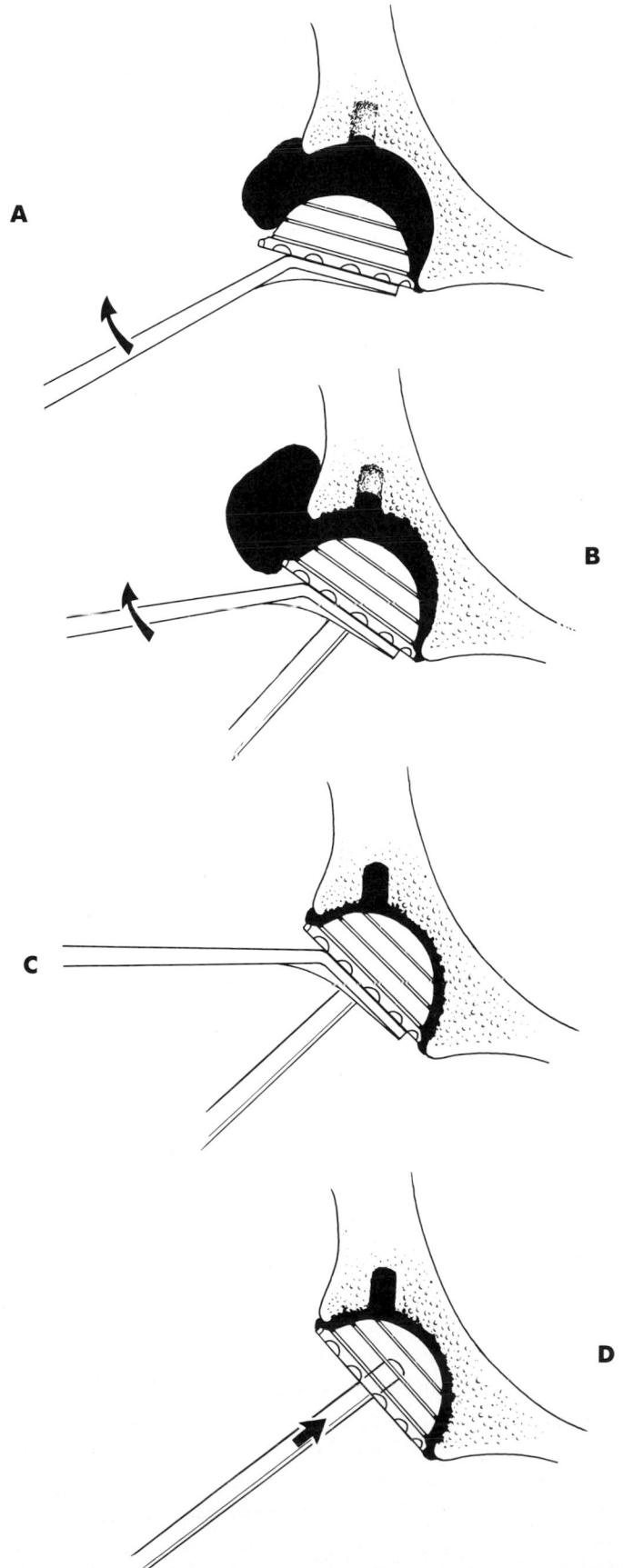

Fig. 15-36. A, Socket clipped to socket holder is pushed into depth of acetabulum pressing onto cement. Socket holder is maintained maximally toward patient's foot. **B,** Socket pusher is positioned into depression in socket holder to keep socket at depth of acetabulum while handle is brought up toward patient's head. NOTE: excess cement being squeezed out of depth of acetabulum toward superior lip. **C,** Handle is brought to final orientation (transverse arm parallel to transaxis of pelvis) and excess cement removed. **D,** Socket holder is removed and pusher is placed into depth of socket, and pressure is maintained until cement fully polymerizes.

4. Excessive proximal positioning of the socket holder (toward the patient's head) and later correction create a space between the weight-bearing portion of the acetabulum and the socket.

5. An unchecked flow of cement into the anterior soft tissues is a potential hazard to the femoral nerve.

6. Poor access to the acetabulum, poor exposure, or any other factor delaying the surgeon may allow cement to harden around the holder and prevent its disengagement from the cup.

7. A steady two-handed grip and absolute attention by the first assistant are essential to allow the surgeon to push the cup firmly into the acetabulum. (No talking at this stage.)

8. Excess cement must be removed before its polymerization and the removal of the self-retaining retractors.

9. A complete evaluation of the periphery of the cup and its relation to the acetabulum must be performed before removing the self-retaining retractors. Note the amount of bone covered by the cup and record it in the operative record.

10. Before removing the retractors attain complete hemostasis and irrigate with jet lavage to remove devitalized tissue and loose cement particles.

11. Search for and excise any significant marginal osteophytes before removing the self-retaining retractors.

12. The retractors must not come in contact with the cement, since this can make their removal difficult.

13. Remove any polymerized cement on the periphery of the acetabulum (cementophytes) by striking a half-inch chisel with hammer blows (see Fig. 15-30).

14. Remove the capsular pin retractors, using the cup pusher to stabilize the pelvis during extraction.

15. Removing the self-retaining retractors completes this phase.

Inserting a Pressure Injection Cup

Inserting a pressure injection cup is similar to but easier than inserting a rimless cup. The cup should be trimmed as previously described (see Figs. 15-32 and 15-33). Before insertion, the surgeon must check the retractors for an unimpeded rehearsal of the pressure injection cup. The cup must fit within the mouth of the acetabulum. There will be less clearance between this cup and the bone than a rimless cup (i.e., standard cup).

Socket alignment with the pressure injection cup should have already been rehearsed. The final positioning of this cup is easier than the rimless cup, since once the superior lobe reaches the acetabular rim, the cup is perfectly positioned. Cement is introduced as previously described. Full penetration of the cup (held in the socket holder) can be facilitated by simultaneously inserting the socket pusher along with the socket holder, forcing the socket into the depths of the acetabulum. A slight deflection of the superior lobe of the socket rim indicates that good pressurization has been achieved. Pressure by the pusher against the neck of the femur must be avoided, since it may tilt the socket. No hammering via the pusher rod is necessary or advisable and can even be harmful. It is important that the pusher continue to exert pressure onto the face of the cup via the socket holder, but the socket holder must remain motionless (see Fig. 15-34).

As the cement stiffens (toward the end of its plastic stage), eject the cup from the cup holder. However, maintain pressure on the cup by placing the pusher concentrically within the cup. The cup may begin to pull away from the room of the acetabulum, creating a space (in the critical superior zone of the acetabulum) between cement and bone. Therefore a thumb or an appropriate instrument must keep the cup in position with the upper lobe and in maximum contact with the roof of the acetabulum.

At the final stage of polymerization, any excess cement or marginal osteophytes may be excised before removing the self-retaining retractors and changing the acetabular exposure. Ectopic bone rarely forms in this region. Copious irrigation of the wound with a jet lavage is essential before removing the retractor.

Testing for Orientation

The trimmed prosthetic cup, held in the socket holder, is introduced. The hemispherical portion of the cup must be well covered by bone. Occasionally this may not be possible anteriorly because of a mild dysplasia. The superior rim must make contact with the roof of the acetabulum, and a good general seal of socket rim is desirable.

Allow no more than 5 degrees anteversion of the cup using a long posterior wall socket (i.e., Ogee or pressurization cups); orient the cup at 45 degrees of abduction. The pusher applied to the cup holder should stabilize the cup in the acetabulum sufficiently for the surgeon to be able to take his or her hand off the holder (see Chapter 19) without changing the position of the cup within the acetabulum.

Drilling Multiple Cement Anchor Holes

Using the acetabular drill and guide, 12 to 16 six mm outer diameter drill holes are evenly distributed in the small acetabula (see Fig. 15-26). In larger individuals these numbers can be increased, depending on the size of the acetabulum. The holes must pierce 1 cm deep the acetabular cancellous bone and are drilled only in the articulating portion of the acetabulum. Additional anchor holes may be placed in large acetabula, using a larger drill (i.e., 12.5 mm outer diameter) in the direction of the ilium, ischium, and pubis. In the left hip, large 12.5 mm holes should be placed at 3 o'clock for the ilium, between 7 and 8 o'clock for the ischium, and between 11 and 12 o'clock for the pubis (Fig. 15-25, A). The corresponding locations for the right hip would be at 9 o'clock for the ilium, between 4 and 5 o'clock for the ischium, and at 1 o'clock for the pubis (see Fig. 15-25, B). One cm penetration is adequate. Never penetrate the inner table of the pelvis with a drill. If this occurs, it should be plugged with a piece of cancellous bone or a cement restrictor (Fig. 5-25, C). Ischial bone is very soft, and subchondral bone is thin. It only requires a gentle pressure from the drill or the use of a curette to create a small cavity in this region.

It is important to protect the sciatic nerve from overpenetration by the drill, since cement may escape and damage the nerve. See Chapter 19 for the position of the drill for large holes in the right and left sides of the acetabulum. Final scraping of bone and cleaning of the drilled cavities are essential steps before cement is introduced.

Irrigation, Brushing, and Applying Hydrogen Peroxide

To clean the socket the acetabulum is thoroughly irrigated, and remnants of soft tissue and bone debris are removed (see Figs. 15-26, 15-27, and 15-28, A). It is important to clean the holes with a curette. A disposable rotary brush with jet lavage should be used routinely (see Fig. 15-27). Any soft tissue remaining after irrigation should be removed using a sharp curette.

It is essential to remove all debris before packing the acetabulum with a hydrogen peroxide–soaked sponge. When it is time to insert the cement, if there is visible blood on the surface of the bone (after removal of the hydrogen peroxide–soaked sponge), the surgeon may choose to irrigate again with Ringer's solution and suck the solution out quickly. A wet bony surface is better than one clotted with blood. Because of the lower viscosity of the irrigating solution compared with that of blood, the fluid can be displaced more easily than if a clot is occupying the perforations in the bone.

POSITIONING AND CEMENTING THE ACETABULAR COMPONENT

The cemented cup, regardless of the design or size of the flange of the inner diameter (22 or 26 mm), should be oriented between 40 and 45 degrees in relation to the transaxis of the pelvis and with no more than 5 degrees of anteversion if the cup has an extended posterior wall.

Insert the cement, and firmly pack it with a flat or round-ended instrument such as a disc and rod or a pressurization device as described by Ling.[15] This step is obviously important to initiate pressurization of the cement into the interstices of the bone. However, this author believes that containment of the cement by the rim of the cup is far more important than pressurization itself. On the other hand, if pressurization is initiated, it must be sustained while the cement is being polymerized. The best time for cement insertion is when it is in its "plastic stage" (no longer adheres to the surgeon's gloves or when wrinkles begin to appear on the surface of the bolus of cement). The initial pressurization is sustained by the rim of the cup. The pressure exerted on the cement must exceed the "bleeding pressure." There must be no motion transferred to the cement-bone interface until the cement is fully polymerized.

Observe the following details:

1. If any impingement prevents the cup from entering the socket, it either must be removed or the socket edge cut away (particularly on the anterior lip). As an alternative, a smaller socket may be used. If the fit is not perfect, the cup may "bottom" or will not be fully inserted when the cement is introduced.
2. To prevent unnecessary damage to the bone, do not drill the anchor holes deeper than 1 cm.
3. Do not routinely drill the pubic hole unless the acetabulum is large and good bony stock is present in that area. Large (12.5 mm outer diameter) anchor holes are unnecessary in severely osteoporotic bone, since curettage alone provides maximum surface for anchoring the cement.
4. Control severe bleeding into the acetabulum from cancellous bone by repeated tight packing with sponges to ensure a dry bed for the cement.
5. The position of the socket holder, the socket, and the edge of the acetabulum must be considered when determining the optimal position of the socket before its fixation by cement.
6. Take time to irrigate and suction the acetabulum, and insert the hydrogen peroxide–soaked sponge into the acetabulum before inserting the cement. Mixing the cement too soon places the surgeon in a hurried and uncontrolled situation, thus compromising the preparation.
7. When the preparation of the acetabulum cannot be completed in some areas using the reamers alone (especially in a large acetabulum), it is recommended that an acetabular gouge or a sharp curette (long-handled Volkmann's spoon) be used. A bone scraper is also invaluable for this purpose. Multiple 6 mm outer diameter drill holes may be made to maximize the fixation.
8. Before inserting the cup, the surgeon must make sure the socket is correctly fixed (clipped) to the cup "holder"* noting the position of the radiographic marker and the posterior extended wall of the cup.
9. Make sure that the self-retaining and pin retractors do not impinge against the handle of the cup holder when it is brought to its final position.
10. Readjust the retractors, if necessary, before inserting the cement.
11. It is essential to make a final inspection of the acetabulum and remove all bone debris before inserting the cement. Irrigating with an isotonic solution is useful in removing bone dust, finding unremoved soft tissue, and cleansing the acetabulum.
12. Before removing the retractors, complete hemostasis must be attained. Flush the area with irrigation solution to remove devitalized tissue and loose cement particles.
13. Search for and excise any significant marginal osteophytes before removing the self-retaining retractors.

FIXATION OF CEMENTLESS CUPS

Reaming is necessary for the interference fit of porous coated cups. For a perfect fit, the cavity must be prepared precisely to allow insertion with maximum contact and security at its initial fixation. The following principles must be observed:

1. Contain the cup within the bony acetabulum.
2. Perform acetabular reaming to bleeding bone while retaining the subchondral bone.
3. Enlarge the acetabulum with power tools such as an air-driven hemispherical graded reamer.

---

* This instrument is also identified as the "inserter."

Manual tools such as chisels, gouges, or curettes are inadequate to perform this task.

4. Use sharp reamers in a direction similar to the final cup positioning.
5. Note that the final reamer size determines the cup size; the press-fit effect at insertion may be enhanced if the selected cup size is 1 to 2 mm larger in its outer diameter than the last reamer used. This is the preferred method when the bone is malleable or the cancellous bone has been exposed during the final reaming.
6. Irrigate the bony acetabulum (without brushing) to reveal any fibrous tissue; carefully remove this tissue before inserting the cup.
7. When large cysts are exposed, remove them with curettes and pack them with cancellous bone before inserting the cup.
8. Two types of porous-coated acetabular components are currently used: (a) those achieving the initial fixation by projections on the cup, that is, AML and PCA, and (b) those with screw fixation, that is, Harris-Galante cup and similar designs by various manufacturers. When screws are used, be particularly careful in selecting insertion sites to avoid damage to the neurovascular structures of the pelvis (see Figs. 16-16 and 16-17).

To avoid injury to the intrapelvic structures not visible to the surgeon at surgery, four acetabular quadrants have been found clinically useful as a guide.[29] A line drawn from the anterosuperior spine through the center of the acetabulum to the posterior fovea forms acetabular halves. A second line drawn perpendicular to the first line at the midpoint of the acetabulum forms four quadrants; the posterior-superior quadrant is the best and the posterior-anterior quadrant the next best choice for safe screw placement and the best location for bone to be used for fixation of the cup. The other two zones, the anterosuperior and the anteroinferior quadrants, must be avoided since placement of the drill bits, depth gauge, and screws in these quadrants may endanger the external iliac artery and the obturator artery, nerve, and vein. Intrapelvic structures at risk because of injudicious reaming during the initial fixation and migration of the total hip arthroplasty are described in Chapter 22.[13]

PREPARATION OF THE FEMUR AND FIXATION OF THE FEMORAL PROSTHESIS
Femoral Exposure

During reaming and fixation of the stem, particularly if cement is used, an unimpeded access to the upper femur is essential. Difficulties are encountered in hips with severe stiffness, shortening, and fixed flexion and adduction deformity. Also, it can be difficult to access the upper femur in a straight line toward the knee in patients with large muscle bulk or who are obese.

1. Perform mobilization of the upper femur after resecting the femoral head and before attempting to prepare the femur (see Chapters 24 and 25).
2. Detach structures from the femur, including the short rotators, the femoral insertion of the gluteus maximus to the femur, the anterior and superior capsule, the psoas tendon, and the anterior capsule, in that order (see Chapters 20 and 25).
3. The surgeon should ensure appropriate positioning of the leg during preparation (see Chapters 16 and 25).

Femoral Preparation for the Use of Cement

The following principles apply to preparation of the femur for a cement stem:

1. The prepared cavity of the femur must be larger than the stem size to allow space for the cement. A minimum of 2 to 3 mm cement thickness is necessary, especially in the highly loaded regions of the femur.[14]
2. Strong cancellous bone must be preserved, but all loose and fragile endosteal trabeculae should be removed; good bony support for cement is essential.
3. Maximum widening of the femur (within its anatomical limits), especially in the presence of

a narrow medullary canal, is necessary to accommodate a standard-size caliber prosthesis.

4. While held in the holder, the stem must be inserted and rehearsed for proper fit and alignment.
5. Centralization of the stem proximally and distally is required (see Chapter 19).
6. Test for stability and range of motion before cementing the component. If the trochanter has been detached, wires are inserted before inserting the cement.
7. An identical orientation of the stem in the canal before and after insertion of cement is mandatory.

Preparation of the medullary canal for stems fixed with or without cement is vastly different. When cement is used, the canal must be reamed more extensively so that it can accommodate both the cement and the stem. With a cementless technique, the femur must be reamed to the precise shape and size of the stem to be inserted.

Preparation of the Medullary Canal for Cemented Stem

Insert a T-handle straight reamer exactly at the site of insertion of the piriformis tendon, which must be cleared off the distal fossa. Use a 6 or 8 mm drill to penetrate the thick cortex. When the trochanter is osteotomized, the site of the opening of the medullary canal is at the junction of the cut surface of the trochanter and the neck of the femur (Figs. 15-37 and 15-38). Aim the tapered T-handle reamer at the knee, thereby defining the medullary canal. It is important to pack a swab behind the femur to prevent reamed marrow from entering the wound, since marrow may be responsible for ectopic bone formation after surgery. Once the reamer is fully inserted, shift it toward the lateral cortex to produce a slightly valgus track. This entails encroachment on the trochanteric bed. The surgeon stabilizes the knee with one hand while guiding the reamer with the other; the second assistant holds the tip in maximum adduction and neutral rotation to aid stabilization. The assistant on the far side of the table holds the tibia vertical so that the amount of anteversion in the femoral neck can be recognized. Check the tapered reamer to be sure it is within the medullary canal and that valgus orientation is maintained. This way the surgeon can be sure that the reamer is not piercing the femoral cortex. Enlarge the aperture by cutting toward the trochanteric bed as the reamer is inserted, making an oval opening for femoral broach in the correct "version." A straight tapered reamer attached to a power drill may be used to enlarge the cavity of the upper femur. The plane of version has already been determined by the tapered pin reamer. To ensure accuracy of the plane of anteversion when a broach is used, the knee is kept at 90 degrees flexion and the tibia perpendicular to the floor. The plane of the broach should also be parallel to the transverse intracondylar axis of the knee if no anteversion or retroversion is required. The use of a boxed chisel facilitates the orientation of the plane of version (see Chapter 16). Make reference to the following anatomical features in guiding broaches and reamers:

1. Patella and the transverse axis of the knee (transcondylar line).
2. Flexed knee at right angles.
3. The size and shape of the greater trochanter.
4. Shape of the upper femur, including the orientation of the lesser trochanter (see Chapters 3, 16, and 18). When broaches are used they should be inserted in a valgus orientation, as if cutting takes place with the convex edge of the broach. Should the broaches impinge against the medial calcar, they must be withdrawn and reinserted: (1) to ensure valgus positioning and (2) to prevent fracturing the calcar femorale.

When the medullary canal is excessively narrow and the isthmus prevents full broaching, further widening may be accomplished by using graded cylindrical reamers, such as the Kuntscher reamers. Broaching may then be completed.

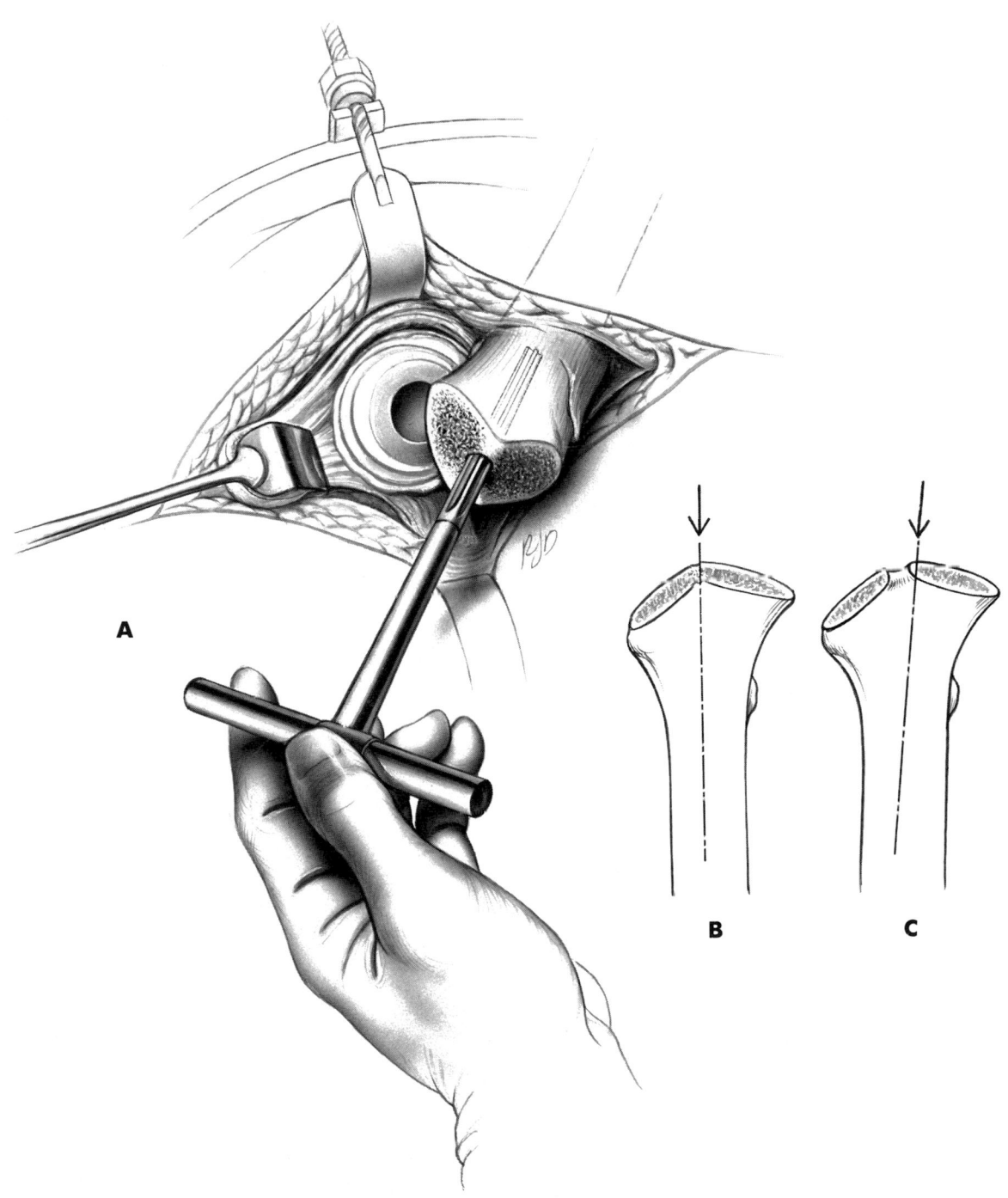

Fig. 15-37. Medullary canal is opened with tapered pin T-handled reamer. Starting point of insertion of tapered reamer is at junction of cut surface of trochanter and cut surface at neck. Direction of insertion of reamer is in slight valgus (to avoid any varus position), thus encroaching into bed of trochanter. Tapered pin reamer enters at somewhat posterior level of cut surface of neck and is aimed at knee joint. **A** and **B** indicate correct and **C** "faulty" insertion. In **C**, bridge between neck of femur and greater trochanteric bed is not removed, thus forcing reamer into varus position. When the trochanter is not removed, the reamers must encroach into the base of the trochanter.

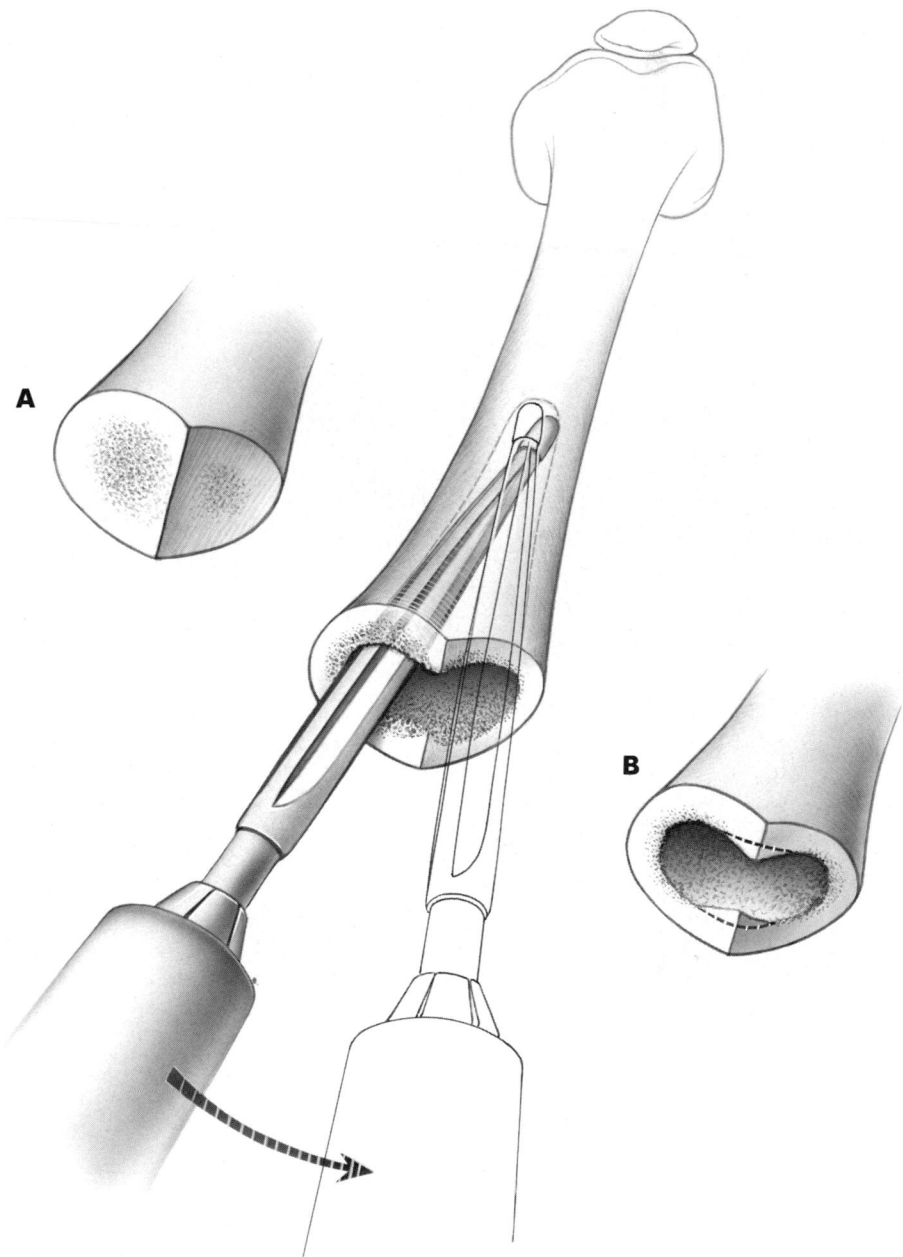

Fig. 15-38. Medullary canal opening is best accomplished by a Charnley T-handled tapered reamer (canal finder) at the junction of the femoral neck and trochanteric bed. **A,** Thus the tapered reamer can be centered within the canal aiming at the patella. The use of a tapered rotary reamer (blunt tip) will prevent accidental perforation of the femoral shaft. The tapered reamer is operated in low speed and shifted from medial to lateral. **B,** The upper femur is enlarged to allow insertion of the provisional prosthesis, which must be loose within the trochanter canal to allow space for the cement. Mediolateral shift of the drill handle removed bone in respective areas of the upper femur. Note, the reamer must be withdrawn for about half of its length before it can effectively remove bone from the top of the femur (encroachment on the trochanter bed has been exaggerated for demonstration).

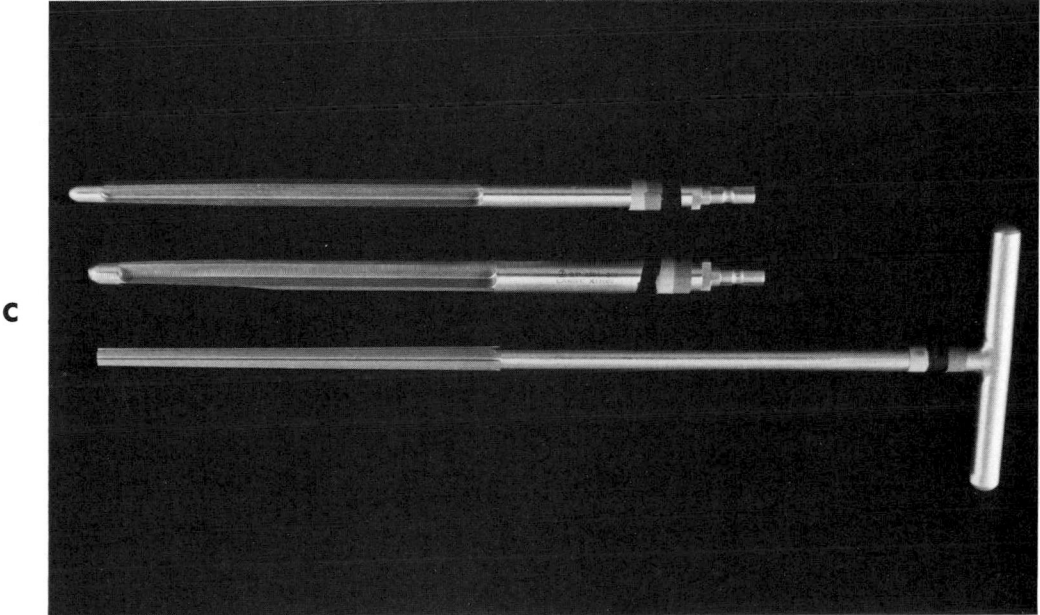

C

Fig. 15-38—cont'd. C, Three key instruments in preparing the medullary canal include Charnley T handle reamer (canal finder) *(top),* Small and large tapered reamers are used with air-driven power tools. These reamers (designed by the author) incorporate a blunt tip for safety to avoid perforating the shaft of the femur when used eccentrically in the medullary canal. (From Eftekhar NS: Total hip replacement: low-friction arthroplasty. In Evarts CM: *Surgery of the musculoskeletal system,* New York, 1983, Churchill Livingstone.)

Test Reduction

Attempt reduction after inserting the test prosthesis. This is achieved in three steps: (1) longitudinal traction, (2) flexing the hip and guiding the head into the cup, and (3) slight abduction to keep the head in.

The first assistant retracts the greater trochanter (when detached) cephalad. The second assistant applies longitudinal traction on the femur. The surgeon may also apply longitudinal traction to the femur while holding the knee in a 90-degree flexed position. Keeping the knee flexed provides grasping power for traction and relaxes the flexor muscles of the hip, especially the iliotibial tract.

1. The surgeon must make sure that the orientation of the femoral prosthesis has not changed within the canal since its insertion. This is accomplished by holding the femoral prosthesis in position with the middle and index fingers (this is especially important if there is an excessively large medullary canal). The Cobra flange usually is stable within the medullary canal and should not rotate during rehearsal for reduction. However, if it is not stable it may indicate that a larger caliber stem might be the preferred choice. If at reduction the stem rotates and drifts into a varus position, either Charnley's neck length jig or this author's technique of centralization of the stem is used (see Chapters 18 and 19). The first assistant holds the greater trochanter in the retracted cephalad position (if osteotomized); no retractors are used since they may interfere with the reduction; and flex the hip no less than 45 degrees without internal or external rotation. In addition to placing longitudinal traction on the limb, the surgeon must determine the location of the socket, and while holding the prosthesis within the femur, direct the head into the socket (Fig. 15-39).

Reduction may be difficult or impossible if: (1) the patient has not been adequately anesthetized and there is insufficient muscle relaxation, (2) the femoral neck is excessively long, (3) the socket has been inserted in a low position, or (4) the soft tissues are excessively tight. If present, correct these impediments, and examine the soft tissue closely to determine what is causing the problem. Attain adequate muscle relaxation, and divide soft tissue contractions, if present, before deciding whether to shorten the femur. If shortening is indicated, it must be done in stages so that excess shortening is avoided.

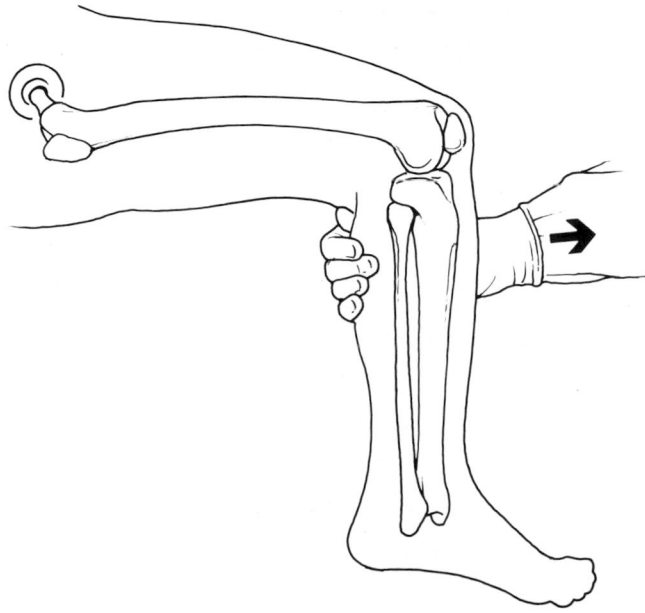

Fig. 15-39. The test for stability of the joint after insertion of provisional prosthesis is demonstrated. The hip is flexed to 45 degrees while the knee is flexed to right angle. With a firm grip on the proximal tibia a longitudinal traction is applied while the surgeon checks for separation of the femoral head prosthesis from the depth of the socket.

Testing for Motion and Stability

After the prosthesis is reduced into the socket, test the hip in flexion, abduction, and adduction, as well as rotation. If full abduction is not achieved, perform an adductor tenotomy (see Chapter 24). Next, while placing strong longitudinal traction on the limb (with the knee slightly flexed), the surgeon inserts his index finger between the prosthetic components to determine the amount of separation attained (no more than 5 mm of separation should be possible) (Fig. 15-40). Evaluate the coverage of the head and its relation to the cup with the hip in neutral position. Finally, determine how much adduction or external rotation produces dislocation. This is the real test of instability and is done with the hip in extension, while testing for "impingement" of the inferior and medial neck against the acetabular margin. By adducting the limb across the table, subluxation and dislocation are observed. Ideally, the prosthesis should not begin dislocating before 40 degrees of adduction (slight flexion is required to allow adduction of the leg across the opposite thigh). If this occurs with less adduction, one must check for impingement of the medial femoral neck against the acetabular rim, vertical placement of the cup, laxity of the joint, or excessive valgus placement of the prosthesis. The cup should be oriented at 40 to 45 degrees to the axis of the body without anteversion or retroversion of either component. If the head is not completely covered by the cup while the leg is in neutral position, it must be assumed that one or both of the components is malpositioned (see Chapter 32).

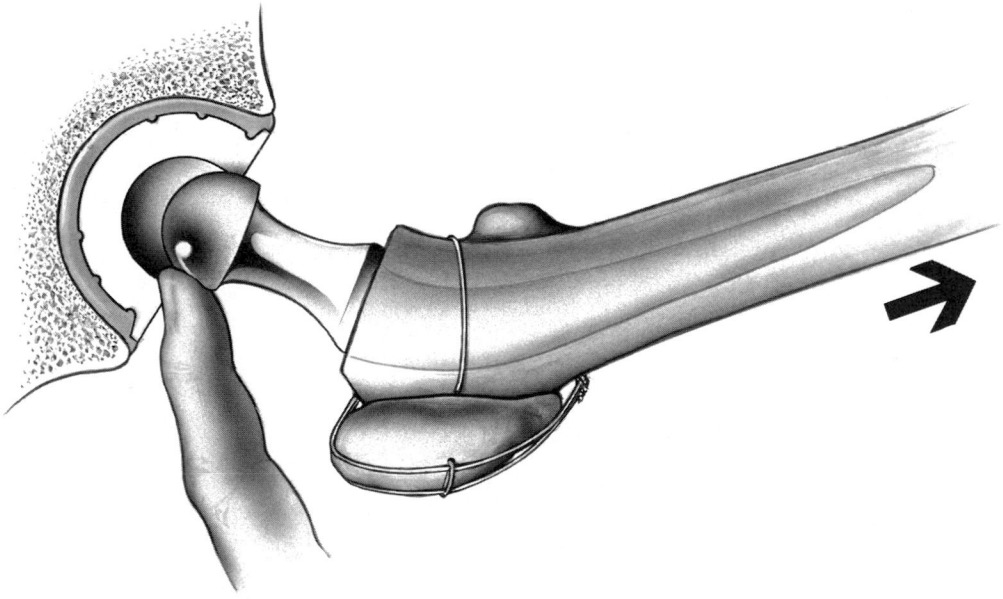

Fig. 15-40. Longitudinal traction must produce only minimum separation between the head of the socket; 5 mm (or equivalent of the surgeon's index finger tip inserted between the components). Excess of 5 mm calls for correction of instability, that is, the use of a longer neck prosthesis.

It is not necessary to test for flexion range if the orientation of the components is satisfactory after reducing the hip. However, the most important test is external rotation in neutral abduction/adduction position. If the hip is unstable in this position, one or more of the following conditions may exist: (1) excess anteversion of the cup or femoral component; (2) anteversion of cup with a long posterior wall socket; and (3) excess laxity of the myofascial sleeve of the thigh, that is, the neck of the prosthesis is too short. External rotation instability cannot be corrected by reattaching the greater trochanter. Therefore the cause of instability must be identified and corrected before cementing the femoral component. The dislocation of total hip arthroplasty caused by malpositioning of the components may be caused by neck socket impingement, especially in patients who gain a large range of postoperative motion (Figs. 15-41 and 15-42).

In summary, when the joint is reduced, several things should be noted.

1. The amount of traction required to locate the head into the socket (reduction) should be determined.
2. Flexion to 90 degrees, abduction to 30 degrees, and adduction to 30 degrees without dislocation should be present.
3. Separation of the two components by longitudinal traction should be no more than 5 mm, that is, the tip of the index finger can barely be positioned between the two components.
4. Full coverage of the prosthetic head by the cup when the hip is in neutral rotation should be noted.
5. Full extension must be possible without any residual fixed flexion deformity.
6. A satisfactory "effective neck length" produced by the prosthesis should render equal leg length. When the limb is placed on the operating table parallel to the opposite side, if both malleoli lie at the same level, that denotes equal leg length (the malleoli can be palpated through the drapes).

An Unsatisfactory Test Reduction

When reduction is not possible, it may be caused by an excessive neck length, unreleased contracted capsule, contraction of the iliopsoas tendon, or inadequate muscle relaxation. On the other hand, instability may be caused by (1) excessive shortening of the neck, (2) a high positioning of the socket, (3) medial and anterior osteophytes or cementophytes about the acetabulum, (4) projecting osteophytes on the upper femur, (5) lack of clearance caused by an excessively deepened acetabulum, (6) previous surgery with subsequent loss of tissue elasticity, (7) sinking of the femoral prosthesis into the medullary canal during rehearsal, (8) rotation of the stem within the canal, and (9) malposition of either component.

Correction of an Unstable Reduction

An unstable reduction resulting from a short neck may be rectified by placing the prosthesis in a more valgus position or by using a long-neck prosthesis. When recognized, faulty orientation of the socket or the femoral prosthesis must be corrected at once (see Chapter 32). Further stability should not be expected from a firm reattachment of the greater trochanter. The hip must be made stable before cementing the femoral component.

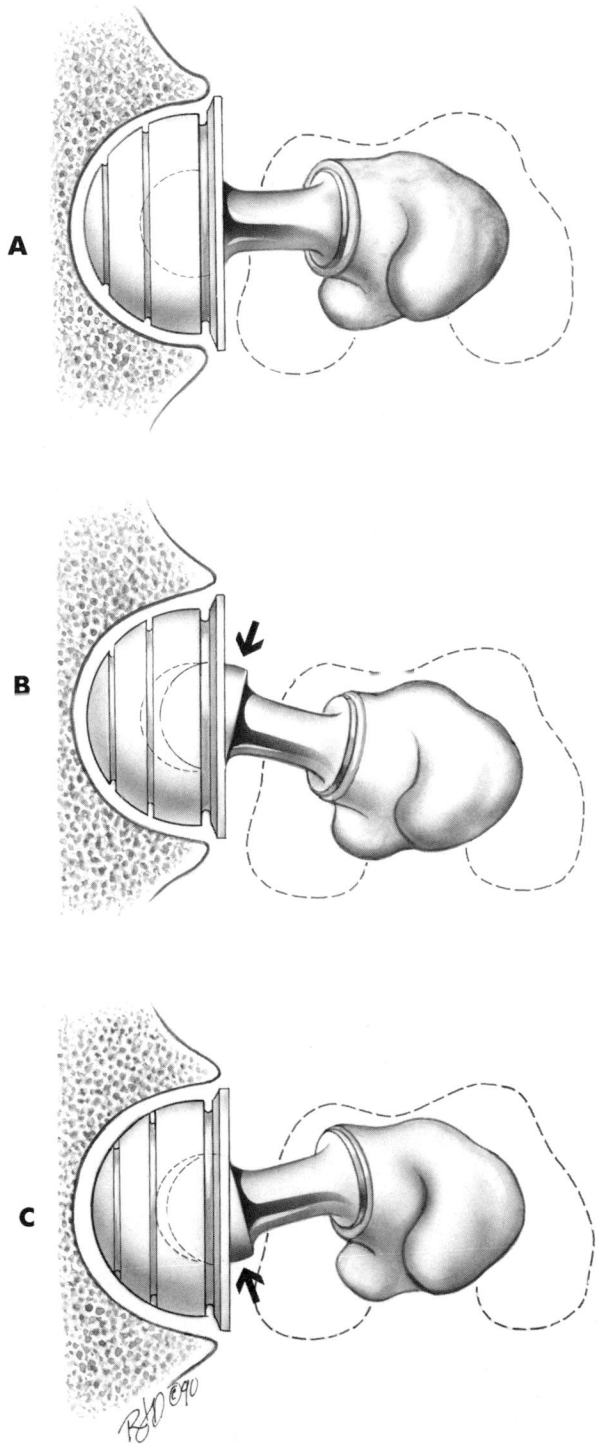

Fig. 15-41. Instability caused by excess anteversion or retroversion of the femoral component is demonstrated. **A,** A complete coverage of the femoral head by the acetabular component (both components are in "neutroversion"). **B,** Excess anteversion leads to partly exposed head *(arrow)*. The hip is prone to dislocate anteriorly postoperatively. **C,** Excess retroversion leading to a partially exposed head. Hip is prone to postoperative posterior dislocation.

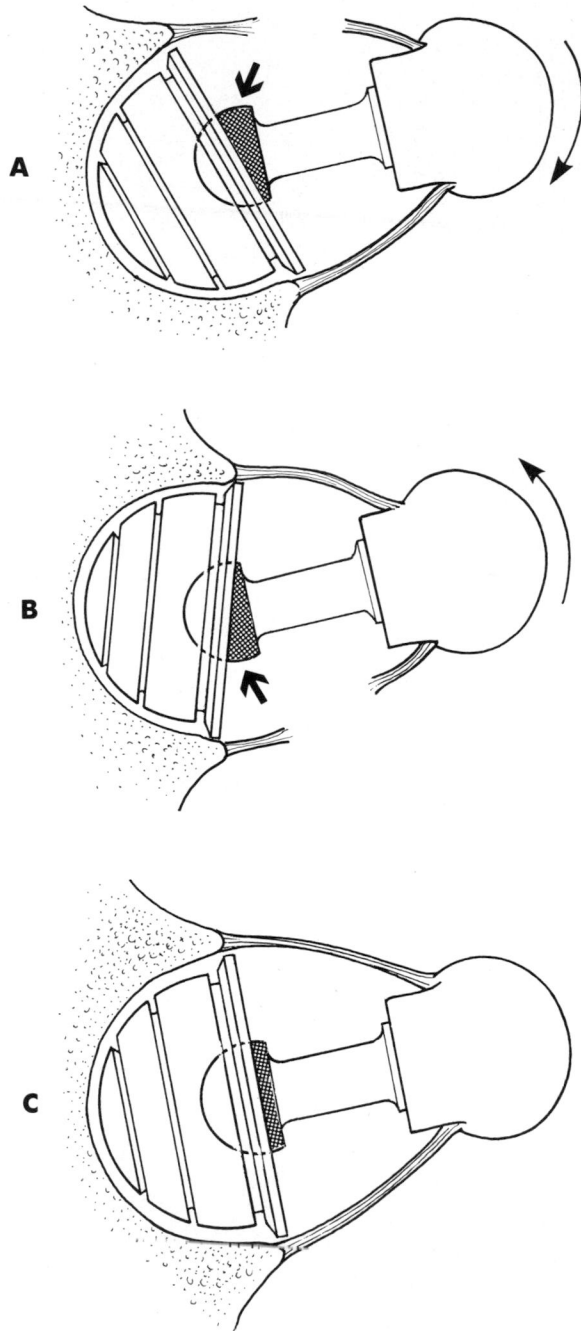

Fig. 15-42. Late cause of anterior or posterior dislocation. **A,** Excess anteversion of the cup or a long posterior wall can render the hip unstable anteriorly resulting from soft tissue stretch; note uncovered femoral head *(arrow)*. **B,** Excess retroversion of the cup with increasing soft tissue "stretch" from excess range of motion of the hip renders the hip unstable in a posterior direction *(arrow)*. **C,** Perfect alignment of both components is critical in preventing dislocation (early or late).

Final Preparation

After testing for motion and stability, dislocate the hip, remove the test prosthesis, and once again, deliver the stump of the femur out of the wound. Pack a clean swab behind the proximal femur to prevent marrow from entering the wound. A Watson-Jones gauge may facilitate delivery. Remove the loose cancellous bone and fatty marrow within the intramedullary canal, especially in the region of the calcar femorale, using a small Volkmann's spoon. Vigorous curettage is unnecessary. Curettage of the calcar area produces a space between the concavity of the stem and bone, thereby ensuring a thick layer of cement at this load-bearing portion of the femur (Fig. 15-43). Apply strong suction within the medullary canal to remove blood and fatty marrow. Irrigate with jet lavage, and brush using a powered rotary brush to facilitate removal of debris, clots, and bone marrow (Fig. 15-44). Insert a dry swab into the canal before inserting the wires (when the trochanter is osteotomized).

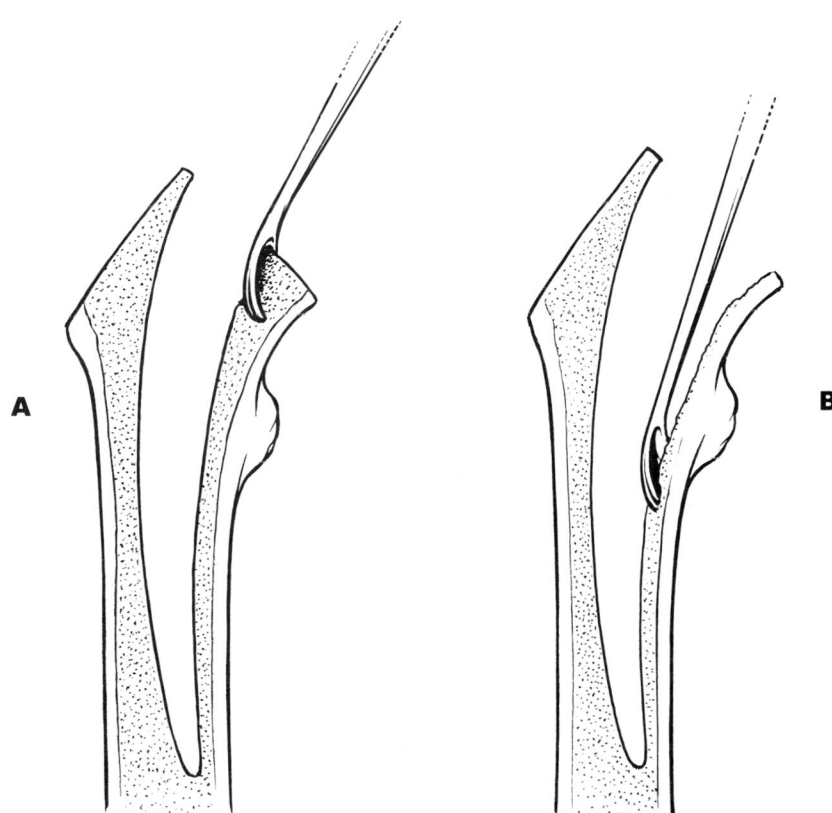

Fig. 15-43. A, Gentle curettage of calcar region produces space between concavity of stem and bone, ensuring thick layer of cement at this load-bearing region of femur. Additionally, strong bone of calcar will support cement. **B,** Severe curettage may remove strong trabeculae available for interdigitation.

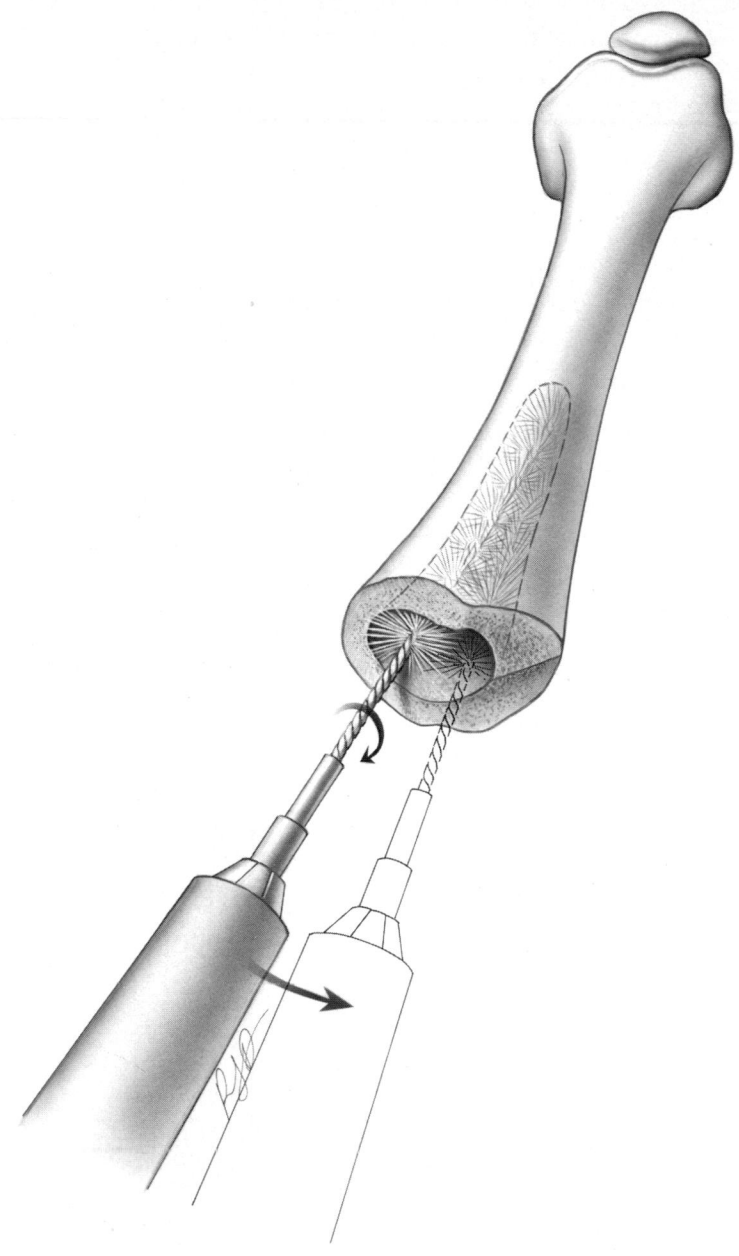

Fig. 15-44. Use a rotary brush attached to power drill while irrigating the canal with pulsating jet lavage (Ringer's solution) to remove clots and bone debris.

Patients Predisposed to Stem Malpositioning

The surgeon must be alert to certain conditions that contribute to malpositioning of the femoral component. These include the following:

1. Excess obesity or hip stiffness.
2. Difficult surgical exposure of the hip.
3. A large medullary canal.
4. Heavily muscled bodies.
5. Pathology of the upper femur, such as in Paget's disease.
6. A small-caliber prosthesis for a large canal.
7. Revisionary surgery.
8. Nontranstrochanteric approaches used in difficult anatomical situations.

Steps Just Before Cementing

Several important steps should be undertaken just before mixing or inserting the cement. They include: (1) testing for stability, (2) curettage of the bone, (3) brushing of the medullary canal, (4) controlling intramedullary bleeding and clots, and (5) plugging the medullary canal.

Testing for Stability

A systematic test for range of motion for all approaches and prostheses is mandatory before cementing the stem. A similar test must be conducted after inserting the actual prosthesis and before reattaching the greater trochanter and closing the wound when cementless components have been used. Single anatomical planes and combinations should be considered:

1. Extension-flexion, 0 to 140 degrees.
2. Abduction-adduction, 0 to 40 degrees.
3. Internal-external rotation, 45 to 45 degrees.
4. Flexion-adduction, 90 to 30 degrees.
5. Flexion-internal rotation, 90 to 30 degrees.
6. Flexion-adduction-internal rotation, 90 to 30 to 30 degrees.
7. Extension-internal rotation, 0 to 30 degrees.
8. Extension-external rotation, 0 to 30 degrees.
9. Flexion-abduction-external rotation, 45 to 30 to 30 degrees.

Curettage of Bone

Long T-handled curettes (Volkmann spoons) with 1 to 1.2 cm diameter spoon size are used to clean out the loose bony trabecular fat, marrow, and bone debris. The T-handle spoon provides a good sense of orientation in the medullary canal and allows a firm grip. However, curettage is not intended to remove all cancellous bone, only fragile or loose trabeculae. With each stroke the curette is brought out, and the content of the spoon is observed. Remove the medial cancellous bone of the neck more vigorously than the cancellous bone of the lateral proximal portion (at the site of the greater trochanter). The medial neck region is an important load-bearing zone of the femur and provides support for the cement.

Controlling Intramedullary Bleeding and Clots

To achieve a microinterlock between cement and bone, blood must be eliminated from the interface. This can be largely accomplished by (1) inducing hypotensive anesthesia, (2) packing the medullary canal with sponges, (3) controlling bleeding with an intramedullary plug (if the source of bleeding is from the distal portion of the femur), (4) using dilute epinephrine to reduce bleeding or hydrogen peroxide to prevent clots,* and (5) continuously suctioning the closed cavity packed with epinephrine or hydrogen peroxide–soaked ribbon gauze (see Figs. 15-45 and 15-46).

PLUGGING THE CANAL Plugging the distal medullary canal has the following advantages: (1) cement is contained within the medullary cavity, and its extension is limited to the level of the plug; (2) pressure is increased, thus cement penetrates substantially into the endosteal surface of the bone, and the cement plug also increases extrusion pressure proximally to a significant degree; (3) plugging prevents increased pressure distal to the stem tip level, which can promote fat embolization (see Chapter 5); and (4) plugging also prevents retrograde bleeding and thus mixing the cement with blood.

Several methods can be used to occlude the medullary canal distal to the stem tip.

CEMENT Four to seven ml of prepolymerized cement is delivered 2 to 3 cm distal to the stem top level by a special two-step syringe. This syringe is larger at one end to facilitate loading with PMMA and has a long, narrow nozzle at the other end that reaches a desired level within the medullary canal distal to the tip of the stem.[24] After delivering the cement, the syringe is rotated 360 degrees clockwise and counter-clockwise to detach the cement from the syringe. The cement must be delivered distal to the tip of the step to avoid interfering with a subsequent insertion of cement.

This method is most effective in occluding the canal; however, it is rather cumbersome because the cement must be mixed in two stages, one for the plug and the other for fixation of the stem, adding to the operating time. Additionally, there is a danger that the cement will be pulled into the canal as the syringe is being removed, thus interfering with the stem insertion.

BONE PLUGS Bone plugs are made from the femoral head removed at surgery[18,30] or from the neck of the femur. A piece of cancellous bone from the patient's femoral head, 1 to 2 cm in length, is shaped and delivered to the appropriate level (just beyond the tip of the stem). Since the bone is taken from the patient's femoral head it is biologically compatible and economical. Sizing using commercially available gauges is necessary to ensure the plug is the correct size. Obviously, when there is an existing plug beyond the tip of the stem, as in revision surgery (see Chapter 25), there is no need to insert a new plug. Therefore the old plug serves as an excellent block for the new cement.

SYNTHETIC PLUGS Several types of synthetic plugs, made of high-density polyethylene or PMMA, are commercially available, each with its appropriate instrumentation to gauge the size of the medullary canal and insertion tool. The primary goal in using synthetic plugs during total hip arthroplasty is to enhance cement fixation by increasing intrusion properties. Such a plug must completely obliterate the medullary canal. Using a scoring system for plug migration, cement leakage, and relative ability to withstand pressure (force of more than 50 psi) during cementing, a great variation in performance has been observed. The PMMA plugs have the highest overall score and can sustain pressures above 100 psi longer than the three other commercially available plugs tested.[1] This author has used PMMA preformed plugs and a centralization plug of his own design, which, in addition to plugging the medullary canal, provides centralization of the distal stem tip within the medullary canal (see Chapter 19).

---

* The use of hydrogen peroxide in a closed cavity may cause cardiac arrest during surgery. A case of cardiac arrest immediately after the use of hydrogen peroxide during preparation of the medullary canal has been reported; the author suggested that this might have been caused by a rapid absorption of oxygen leading to gas embolization and the sudden loss of cardiac output. Although the actual mechanism of cardiac arrest may be related to other causes (see Chapter 5), the release of oxygen gas can be circumvented by using a venting catheter to change the closed cavity to an open cavity.

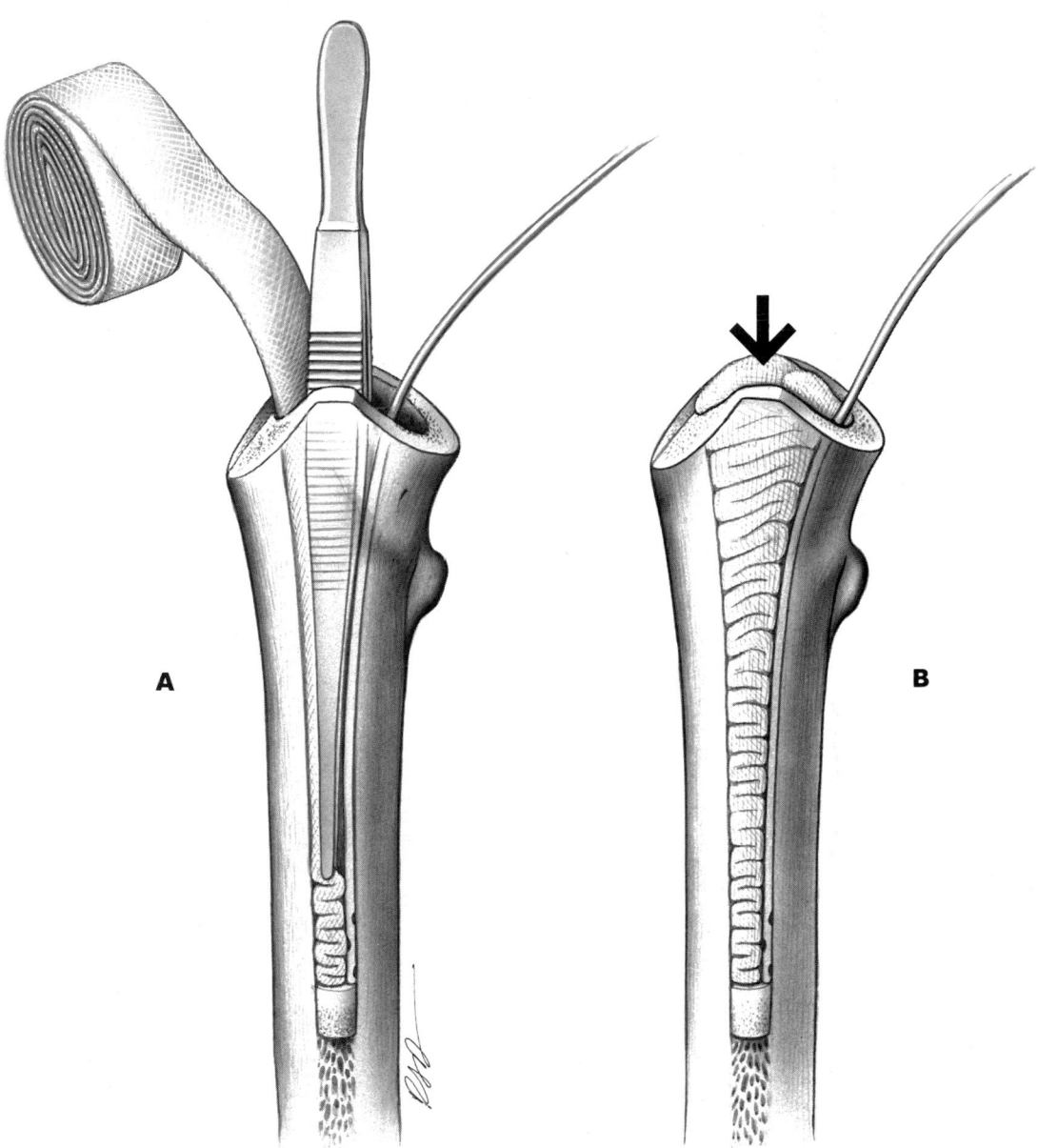

Fig. 15-45. A, While cement is being mixed, a 2 cm wide ribbon gauze (soaked in hydrogen peroxide) is inserted after a thorough irrigation of the canal. Note a small-lumen polyethylene tube is in place, which is connected to suction. Note also that packing is accomplished from the depth of the canal toward the opening. **B,** Fully packed canal just before insertion of cement.

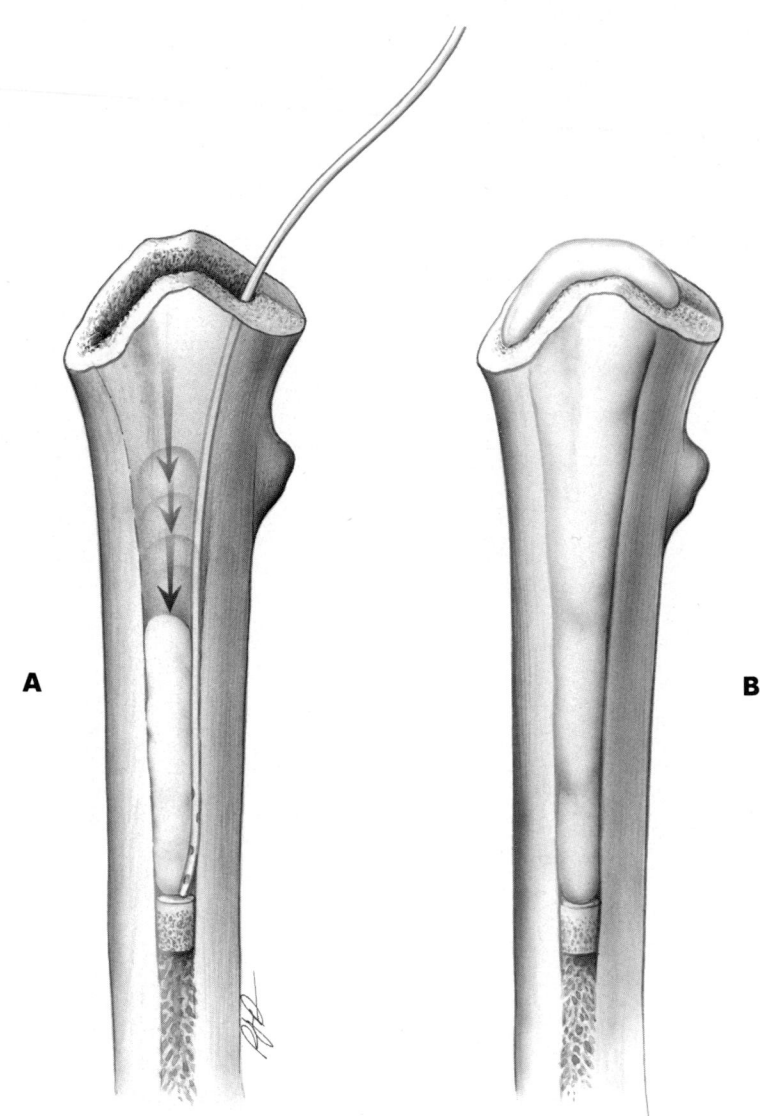

Fig. 15-46. A, The ribbon gauze has been removed while the polyethylene tube remains in place while cement is delivered into the medullary canal. **B,** After the canal is filled with half of the cement, the remaining cement should be inserted only after removal of the polyethylene tube.

Inserting Wires

When trochanteric osteotomy is performed (see Chapters 18 and 19), insert wires for subsequent reattachment of the greater trochanter, unless the surgeon chooses to use extraosseous methods for reattachment.

Rehearsal of Prosthesis Insertion

A deliberately slow and staged rehearsal (without cement) enables the surgeon to determine the correct orientation of the femoral prosthesis within the medullary canal. The prosthesis should be secured in valgus* and neutral rotation.

Observe the following:

1. Note the longitudinal axis of the femur, position of the knee and patella, and tibia for reference.
2. Observe the amount of valgus* orientation of the stem as it is being inserted into the femoral canal.
3. Note the axial orientation of the prosthesis (anteversion-retroversion) within the medullary canal.
4. Observe the fit of the stem. The prosthesis must be inserted with ease.
5. Observe the location and relation of the wires (when used) to the prosthesis. They must not interfere with the insertion of the prosthesis.
6. Observe and remove marrow tissue and soft cancellous bone as indicated without disturbing the position of wires when used.

Irrigating, Brushing, and Packing the Canal

The medullary canal must be free of all debris, such as marrow, fat, bone fragments, clots, and fibrous interface membrane. After using the long T-handled Volkmann spoon, a stiff bottle-type brush, used with a power tool, or a hand brush is twisted, turned, withdrawn several times in a plugged canal: a hand brush can accomplish this task satisfactorily. The cross-legged position produces access to the top of the femur. Irrigate the canal with pulsating jet lavage, and use a rotary brush as needed. Place a 4 mm outer diameter polyethylene tube, connected to suction, deep into the medullary canal while 2 cm wide ribbon guaze, soaked in hydrogen peroxide, is packed into the medullary canal.† Use a long-handled, smooth forceps to pack the ribbon deep into the canal, thus packing the canal from bottom to top (see Fig. 15-45). This detail is important since the tendency is to pack the ribbon from the top, which leaves behind a large cul-de-sac filled with blood.

---

* The term *valgus* denotes avoidance of any "varus" positioning. Ideally, at the final step, the stem should be centered in the canal without any varus or valgus orientation.

†The hydrogen peroxide is advantageous in preventing blood from unclotting. Unclotted blood with a lower viscosity is more readily displaced than the viscous blood clot.

Inserting the Cement

Observe the following details during this important phase of the operation:

- Isolate the neck of the femur so it is not contaminated with blood or fat.
- Pack a gauze sponge into the acetabulum and behind the neck. Drape the neck with a fenestrated towel.
- Prepare and use 40 gm cement (2 packets of 20 gm) routinely. A large portion of this cement is unnecessary, since the surgeon must have an adequate amount of cement for each insertion.
- Avoid using cement that sticks to the glove. Use of a low-viscosity cement is not desirable, since it is difficult to handle and can cause tissue damage (see Chapter 5).
- Deliver the cement in doughy stage manually or by a cement gun, but pack the cement by digital pressure (Fig 15-47).
- A "double thumb" technique exerts forceful pressure and advances the cement. The thumbs must work like pistons in pressurizing and advancing the cement.
- Place one thumb against the opening of the canal while the other partially obliterates the opening into the trochanter.
- Avoid a delicate and gentle use of a digit, since poking with the finger tips does not advance the cement into the canal or pressure it.
- Avoid glove tears or contamination of cement with blood. Use a third pair of gloves for delivery and pressurization of cement.

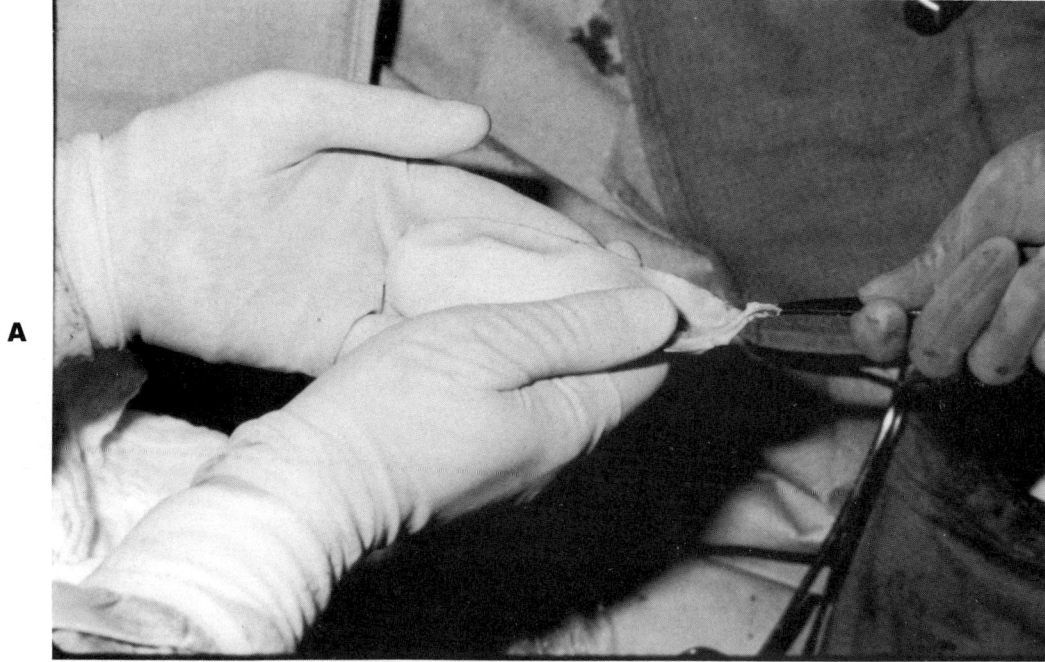

Fig. 15-47. A, Cement is collected with a spoon when it no longer adheres to the surgeon's glove. **B,** Cement is shaped like sausage and ready to be inserted. **C,** "Double-thumb" technique used for inserting the cement.

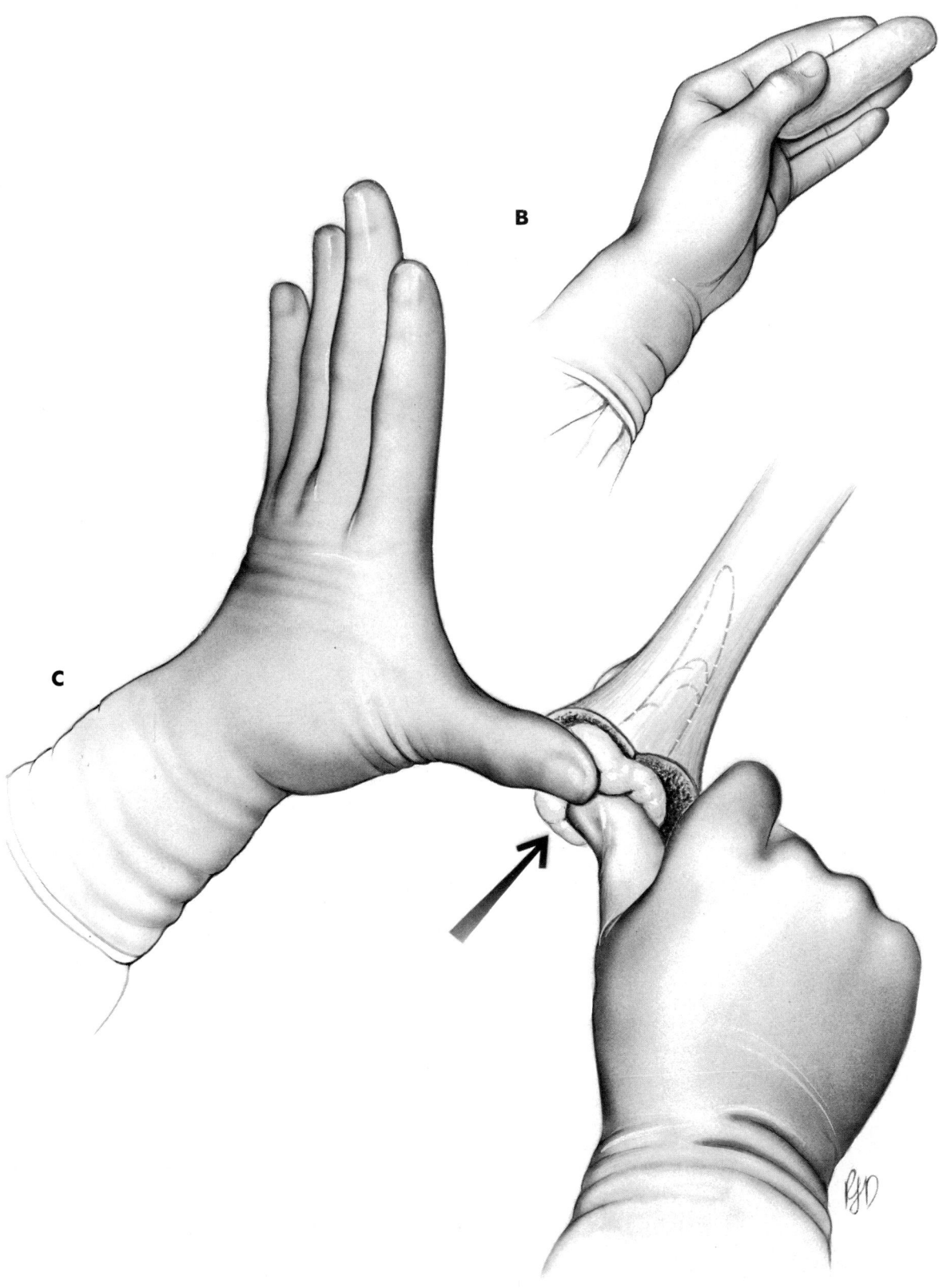

Fig. 15-47, cont'd. See legend on opposite page.   *Continued.*

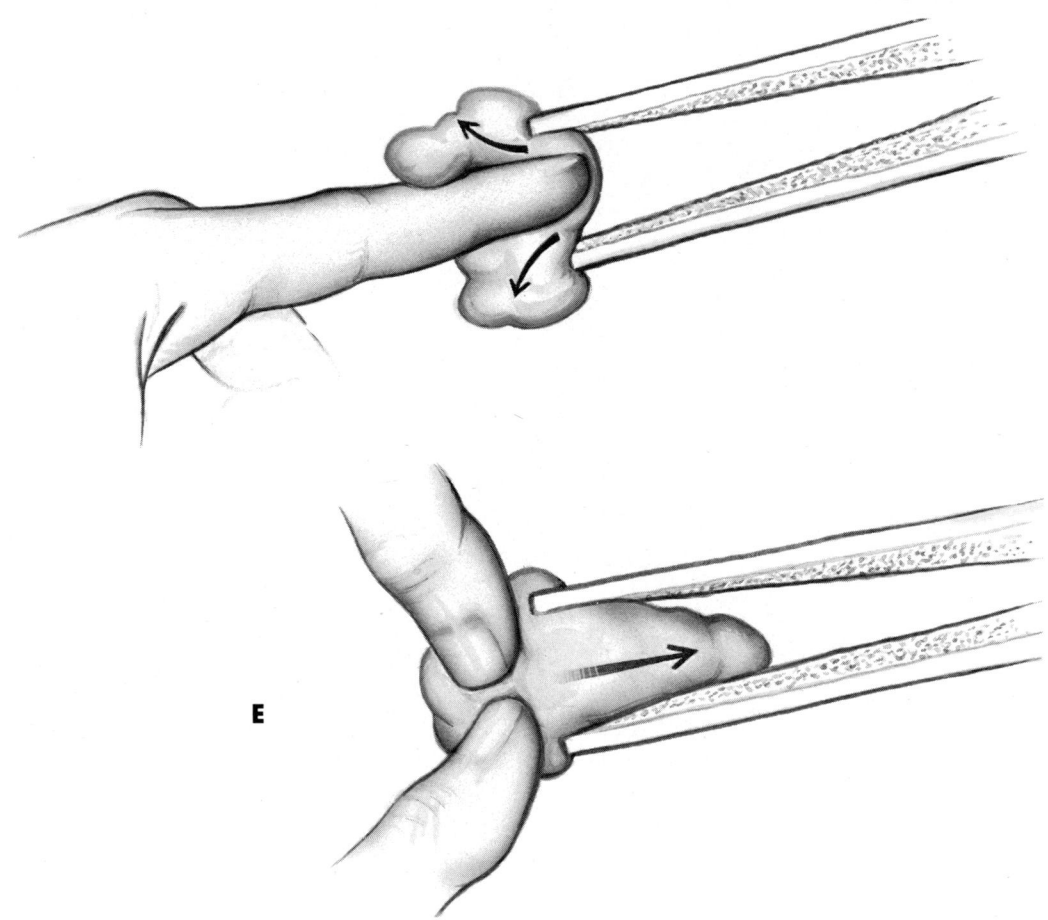

E

Fig. 15-47—cont'd. D, Little progress is made by using index finger singly to drive cement inside medullary canal. **E,** Effective force is created by double-thumb technique.

Inserting the Prosthesis

Insert the prosthesis in neutroversion while it is held by the holder. The term *neutroversion* has been applied to the positioning of the femoral component. It means that anteversion or retroversion must be avoided. However, experience suggests that in many instances, especially patients with a narrow medullary canal, 5 degrees of anteversion will allow the cement to be better distributed in the upper femur. Also the possibility of contact between the metal (upper stem) and the posterior wall of the femoral canal (Fig. 15-48) is eliminated. While up to 5 degrees of anteversion may be beneficial, the prosthesis should never be oriented in retroversion because that position may affect the stability of the hip.

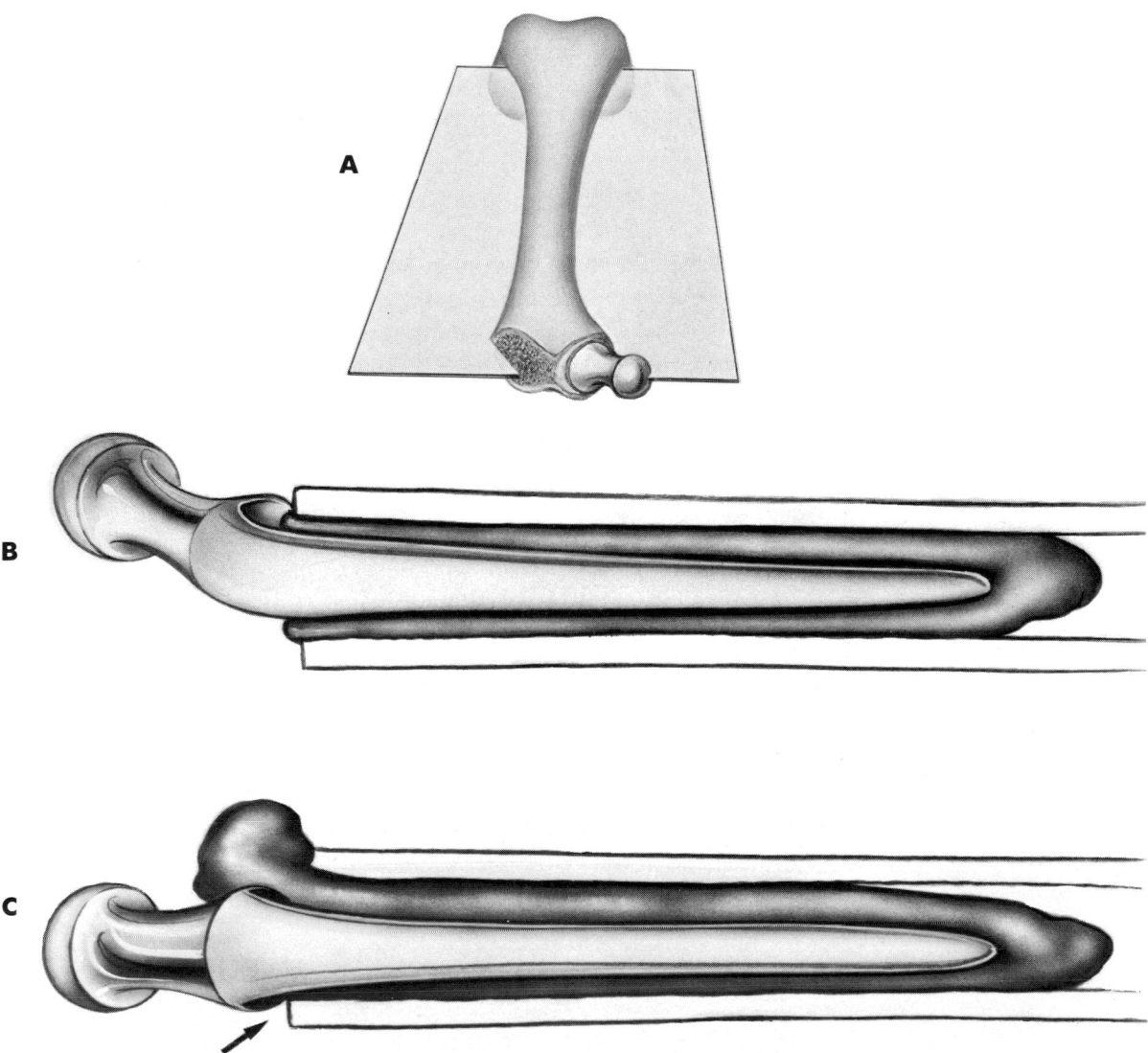

Fig. 15-48. Femoral component (of Charnley prosthesis) is inserted in neutroversion; however, slight anteversion (no more than 5 degrees) would allow better distribution of cement within upper end of femur. **A,** Plane of neutroversion. **B,** 5 degrees anteversion. NOTE: optimal thickness of cement between prosthesis and posterior cortex. **C,** Absolute neutroversion (no anteversion or retroversion) brings stem close to posterior cortex (caused by normal anteversion of femoral neck), thus eliminating thickness of cement in that region *(arrow).*

As in rehearsal, the position of the knee is demonstrated by the second assistant. The tip of the stem is introduced into the prepared canal at the junction between the trochanter and the neck into the cement. The prosthesis (firmly held in the holder) is slowly, deliberately inserted in neutroversion. Place it in a straight line in a valgus position relative to the shaft. This valgus orientation is maximized by holding the prosthesis back against the cancellous bone area of the bed of the trochanter and the lateral aspect of the femur (Fig. 15-49). The surgeon or the first assistant blocks the opening of the medial aspect of the neck to resist the flow of cement out of the medullary canal, which increases medullary cement pressure. Slow and deliberate action is essential while the insertion progresses. This maneuver also packs cement in the area between the concavity, the femoral canal, and the prosthesis. Avoid rotation (anteversion-retroversion) or mediolateral (varus-valgus) change in direction, since it results in a large track being made in the cement, which can lead to later loosening and should be avoided. In short, the surgeon must be able to reproduce the precementing orientation of the stem after insertion of cement.

Hammering is unnecessary if full insertion is easily achieved, as evidenced by the neck of the prosthesis resting flush with the entrance of the medullary canal. Keep the holder on the prosthesis without changing orientation, and detach it only after the cement is fully polymerized. Maintain the valgus position until full polymerization. Remove excess cement with a curette, again taking care not to move the prosthesis (see Chapter 18). Observe the following details:

1. Remain immobile during the final stages of polymerization of cement, since any motion of the limb may change the orientation of the prosthesis within the medullary canal. Retain maximum adduction of the leg in the cross-leg position.
2. Avoid damaging the femoral head if it is not protected by a plastic cover.
3. Avoid removing the holder before the cement is fully polymerized.
4. Test the cement for hardness at the neck level before attempting reduction of the prosthesis.
5. Do not push the prosthesis into a varus position during the polymerization phase.
6. Do not remove the holder too early or apply the pusher to the head, since it may change the "version" or cause a varus tilt of the stem while the cement is being polymerized.
7. All cement must be curetted away from the trochanteric region before hardening. Detach the holder just before final hardening of the cement.
8. The second assistant must stabilize the femur to ensure slow but deliberate insertion of stem in a prerehearsed alignment.
9. Avoid changing the mediolateral or internal-external direction as the stem insertion progresses.
10. Do not remove the holder until cement is fully polymerized.
11. Do not hammer the prosthesis into the canal unless the femur is very narrow and a portion of stem cannot be fully inserted.
12. An excessively slow insertion of the cement and stem can be disastrous, since the cement may harden inside the canal before the surgeon has fully inserted the prosthesis.
13. Using a light grip on the holder, maintain the position of the stem in a valgus direction. The second assistant must not move while the cement sets up.
14. Remove excess cement before setting.

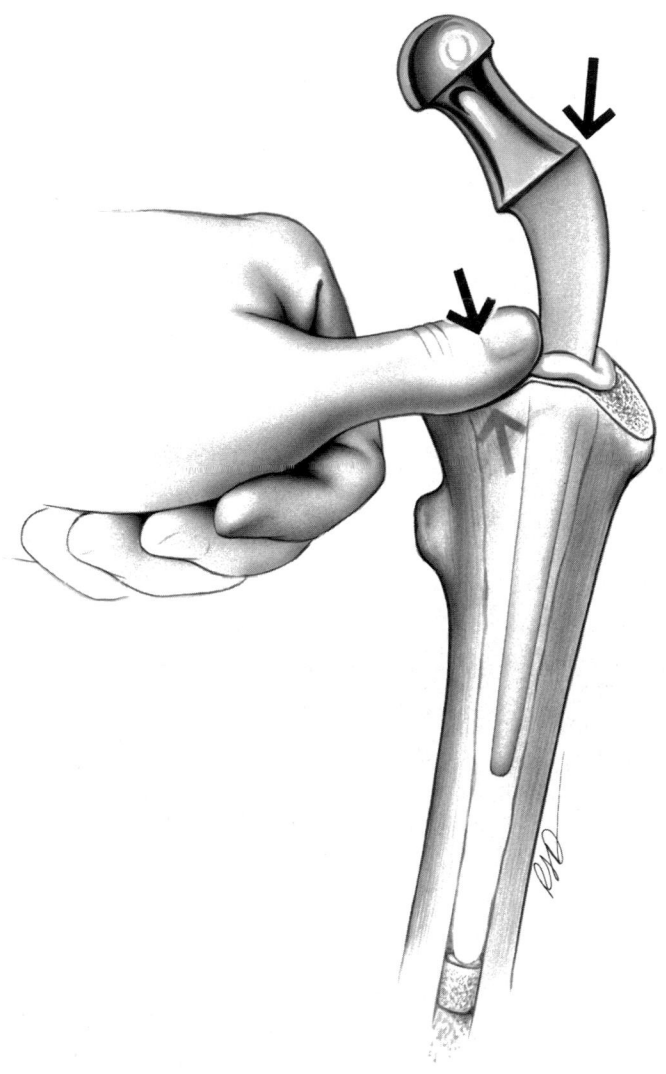

Fig. 15-49. Entry of the stem into the cement within the canal produces maximum pressure. A seal created at the opening should assist in containing the cement, thus increasing pressurization. Surgeon's thumb can achieve this over the medial side of the neck while the stem advances to its final position.

Reduction

Perform reduction after absolute hemostasis is achieved and all cement debris is removed from the wound. Irrigate the wound copiously. Remove cement particles and devitalized portions of muscle (usually found in the posterior aspect of the wound). Check and control posterior capsular bleeding before reattaching the greater trochanter (see Chapters 18 and 19) or reattaching the short rotators (see Chapter 16).

Test the range of motion and stability at this point. The surgeon must be certain that the two components are in a satisfactory relationship relative to each other. The hip must be stable before reattaching the greater trochanter if it has been osteotomized. Ideally, the orientation of the components relative to each other should be exactly the same as noted before the cementing of the femoral component.

Some Technical Details

Since technical cementing depends on firm injection of the cement into the femoral canal, delicate handling should be avoided. Double-thumb or single-digit forceful but steady pressure results not only in excellent distal filling but also in injection into the peripheral cancellous bone. Wide exposure, especially at the proximal end of the wound, full mobilization of the upper femur, and adequate retraction of the trochanter (if osteotomized) provide the surgeon optimal access to the medullary opening during cement insertion.

Beginners are usually concerned about the "working time" of the cement and, as a result, may use it too soon after mixing. This only makes the process of insertion difficult and actually prolongs insertion time, since the cement adheres to the gloves. Likewise, hasty insertion with short rapid strokes does not move the cement down the canal as well and results in a greater admixture of blood. The temptation to pick up the cement from the mixing bowl too early, while it is still at the tenacious stage (when it sticks to the surgeon's glove), must therefore be avoided. Allowing the cement to stiffen slightly not only minimizes absorption of monomer by the patient but also makes insertion easier, although it reduces the flow characteristics of the cement. The surgeon must be aware of the room temperature and observe the 10-minute check for "setting time"; the temperature of the mixing bowl and storage area should be checked, since this has a profound influence on the setting time of the cement (see Chapter 5). The cement is ready when it no longer sticks to the gloves. Check the stage of polymerization of cement based on excess (unused) cement.

A full coordination of the tasks performed by the assistants is essential so that the entire process can be executed in an organized fashion with minimal effort. Excessively slow insertion of the cement or the prosthesis can be disastrous, since the cement may harden inside the canal before the surgeon has fully inserted the prosthesis.

Some surgeons use low-viscosity cement and deliver it via a cement gun. Then, a second batch cement at a further or stiffer stage of polymerization is introduced by thumb. The use of low-viscosity cement delivered by cement gun, the use of the cement compactor, and effects of centrifugation of cement have been previously discussed.

Preparing the Canal for Cementless Stem

As stated in Chapter 11, each cementless stem design is supplied with an appropriate template for sizing. Templates are used as guides to determine (1) the approximate level of cut for the neck of the femur, (2) the approximate location of the site and the amount of socket deepening necessary to accommodate and contain the cup, (3) the approximate size and length of the stem, and (4) the patient's leg length.

Preoperative templating helps the surgeon judge the potential size of an off-the-shelf prosthesis and is strongly recommended. X-ray magnification of 15% to 20% is generally recorded on transparencies supplied by the manufacturers. Manufacturers also supply instructions for templating, but the following principles are applicable to all prosthetic designs and their templates:

1. Template the acetabulum first.
2. Template the femur for proximal and distal fit.
3. Estimate the head size for the femoral component.
4. Estimate and mark the site of neck resection for length.
5. Consider a small-sized, 22 mm femoral head for acetabula smaller than 46 mm outer diameter and 26 mm or 28 mm for larger acetabula.
6. Use templating to assist in sizing the stem in the lateral projection (frog lateral) to determine the amount of anterior bowing of the femur.
7. Be prepared for upsizing or downsizing despite the use of templates. Remember that templating is used only as a guide; the actual and precise sizing is determined at surgery.
8. Follow specific instructions for each system. Techniques used in inserting on a prosthetic system may not apply to another.

Inserting the Cementless Stem

To insert a cementless stem, a technique without osteotomy of the trochanter is preferred (see Chapters 3 and 16). The hip can be dislocated anteriorly (see Chapter 16) or posteriorly. Severely deformed hips require a capsulectomy to mobilize the upper femur. The abductors must be protected during reaming and broaching. The posterior approach is the least traumatic to the abductor muscles. Protect the tendinous attachment of the abductors to the greater trochanter when inserting tapered reamers. It is recommended that the surgeon use broaches to lateralize the stem; they are available for most cementless techniques. In some techniques, overreaming is preferred to avoid a tight fit of the implant at the level of the distal stem. Use broaches of approximate size for proximal preparation. Insert them by 1 mm increments until the rasp no longer advances with each blow of the hammer. The goal is to obtain a "press fit" for the stem in the conical shape of the metaphysis and a fit only 1 mm undersized in cylindrical diaphysis. Trial reduction is carried out as previously indicated. Two developmental issues are currently under study: (1) prophylactic wiring of the femur to prevent fractures of the femur during broaching and insertion of the cementless stems, and (2) applying a torque wrench to the rasp handle to determine stability of the stem in the canal of the femur.

WOUND CLOSURE AND APPLICATION OF DRESSINGS, STOCKINGS, AND SPLINTS
Closure of Fascia

Insert two Hemovac drains into the joint space, one anterior and the other posterior to the prosthesis. Use nonabsorbable sutures, such as one monofilament (Mexan) or one multifilament (Teftek). Achieve a perfect, watertight closure of the fascia. The deep fascia, which separates the superficial layers of the wound from the artificial joint, must be repaired in a "water-tight" fashion to restore the function of the tensor fascia lata and prevent communication should superficial infection develop. The first assistant retracts the proximal corner of the wound; the hip is placed in some abduction to provide relaxation of the fascia. Fascia closure begins proximally and proceeds distally. Just before tying the most distal stitch, the surgeon can verify the position of the drains in relation to the sutures along the line of the repaired fascia. This author prefers interrupted figure-8 stitches. Special care must be taken to avoid inadvertent inclusion of the drains in the closure. With the hip in abduction at the time of fascial closure, stability is enhanced and the fascia is relaxed, thus easing closure.

Fat Closure

Pull-out retention sutures are a popular and excellent method of wound closure.[3] The importance of good fat closure cannot be overemphasized; it is crucial in preventing hematoma formation and infection. The full thickness of the skin and fat are brought together with five stitches using number 1 nylon. The needle is passed on either side from within the wound outward. The large, curved needle is introduced at the deepest level of the fat and brought out through the skin 1-inch lateral to the skin edge (Fig. 15-50). The depth and level of the sutures must be the same on both sides so that no dead space is left behind. In a thin person, the sutures must be brought out closer to the edge of the skin, that is, 1.5 to 2 cm away from the edge so that the wound will not be excessively everted after fastening the retention sutures over the sponges. A second pair of Hemovac drains is placed deep in the subcutaneous tissue to prevent hematoma formation in both very obese and extremely thin individuals.

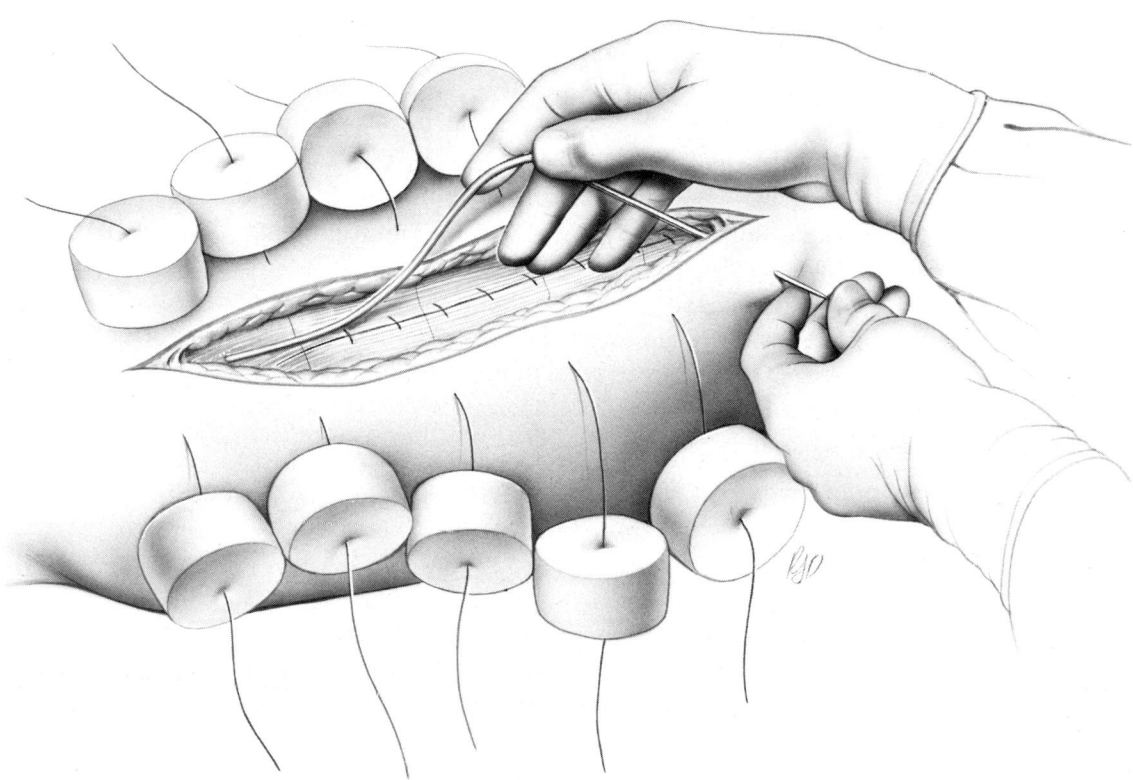

Fig. 15-50. Fascia lata is closed with interrupted nonabsorbable sutures. Deep drains (deep to fascia; not seen in this figure) are inserted. Second set of drains (if used) is placed superficial to fascia. Pull-out fat sutures are U-shaped and can be seen at depth of wound.

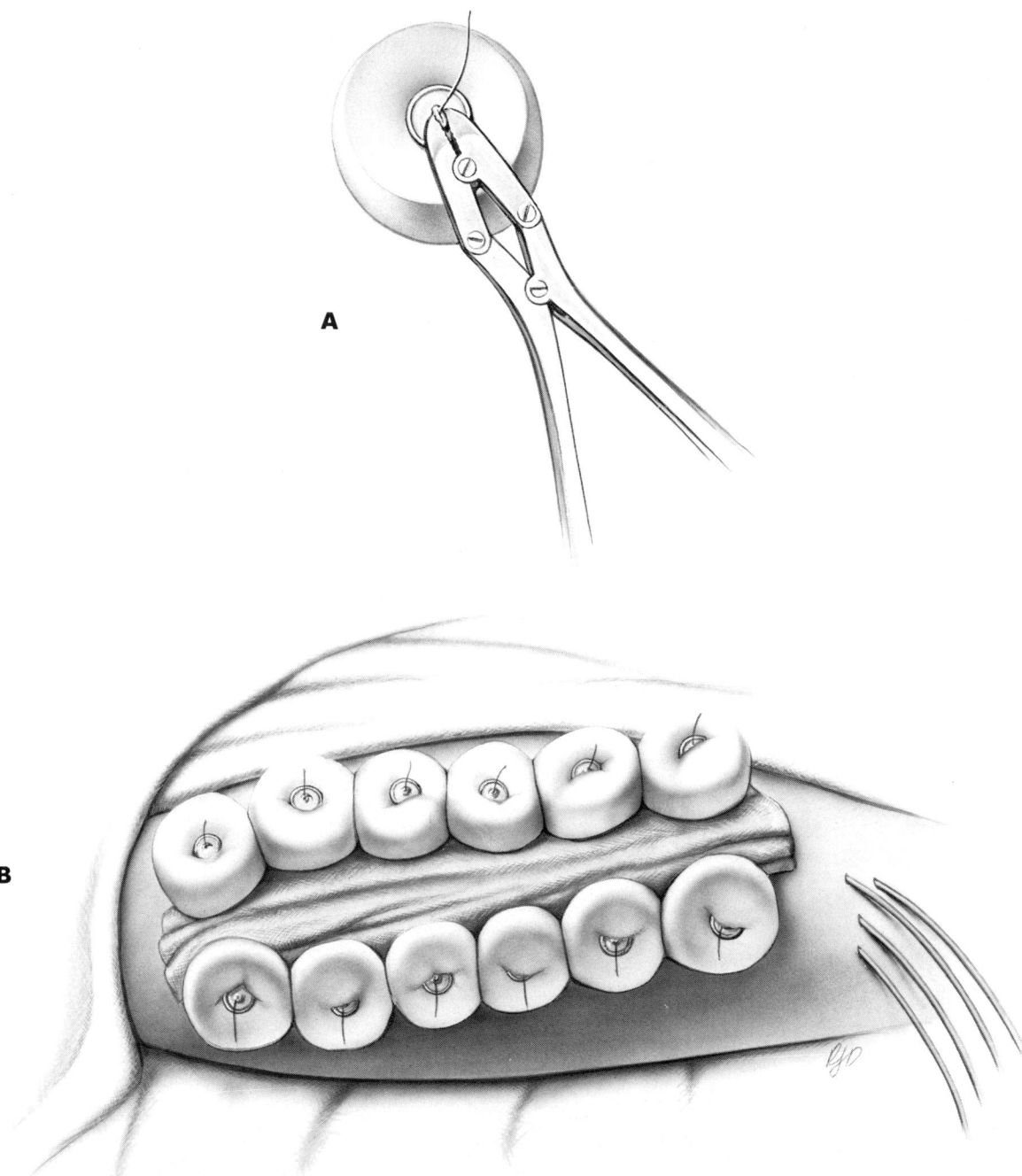

Fig. 15-51. A, Aluminum button is crushed to secure suture over foam pads used in retention sutures. **B,** Final dressing held in position by pressure pads. Position of drains in lower end of wound is shown. NOTE: only half of thickness of pressure pads has been compressed to allow swelling of wound without undue pressure necrosis on skin.

Skin Closure

Before tightening the retention sutures, the skin is meticulously closed with a running 3-0 Dermalon mattress stitch. This author uses three single, interrupted mattress stitches evenly distributed to reduce tension and then staples for the entire length of the skin. The fat layer retention sutures are then fastened over pressure foam pads; the retention sutures are passed through the center foam pads and suture buttons. The buttons are fixed to the nylon traversing the wound and held in place using a "button crusher" (Fig. 15-51). The foam pads should be compressed to only half their thickness to allow adjustment of the wound postoperatively without skin necrosis. A Hibbs strip soaked in povidine-iodine (Betadine) solution is applied over the suture line. Finally, the entire wound area is covered by a compression dressing with the drainage tubes exiting from the distal and posterior ends of the incision (see Fig. 15-51). The drainage tubes are not sutured in place but are secured with adhesive tape along with the rest of the dressing so that they can subsequently be removed without disturbing the dressing. Fig. 15-52 illustrates the method for removing retention sutures.

Application of Antiembolic Stockings and Abduction Splint

While the patient is still under anesthesia, elastic bandages (e.g., Ace bandages or antiembolic stockings) and an abduction splint are applied. The surgeon and first assistant should supervise transfer from the operating room table to bed with special care being taken to avoid dislocating the hip while the patient is still under the muscle relaxing effect of anesthesia.

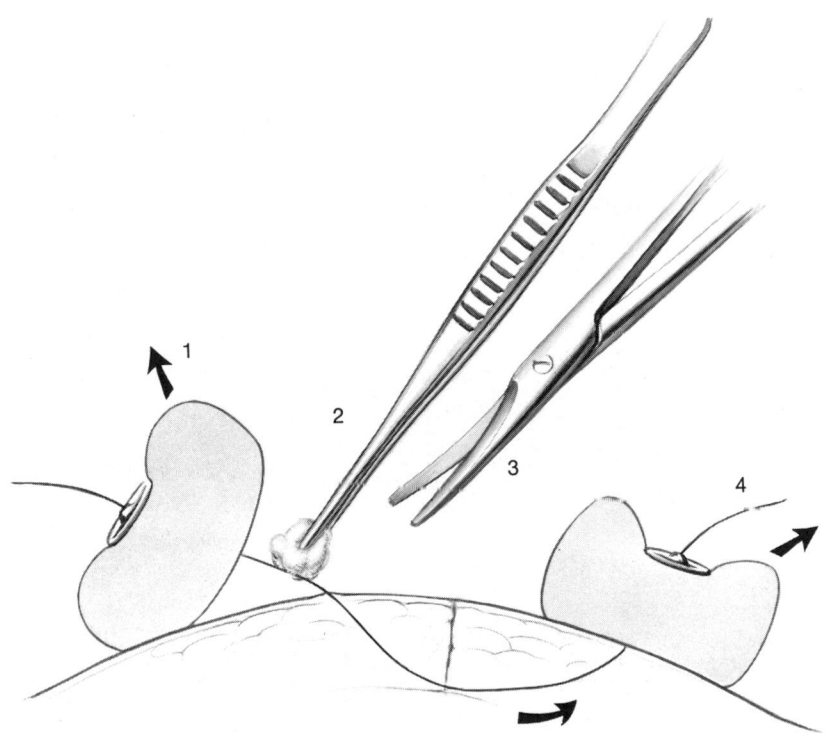

Fig. 15-52. Pressure pads and skin sutures are removed 13 to 14 days postoperatively. Remove retention sutures by (1) pulling on one end of suture, (2) using iodine swab to clean emerged suture from skin, (3) cutting suture, and (4) removing opposite end of suture.

PRACTICAL ASPECTS OF THE USE OF ACRYLIC CEMENT

As stated in Chapters 4 and 5, the success of cement fixation depends solely on the secure initial bonding between cement and bone. The fundamental issues here are (1) a clean and strong trabecular bone to receive cement and (2) adequate pressurization of contained cement in a closed cavity. By blocking the medullary cavity, considerable pressure can be generated, which drives the cement into small intratrabecular spaces to produce a microinterlock; the advantages are that the cement can be pressurized and the pressure can be sustained through pressurization.[22,23,26]

The Mechanical Properties of PMMA

PMMA is considered the weakest link in total hip arthroplasty because of its mechanical properties; the surgeon must be aware of its shortcomings (see Chapter 5). Acrylic cement is mechanically weak in tension, and when it is used as a thin layer, its fatigue life becomes extremely critical in determining its longevity under cyclic load. PMMA is expected to undergo an average of 1 million cycles per year under normal load. Others have suggested that, in part, late failures of cemented total hips may be caused by fatigue failures and not how they perform under static conditions.[7] Several variables that can affect the basic mechanical properties of the cement are discussed in Chapter 5. The surgeon is well advised to remember that some of the mechanical changes to the cement are within the surgeon's control and can directly or indirectly influence the longevity and long-term results of total hip arthroplasty. Several factors introduced by the surgeon can substantially reduce the mechanical properties of cement include (1) applying a thin layer of cement for load-bearing areas; (2) including fat, blood, and debris in cement; (3) rapidly beating the cement; (4) layering cement at application; (5) using additives, such as antibiotics, in large quantities; (6) using solutions or poorly mixed additives; (7) applying unconstrained cement, built-up outside the bone; (8) using a prosthesis with stress risers (sharp corners); (9) choosing a too porous brand of cement; (10) chilling the cement (for centrifugation or vacuum before application), which has been shown to substantially reduce the fatigue strength of PMMA.[4–6]

Fatigue testing data supplied by manufacturers for simplex P (Howmedica), Palacos R (R.E. Mark, Germany), low-viscosity cement (Zimmer), regular (Zimmer), and CMW (North Hill Plastic, UK) are 15,147; 11,500; 2575; 897; and 7043 cycles to failure, respectively. Evidently, the fatigue life of simplex P cement is significantly better than that of the other brands as tested under laboratory conditions.[8]

The fatigue life of each brand of cement is independent and not related to porosity. A significant increase in the fatigue life of most types of cement has been demonstrated if it is centrifuged to reduce its porosity. For example, reducing porosity in simplex P to 4.3% increased its mean fatigue life to 71,749 cycles.[6] Chilling the monomer also has been shown to increase the porosity, resulting in a markedly diminished fatigue life. Therefore cement mixed with a chilled monomer should be centrifuged to decrease its porosity.[8] If two packs of Simplex cement mixed with chilled monomer are centrifuged at full speed for 60 seconds, its fatigue life increases by a factor of nearly 5 and is 15 times stronger than some of the other brands of cement marketed for use without centrifugation.[8]

The Viscoelasticity of Cement

For practical purposes, the surgeon should consider PMMA polymer mixed with monomer to have varying physical characteristics when applied to surgery. It changes its physical form during at least four major stages: (1) liquid stage, (2) plastic stage, (3) elastic stage, and (4) solid stage.

Stage 1: Liquid Form (Must Be Delivered by Syringe)

During the liquid stage, because its low-viscosity PMMA flows and cannot be handled by gloved hands. It can be delivered to the bone only by a syringe or cement gun. Its penetration characteristics are excellent when pressurized. However, it contains a high level of free monomer that can be toxic to the cells and can perhaps cause sudden cardiopulmonary collapse if rapidly absorbed (see Chapter 5). It is difficult to maintain uninterrupted pressure in a closed cavity to resist bleeding pressure, and it is not possible to maintain orientation of the prosthesis within the canal while awaiting full polymerization of the cement. Low-viscosity cement has been shown to have a low fatigue property.

Stage 2: Plastic Form (Delivery Possible by Hand or Cement Gun)

At this stage the cement can be delivered by a cement delivery gun or by hand. This state is ideal for delivery and pressurization. It is deformable, thus displaceable, and it requires relatively small amounts of sustained pressure for displacement, by digital pressure or pressurization devices. It is easily delivered to bone, can conform and interdigitate with interstices of trabecular bone, and can resist bleeding pressure when applied with relatively small amounts of pressure. Because it can be displaced, minor adjustments to the position of the prosthesis are possible to fully insert the stem.

Stage 3: Elastic Form (Delivery Possible by Hand but Not Cement Gun)

During the elastic stage the cement becomes stiffer and can be displaced only under manual pressure. Within a short while it becomes so elastic that it is nondisplaceable and thus can no longer be pushed into the bony trabeculae, although it remains deformable. Eccentric pressure applied from the prosthesis onto the cement can drift the stem to one side during the terminal phase of setting, causing the stem and the cement to separate. Containment of the cement and steadiness of the component are mandatory: space created between the cement and bone will not be recovered by further pressure onto the component. It is critical during this phase that the stem not be driven into its bed by hammer blows, which will make the stem bounce off the cement because of the cement's elasticity.

Stage 4: Solid Form (Cannot Be Delivered)

The solid phase is determined by a small sample of cement outside the wound. Once the cement is no longer deformable, the surgeon ceases to hold the prosthesis. Because it is brittle, the unremoved cement can be excised only by a chisel or an osteotome. Sharp strokes are used to detach the excess cement from the bone. Cement in the body solidifies 30 to 60 seconds faster than that at ambient temperature.

MIXING AND DELIVERING CEMENT

Delivery of cement into the medullary canal can be accomplished without admixture with blood, providing that the following several conditions prevail: (1) the cement is in a doughy state (the plastic phase), (2) the cement retains its sausage shape at the time of insertion and does not adhere to the gloved finger, (3) the surgeon has obtained exposure of the upper femur, and there is unimpeded access to the upper femur, and (4) the surgeon is experienced in using acrylic cement. Venting is necessary during insertion to rid blood distal to the advancing cement. Venting also facilitates delivery of the cement. The surgeon will add cement after removing the vent tube (see Figs. 15-45 and 15-46). Delivery by hand allows the surgeon to control the exact timing or delivery of cement, thus reducing the length of the interval between inserting the cement and inserting the stem. This critical interval, which results when high-viscosity cement has been inserted, reduces the chance of bleeding. Although low-viscosity cement can penetrate into the cancellous bone better than high-viscosity cement, it is less resistant to bleeding pressure than the latter[19] (Fig. 15-53). Additionally, high-viscosity cement has a low free-surface monomer that is less toxic to the bone cells and is less likely to cause fat embolization (see Chapter 5).

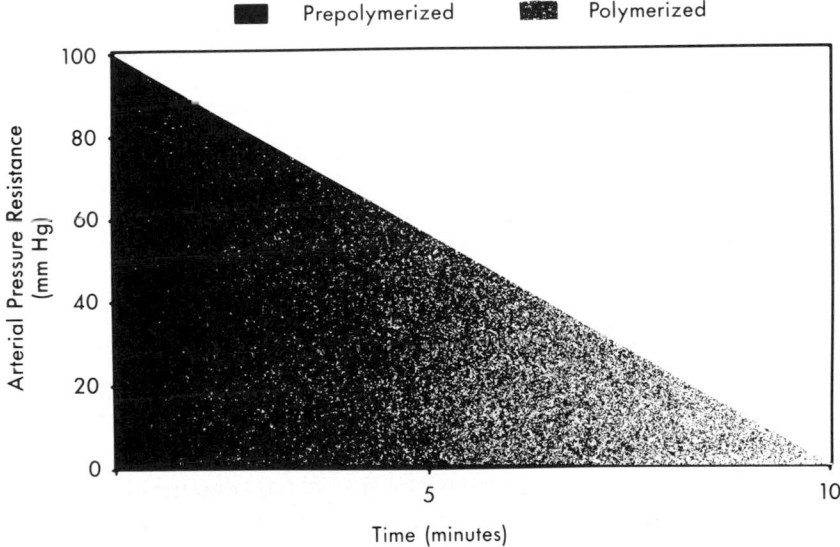

Fig. 15-53. A schematic representation of progressive "stiffening of cement" (x axis) against "arterial bleeding pressure" (y axis) is demonstrated. The surgeon must apply adequate pressure (greater than arterial blood pressure) at varying stages of cement polymerization to prevent bleeding between the bone and cement interface. This drawing assumes that cement is fully polymerized 10 minutes after mixing.

MIXING CEMENT AT SURGERY

The outer surface of the ampule of the liquid cement is supplied sterile. Keep the ampules of monomers in a storage facility near the operating room and at a constant temperature. The outer surface of the packet containing the powder component is sterilized at the time of packaging and double-wrapped for safety and ease of delivery to the surgical field (Fig. 15-54).

To prepare one dose, mix the entire contents of one packet of powder (a mixture of PMMA, styrene copolymer, and barium sulfate) 40 gm, and one ampule of the liquid monomer (MMA), 20 ml. Depending on the surgical procedure and technique, one or two doses are required. Mix each dose separately when used sequentially.

To mix, empty the entire contents of the packet containing the powder component into a disposable plastic, porcelain, or stainless steel mixing bowl. Add the entire contents of the ampule containing the liquid component. Add the liquid component to the powder, not the powder to the liquid (except in the case of Palacos cement, in which the powder is added to the liquid). Continue stirring until a doughlike mass forms that does not stick or adhere to the operator's rubber gloves.

The doughlike mass (at completion of doughing time) is then ready for manipulation. The mixing and manipulation process should last at least 4 minutes for Simplex P radiopaque cement. Earlier experience will help the surgeon to judge the mixing and kneading time required to obtain a proper consistency for application to bone. Continue mixing if cement adheres to the rubber glove. Make sure all the cement is removed from the bowl. If more than one unit of cement (40 gm powder and 20 ml liquid) is needed, empty the contents of two packets of powder into the mixing bowl, then empty two ampules (20 ml each) simultaneously into the powder, thus using 40 ml of monomer.

When adding antibiotic powder, mix it thoroughly with the polymer before adding the monomer.

There are two stages of setting time: doughing time and working time. Doughing time begins when the cement can be made into forms by digital manipulation. Working time begins when the dough is no longer "sticky" and ends when it is "hard set." Reducing setting time by reducing the monomer amount will reduce working time at the expense of increasing the doughing time. An informed surgeon is not likely to be caught by surprise if a sloppy mixing technique results in loss of 3 or 4 ml of monomer.

The ambient temperature significantly affects the setting time and working time of PMMA, but the polymerization process can also be influenced by the temperature of the mixing bowl and spoon or a "preheated prosthetic stem". Dall and associates,[3a] in an experimental model, have shown the effectiveness of a preheated prosthesis in reducing the polymerization time of acrylic cement. They also found coincidental changes in the mechanical properties of the cement and the bone-cement interface temperature resulting from insertion of a preheated prosthesis. The time required for cement to polymerize was reduced from 7½ minutes at a room temperature of 23.5° C to 5 minutes for a stem temperature of 50° C, thus demonstrating a 33% reduction of total curing time in in-vitro tests, which equates with a 50% time reduction from the start of the mix. They observed some increase in maximum temperature in the interface from preheating of the stem. When they inserted the stem that was at room temperature (with the thickest cement mass), the increased temperature reached 50.5° C, but they recorded a maximum temperature of 57° C when they preheated the stem to 50° C. The increased temperature in-vivo is less a result of the better conductivity of bone than the Teflon used to perform the simulated tests. A slight reduction in maximum compressive strength of PMMA occurred, from 98 MPA (at 23.5° C) to 90 MPA (at 50° C), which is well above the recommended minimum compressive strength for PMMA used by ASTM standards.

Manual Delivery of Cement (PMMA)

The surgeon receives the cement in its prepolymerized form, shaped like a sausage and ready for stuffing down the femoral canal (see Fig. 15-47, *B* and *C*). At room temperature (19° C), working time for CMW cement is 3 to 4 minutes; for Simplex P radiopaque, 5 to 6 minutes (see Chapter 5). A two-thumbed pressure insertion technique is preferable when possible. Portions are advanced

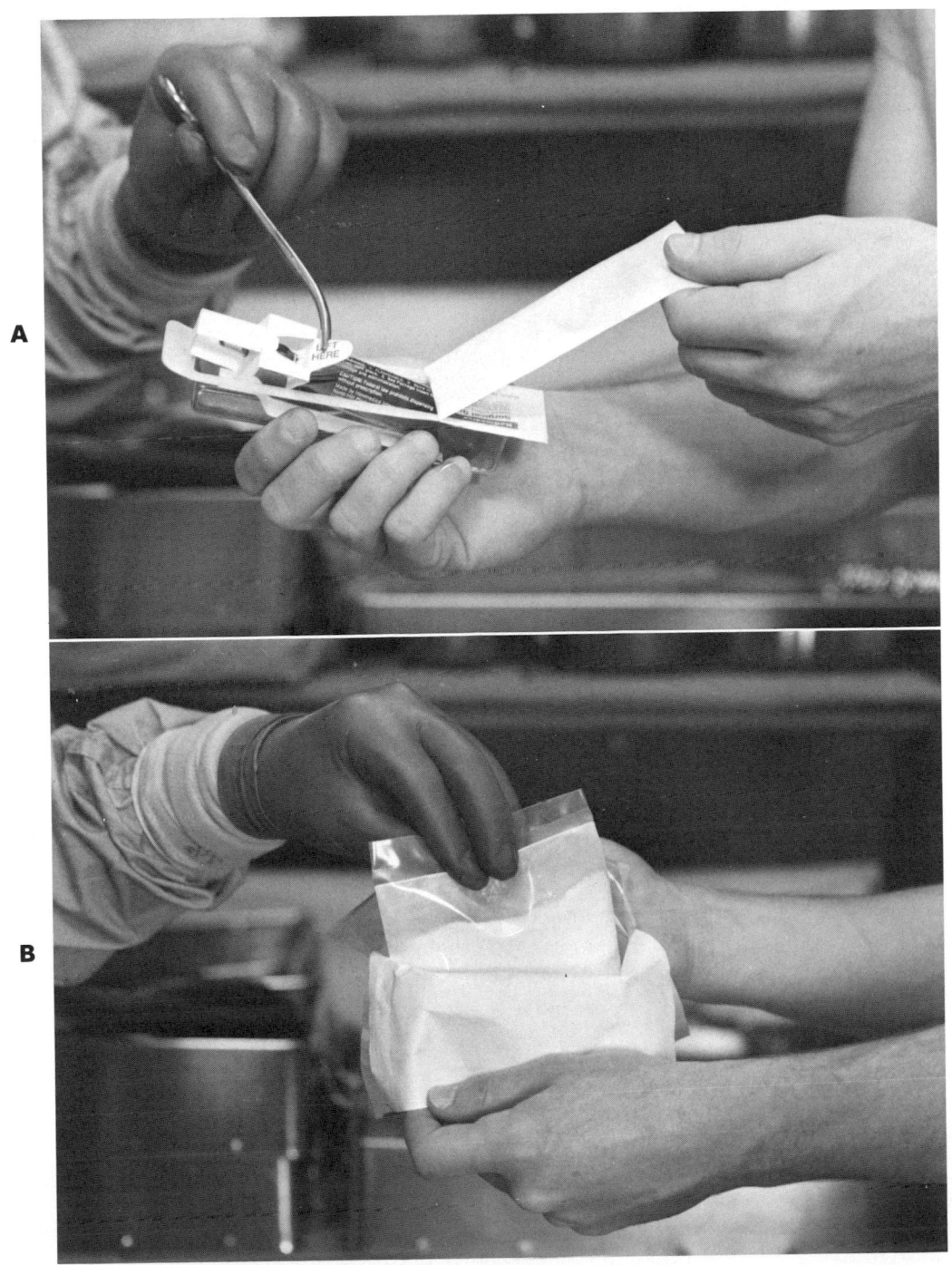

Fig. 15-54. A, Removal of liquid (monomer) of PMMA. Outer package is opened by "peeling off" seal. Operating nurse, wearing sterile gown and gloves, removes the liquid. **B,** Hand delivery of heat-sealed packet of PMMA powder. Note that circulating nongloved hand peels package open while sterile gloved hand of scrub nurse removes inner package.

into the canal, with 1- or 2-second pauses between each inserting motion. With each stroke, part of the cement is advanced down the canal, and the pause aids its progress. Complete obstruction of the opening of the femur by the thumbs maximizes pressure behind the column of cement, thus advancing the cement within the canal. Admixture of blood with cement should be avoided. A total of 10 to 15 strokes usually enables the entire batch to be inserted. All of the cement is used.

Delivery by Cement Gun

Several authors have advocated the use of a cement gun for delivery and pressurization of cement.* In all cement delivery systems the cement is discharged in a retrograde fashion from the distal plug toward the neck of the femur. Advocates claim that the cement gun can easily apply a relatively low-viscosity cement, thus reducing voids and defects, layering and thus reducing the admixture of blood commonly associated with finger packing. The use of a cement gun is obviously attractive for the delivery of either low-viscosity cement or standard cement, the latter during low-viscosity phase. In this situation, a longer period of sustained pressure on the liquid cement is required to resist arterial and venous bleeding pressure.

When the cement gun is used, it is essential to contain the cement and prevent "running out" by using a sealer such as a silicone disc or a compactor as described by Harris and Oh.[24] Cement must be pressurized adequately and uninterruptedly until it becomes doughy. This technique is demanding, since the surgeon must control the bleeding pressure and maintain pressure via the gun (while the cement is contained) until the cement becomes doughy and stiff. As laboratory work has shown, if the cement gun is used, delivery and pressurization of cement certainly result in a higher medullary pressure and intrusion distally. However, the proximal fixation (the most important part of the fixation) requires careful sealing of the proximal femur when the low-viscosity cement is inserted. Digital impaction of cement creates considerable pressure in the proximal femur if the surgeon's thumb is placed so as to act as a piston covering the opening of the neck of the femur.

CEMENT PRESSURIZATION

Laboratory studies have indicated that large stems also produce significantly higher extrusion pressures.[24] A maximum cement pressurization is generated when the stem is inserted. Therefore for optimal stem fixation the stem caliber must be as large as possible while still allowing ease of insertion. The stem should never fit so tightly that hammering is necessary for its insertion into the cement, even at the final stages of setting. The Charnley stem design, with its dorsal flange (Cobra), is superior to the nonflanged stems. It allows progressive medial compression of the cement while it is being introduced into the medullary canal. Although it does not have a formal collar, it is stabilized at the final stage of insertion, keeping the cement under boundary compression in the proximal femur.[3] Before the last 1 to 2 cm of the stem sinks into the medullary cavity, the surgeon must pack the cement into the flanges of the prosthesis.[3] The medial femoral neck deserves special attention, since the stem penetrates deeply into the canal. If a noncollared prosthesis is used, digital pressure can block the proximal neck and reduce the cement escape by directing it toward the medial, anterior, and posterior neck regions (see Fig. 15-49).

Inserting the stem into the cement within the medullary cavity will generate greater pressurization of cement. The prosthesis is best held in a prosthesis holder with control in a rehearsed direction. Insertion must be in a direct line and straight from the point of entry of the tip of the stem to the full insertion of the dorsal flange of the prosthesis into the medullary canal of the femur.

---

*References 9, 10, 16, 17, 24.

OPTIMUM CEMENT MANTLE

As reported in recent years, failure has exceeded success 20-fold after a cemented femoral component. This is primarily related to the technique, a poor understanding of the use of cement and its mechanical behavior under loading condition, and the use of unacceptable femoral component designs. The following can contribute to the failure of a procedure:

1. Deficiencies in the cement mantle (that is, direct contact of metal with bone). In one series, 76% of defective mantles developed associated bone resorptive cysts.[11] This has also been observed by others.[27, 28]
2. Interruption of the cement mantle resulting from severe varus or valgus, which causes bone-stem contact.[20]
3. Increased internal stress within the cement mantle. It has been suggested that by controlling the mantle geometry, the stress within the mantle can be reduced by 50% to 90%, whereas a relatively modest enhancement of the mechanical properties of cement may only reduce stress by 20% to 30%.[20]
4. Correlation of cement thickness with stress generated (at various zones of load transmission) varies, indicating that the stress borne by cement is indeed uneven. The maximum stress is at the proximal, medial, distal, and lateral stem tip levels where the cement thickness and continuity of the cement mantle are essential.[12]

This uneven geometry of the cement mantle is controlled by stem geometry and stem alignment in the canal. For example, a tight fit of the stem proximally may reduce the cement mantle at the heavily loaded medial neck, and a tight fit distally eliminates the cement distally from the high-stress zone of the femur. A compromise has been recommended in which the prosthesis fills 70% to 80% of the medullary canal, thus leaving a 1 to 2 mm thickness for the distal mantle.[20]

OPTIMUM STEM DESIGN FOR CEMENT

When used in conjunction with cement, the intramedullary stem of a hip prosthesis must have the following characteristics:

- A configuration and size that will fit the anatomical shape of the upper femur.
- Dimensions that do not exceed the narrow segment of the shaft of the femur.
- Biplane or single plane tapering to facilitate cement injection at insertion.
- Adequate tapering angle to resist rotational and compressive force.
- Size variation to allow adaptation in all cases.
- Sufficient static and fatigue strengths to withstand cyclic load equivalent of biological demand without failure.
- Composition and metallurgical processing compliant with today's technological standards.

Because most stems have a fixed offset (center head to center shaft distance), it would be advantageous to preserve the predetermined offset angle designed in a given prosthesis by centralizing it within the shaft of the femur. Any prosthesis must be somewhat loose within the femoral canal before cementing so that an adequate thickness of cement on the concave side of the prosthesis, as well as on the lateral distal end, can be provided (see Chapter 11).

To provide an optimal fit, various stem sizes should be available to accommodate the geometrical shape variations of the femur (see Chapter 11). Most femora fall within a distribution of flare index that is considered normal (flare index = the ratio of the metaphysis to diaphysis) (see Chapter 6). However, with a reduced flare index in older patients and an increased flare index in younger individuals, various designs and geometrical proportions might be required to optimize the stress within the cement mantle. As has been pointed out, a loose relationship exists between the size of the canal and its contours; the smaller bones tend to become more fluted while larger bones tend to become stovepipe in shape.[21] As suggested by Noble, when components of average shape are implanted, a shape mismatch between the stem and bone becomes inevitable.[21] This suggests that those with an abnormal femoral shape may require a specially designed prosthesis (see Chapters 6 and 11). Similarly, the length of the stem, based on the shape of the femur (degrees of anterior and lateral bow), may ideally call for more variation in size and geometry. Currently, we feel that a customized stem for use with cement may be indicated in certain situations.

This author's technique for centralizing the stem proximally and distally has been successful in his practice during the past 15 years (see Chapter 19). Other methods of centralization that prevent impingement of the stem against that bone proximally and distally have also been used in clinical practice with technical success.[28] While the long-term beneficial effects of stem centralization is not available, the surgeon must strive to orient the stem as centrally as possible within the medullary cavity of the femur. If the stem is inadvertently positioned in a valgus, it is preferable to any varus positioning that must be avoided. The use of PMMA centralization is advantageous, since it allows accurate positioning while the stem incorporates into the cement mantle, avoiding stress risers caused by other methods.

SUMMARY OF ESSENTIALS

- When inserting a cemented prosthesis, it is important to achieve microinterlock by exposing the firm trabecular bone free of debris and clots, improve intrusion of the cement into the trabecular bone, pressurize the cement after containment, and check the bleeding pressure by sustained pressure of cement while it is being polymerized.

- When inserting a cementless prosthesis, it is important to create a bony cavity that conforms to the precise shape of the prosthesis, produce a maximum surface area conforming to the shape of the prosthesis, and maintain initial rigid fixation long enough to achieve bony ingrowth or ongrowth.

- Regardless of the surgical approach, time spent developing a good view of the acetabulum and delivering the upper femur will provide a straight entry to the femur, thus ensuring the safety and accuracy of the bone preparation and component placement while avoiding damage to the hip. With proper surgical training and appropriate instrumentation, most total hip arthroplasty procedures can be performed without osteotomy of the greater trochanter. However, the hip surgeon must learn the technique for detaching and reattaching the trochanter, since it may be necessary in difficult primary and most revision surgeries. Careful planning and execution are necessary to avoid complications related to trochanteric osteotomy.

- Guidelines for organizing the operating suite and positioning and preparing the patient have been established to make the procedure safe. The surgeon must be responsible for positioning the patient correctly, since it is essential for orientation of the components, as well as safety of the upper and lower extremities. A faulty positioning technique may cause neurovascular embarrassment of the upper or lower extremities. The safety of the brachial plexus and the down leg (in lateral decubitus position) must be the foremost concern of the surgeon.

- Based on the surgeon's experience and the surgical approach to be used, the patient may be placed in a supine or lateral decubitus position. With only a minor modification, the techniques for draping for both positions are similar, but the surgeon must avoid restricting the exposure because of limitations imposed by the draping technique.

- Disposable drapes and suction hoods (helmet aspirator) are essential in performing total hip arthroplasty.

- The importance of a properly placed incision of adequate length cannot be overemphasized. Undue trauma to soft tissue and bone resulting in complications certainly can be more damaging than a longer skin incision. Insulate the skin edges with towels, and use adhesive plastic sheets. Ensure adequate length of the incision before deepening the exposure into the fat and fascial layers.

- While the fat layer is incised along the incision, an optimal level of incision of the fascia is essential. Use self-retaining retractors to expose the fascia. With proper exposure, the wound opens in a diamond shape with the greater trochanter appearing at the center of the wound.

- Leg length equalization must be practiced in all total hip procedures. Several methods available to the surgeon must be used in combination to assist in equalizing leg length during surgery. They include preoperative clinical leg length measurements, preoperative templating using x-ray, with known magnification, intraoperative measurements through drapes, and intraoperative measurements between two fixed points on the pelvis and femur.

- Intraoperative measurements of leg length changes during surgery can be accomplished as follows. Insert a pin retractor proximal to the hip of the acetabulum, mark a fixed point on the femur, and measure the distance between the two. Repeat the same measurements between the two points after inserting the component at test rehearsal and finally, repeat the same measurements after the actual prosthesis is inserted. The leg position on the operating table during the measurements must remain unchanged.

- Before dislocating the hip, instruct the assistant to avoid severe rotational forces on the limb and release remaining constricting capsule and labrum. Sever the ligamentum teres, and excise the osteophytes, which may prevent the head from dislocating. Further, place a flat instrument between the head of the femur and the acetabulum to assist in levering the head out while the hip is being adducted. Successive flexion and extension of the hip will break the vacuum within the joint, and excision of the overhanging acetabular margin will facilitate dislocation. When dislocation is impossible, transect the neck of the femur, and remove the head in a retrograde fashion.

- Acetabular preparation should be based on the existing acetabular morphology: normal acetabular configuration, medial pole migration, upper pole arthritis, or mild acetabular dysplasia.

- When preparing the acetabulum, the surgeon should strive to: (1) produce a cavity large enough to accommodate the acetabular component and cement; (2) protect the integrity of the acetabulum by preserving the subchondral bone of the roof of the acetabulum, thus providing a bony cavity after reaming that can contain the cup and cement with full bony support from the ilium, ischium, and pubis; (3) locate the center of rotation at the original site of the normal acetabulum; and (4) provide a precise hemispherical cavity to accommodate the cup when a cementless cup is used.

- Two methods of preparation are recommended: (1) in situ preparation for types I and II acetabular pathology, and (2) preparation in lower position for types III and IV acetabular pathology. Preparing the acetabulum for cementless cups demands precision in cavity preparation while the subchondral bone is retained. A maximum contact between the bone and the porous-coating surface of the cup is essential. When preparing the acetabulum for a cemented cup the cavity must be larger than the size of the cup to accommodate the cement thickness. The surgeon must be sure that the flange of the cup seals the acetabular cavity, the use of adequate anchoring holes are producing added surface area for cement, irrigation and brushing facilitates cause bonding between cement and bone, and the cup is supported throughout the acetabular walls and is contained within the acetabular cavity.

- Perform gauging for socket size. For the socket to be positioned in appropriate alignment, it should be completely contained within the bone of the acetabulum. Choose 22 or 26 mm inner bearings based on the size of the prepared acetabular cavity. Ensure adequate cement thickness when cement is used. Use a flanged cup routinely.

- The flanged cup allows retention of the cement within the acetabulum. It allows pressurization at insertion and enables the surgeon to locate the center of the rotation of the hip at the desired level. Observe the details of cementing technique for the socket.

- Inserting a pressure injection cup requires a precise tailoring of the cup rim to fit the acetabular cavity at rehearsal that is reproduced after inserting the cement with the cup. Multiple anchor holes, brushing, and irrigating the acetabulum are routine before inserting the cement and cup. Excess cement must be removed before preparing the femur.

- A precise reaming for a cementless porous-coated cup is necessary. Observe the following principles: the cup must be contained within the bony acetabulum; bleeding bone must be exposed while retaining the subchondral bone; the bone should be reamed in a direction similar to the position of the cup; and the final reamer used is a guide for selecting the cup (1 or 2 mm larger than the last reamer used). To prevent injury to the intrapelvic structures, the surgeon must not insert drills, screws, and depth gauges toward the anterior and inferior quadrants of the acetabulum.

- Preparation of the femoral canal begins by inserting a T-handled straight reamer exactly at the site of the insertion of the piriformis tendon in the digital fossa of the femur. The subsequent reamers are inserted to enlarge the metaphyseal area and expand the diaphyseal zone of the femur. Preparation of the canal for a cemented device is different from that of a cementless device. When using cement, the cavity must be larger than the size of the prosthesis to accommodate the thickness of cement. For a cementless device, a cavity the precise size of the prosthesis is essential to maximize the contact between the prosthesis and bone. Most contemporary cementless designs are produced with broaches of similar sizes for proper reaming to match the size of the prosthesis.

- Because cementless devices are still in the evolutionary stage, the surgeon interested in these devices should study and follow the principles involved in each design before their use. A reduction test is mandatory to show that all prostheses will be stable and produce equal leg length after insertion. A reduction may be difficult or impossible when the patient has not been adequately anesthetized, the femoral neck is excessively long, the socket has been inserted in a low position, or the soft tissues are excessively tight. During reduction, observe the following details: (1) determine the amount of traction required to locate the head into the socket, (2) determine the full range of motion of the hip, especially in positions of function, (3) do not separate the two components by longitudinal traction more than 5 mm, (4) secure a full coverage of the prosthetic head by the cup with the hip in a neutral rotation, (5) make full extension possible without any residual fixed flexion deformity.

- The effective neck length must produce equal leg lengths and stability for the hip. On the other hand, intraoperative instability may be caused by excessive shortening of the neck, a high positioning of the socket, medial and anterior osteophytes, projecting osteophytes on the upper femur, lack of clearance caused by an excessive deepened acetabulum, previous surgery with loss of tissue elasticity, sinking of the femoral prosthesis into the medullary canal during rehearsal, rotation of the stem within the canal, and malpositioning of either component.

- When using a cemented device, the following principles must be observed. The prepared cavity of the femur must be larger than the stem size to allow space for cement. Strong cancellous bone must be preserved, but all loose and fragile endosteal trabeculae should be removed. Maximum widening of the femur must be carried out to accommodate standard size caliber prostheses. Insertion of the stem should include centralization of the stem proximally and distally, and testing for stability and range of motion must always be done before cementing the component, since an identical orientation of the stem in the canal before and after insertion of cement is mandatory. A high-implant/canal and stem/canal ratio should be the surgeon's goal.

- To achieve microinterlock between cement and bone, eliminate blood from the interface by the following methods: inducing hypotensive anesthesia; packing the medullary canal with sponges; controlling bleeding with an intramedullary plug; using dilute epinephrine to reduce bleeding or hydrogen peroxide to prevent clots; and using continuous suction in a closed cavity packed with epinephrine or hydrogen peroxide to eliminate the blood. Plugging the medullary canal has several advantages. This prevents the cement from flowing to a long distance beyond the stem tip, increases pressurization and thus intrusion of the cement into the trabeculae of the femur, and decreases fat embolization. It also prevents retrograde bleeding and blood admixture with cement. Plugs made of prepolymerized cement, bone plugs, and plastic plugs are all effective in obliterating the medullary canal.

- When the trochanter has been detached, insert the wires before inserting the cement.

- While inserting the prosthesis it is important to achieve a neutral (centered) position in the femur. Allow no more than 5 degrees of anteversion when using a cup with an extended posterior wall. If a posterior wall cup is not used, allow no more than 15 degrees of anteversion, since it may predispose the hip to anterior dislocation. When inserting the stem, avoid hammering on the prosthesis. The surgeon should remain immobile during the final stages of polymerization of cement. Avoid damaging the femoral head. Do not remove the holder from the prosthesis before the cement is fully polymerized. Test the cement for hardness at the level of the neck before attempting to reduce the prosthesis. Do not push the prosthesis into a varus position during the polymerization phase. Remove all excess cement. All the details regarding the use of cement and insertion of the prosthesis are essential.

- In preparing the canal for cementless stems, preoperative templating of the femur is essential. When considering x-ray magnifications of 15% to 20%, use the manufacturer's instruments for the technique and their templates for measuring the femoral canal. Template the acetabulum first, then the femur for proximal and distal fit. Estimate the head size of the femoral component, and mark the site of neck resection for length. Consider a small sized (22 mm) femoral head for acetabula smaller than 46 mm outer diameter and 26 or 28 mm for larger acetabula. Use templates also based on the lateral projection films to determine the amount of anterior bow of the femur. Be prepared for upsizing or downsizing despite the use of templates. Remember that templating is used only as a guide; the actual and precise sizing is determined at surgery. Follow specific instructions for each system. Techniques used in inserting one prosthesis system may not apply to another. The posterior lateral approach is the most suitable for inserting a cementless femoral component, although other approaches can be used equally well.

- Wound closure consists of a water-tight closure of the fascia using nonabsorbable suture materials. Be careful to avoid inadvertent inclusion of the drains in the closure. For closure of fat, pull-out retention sutures are the best. Retention sutures and entrapped sutures or metallic clips provide adequate closure.

REFERENCES

1. **Beim GM, Lavernia C, Convery FR:** Intramedullary plugs in cemented hip arthroplasty, *J Arthroplasty* 4(2):139, 1989.
1a. **Benjamin JB, et al:** Cementing techniques and the effects of bleeding, *J Bone Joint Surg* 69[Br]:620, 1987.
2. **Blacker G, Charnley J:** *Long-term study of changes in the upper femur after low-friction arthroplasty.* Internal Publication No. 62, Centre for Hip Surgery, Wrightington Hospital, 1976.
3. **Charnley J:** *Low-friction arthroplasty of the hip: theory and practice,* Berlin, 1979, Springer-Verlag.
3a. **Dall DM, Miles AW, Juby G:** Accelerated polymerization of acrylic bone cement using preheated implants, *Clin Orthop* 211:148, 1986.
4. **Davies JP, Harris WH:** Optimization and comparison of three vacuum mixing systems for porosity reduction of Simplex, *Clin Orthop,* in press.
5. **Davies JP, O'Connor DO, Burke DW, et al:** Comparison and optimization of three centrifugation systems for reducing porosity of Simplex P bone cement, *J Arthroplasty* 4:15, 1989.
6. **Davies JP, Jasty M, O'Connor DO, et al:** The effect of centrifuging bone cement, *J Bone Joint Surg* 71[Br]:39, 1989.
7. **Gates EI, Carter DR, Harris WH:** Comparative fatigue behavior of different bone cements, *Clin Orthop* 189:294, 1984.
8. **Harris WH, Davies JP:** Why cement is weak and how it can be strengthened, *AAOS: Instructional Course Lectures* XL:141, 1991.
9. **Harris WH, McCarthy JC Jr, O'Neill DA:** Femoral component loosening using contemporary techniques of femoral cement fixation, *J Bone Joint Surg* 64:1063, 1982.

10. **Harris WH, McGann WA:** Loosening of the femoral component after use of the medullary-plug cementing technique. Follow-up note with a minimum five-year follow-up, *J Bone Joint Surg* 68:1064, 1986.

11. **Huddleston HD:** Femoral lysis after cemented hip arthroplasty, *J Arthroplasty* 3:285, 1988.

12. **Huiskes R:** Some fundamental aspects of human joint replacement. Analyses of stresses and heat conduction in bone-prosthesis structures, *Acta Orthop Scand (Suppl)* 185:1, 1980.

13. **Keating EM, Ritter MA, Faris PM:** Structures at risk from medially placed acetabular screws, *J Bone Joint Surg* 72:509, 1990.

14. **Kwak BM, et al:** An investigation of the effect of cement thickness on an implant by finite element stress analysis. *International Orthopaedics (SICOT)* 2:315, 1979.

15. **Ling RSM:** Prevention of loosening of total hip components. In The Hip Society: *The hip: proceedings of the eighth open scientific meeting of The Hip Society,* St Louis, 1980, Mosby–Year Book.

16. **Miller J, et al:** Improved fixation of knee arthroplasty components by the injection of acrylic cement into cancellous bone surfaces, *J Bone Joint Surg* 61[Br]:515, 1979.

17. **Miller J, et al:** Pathophysiology of loosening of femoral components in total hip arthroplasty: clinical and experimental study of cement fracture and loosening of the cement-bone interface. In The Hip Society: *The hip: proceedings of the sixth open scientific meeting of The Hip Society,* St Louis, 1978, Mosby–Year Book.

18. **Miller J, et al:** Implant fixation. In Turner RH, Scheller AD Jr, editors: *Revision total hip arthroplasty,* New York, 1982, Grune & Stratton.

19. **Nelson CL, et al:** Device and method for controlling cement thickness, *Clin Orthop* 151:160, 1980.

20. **Noble PC, Tullos HS, Landon GC:** The optimum cement mantle for total hip replacement. Theory and practice, *Instructional Course Lectures,* St Louis, 1991, Mosby–Year Book.

21. **Noble PC, Alexander JW, Lindahl LJ, et al:** The anatomic basis of femoral component design, *Clin Orthop* 235:148, 1988.

22. **Oh I, Bourne RB, Harris WH:** The femoral cement compactor. An improvement in cementing technique in total hip replacement, *J Bone Joint Surg* 65:1335, 1983.

23. **Oh I, et al:** Improved fixation of the femoral component after total hip replacement using a methyacrylate intramedullary plug, *J Bone Joint Surg* 60:608, 1978.

24. **Oh I, Harris WH:** A cement fixation system for total hip arthroplasty, *Clin Orthop* 164:221, 1982.

25. **Oh I, Merckx DB, Harris WH:** Acetabular cement compactor. An experimental study of pressurization of cement in the acetabulum in total hip arthroplasty, *Clin Orthop* 177:289, 1983.

26. **Rey RM Jr, Paiement GD, McGann WM, et al:** A study of intrusion characteristics of low viscosity cement Simplex-P and Palacos cements in a bovine cancellous bone model, *Clin Orthop* 215:272, 1987.

27. **Sarmiento A, Gruen TA:** Radiographic analysis of a low-modulus titanium-alloy femoral total hip component. Two to six-year follow-up, *J Bone Joint Surg* 67:48, 1985.

28. **Scheller A, et al:** *A comparative analysis of total hip component position and cement technique.* Presented at the 56th Annual Meeting of the American Academy of Orthopaedic Surgeons, Las Vegas, 1989.

29. **Wasielewski RC, Cooperstein LA, Kruger MP, et al:** Acetabular anatomy and the transacetabular fixation of screws in total hip arthroplasty, *J Bone Joint Surg* 72:501, 1990.

30. **Wroblewski BM, van der Rijt A:** Intramedullary cancellous bone block to improve femoral stem fixation in Charnley low-friction arthroplasty, *J Bone Joint Surg* 66[Br]:639, 1984.

ADDITIONAL READINGS

Bocco F, Langan P, Charnley J: Changes in the calcar femoris in relation to cement technology in total hip replacement, *Clin Orthop* 128:287, 1977.

Carter DR, Gatcs EI, Harris WH: Strain-controlled fatigue of acrylic bone cement, *J Biomed Mater Res* 16:647, 1982.

Eftekhar NS: Total hip replacement using principles of low-friction arthroplasty. In Evarts, editor, *Surgery of musculoskeletal system,* London, 1983, Churchill Livingstone.

Eftekhar NS: Centralization of the femoral stem in total hip replacement. A scientific exhibit (booth #1710) presented at the 49th Annual Meeting, American Academy of Orthopaedic Surgeons, New Orleans, 1985.

Eftekhar NS, Pawluk RJ: Role of surgical preparation in acetabular cup fixation. In The Hip Society: *The hip: proceedings of the eighth open scientific meeting of The Hip Society,* St Louis, 1980, Mosby–Year Book.

Gerish SP: Gas embolism due to hydrogen peroxide, *Anaesthesia* 40:1244, 1985.

Gruen TA, Markof KL, Amstutz HC: Effects of laminations and blood entrapment on the strength of acrylic cone cement, *Clin Orthop* 119:250, 1976.

Halawa M, et al: The shear strength of trabecular bone from the femur, and some factors affecting the shear strength of the cement-bone interface, *Arch Orthop Trauma Surg* 92:19, 1978.

Harris WH: Total hip replacement: technical considerations of femoral component insertion. In The Hip Society: *The hip: proceedings of the eighth open scientific meeting of The Hip Society,* St Louis, 1980, Mosby–Year Book.

Hyland J, Robins RHC: Cardiac arrest and bone cement, *Br Med J* 4:176, 1970.

Knight WE: Accurate determination of leg lengths during total hip replacement, *Clin Orthop* 123:27, 1977.

Lazansky MG: Preparation of the femoral shaft for total hip replacement. In The Hip Society: *The hip: proceedings of the sixth open scientific meeting of The Hip Society,* St Louis, 1978, Mosby–Year Book.

Lee AJC, Ling RSM: A device to improve the extrusion of bone cement into the bone of the acetabulum in the replacement of the hip joint, *Biomed Eng* 9:522, 1974.

Lee AJC, Ling RSM, Vangala SS: The mechanical properties of bone cements, *J Med Eng Technol* 1:137, 1977.

Lee AJC, Ling RSM, Vangala SS: Some clinically relevant variables affecting the mechanical behaviour of bone cement, *Arch Orthop Trauma Surg* 92:1, 1978.

Lee AJC, Wrighton JD: Some properties of polymethylmethacrylate with reference to its use in orthopedic surgery, *Clin Orthop* 95:281, 1973.

Ling RSM, editor: *Complications of total hip replacement,* New York, 1984, Churchill Livingstone.

Ling RSM, James ML: Blood pressure and bone cement, *Br Med J* 2:404, 1971.

Mallory TH: A plastic intermedullary plug for total hip arthroplasty, *Clin Orthop* 155:37, 1981.

Markolf KL: In vitro and technical considerations in femoral component insertion. In The Hip Society: *The hip: proceedings of the eighth open scientific meeting of The Hip Society,* St Louis, 1980, Mosby–Year Book.

Markolf KC, Amstutz HC: Penetration and flow of acrylic bone cement, *Clin Orthop* 121:99, 1976.

Shaw A, Cooperman A, Fusco J: Gas embolism produced by hydrogen peroxide, *N Engl J Med* 277:238, 1967.

Smith JW, Pellicci PM, Sharruck N, et al: Complications after total hip replacement. The contralateral limb, *J Bone Joint Surg* 71A:528, 1989.

Timperley AJ, Bracey DJ: Cardiac arrest following the use of hydrogen peroxide during arthroplasty, *J Arthroplasty* 4(4):369, 1989.

Weber BG: Technique and results of primary and revision arthroplasty of hip joint: pressurization of bone cement. In: *Progress in cemented total hip surgery and revision,* Amsterdam, 1983, Excerpta Medica.

Weber BG: Pressurized cement fixation in total hip arthroplasty, *Clin Orthop* 232:87, 1988.

Weber BG, Stühmer G: Improvements in total hip prosthesis implantation technique. A cement-proof seal for the lower medullary cavity and a dihedral self-stabilizing trochanteric osteotomy, *Arch Orthop Trauma Surg* 93:185, 1979.

See Chapters 5, Acrylic Cement: Properties and Application; 16, Posterolateral Approach; 18, Transtrochanteric Approach (Modified Charnley); 19, Transtrochanteric Approach (Author's Method); and 25, Revision in Absence of Infection for additional information.

CHAPTER SIXTEEN

Posterolateral Approach

- The object of total hip replacement is to build well for 20 years; it is not for sensational short-term results.
  Sir John Charnley

The operation is described in seven phases.

PHASE I: POSITIONING, PREPARATION, AND DRAPING

For positioning, preparing, and draping the patient see Chapter 15.

PHASE II: SURGICAL EXPOSURE OF THE HIP AND LEG LENGTH MEASUREMENTS

During this phase the surgeon stands behind the patient.

Skin Incision and Insulation

Make the skin incision with the limb placed in anatomical position; some adduction is inevitable. The landmarks to be defined are the anterior-superior spine, the vastus lateralis ridge, and the posterior-superior iliac spine. Center the distal section of the incision over the shaft of the femur, extending from a point 6 to 8 cm distal to the vastus lateralis ridge to the top of the greater trochanter. Then incline the proximal limb of the incision posteriorly toward the posterior-superior iliac spine for a distance of 8 to 10 cm (Fig. 16-1). The incision is Marcy and Fletcher's[3] modification of Gibson's[1] approach based on von Langenbech and Kocher's[5] approach to the hip. This author finds it convenient to flex the hip to approximately 60 degrees and make the incision in a straight line, which automatically inclines the incision toward the posterior-superior iliac spine once the leg is placed in the anatomical position. Positioning the incision toward the posterior inferior spine places the incision too far posteriorly because the gluteus maximus muscle split will occur in its deeper portion (third or fourth bundle) along the line of posterior approach described by Moore.[4] Anatomically, the surgeon must have access distally to the entire length of the tendinous attachment of the gluteus maximus to the femur and proximally reaching to the level of the acetabulum. In this way the incision will be located along the midportion of the iliotibial band and along the posterior border of the gluteus medius and mimimus. Additional lengthening of the incision may be necessary in obese patients or difficult anatomical pathological situations. Faulty draping or high positioning of the posterior support (clamp) may cover a portion of the incision area, producing a short proximal limb of the incision. This may make it difficult to expose the acetabulum during surgery. The skin edge towels are either attached or sewn to the wound edge and soaked with Betadine solution.

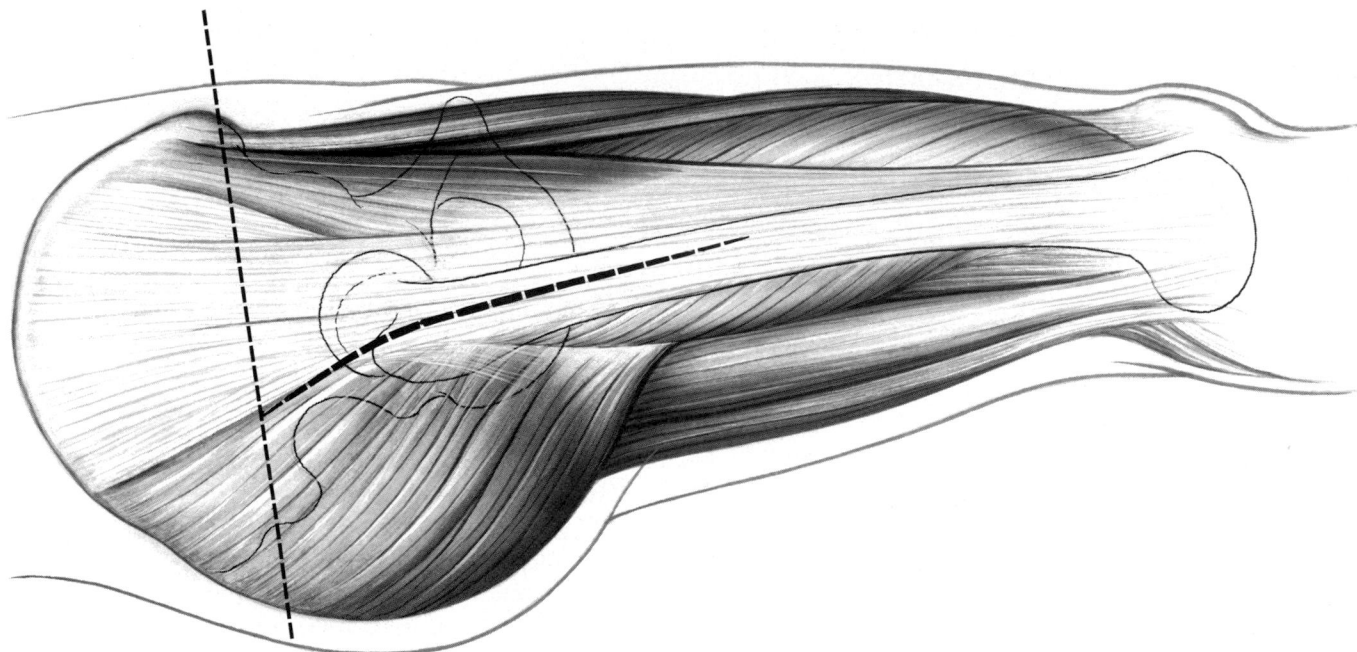

Fig. 16-1. The skin incision is centered distally over the shaft of the femur and slightly posterior to it, extending from a point 6 to 8 cm distal to the vastus lateralis ridge to the top of the greater trochanter. Proximally it is inclined posteriorly for a distance of 8 to 10 cm toward the posterior superior iliac spine.

Fascial Incision

Incise the fascial layer along the line of incision. Adjust the fascial incision if the original skin incision was not accurate; that is, undermine the fat to expose the fascia, thus relocating the fascial incision. Note the following anatomical observations:

1. Distal to the trochanteric ridge the fascia is thick and fibrous, composed of fibers of the iliotibial band, which are parallel.
2. Proximally, the fascia progressively becomes thin and gradually blends into the gluteus maximus aponeurotic layer. Open the fascia distally, and split the fibers to the midpoint of the vastus lateralis ridge. Then carefully open without cutting into the gluteus maximus muscle bundles proximally (Fig. 16-2). Gentle, blunt finger dissection of the gluteus maximus is the best method for deepening the incision to the level of the short rotators. At the uppermost bundle, open the gluteus maximus along the posterior border of the gluteus medius and minimus muscles. Note that both the gluteal bursa and short rotators remain undisturbed until, by blunt dissection, the fascia is mobilized from surrounding muscle planes, that is, the vastus lateralis, short rotators, and gluteus maximus tendon. Center the Charnley initial incision retractor at the level of the trochanteric ridge (Fig. 16-3).

Detaching the Gluteus Maximus Tendon

Detaching the gluteus maximus tendinous insertion to the linea aspera of the femur can enhance surgical exposure considerably. In doing so observe five points:

1. Place the limb in as maximal internal rotation as possible to produce a taut tendon for ease of detachment.
2. Carefully cauterize perforator vessels if they are cut; they are a possible source of troublesome bleeding.
3. If an electric knife is used, guard the sciatic nerve, which is within the vicinity of the tendon.
4. Note that in thin patients (especially the elderly) with less muscle bulk and in individuals with good joint mobility, exposure may be adequate without detaching the gluteus maximus tendon. However, if difficulties are encountered in mobilizing the upper femur, this step of the operation may be necessary.
5. While detaching the gluteus maximus tendon, leave 5 to 8 mm of the broad attachment of this tendon to the femur for subsequent repair.

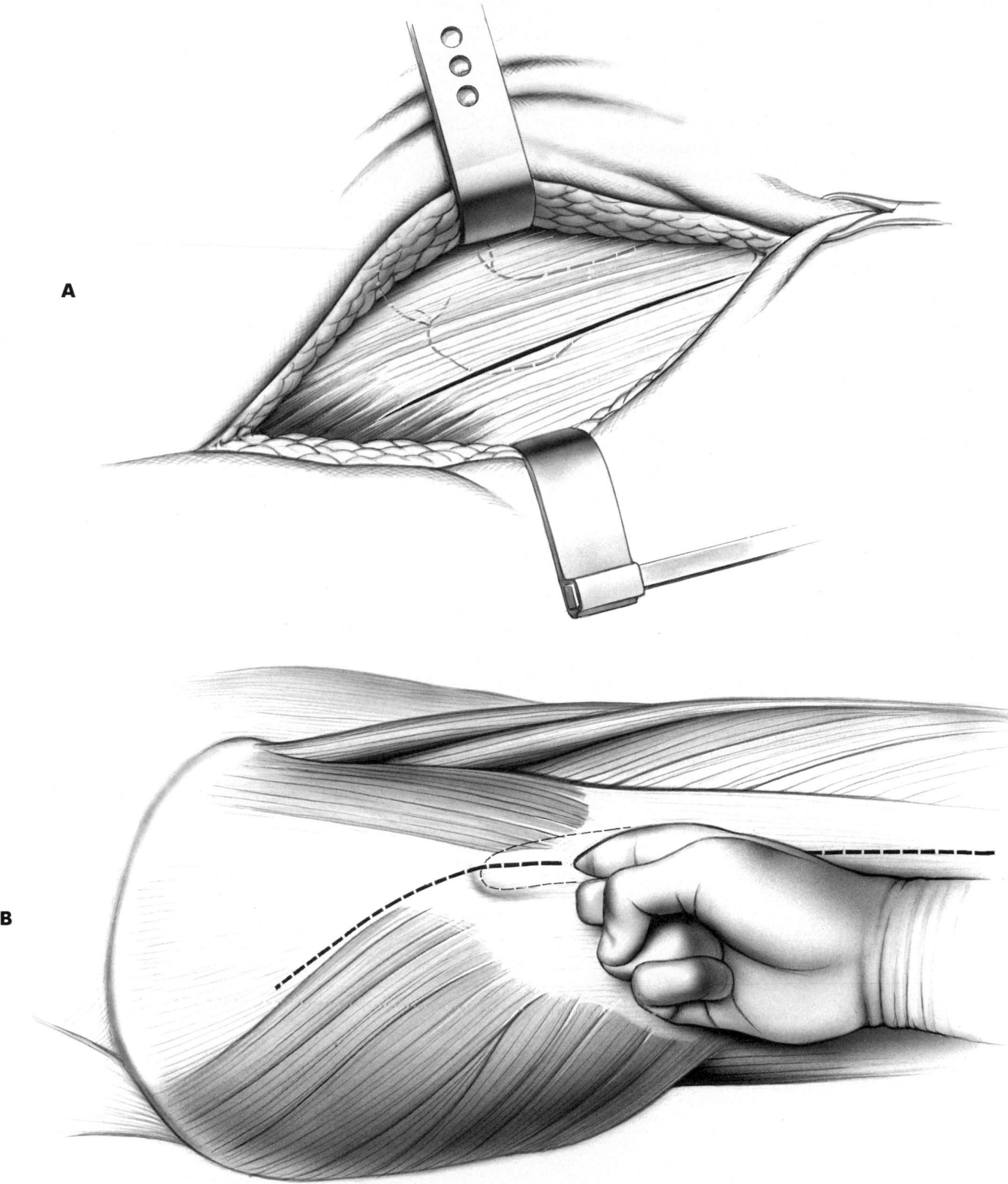

Fig. 16-2. A, Fascial incision is made along the skin incision as centered over the iliotibial band distally and further proximally located along the superior border of the gluteus maximus. **B,** An index finger lifts up the fascia outwardly as the incision is made along the uppermost bundle of the gluteus maximus, a technical detail that prevents cutting into tensor fascia femoris muscle fibers.

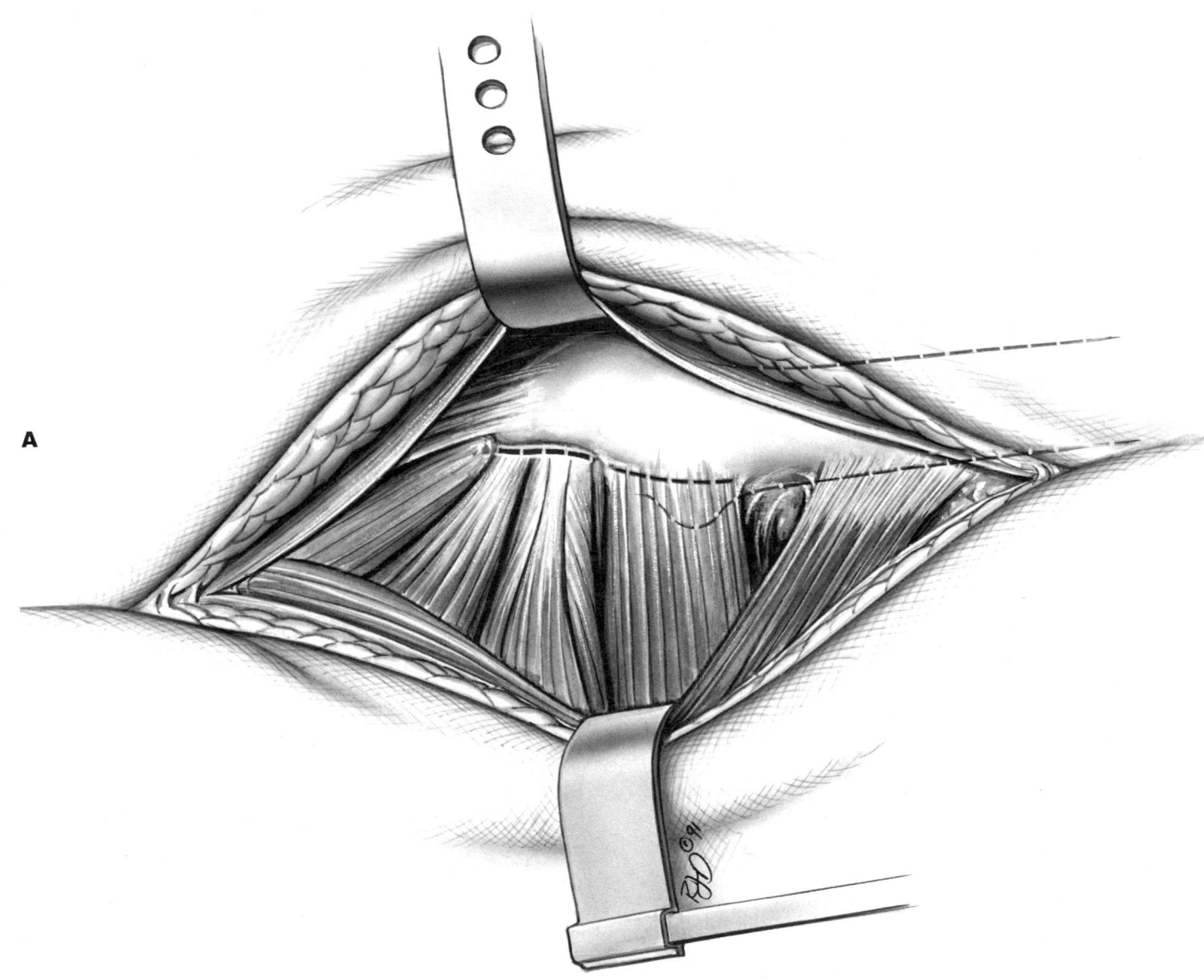

A

Fig. 16-3. A, The short rotators are best visualized by wiping off the areolar tissue and bursa from the trochanteric region to identify the "key" muscle in this region, the piriformis. Outline the extent of the detachment of the short rotators from the bone and the capsule. Detach the quadratus (the lowest muscle) only if necessary. Also detach the gluteus maximus from the femur to improve the exposure.

Continued.

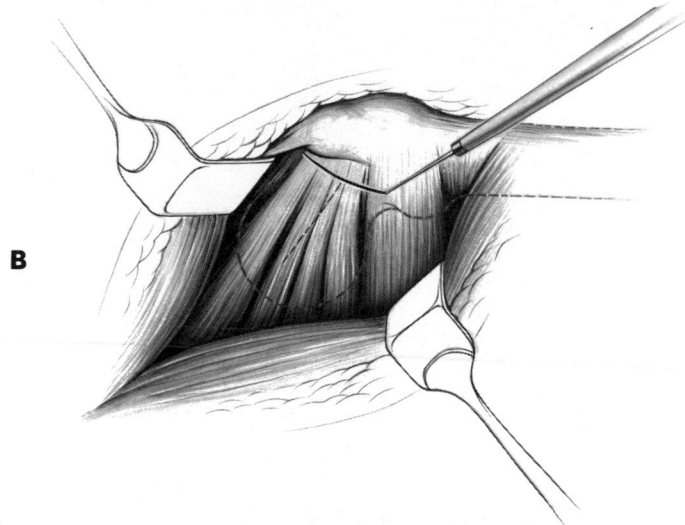

B

Fig. 16-3, cont'd. B, Inset, The short rotators are detached using an electrocautery knife. Detach the muscle as closely as possible to their insertion on the femur.

Detaching the Short Rotators

Use a swab and a periosteal elevator, and gently remove the fatty and areolar tissue to expose the attachment of the short rotators to the femur. Identify the uppermost one, the piriformis with its distinct slender tendon attached to the digital fossa. It is a "key muscle"[2] in the region and the following help to identify it:

- It is attached to the digital fossa of the trochanter.
- Its upper margin borders gluteus medius muscle and tendon.
- Its inferior and anterior margin borders the gluteus minimus muscle.
- The sciatic and inferior gluteal nerve, artery, and vein emerge inferior to it, and the superior gluteal nerve, artery, and vein emerge superior to it as they appear in the buttock region (see Chapter 2).

Isolate and detach the piriformis from its attachment to the digital fossa of the trochanter as close to the bone as possible. Cauterize its vascular bed. Tag the tendon with a nonabsorbable suture such as #1 Tevdek (Fig. 16-4). Detach short rotators, inferior and superior gemelli, and obturator internus from the femur using an electric knife as the second assistant internally rotates the femur. The quadratus femoris may remain undisturbed but may also be partially or totally detached from the femur as needed to obtain exposure. Separate the piriformis tendon from other short rotators and from the joint capsule (see Figs. 16-3, *B* and 16-4).

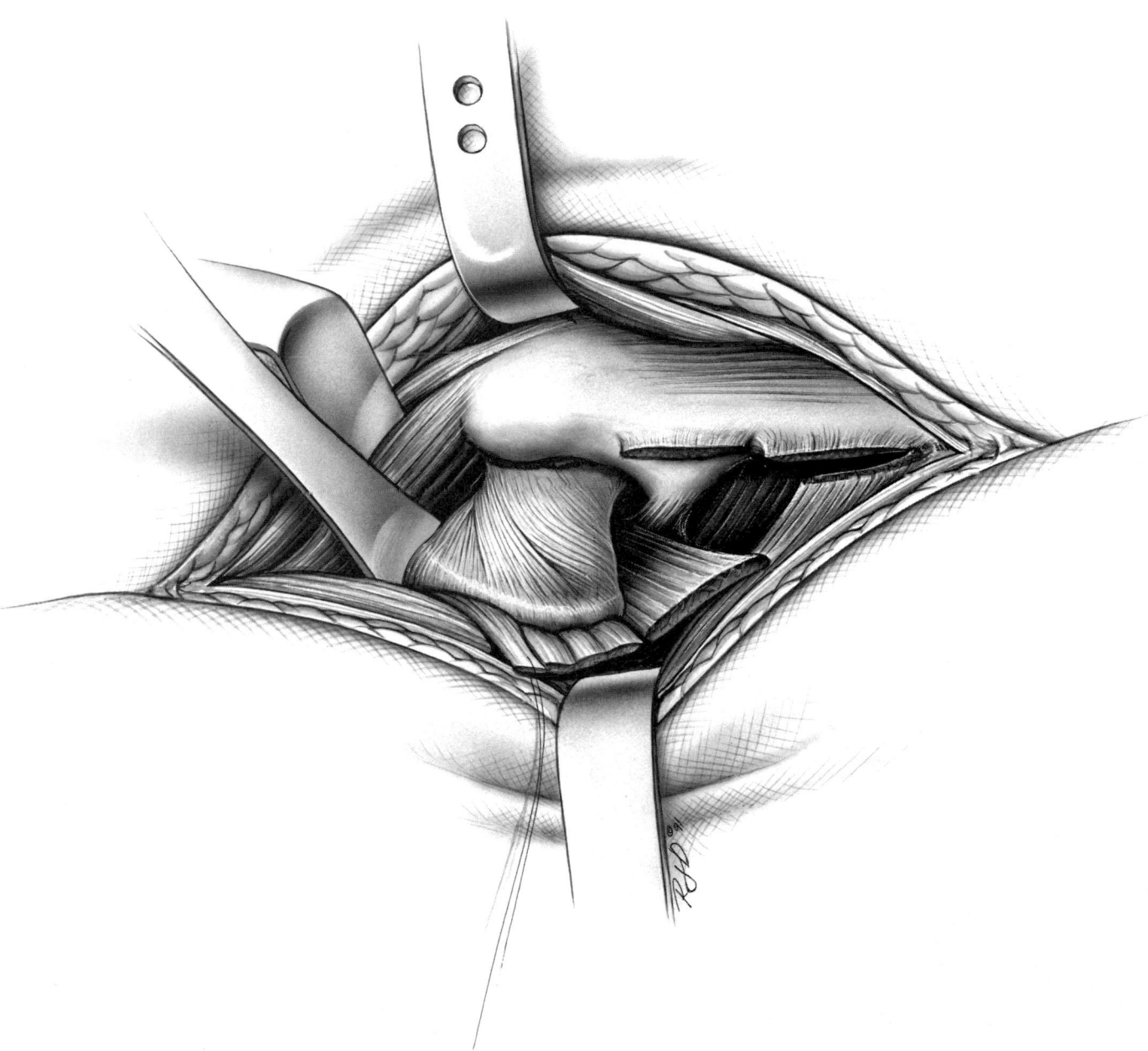

Fig. 16-4. The piriformis has been identified, tagged, and retracted posteriorly. Locate the sciatic nerve, but do not dissect around it. Visualize the posterior capsule by reflecting the short rotators. Using an elevator, separate the capsule from the gluteus minimus to define the superior margin of the acetabulum. Note detachment of the quadratus femoris and gluteus maximus from the femur.

Detaching the Capsule

Before incising the capsule, lift the gluteus minimus origin and its often-present attached muscular fibers from the superior margin of the acetabulum and capsule for a distance of 2 to 3 cm. Develop the plane of the separation just above the margin of the piriformis (which has just been detached) using a Cobb's elevator. Use a small Hohmann retractor to retract the gluteus minimus muscle as a capsulotomy is being performed circumferentially along the capsular attachment to the femur. Two radial incisions (superiorly and inferiorly, Fig. 16-5) permit freedom of the capsule, which can then be reflected posteriorly (Fig. 16-6). Now replace the Hohmann retractor with a Charnley pin retractor to expose the upper margin of the acetabular rim. The pin retractor attached to a T-handled insertor-extractor is driven bit by bit as the handle of the instrument assumes a perpendicular position to the floor (parallel to the transaxis of the pelvis) from a horizontal position (parallel to the floor). The ideal position of the pin retractor is midanteroposterior and 2 cm proximal to the rim of the acetabulum (Fig. 16-7).

The pin retractor has a dual function. It is used for retraction and reference for leg length measurement. The following details must be observed to insert the pin properly:

1. Do not place the pin too close to the acetabular cavity because it will interfere with the reaming.
2. The pin is engaged to both cortices of the pelvic bone; thus, the test by "rocking" the pin back and forth does not indicate loosening of the pin.
3. Hammer the pin in at an angle perpendicular to the floor (this also serves as a reference for aligning the cup).
4. Use a pin retractor extender to avoid burying the pin within the abductor muscles.
5. Place the pin so as not to obstruct access to the top of the femur during the femoral preparation.
6. Last, but not least, this pin, which has been inserted before dislocation of the hip, must remain undisturbed until both components are inserted and leg length measurements are carried out during surgery.

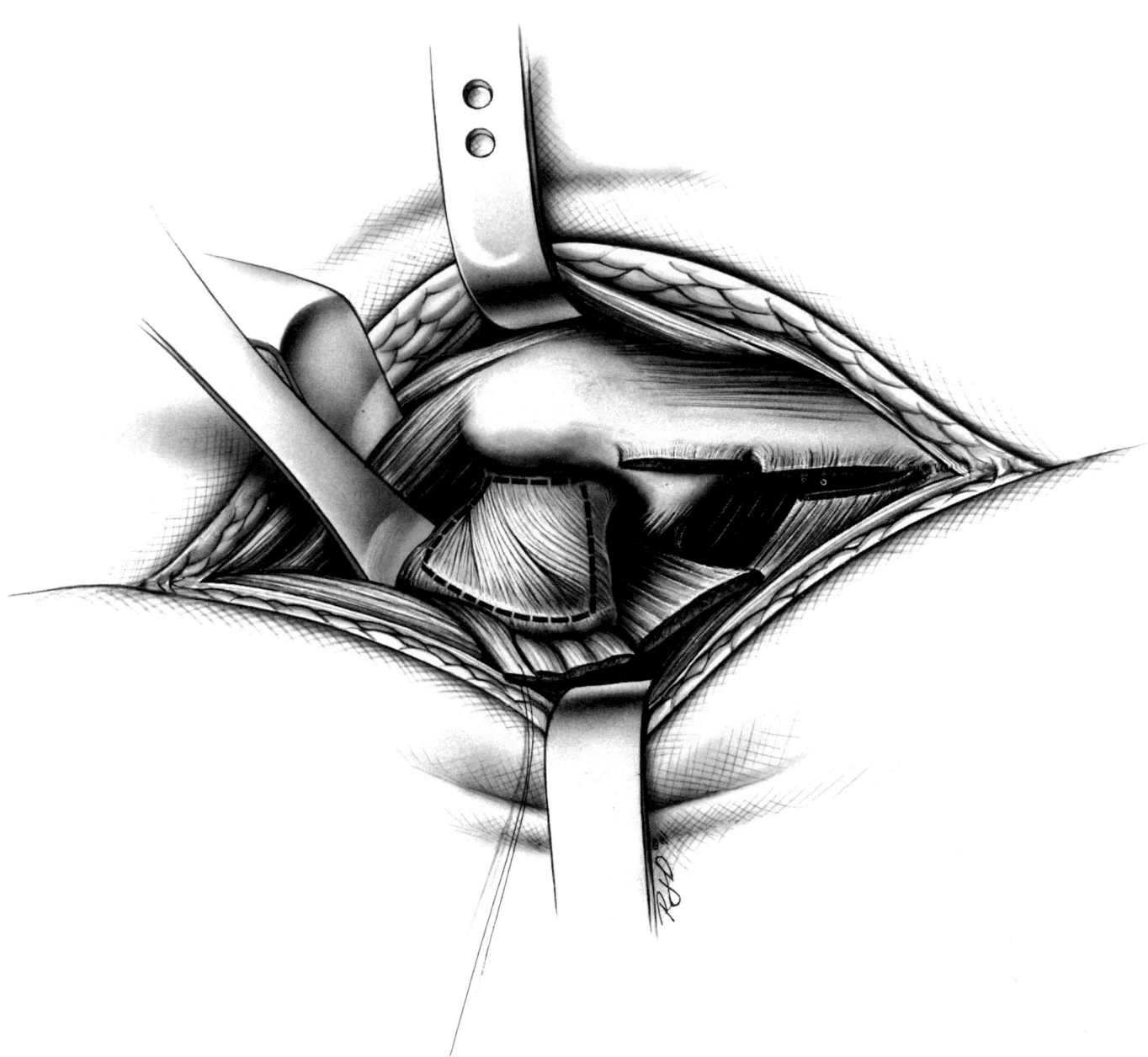

Fig. 16-5. Incise the capsule along the superior and inferior margins of the neck, and reflect it along the rim of the acetabulum as it is detached from the femur *(dotted lines).* Excise the capsule only if required to obtain exposure in stiff and deformed hips.

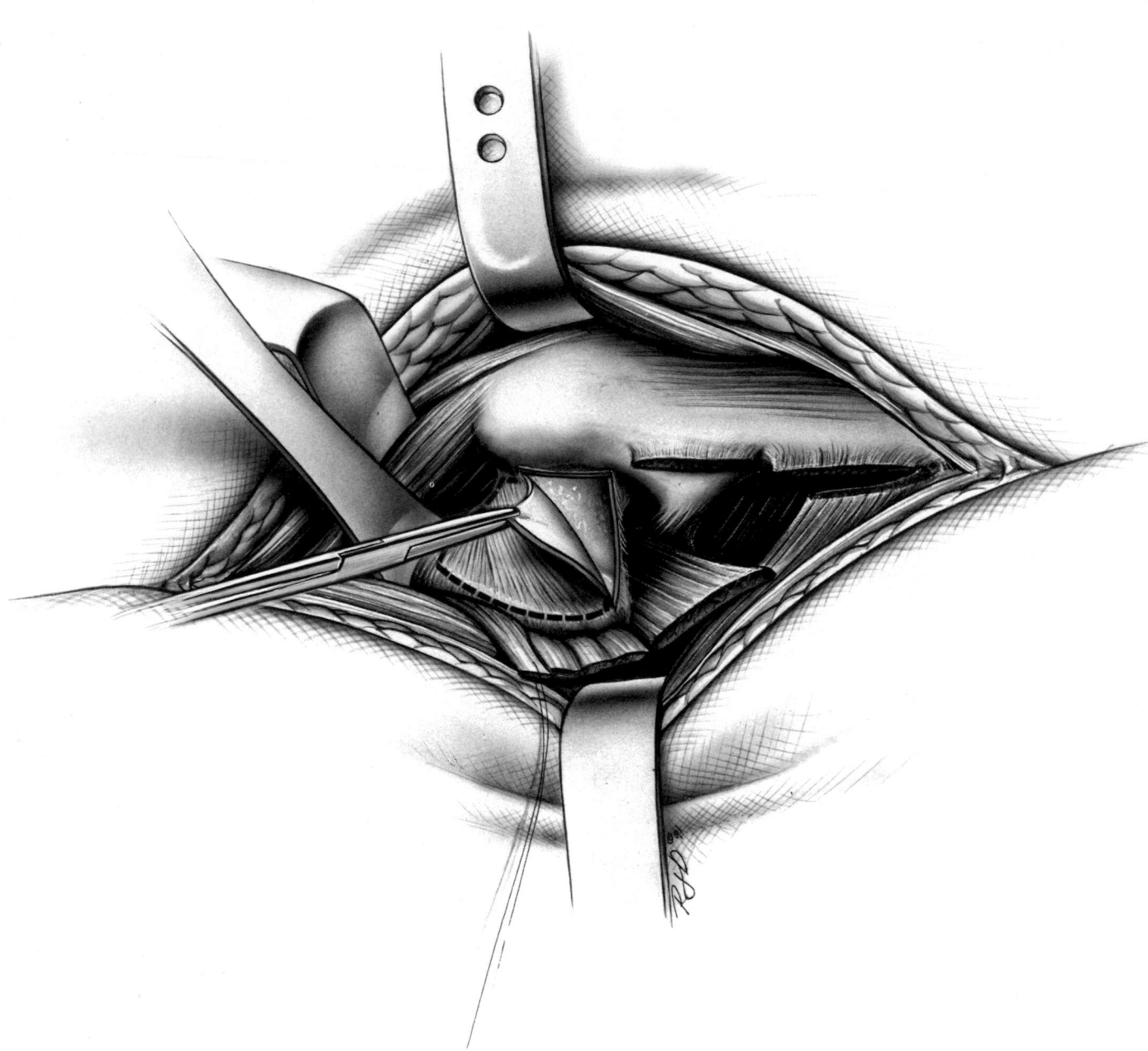

Fig. 16-6. Lift the capsule off the femur, and protect it so that it can be repaired later at the completion of the procedure.

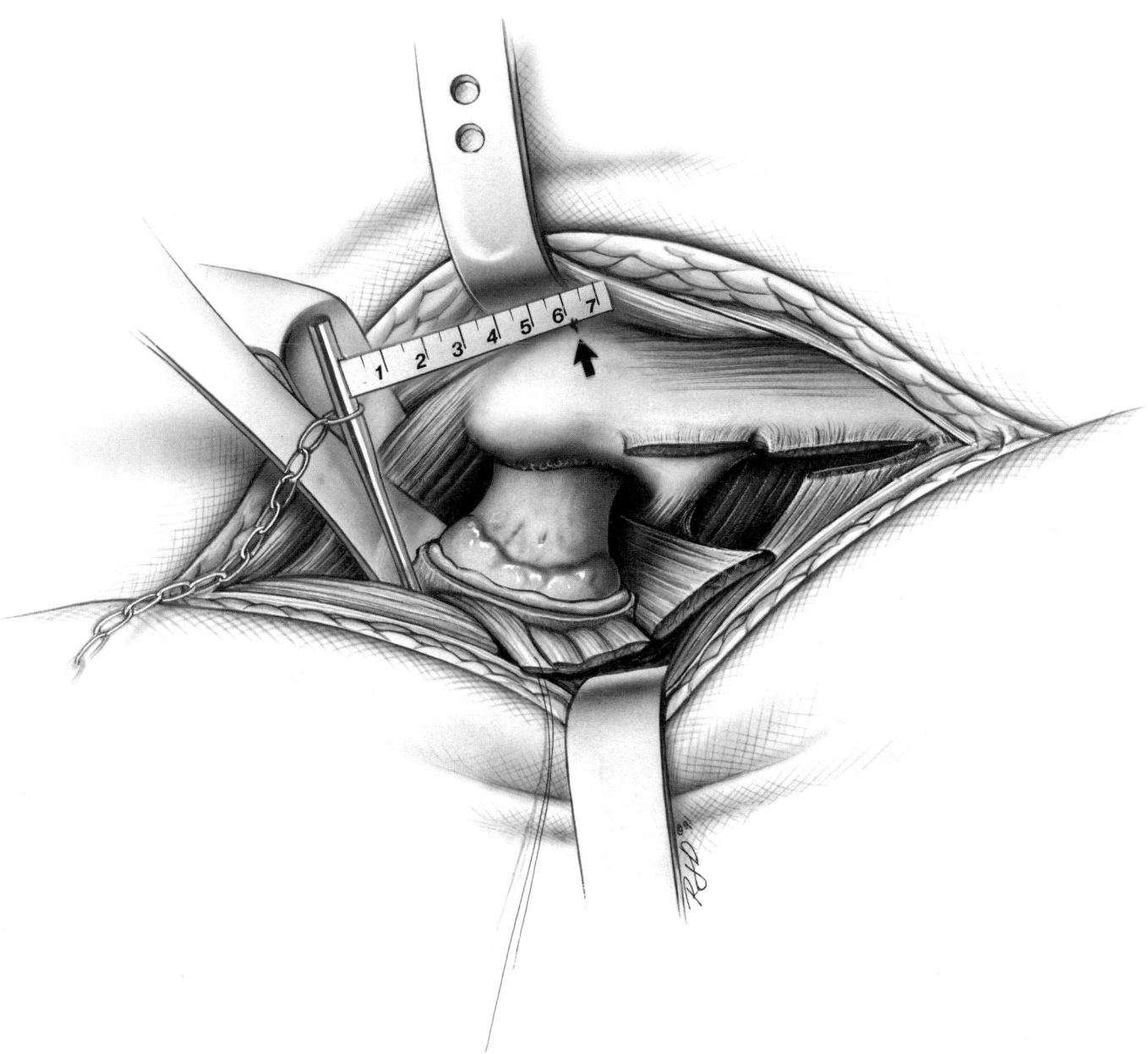

Fig. 16-7. Before dislocating the hip, insert the superior acetabular pin retractor to the ilium to retract the gluteus medius and minimus. It serves a dual function as a retractor and marker. It is used to carefully measure the distance between the acetabulum and femur. Arrow indicates a fixed point marked on the femur by a cautery and a stay suture. The capsule of the joint has been excised in this case.

PHASE III: DISLOCATING THE HIP, INCISING AND MOBILIZING THE CAPSULE, EXPOSURE BY PERIACETABULAR RETRACTORS

Before dislocation do the following:

- Perform leg length measurements as described in Chapter 15.
- Perform a complete capsulotomy by cautery knife posterosuperiorly, as the labrum is cut radially and the bony margin of the acetabulum becomes visible.
- Control posterior capsular bleeders.
- Retract the tagged short rotators and capsule to visualize the rim of the acetabulum. Verify the location of the sciatic nerve by palpating the nerve through its fatty bed. I do not visualize the sciatic nerve by dissecting around it, nor do I place any retractors about the nerve.

Dislocating the Hip by Adduction and Internal Rotation

Dislocation must be done with care to avoid fractures. The second assistant is instructed to adduct the hip with no more than 20 to 30 degrees' flexion. Internal rotation and axial traction facilitate dislocation (Figs. 16-8 and 16-9). Dislocation may be difficult because of the following factors:

1. Inadequate capsular release or excision of the labrum or of marginal osteophytes.
2. The vacuum created as the head is moved out of the depth of the socket.
3. Marginal osteophytes or a deep-seated head, resulting from protrusion acetabuli.
4. Ankylosis of the hip joint without any bony fusion.
5. Coxa magna senilis with osteophytes in a large-muscled person.
6. Intact ligamentum teres.
7. Excess traction on the limb during dislocation.

When dislocation is not possible despite adequate capsular release, do one or more of the following steps:

1. Place the hook under the neck, and bring the head out of the acetabulum.
2. Use a "skid" such as an acetabular skid or a flat gouge (such as a Watson-Jones) intraarticularly, and pry the hip out of the depth of the socket. However, if dislocation is difficult and necessitates excess force, it is advisable to osteotomize the neck in situ and remove the head in a retrograde fashion to avoid fracturing the femoral shaft. A T-handled corkscrew is necessary to facilitate removal of the head.

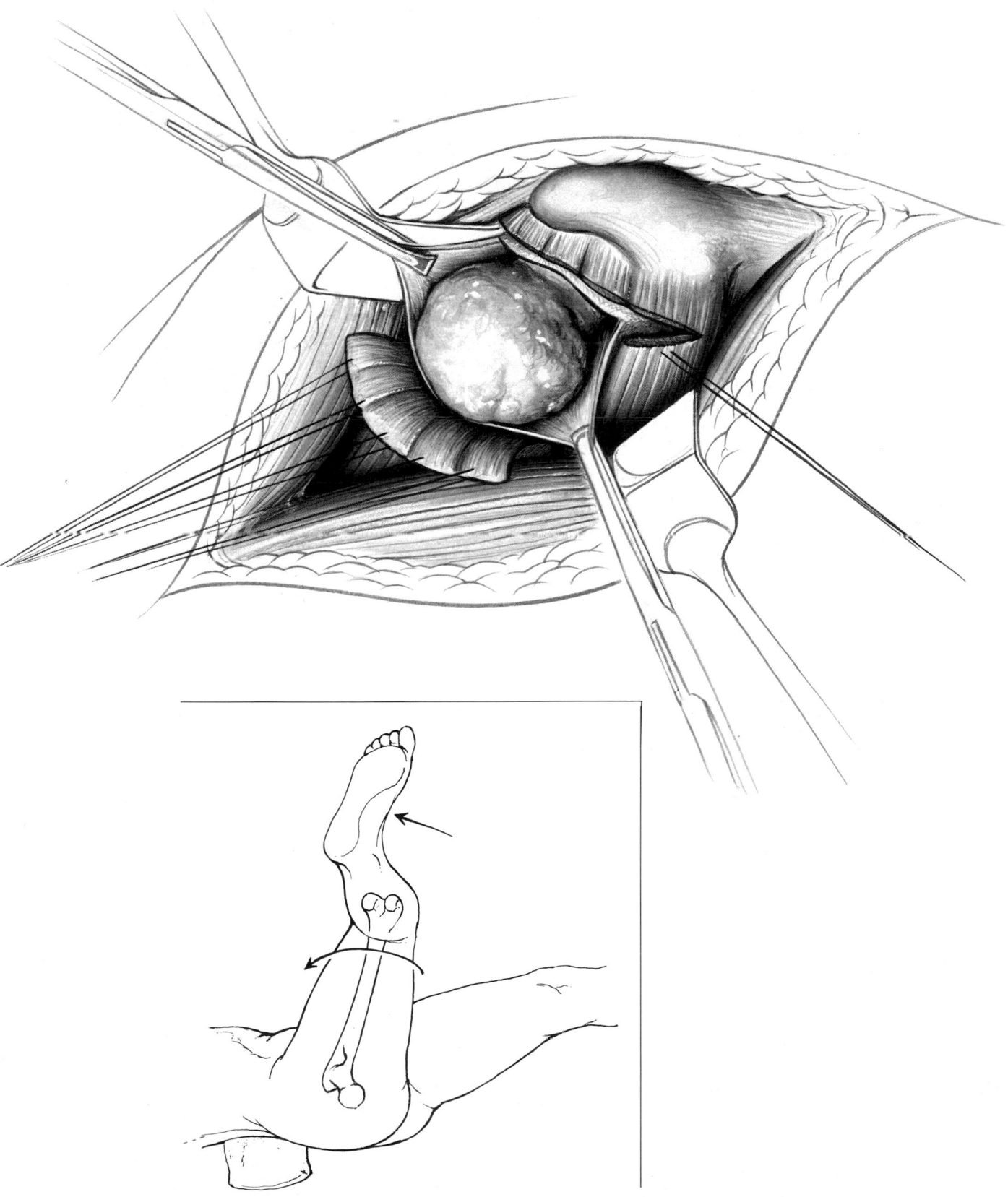

Fig. 16-8. Dislocation is accomplished by adduction, internal rotation, and some flexion. Note that some capsular release may be necessary to mobilize the head and femur out of the depth of the wound. Inset, The position of the hip at dislocation. The acetabular pin retractor is not shown.

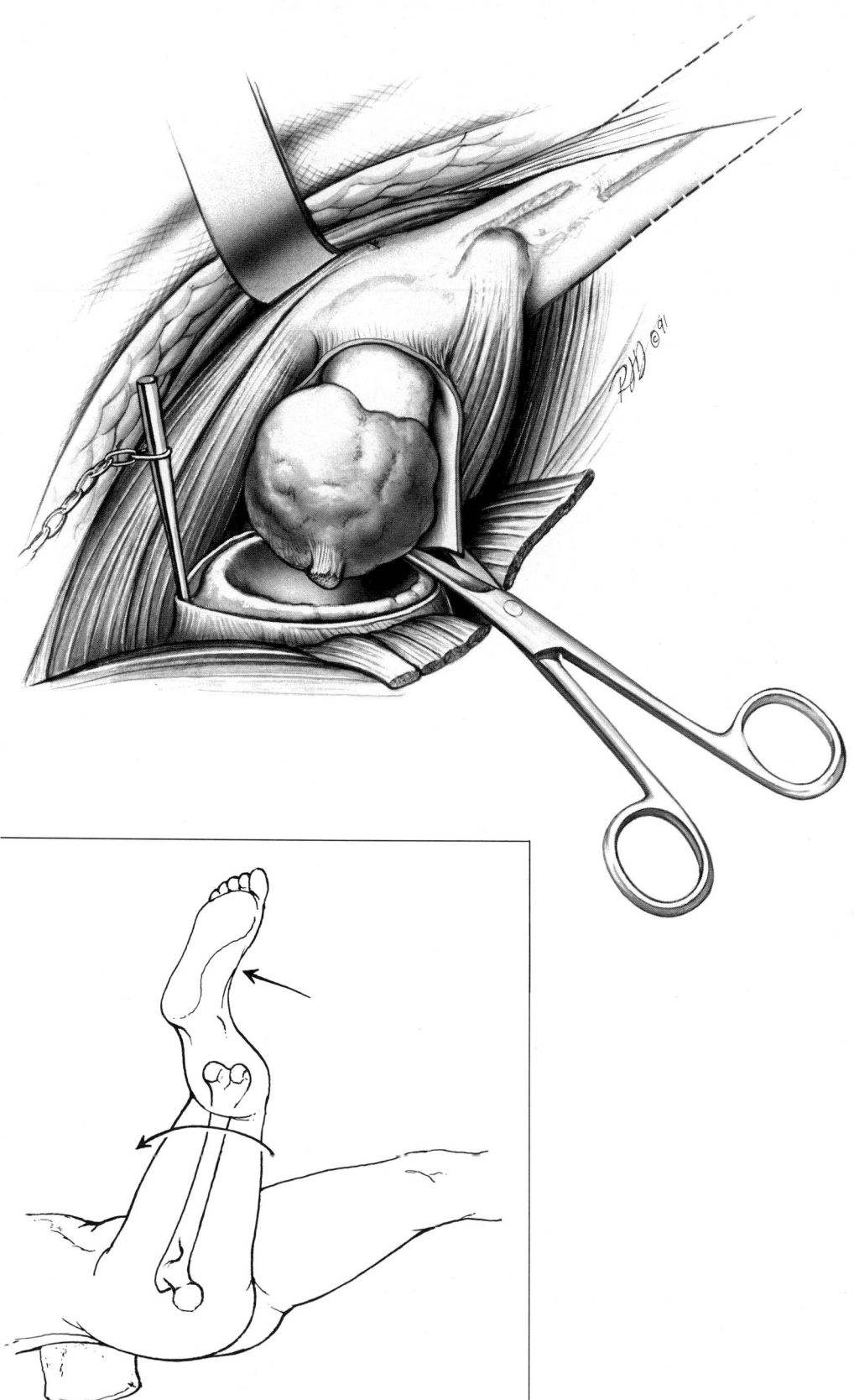

Fig. 16-9. To improve the exposure a partial incision of the inferior or superior capsule may be required. The extremity must be progressively internally rotated to facilitate the capsular release (inset) during this procedure.

Amputation of the Femoral Head

Before sectioning the neck, divide any remaining tight synovial or capsular tissue between the neck and femur if the hip cannot be rotated internally to 90 degrees. Additionally, measure the offset of the femoral head, the distance between the center of the head and the axis of the shaft of the femur. Record this for subsequent reference after implantation of the trial and actual prostheses. When 90 degrees of internal rotation of the hip is not possible, perform an inferior capsular and a psoas release as needed.

The 90-degree internally rotated limb places the posterior neck upward as the 90-degree-flexed knee places the tibia vertical to the table (floor). Place two narrow flat Hohmann-type retractors, one inferior and one superior to the neck, while removing the head at an appropriate level (see Chapter 15). This appropriate level of neck section is based on previous templating and required postoperative leg length, as well as the type of prosthesis used (Fig. 16-10).

The level of the cut must be marked and cut by the saw. During sectioning of the neck it is best to have the second assistant abduct the leg to a neutral position because the leg tends to drift the adduction and flexion by gravity.

Observe the following:

1. The saw blade must never encroach upon the trochanter. The blade must be placed so as to start at the desired level medially and extend toward the junction of the neck and the trochanter laterally.
2. Exposure must be sufficient to avoid damage to the abductor muscles; it is best to release the capsule as needed to free up the femur. Saw in a perpendicular plane so that the anterior and posterior neck are cut at the same level.
3. When making the first cut, it is best to retain a longer neck than a shorter one; further adjustments are easy to make later on.
4. Avoid damage to the soft tissue by placing the Hohmann retractors properly while bone is being cut.
5. Do not discard the femoral head if the surgeon plans to use it for an intramedullary plug or bone graft to the acetabulum.

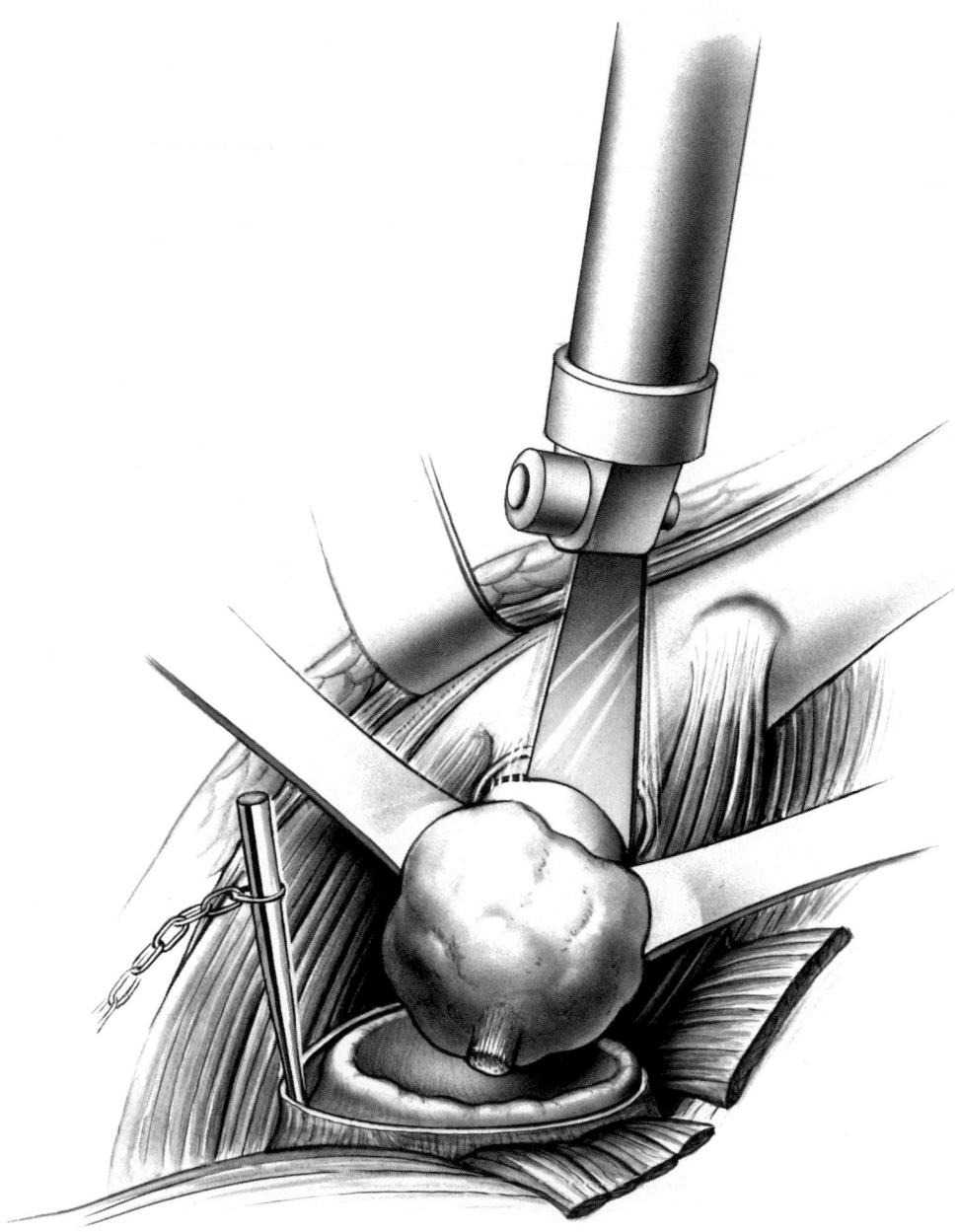

Fig. 16-10. The two narrow Hohmann retractors are placed one superiorly and one inferiorly along the neck. The neck is being resected at an appropriate level.

PHASE IV: ACETABULAR EXPOSURE, PREPARATION, AND FIXATION OF THE ACETABULAR COMPONENT

For this phase of the procedure the surgeon stands in front of the patient.

Maximizing Exposure

The principle of acetabular exposure by this approach is to displace the upper femur anterior to the acetabulum. Accomplish this by using a small-pointed Hohmann or a similar retractor anteromedially over the iliopubic ramus. Further capsular release anteriorly is often necessary to mobilize the femur. This is best accomplished by inserting a curved clamp anterior to the capsule along the margin of the acetabulum (Fig. 16-11). The best site for insertion is proximal and over the bulky and strong portion of the anterior rim at the junction of the rim with the ilium near the insertion of the iliofemoral ligament attached to the pelvis. This site is at one to two o'clock for the left and between ten and eleven o'clock for the right hip as the surgeon views the acetabulum from the posterior aspect of the hip. The following details must be observed:

1. The leg must be positioned so as to relax the anterior capsule; apply adduction, internal rotation, and flexion.
2. Internally rotate the hip, place the thigh on the opposite thigh, and support the lower leg over the bulk of folded sheets to maintain internal rotation of 20 to 30 degrees.
3. Place one hook under the femoral neck to facilitate the insertion of the anterior pointed Hohmann retractor.
4. Pierce the capsule with the tip of a Hohmann retractor at the site of the insertion. Use electrocautery to make an opening into the capsule if insertion of the pointed Hohmann is difficult.
5. Make sure the tip of the retractor is well engaged before the second assistant retracts the femur forward (Fig. 16-12).
6. Use care to keep the tip of the retractor as close to the bone as possible to avoid accidental injury to the neurovascular structures located within the vicinity of the anterior capsule at this level.
7. In a severely contracted and thickened capsule, detachment of the anterior capsule (especially in stiff hips) from the rim of the acetabulum may be required before either insertion or retraction of the femur is possible (see Fig. 16-11).
8. To be most effective and safe, engage the flat portion of the back of the handle of the retractor against the femur at the distance between the medial neck and lesser trochanter to displace the femur forward.

Note of Caution when Retracting the Femur

- Never retract the abductors by the anterior Hohmann retractor, since damage to the muscles or its tendon is inevitable.
- Do not remove and reinsert the Hohmann retractor; such a maneuver can be potentially damaging to the bone and soft tissue structures.
- Always place the anterior Hohmann retractor as proximal as possible (near the iliopubic junction) because the bone is strongest near the ilium.
- Do not engage the tip of the retractor at the midportion or lower portion of the iliopubic ramus, since it can fracture the weak anterior wall, especially during reaming of the acetabulum.
- Do not begin retracting the femur before the tip is well engaged.

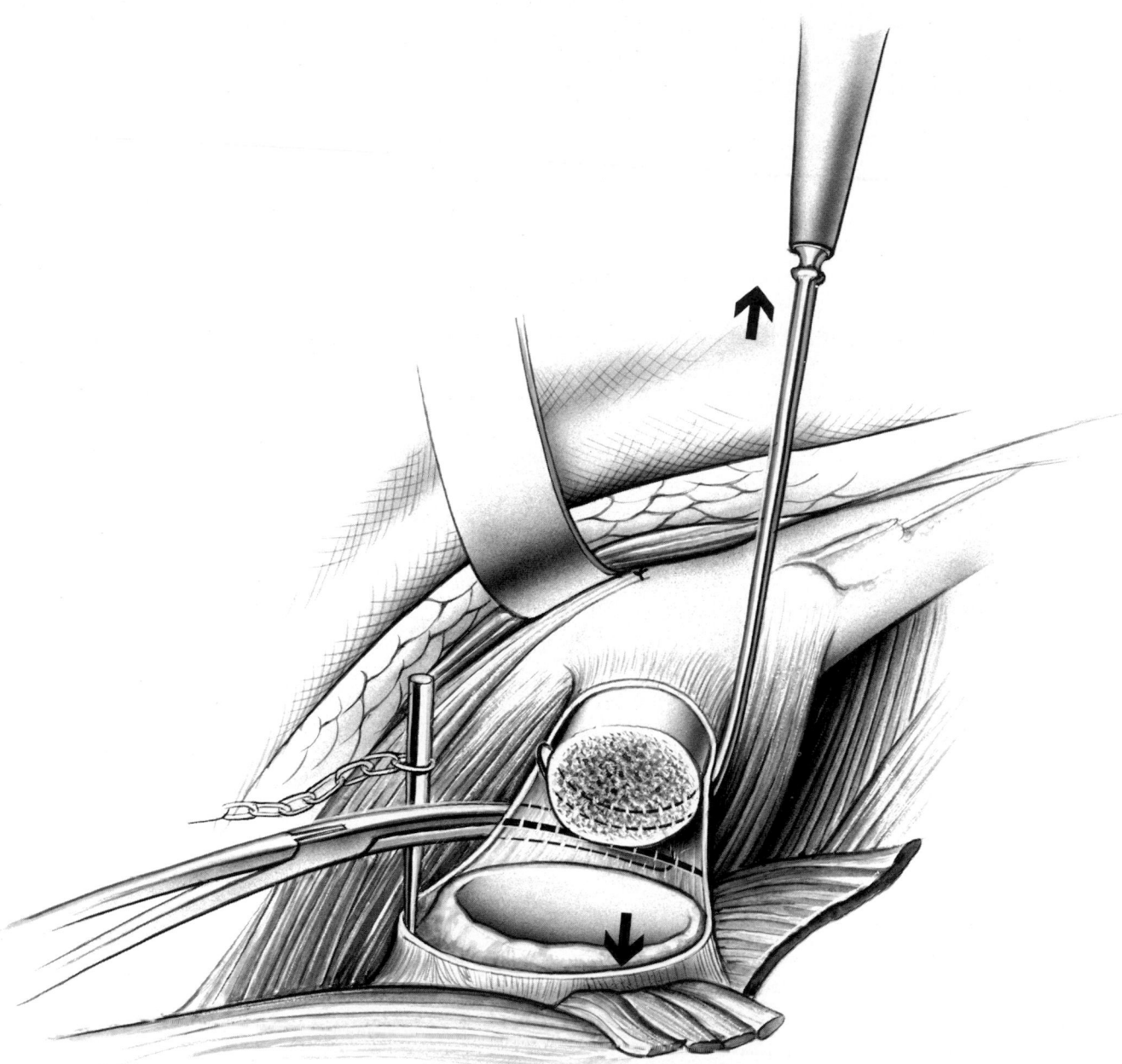

Fig. 16-11. Anterior capsular release is best accomplished by lifting the neck of the femur in an upward direction using a bone hook. Note that inserting a curved clamp makes the mobilization and removal of the capsule from the margin of the acetabulum safe. Lower arrow in this figure illustrates the site of insertion of the second (posterior) capsular pin retractor (not shown in this illustration).

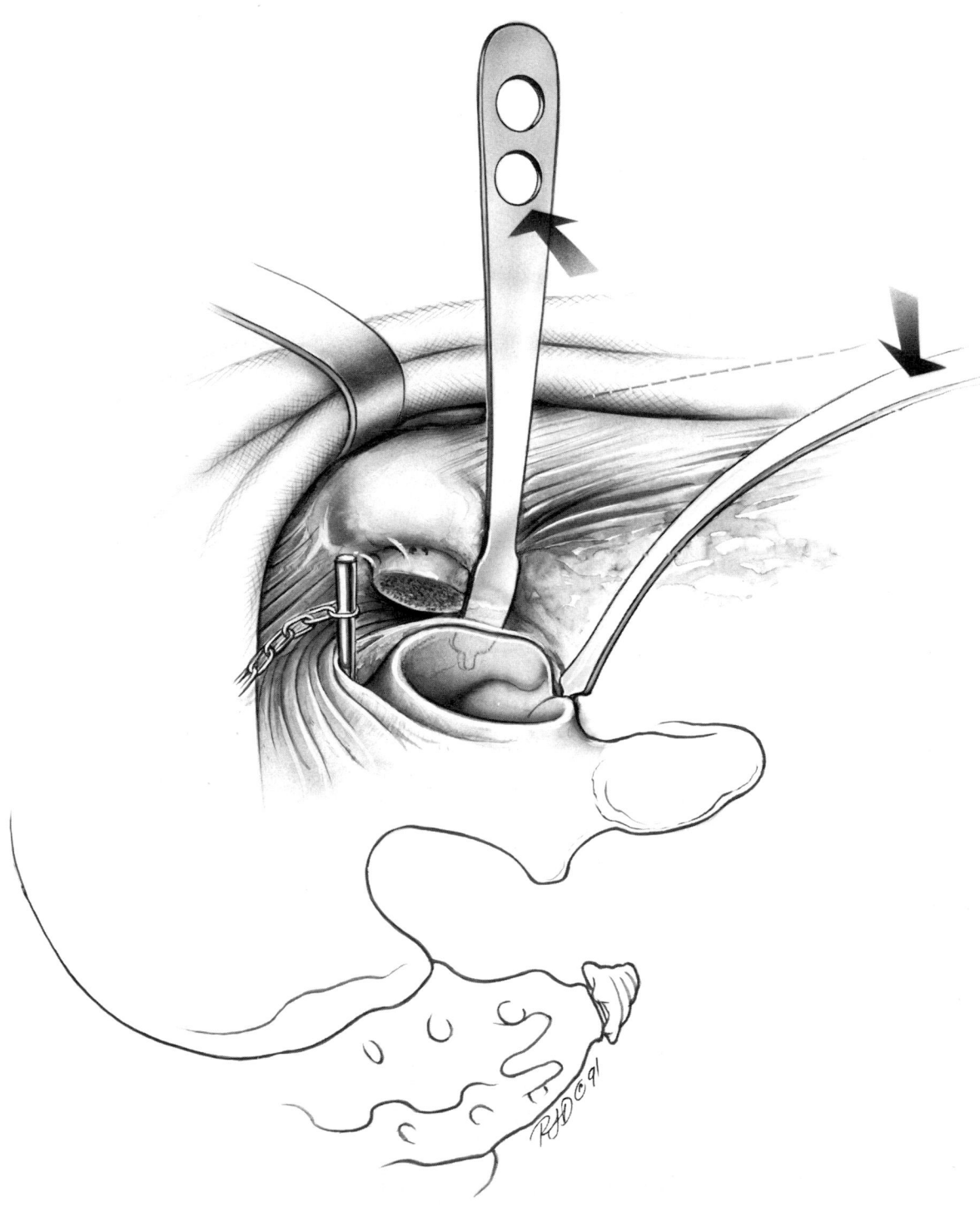

Fig. 16-12. Exposure of the acetabulum is maximized by an anterior retractor placed so as to retract the femur in a forward direction. Soft tissue mobilization is essential in producing a good exposure. A second retractor (triangular Hohmann) is placed under the transverse acetabular ligament beneath the intercotyloid notch of the acetabulum. Arrows indicate the direction of retraction by the two Hohmanns shown here.

Visualizing the Acetabular Rim

First expose the entire bony rim of the acetabulum by excising the labrum and redundant capsule. Retain the posterior capsule, which can protect the sciatic nerve (during the insertion of the second pin retractor) and also for subsequent repair along with the short rotators to produce posterior stability for the hip. To expose the posterior rim and retain the exposure of the acetabulum posteriorly, insert a second pin retractor intracapsullarly to retract the posterior capsule (see Fig. 16-11). Engage this pin to the bone of the ilioischial ramus with care to avoid injury to the sciatic nerve. Insert the second pin to the handle of the insertor, tilt the handle forward while the tip is in contact with the bone, then incline the handle in a backward direction to retract the capsule while the pin is being driven to the bone. The pin must engage into the inner cortex to be firmly attached. Remove the T handle from the pin.

Second, define and expose the lower margin of the acetabulum. To expose and maintain the exposure of the inferior margin of the acetabulum insert a broad triangular-shaped Hohmann retractor inferiorly and distal to the transverse ligament or under the cotyloid notch at the top of the obturator foramen. The retractor should be held in position by the second assistant. It is often necessary to make a radial cut in the inferior capsule to retract the inferior capsule with this retractor (see Fig. 16-12).

Exposing the Pulvinar, Nonarticulating Portion of the Acetabulum

It is fundamental to expose the "true" medial wall of the acetabulum by removing the overhanging medial and inferior osteophytes, ligamentum teres, and fibrofatty tissue from this region. Use a T-handled long Volkmann spoon to expose the cortical-like floor (medial wall) acetabulum. Control bleeders from the lower margin (branches of obturator vessels to the ligamentum teres). Using cautery, excise the transverse ligament in part or completely to expose the bony margin of the cotyloid notch. Unroof the fused osteophytes when the ligamentum teres is completely covered (see Chapter 15). Exposure of the pulvinar is the limit to which the acetabulum can be safely deepened without violating its medial wall. This must be done before reaming the acetabulum. If the lower margin of the true acetabulum is not exposed, it may be difficult to locate the socket low at the anatomical position.

Preparing the Acetabulum

Ream the acetabulum in two steps. First, ream inferiorly (low position), then ream for expansion and deepening.

For inferior reaming, use a small acetabular debris-retaining reamer that has a 40-cm outer diameter, and place it low in the socket to remove reactive osteophytes from the lower margin of the acetabulum. This reaming also helps to show the pulvinar. Take care to avoid excess deepening at this level since the reamers can penetrate the acetabulum, which is thin at this level. For subsequent reaming, use graded debris-retaining reamers directed at an angle of 40 to 45 degrees to the longitudinal axis of the body (or transverse axis of the pelvis). Accommodate 15 to 20 degrees of anteversion as reaming is being done (Fig. 16-13).

In reaming the acetabulum with this exposure several details must be observed.

1. Make sure that the second assistant maintains adequate forward displacement of the femur to produce a satisfactory insertion and removal of the reamers. When additional adjustment is necessary it should be done before reaming has begun.
2. The strong and massive bone of the ischium and ilioischial ramus (as opposed to the less developed and often weak iliopubic ramus) often shifts the reamers toward the anterior wall of the femur of the acetabulum, leading to an eccentric preparation and increased damage to the commonly defective anterior wall of the acetabulum.
3. When the anterior wall is defective it is necessary to push the reamers posteriorly to keep them away from the anterior wall. Use the opposite hand to hold the sleeve of the reamer for this

purpose. Use a one- or two-size-smaller reamer to remove dense and thick posterior bone, thus avoiding damage to the iliopubic ramus.

4. Check frequently and after each reamer size is used to avoid accidental damage to each wall of the acetabulum.
5. Protect and retain the subchondral bone of the roof of the acetabulum as much as possible (see Chapter 15).

Acetabular Preparation vs. Socket Fixation

As noted in Chapter 15, the method of acetabular preparation differs for cemented and cementless cups. In the former a precise fit is not desirable, since room must be created not only for the cup but also for the cement. In the latter, the prepared acetabulum must be precisely reamed to create maximum contact between the bone and the porous surface of the cup. The press-fit sockets with porous-coated surfaces require porous bleeding corticocancellous bone for ingrowth, whereas the supportive cortical-like subchondral bone may remain intact because multiple drill holes provide increased surface area for fixation by cement. In both types of sockets, the cup must be contained within the bone of the acetabular cavity. The load bearing and the central rotation must be placed as close to an anatomical position as possible (see Chapter 15).

Positioning the Cup

As stated in Chapter 3, one disadvantage of the posterolateral approach is the difficulty in assessing the exact position of the pelvis intraoperatively as the patient is positioned in a lateral decubitus position. This is in spite of proper positioning and securing of the patient on the table (see Chapter 15).

As has been observed, the amount of anteversion of the acetabulum may vary from lateral decubitus to standing, affecting the cup position and thus postoperative hip stability (see Chapter 33). Although the angle of abduction is usually reproducible with this approach, the exact amount of anteversion is difficult to assess. To avoid placing the cup in an excessively retroverted position, most surgeons place the cup in a 20- to 30-degree anteverted position. This naturally may cause an anterior dislocation postoperatively.

The following details are helpful in reducing malpositioning resulting from the lateral decubitus positioning of the patient.

1. Check the position of the patient on the table; the trunk and the pelvis must be secure so that the transaxis of the thorax and pelvis remains perpendicular to the operating table (see Chapter 15). Check the position and firm fixation of the pubic and sacral pads before draping.
2. Flex the down leg to 90 degrees at the knee and up to 60 degrees at the hip to stabilize the patient on the operating table. Flexion of the hip also reduces the amount of lumbar lordosis and thus the extension of the pelvis. Locate the patient's loin after draping by palpating through the drapes. Draw an axial line over the drape to indicate a reference for the angle of anteversion formed between this line and the vertical bar of the cup holder (Fig. 16-13, C).
3. Antevert the cup 20 to 30 degrees for cups without an extended long posterior wall. When a cup with 15 degrees anteversion is used, no more than 15 to 20 degrees of anteversion should be allowed.
4. Familiarize yourself with the design of the cup and recommended manufacturing instructions; some cup holders automatically dial 15 to 20 degrees anteversion into the positioning holder (Fig. 16-13, C). In this case no additional anteversion should be allowed.
5. When a long posterior wall is used, make sure that at test rehearsal for stability, with the hip in extension and external rotation, the longer posterior wall does not impinge against the neck of the prosthesis.
6. When a cemented cup is used, the final position (with cement) must be similar to the one used at test rehearsal.

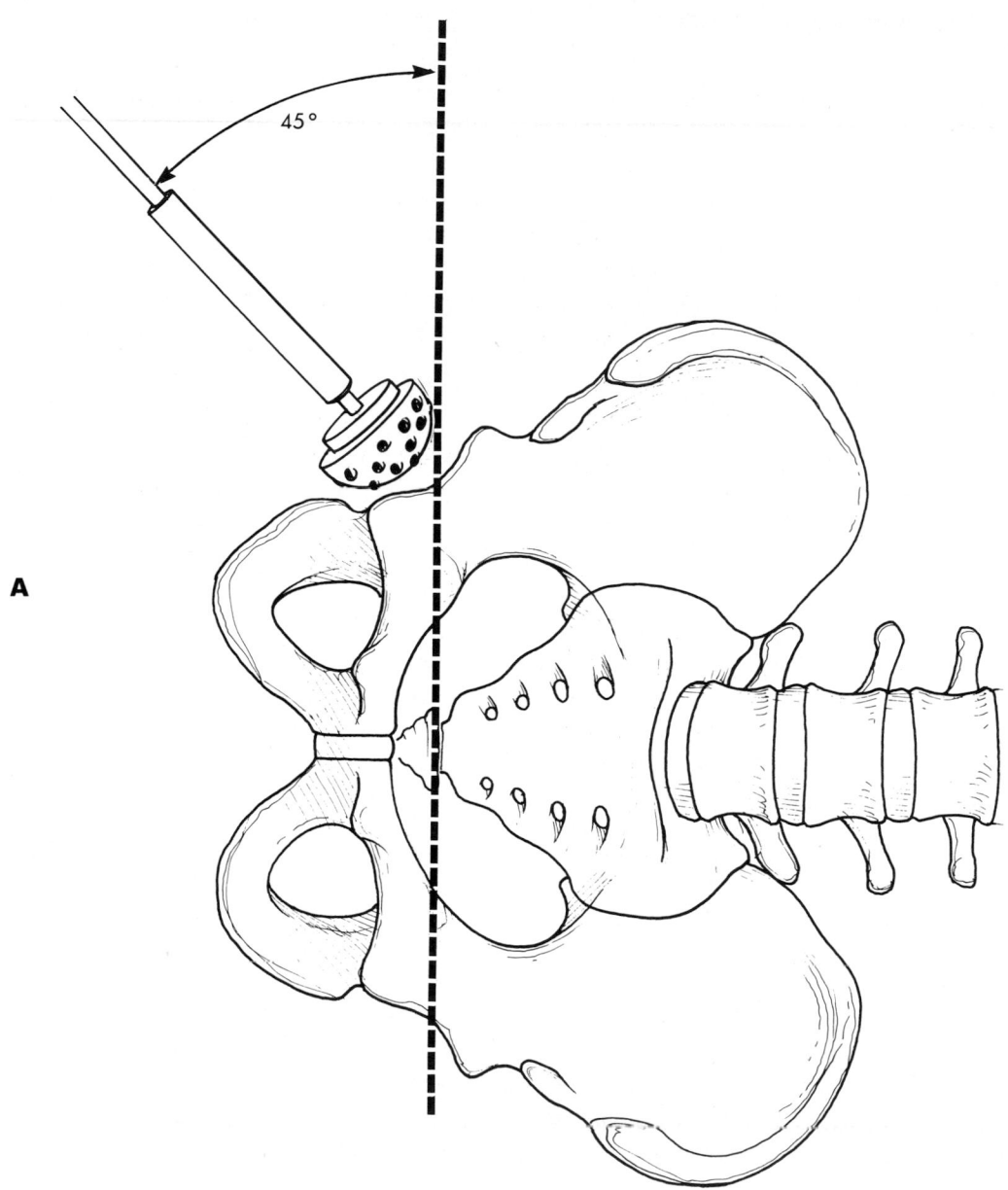

45°

A

Fig. 16-13. A, Demonstrates a 45-degree angle of the reamers to the transaxis of the pelvis (as viewed anteroposteriorly) as designated by a vertical plumbline.

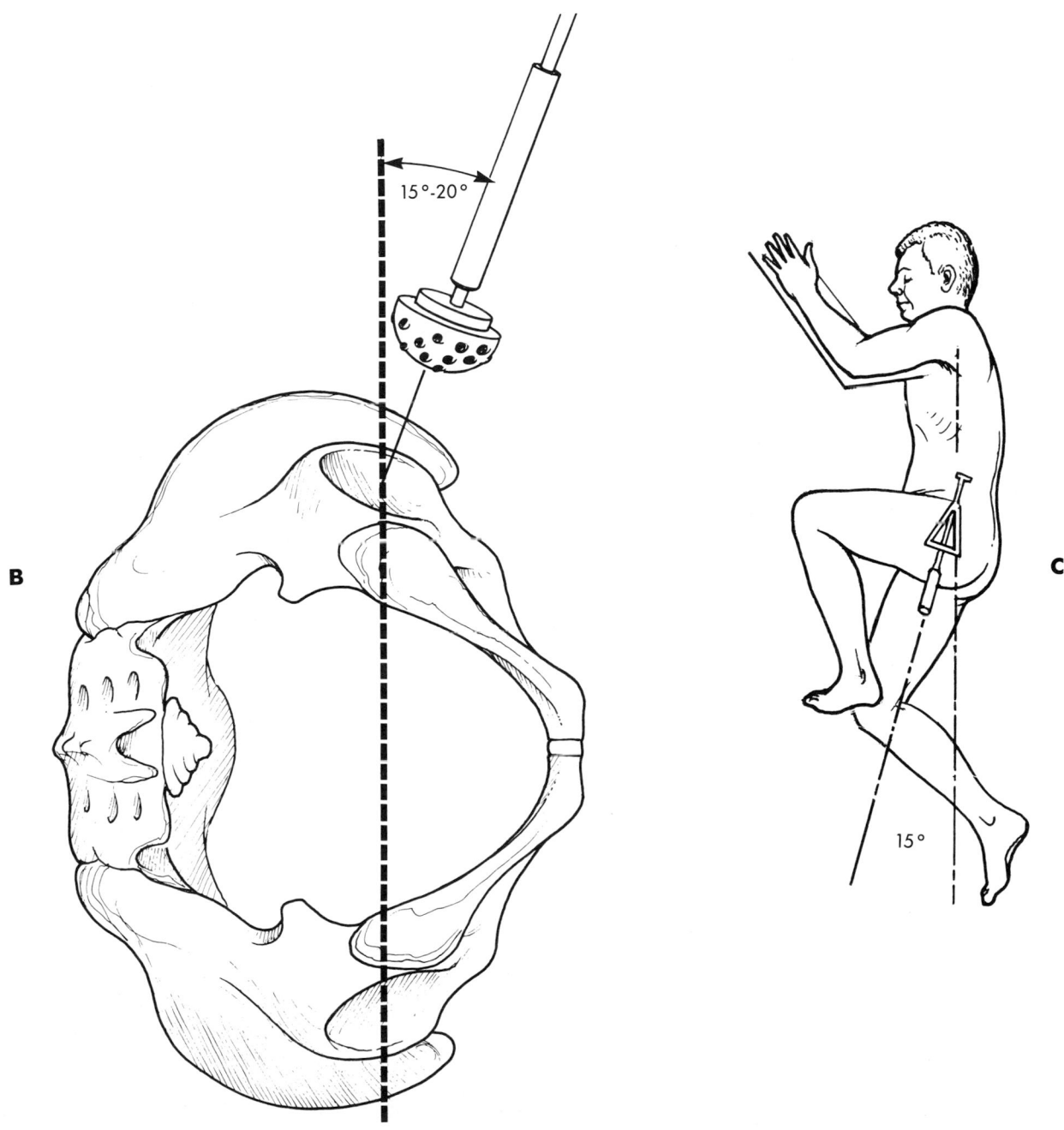

15°-20°

B

C

15°

Fig. 16-13—cont'd. B, Axial view of the pelvis in lateral decubitus demonstrating the angle of anteversion. By a forward tilt of the handle of the reamer to the vertical line (parallel to the transaxis of the pelvis) 15 to 20 degrees anteversion is incorporated. **C,** Most vendors of prostheses offer a "jig" to be used as a guide to properly orient the cup. In some designs, when the guide is properly aligned for the angle of abduction (see **A**), the instrument shows the degree of the anteversion of the cup as well. Note that an imaginary line of the patient's body axis is defined, which must be drawn on the drapes, for reference.

Sizing for Socket Selection and Fixation

The second assistant retracts the femur forward while the surgeon inserts the cup gauges into the acetabulum for sizing. The sizing for a cementless, porous-coated cup must be identical to the one used for gauging. However, the use of cement requires a larger cavity to accommodate both cup and cement. Additionally, during the test for the best fit of the cup, the surgeon must test the trimmed pressure injection cup within the acetabular cavity as it is oriented in the proper alignment (see Chapter 15). In the posterolateral approach, the angle of abduction is easy to determine when it is carried out as follows:

1. Attach the cup to the holder, and align the transverse bar of the holder (the bar adjacent to the cup) parallel to the transaxis of the pelvis, which automatically locates the vertical handle (bar) of the holder parallel to the patient's body axis (Fig. 16-14).
2. Correct anteversion of the cup may be more difficult to estimate in the lateral decubitus position used in this approach. It has been suggested that 15 to 20 degrees of anteversion is desirable to avoid any retroversion. To dial 15 to 20 degrees of anteversion, the vertical bar of the holder must form an angle with the axis of the body. Define the body axis through the drapes, and draw a line on the drapes to define it (as stated previously). Rotate the vertical limb of the cup holder to form an angle with the defined axis of the body. Note that some cup positioners automatically establish the amount of required forward flexion (anteversion) of the cup by aligning the axis of the positioner parallel to the axis of the body. In this way the cup is automatically positioned in 15 to 20 degrees of forward flexion (see Fig. 16-13, C). The cups with a long post wall should never be anteverted more than 15 degrees.

Fixation of the Acetabular Component

Cementing the Cup

FINAL PREPARATION AND ANCHOR HOLES Multiple 6-mm outer-diameter drill holes are drilled throughout the articulating portion of the acetabulum. Large holes (12.5 mm outer diameter) of 1 cm depth are only used in large bony individuals (see Chapter 15). Brush the acetabular cavity using a rotary brush and copious irrigation to remove debris (see Fig. 15-31). Clean the anchor holes with a curette. Before cementing the socket, plug with bone or cement any anchor holes that have inadvertently perforated into the pelvis.

Firmly pack the acetabulum with a large gauze sponge soaked with hydrogen peroxide (see Fig. 15-32, A).

INTRODUCING THE CUP AND CEMENT Make sure that the cup is properly oriented on the cup holder and is clean. Also make sure that insertion of cement and cup remains unimpeded. Insert the cement when it no longer adheres to the surgeon's glove and wrinkles appear on the surface of cement mass (see Chapter 15). Pressurize the cement with a pressurization disk or device, and then insert the cup in a prerehearsed position. Remove the cup holder early if stabilization of the holder cannot be guaranteed. Replace it with a pusher, which is maintained in place until full polymerization occurs. Remove excess cement (see Chapter 15). The following details must be observed:

1. Instruct the second assistant to retract the femur forward to allow easy access to the acetabulum.
2. Insert the inferior margin of the cup into the acetabulum to ensure deep penetration.
3. Make certain that no blood clot is present when inserting the cement. Use suction and irrigate just before inserting the cement (see Chapter 15).
4. When the cup holder is detached and replaced by the pusher, use thumb pressure to maintain the contact between the superior lobe of the flanged cup and bone, since the cup has a tendency to tilt downward during polymerization.
5. Detach the cup holder gently to avoid separating the cement from the bone, especially in the region of the ilium.
6. Insert and remove all fragments of cement before the retractors and the ischial pin retractor are removed.

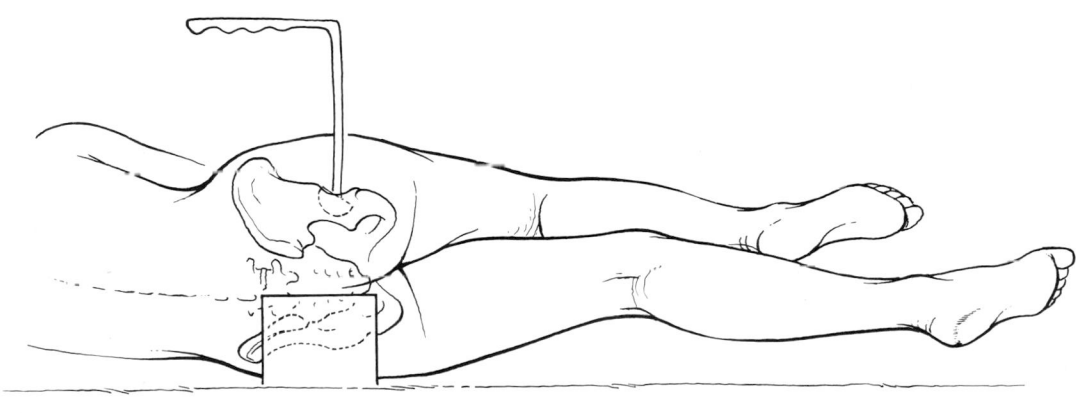

Fig. 16-14. Alignment of the cup in relation to the patient is checked by keeping the transverse bar of the holder parallel to the transaxis of the pelvis, which automatically locates the vertical handle of the holder parallel to the patient's body axis. As such the cup will be automatically oriented at a 45-degree angle in relation to the transaxis of the pelvis and the body axis. (Charnley cup holder is shown for use with a cemented hip system.)

Fixing the Cup by Interference Fit

At this time porous-coated metal shells lined with HDP are favored because of improved clinical results over threaded acetabular cups. The initial fixation of the porous-coated cups is either by interference fit alone* or by adding one or more screws.† Most vendors now produce both types since the indications and advantages of the two types are not well defined. The porous-coated cups are attached to a holder and driven into the bone by impaction in a prerehearsed orientation. The posterolateral approach permits an excellent exposure for inserting the cup and screws (Fig. 16-15). The following details must be observed:

1. Avoid inserting the screw in the anteromedial quadrants of the pelvis to avoid injury to major vascular structures.
2. Follow the manufacturer's instructions regarding the use of instruments and cups. Recommended orientation for most cups is 40 to 45 degrees abduction and 15 to 20 degrees anteversion.
3. Use a flexible (or angulated) drill to allow angulation with its attached drill bit and a variable-axis screwdriver to fix screws of the appropriate length into the cup and bone (Fig. 16-16).
4. The best screw fixation is in the region of the superior and posterior quadrants (Fig. 16-17) (see Chapter 15).
5. Use the insertor and impactor to seat the HDP liner into the metal cup. Ensure a full seating of the liner. Insertion of the threaded acetabular cup is similar to the press-fit cup except for the holder-driver mechanism. The cup attached to the cup is screwed into the acetabulum in a predetermined direction, that is, 40 to 45 degrees of abduction and 15 to 20 degrees of anteversion. Threaded acetabular cups vary in their design: they may be hemispherical, truncated, or have partially porous-coated surfaces. When they are used, the manufacturer's guide must be strictly followed.

---

* Original AML DePuy U.S.A. and PCA (Howmedica International).
† Harris-Galante (Zimmer U.S.A.)

Text continued on p. 772.

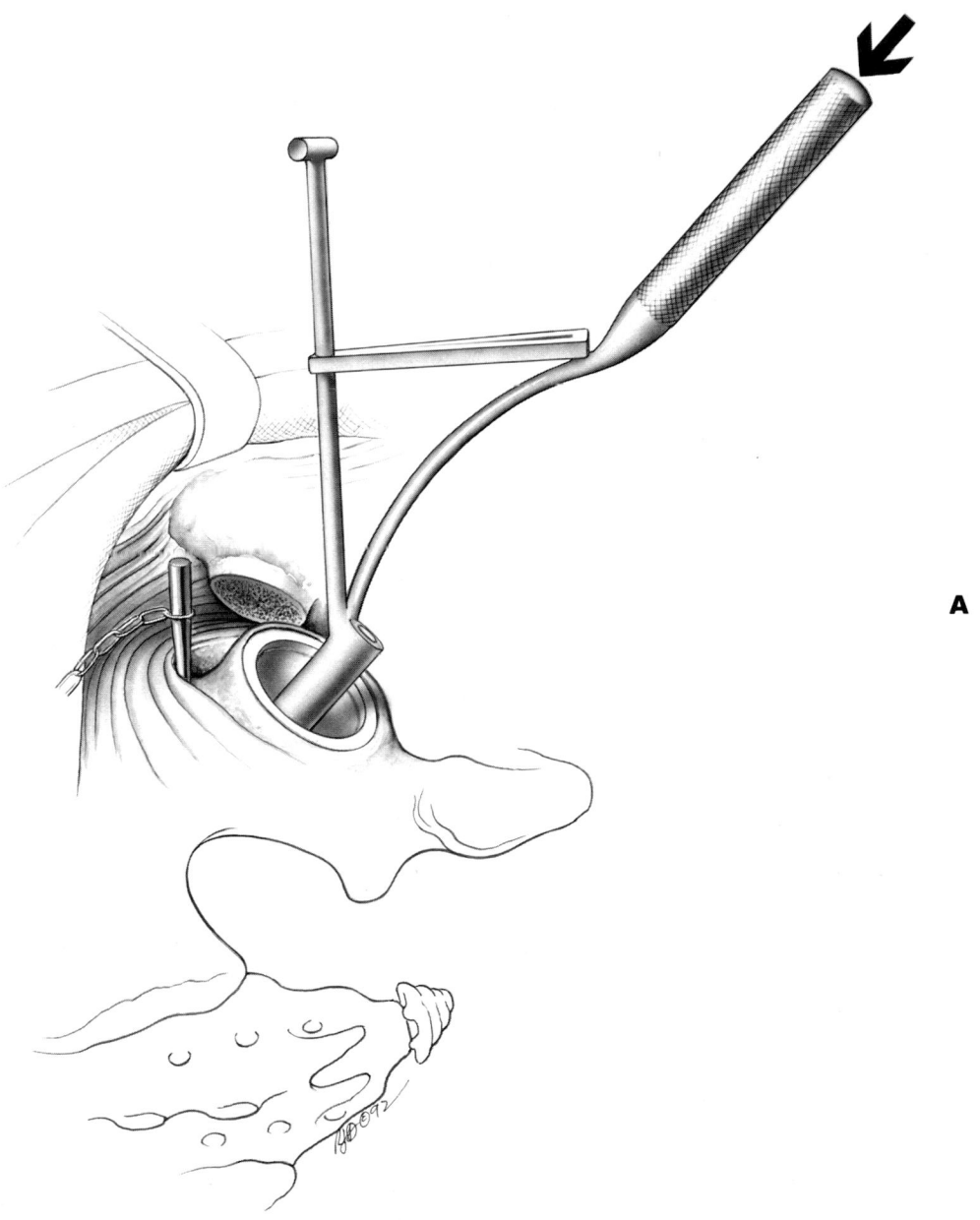

A

Fig. 16-15. A, The positioning of a cementless cup using a more complex cup-holder system. In this cup holder the angle of anteversion has been dialed into handle of the cup holder. Thus, abduction angle also determines 15 to 20 degrees of anteversion of the cup (cup holder designed for Harris-Galante system).

Continued.

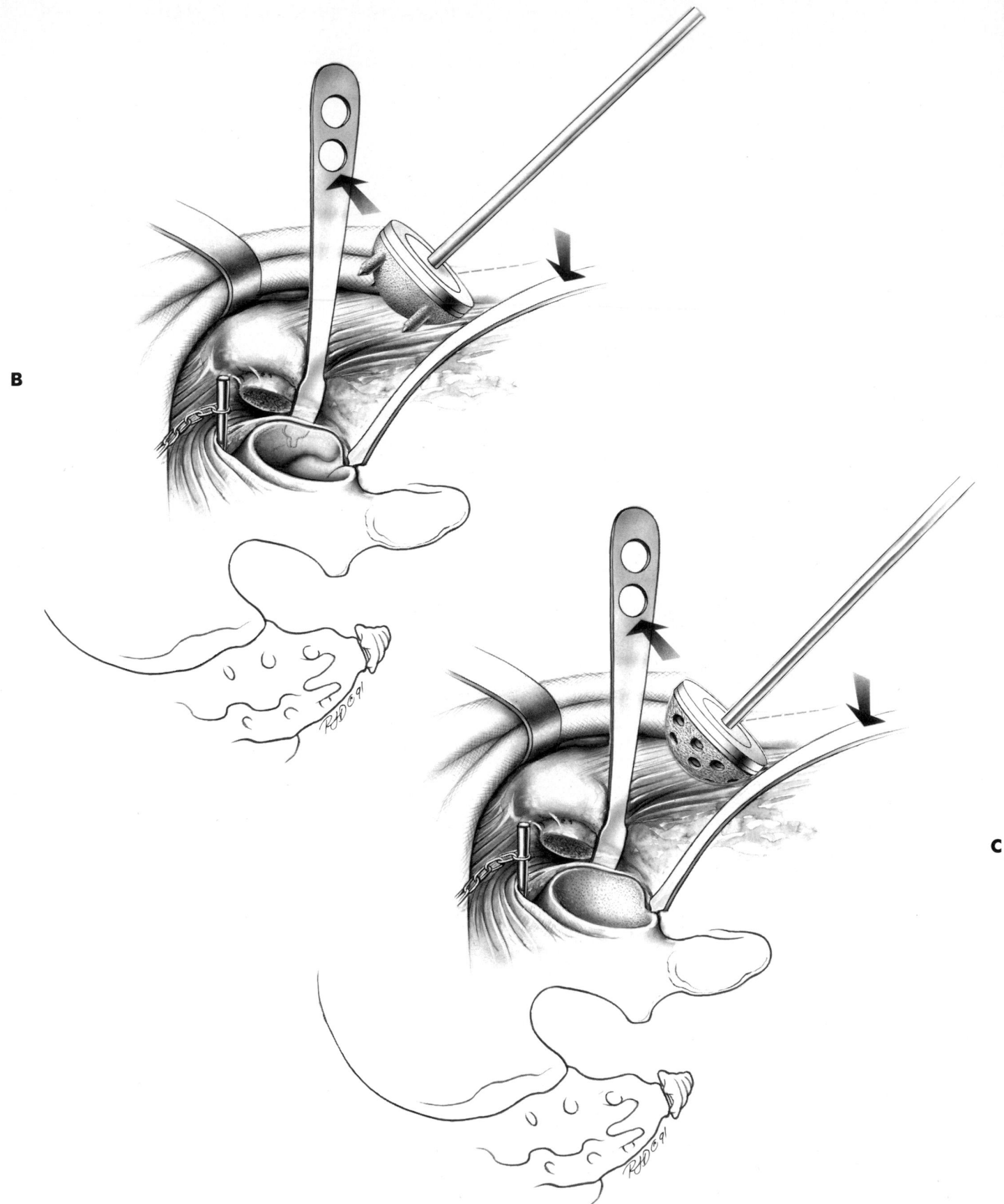

Fig. 16-15—cont'd. B and **C,** The insertion of two contemporary cementless cups. Note that the anterior and posterior retractors need careful and deliberate adjustment to allow unimpeded entry of the cup into the opening of the acetabulum (rim). For demonstration purposes the cup holder is not shown in this illustration.

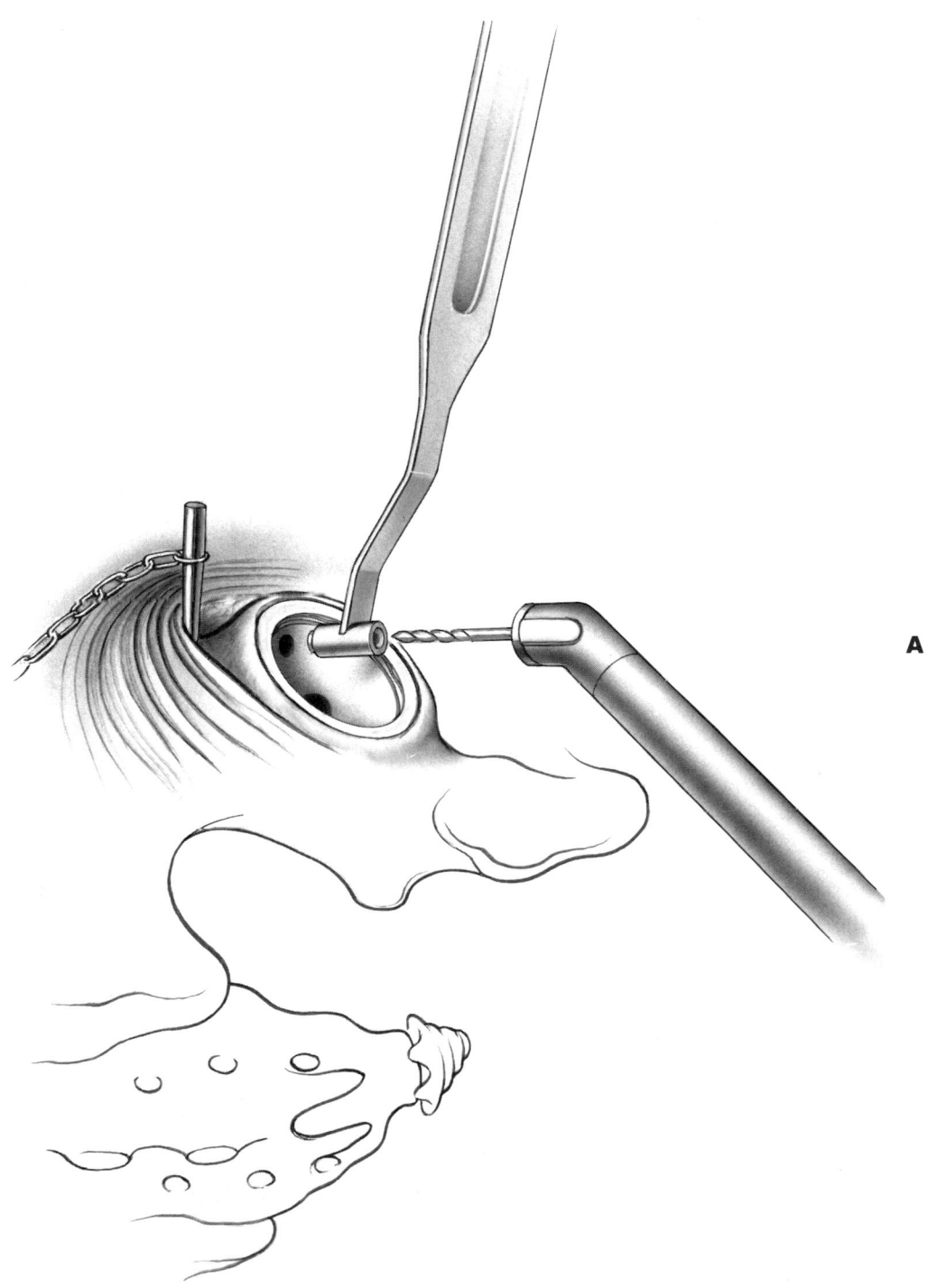

Fig. 16-16. A, For the initial flexion of the cup, occasionally one to three screws are used. An angulated drill is required. Ideally, the screws (two or three) must be located in the superior and posterosuperior region of the acetabulum, never in the anterosuperior or anteromedial quadrant because they can potentially cause intrapelvic damage.

Continued.

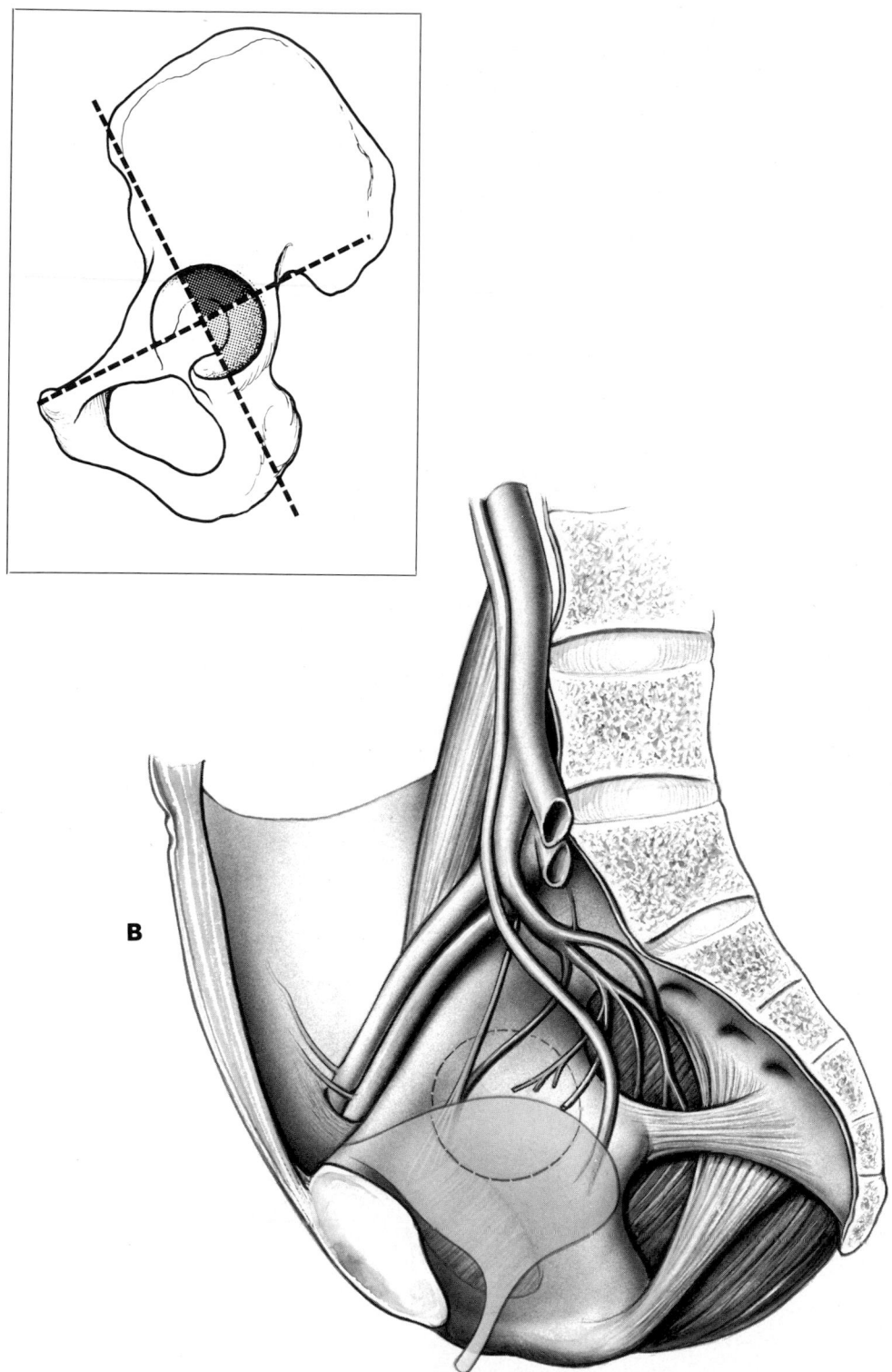

B

Fig. 16-16—cont'd. B, Medial wall of pelvic minor as viewed from opposite side. The corresponding medial wall of the acetabulum is identified by a circle. NOTE: proximity of neurovascular structures to medial wall of acetabulum. **Inset,** Two safe zones for insertion of screws—anterior and posterior—used to fix porous-coated acetabular component *(shaded area).* The other two zones—anterior and inferior quadrants—are unsafe because penetration by drill, depth gauge, or screws may be unavoidable.

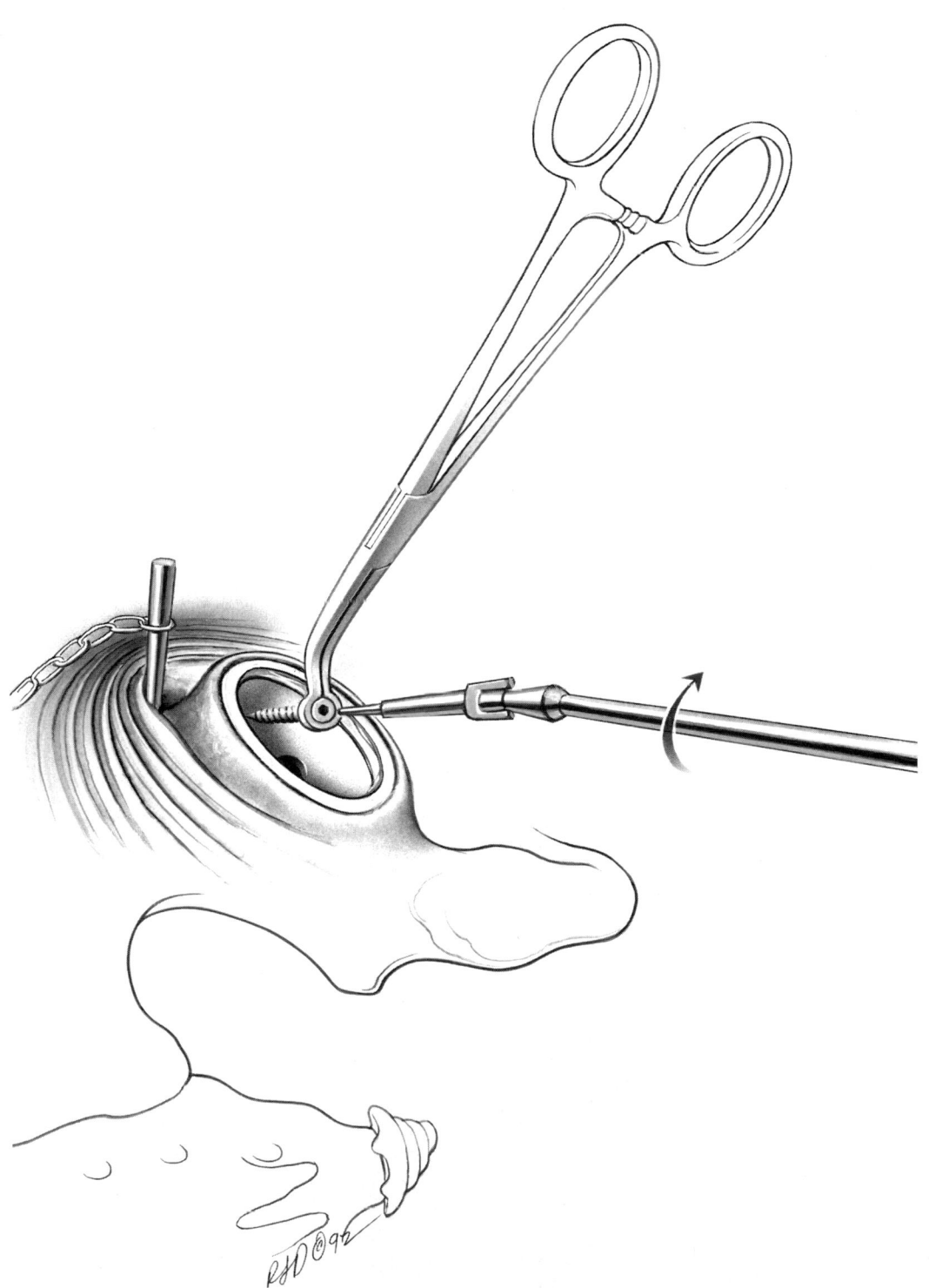

Fig. 16-17. An appropriately sized screw (determined by using a depth gauge) is inserted using a variable-angle screwdriver held by an angulated screw clamp.

PHASE V: PREPARATION OF THE FEMUR, SELECTION OF THE FEMORAL COMPONENT, TEST REDUCTION FOR STABILITY AND LENGTH MEASUREMENTS

For this phase of the procedure the surgeon stands behind the patient.

Delivering the Stump of the Upper Femur

1. Place a clean sponge gauze into the acetabulum and behind the femur to prevent debris and marrow from entering the acetabulum.
2. Protect the skin edge (posterior flap) with a towel.
3. Position the leg across the table (away from the surgeon) with the knee at a right angle. The hip is flexed 60 to 80 degrees as the lower leg (tibia) is held by the second assistant at a right angle to the floor (Fig. 16-18).
4. Release capsule, iliopsoas tendon, or both to mobilize the femur as needed. Detachment of the gluteus maximus insertion to the femur may also be required.
5. Place the femoral neck retractor under the neck to present the stump of the upper femur out of the wound.

The femoral neck retractor (see Fig. 16-18) is designed to be engaged to the neck by a specially designed tip. By exerting a fair amount of pressure on the retractor, the second assistant can produce a good exposure of the end of the femur. The following details must be observed:

- The surgeon should be positioned just proximal to the hip as he or she works on the femur.
- Avoid excess force, which can damage the bone or soft tissue.
- Adjust the amount of hip flexion until good access to the femur becomes possible.
- The second assistant must keep the leg stationary; otherwise the femoral retractor can disengage.

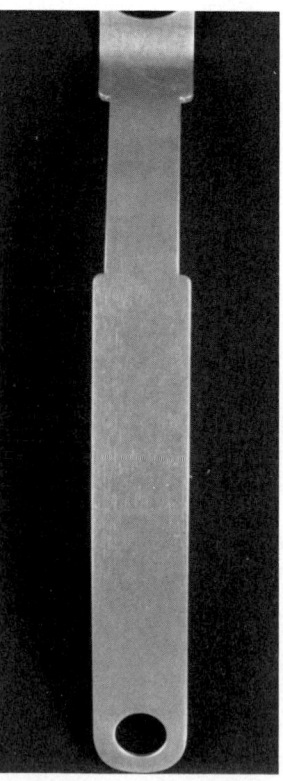

Fig. 16-18. See legend on opposite page.

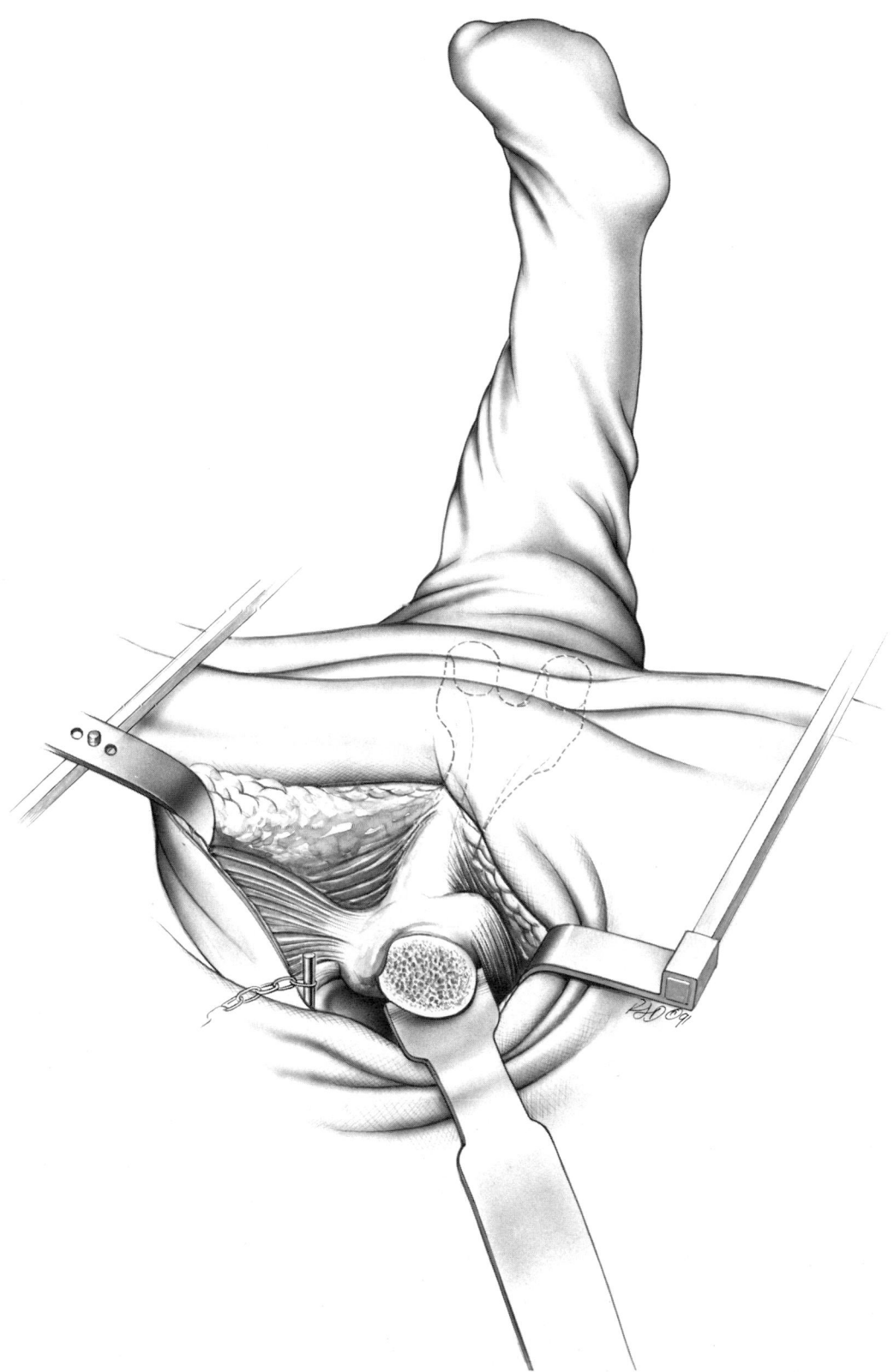

Fig. 16-18. In preparing the upper femur the leg must be internally rotated to 90 degrees and the stump of the femur must be delivered out of the wound by a femoral retractor. It is necessary to mobilize the femur by soft tissue release before preparing the femur.

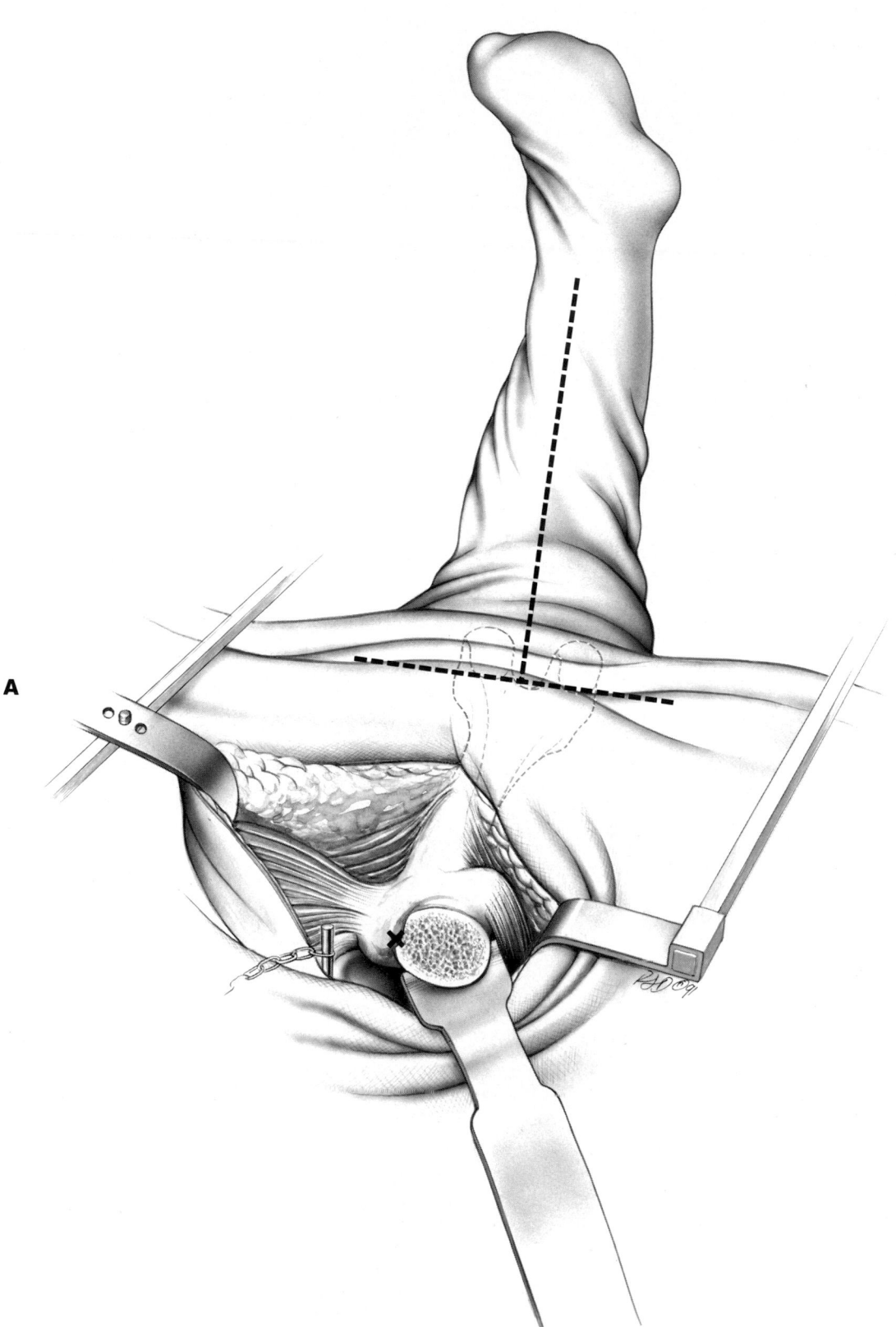

Fig. 16-19. A, The right angle of the leg in relation to the transcondylar line as viewed by the surgeon. The cross on the top of the femur shows the point of entry to the femur at the site of the digital fossa of the greater trochanter.

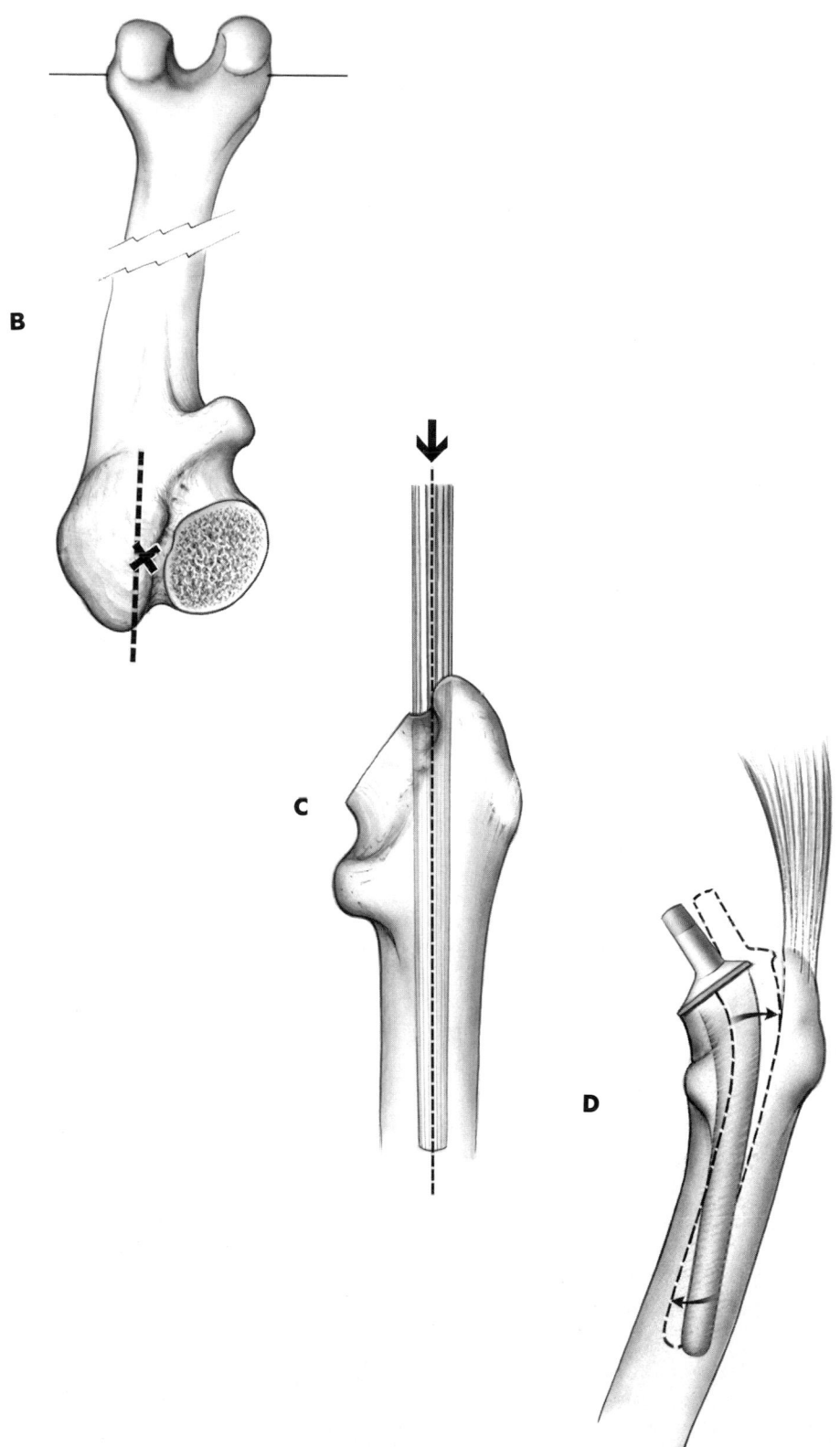

Fig. 16-19—cont'd. B, The overhang of the greater trochanter, which must be removed to enter the medullary canal. **C,** Note the encroachment into the bed of the trochanter to directly access the medullary canal, **B. D,** The importance of preparing the canal correctly by beginning at the digital fossa, **A,** and entering the medullary canal as lateral and posterior as possible, **B.** If a special effort is not made to lateralize the entry to the femur, a varus positioning is inevitable. Arrows indicate the correct placement of the stem *(dotted line).*

Preparing the Medullary Canal

Locate and remove all the soft tissues, including the stump of the piriformis tendon, from the digital fossa using an electrocautery knife before preparing the bone. Note the relationship of the tip of the greater trochanter to the neck, and become familiar with the reverse position of the femur (as viewed from the surgeon's vantage point upside down). This is caused by the lateral position of the patient and the 90-degree internally rotated limb (Fig. 16-19, *A*). Make sure that the upper femur is accessible and that the superior acetabular pin retractor does not interfere with the insertion of the reamers and broaches.

Find the medullary canal by inserting a quarter-inch (6 mm outer diameter) drill bit just anterior to the digital fossa but as lateral as possible into the base of the trochanter (Fig. 16-19, *A* to *D*). Trim away the tip of the trochanter using a rongeur or a burr (which prevents entry of the femur in a lateral position as needed). Enlarge the drill hole by rotating the drill handle concentrically to allow insertion of a T-handle tapered pin canal finder. The correct entry is very important when preparing for most cementless prostheses, because the track of the predrilled entry forms a path for subsequent larger straight reamers (see Chapters 11 and 15).

To prepare the metaphysis of the femur, use a boxed chisel (also known as *cookie cutter*) to map and remove the cancellous and cortical bone from the top of the femur. This is the first step in the mediolateral reaming of the medullary canal. Observe the following details:

1. Place the leg with the knee at a right angle to be sure that the femur is internally rotated and the lower leg is perpendicular to the floor (ignore the position of the foot) (see Fig. 16-19, *A*).
2. Place the boxed chisel in the correct position to map the desired anteversion for the prosthesis (Fig. 16-20). The boxed chisel must include the drill hole and be placed as lateral and as close to the rise of the trochanter from the neck of the femur as possible. Use a rongeur or burr as indicated to remove bone from the tip of an overhang trochanter to ensure lateral placement of the boxed chisel. Dial 10 to 15 degrees of anteversion, which generally corresponds to the anteversion of the neck of the femur (Fig. 16-20, *A*).

    While hammering the boxed chisel be sure it is well laterally and posteriorly orientated. Correctly remove a small wedge of bone posteriorly and laterally along the line of the orientation of the medullary canal.
3. Initiate the valgus and correct plane of anteversion by appropriate positioning of the boxed chisel.

Expanding the Isthmus and Metaphysis

To accommodate the prosthesis, the fit of the stem proximally (metaphysis) and distally (diaphysis) must be considered independently. Preparation of the femur for cemented or cementless devices (both anatomical and straight stems) varies. Designs and concepts for fixation of cementless devices change constantly, so careful study of the newer implants is required. The related techniques (as described by the originator of the design and in the manufacturer's recommendation) must be individually followed (see Chapters 11 and 15).

Reaming and Preparing Cemented Stem

Pack the acetabulum behind the femur with a swab to prevent reamed marrow from entering the wound.

A rotary reamer with a blunt tip attached to the powered reamer is directed straight into the femur from the lateral opening of the medullary canal (the site of the digital fossa). Penetrate the reamer to its full depth (14 cm), then ream in a medial direction toward the neck of the femur. Expand also in an anteroposterior direction to accommodate the flanged prosthesis (see Chapter 15). Use a curette to remove all loose cancellous bone, especially from the proximal, medial, and calcar region of the neck.

Use a curved broach or a large curette to remove cancellous bone from the lateral aspect of the femur to accommodate the convexity of the stem and flange in the region of the greater trochanter.

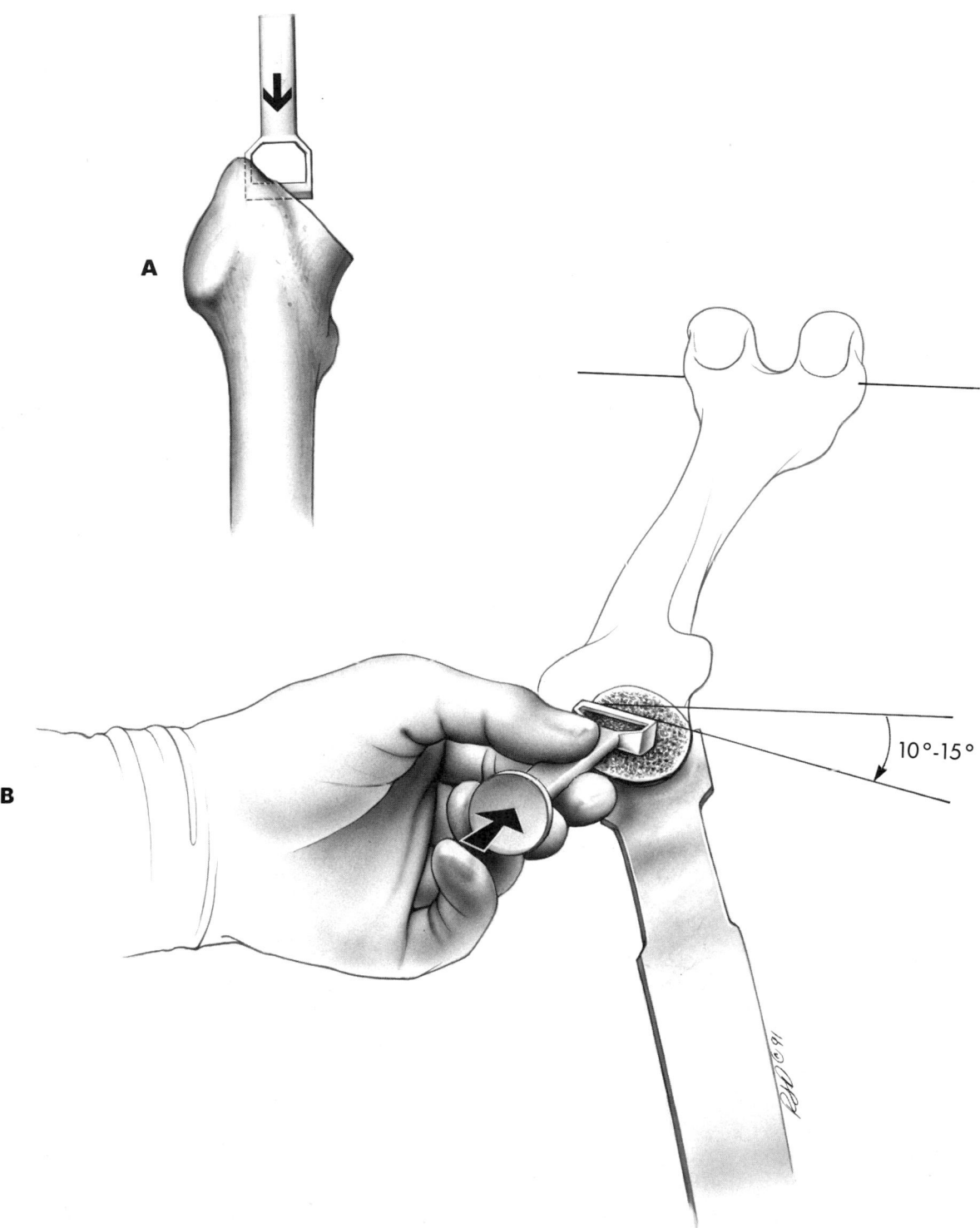

Fig. 16-20. A, Place the boxed chisel so as to map *(dial)* the desired anteversion for the prosthesis *(arrow).* The boxed chisel must be as laterally placed as possible to include the site of entry by the drill at the digital fossa of the greater trochanter. **B,** Note that the transcondylar line of the femur with the knee at a right angle is the only reference by which a correct angle of anteversion can be dialed.

Use broaches for sizing and final preparation as desired.

1. Ensure good quality of bone endosteally for fixation in high-priority areas (critical load-bearing zones): proximal, medial, and distal lateral.
2. Reduce the test prosthesis as it is entered proximally and distally, avoiding any varus or retroversion of the stem.
3. Prevent fracture of the femur by careless rotation of the femur before placing the head into the socket at reduction, especially in severely osteopenic femurs.
4. Use a pusher to guide the head into the acetabulum while the assistant applies longitudinal traction along the femur.

Preparing to Insert the Stem Without Cement

The technique for prosthesis fixation by interference fit varies based on the design of the prosthesis, which should have one of the following features:

1. Only proximal fit
2. Proximal and distal fit
3. Anatomical fit (curved stems)
4. Nonanatomical fit (straight stems)
5. Identical fit (customized)

The posterior approach is suitable for preparing and inserting all types of stems. The instrumentation and insertion technique of most designs are well developed and vary little from manufacturer to manufacturer (see Chapter 15).

Selection of Prosthesis and Sizing

Based on various factors, the surgeon may choose a cemented, porous ingrowth, or mechanical interference fit prosthesis. The rationale and scientific basis for selection of the stem were discussed in Chapters 6, 11, and 15. The surgeon may change his or her mind intraoperatively as to the type of prosthesis, based on pathological findings such as osteoporosis of bone, bone defects, and so on. At times, it may be difficult to achieve a good fit and fill of the stem in the cavity of the femur. Therefore regardless of the patient's age, sex, or weight, the choice may be weighed toward the use of cement. Most prostheses currently available (cemented or cementless) can be conveniently inserted through a posterolateral approach. Cementless devices in particular require less exposure of the top of the femur. Therefore the routine use of the posterolateral approach is highly recommended for this type of prosthesis.

Test Reduction

Because the posterolateral approach (without detachment of the trochanter) is more prone to postoperative dislocation than other approaches, a careful test rehearsal should be made before cementing or inserting cementless devices. Testing for dislocation in vulnerable positions (that is, flexion and adduction, flexion and internal rotation, and extension and external rotation) is mandatory when using the posterolateral approach. The ability to flex to 120 degrees and adduct to 30 or 40 degrees (with slight flexion) and externally rotate to 40 degrees without dislocation indicates stability. Additionally, the hip should be stable in combinations of 90 degrees of flexion and 45 degrees of adduction or internal rotation without neck-socket impingement or anterior dislocation (see Chapter 15). Any stability observed and attributable to malpositioning of either component must be corrected by a reorientation of the prosthetic component. An added long posterior wall feature to the cup and the use of a longer neck prosthesis can also be considered.

Measure the leg length (the distance between the superior acetabular pin and the point marked for reference on the femur), avoiding any lengthening on the leg if hip stability can be ensured* (see Chapter 32).

---

* Regrettably, overlengthening of the ipsilateral limb by this approach is occasionally unavoidable.

At test rehearsal the following details must be observed:

1. Note the relationship of the neck of the prosthesis to the femoral neck. In wide medullary canals or when an undersized prosthesis is used, the stem tends to be unstable and drifts into a varus position. A flanged stem is more stable than a nonflanged stem (inside the medullary canal). A nonflanged stem or an undersized stem may subside within the medullary cavity during test reduction, thus producing a false impression regarding the true neck length and the stability of the prosthesis.
2. Prevent axial rotation of the stem within the canal, which may produce a false impression regarding the proper axial orientation (anteversion/retroversion) of the stem.
3. Observe the coverage of the prosthetic head by the cup while the hip is positioned in a neutral and anatomical position for abduction/adduction, flexion/extension, and internal/external rotation (see Chapter 15).
4. Any instability in flexion and internal rotation or extension and external rotation should alert the surgeon to the possibility of malalignment or a short neck.
5. Determine the soft-tissue tension by applying strong traction to the hip (with knee flexed), and observe the separation of the two components. No more than 5 mm separation should be accepted (see Chapter 15).
6. Measure the distance between the acetabular pin retractor and the femur. Note the changes in the leg length produced by the prosthesis.

Final Preparations

As in all other approaches, curettes must now be used to remove all remaining marrow and bone debris from the medullary canal. Also remove loose cancellous bone from the medial neck, and plug the medullary canal with a bone block after brushing and irrigating the canal (see Chapter 15). Now organize the required instruments, including the prosthesis, and stage the process of insertion of the stem and cement (when used).

PHASE VI: REHEARSAL AND INSERTION OF CEMENT, STEM, AND REDUCTION
Rehearsal Before Introducing Cement

Because of limited exposure of the top of the femur before introducing cement, follow the following steps:

1. Place a clean swan (sponge) into the acetabulum, and pack one behind the femur.
2. Flex the knee to 90 degrees, and maximally rotate the femur internally.
3. Deliver the stump of the femur out of the wound with the femoral neck retractor while the first assistant maintains the position of this retractor.
   With the prosthesis inserted into the holder, rehearse inserting the stem into the canal, noting the desired centering of the stem proximally and distally (see Chapter 15 and 17).
4. Drape the stump of the femur with a fenestrated towel, and insert the medullary venting tube (if a cement gun is not used). Pack the canal with a 5-cm-wide gauze ribbon soaked with hydrogen peroxide (see Chapter 15).

Observe the following details:

- Wear a third pair of gloves before handling the cement.
- Prosthesis must be held firmly in the holder.
- Note that the correct size (stem and neck) has been applied to the holder.
- Note orientation of the stem in the holder.
- Remove sharp bony spicules from the opening of the femur.
- Ensure that the prosthesis can be easily inserted without impediment. Observe the amount of space between the medial side of the neck and the prosthesis.
- The second assistant must be instructed to maintain the position of the leg by supporting the knee and resist the force the surgeon uses as the cement or stem is inserted into the medullary cavity.

Inserting the Cement
Delivering the Cement by Syringe (Cement Gun)

Routinely use two packets of cement (40 ml) when cementing the femoral component. Pressurize the cement using thumb pressure or a device such as a cement compactor, remembering that maximum pressurization is generated when the stem is being inserted (see Chapter 15).

Observe the following details:

1. Avoid mixing blood with cement. In the posterolateral approach, inserting cement by thumb pressure can be difficult, so delivery by a cement gun may be advantageous.
2. When cement is inserted by thumb pressure, use the fleshy part of the thumb against the opening of the femur to act as a piston. Careful hemostasis in the abductor region is necessary to avoid contamination of the cement with blood.
3. The second assistant must be instructed to hold the knee and resist the force the surgeon applies to the femur while cement is being inserted.

Inserting the Stem

Organize the required instruments and prosthesis before inserting the cement. Do not allow anyone to handle the stem in the holder. Inappropriate handling such as dropping the stem off the table or soiling it with bloody hands can be disquieting because the cement must be immediately removed before it is polymerized. Insert the stem deliberately in the prerehearsed alignment while the femur is kept in the prerehearsed position of 90 degrees to the floor. Insert the stem steadily, and maintain the proper orientation (for valgus and rotational alignment), without changing the position after half of the stem has been inserted. Inclining the holder toward the greater trochanter is preferred because it is usually corrected at full insertion. Never attempt to force the stem into a valgus once it has been fully inserted. Maintain the position of the stem with a lightweight holder until the cement is completely set.

Note the following details:

1. Because access to the top of the femur is limited, slowly inserting the stem into the cement, especially in a narrow medullary canal, can be disastrous since the cement may harden before the surgeon can insert the stem fully into the canal. Use the cement while it is less polymerized for the narrow canals.
2. When the stem meets severe resistance, change the direction of insertion slightly to facilitate insertion.
3. Use a hammer when more than half the length of the stem is in the canal and it resists further advancement. Hammer blows must be gentle. The direction of the stem is controlled with the operator's opposite hand.
4. Keep the holder attached to the prosthesis until cement is fully polymerized (see Chapter 15).
5. Remove excess cement before full polymerization.

Performing Reduction

Before reduction, ensure that no foreign matter is in the acetabular cavity and that irrigation precedes reduction. For reduction, adequately retract the soft tissue to allow unimpeded delivery of the head into the depth of the socket. Avoid contact between the femoral head and metallic instruments to prevent damage and the resulting rapid wear of the HDP cup. Hip reduction must reveal a stability similar to that achieved at trial. A push-pull test with heavy traction should reveal no more than 5 mm separation between the two components. Copiously irrigate and debride devitalized tissue about the hip before inserting drains and performing wound closure.

PHASE VII: SHORT ROTATOR REATTACHMENT; CAPSULAR REPAIR; CLOSURE OF FASCIA, FAT, AND SKIN; APPLICATION OF DRESSING AND SPLINT

Reattaching the Short Rotators

Place the operated leg on the contralateral limb side. By internally rotating the leg, visualize the stump of the short rotator tendons. Insert three to four stay sutures (each with a double entry and exit) to the detached short retractors (as piriformis is already tagged). Clamp the end of each pair of sutures with a hemostat.

Drill four holes (using a 2-mm outer diameter bit) 10 to 15 cm apart onto the trochanteric crest in a lateral to medial direction (Fig. 16-21). Mark each hole with a marking pen. Pass a 1.5-mm crochet hook to retrieve each pair of stay sutures from the back of the femur (Fig. 16-22). Insert two medium-sized drains, from distal to proximal, into the joint before fastening the short rotators or capsule to the femur. Fasten the sutures while the leg is placed into neutral without abduction or adduction and is maximally externally rotated (Fig. 16-23).

Observe the following details:

• Consider including all or a portion of the capsule in the repair when a good layer of capsule is available.
• Do not excise the capsule if it was not repaired; it will scar in place.
• Protect the sciatic nerve using a Watson-Jones gauge while the drilling is done or the crochet hook is being inserted to retrieve the sutures.

Reattaching the Gluteus Maximus Tendon

Place one or two additional sutures to attach the gluteus maximus tendon to its stump on the femur. Do not tie these until the Charnley initial incision retractor is removed.

Closure and Postoperative Care

For details of closure of fascia, fat, and skin, see Figs. 15-54 to 15-56. Postoperative care is discussed in Chapter 13.

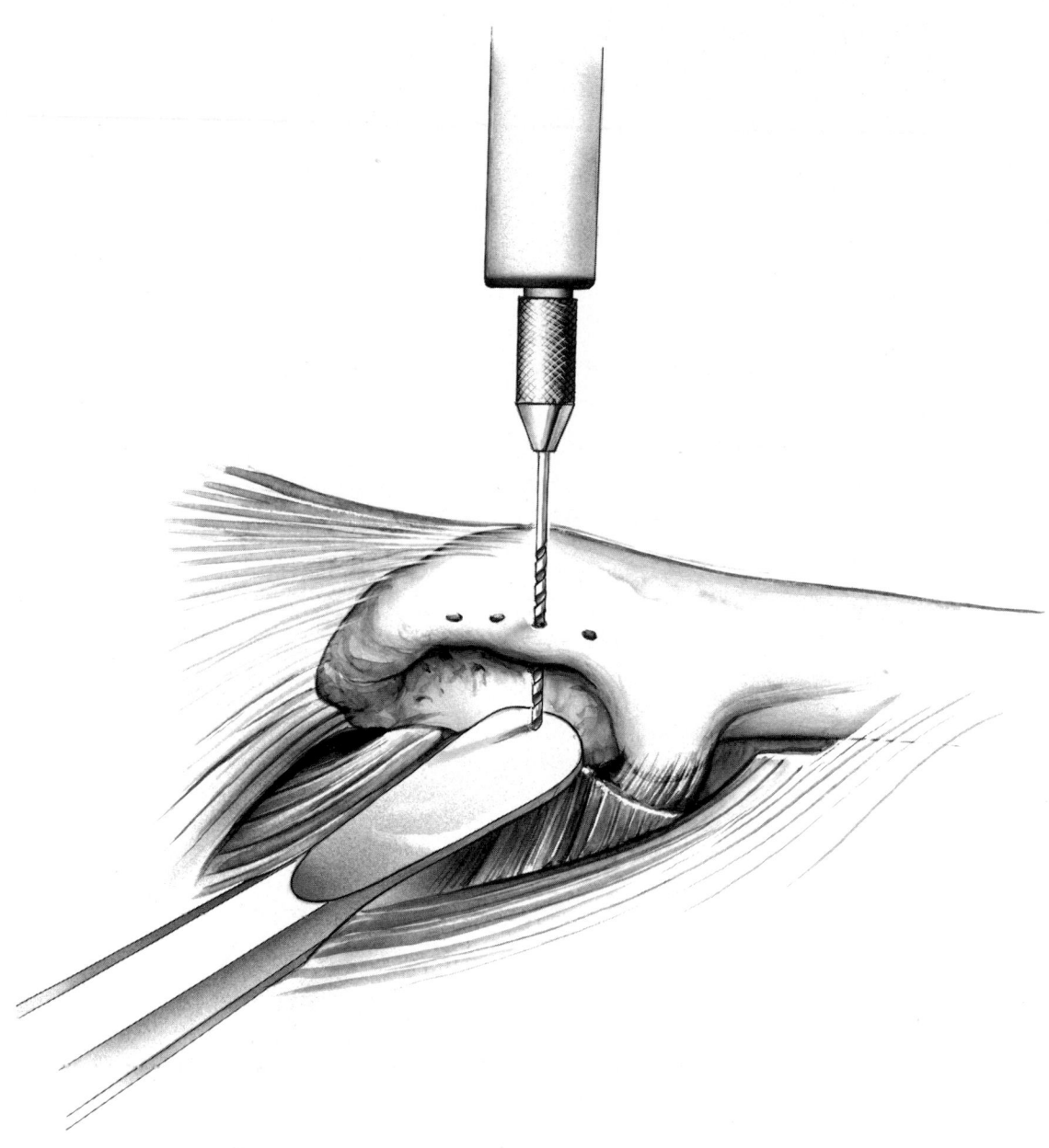

Fig. 16-21. Three or four drill holes are used to fasten the short rotators back to the crest of the trochanter.

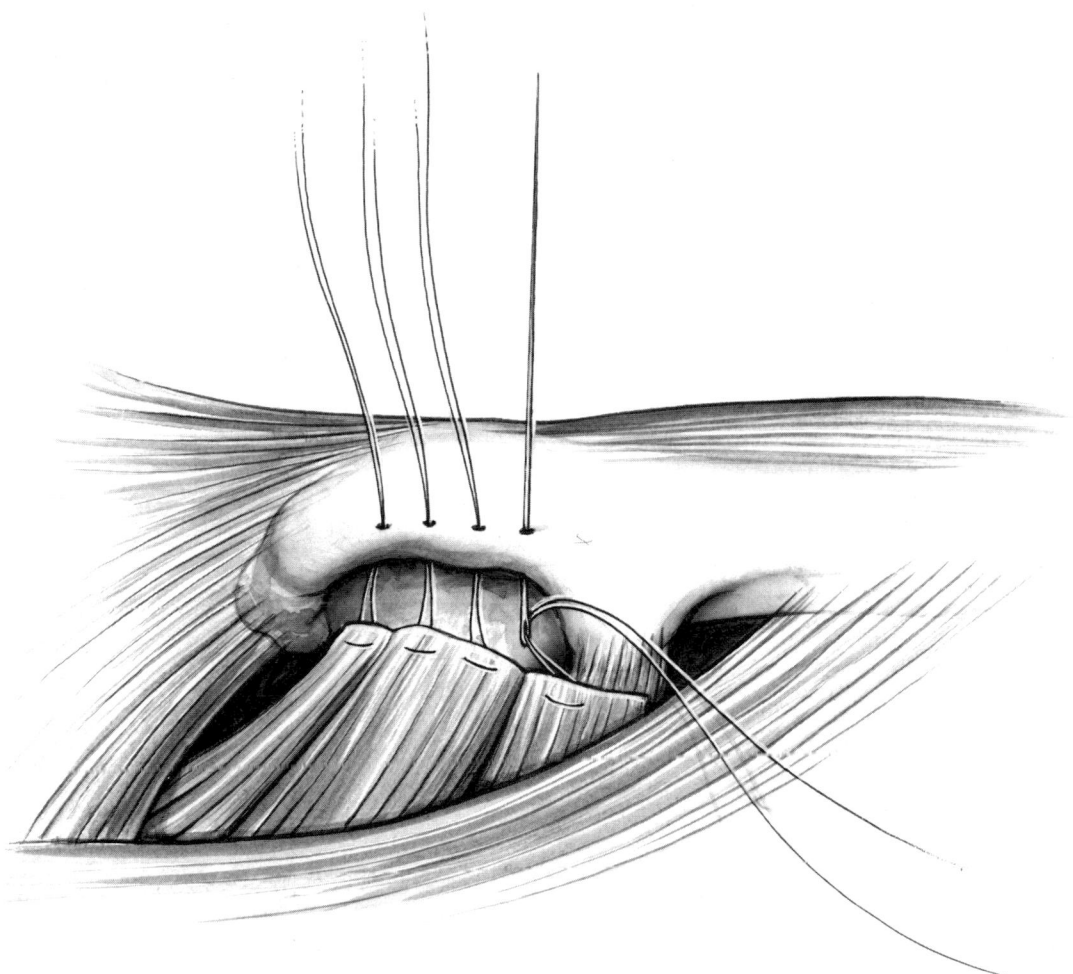

Fig. 16-22. The sutures attached to the short rotators are passed through the holes previously drilled.

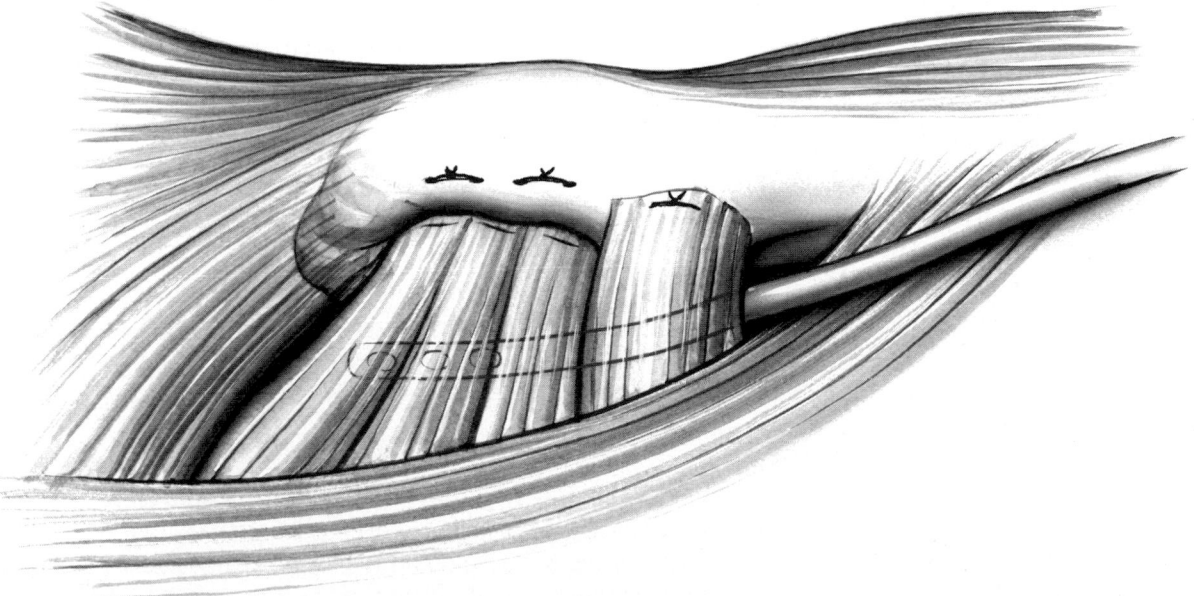

Fig. 16-23. The sutures are tied over the bone after inserting the drain into the posterior aspect of the joint. The detached gluteus maximus tendon is now reattached to the femur (not shown).

SUMMARY OF ESSENTIALS

- Phase I includes positioning. Preparation and draping are described in Chapter 15.

- Phase II begins with the surgical exposure. Center the skin incision over the femur distally, and extend from a point 6 to 8 cm distally to the vastus lateralis ridge to the top of the greater trochanter. Proximally incline the incision posteriorly toward the posterior superior iliac spine for a distance of 8 to 10 cm. Open the fascia along the skin incision, which should locate the exposure along the posterior margin of the gluteus medius and minimus and the midportion of the upper femur.

- Detach the gluteus maximus tendon insertion to the femur as distal as needed to mobilize the femur. Detach the short rotators from the femur by first identifying the key muscle in this region, the piriformis.

- Elevate the short rotators to expose the posterior capsule. Incise the capsule superiorly and inferiorly, but reflect it posteriorly toward the rim of the acetabulum, and insert the pin to retract the abductors. The pin will also act as a landmark for leg length measurement intraoperatively. Mark a fixed point on the femur within the vicinity of the vastus tubercle. Measure the distance between the fixed point of the pelvis and the femur before dislocating the hip.

- Begin to dislocate the hip by adducting, flexing, and internally rotating the hip. Be sure that a complete capsular release is carried out, avoiding undue force on the femur to prevent fracturing the femur. Amputate the femoral head at a preplanned level based on the template measurements as the femur is held at 90 degrees internal rotation and two narrow flat Hohmann retractors are placed, one inferiorly and one superiorly, at the neck of the femur. Avoid damaging the soft tissue and shortening the femur too much. The correct neck length adjustment can be made later.

- Phase III includes dislocating the hip, incising and mobilizing the capsule, and exposing the femoral neck using periacetabular retractors. Dislocation is carried out by adduction and internal rotation only after mobilization of the femur. This phase will be completed after amputation of the femoral head at an appropriate level.

- Phase IV includes acetabular exposure, preparation, and fixation of the acetabular component. During this phase the surgeon stands in front of the patient as he or she works on the acetabulum. Further capsular release may be required to mobilize the femur, which is best accomplished by inserting a clamp along the margin of the acetabulum and detaching the capsule from the pelvis.

- To maximize the exposure of the acetabulum, insert a Hohmann retractor onto the iliopubic ramus near the ilium, and retract the femur forward. This maneuver can be facilitated by proper positioning of the limb. Avoid damage to the iliopubic ramus by placing the tip of this retractor closer to the ilium than pubis.

- Expose the entire bony rim of the acetabulum by excising the labrum and redundant capsule. Then expose the posterior rim by retracting the retained capsule by inserting a second pin engaged to the ilioischial ramus.

- Define and expose the lower margin of the acetabulum by inserting a second Hohmann retractor under the transverse acetabular ligament within the intracotyloid notch of the pelvis.

- Exposing the pulvinar is of fundamental importance to delineate the true medial wall of the acetabulum. Remove the medial osteophytes and ligamentum teres using a long-handled Volkmann spoon.

- Ream the acetabulum in an inferior position to medialize it, then perform general reaming to expand and deepen the acetabulum as needed. A precision fit is a prerequisite for a cementless device. If a cemented device is used, a larger acetabular cavity is created to accommodate the cement and the cup. Prepare the final anchoring holes, and do final refinement for insertion of the acetabular component. Brush and irrigate the acetabulum if cement is used.

- In a cementless device, a good bleeding surface should be provided to promote bony ingrowth into the porous surface of the cup. With the patient in a lateral decubitus position, positioning the cup at 40 to 45 degrees abduction poses no difficulty. However, special care is required to produce adequate anteversion for the cup. A 20- to 25-degree anteversion has been recommended in this approach, which must be dialed into the cup holder at insertion. A long posterior wall cup may be used if the hip is not stable with flexion and adduction of the hip. Careful positioning of the cup in the lateral decubitus position is very important, since the hip may be more prone to dislocate posteriorly with this approach than with any other. The details of cup fixation with and without cement are similar to other approaches described in this text (see Chapter 15).

- Phase V includes preparing the femur, selecting the femoral component, and performing test reduction for stability and length.

- Deliver the stump of the upper femur out of the wound. Position the leg across the table away from the surgeon's side as the surgeon stands behind the patient. Release the capsule and the restrictive connective tissue, including the iliopsoas tendon to mobilize the upper femur if needed. Place the femoral neck retractor under the neck to present the stump of the upper femur out of the wound.

- Locate the digital fascia of the trochanter, and insert a 6-mm drill hole to locate the entry to the femur as lateral and posterior as possible. Trim away the tip of the trochanter if it prevents correct entry to the femur. Use a box chisel with proper anteversion for insertion. Locate the box chisel as lateral and posterior as possible to create proper alignment for inserting the prosthesis. Expand the isthmus and metaphysis until the largest-caliber prosthesis can be inserted. Use rotary reamers to expand the upper femur if a cemented stem is used. Use appropriate broaches to expand the medullary canal for cementless devices.

- Phase VI includes rehearsal and insertion of cement/stem and reduction.

- Select the correct size stem. Insert a provisional prosthesis to test for stability and leg length. A careful test rehearsal before cementing or definitive insertion of the cemented device is mandatory. The hip must be stable in extreme degrees of flexion, adduction, and internal rotation, as well as extension and external rotation. Measure and determine the elongation or shortening of the limb.

- Perform the final preparation of the medullary canal by curetting, brushing, irrigating, and packing the canal before inserting the cement. For a cementless stem, also ensure that the debris is removed and a proper orientation of the stem is rehearsed before insertion. Insert a medullary plug before cement insertion.

- Deliver the cement with a cement gun or manually. Pressurization is achieved by thumb pressure, a compactor, or both. Final pressurization is achieved by inserting the stem. Be sure that the prosthesis is held firmly in the holder. Note correct orientation at insertion, and maintain the position of the leg as the stem is introduced. The assistant must block the opening of the canal to prevent extrusion of cement. Cement must not adhere to the surgeon's glove at delivery. Remain immobile until the cement is fully polymerized. Remove excess cement, and perform a test reduction for stability and range of motion of the hip.

- Phase VII includes reattachment of short rotator and capsule and wound closure. Reattach the short rotators through drill holes to the back of the femur, insert drains, and close the fascia, fat, and skin. Also use a superficial drain and retention sutures at closure.

REFERENCES

1. **Gibson A:** Posterior exposure of the hip joint, *J Bone Joint Surg* 32[Br]:183, 1950.
2. **Henry AK:** *Extensile exposure*, Edinburgh, 1960, E & S Livingstone.
3. **Marcy GH, Fletcher RS:** Modification of the posterolateral approach to the hip for insertion of femoral head prosthesis, *J Bone Joint Surg* 36:142, 1954.
4. **Moore AT:** The self-locking metal hip prosthesis, *J Bone Joint Surg* 39:811, 1957.
5. **von Langenbech B:** Vorstellung cines falles von geheilter enterotomie verhandl, *Deutsch Gesellesch Chir* 740, 1878.

See Chapters 11, Choice of Implants and Customization; 13, Postoperative Management; 15, Principles Common to all Surgical Approaches; and 17, Anterolateral and Transgluteal Approaches for additional information.

CHAPTER SEVENTEEN

Anterolateral and Transgluteal Approaches

- If the right instruments are used and if some points of technique during the operation are carefully considered, you will be soon able to do 80% to 90% of THRs without removal of the greater trochanter. The operation is much easier and quicker.

Maurice Müller

ANTEROLATERAL APPROACH

- The operation is described in seven phases.

PHASE I: POSITIONING, PREPARATION, AND DRAPING

See Chapter 15.

PHASE II: SURGICAL EXPOSURE OF THE HIP
Skin Incision

Place the incision straight laterally for approximately 15 to 20 cm just anterior to the greater trochanter and centered over the trochanteric ridge (tubercle).[2] Some surgeons prefer a curved incision. Begin 2 to 3 cm posterior to the level of the anterosuperior iliac spine, then curve the incision anteriorly and laterally to the trochanter. Extend it 4 to 6 cm to the level of the vastus lateralis ridge (Fig. 17-1) on the lateral surface of the femoral shaft.

Fascial Incision and Exposure

Open the fascia along the skin incision and iliotibial band. Separate it from the underlying vastus lateralis distally and the gluteal fascia proximally, revealing the gluteus medius muscle fibers. This is best accomplished by blunt dissection. The anterior border of the gluteus medius is the landmark while it inserts into the trochanter over a relatively wide area. Loose areolar tissue and fat facilitate blunt dissection between the gluteus medius and tensor fascia femoris muscle, where the anterior capsule can be visualized. A self-retaining retractor, such as a Charnley initial retractor, facilitates and maintains the exposure throughout the operation.

Detaching the Gluteus Medius and Minimus

Retract the anterior fibers of the gluteus medius proximally with a Richardson retractor. Sharply divide the anterior attachment of the gluteus muscle from the femur. Identify and sharply divide the tendon of the gluteus minimus with a curved clamp, place tension on the tendon, and retract it away from the femur. Detaching both the gluteus medius and minimus requires subsequent repair. Cut the tendon of the gluteus minimus 1 cm proximal to its attachment to the anterior surface of the trochanter (see Chapter 2), and tag it with a "stay suture" for subsequent repair. Alternatively, a small fragment of bone may be detached with the tendon and secured using a single screw.

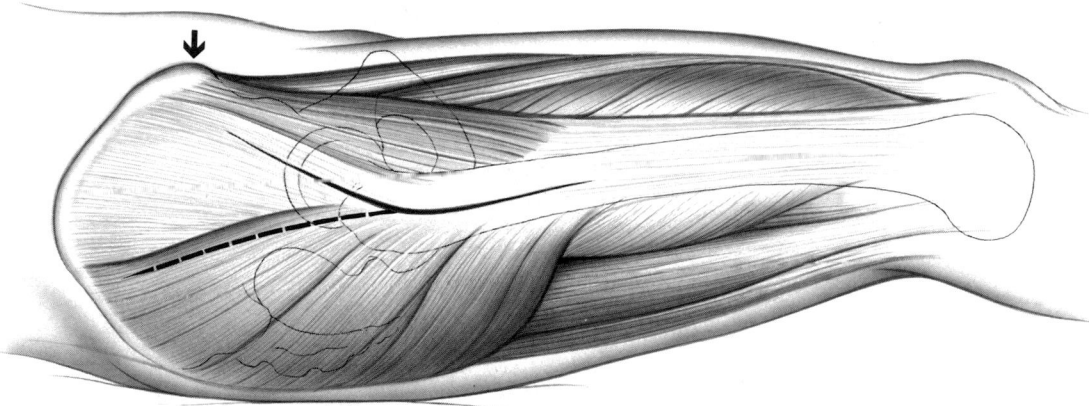

Fig. 17-1. Place the patient on the operating table in supine position. Anterolateral approach to the hip (described by Watson-Jones) uses a curved incision with its proximal limb extending toward the anterosuperior iliac spine. This line of skin incision facilitates the exposure of the interval between the tensor fascia femoris medially and the anterior border of the gluteus medius posteriorly. NOTE: in performing total hip arthroplasty, a straight incision is preferred because it is more extensile than a curved one. It should be located along the anterior border of the femur distally and extended toward the posterior superior iliac spine.

Capsulotomy and Capsulectomy

Anterior capsulectomy is performed after three pointed retractors are inserted, one inferior to the neck, one superior to the neck, and the third medially over the anterior rim of the acetabulum. Before inserting the pointed Hohmann retractors, use a broad and sharp periosteal elevator or a sharp 1-inch curved osteotome to peel off the soft tissue and visualize the capsule in preparation for capsule excision. A note of caution is indicated here; the anterior retractor must be judiciously inserted because the femoral nerve and vessels can be damaged if the tip of the retractor is not fully engaged to the iliopubic ramus and if it is placed into the soft tissue away from the bone (see Chapters 33 and 34).

A capsulotomy is performed using a T incision along the periphery of the acetabulum and medial portion of the neck (Fig. 17-2).

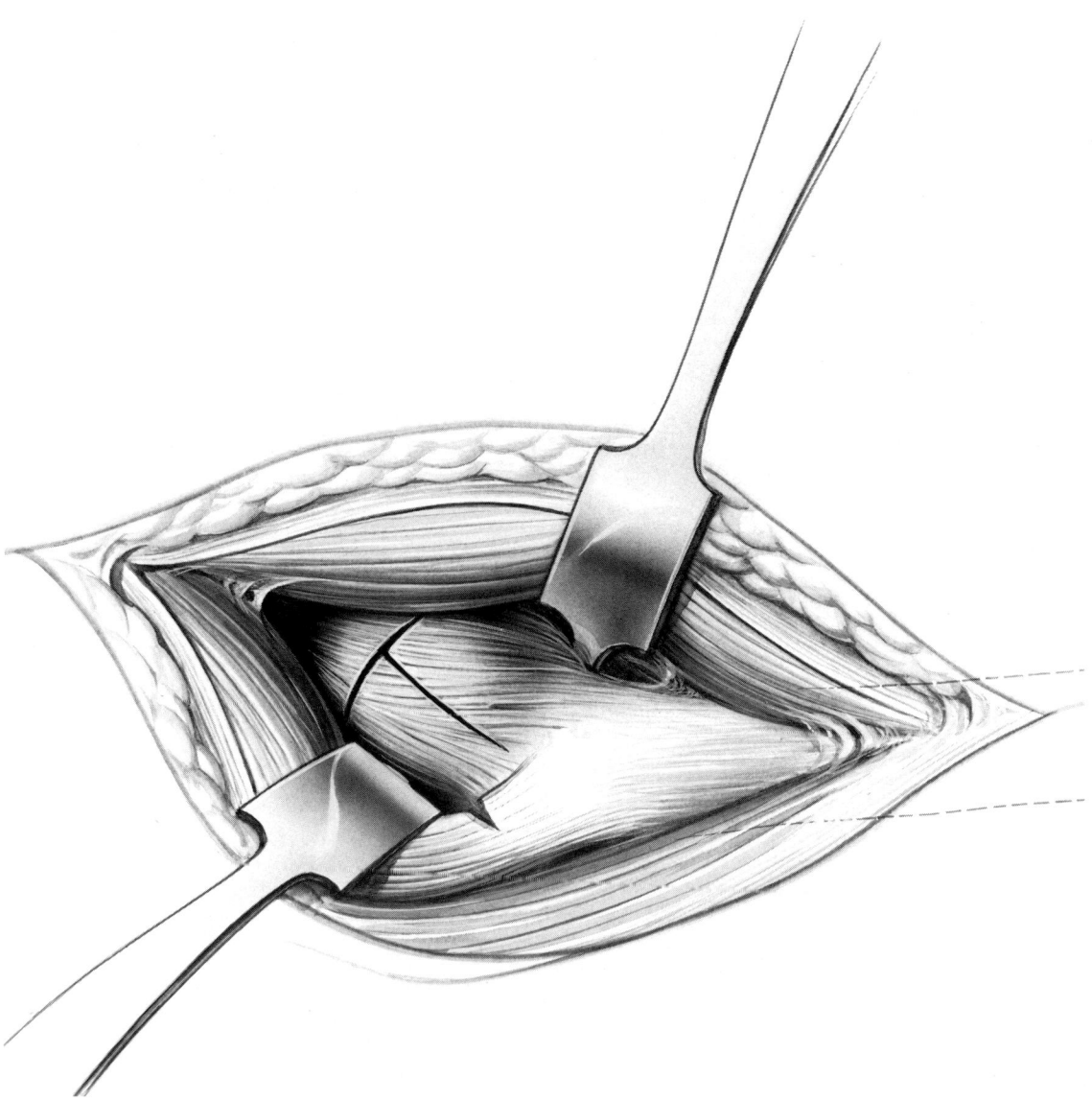

Fig. 17-2. The anterior capsule is exposed by retracting gluteus medius posteriorly and tensor fascia femoris anteriorly. Heavy retraction of gluteus medius and minimus is necessary to visualize width of neck and periphery of capsule. A portion of gluteus medius and minimus tendon may have to be detached to provide exposure. T-shaped incision of capsule facilitates complete capsulectomy, which is necessary for this exposure.

Excise the anterior capsule using a heavy-jawed Kocher for retraction and a knife or heavy-duty cartilage scissors. The surgeon must constantly be aware of potential injury to the femoral nerve, artery, vein, and the psoas tendon, which may lie very close to the anterior and inferior capsule (Fig. 17-3).

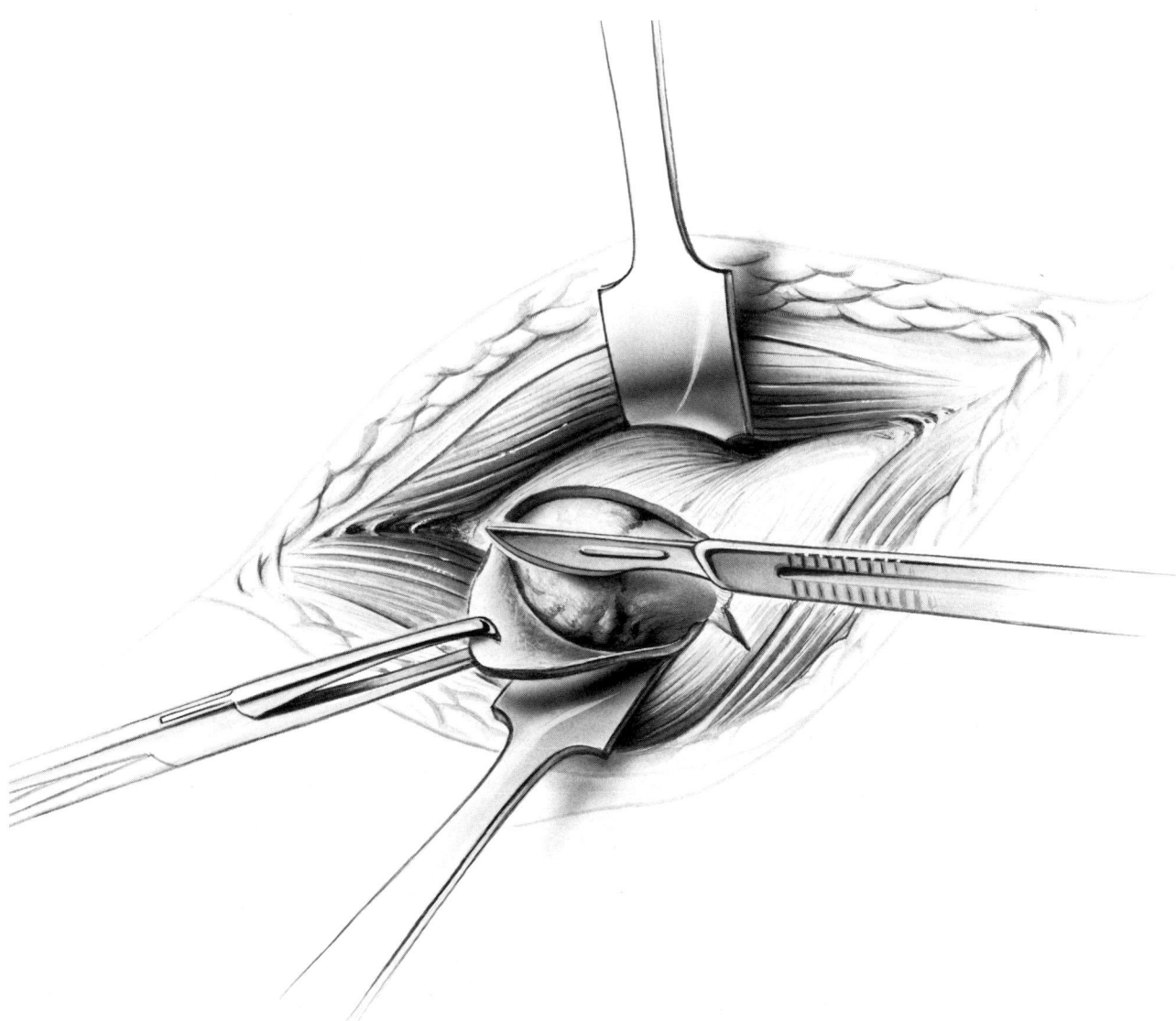

Fig. 17-3. Complete capsulectomy is essential to visualize head and periphery of acetabulum. Leg is positioned in somewhat external rotation. A heavy-jawed Kocher clamp retracts the capsule while capsulectomy is performed.

PHASE III: DISLOCATING THE HIP

Before dislocating the hip, make sure that a complete capsulectomy is done to provide a good view of the anterior margin of the acetabulum. Remove the anterior or superior marginal osteophytes when present. Instruct the second assistant, on the opposite side of table, to dislocate the hip by adduction, external rotation, and extension. Use of excessive force may fracture the femur, especially in stiff hips with marked osteoporosis. Place a hip skid such as a Watson-Jones gouge between the head and the roof of the acetabulum to facilitate dislocation. When dislocation is difficult, consider osteotomy of the trochanter (see Chapters 18 and 19), or remove the head in a retrograde fashion after in-situ osteotomy of the neck to avoid fracturing the femur (Figs. 17-4 and 17-5).

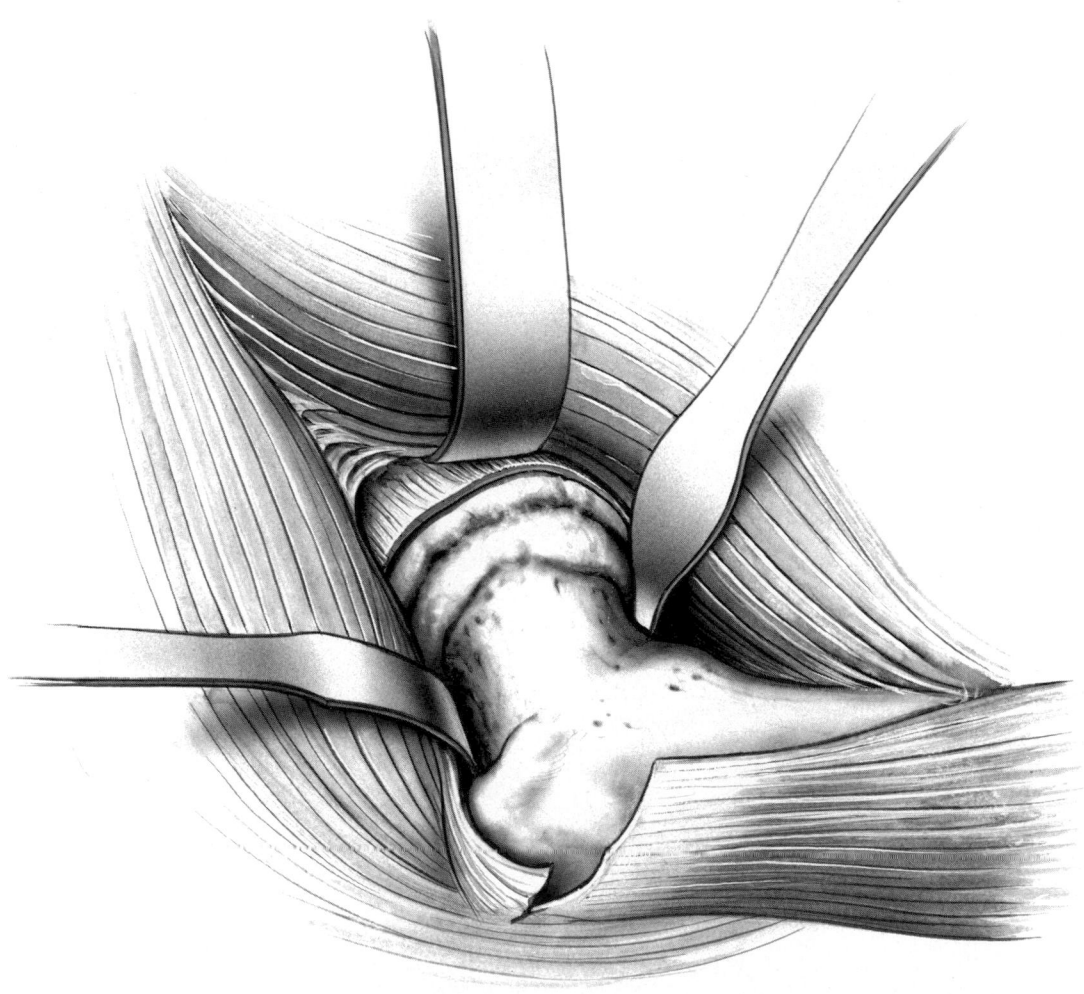

Fig. 17-4. After a complete anterior capsulectomy, heavy retraction of the glutei is required to expose the neck. NOTE: unless a portion of the gluteal attachment is released from the femur, severe damage to the anterior fibers of gluteus medius and damage to the superior gluteal nerve to the tensor fascia femoris may occur. By placing two Hohmann retractors (one inferior and one superior to the neck), damage to the gluteus medius and tensor fascia femoris can be avoided.

In-Situ Osteotomy of the Neck

After a complete capsulectomy, place two Hohmann retractors, one superior and the other inferior to the neck, to protect the soft tissues. Use an oscillating saw to cut the neck at a desired level, which is determined based on preoperative templating (see Fig. 17-5). When severe shortening is present, osteotomy of the neck may be carried out in two steps: (1) section the neck high at the subcapital level, and (2) readjust the neck length by shortening it based on the desired neck length to accommodate the soft tissues, required neck length, and stability of the joint.

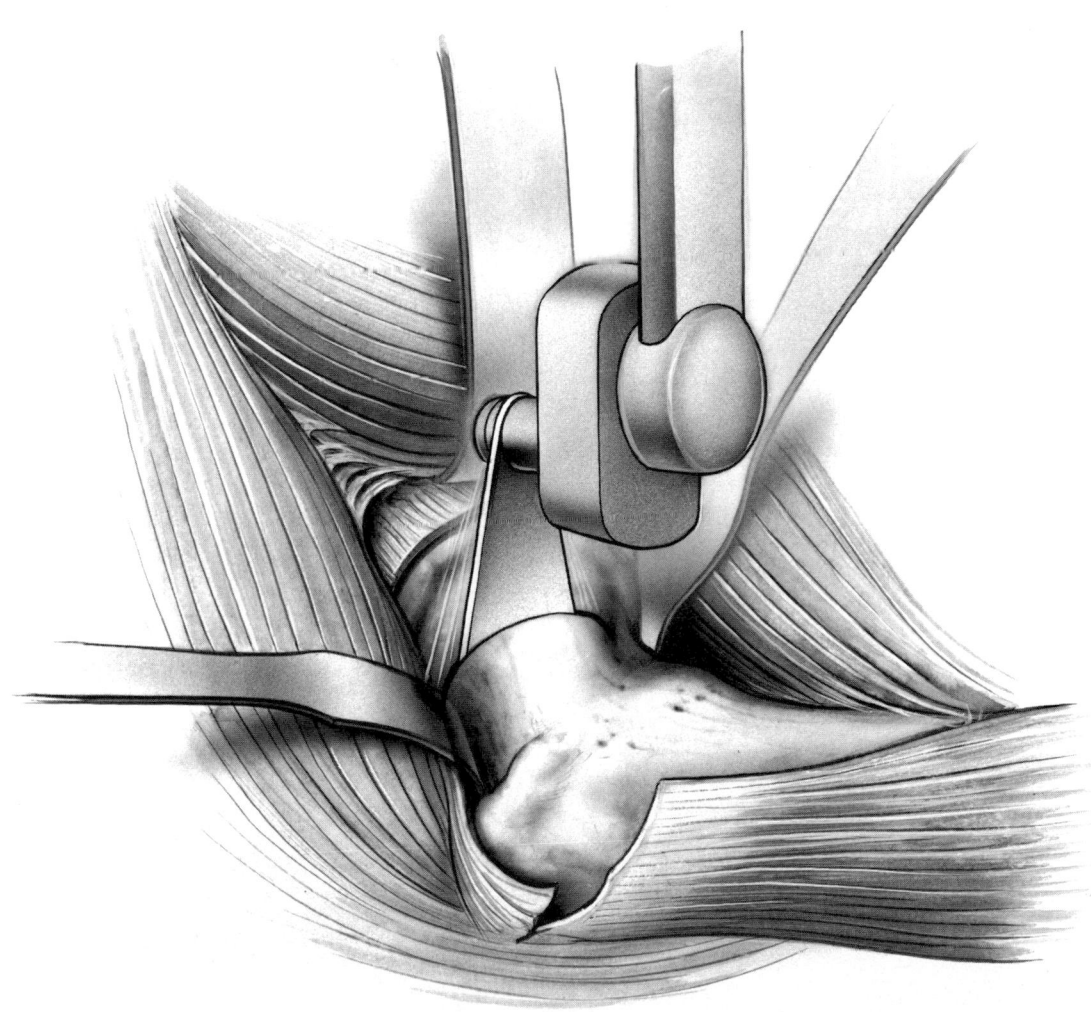

Fig. 17-5. An in-situ amputation of the neck is carried out using an oscillating saw. The femoral neck should be transected to leave a long neck on the femur. This can be revised (shortened) as needed at a subsequent step in the operation. Note the position of Hohmann retractors during the amputation of the head. The hip must be positioned in 10 to 15 degrees of abduction and maximum external rotation.

Removing the Femoral Head

Lever the head out of the acetabulum after separating the neck and the head with an osteotome (Fig. 17-6). Extract the femoral head in a retrograde manner by inserting a "corkscrew"-type instrument into the head (Fig. 17-7).

When dislocating the hip by this approach, observe the following principles:

1. Never apply a forced torsion to the femur for fear of fracturing the femur.
2. In osteopenic patients with rheumatoid arthritis, osteotomize the neck in-situ, and remove the femoral head in a retrograde fashion before dislocating the hip.
3. When protrusio acetabuli or extreme stiffness is present, use a transtrochanteric approach.
4. Train the second assistant carefully in the correct position of the leg and the amount of force to produce dislocation.

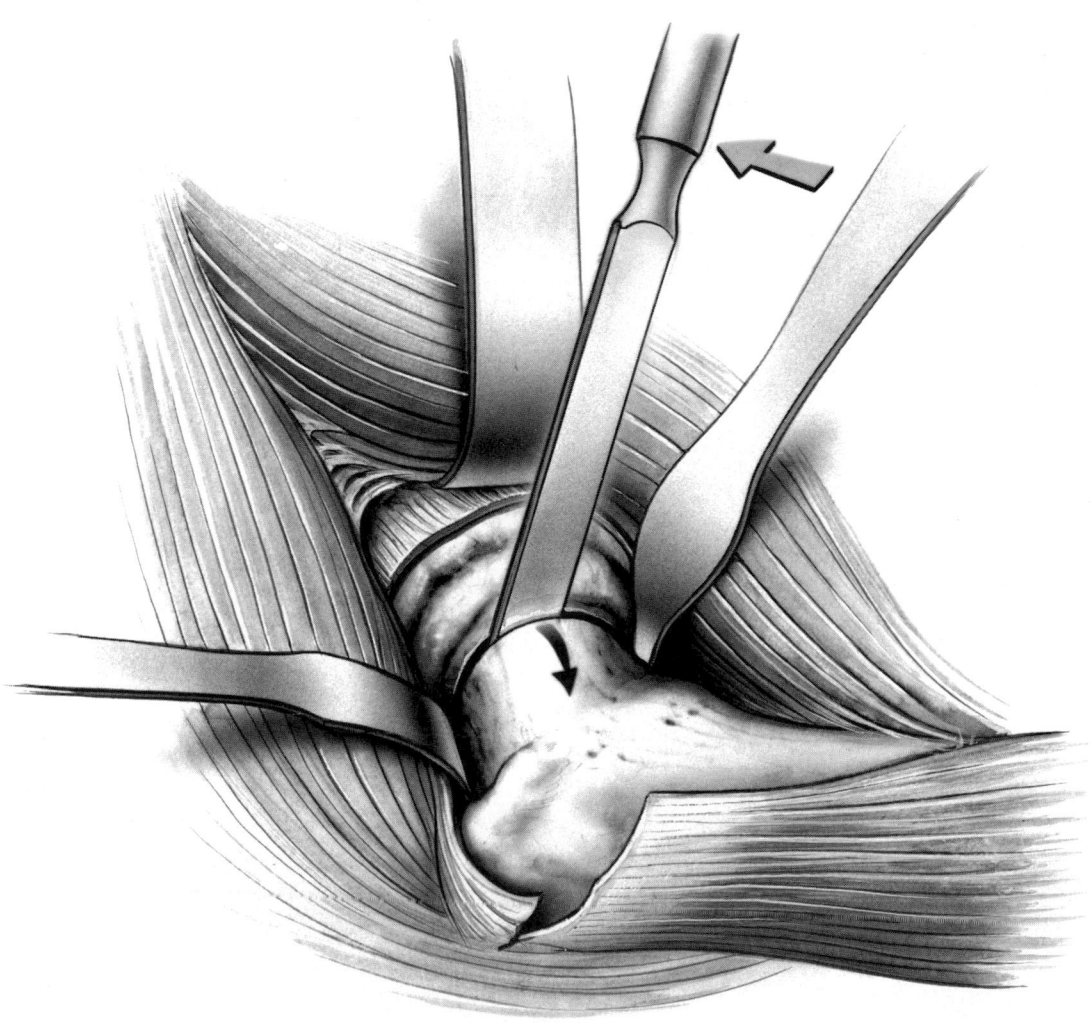

Fig. 17-6. After completion of femoral neck osteotomy, separation of the neck from the head can be facilitated using a 2.5-cm-wide osteotome.

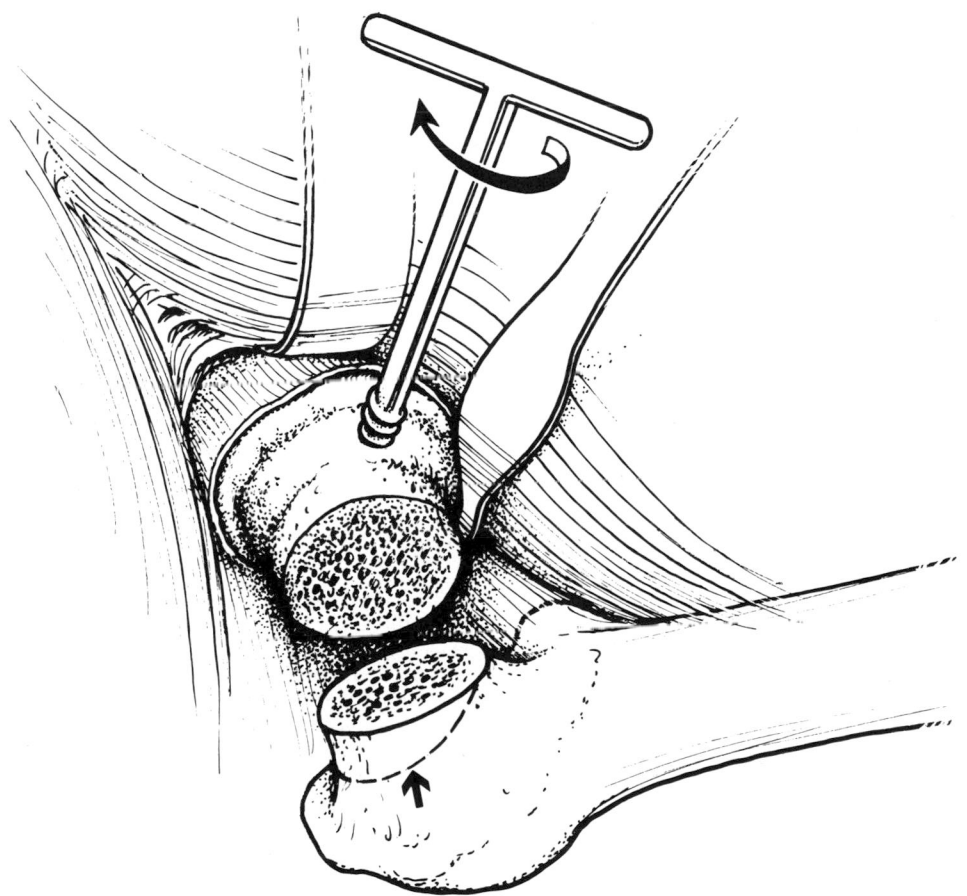

Fig. 17-7. A retrograde removal of the head is accomplished using a T-handled corkscrewlike instrument. Arrow indicates revision of the neck length as required (based on template measurements).

PHASE IV: ACETABULUM EXPOSURE AND PREPARATION, AND FIXATION OF THE ACETABULAR COMPONENT
Maximizing Exposure

Excise the remaining capsule, labrum, loose fibrocartilage, and osteophytes while applying a bone hook to the femur and pulling the femoral head toward the operating surgeon. This further facilitates the detachment of the capsule from the posterior neck of the femur and release of the short rotators as needed.

Four retractors are used to provide acetabular exposure: (1) an anterior (curved iliopubic) retractor (Fig. 17-8), (2) a posterior (femoral) retractor (Fig. 17-9), (3) an inferior notch (intracotyloid) retractor, and (4) a superior acetabular "pin" retractor.

The femoral retractor is uniquely designed for this exposure. It must be carefully engaged to the posterior inferior margin (rim) of the acetabulum (see Fig. 17-9). Tap this straight (with 45 degrees offset) double-pointed retractor in place with a hammer, engaging it to the bone while the femur is positioned in some flexion and adduction. It is essential that the teeth of this retractor be properly engaged to the femur while it is being retracted in a backward direction. Müller advocated applying a weight to this retractor to eliminate the need for retraction by an assistant (see Fig. 17-9). Then place the long-handled curved retractor's pointed end against the anterior lip of the acetabulum to retract the iliopsoas and the neurovascular structures medially. It is important to place the point of this retractor against the bone to avoid accidental injury to the femoral nerve, artery, and vein. The third pointed triangular Hohmann retractor is placed inferiorly under the transverse ligament of the acetabulum while a pin retractor or a sharp-pointed Hohmann retractor retracts the superior capsule and abductors as needed. Expose the entire rim of the acetabulum by appropriately placing and readjusting the retractors and excising or incising the remaining capsule as necessary to provide a 360-degree visualization of the acetabulum.

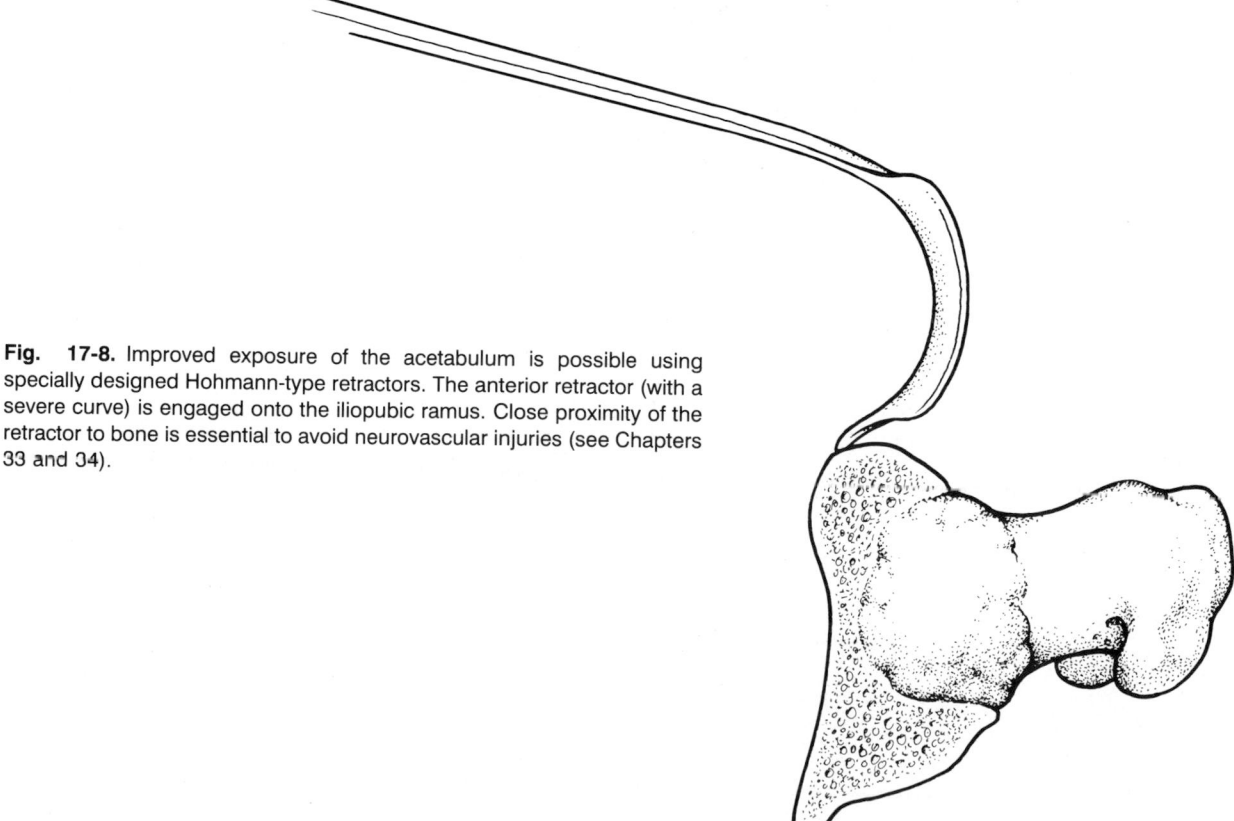

Fig. 17-8. Improved exposure of the acetabulum is possible using specially designed Hohmann-type retractors. The anterior retractor (with a severe curve) is engaged onto the iliopubic ramus. Close proximity of the retractor to bone is essential to avoid neurovascular injuries (see Chapters 33 and 34).

Expose the pulvinar (nonarticulating portion of the acetabulum) using a curette and acetabular gouges as required. Removed overhang inferior osteophytes to view the true medial wall of the acetabulum (Fig. 15-2).

Preparing the Socket and Fixation with Cement

The principles and techniques of acetabular preparation, insertion of cement, and insertion of the cup are similar to those described in Chapters 15 through 19.

Socket Fixation Without Cement

The principles and techniques of acetabular preparation and insertion of cementless cups are similar to those described in Chapter 15.

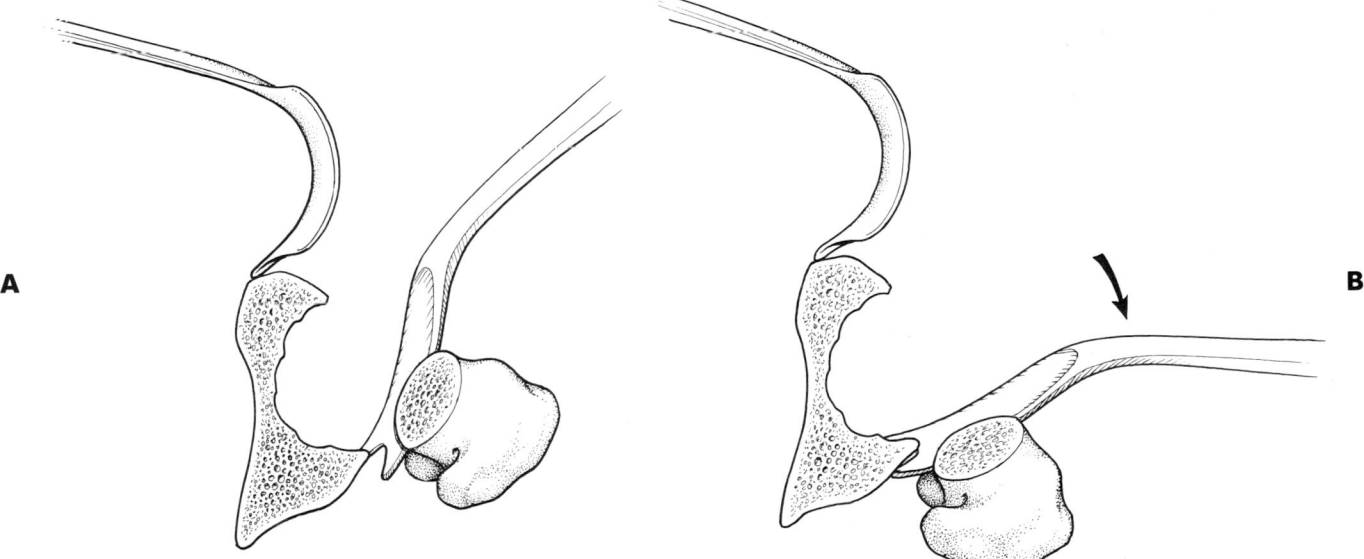

A   **B**

Fig. 17-9. A posterior retraction of the femur during acetabular exposure and preparation. **A,** Engaging the femoral (lever-type) retractor to the ilioischial ramus. **B,** Retracting the femur — maintaining the position of the retractor using a weight applied to its handle (not shown).

PHASE V: PREPARING THE FEMUR
Mobilizing the Upper Femur

The most important step in preparing the femur and inserting the femoral component with this approach is to obtain direct access to the top of the femur to facilitate the insertion of reamers, broaches, and stem. The following details must be observed:

- Remove the acetabular retractors.
- Mobilize as much capsule as possible by incision or excision close to the femur or the periphery of the acetabulum.
- Detach the piriformis from the digital fossa, and sever other short rotators near the femur to correct preexisting fixed external rotational deformity.
- Protect the sciatic nerve.
- Perform a psoas tenotomy when severe fixed flexion deformity requires it.
- Control all troublesome bleeders, especially branches of the medial circumflex vessels.
- Protect the abductor muscles by gentle handling, placing the femoral retractors underneath the greater trochanter. Place another pointed Hohmann retractor medial to the neck to protect the psoas tendon.
- Shorten the neck as required, but never before adequate soft tissue correction and evaluation of leg length.
- Ensure anterior stability of the hip after inserting the femoral component.

Preparing the Medullary Cavity

Insert the femoral retractor behind the trochanter to deliver the proximal femur. First internally rotate, extend, and abduct the leg, and place the femoral retractor underneath the greater trochanter. Now have the second assistant externally rotate, flex, and abduct the hip to view the opening of the upper femur.

Preparation of the medullary cavity begins only after the upper femur is adequately mobilized by soft tissue release (as previously indicated) facilitated by the femoral retractor. Note that despite partial detachment of the gluteus medius and detachment of the gluteus minimus, this approach does not offer sufficient exposure of the upper femur to allow direct access for inserting straight reamers. This is caused by the remaining mass of the abductor muscles, which can be significant in large-muscled individuals.

Begin the preparation with gouges, which should remove bone from the top of the neck near the digital fossa at the base of the trochanter. Starting laterally enables the surgeon to use broaches more laterally, thus avoiding a varus alignment or perforation of the lateral cortex of the femur. Using rotary straight reamers with this approach is awkward and can result in significant damage to the abductors. Use femoral broaches to engage laterally into the trochanteric cancellous bed, thus achieving a valgus orientation of the stem (Fig. 17-10). Use the transcondylar line of the knee as a reference for anteversion. Clear the medullary canal using a rotary brush and irrigation. Insert the test prosthesis to determine the required stem size and neck length.

Testing Reduction, Stability, and Leg Length Measurement

Reduction is carried out with longitudinal traction on the femur while the hip is reduced by internal rotation after initial adduction. Make sure that the hip is stable in adduction but also in external rotation and extension before inserting the actual prosthesis using the anterolateral approach. When the hip is unstable, resulting in anterior dislocation, it is commonly the result of (1) excessive anteversion of the cup or femoral component, (2) excision of the anterior capsule and the removal of the iliofemoral and pubofemoral ligaments (Y ligament of Bigelow).

Measure the leg length by bringing the legs together and palpating the medial malleoli through the drapes. Also measure the length directly, measuring the distance between fixed points on the pelvis and on the femur (see Chapter 15).

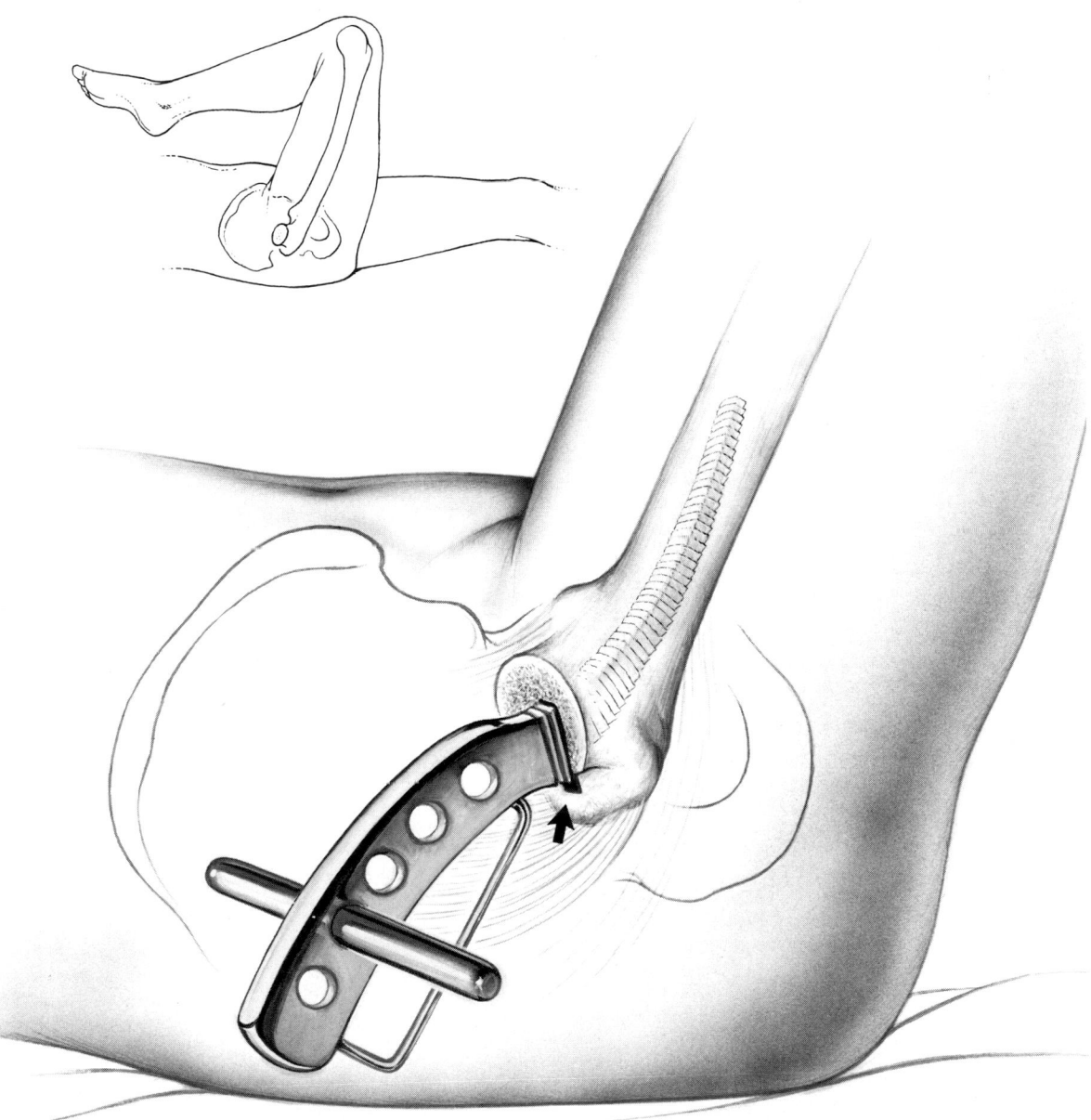

Fig. 17-10. Insertion of broaches in appropriate attitude is not feasible with the anterior approach unless the hip is maximally adducted, flexed, and externally rotated. This position is dangerous because of possibility of fracture of the femur in an osteoporotic person. Transcondylar axis of the knee serves as reference for orientation of broaches and prosthesis. NOTE: valgus orientation of the prosthesis is possible only if broaches are inserted to encroach onto the greater trochanteric bed *(arrow),* but performing the operation may damage fibers of the gluteus medius and its tendon. To achieve a valgus orientation, a small gouge may be used before inserting the broaches *(arrow).*

PHASE VI: INSERTING CEMENT AND FEMORAL COMPONENT
Rehearsal

Before inserting cement, the following steps should be taken:

1. Position the leg in adduction, flexion, and external rotation after reinsertion of the femoral retractor to deliver the upper femur.
2. Place a sponge in the acetabular cavity after irrigating the wound copiously.
3. Obtain an appropriate size bone block, or use a prefabricated synthetic medullary plug and deliver it into the medullary cavity to an appropriate level (see Chapter 15).
4. The second assistant (leg holder) is instructed to place the hip in the desired degree of adduction, flexion, and external rotation while the surgeon rehearses the unimpeded, full-length insertion of the femoral component before inserting the cement.

Inserting the Cement and Prosthesis

Use a cement gun to deliver the cement into the medullary cavity. Finger packing of the canal may be difficult and the mixing of cement with blood unavoidable.

Cement is delivered when it no longer adheres to the surgeon's gloves. Then insert the stem, to its full length, in the canal. Note the following details as related to anterolateral approach:

- Because the bulk of the abductor muscles may preclude good access to the top of femur in this approach, the cemented prosthesis can drift into a varus alignment while it is being fully inserted.
- The prosthesis must be inserted with a lateral thrust to prevent the tip from coming in contact with the lateral cortex, which will make insertion difficult.
- Keep the prosthesis in a valgus alignment while it is fully penetrated into the canal.
- Avoid pushing on the head by inadvertently rotating the leg. Do not change the direction of the force applied to the head of the prosthesis. This can lead to excess anteversion or retroversion.

Inserting a Cementless Stem

As noted in Chapters 6 and 15, precise cavity preparation is essential for cementless components. Inserting a cementless prosthesis through this approach is not difficult. The stem is directed to the prepared canal in a predetermined direction and seated with a neck punch.

PHASE VII: WOUND DEBRIDEMENT, REATTACHING THE GLUTEI, AND WOUND CLOSURE

Carefully debride any devitalized tissue, and remove bone and cement at this stage to avoid potential damage to the anterior portion of the abductors. Recheck the range of motion for stability. Reattach the gluteus minimus tendon to the femur with a "stay suture" through a drill hole. Repair the portion of the gluteus medius that was detached from the trochanter as follows:

- Place two to four stay sutures of nonabsorbable material, such as Tevdek, through the muscle fibers.
- Drill two to four holes with a 2.3-mm drill bit through the anterior border of the greater trochanter. Pass the sutures, and firmly attach the gluteus medius insertion to the trochanter.
- Irrigate the wound copiously, and insert two deep drains into the joint.

Perform a tight repair of the fascia, inserting a second pair of drains superficial to the fascia. Repair the fat layer using retention sutures as described in Chapter 15.

TRANSGLUTEAL APPROACH

- The operation is described in seven phases.

PHASE I: POSITIONING, PREPARATION, AND DRAPING

For a transgluteal approach, either a supine or a lateral decubitus position may be used (see Chapter 15.)

PHASE II: SURGICAL EXPOSURE OF THE HIP AND LEG LENGTH MEASUREMENT
Skin Incision

Identify the bony landmarks, which include the anterosuperior and the posterosuperior iliac spine, the midshaft of the femur, and the vastus lateralis ridge (tubercle).

The incision begins along the midline of the femur for a distance of 10 to 15 cm to the ridge and is extended proximally for a distance of approximately 8 to 10 cm (Fig. 17-11). The length of the incision varies depending on the patient's size, the thickness of the fat, the stiffness of the hip, and so on. A longer incision both proximally and distally is advisable in obese patients. Although originally a posterior inclination of the proximal limb of the incision was advocated, a straight incision is more versatile and can be conveniently extended in both directions. A straight incision is preferred because it allows optimal access to the anterior and posterior acetabulum and the femur. For difficult pelvic and acetabular reconstruction, the incision should be longer proximally.

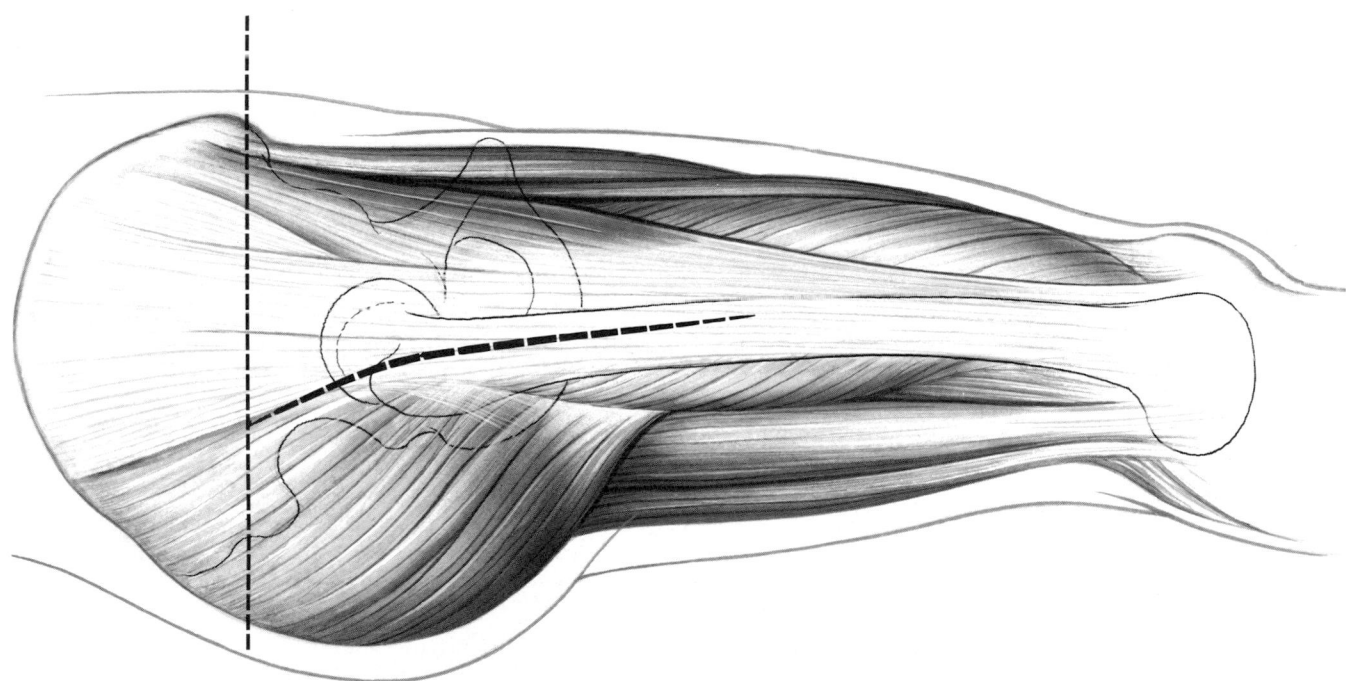

Fig. 17-11. For a transgluteal (direct lateral) approach, a supine position is preferred—the skin incision transverses along the anterior border of the femur and is directed toward the posterosuperior iliac spine. Proximally, the incision must be extended beyond the level of the anterosuperior iliac spine.

Fascial Incision

For the fascial incision, the parallel fibers of the iliotibial band are incised at midfemur, and the incision is then extended proximally toward the posterosuperior iliac spine. In this line, the anterior border of the gluteus maximus muscle fibers is split proximally, and mobilization of the fascia by blunt dissection separates the vastus lateralis muscle distally and the gluteus medius proximally. Place the Charnley initial incision retractor at the midpoint of the two ends of the fascial incision. Place the posterior claw of the retractor just proximal to the deep insertion of the gluteus maximus tendon to the linea aspera, which corresponds to the level of the lesser trochanter. Then retract the gluteus maximum posteriorly while the anterior member of the retractor retracts the tensor fascia femoris anteriorly. Cut the tensor fascia in a T fashion when exposure is inadequate. Also detach the insertion of the gluteus maximus to the femur as required to widen the exposure. At completion of the fascial opening the wound is exposed widely and is diamond shaped, with the greater trochanter presenting itself at the center of the wound.

Splitting the Abductors and Vastus Lateralis

The principle involved in this surgical approach is mobilization of the anterior insertion of the gluteus medius and minimus to the femur as continuity of the two muscles is preserved. To accomplish this, perform the following:

- Excise the trochanteric bursa, and develop the line of transgluteal incision in the aponeurosis and through the vastus lateralis and the gluteus medius and minimus.
- Proximally the incision starts at the junction of the anterior two thirds with the posterior third of the gluteus medium muscle. This line can be located at the interval between the anterior muscle section of this muscle (two thirds) and the posterior tendinous portion of the muscle (one third) of the gluteus medius attachment to the greater trochanter (Fig. 17-12).

  By extending the incision deep into the vastus aponeurosis in a slightly forward medial direction, a continuous musculotendinous flap will develop. Using an electrocautery knife (adjusted to the proper intensity to avoid charring the muscle), the incision is deepened to the femur distally and to the anterior portion of the greater trochanter proximally. Extend the incision proximally along the anterior tendon of the gluteus medius, being careful not to cut the tendon. The fibers of the gluteus medius may be split bluntly proximal to the tip of the greater trochanter for a distance of 6 to 8 cm. Split the gluteus medius in the direction of its fibers, avoiding damage to the muscle. Develop and mobilize the anterior flap as follows:

- Split the vastus near its anterior border distally while the hip is slightly flexed. Control bleeding from the vastus lateralis (branches of lateral circumflex).

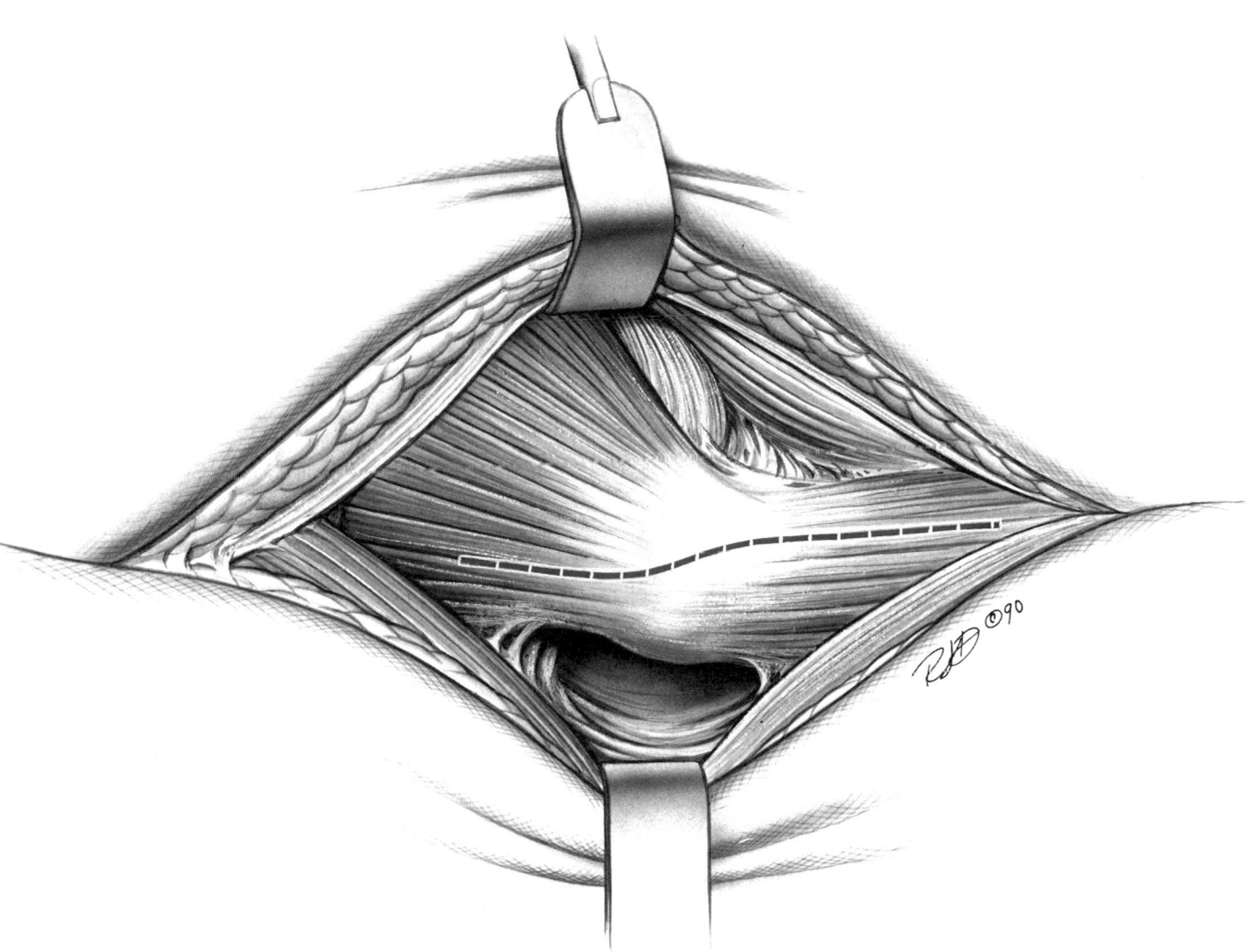

Fig. 17-12. The ''nonanatomical'' muscle-splitting incision *(dotted line)* includes a line along the femur located at the junction of medial third and lateral two thirds of the vastus lateralis muscle fibers distally. This line of incision is curved posteriorly at the level of the tip of the trochanter so that it is located at the junction of two thirds (anteriorly) and one third (posteriorly) over the gluteus medius and minimus.

- Elevate sharply from the femur the anterior fibers of the gluteus medius and the tendinous attachment of the gluteus minimus (Fig. 17-13). Begin this with a sharp knife or a cautery. A sharp Cobb's elevator or a 2.5-cm osteotome is especially useful. It is important to keep the tip of the elevator as close to the bone as possible to avoid added damage and excess bleeding, thus minimizing formation of heterotopic ossification.
- Define and separate the anterior capsule from the abductors while the hip is flexed and externally rotated by the second assistant. Insert two narrow Hohmann retractors, one proximal and one distal to the neck, to define the boundary of the entire anterior capsule. Avoid excess mobilization of the abductors from the pelvis, since stripping can damage the superior gluteal nerve in this region (Fig. 17-13, inset).

Anterior Capsulotomy or Capsulectomy

Incise the capsule radially along the rim of the acetabulum. Extend the capsular incision along the superior and inferior margins of the acetabulum to facilitate exposure and dislocation. While a routine anterior capsulectomy is not recommended, a partial or total capsulectomy may be required to dislocate the hip.

Leg Length Measurement

Measure the leg length before dislocating the hip using two fixed points, one on the femur and the other on the acetabulum, as previously described (see Chapter 15).

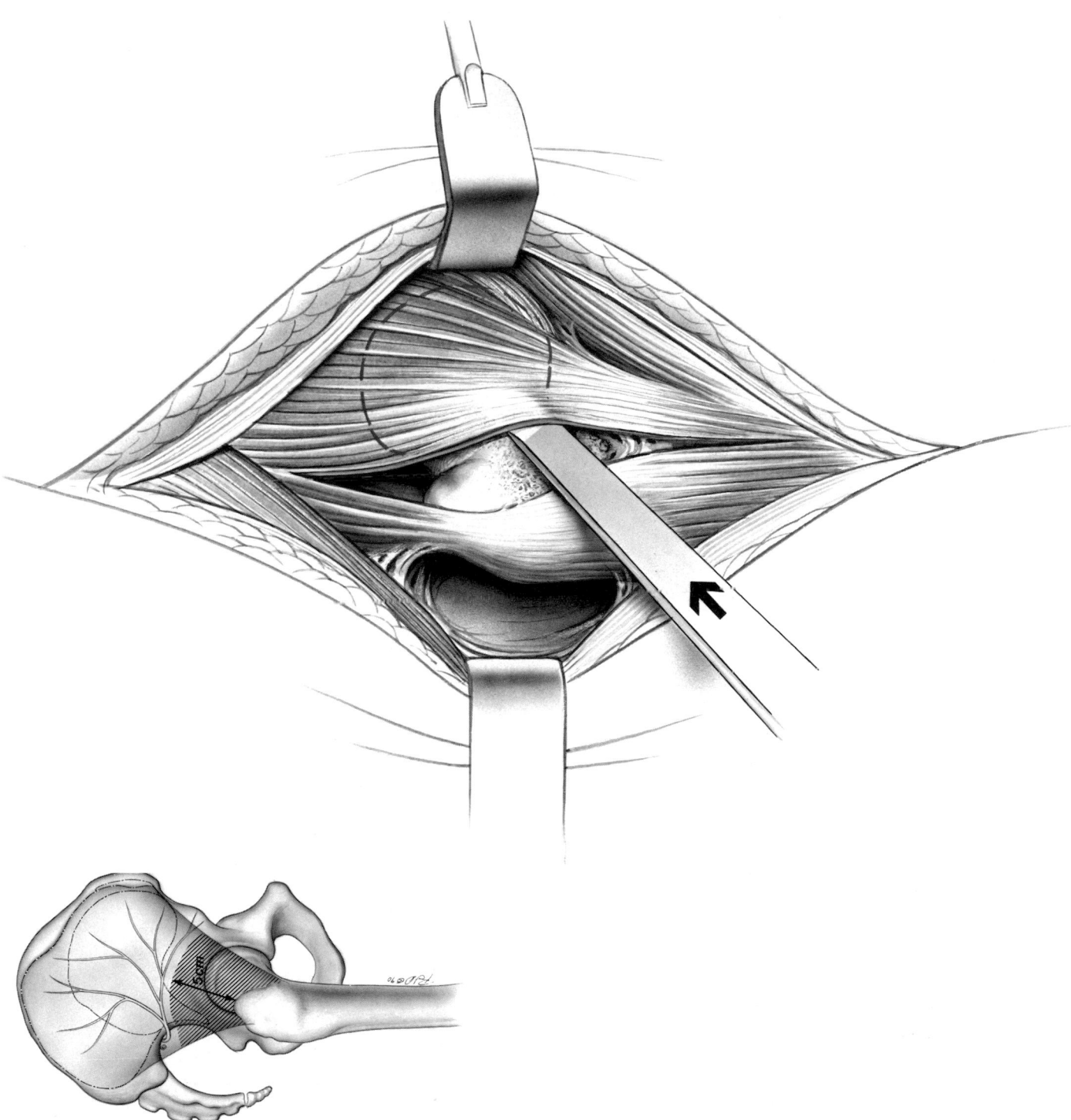

Fig. 17-13. Muscle-splitting incision is carried out using a sharp osteotome, detaching the insertion of the gluteus minimus tendon (proximally) and fibers of the vastus lateralis distally. The interval between the anterior capsule and the glutei is entered to develop the anterior flap of the conjoint tendon. Inset illustrates the location of the superior gluteal nerve in relation to the tip of the trochanter and acetabular margin. The safe limit (shaded area) must be kept in mind while developing the exposure.

PHASE III: DISLOCATING THE HIP

As in the anterolateral approach, a second assistant dislocates the hip by flexing, adducting, and externally rotating the femur. Use a large bone hook, and place it medial to the neck to dislocate the head out of the socket depth. When difficulty is encountered, release the capsule, remove the marginal osteophyte if present, or remove the head in a retrograde manner. Place two narrow Hohmann retractors, one inferior and one superior to the neck, and remove the head by osteotomy of the neck at the appropriate level based on preoperative planning. Osteotomy is best accomplished using an oscillating saw.

PHASE IV: ACETABULAR EXPOSURE AND PREPARATION AND FIXATION OF THE ACETABULAR COMPONENT
Exposing the Acetabular Rim

A circumferential exposure of the rim is best accomplished using a curved Hohmann retractor similar to one used for the anterolateral exposure (see Fig. 17-8). Puncture the anterior capsule close to the bone and near the ilium along the iliopubic ramus. Insert the tip of the retractor, and gently retract the anterior half of the split muscle flap medially. Use an additional Hohmann retractor, and properly position one inferiorly to visualize the margin of the acetabulum and one posteriorly to visualize the posterior rim. Enhance the superior marginal exposure using a Charnley pin retractor (see Chapter 18) or the author's acetabular staple retractor (see Chapter 19). The pin retractors also serve as a reference point for intraoperative leg length measurements. To improve the exposure of the acetabulum, separate a portion of the origin of the gluteus minimus attachment to the superior capsule and the acetabulum and detach the insertion of the rectus femoris to visualize the acetabular rim. Guard against damage to the abductors and the anterior divisions of the superior gluteal nerve to the tensor fascia femoris. Avoid heavy retraction of the glutei, which can cause fibrosis and heterotopic ossification. The superior gluteal nerve is located approximately 5 cm proximal to the rim of the acetabulum, which can be directly damaged as a result of excess traction.

Inferior retraction is achieved using a triangular Hohmann retractor with its tip placed under the transverse ligament. This retractor is effectively inserted when the inferior capsule is radially incised and the femur is retracted in a distal and posterior direction. To expose the posterior margin of the acetabulum, a posterior sharp-pointed Hohmann retractor or a second pin retraction facilitates retraction of the capsule. Capsulotomy or capsulectomy may also be required. Most surgeons[1] prefer to place the leg across the table (the opposite side) during socket preparation with the tibia vertical to the floor and the leg in a pouch (for sterility). The leg can also be conveniently placed on the table in a position of slight flexion, moderate adduction, and external rotation. Posterior acetabular retraction can then displace the femur posteriorly as seen in Fig. 17-9.

Exposing the Pulvinar

The nonarticulating portion of the acetabulum is curetted out to expose the medial wall of the acetabulum. For details of this technique, see Chapter 15.

This approach provides a good view of the acetabulum and facilitates the preparation, gauging, and insertion of the acetabular component. These procedures are similar in principle to those described for the anterolateral approach described in this chapter and Chapter 15.

PHASE V: PREPARING THE FEMUR
Mobilizing the Femur

Release the capsule as necessary, and place a two-prong straight retractor behind the trochanter (while the leg is externally rotated and abducted). The second assistant then brings the stump of the femur into view by flexing, adducting, and externally rotating the hip. Prepare the medullary cavity with appropriate broaching, making sure that the orientation of the stem is correct for centralization of the stem (and for the use of cement). Insert the femoral prosthesis in a manner similar to the anterolateral approach.

Testing for Stability

Before inserting the actual femoral component, the stability test (either via a trial head/neck/broach assembly or trial test prosthesis) must confirm the stability of the joint in flexion, adduction, and rotation. With this approach, the test must ensure anterior stability, since anterior dislocation can occur as a result of anterior capsulectomy or detachment of the abductors during exposure, both of which are unrelated to the orientation of the component. Soft tissue stability is restored after repair of the conjoint tendons of the gluteus/vastus lateralis at the end of the procedure.

PHASE VI: INSERTING CEMENT AND THE FEMORAL COMPONENT

As in the anterolateral approach, the surgeon must obtain access to the top of the femur to insert the cement and stem. The cement is ready when it no longer adheres to the glove. Insert cement with a cement gun after brushing and removing the debris as in other techniques. As in the anterolateral approach, manual insertion of cement may be difficult because of the limited exposure. Use a medullary bone or synthetic plug, then insert the stem to maintain a central location in the femur, avoiding mediolateral or axial malpositioning (see Chapters 15 and 19).

PHASE VII: REATTACHING THE GLUTEUS MINIMUS AND CAPSULE, REPAIRING THE CONJOINT TENDON, AND FASCIAL REPAIR AND CLOSURE
Reattachment of the Gluteus Minimus and Capsule

When the anterior capsule and Y-ligament of Bigelow have been adequately preserved, this structure, along with the gluteus minimus tendon, is firmly reattached to the femur at the anterior trochanteric line. Drill three or four 2.5-mm holes. Identify and place stay sutures in the gluteus minimus and capsule. Bring the sutures through the holes, and tie them firmly to the bone. The ease and accuracy of repair depend on the properly planned detachment of the tendon and capsule at the beginning of the operation and on the availability of tissue. Insert deep drains now.

Repair of Conjoint Tendon

Repair the musculotendinous incision of the gluteus medius and vastus while the hip is kept in an abducted position (Figs. 17-14 and 17-15). This repair is important for the function of the abductors and stability of the hip. Use strong nonabsorbable suture material, such as no. 2 Tevdek. When the anterior flap of the gluteus medius is inadequate because of a misplaced incision, the repair must

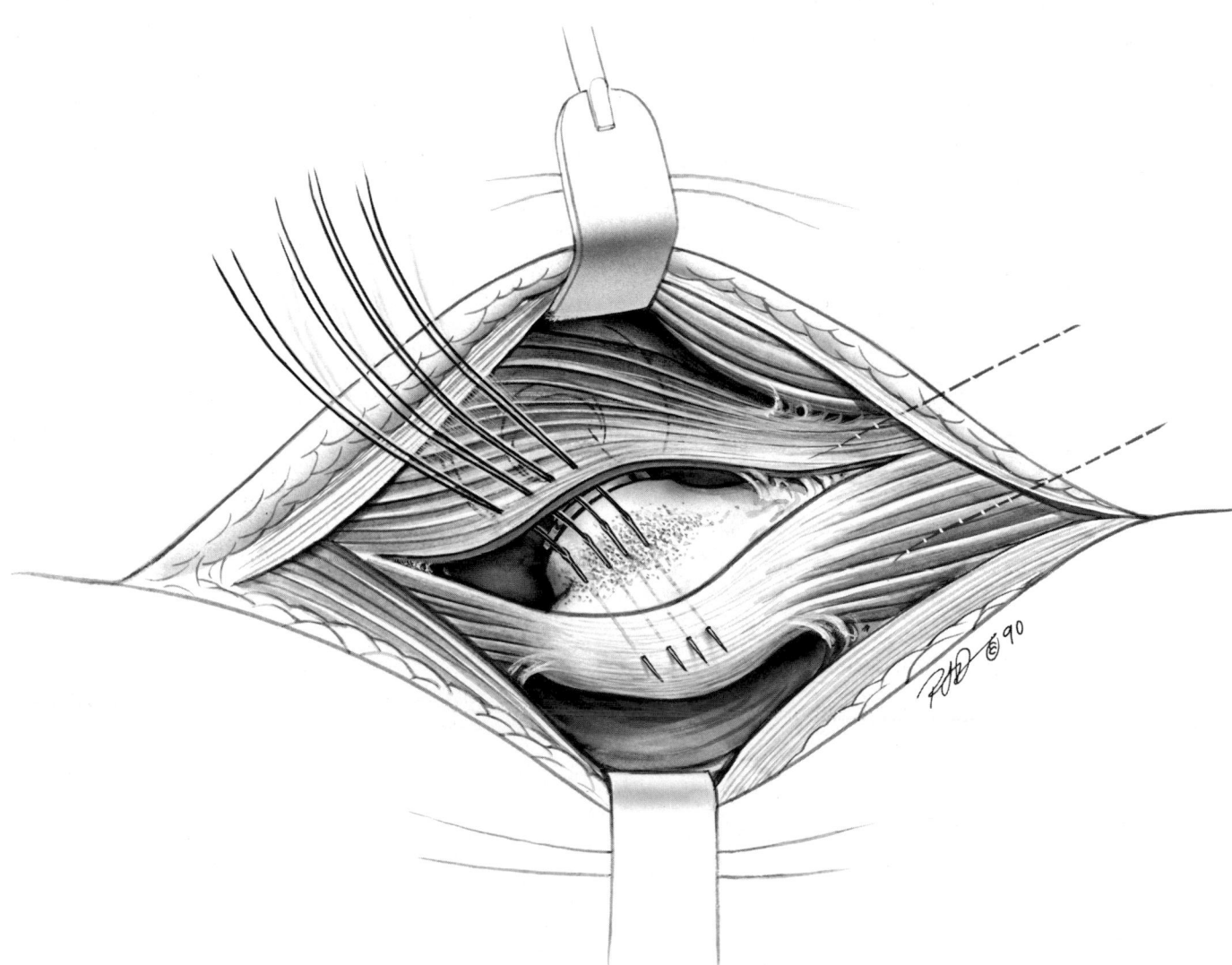

Fig. 17-14. Repair the conjoint tendon by applying "stay sutures" to affix the detailed gluteus minimus tendon and available capsule to the intertrochanteric line of the femur through drilled holes. Nonabsorbable monofilament sutures are used.

be augmented by direct attachment of the anterior fibers of the gluteus medius to the trochanter via several holes drilled into the trochanter as described for the gluteus minimus tendon (see Fig. 17-14). Repair of the conjoint tendon must be complete proximally and distally (see Fig. 17-15). The seam of the repair must be strong enough to allow early ambulation and to ensure stability of the hip. A weak repair may result in herniation and weakness, and thus a functional loss of abductors.

Closure of Fascia, Fat, and Skin

As in other approaches previously described, the fascial closure must be watertight. Nonabsorbable interrupted sutures are used with the hip in the abducted position. The technique for fat and skin closure has been described (see Chapter 15).

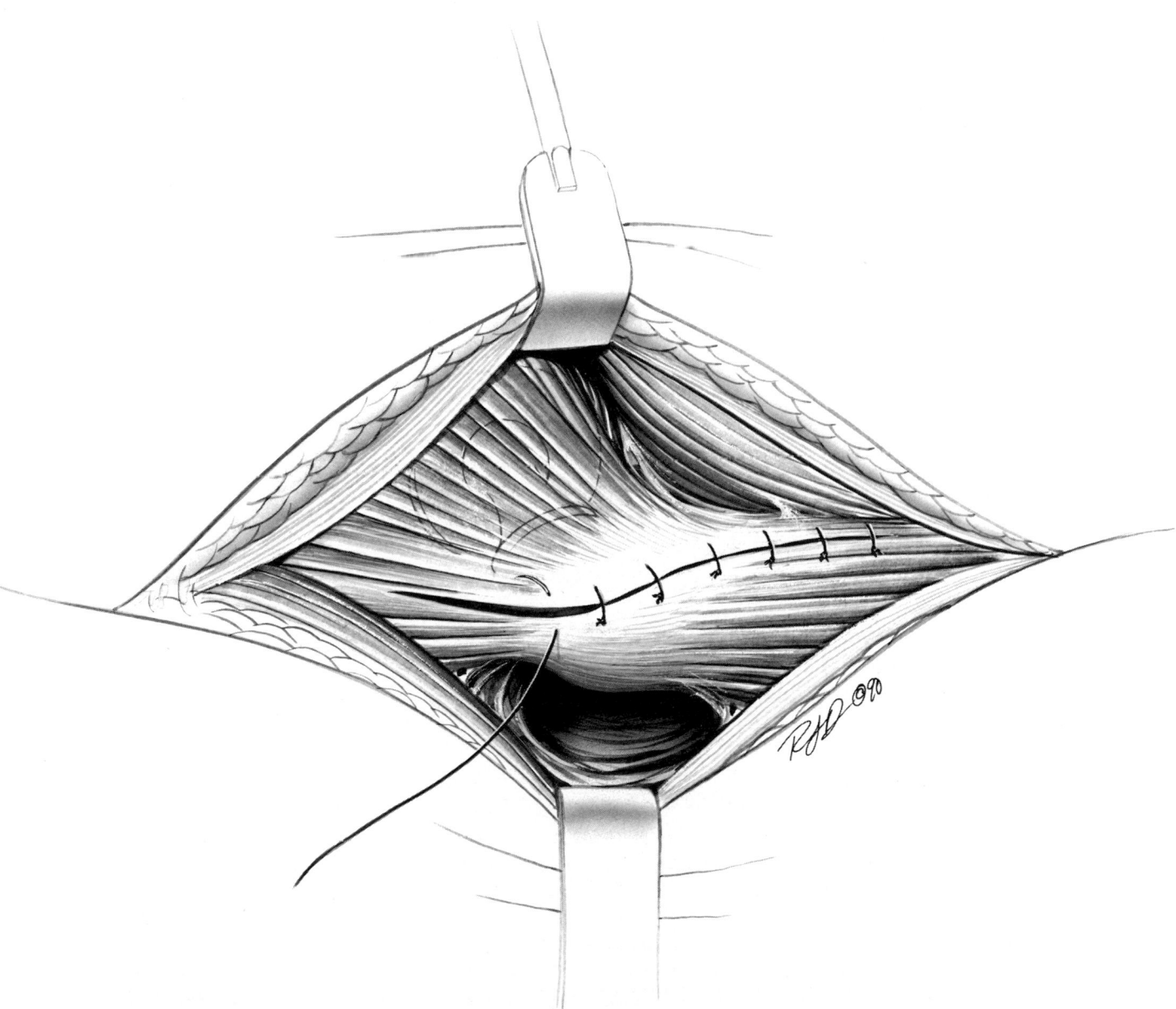

Fig. 17-15. The repair of conjoint tendon (myotendinous continuity) is augmented by interrupted sutures placed along the splitting incision.

SUMMARY OF ESSENTIALS

- Total hip arthroplasty techniques using an anterolateral and transgluteal approach have the same advantages and disadvantages. The abductor mechanism is partly released from the femur or lifted off the femur, which results in partial damage to the abductors. In both, an anterior capsulectomy must be performed to allow dislocation. Also, the femur must be externally rotated forcefully to allow dislocation and exposure of the upper femur. The superior gluteal nerve and major neurovascular structures about the hip are endangered by their proximity and the need for retraction. In both approaches the patient should be placed in a supine position on the operating table.

- The anterolateral approach originally described by Watson Jones was advocated by Müller and is popular in some parts of the world. The surgeon must have special experience with this approach to avoid damaging the neurovascular and muscular structures of the hip.

- Enter the interval between the tensor fascia femoris and glutei, then perform a complete capsulectomy of the joint. Detach the anterior fibers of the gluteus medius, and sharply divide the gluteus minimus tendon from the femur to improve the exposure.

- Perform an in-situ osteotomy of the neck, and remove the head in a retrograde fashion if it cannot be dislocated. Excessive force by adduction, external rotation, and flexion may fracture the femur.

- Avoid injuring the neurovascular structures with the tip of the pointed retractor used to expose the anterior rim of the acetabulum.

- Make a straight incision laterally for approximately 15 to 20 cm just anterior to the greater trochanter, and center it over the trochanter ridge. Make the fascial incision along the skin incision, and apply a self-retaining retractor to expose the fascia.

- Detach a portion of gluteus medius and minimus tendon sharply from the anterior trochanter, and then perform a complete capsulectomy of the hip. Dislocate the hip by flexion, external rotation, and adduction. Use caution to avoid fracturing the femur. When dislocation is difficult, perform an in-situ osteotomy of the neck of the femur, and remove the head in a retrograde fashion.

- Maximize the exposure by excising the remaining capsule, labrum, and osteophytes as necessary while applying a bone hook to the femur to expose the acetabulum. Mobilize the femur by detaching the capsule as necessary, and place four Müller retractors specially designed for this approach. Two of the retractors are unique, the posterior (femoral) and anterior (curved iliopubic). The first retractor forces the femur in a backward direction as it engages the posterior rim of the acetabulum. The second retractor engages the anterior lip of the acetabulum to retract the remaining anterior capsule and iliopsoas muscle.

- Expose the pulvinar to determine the depth of the acetabulum, and readjust the retractors as needed to fully expose the acetabulum.

- Acetabular preparation, testing for sizing, and inserting the cup (with and without cement) are similar to procedures described in Chapter 15. As noted, the acetabulum can be fully visualized 360 degrees with the proper use of Hohmann-type retractors. The acetabular components (cemented or noncemented) can be inserted with ease, and the component can be properly oriented while the patient is in a supine position.

- Mobilize the upper femur by detaching the remaining capsule as necessary after removal of the acetabular retractors. Mobilize the femur to allow access to the top of the femur for detaching the piriformis and part of posterior capsule as needed while protecting the abductor muscles by gentle retraction. Prepare the medullary cavity by inserting the femoral retractor behind the greater trochanter to deliver the proximal femur. Access to the top of the femur is somewhat restricted with this approach but can be facilitated by the femoral retractor as it pushes the top of the femur forward and as the assistant exaggerates the external rotation and adduction of the hip.

- Begin preparation with the gouges, remove as much bone as needed in a lateral position in relation to the center of the medullary canal, and lateralize the prepared channel into the bed of the trochanter. Use femoral broaches to engage laterally into the trochanteric bed while avoiding damage to the abductor muscles.

- Perform test reduction using the test prosthesis. Reduce the femoral component into the acetabular component while the hip is maneuvered by traction, adduction, and internal rotation. Make sure the hip is stable by traction, especially in the extension and external rotation position. Any instability must be corrected at this stage. Measure the leg length. Adjust for length and stability by using a prosthesis with appropriate neck length or resection of the femoral neck.

- Before inserting the femoral component or cement, observe the position of the leg (in adduction, flexion, and external rotation). Deliver the upper femur out of the wound as much as possible to avoid restriction by the abductor muscles. Place a sponge inside the acetabular cavity, and insert the medullary plug. Insert the cement after copious irrigation. Use an intramedullary tube for venting, and deliver cement after removing the packing from the medullary canal. Use the cement when it no longer adheres to the surgeon's glove. Inserting the stem may be difficult if the cement is too viscous, so allow ample time. Protect the alignment of the stem by avoiding a tilt toward a varus position.

- Inserting a cementless stem through this approach is easier than a cemented stem since the femoral component finds its prepared channel while it is hammered in place. Irrigate the wound copiously, and insert two Hemovac drains into the joint.

- Remove damaged muscle fibers or devitalized tissue. Place two to four stay sutures of nonabsorbable material through the glutei muscle fibers, and drill holes made in the femur. Irrigate the wound copiously, and proceed with the wound closure.

- Perform a tight closure of the fascia, inserting a pair of drains superficial to the fascia. Repair fatty layer by retention sutures.

- Transgluteal approach, originally described by McFarland and Osborne and used for total hip arthroplasty by Harding, uses a nonanatomical plane to the hip joint. It is based on splitting the gluteus medius proximally and the vastus lateralis distally. It requires maintaining the continuity of the vastus lateralis and gluteal muscles to secure continuity of the abductors. This is accomplished by a tight repair of the conjoint tendon of the gluteus medius and vastus lateralis. The risk of this approach, in addition to potential damage to the abductors, is of heterotopic ossification and damage to the superior gluteal nerve branch to the tensor fascia femoris and abductors.

- Identify the bony landmarks, and make an incision 10 to 15 cm long beginning at the midline of the femur, extending for a distance of 8 to 10 cm proximally. Use a longer incision both proximally and distally in obese patients and heavy and muscular individuals.

- Incise the fascia along the skin incision by splitting the iliotibial band distally parallel to the femur while the fascia is incised proximally, inclined posteriorly. Use the Charnley initial incision retractor to maintain the exposure. Expose the hip by a splitting incision through the abductors and vastus lateralis. Develop this transgluteal incision carefully so that the incision starts proximally at the junction between the anterior two thirds and the posterior third of the gluteus medius muscle. Extend this incision distally deep into the vastus lateralis aponeurosis in a slightly forward and medial direction; develop a continuous musculotendinous flap. Deepen this incision to the femoral bone distally and to the anterior portion of the greater trochanter proximally. Extend the incision proximally for a distance of 6 to 8 cm, and split the vastus lateralis near its anterior border, and elevate the gluteus minimus sharply from the femur. Begin with a sharp knife or cautery, but use a sharp osteotome to elevate the muscle off the bone along the anterior intertrochanteric line. Define and separate the anterior capsule, and place retractors superiorly and inferiorly to the neck to define the entire capsule. Then perform an anterior capsulectomy as required. Perform leg length measurements before dislocating the hip.

- Dislocate the hip while the second assistant externally rotates, adducts, and extends the hip from a slight flexed position. Deliver the head of the femur out of the wound by preparing for osteotomy of the neck. Ostetotomize the neck of the femur at the appropriate level.

- Expose the acetabular rim as much as possible using Hohmann-like periacetabular retractors similar to the ones used in the anterolateral approach. Puncture the anterior capsule as close as possible to the bone and near the ilium along the iliopubic ramus. Retract the anterior half of the split muscle flap medially, in addition to the marginal retractors inferiorly and posteriorly. Enhance the superior marginal exposure by using a pin retractor. Guard against damage to the abductors and the superior gluteal nerve along the superior margin of the acetabulum. Expose the pulvinar, and readjust the inferior retractor to define the inferior margin of the acetabulum, thus visually gauging the amount of bone to be removed by deepening.

- Mobilize the femur as necessary to allow the insertion of the femoral component. Deliver the top of the femur out of the wound while the leg is crossed to the opposite side, and visualize the proximal opening of the femur. Begin preparation as laterally as possible on the top of the femur, and use broaches or rotary reamers as required to create a centered cavity for inserting the prosthesis. Insert the test prosthesis, and perform test reduction to verify the stability of the joint and leg length. Select the prosthesis with the correct size and design. Copiously irrigate the wound. Note that preparation and insertion of broaches and rotary reamers are much easier through this approach than through the anterolateral one because of the splitting of the gluteus medius, a major part of which is located anterior to the femur. Therefore there will be less damage to the anterior fibers of the gluteus medius and gluteus minimus tendon.

- Deliver the cement by hand or gun after brushing and irrigating the medullary canal. Deliver a plug to the appropriate level, and avoid mixing the cement with blood and debris. Insert the stem in an appropriate alignment. Cementless insertion can be achieved without any difficulty with this exposure.

- Reattach the gluteus minimus and capsule firmly to the anterior femur using three or four 2.5-mm holes. Insert deep drains, then repair the conjoint tendon of the gluteus medius and vastus lateralis. Repair this layer with care using nonabsorbable suture materials. A weak repair may result in herniation and weakness, and thus a functional loss of the abductors.

- Close fascia, fat, and skin in a manner similar to that used in previous approaches using retention sutures for the fat layer.

REFERENCES

1. **Hedley AK, Hungerford DS, Habermann ET, et al:** *Howmedica, surgical techniques, the P.C.A. total hip system surgical technique.* Rutherford, NJ, no date, Orthopaedic Division, Howmedica.
2. **Müller ME:** Total hip reconstruction. In Evarts, editor: *The surgery of the musculoskeletal system,* vol 3, New York, 1983, Churchill Livingstone.

See Chapters 15, Principles Common to all Surgical Approaches; 16, Posterolateral Approach; 18, Transtrochanteric Approach (Modified Charnley); and 19, Transtrochanteric Approach (Author's Method) for additional information.

CHAPTER EIGHTEEN

Transtrochanteric Approach (Modified Charnley)

- Strictly speaking [this] surgical procedure should be seen as an exercise in practical mechanical engineering. Seen in this way the rate of mechanical failure ought to be as low as after any well-tried engineering routine.

  Sir John Charnley

PHASE I: POSITIONING, PREPARATION, AND DRAPING

Throughout the procedure the patient is in a supine position and the surgeon seated. For details, see Chapter 15 and Fig. 18-1. Delivering prewrapped sterile instrument trays to the operating room enclosure and using them in sequence facilitates transitions to various phases of the operation and saves time (see Appendix I and Fig. 18-30).

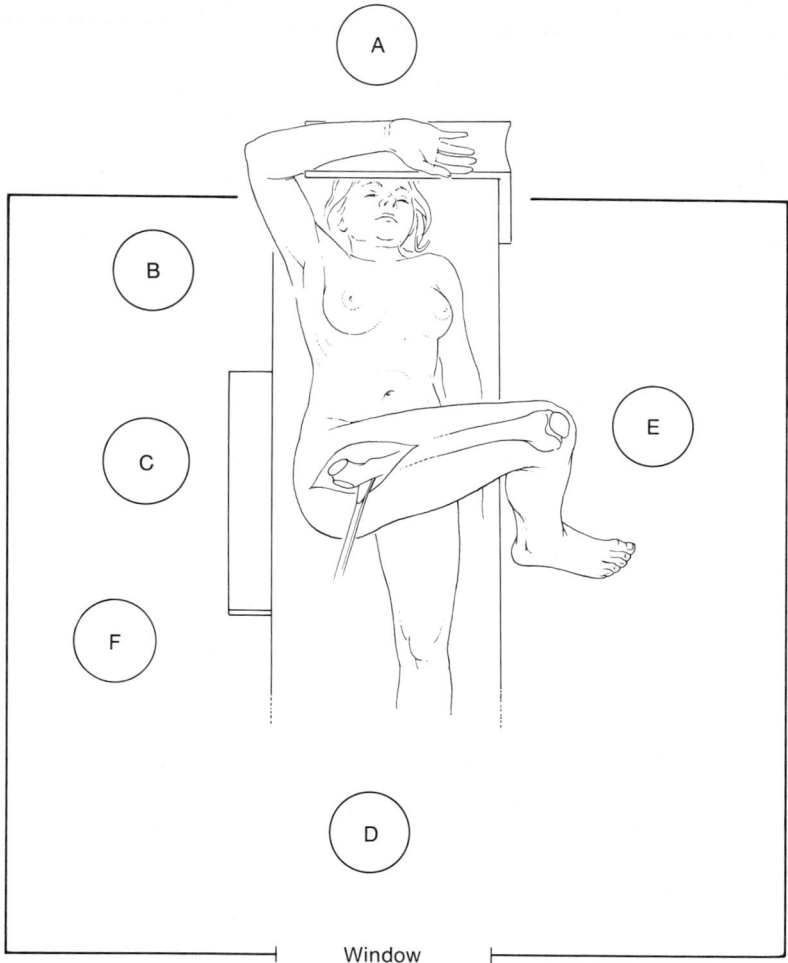

Window

Fig. 18-1. General view of enclosure *(solid lines)*, position of patient, operating table, position of personnel, and their relationship to operating and instrument tables. *A,* Anesthetist; *B,* first assistant; *C,* surgeon; *D,* nurse; *E,* second assistant. Second assistant may move to position *F* after application of self-retaining retractors to observe operation. Rectangular space attached to operating table in front of surgeon, *C,* is surgeon's instrument table. This table is used to place instrument trays as they arrive in enclosure.

PHASE II: SURGICAL EXPOSURE
Skin Incision and Insulation

Palpate the vastus lateralis ridge through the skin with the index finger to locate the center of the incision. The proximal end of the incision is posteriorly inclined 2 to 3 cm in relation to the distal limb of the incision, which is along the anterior border of the femur shaft. Even though the shaft of the femur can be palpated through the skin by the index finger, the hollow area indicating the iliotibial band is always a good landmark and should be observed (see Chapter 2). The distal limb of the incision travels from the trochanteric ridge along the shaft of the femur for approximately 10 to 15 cm. (The incision may be as long as 30 cm, depending on the size of the patient) (Fig. 18-2). Extend the incision proximally for the same distance.

Extend the incision at least 2.5 to 3.0 cm proximal to the level of the anterosuperior iliac spine to provide adequate access to the acetabulum and greater trochanter.

Make the skin incision with the hip in only 5 to 10 degrees of flexion and approximately 10 to 15 degrees of adduction and with no (internal or external) rotation. Avoid misplacement of the incision, caused by excessive flexion of the hip, faulty draping (usually obstructed proximal end of the incision), or excessive internal rotation of the hip. Attach the skin-edge towels to insulate the skin edges from the wound. Apply Betadine solution to the towels at skin edges (Fig. 18-3).

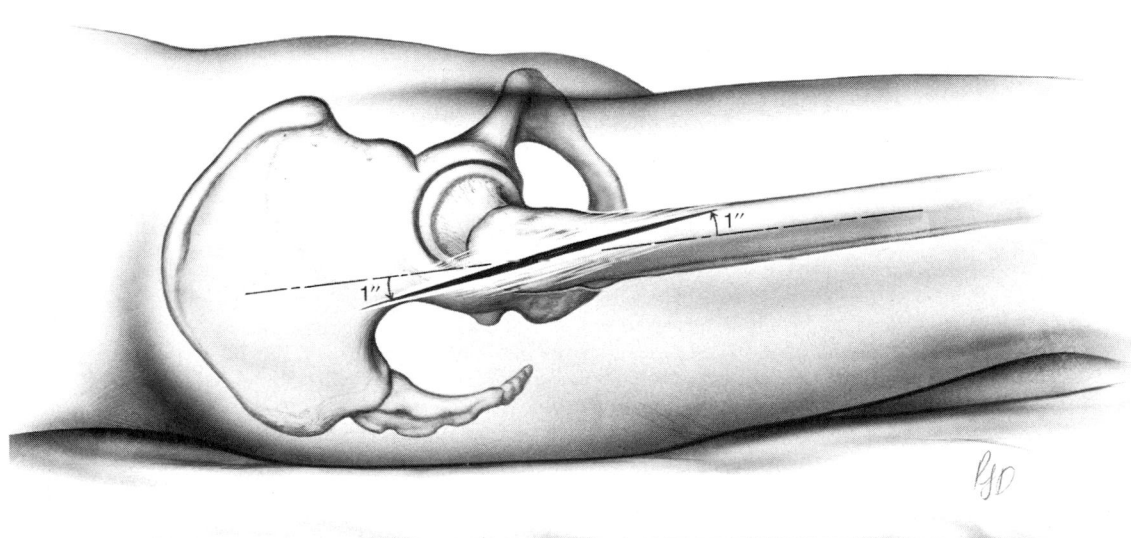

Fig. 18-2. Placement of incision is determined in reference to an imaginary midtrochanteric horizontal line. The incision traverses this line at the trochanteric tip, with the proximal incision end 1 inch posterior to it and the distal end 1 inch anterior to it. Incision is approximately 6 inches long, and proximal end should reach level of anterosuperior spine to provide sufficient room above greater trochanter.

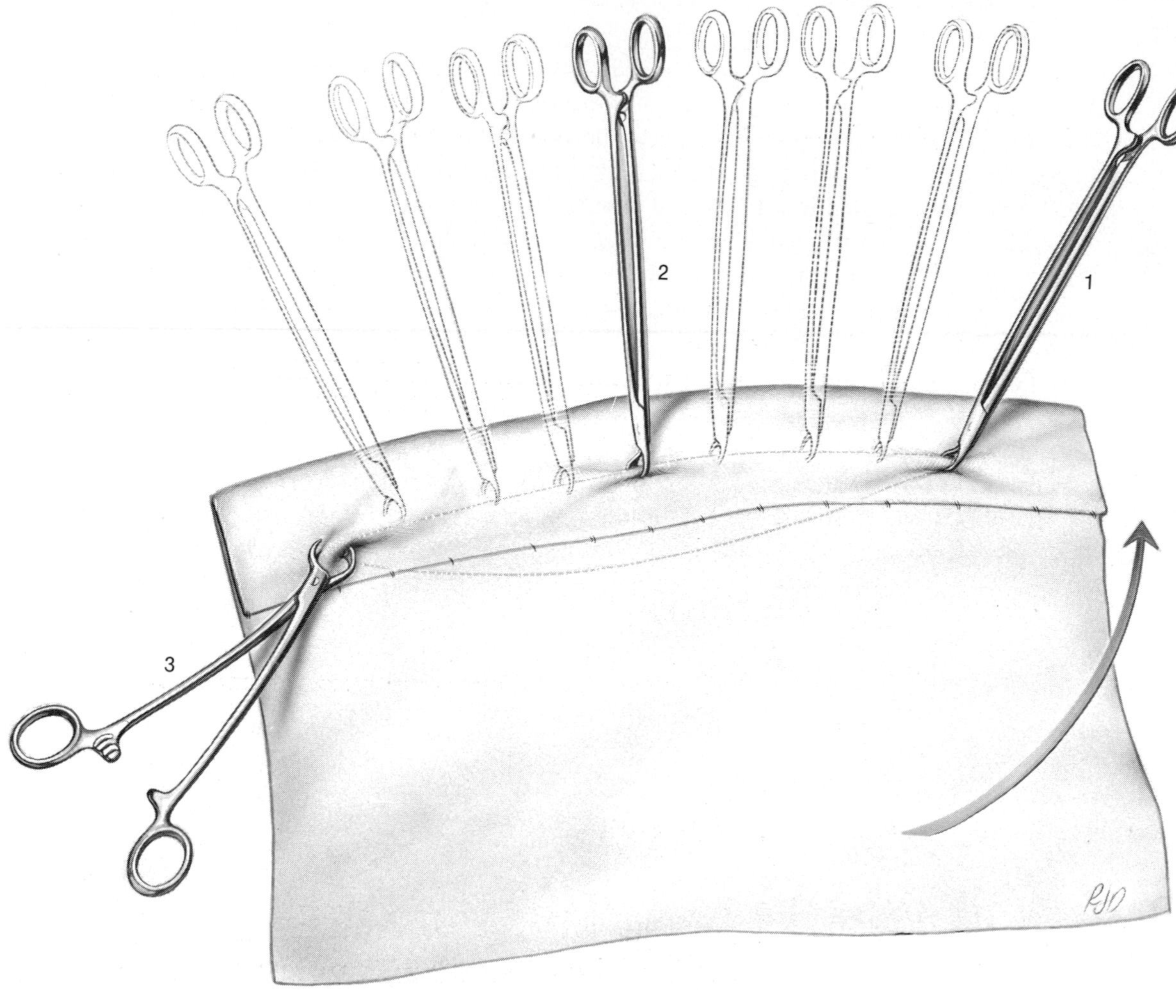

Fig. 18-3. Skin edge towels are attached to isolate cut edges of skin, each towel secured by nine Moynihan clamps. Skin protection by adhesive plastic sheet alone is not considered adequate. There is a possibility of contamination from cut edges of skin. Anterior skin edge towel is applied first. By centering it over wound edge, distal, middle, and proximal towel clips are applied in such a way as to stretch towel throughout its full length, using three clips. Remainder of skin edge is then clipped onto towels by six more clamps equally spaced along edge of wound. Forceful compression of skin edge in clamps results in skin necrosis and should be avoided.

Fascial Incision

Incise the fascia with the hip flexed to 20 degrees. Place the line of incision along the line of the skin incision. The incision begins just anterior to the trochanter. First a small opening is made to allow the surgeon to use the index finger to locate and identify the level of insertion of the tensor fascia femoris muscle to the iliotibial tract (ITT). This is done to avoid cutting fibers of the tensor fascia femoris muscle distal to the trochanteric ridge (Fig. 18-4). Because the fibers of the ITT are parallel, the ITT can be conveniently split distal to the trochanteric ridge.

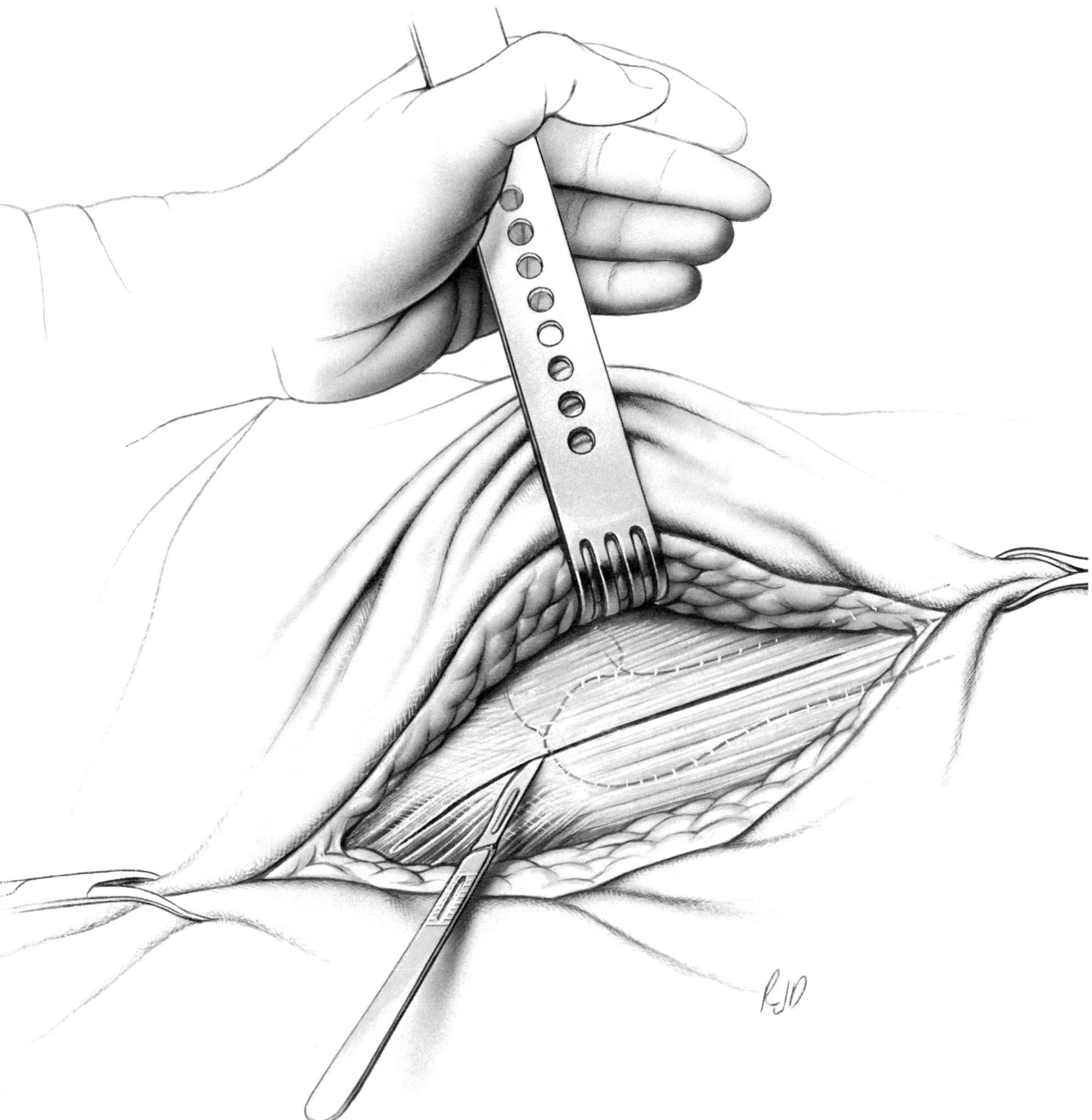

Fig. 18-4. A, Incision must be centered over greater trochanter. Fascia should be opened sharply with knife, avoiding deep cutting into underlying vastus lateralis distally and gluteus maximus proximally. Incision is extended from tip of trochanter proximally to area of approximately 3 inches. NOTE: initial wound retractor, used by first assistant, holds fat to expose fascia.

Continued.

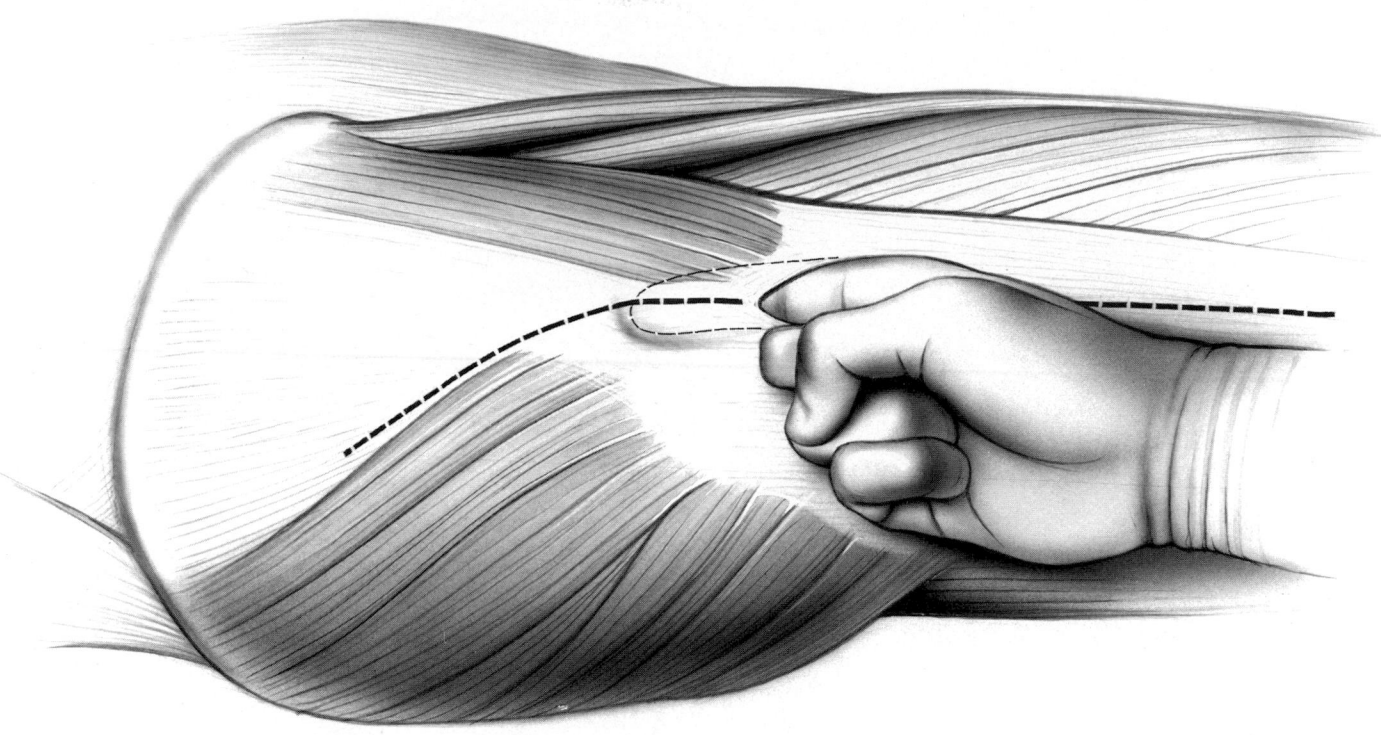

Fig. 18-4 — cont'd. B, How to avoid cutting fibers of tensor fascia femoris. Make an opening in the fascia distal to the trochanteric ridge, then place the index finger to palpate the level of the insertion of the tensor fascia femoris to iliotibial tract, thus avoiding excess anterior placement of the incision and damage to the tensor fascia femoris muscle. (**B** from Eftekhar NS: Total hip replacement: low-friction arthroplasty. In Evarts CM: *Surgery of the musculoskeletal system,* ed 2, 1983, Churchill Livingstone.)

Arthrotomy

The anteromedial border of the gluteus medius and minimus and posterolateral border of the tensor muscle are effective landmarks for this procedure (Fig. 18-5). Press your thumb against the anterior border of the gluteus medius and minimus, and apply a medium-sized retractor while externally rotating the hip maximally. The interval between the tensor fascia femoris and the abductors can conveniently be entered. Flex the hip, and externally rotate no more than 30 degrees; the hip should also be slightly abducted. Precapsular fat may be removed after incising a membranous layer stretching across the space between the two muscles. Place a deep retractor (the blade of this retractor must be 8 cm long and 3 cm wide, i.e., a broad Hibbs or Durham's retractor) medially to retract the tensor fascia femoris and iliopsoas medially and cephalad. The first assistant places a shallow retractor (i.e., Morris or Richardson) to retract the abductors laterally and cephalad, thus rendering the capsule available to the surgeon. Facilitate this exposure by adjusting the retractors as necessary (Fig. 18-6). Cauterize the ascending branches of the lateral circumflex, the transverse circumflex, and the superior gluteal vessels contributing to the anterior capsule before arthrotomy. Incise the capsule along the inferior margin of the neck since it facilitates the insertion of the cholecystectomy clamp (see Fig. 18-6).

Arthrotomy must be complete. Flow of synovial fluid is an indication of arthrotomy. Control capsular bleeders before attempting to insert the cholecystectomy clamp; it is futile to attempt to pass this clamp before actually seeing the synovial lining of the joint. Do not pass the clamp without being certain that it is intraarticular. Pick up the superior edge of the capsular incision with a forceps to facilitate insertion.

Passage and Retrieval of Gigli's Saw

Accomplish this in four steps (Fig. 18-7):

1. Lift the superior edge of the capsular incision with a thumb forceps, and insert the tip of the cholecystectomy clamp into the joint cavity.
2. Pass the tip of the clamp superiorly over the neck with the concave side of the clamp facing the superior neck of the femur.
3. With the tip completely in contact with the neck (without digging into the bone of the trochanter), bring the handle toward the patient's head, directing the tip toward the posterior aspect of the neck.
4. Feel the tip of the clamp protruding.

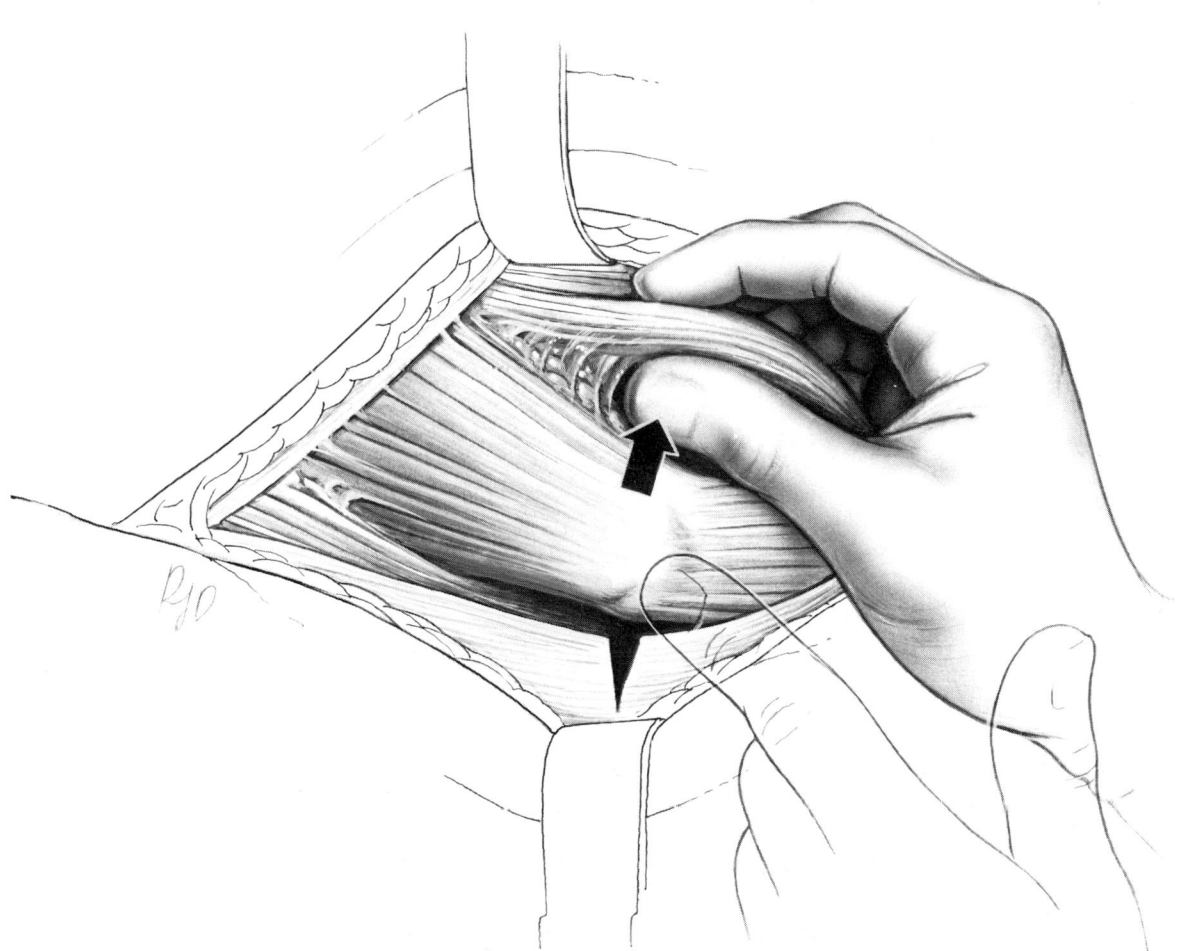

Fig. 18-5. Additional mobilization of fascia may be achieved by placing thumb onto edge of fascia anteriorly and mobilizing it from adhesions and intramuscular septa between tensor fascia femoris and gluteus medius. In this drawing, tensor fascia femoris is held between thumb and index finger (for demonstration). Arrow indicates direction of thumb opening space that leads to precapsular fat and capsule. Phantom finger points to vastus ridge. Tensor fascia femoris is T'ed but not held by retractor (for demonstration).

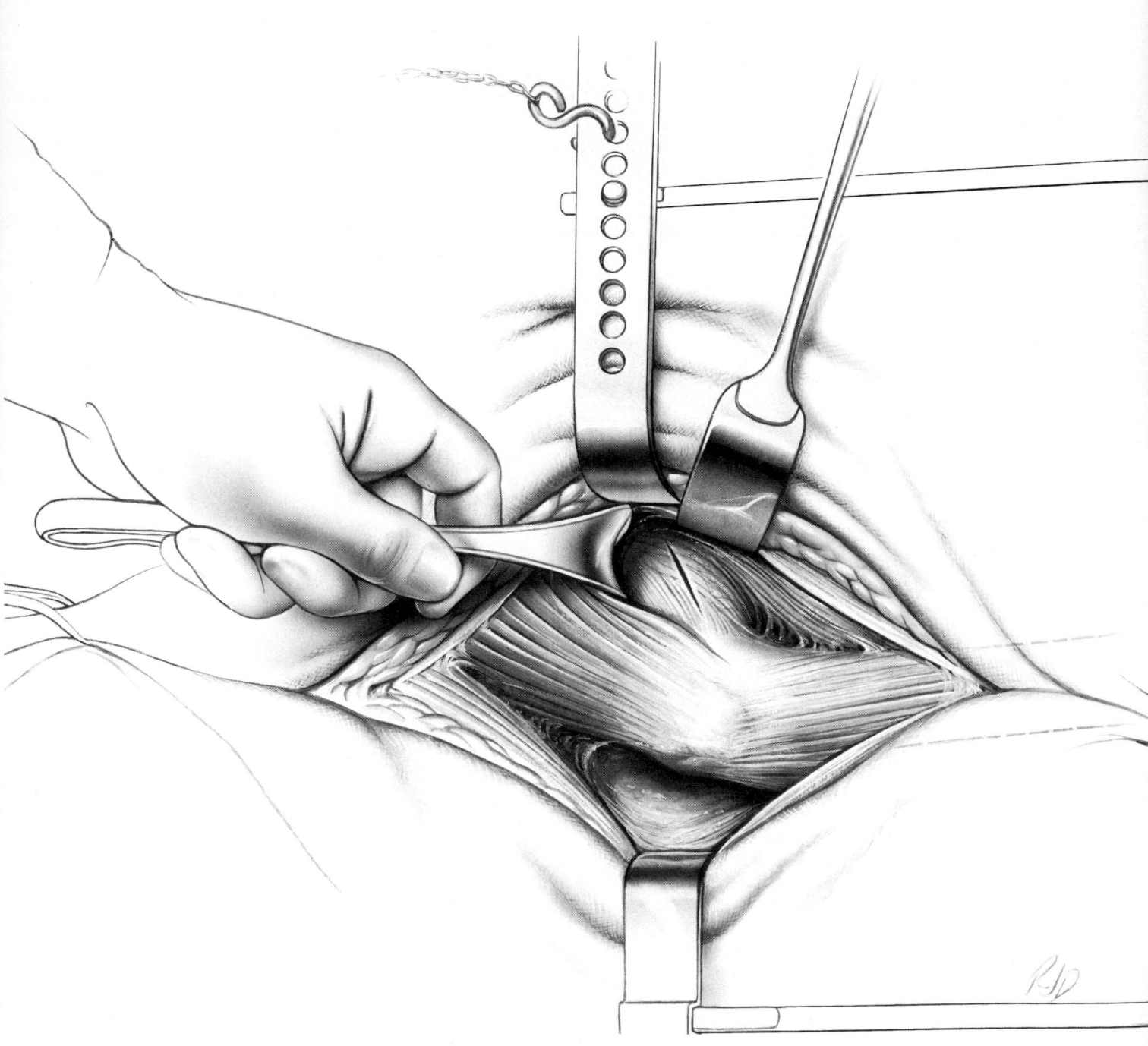

Fig. 18-6. Initial incision retractor holds cut edges of fascia lata apart. Initial incision retractor must be placed carefully to open wound in diamond shape with equal exposure proximal and distal to trochanter. Ideally, approximately 2½ to 3 inches of abductor muscle with its tendinous insertion and about 2 to 3 inches of vastus lateralis muscle should appear in wound, cantered by greater trochanter. Chain and hook carrying weights are applied to perforation of upper jaw of initial incision retractor to provide somewhat horizontal plane for this retractor. Small retractor (Richardson's) pulls back anterior edge of gluteus medius and minimus, and deep retractor draws tensor and psoas muscle medially, exposing front surface of capsule of hip joint. Incision into capsule is made carefully parallel to neck of femur but somewhat distal in regard to width of neck. Synovial cavity of joint is now exposed.

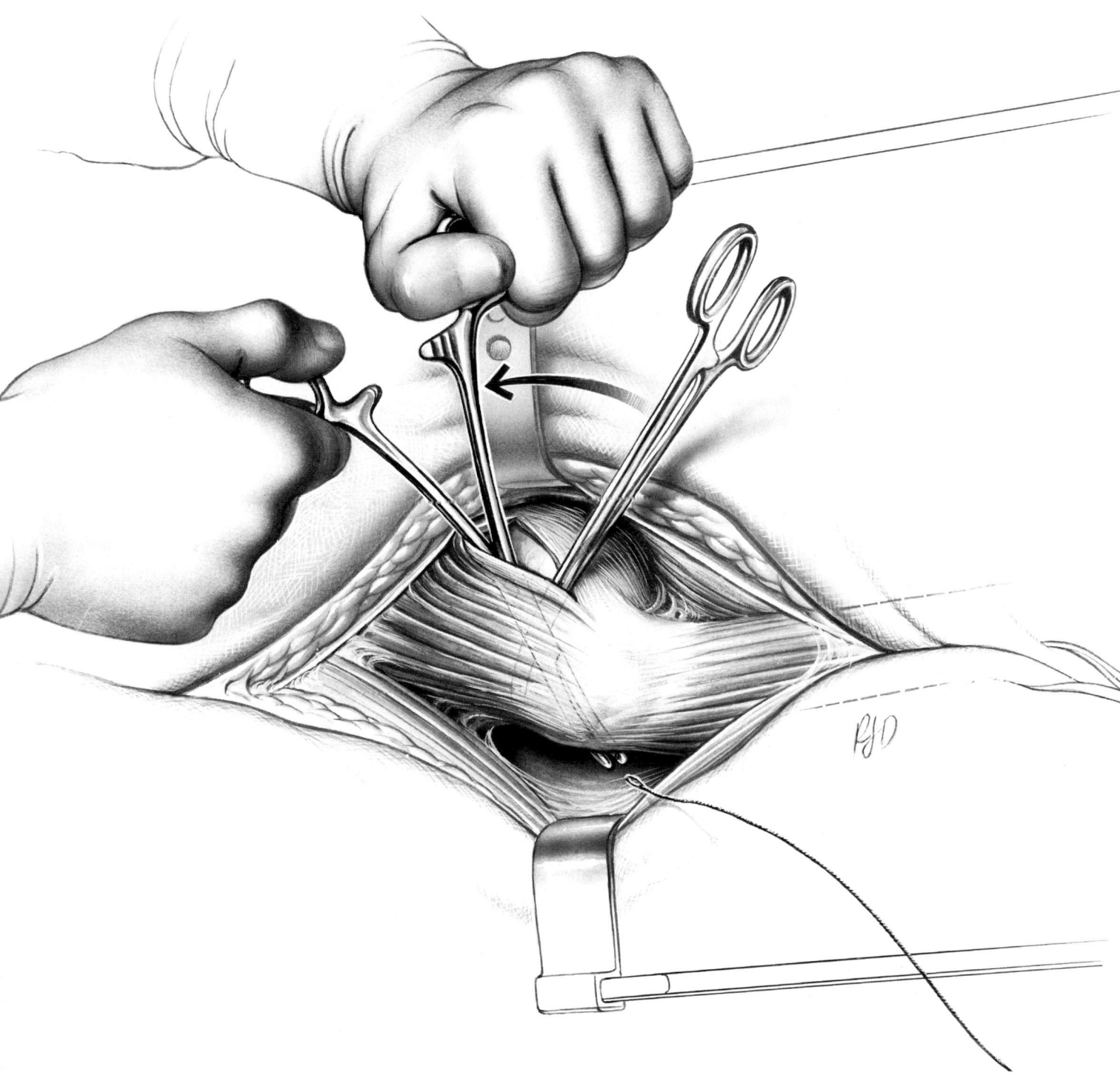

Fig. 18-7. Cholecystectomy forceps are inserted into synovial cavity of joint to pass above neck of femur and to reach posterior part of joint behind neck to retrieve Gigli's saw. Tip of cholecystectomy clamp is forced through and out of posterior capsule of joint. End of Gigli's saw wire is then caught in jaws of cholecystectomy forceps and pulled back through synovial cavity of joint. NOTE: first assistant has turned handles of cholecystectomy clamp to face surgeon. Jaws must be spread apart by first assistant using both hands.

Detachment of Trochanter

Determine the size of the portion of the trochanter to be osteotomized. As indicated in Fig. 18-8, the plane and level of osteotomy are controlled by the point of exit of the saw on the femur (Fig. 18-9, *A*). If the trochanter is normal, that is, if there is no deformity of the upper femur, the Gigli's saw should exit on the lateral aspect of the femur, through the vastus ridge or tubercle. This leaves adequate trochanter for subsequent reattachment.

After the surgeon has passed the Gigli's saw, make certain that the following occur:

1. The limb is in the neutral position without external/internal rotation or adduction/abduction.
2. The saw is in the correct position with respect to the greater trochanter and the femoral neck.
3. The sciatic nerve remains medial to the saw. Verify this by palpating the point of emergence of the saw (see Fig. 18-8).
4. Neither subcutaneous fat nor the anterior border of the gluteus medius are in the path of the saw. The fat is retracted as needed using a Watson-Jones gouge.
   After passing the Gigli saw and verifying its position, it is often tempting to remove the trochanter without reassessing the points just outlined, but this should not be done.
5. Next, place the knee at right angle to the floor with the hip maximally adducted (Fig. 18-9). The saw must be directed first toward the patient's foot so that it engages against the inner aspect of the base of the trochanter. The hands and arms must be kept well apart while holding the saw. Perform the osteotomy with a smooth reciprocal motion. The first stroke must be gentle and at an acute angle to the shaft of the femur (almost parallel to the femur and thigh) so that the saw is engaged to the trochanter at its base (neck-trochanter junction).
6. After the osteotomy has been started, the saw is directed toward the exit point through the vastus lateralis ridge. One half of the ridge remains on the shaft for the subsequent reattachment of the trochanter. If the saw is caught in the bone and unable to pass, it may be the result of (1) entering the bone at an acute angle, by not keeping the hands sufficiently apart while sawing, or (2) excessive and hasty pull, engaging the saw deep into the bone before actual cutting.
7. Before completing the cutting (emergence of the saw), the surgeon must detach the remaining vastus lateralis muscle from the ridge circumferentially; failure to do this will cause this muscle to be torn off the ridge and the shaft of the femur as the saw disengages from the bone.

Leg Length Measurements

Conduct leg length measurements according to the technique described in Chapter 15.

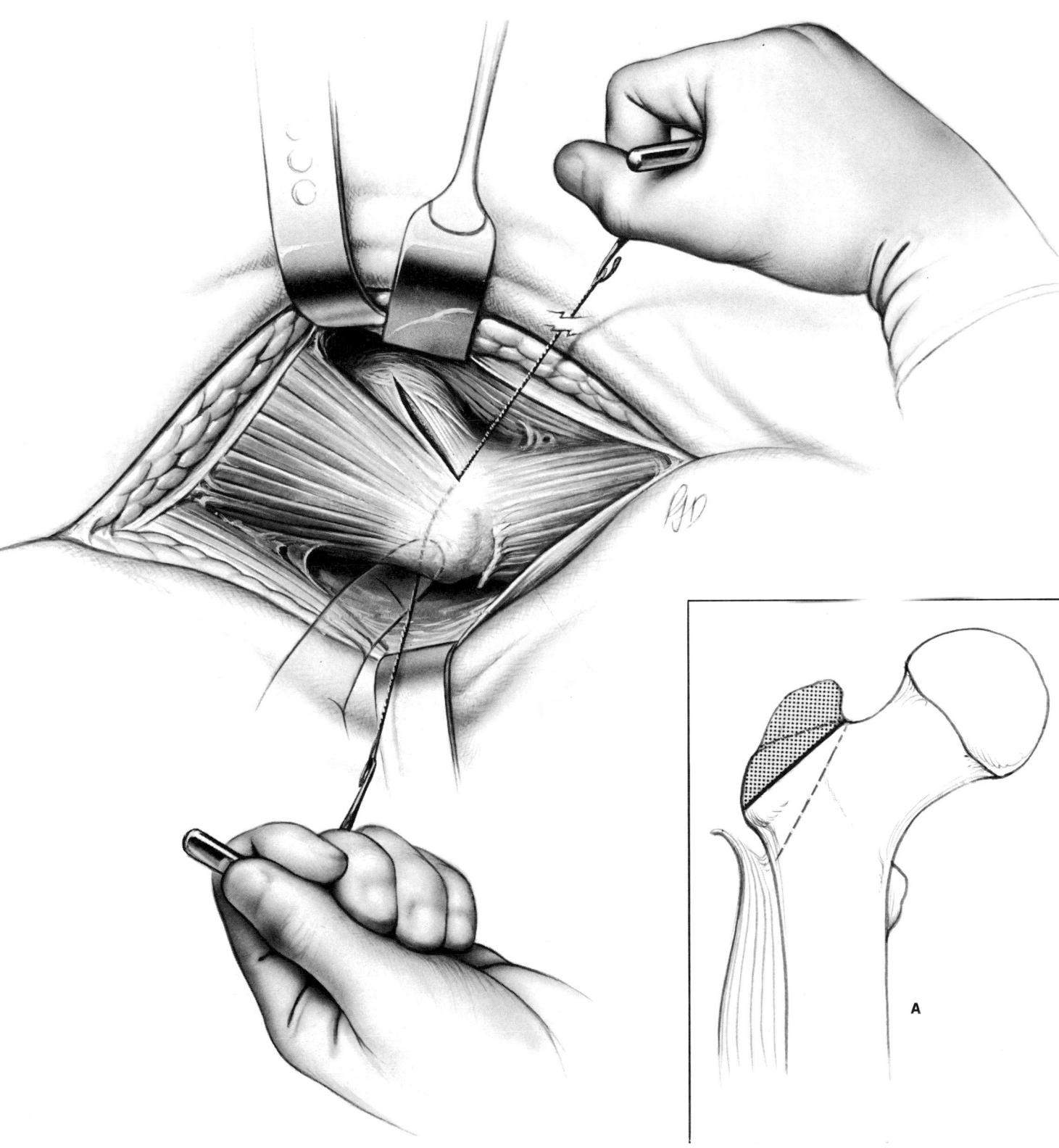

Fig. 18-8. Once Gigli's saw is passed, it is laid aside for a moment and the surgeon palpates the emergence of the saw at posterior aspect of greater trochanter and ascertains its relation to crest of trochanter. Surgeon also assures that sciatic nerve does not lie between saw and bone (phantom finger). Incision is now made onto periosteum over lateral surface of greater trochanter to detach approximately 1 cm of vastus lateralis from ridge and 0.5 to 1 cm of periosteum over lateral surface of greater trochanter proximal to ridge. This exposes vastus ridge and determines point of exit of saw. Direction of Gigli's saw is first toward patient's foot and then changes to cut laterally so that it emerges just proximal to vastus lateralis ridge. Inset **A,** optimal section of trochanter to be removed. Saw must emerge just above vastus lateralis ridge. Solid line illustrates optimal site, and interrupted lines show incorrect sites of removal.

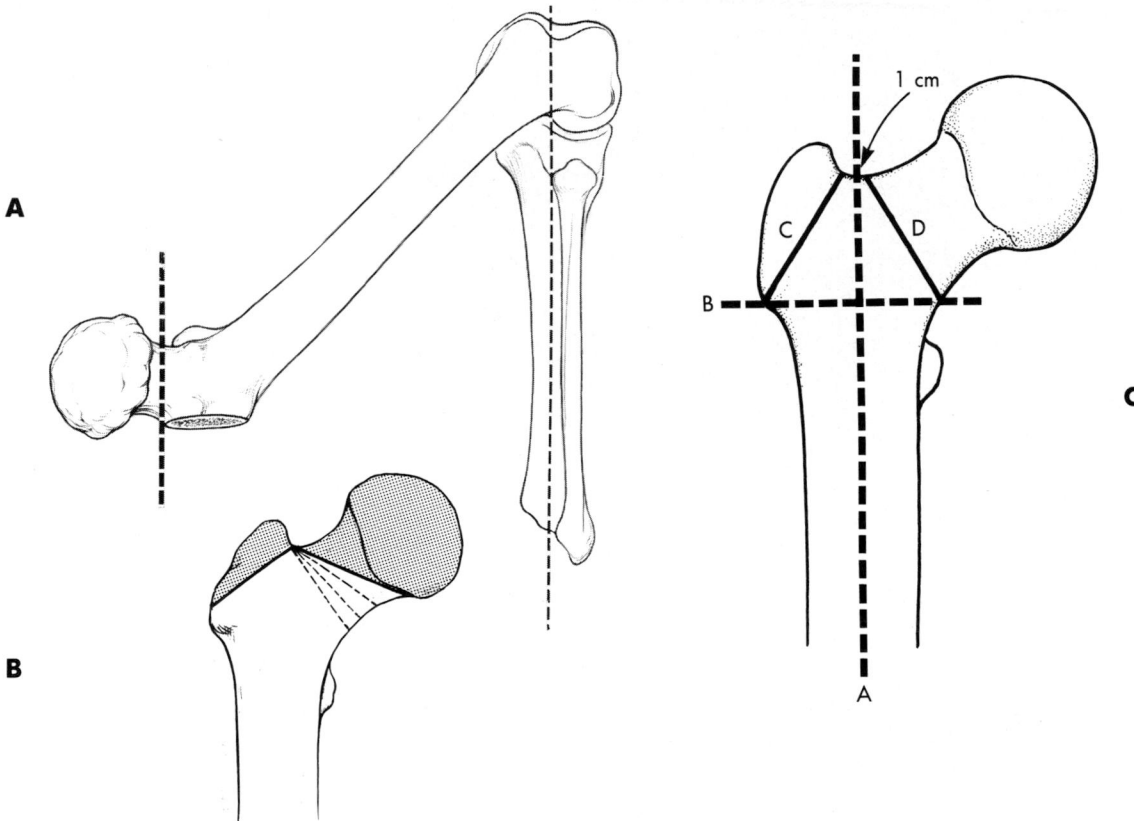

Fig. 18-9. A, Plane of section of neck is judged in relation to vertical position of tibia. This plane of section of neck ignores any anteversion or retroversion that may be present in neck of femur. **B,** Femoral head is divided by Gigli's saw at "meeting point" of cut surface of greater trochanter with femoral head. Several optional lines *(dashed lines)* show meeting points. These optional lines indicate further shortening of neck of femur when it becomes necessary. **C,** The neck-section level on the medial neck is determined by a perpendicular line drawn from the vastus lateralis ridge to the medial femoral cortex. A second line is drawn from this point on the femur to a point separating it 1 cm from the cut surface of the trochanter.

Completion of Capsulotomy Before Dislocation

Before any attempt at dislocation, three steps must be taken.

Retraction of Trochanter

The first assistant pulls the greater trochanter cephalad using a Morris or a Hibbs retractor. If the trochanter is severely externally rotated and requires release, it should be done at this stage (Fig. 18-10, A). The detached trochanter is retracted by a sharp hook to put the external rotators under tension. The external rotators stretch between the posterior parts of the greater trochanter and the hip joint. The tip of the cholecystectomy forceps is passed from behind forward around the external rotators. The cholecystectomy forceps are chosen because of their acute curvature. They are used at this stage like a hook. A scalpel is then used to divide the rotators. This step is rarely indicated in rheumatoid hips and should be performed judiciously in patients with osteoarthritis with fixed external rotation deformity.

Note that only the external rotator tendons are divided. The superior and anterosuperior parts of the capsule of the hip joint are left intact. This part of the capsule connects the detached trochanter to the superior lip of the acetabulum. The lateral and superior capsule is a very important connection between the detached trochanter and the acetabulum. It prevents dislocation of the joint when it is correctly tensioned during reattachment of the trochanter.

Control of Posterior Capsular Vessels

The hip is flexed, adducted, and internally rotated to expose the posterior capsule to view (Fig. 18-10, B). Retinacular bleeders commonly found there must be controlled at this stage. With the hip in this position, the sciatic nerve is protected in its bed of fatty tissue by a Watson-Jones retractor held by the first assistant (see Fig. 18-10, B). The posterior capsule is palpated against the head of the femur deep in the wound to determine where the capsular incision will be made.

Completion of Capsular Release

The posterior capsulotomy is then performed over the posterior aspect of the neck of the femur (at about a 6 o'clock position) (Fig. 18-10, C). Further diathermy of the brisk bleeders may be necessary at this stage before changing limb position. If contracted external rotated capsules attached to the greater trochanter require release, they are sharply divided at this point close to the trochanter. While the capsulotomy is performed, the sciatic nerve is protected by the Watson-Jones gouge to visualize the posterior rim of the acetabulum.

In summary, follow these steps before attempting to dislocate the hip. (1) Retract the trochanter cephalad. (2) Complete capsular and piriformis release as necessary. (3) Excise marginal osteophytes (if present). (4) Control bleeding of posterior capsular vessels.

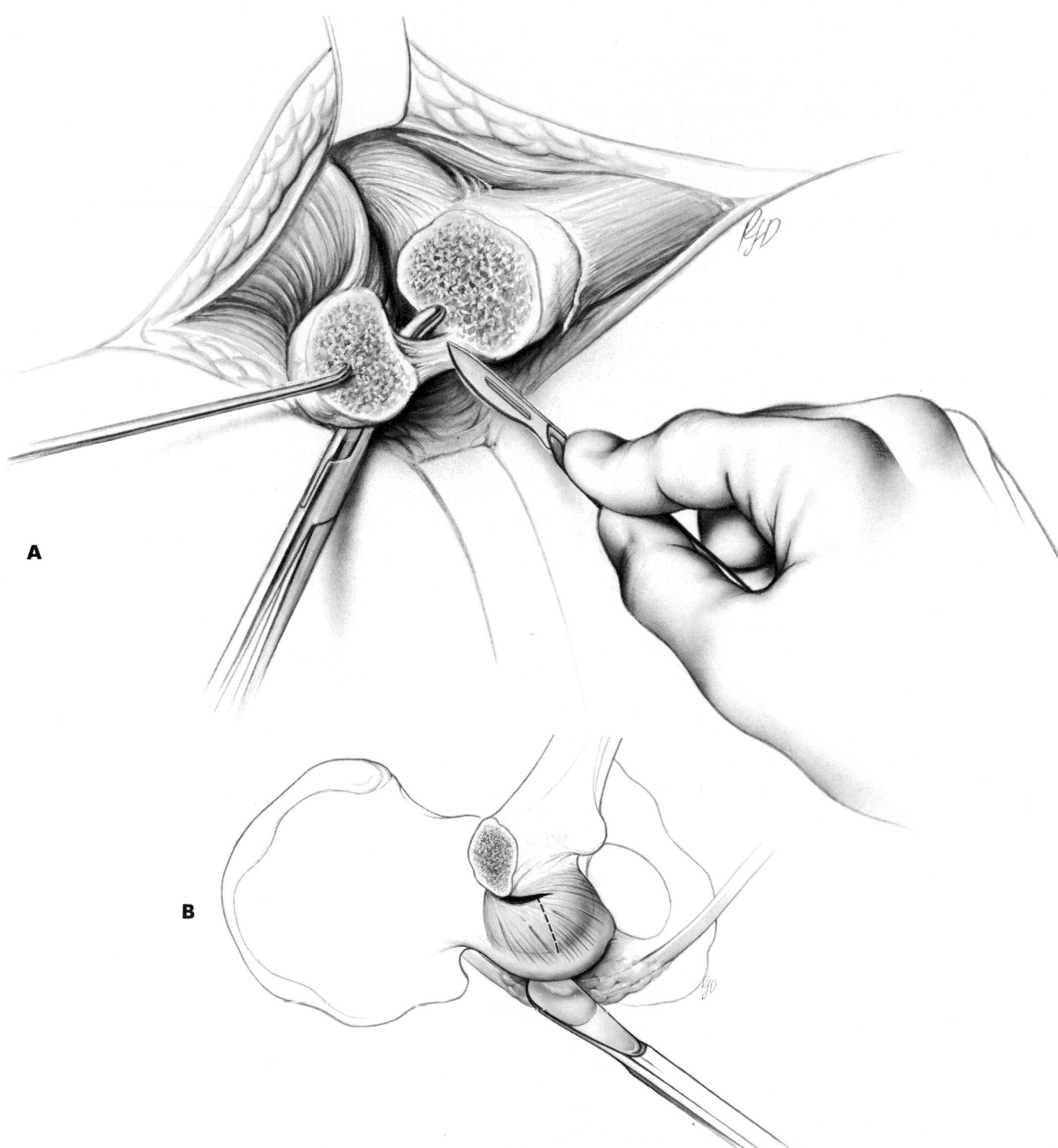

Fig. 18-10. A, External rotators are divided when trochanter is severely externally rotated. Cholecystectomy forceps have been passed behind external rotators (piriformis), and scalpel is in position to divide it. **B,** Before attempting dislocation, posterior capsulotomy must be completed. Posterior capsulotomy is done over flexed and internally rotated head of femur at about 6-o'clock position from surgeon's perspective. While capsulotomy is performed, sciatic nerve is protected by Watson-Jones gouge to visualize posterior rim of acetabulum.

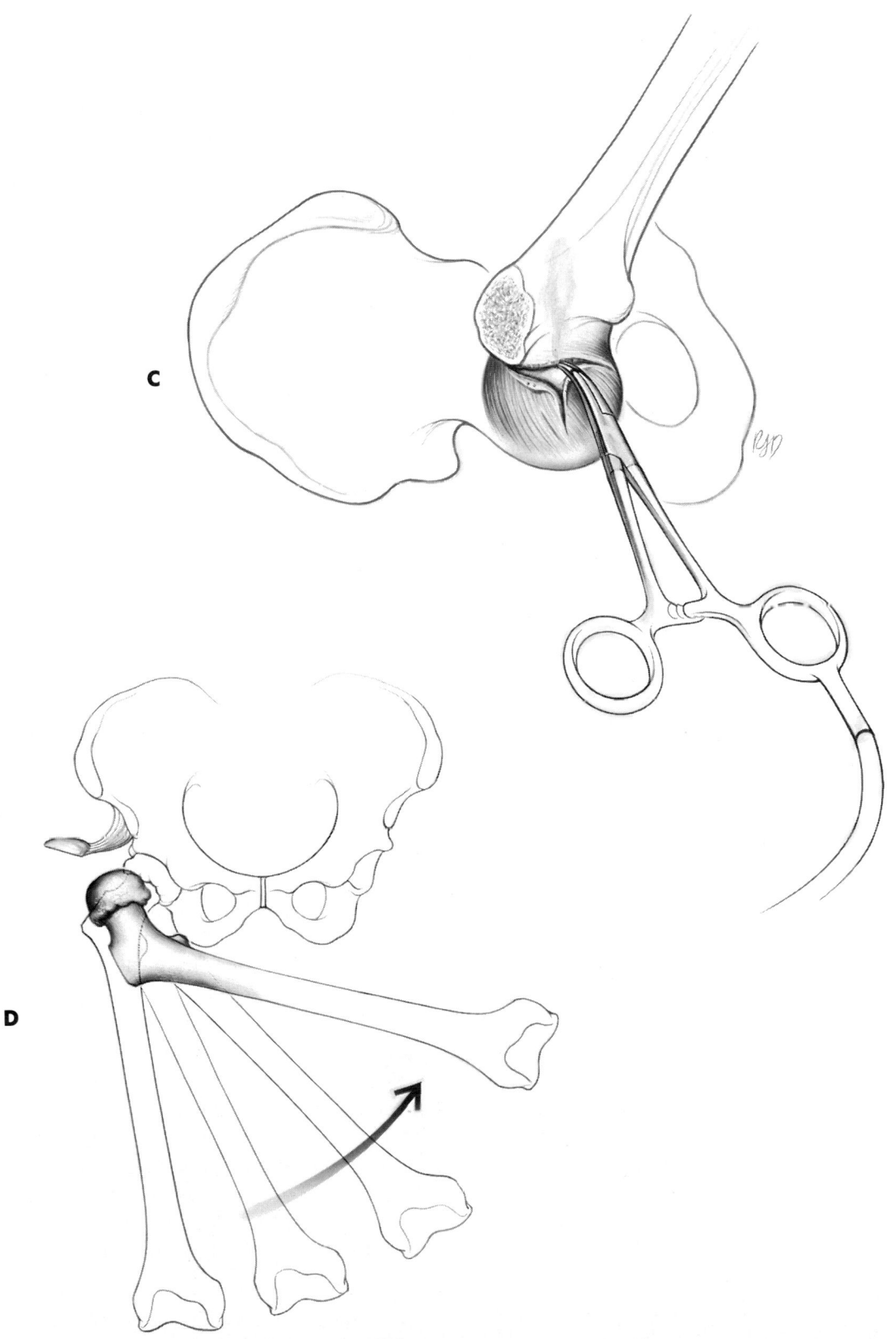

Fig. 18–10 — cont'd. C, Posterior retinacular capsular bleeders are controlled with hip in flexion, internal rotation, and adduction. With hip in this position, sciatic nerve must again be protected in its bed of fatty tissue, while cautery forceps are used. **D,** Dislocation is accomplished by adducting limb without external rotation to bring head out of socket.

Continued.

PHASE III: DISLOCATING THE HIP

The second assistant adducts the limb *without* external rotation to bring the head out of the socket (Fig. 18-10, *D*). No external rotation force must be applied before the head is out of the acetabulum because it may cause a spiral fracture of the femur. Resistance may occur from the following:

1. The vacuum created when the head is moved from the depth of the socket.
2. Persistent posterosuperior or anterior capsular attachments.
3. A peripheral osteophyte or an excessively deep acetabulum, that is, protrusio acetabuli.
4. A coxa magna senilis larger than the opening of the acetabulum restricted by capsule and labrum.
5. Residual ligamentum teres.
6. A hypertrophied labrum.

Complete dislocation and delivery of the head into the wound may be facilitated by the following:

1. Placing the Watson-Jones bone gouge between the head and the acetabulum and levering the head out as the hip is adducted (Fig. 18-10, *E*).
2. Successively flexing and extending the hip to break the vacuum.
3. Further release of residual capsular and ligamentous structures.
4. Removal of overhanging acetabular osteophytes if present.
5. Incising the labrum along the superior acetabular rim.
6. Most important, maximal posterior capsular release (see Fig. 18-10, *C*).

An excessively flexed hip in an adducted posture is more difficult to dislocate. An experienced second assistant is valuable at this stage of the operation; however, the surgeon is fully responsible for the "act of dislocation."

In summary, dislocation is achieved by maximum adduction without external rotation or flexion. External rotation can cause a spiral fracture of the femur if the head is still in the acetabulum.

Amputating the Femoral Head

Before amputating the femoral head, the surgeon should divide any tight synovial or capsular bands remaining between the inferior neck and the acetabulum. Maximum adduction of the hip must be possible to allow the surgeon to pass the Gigli's saw over the head and around the neck; proximal retraction of the greater trochanter is necessary to allow passage of the saw over the head.

The line of amputation is directed toward the proximal edge of the greater trochanteric osteotomy site (Fig. 18-10, *F*). Unless the surgeon deliberately plans to cut the neck shorter or longer for shortening or lengthening of the extremity, the level of the cut must be determined by radiographs with appropriate magnifications as guided by radiograph templates. However, in a normal situation the neck sectioning begins at the point of the XY axis through the vastus tubercle (perpendicular to the longitudinal axis of the femur). The saw then meets at a point 1 cm medial to the cut surface of the trochanter proximally (see Fig. 18-9, *C*). During the amputation of the head the second assistant keeps the knee flexed and the tibial shaft perpendicular (90 degrees) to the floor (see Fig. 18-9). The plane of section of the neck is judged in relation to the vertical position of the tibia. It ignores any anteversion or retroversion that may be present in the femoral neck. The first assistant holds the head with a sponge to resist the pull of the Gigli's saw. This prevents undue stripping of the capsule and detachment of the femur from the pelvic wall (especially in fragile rheumatoid patients), while the surgeon performs the amputation with a gentle reciprocating motion (Fig. 18-10, *F*).

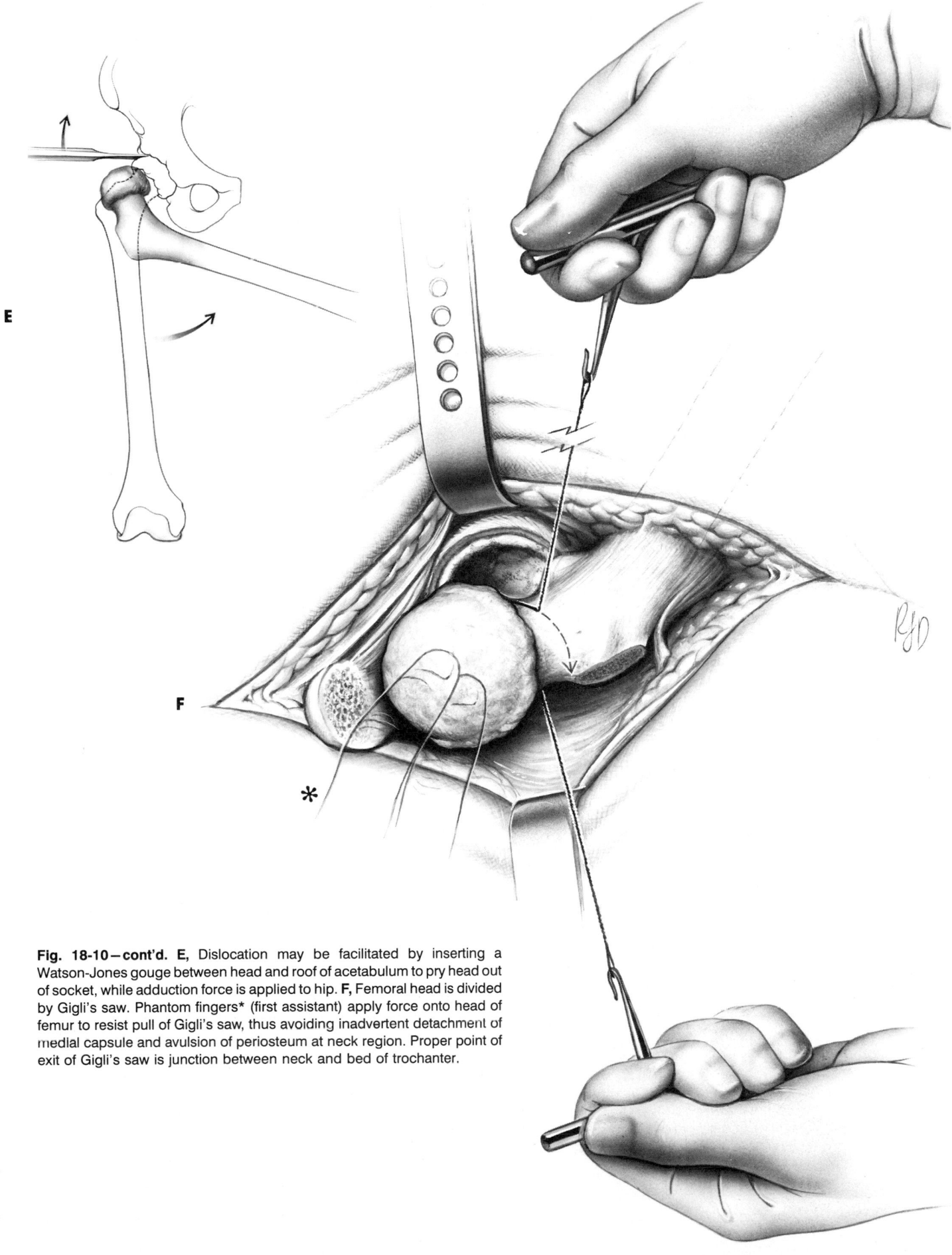

Fig. 18-10—cont'd. E, Dislocation may be facilitated by inserting a Watson-Jones gouge between head and roof of acetabulum to pry head out of socket, while adduction force is applied to hip. **F,** Femoral head is divided by Gigli's saw. Phantom fingers* (first assistant) apply force onto head of femur to resist pull of Gigli's saw, thus avoiding inadvertent detachment of medial capsule and avulsion of periosteum at neck region. Proper point of exit of Gigli's saw is junction between neck and bed of trochanter.

PHASE IV: PREPARING THE ACETABULUM AND FIXING THE ACETABULAR COMPONENT
Maximizing Exposure

Adduct the hip maximally across the table, and place the Charnley self-retaining retractors to give an adequate view of the acetabular cavity; sometimes additional soft tissue release is necessary to apply them properly.

The insertion sites of the jaws of the "east-west" and "north-south" retractors must be carefully selected (Fig. 18-11). The east-west retractor is used to hold the trochanter cephalad and the femur caudad. A screw jack attached to the retractor provides the added force required to separate the retractor jaws (Fig. 18-11, *A*, inset). Use the north-south retractor to hold the tensor fascia femoris muscle anteriorly and the posterior capsule posteriorly to expose the periphery of the acetabulum. Engage the proximal jaw of the east-west retractor into the strap of the superior capsule proximal to the trochanter. Avoid fracturing the trochanter by careless placement of the proximal jaw into an osteoporotic bone. Place the distal jaw across the intramedullary canal of the osteotomized femoral neck. NOTE: the posterior jaw of the north-south retractor is engaged into the posterior capsule (taking care to avoid the sciatic nerve) and the anterior jaw into the anterior capsule (under the psoas and tensor muscles). These retractors (1) must produce maximum exposure of the acetabulum; and (2) must not be engaged into the periphery of the bony acetabulum or the labrum; use a Hohmann-type retractor engaged onto the anterior rim of acetabulum when full exposure of the anterior wall of the acetabulum is not feasible with a north-south retractor (Fig. 18-12).

Drive one or two "pin retractors" into the ilium just superior to the acetabular rim and external to the labrum (but intracapsularly) to allow visibility of the superior bony periphery (see Fig. 18-12). The pins must first be directed craniad at about a 45-degree angle to the axis of the body; then as they are hammered into place, the pin handle is brought craniad to a line perpendicular to the body's axis. Ideally, when fully engaged, they also hold the greater trochanter cephalad, exposing the superior acetabular rim (see Fig. 18-12).

If exposure is not satisfactory, do the following:

1. Detach contracted external rotators from the posterior aspect of the femur.
2. Perform tenotomy of piriformis if contracted.
3. Increase flexion and adduction of the extremity.
4. Reposition the limb (by even a few degrees), as directed by the surgeon.

Preparing the Socket

As noted in Chapter 15, the type of socket preparation depends largely on whether cement is used and on the morphological pathology of the acetabulum. Preparing the acetabulum according to Charnley's recommended technique requires drilling a 12.5-mm hole through the floor of the acetabulum into which deepening and expanding reamers are engaged as follows*:

- Drill a pilot hole after marking the acetabular floor as shown in Figs. 18-11 and 18-13. Use a collared 12.5-mm drill, carrying the centering ring to drill the spigot hole for deepening and expanding reamers. Depending on the pathology of the acetabulum, a high or low position for drilling the spigot hole may be selected (Fig. 18-13).
- Engage the spigot of deepening and expanding reamers to prepare the acetabulum (Figs. 18-13 to 18-15). Deepen only to the level of the nonarticulating portion of the acetabular wall (corresponding to the outer table of the medial acetabular wall; the teardrop sign) (see Chapter 15).

---

*This author no longer uses Charnley's technique to prepare the acetabulum because it may excessively damage the medial wall of the acetabulum and requires the use of a cement restrictor to limit the flow of the cement into the pelvis.[1-4]

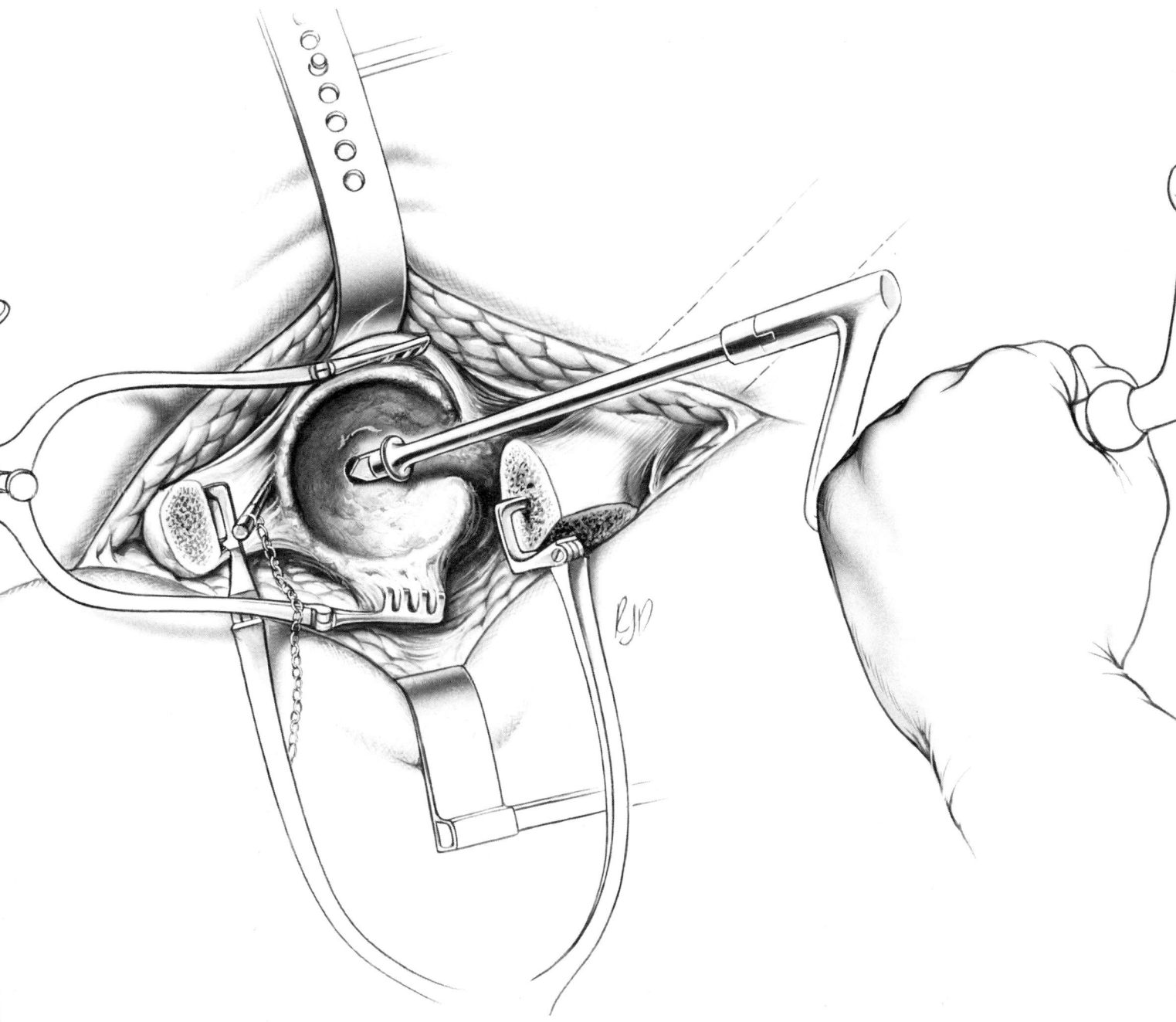

Fig. 18-11. East-west and north-south retractors are in place. Nail retractor with safety chain and detachable handle is used to complete exposure of superior rim of acetabulum. Nail retractor holds capsule in headward direction to make sure that bony margin of acetabulum is clearly visible throughout subsequent steps of operation. This visualization is most important to make surgeon sure that hip socket will be completely contained inside superior lip of acetabulum when cemented in position.

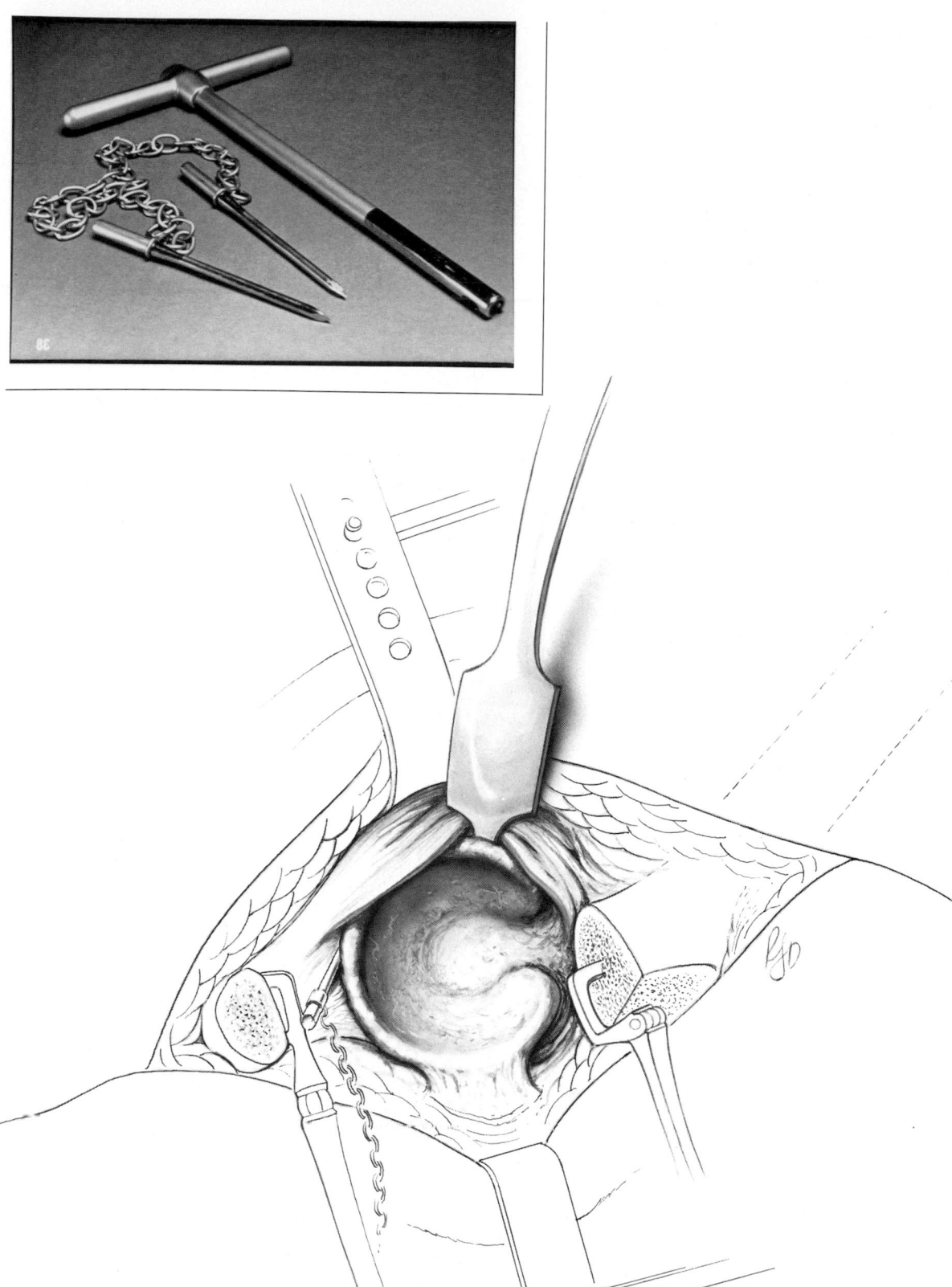

Fig. 18-12. Same visualization of acetabulum as shown in Fig. 18-11. North-south retractor has been replaced by Hohmann retractor to visualize anterior lip of acetabulum. In addition, a similar retractor may be placed inferior to acetabulum at level of intercotyloid notch if necessary. Inset shows Charnley acetabular pins with "T" handle insertor/extractor.

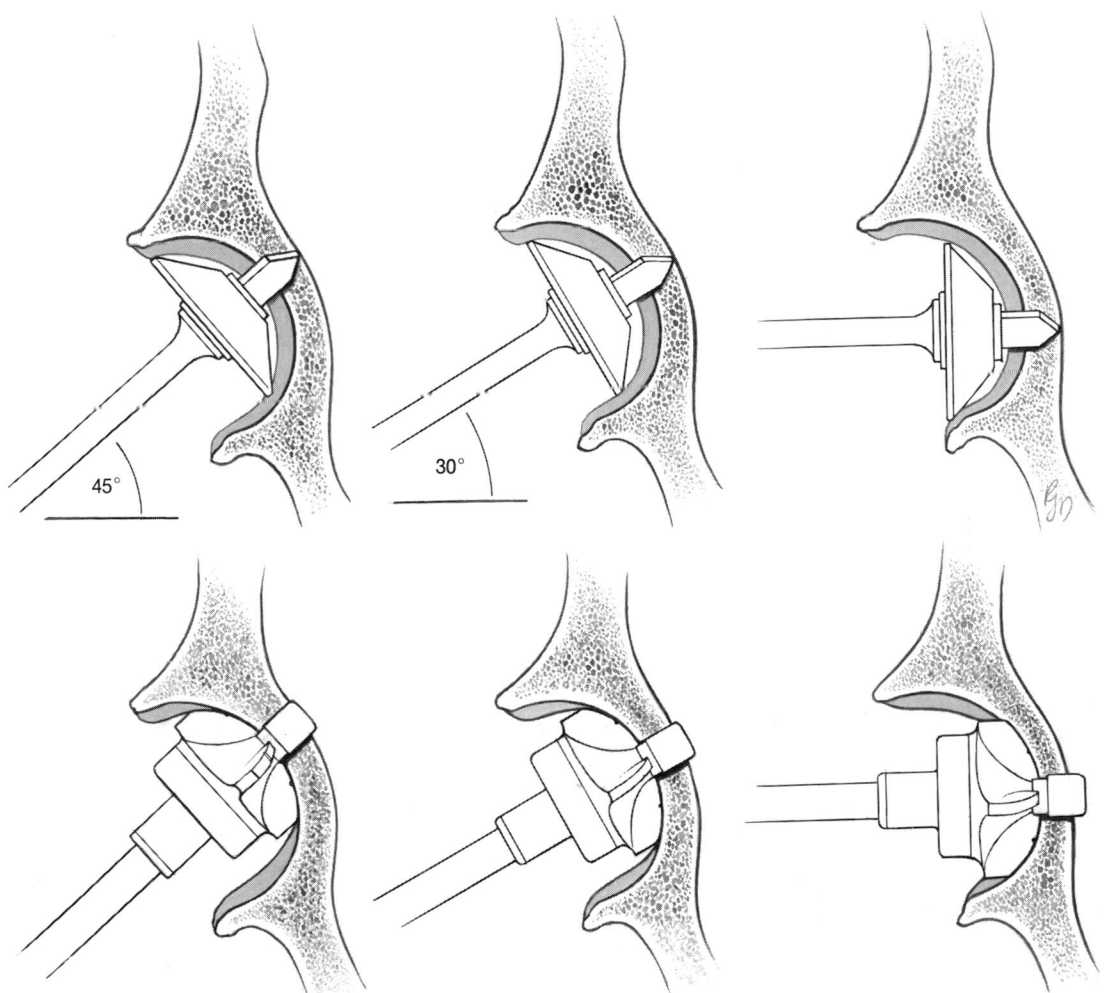

Fig. 18-13. Top shows centering drill with centering ring used to locate center of acetabulum where maximum deepening will be accomplished. NOTE: orientation of drill at 45 degrees, 30 degrees, and 0 degrees in relation to transaxis of pelvis. NOTE: with marking of pelvis in 45 degrees, preparation will be accomplished "high" in acetabulum; with 30 degrees preparation is "intermediate" parallel to the transaxis it is "low." Note also, deepening and expanding will occur where pilot hole is drilled. It is therefore essential to determine the appropriate preparation of the acetabulum and place the pilot hole accordingly at desired angle.

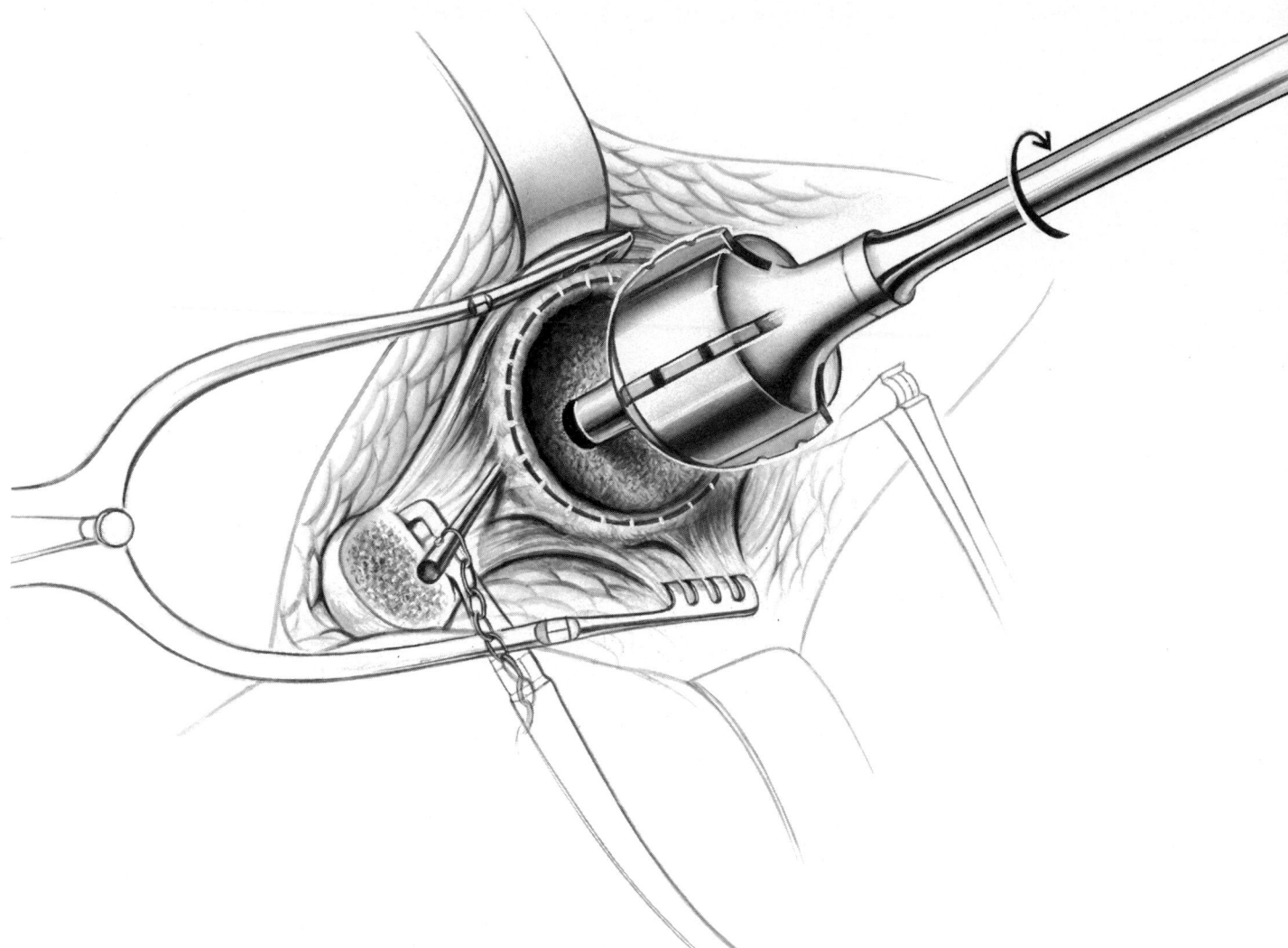

Fig. 18-14. After use of deepening reamer, expanding reamer is used at an angle similar to that in Fig. 18-13.

Drilling Pilot Hole at 30- to 45-Degree Angle (High Position)

The acetabular floor must be marked for placement of the pilot hole. When the acetabulum is small or the head has migrated concentrically medialward at a 30- to 45-degree angle, the centering drill carrying the "centering ring" is placed at the depth of the acetabulum at a 30- to 45-degree angle to the transaxis of the pelvis (see Fig. 18-13), which is about the same angle as the neck-shaft angle when the hip is on a 0-degree abduction/adduction position. The handle of the drill is slightly elevated (5 to 10 degrees) to compensate for the tilt of the patient on the operating table toward the second assistant. After removing the centering ring, the marking must be checked to be sure that it is clearly visible and appropriately placed before actual drilling; if not, a second marking may be called for. The floor of the acetabulum is then perforated at the same angle using the 12.5-mm drill. Drilling the pilot hole is a singularly important step since misplacement directs the reamers improperly and damages the walls of the acetabulum. The direction of the drill in relation to the transaxis line of the pelvis must be constantly observed; minor deviation is permissible but must be deliberate and intentional.

Drilling Pilot Hole at 90-Degree Angle (Low Position)

This method is typically used for dysplastic acetabuli or acetabuli that have migrated proximally; in both situations the desire is to lower the socket to the anatomical level. It is also necessarily used in cases of a wandering acetabulum with proximal migration of the head; in upper pole osteoarthritis and proximal migration in a large, bony man (broken Shenton's line on radiograph); or with a large, inferior osteophyte formation and a short limb (usually accompanied by fixed adduction deformity with occasional dysplasia). The centering device is usually placed against the floor of the acetabulum with the drill perpendicular to the axis of the body. Again, the handle is elevated (as much as 5 to 10 degrees) to compensate for the tilt of the pelvis toward the second assistant. Inadvertent placement of the marking device excessively cephalad leads to removal of important superior acetabular bone. Excessive caudal placement of the marker makes it difficult to remove the cartilage from the roof of the acetabulum and causes unnecessary lengthening of the limb. Schematic drawings (see Fig. 18-13) illustrate the effects of change in direction of the centering tool on the final shape and direction of the prepared acetabulum.

Gauging for the Cup Size and Rehearsal

See Chapter 15.

Trimming and Rehearsal of Pressure Injection Cup

See Chapter 15.

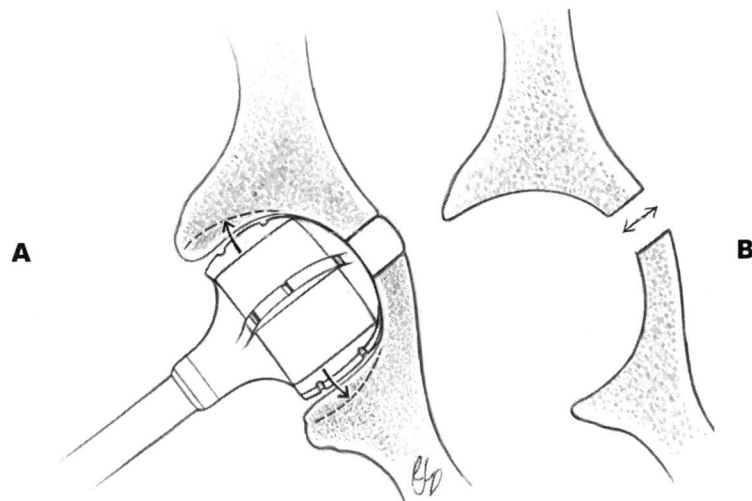

Fig. 18-15. **A** shows amount of bone to be shaved by expanding reamer. **B**, thickness of floor may be judged by thickness of pilot hole made at floor of acetabulum in addition to observing level of pulvinar. NOTE: usually pelvis is rolled away about 10 degrees so that handle of brace has to be elevated about 10 degrees above horizontal line. This means simply that one must elevate brace to compensate for elevation of pelvis from table on surgeon's side.

Positioning and Fixing the Cup

Observe the following:

1. In Charnley's technique no anteversion is allowed (Fig. 18-16). However, Charnley recommends 5 degrees of anteversion to compensate for the patient's pelvic tilt away from the surgeon (since the pelvis is often rolled to the opposite side by the second assistant holding the leg). Confirm the absence of anteversion by holding the horizontal limb of the socket-holder parallel to the floor. Indeed, the extended posterior wall effectively creates about 15 degrees anteversion. Any added anteversion at surgery risks anterior dislocation.

2. Use (ideally) a PIJ cup or an OGEE* cup. Trim to fit the opening of the acetabulum as described in Chapter 15.

3. Use cement at a high-viscosity stage of polymerization immediately after removing the packing from the acetabulum.

4. Immediately detach the socket holder from the face of the cup after final positioning. Maintain a concentric pressure on the cup with a pusher rod.

5. Stabilize the socket by keeping thumb pressure against its superior lobe until the cement is set, because upon removing the socket holder the flanged socket may begin to tilt away from the roof of the acetabulum.

---

*OGEE cup is a variation of the PIJ cup with its posterior flange in an opposite direction of the anterior flange. (see Chapter 11.)

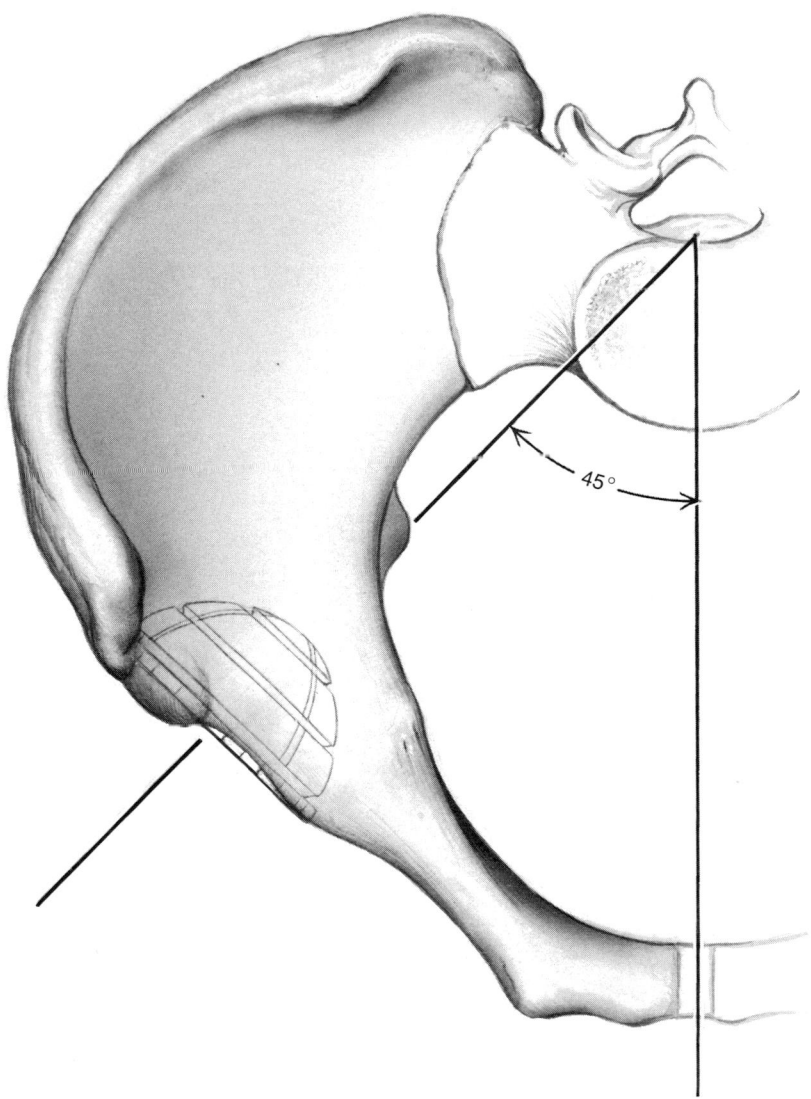

Fig. 18-16. In transpelvic view (inlet), orientation of socket reveals no anteversion.

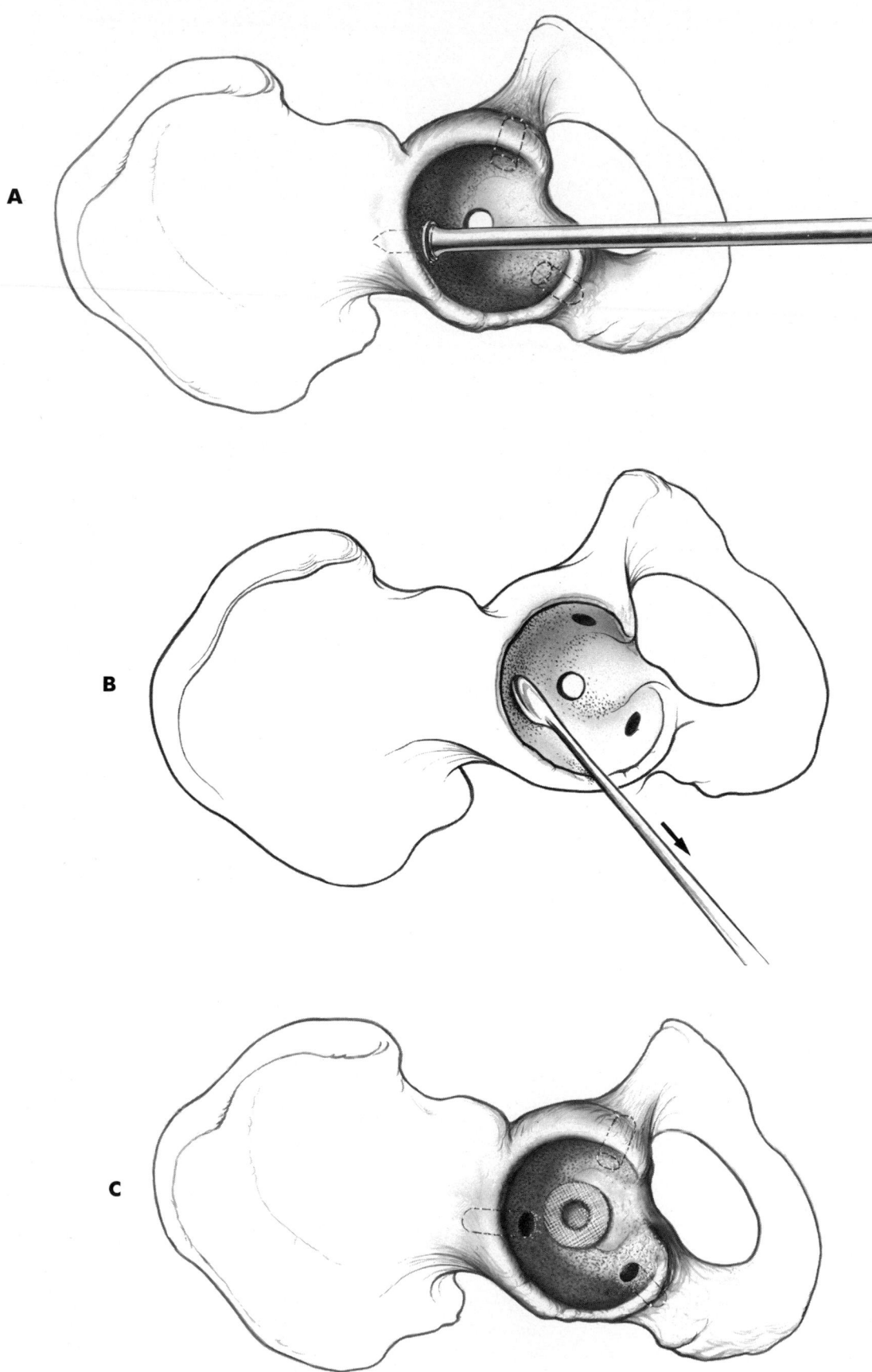

Fig. 18-17. See legend on opposite page.

Final Preparation, Anchor Holes, and Cementing of the Acetabular Component

Specific to Charnley's technique is the use of three large anchor holes (12.5 mm) in addition to multiple 6-mm drill holes. A cement restrictor also is used at the site of the pilot hole to prevent cement intrusion into the pelvis. A large-gauge sponge soaked with hydrogen peroxide is packed into the acetabulum before cement is introduced. Fig. 18-17, *A* to *D,* illustrates the anchor hole sites and Fig. 18-17, *E,* the packing of the acetabulum. For details of cementing of the acetabular component, see Chapter 15.

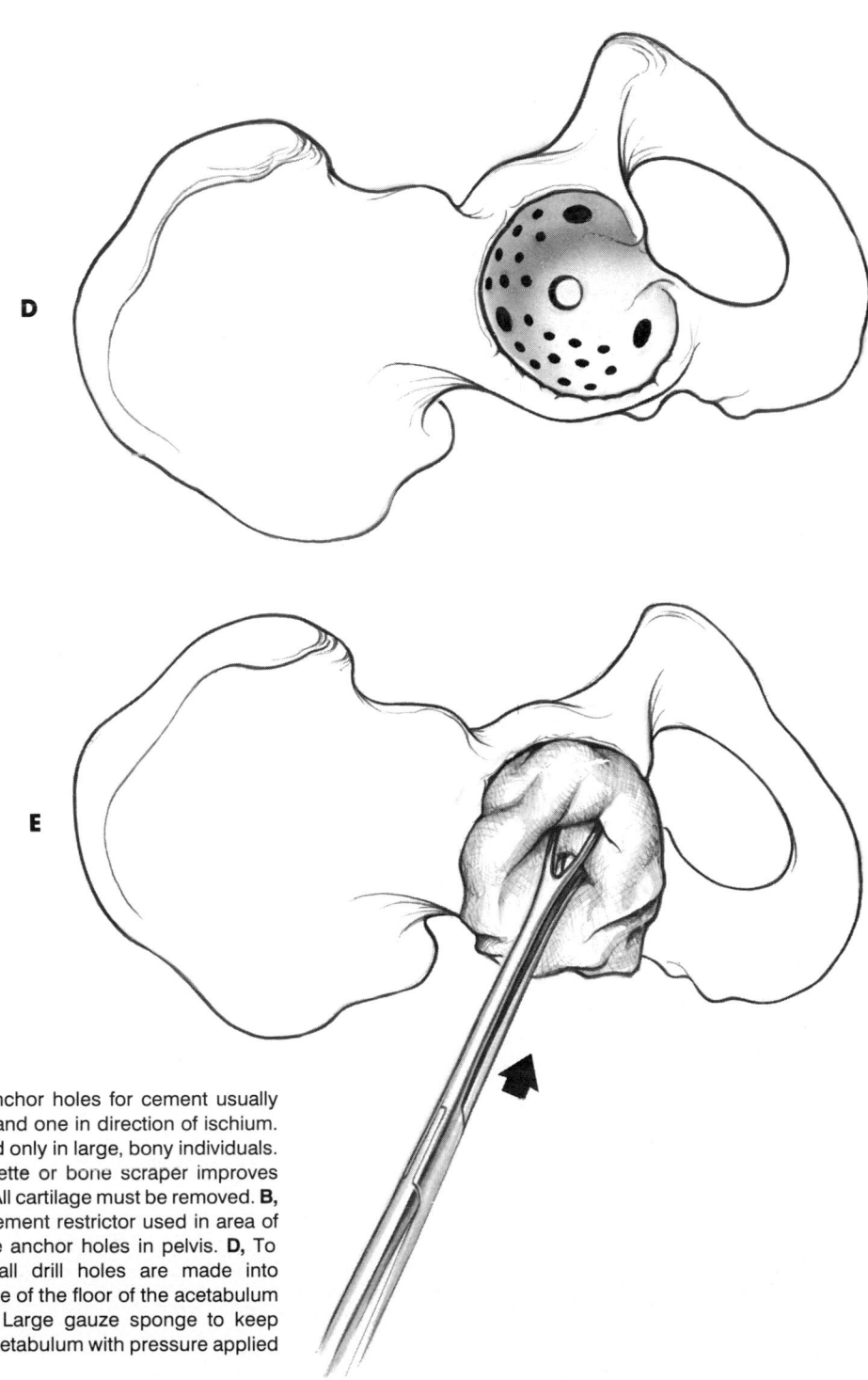

Fig. 18-17. A, Two 12.5 mm anchor holes for cement usually suffice, one in direction of ilium and one in direction of ischium. Anchor hole toward pubis is used only in large, bony individuals. Use of sharp, long-handled curette or bone scraper improves final preparation of acetabulum. All cartilage must be removed. **B,** Use of Volkmann's spoon. **C,** Cement restrictor used in area of pilot hole. NOTE: position of three anchor holes in pelvis. **D,** To maximize fixation, multiple small drill holes are made into subchondral bone when the bone of the floor of the acetabulum is sclerotic and nonporous. **E,** Large gauze sponge to keep acetabulum dry is packed into acetabulum with pressure applied by first assistant.

PHASE V: SELECTION OF FEMORAL COMPONENT, TEST REDUCTION FOR STABILITY AND LENGTH, AND INSERTING WIRES
Delivery of Stump of Upper Femur

With the self-retaining retractors removed, the stump of the proximal femur is now delivered out of the wound for preparation; excessive force is to be avoided. The stump is best delivered by maximal adduction of the hip without flexion by the second assistant, who supports the knee flexed at 90 degrees and places the femur across the opposite side of the table and the opposite thigh. Any medial and posterior soft tissue attachments that remain may be released if necessary at this stage. The second assistant demonstrates the knee axis and the axis of the femur to the surgeon, who can now fully assess the direction of the femur in reference to the transcondylar line and the lesser trochanter.

Further delivery from the wound can be achieved by using a posteriorly placed Watson-Jones gouge, to lever the proximal end of the femur (Fig. 18-18). The position of the instrument is maintained by the first assistant (Fig. 18-18, inset), while the leg position is maintained by the second assistant. The Watson-Jones bone gouge further mobilizes the iliotibial tract medially and posteriorly in relation to the femur to assist in bringing the femur out of and away from the depth of the wound. Occasionally, detachment of the iliopsoas and the remainder of the contracted medial and posterior capsule may be needed, as in muscular and heavy men or obese patients or in difficult situations where persistent adduction and flexion deformity exist. Unless complete mobilization and maximal delivery of the stump are attained, preparation of the upper femur may be severely hindered; complications such as misorientation, poor sense of direction, or perforation of the shaft may result. This delivery is also essential for a valgus preparation and a valgus orientation of the prosthesis.* During this stage of the operation, the greater trochanter is turned into the acetabulum by folding the tendon of the gluteus medius and minimus. Alternatively, the trochanter is pulled proximally by the first assistant — using a Hibbs or similar retractor — carefully to avoid fracture and fragmentation.

---

*The term *valgus* as used in this section implies and stresses avoidance of a *varus* positioning. An exaggerated valgus positioning should also be avoided.

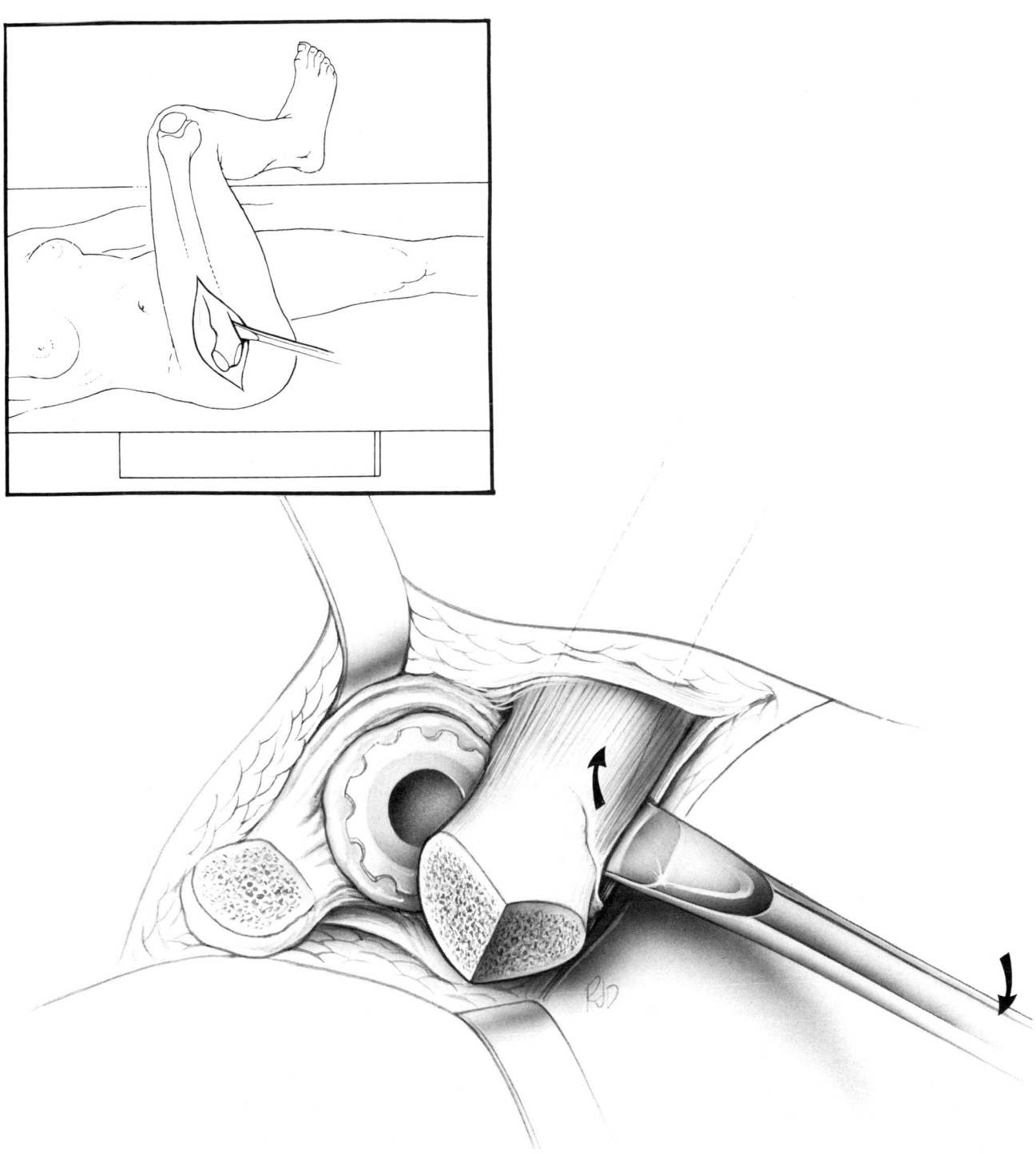

Fig. 18-18. Stump of upper femur is delivered out of wound and assisted by Watson-Jones gouge and maximal adduction of hip. With leg crossed to opposite side of table, surgeon now has complete access to top of femur. Inset illustrates cross-table position of limb during preparation of femur.

Preparation of Femur

The medullary canal is opened with a tapered pin T-handle reamer (Fig. 18-19). The starting point is the junction of the cut surfaces of the trochanter and the neck. The cortical bridge dividing the stump of the neck from the site of the osteotomized greater trochanter is removed with a rongeur, unless it was removed after the resection of the femoral head. The tapered pin T-handle reamer is aimed at the knee, thereby defining the medullary canal (Fig. 18-19, inset). Once the reamer is fully inserted, it is shifted toward the lateral cortex to produce a slightly valgus track. This entails encroachment on the trochanteric bed. The surgeon stabilizes the knee with one hand while guiding the reamer with the other; the second assistant holds the hip in maximum adduction and neutral rotation to aid stabilization. The assistant on the far side of the table holds the tibia vertical so that the amount of anteversion in the femoral neck can be recognized. The tapered reamer must be checked to assure that it is within the medullary canal and that valgus orientation is maintained. In this way the surgeon ascertains that the reamer is not piercing the femoral cortex. The aperture is enlarged by cutting toward the trochanteric bed as it is inserted, making an oval opening for femoral broach in the correct "version." A tapered reamer attached to a wide-throw brace may be used for this purpose instead of a T-handle tapered reamer.*

The straight femoral broach is then hammered into the medullary canal while being held in a valgus orientation. This is best accomplished by inserting a tommy bar into the broach handle and pulling the broach toward the outer cortex (Fig. 18-20). The plane of "version" has already been determined by the tapered pin reamer. To ensure a neutral version plane, the tommy bar should be perpendicular to the floor, while the knee is in 90 degrees flexion and the tibia perpendicular to the floor. The plane of the reamer should also be parallel to the transverse intracondylar axis of the knee. In this way, there are at least four points of reference for orientation:

1. Patella and the transverse axis of the knee (transcondylar line)
2. Operating table or floor
3. Flexed knee at right angle
4. Shape of the upper femur, especially in reference to the lesser trochanter

The curved broach is hammered down the medullary canal maintaining the same orientation (Fig. 18-20). The broaches are hammered in a valgus orientation, as if cutting takes place with the convex edge of the broach (Fig. 18-20, inset). Should the broaches impinge against the medial calcar, they must be withdrawn and reinserted (1) to ensure valgus positioning and (2) to prevent fracture of the calcar femorale. When the medullary canal is excessively narrow and the isthmus prevents full broaching, further widening may be accomplished by using graded reamers, such as the power-driven rotary reamers; broaching may then be completed. The surgeon may only use the rotary reamers (Fig. 18-21) and long-handled curettes as described in Chapter 15. The broaches should not be driven in with excessive force, since this may shatter the upper femur. Instead, the broaches are repeatedly inserted and removed to accomplish their purpose. When the broach is jammed in the canal, it is withdrawn and the rasp action repeated using the tommy bar and oscillating motions in external and internal rotation, followed by reinsertion of the broach. The correct orientation of the broaches relative to the leg is constantly checked. The channel is satisfactorily prepared when the broaches can be freely inserted to their full length in optimal orientation. Ideally the channel should not be in more than 5 degrees of anteversion and should accommodate a standard (or heavy, if the medullary canal is large) prosthesis. With experience the channel may be created without the use of broaches, using the tapered pin reamer and power tools.

---

* A tapered pin reamer attached to a power drill may be used (when power tools are used) to enlarge the cavity of the upper femur.

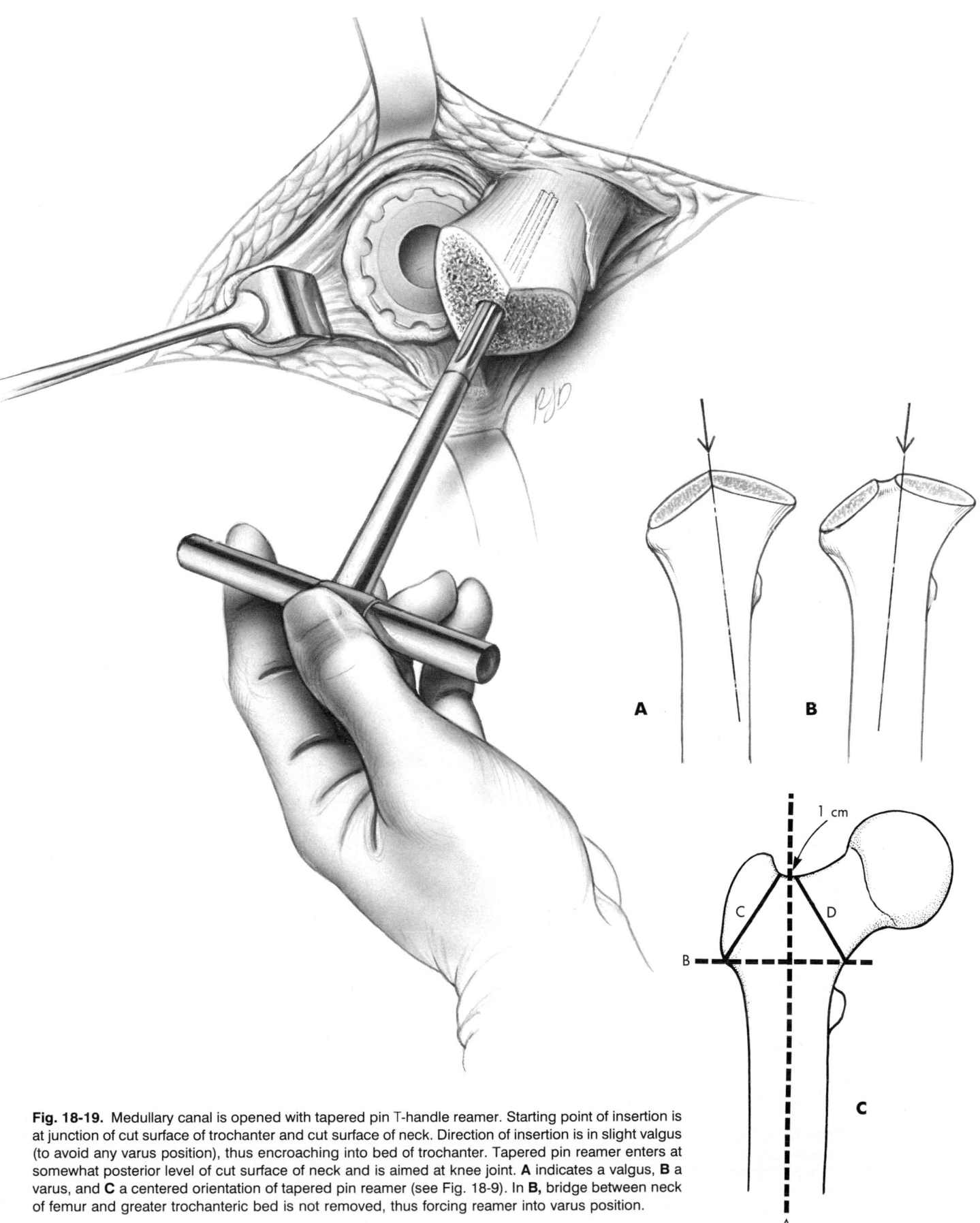

Fig. 18-19. Medullary canal is opened with tapered pin T-handle reamer. Starting point of insertion is at junction of cut surface of trochanter and cut surface of neck. Direction of insertion is in slight valgus (to avoid any varus position), thus encroaching into bed of trochanter. Tapered pin reamer enters at somewhat posterior level of cut surface of neck and is aimed at knee joint. **A** indicates a valgus, **B** a varus, and **C** a centered orientation of tapered pin reamer (see Fig. 18-9). In **B**, bridge between neck of femur and greater trochanteric bed is not removed, thus forcing reamer into varus position.

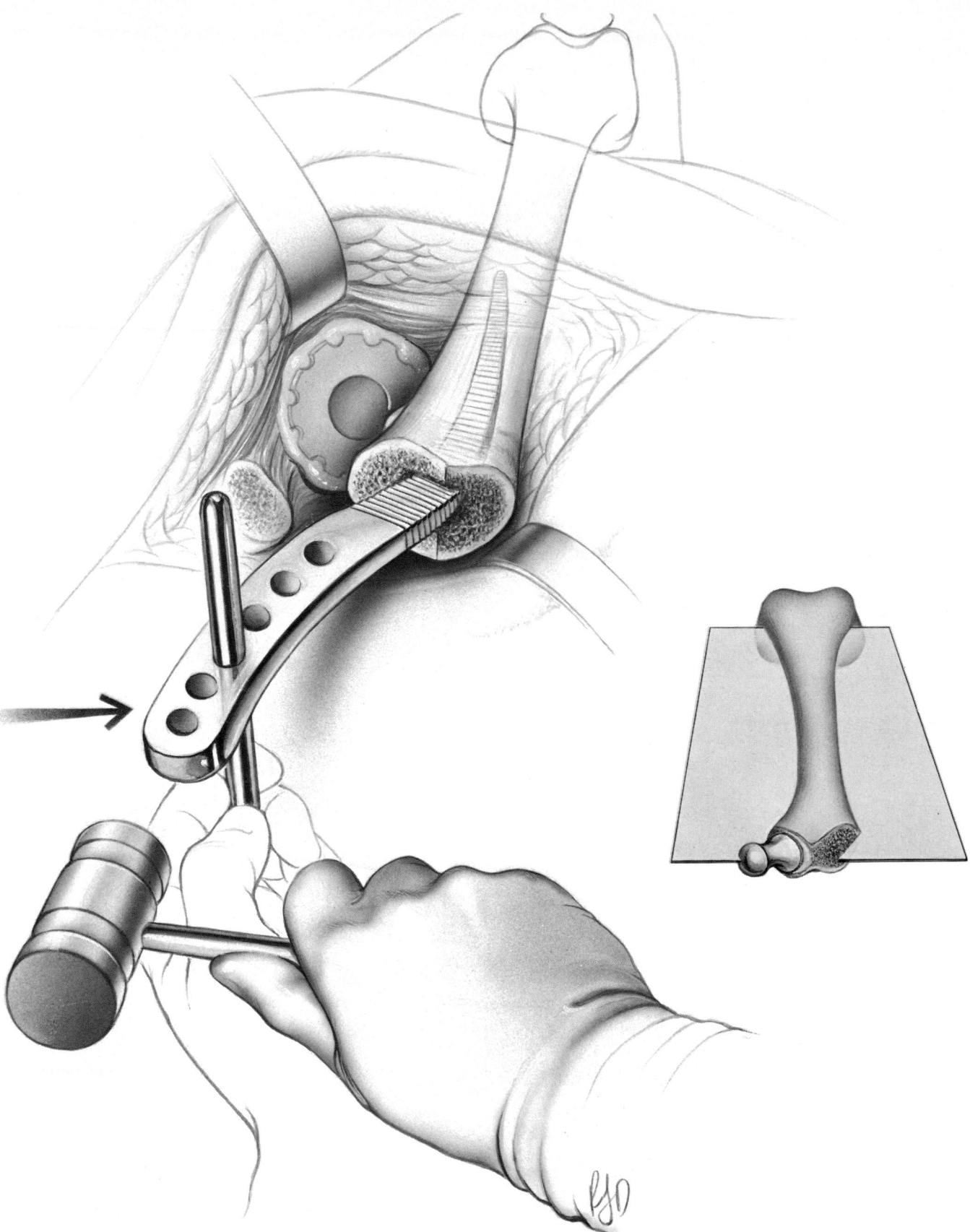

Fig. 18-20. Leg is in cross-table position with patella and flexed knee as point of reference. Transcondylar line of femur and degrees of anteversion of femoral neck *(inset)* determine correct plane of insertion of femoral broach. The bar inserted through broach handle is perpendicular to transcondylar line. Arrow indicates that the surgeon's left hand (phantom) thrusts broach into valgus orientation while it is being driven into medullary canal. This ensures that femoral prosthesis will not lie in varus position.

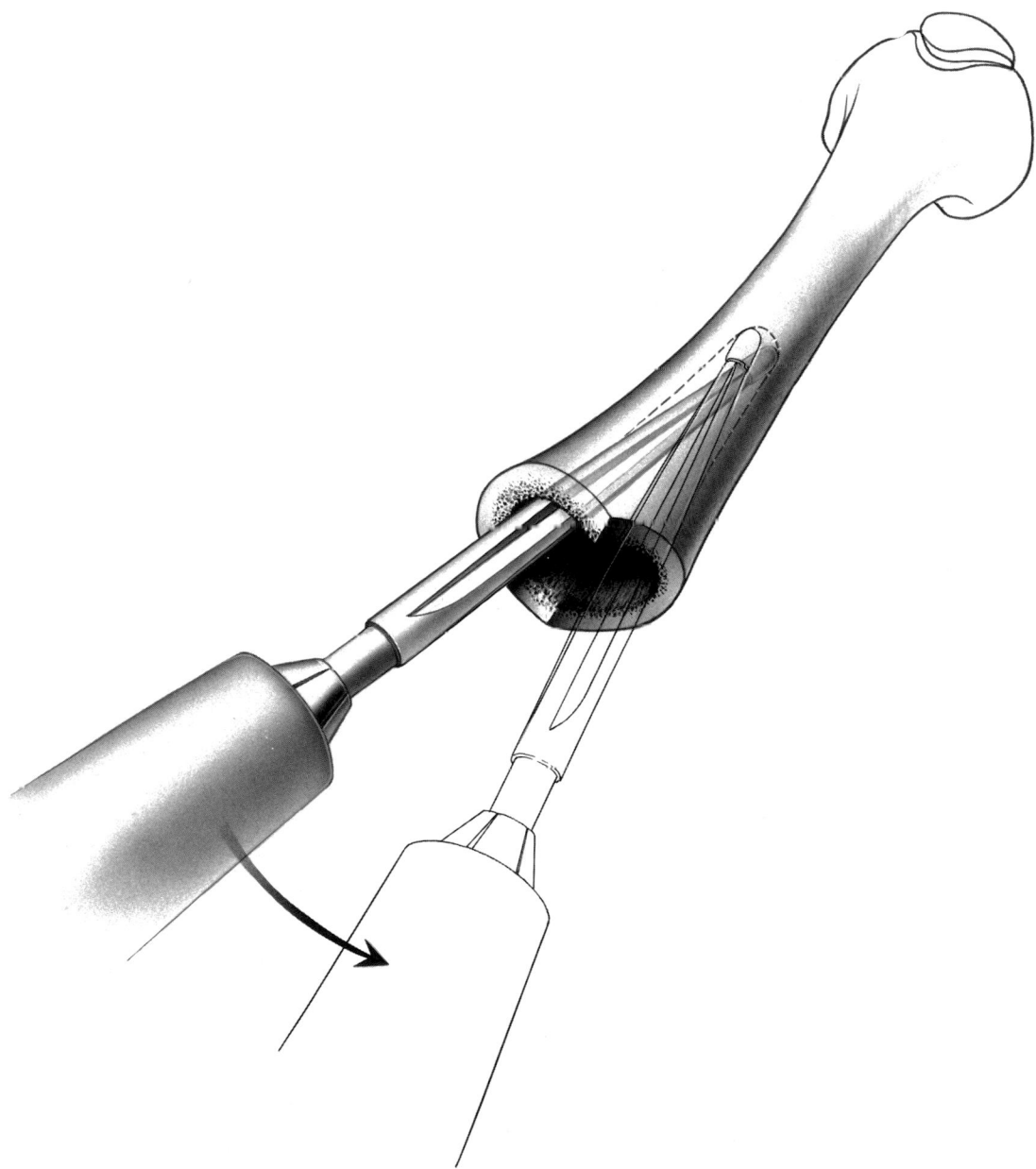

Fig. 18-21. Proximal femoral expansion with a rotary reamer. NOTE: encroachment of the reamer into the bed of trochanter. The opening of the femur is also necessary in an anteroposterior direction to accommodate a large-caliber prosthesis and a flanged stem.

Selection and Insertion of Test Prosthesis

Charnley used a neck-length jig[4] to determine the stability and length. A test prosthesis can also be used to test for length and stability. Unless the second broach could not be inserted, a standard or heavy prosthesis is tested. If the narrow segment of the canal (usually at the isthmus) does not allow penetration of the curved broach, a straight narrow stem may be used. The selected test prosthesis is inserted to its collar in the broached canal. The stem must fit loosely, and full insertion must be easily accomplished. If the posterior cortex of the neck is longer than the anterior, the prosthesis will be forced into anteversion; the converse is also true. Errors in orientation may also be made if the canal is excessively large, allowing unrestricted rotation of the stem in the shaft.

After insertion of the test prosthesis, reduction is attempted. This is achieved in three steps: (1) longitudinal traction, (2) flexing the hip and guiding the head into the cup, and (3) slight abduction to keep the head in. First, the greater trochanter is retracted cephalad by the first assistant. The second assistant applies longitudinal traction onto the femur; the surgeon preferentially may also apply longitudinal traction to the femur while holding the knee in a 90-degree flexed position. Keeping the knee flexed provides grasping power for traction and relaxes the flexor muscles of the hip, especially the iliotibial tract. The surgeon must make sure that: (1) the orientation of the femoral prosthesis has not changed within the canal since its insertion, which is accomplished by holding the femoral prosthesis in position with the middle and index fingers (this is especially important if there is an excessively large medullary canal); (2) the greater trochanter is held adequately cephalad by the first assistant (no retractors are used since they may interfere with the reduction); and (3) the hip is flexed no less than 45 degrees. No internal or external rotation is required. In addition to placing longitudinal traction on the limb, the surgeon must determine the location of the socket and while holding the prosthesis within the femur, direct the head into the socket.

Reduction may be difficult or impossible if (1) the patient has not been adequately anesthetized, and there is insufficient muscle relaxation, (2) the femoral neck is excessively long, (3) the socket has been inserted in a low position, or (4) soft tissues are excessively tight. If present, these impediments must be corrected and the soft tissue then examined closely to ascertain the cause of the difficulty in reduction. Adequate muscle relaxation must be attained, and soft tissue contractions should be divided, if present, before the decision to shorten the femur. If shortening is indicated, it must be done in stages so that excess shortening is avoided (see Chapter 15).

Testing for Motion and Stability

After reduction of the prosthesis into the socket, the hip is tested in flexion, abduction, and adduction, as well as rotation. There is to be no danger of damage to the plastic socket by the test prosthesis. The anterosuperior iliac spines are demonstrated by the first assistant to define the position of the hip. If full abduction is not achieved, an adductor tenotomy should be performed (see Chapter 24). Next, while placing strong longitudinal traction on the limb (with the knee slightly flexed), the surgeon inserts the index finger between the prosthetic components to determine the amount of separation attained (no more than 5 mm of separation should be possible). The coverage of the head and its relation to the cup is then evaluated with the hip in neutral position. Finally, one must determine how much adduction produces dislocation—this is the real test of instability and is done with the hip in extension, including testing for "impingement" of the inferior and medial neck against the acetabular margin. By adducting the limb across the table, subluxation and dislocation are observed. A well-fitted prosthesis should not begin dislocating before 30 degrees of adduction (minimal flexion is required to allow adduction of the leg across the opposite thigh). If this occurs with less adduction, one must check for impingement of the medial femoral neck against the acetabular rim, vertical placement of the cup, laxity of the joint, or excessive valgus placement of the prosthesis. A satisfactory position of the components includes a cup oriented at 45 degrees to the axis of the body without anteversion or retroversion of either component. When the head is not completely covered by the cup while the leg is in neutral position, it must be assumed that one or both of the components are malpositioned.

For further details regarding instability and its causes and remedies, see Chapter 15.

As stated before, reduction as just outlined may not be possible if there is excessive neck length, unreleased contracted capsule, severe contraction of the iliopsoas tendon, or inadequate muscle relaxation. On the other hand, the reduction may be unstable if there are (1) excessive shortening of the neck, (2) high positioning of the socket, (3) medial and anterior osteophytes or "cementophytes" about the acetabulum, (4) projecting osteophytes on the upper femur, (5) lack of clearance caused by an excessively deepened acetabulum, (6) previous surgery with subsequent loss of tissue elasticity, (7) sinking of the femoral prosthesis into the medullary canal, (8) rotation of the stem within the canal, and (9) malorientation of either component.

An unstable reduction resulting from a short neck may be rectified by placing the prosthesis in a more valgus position or by using a long-neck prosthesis. When recognized, faulty orientation of the socket or the femoral prosthesis must be corrected at once (for further details see Chapter 32). Further stability can be achieved by a firm reattachment of the greater trochanter and, in some instances, by applying a hip spica cast after surgery (see Chapters 15 and 32).

After testing for motion and stability, the hip is dislocated, the test prosthesis removed, and the stump of the femur once again delivered out of the wound. A Watson-Jones retractor may facilitate delivery. The loose cancellous bone and fatty marrow within the intramedullary canal, especially in the region of the calcar femorale, must be removed using a small Volkmann's spoon. Vigorous curettage is unnecessary. Curettage of the calcar area produces a space between the concavity of the stem and bone, thereby ensuring a thick layer of cement at this load-bearing portion of the femur (Figs. 18-22 and 18-23). Strong suction applied within the medullary canal also removes blood and fatty marrow. Finally, the medullary canal is packed tightly as described in Chapter 15, before inserting cement.

Irrigate the medullary canal, and use a power-driven brush to remove debris and clots (see Chapter 15). Inserting trochanteric wires is the last step before cement is introduced.

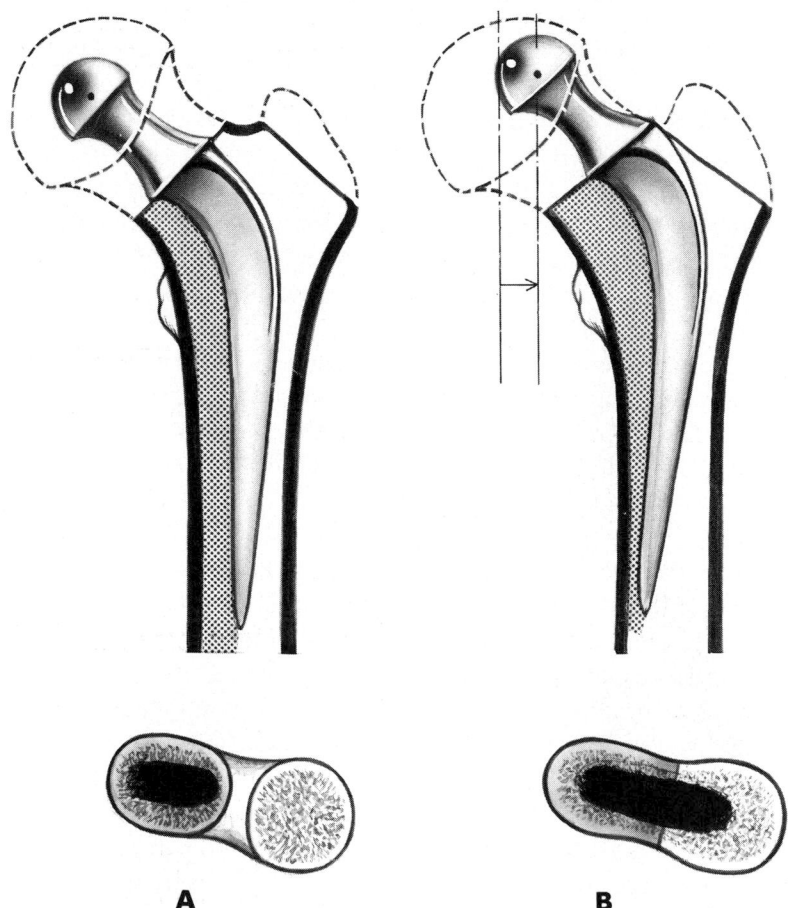

A   **B**

Fig. 18-22. During preparation of canal or rehearsal, femoral axis guide and broach must be pointing slightly medial to patella to avoid any varus position of stem. **A,** When bridge of bone between neck and trochanteric bed is not removed, it is not possible to place stem into any degree of valgus. In **A,** canal is large and central placement was achieved. **B,** Creating good space between concave side of prosthesis and calcar by placing stem in valgus after removal of bridge between neck and trochanter. (Modified after Charnley.)

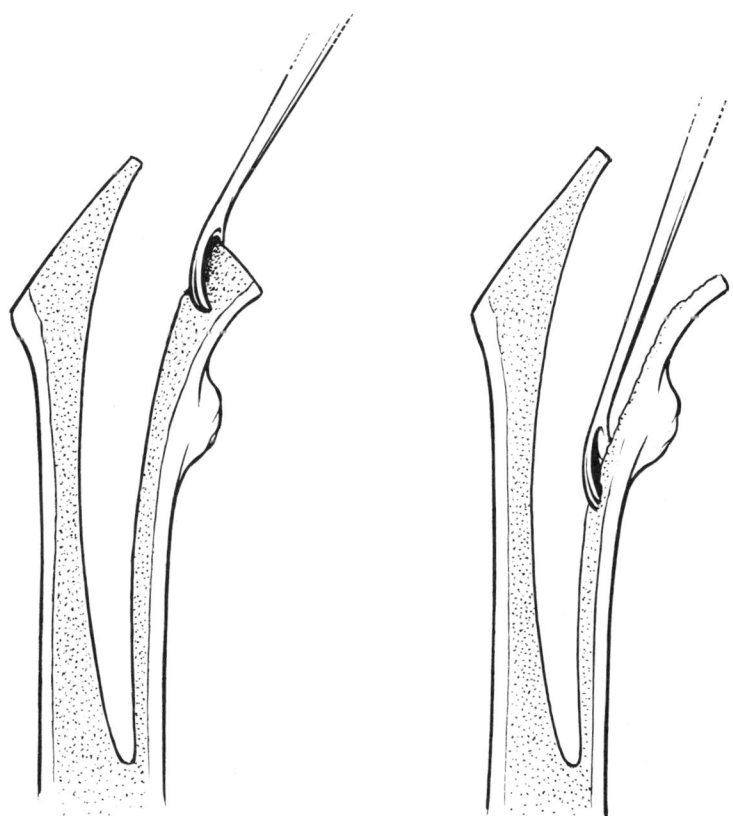

Fig. 18-23. Gentle curettage of calcar region produces space between concavity of stem and bone, ensuring thick layer of cement at this load-bearing region of femur. Additionally, strong bone of calcar supports cement.

Inserting Wires

In Charnley's technique for wiring the trochanter, two independent systems are created: a "double vertical" and a "cruciate" system. Each system is independently tightened over the trochanter after insertion of cement and stem. They produce a six-point fixation for the trochanter.

Inserting Double Vertical Wire

After stripping the vastus lateralis, use a 3.2-mm drill bit entered at the midlateral surface of the femur to drill a hole 3 cm distal from the cut surface of the trochanter. The hole can also be made by pressing a cholecystectomy clamp hard against the muscle (to prevent the drill from picking up muscle and fibrous tissue) and drilling through the muscle. Pass the double end of the vertical (18 swg) wire (38 cm) through the hole. Observe the following details:

1. Pack a sponge into the medullary canal, and insert the vertical wire while the hip is flexed and internally rotated.
2. When you pull the sponge out, the two ends of the wire are pulled out of the canal.
3. Grasp the two ends of the wires, each with a color-coded (gray) wire-holding forceps, and place them against the posterior wall of the medullary canal. This author prefers to separate the two wires and place one against the posterior and one against the anterior wall of the femur.
4. Make sure the loop neither disappears into the canal nor is left too long outside the cortex of the femur while it is being pulled toward the opening of the medullary canal.

Inserting Medial and Lateral Wires (Cruciate System)

Drill two separate 3.2-mm holes from front to back, one medial and the other lateral to the trochanteric bed (Figs. 18-24 to 18-28). Place a Watson-Jones gouge posterior to the femur while the femur is being held maximally adducted. The instrument will prevent accidental damage to the sciatic nerve by the drill bit.

Insert two single 45-cm (18 swg) wires from front to back into the holes, grasping each end of the wires with color-coded (silver and green) wire-holding forceps. Insertion of medial and lateral wires is facilitated by maximum adduction of the femur. Rotate the femur internally while pulling the medial and lateral wires out from the posterior aspects of femur. The length of wire should be equal in front and in back of the femur.

The position of the wires before packing the canal is shown in Fig. 18-28, *A*. A test prosthesis is inserted to ensure that the stem insertion is unimpeded and that the wires are not at risk of being displaced by the stem.

Text continued on p. 856.

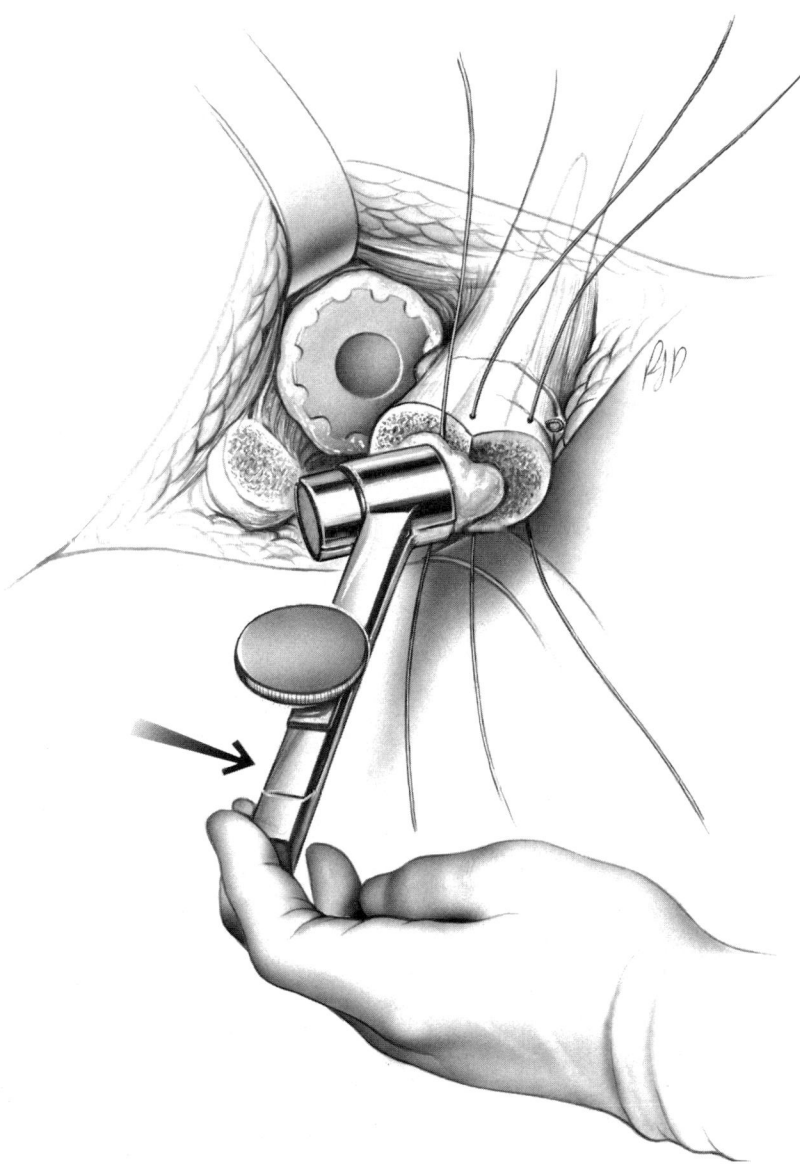

Fig. 18-24. Prosthesis is now at its full depth within medullary canal. Slight valgus position is ensured by maintaining direction of tip of stem toward medial cortex. Slight valgus position ensures that prosthesis is not in varus position and that thick layer of cement intervenes between concave surface of prosthesis and bone of calcar of femur. Holder may be detached just before full polymerization of cement.

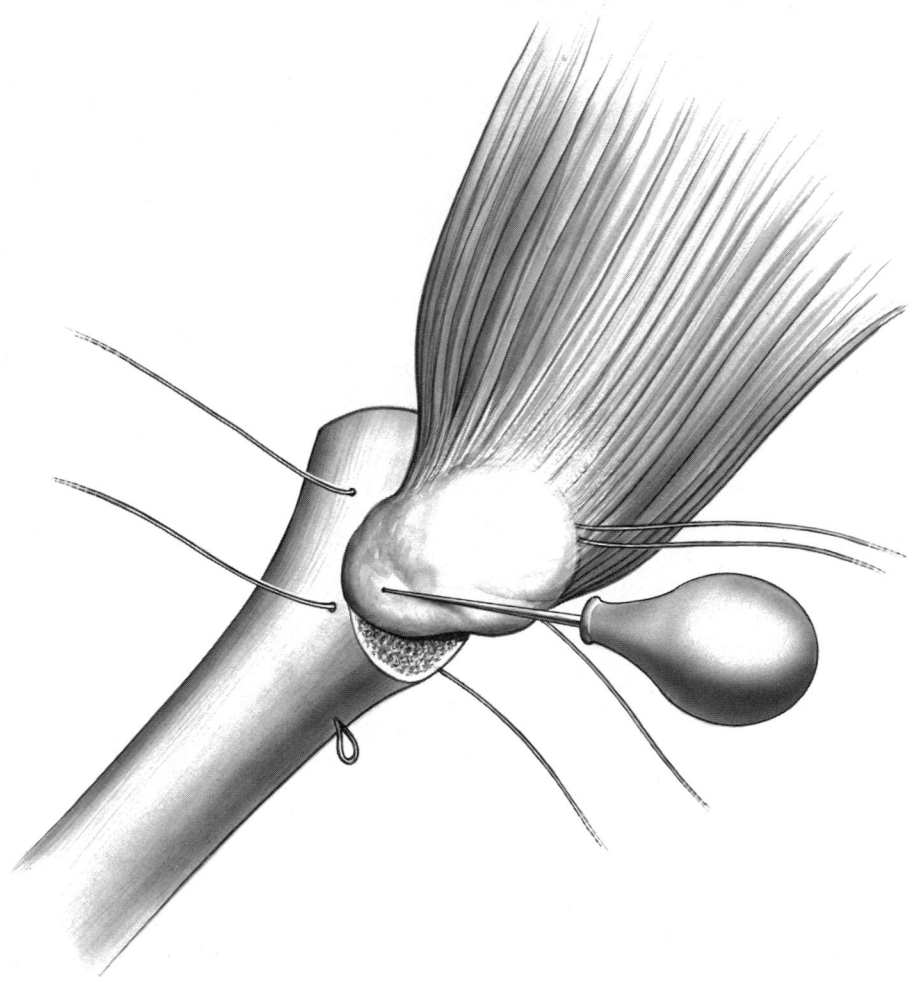

Fig. 18-25. Regardless of the plane of osteotomy (biplane or flat), trochanteric fragments tend to rotate forward despite capsular release. Note the position of the awl and wires. An alternative to placement of the awl would have been to flex the femur against the trochanter.

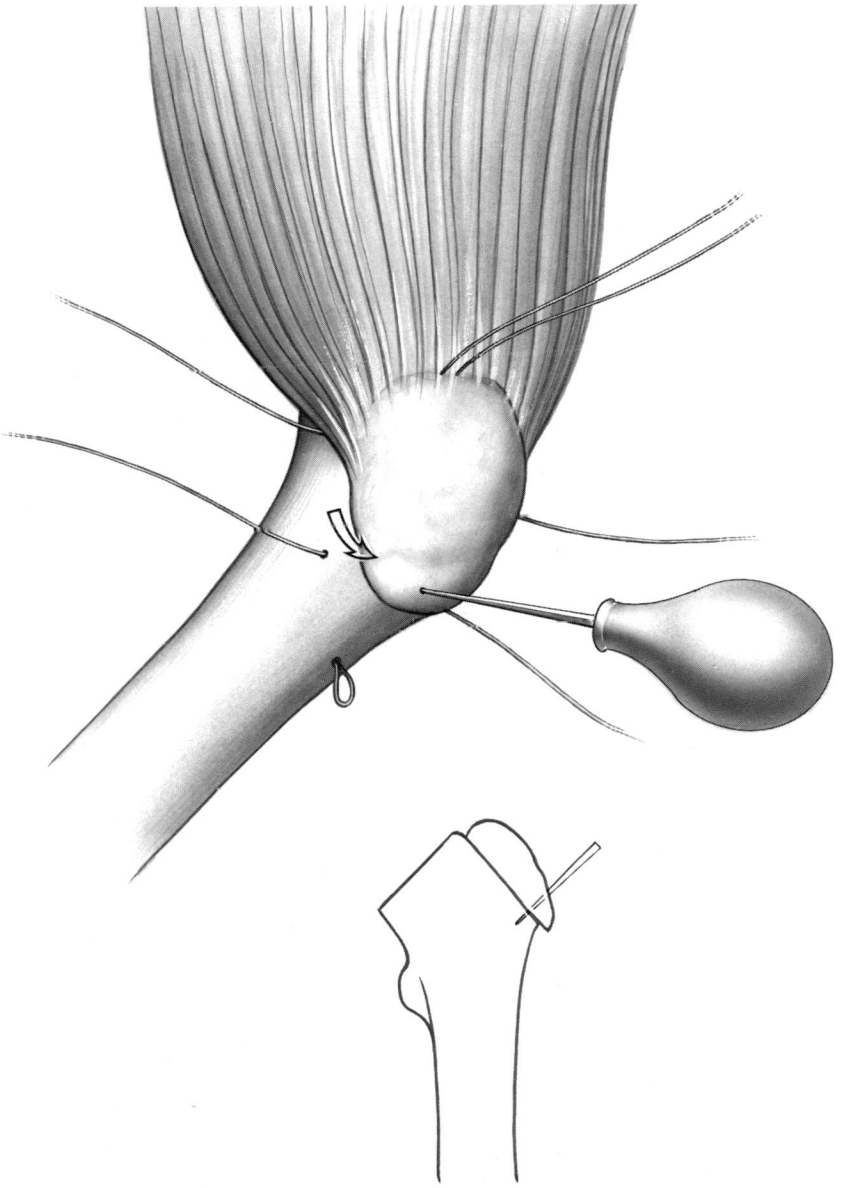

Fig. 18-26. Trochanter is derotated and held in place and an awl (inset) is pegging the trochanter onto its bed.

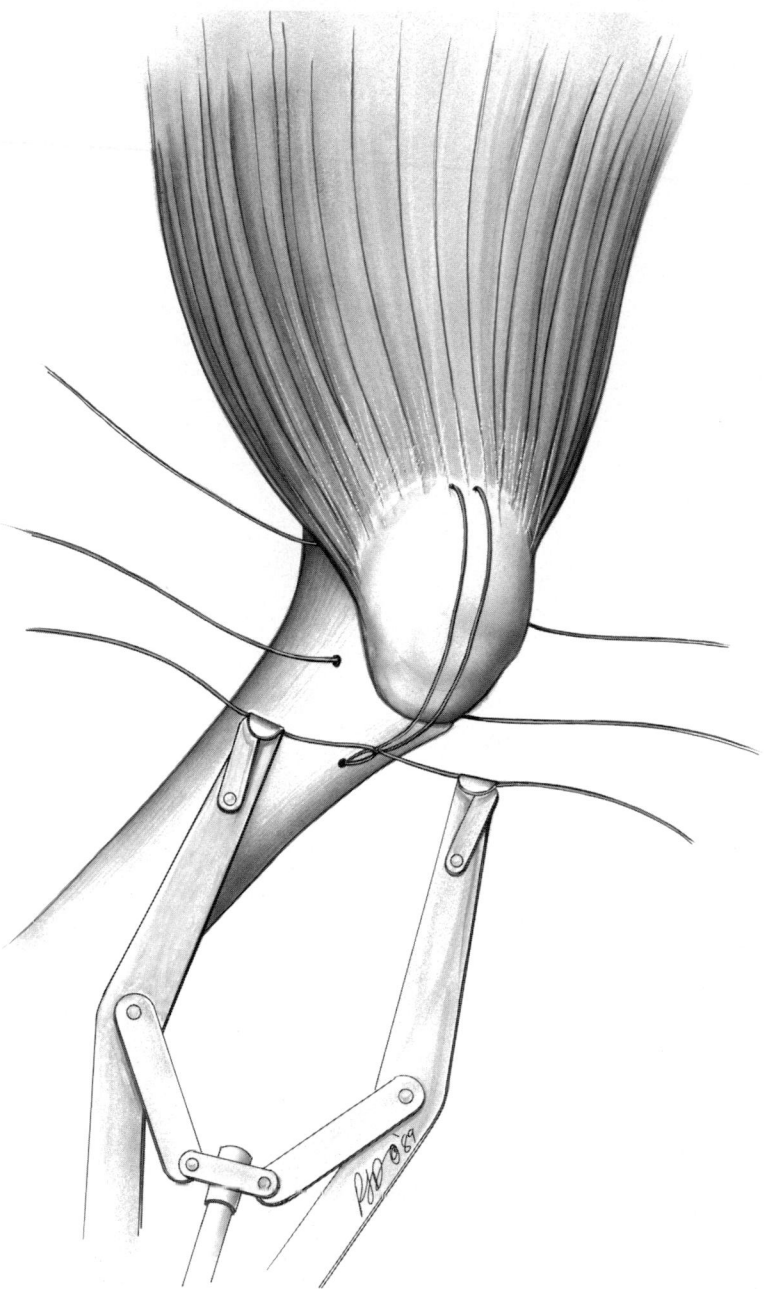

Fig. 18-27. Longitudinal wire is being tightened (awl has been removed). The posterior strand of medial wire (to form pulley later) is drawn through the abductor muscles.

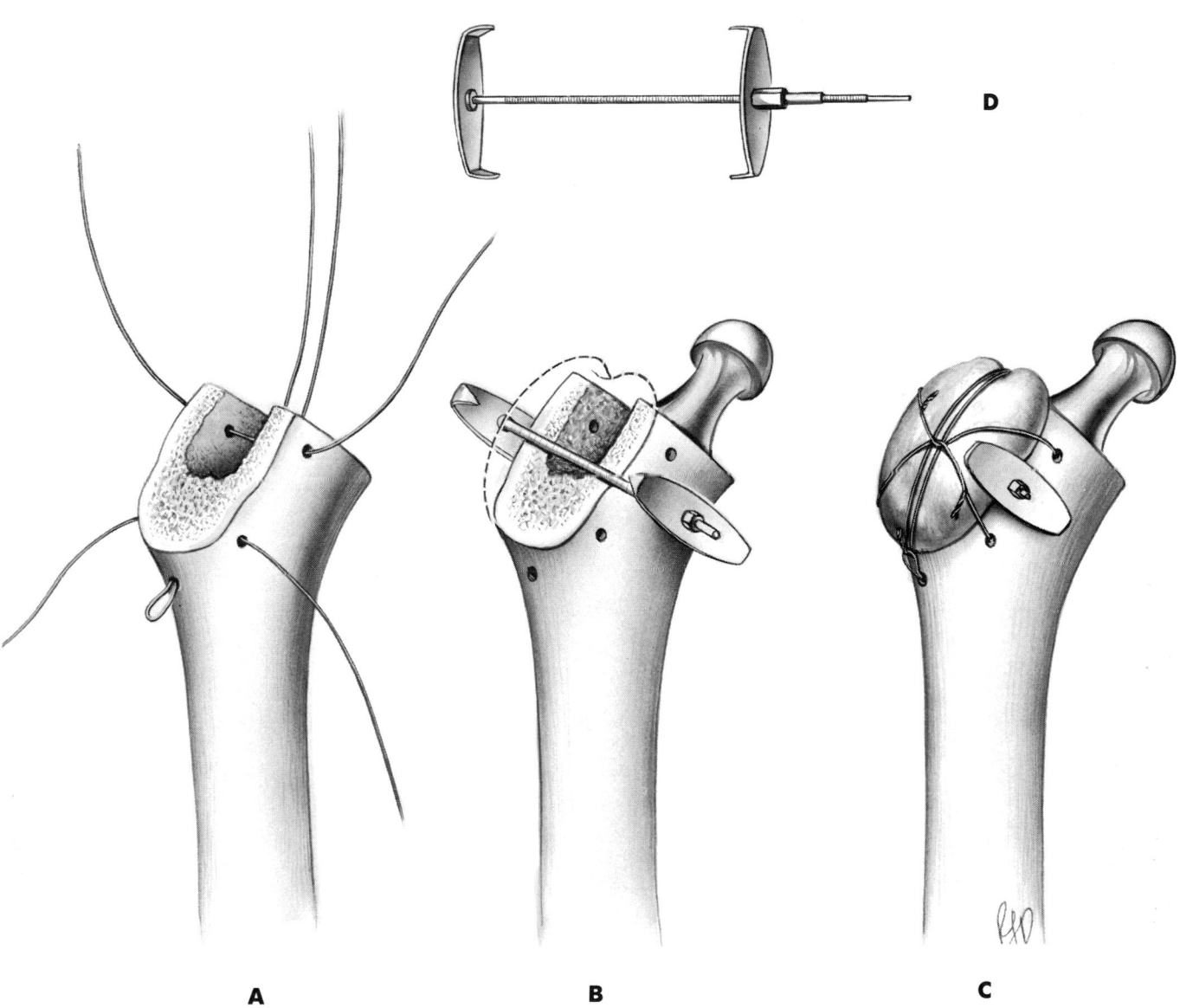

A   **B**   **C**

Fig. 18-28. A, Site of insertion of two transverse wires and one vertical double wire. Medial transverse wire passes through canal, but lateral transverse wire remains within lateral wall of femur. NOTE: both transverse wires are parallel, and vertical wire is passed through hole in medullary canal of femur. **B,** Site of application of staple clamp and orientation of greater trochanter in relation to staple. **C,** Configuration of wires at completion of tightening. NOTE: cruciform arrangement of wires and final position of staple. (Posterior staple clamp is not seen in this figure.) **D,** Staple clamp designed by Charnley.

PHASE VI: REHEARSAL, INSERTING CEMENT AND PROSTHESIS, AND REDUCTION

Before mixing cement, the following steps facilitate the correct insertion of cement and stem.

Test and Rehearsal, and Insertion of Medullary Plug

A deliberately slow and staged rehearsal (without cement) enables the surgeon to determine the correct orientation of the femoral prosthesis within the medullary canal and to ascertain that the prosthesis can be easily inserted with the wires in place. The aim is to be able to secure the prosthesis in valgus* and neutral rotation, centered in the femur.

After the general position of the wires is assessed, the limb is once again placed in the "cross-table position," ready to receive the prosthesis. The longitudinal axis of the femur, position of the knee and patella, perpendicular orientation of the tibia to the floor, and the relationship of the stump of the neck to the lesser trochanter are noted by the surgeon. The direction and the amount of valgus orientation are estimated, and the prosthesis is inserted into the femoral canal, rehearsing the action that will take place at insertion (after cement insertion). The position of the handle of the femoral prosthesis holder is observed. Note the longitudinal axis of the shaft of the femur and the rotational orientation of the prosthesis within the medullary canal. (Is the canal excessively large, or does the prosthesis fit snugly?) Observe the space between the medial calcar and the medial border of the prosthesis, which has to be filled with cement (wedge-shaped). It also must be ascertained that the vertical intramedullary wires are pulled tightly against the inner wall of the lateral femoral cortex so that they do not interfere with the insertion of the prosthesis. Gentle curettage of the calcar femorale to remove marrow tissue and soft cancellous bone may be repeated at this point if necessary. Insert the medullary plug as discussed in Chapter 15. After this, the medullary canal is repacked with a 4- to 5-cm wide gauze ribbon soaked with hydrogen peroxide using a vent tube to remove blood and fluids while cement is being prepared (see Chapter 15). Neither the prosthesis nor the packing should displace the wires. Insertion of the prosthesis in the correct orientation must be accomplished with ease before cementing, and a tight fit should be avoided. It must be noted that the vertical wires obviously occupy space within the medullary canal; thus broaching must take their presence into account (slightly oversize broaching).

Before the actual insertion of the cement, the following are to be noted:

1. Whether the prosthesis is held firmly in the holder with its stem parallel to the handle. (The surgeon must check to verify that the prosthesis placed in the holder is the same as that chosen after the trial insertion, for example, regular-stem or straight-stem.)
2. The orientation of the prosthesis in reference to the holder, the longitudinal axis of the femur, and the perpendicular line of the tibia to the floor.
3. The neck of the femur's complete freedom from spicules that may puncture the surgeon's gloves during the packing of the femoral canal with cement.
4. That the collar of the prosthesis is flush with the neck when fully inserted. (The neck may be trimmed anteriorly or posteriorly as needed using bone-cutting forceps.)
5. Whether the prosthesis head is protected from damage when the holder is applied to it. (The plastic cover is not removed until after cementing.)
6. That valgus orientation can be maintained and that the space between the medial curvature of the prosthesis and the calcar can be filled with cement.

    The second assistant is now instructed to hold the leg steady in the desired position (cross-table position).
7. Make sure that the medullary plug does not prevent full-length insertion of the stem.

---

*The term *valgus* denotes avoidance of any *varus* positioning. Ideally, at the final step, the stem should be centered in the canal without any varus or valgus orientation.

Inserting the Cement

The cement is now mixed, and the surgeon puts on a third pair of gloves. It is essential that the instruments for this phase of the procedure (that is, the prosthesis itself in the holder, the long-handled curette, hammer, and prosthetic pusher) have been previously arranged on the table. The scrub nurse begins mixing the cement while the surgeon once again checks the position of the extremity (for details see Chapters 5 and 15). The second assistant is instructed to maintain the cross-table position, and the cut surface of the neck is rechecked for bone spicules. Final repacking of the canal is done by the first assistant using a fresh sponge, taking care not to interfere with the wires. If further curettage of the calcar and neck is necessary, it is done at this point. The surgeon must make sure, with several rehearsals, that the femoral stem passes smoothly and fully down the canal in the proper orientation. The novice is advised to make this determination before mixing the cement. If this precaution is not taken, malorientation or partial insertion may result. The greater trochanter must be retracted proximally during the insertion of the cement. Alternatively, it may be placed between the medial femoral shaft and the acetabulum. Every effort must be made to provide adequate access to the proximal end of the femur so that both thumbs can forcefully drive the cement down the canal. This is best accomplished by having the second assistant hold the leg in maximal adduction.

The surgeon receives the cement in its prepolymerized form, shaped like a sausage and ready for stuffing down the femoral canal (see Chapter 15). A two-thumbed pressure insertion technique is preferable when possible. Portions are advanced into the canal, with 1- or 2-second pauses between each inserting motion. With each stroke, part of the cement is advanced down the canal, and the pause aids its progress. Complete obstruction of the opening of the upper femur by the thumbs maximizes pressure behind the column of cement. Admixture of blood with cement should be avoided. A total of 10 to 15 strokes usually enables the entire batch to be inserted. Cement should not be allowed to extravasate into the soft tissues, especially posteriorly. The surgeon must continually check for possible glove tears during insertion. A delicate and gentle use of fingers does not produce adequate pressure to advance the cement column inside the shaft.

A catheter is used to vent the femur and prevent possible air embolization, which can be caused by the hydrogen peroxide–soaked gauze ribbon. After the ribbon is removed and 80% to 90% of the canal is filled with cement, the vent should be removed by the first assistant to facilitate delivery of the remaining cement.

Inserting the Prosthesis

Insert the stem centered in the canal. Avoid anteversion or retroversion. However, experience suggests that in many instances, especially in patients with a narrow medullary canal, 5 degrees of anteversion, cement is better distributed in the upper femur to eliminate the possibility of contact between the metal (upper stem) and the posterior wall of the femoral canal (Fig. 18-29; see Chapter 15). While up to 5 degrees of anteversion may be beneficial, the prosthesis should never be oriented in retroversion because that position may prejudice the stability of the hip.

As in the rehearsal, the position of the knee is demonstrated by the second assistant. The tip of the stem is introduced into the prepared canal at the junction between the cut surface of the trochanter and the neck. The prosthesis (firmly held in the holder) is slowly, deliberately inserted in "neutroversion" toward the medial cortex to place it in a valgus position relative to the shaft. This valgus orientation is maximized by holding the prosthesis back against the cancellous bone area of the bed of the trochanter (see Fig. 18-24). The degree of valgus is the same as that decided upon at rehearsal. An extreme degree of valgus is undesirable, especially in a very large canal. Slow and deliberate action is essential while the insertion progresses. With repeated reaming of the cement in the area between its concavity and the femoral canal, maximum cement should be present in the region of the calcar femorale. Rotation (anteversion-retroversion) or mediolateral (varus-

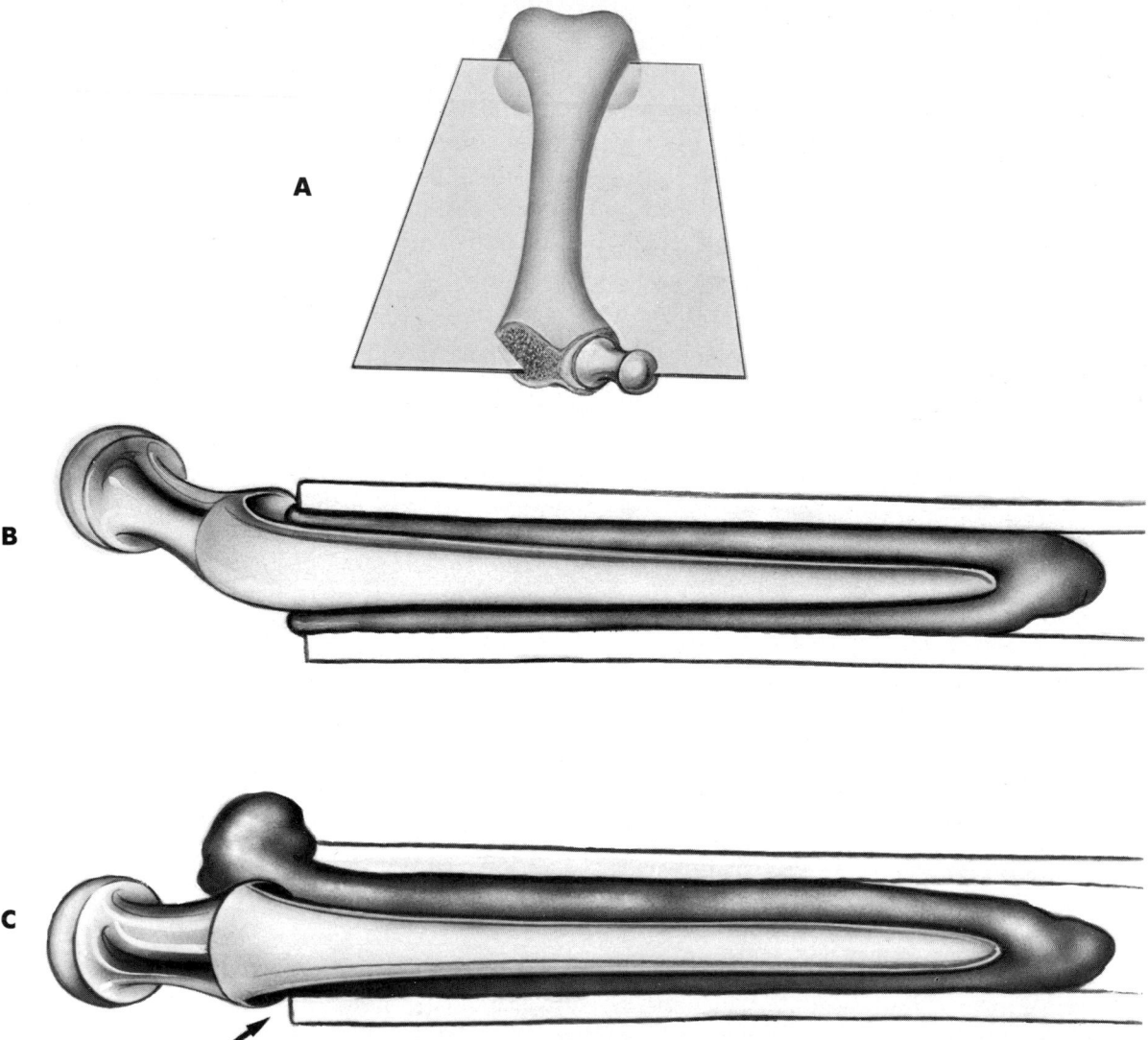

Fig. 18-29. In principle, femoral component (of Charnley prosthesis) is inserted in neutroversion; however, slight anteversion (no more than 5 degrees) would allow better distribution of cement within upper end of femur. **A,** Plane of neutroversion. **B,** 5 degrees anteversion. NOTE: optimal thickness of cement between prosthesis and posterior cortex. **C,** Absolute neutroversion (no anteversion or retroversion) brings stem close to posterior cortex (because of normal anteversion of femoral neck), thus eliminating thickness of cement in that region (arrow).

valgus) change in direction results in a large track being made in the cement, which can lead to later loosening and should be avoided. It must also be recognized that in an extremely large medullary canal excessive valgus placement can be inadvertently produced, resulting in overlengthening of the extremity and difficulty in reducing the hip. A very large canal also may allow the prosthetic stem tip to reach the medial cortex without any cement in the region, and a prosthesis placed in an excessive valgus position can also result in deficient coverage by the acetabular component. In summary, the prosthesis must be inserted in the rehearsed orientation.

Generally speaking, Charnley's cobra design (flanged stem) centers itself proximally as it is being inserted into the medullary cavity of the femur. However, the opening of the canal must be large enough to accommodate the flange. It is important to have the opening of the femur overly reamed to allow easy penetration of the flanges; failure to do so causes the orientation of the stem on the shaft to change while the flange contacts the opening of the upper femur. When a heavy or extra-heavy stem prosthesis is used (Charnley's "cobra" prosthesis), the relationship of the flange to the opening of the medullary canal should be observed to ascertain that the correct degree of valgus orientation has been achieved.

No hammering is necessary if full insertion is easily achieved, as evidenced by the neck of the prosthesis resting flush with the entrance of the medullary canal. The holder must be carefully removed without changing the orientation of the prosthesis while the prosthesis is held in place with the pusher. The holder may be detached just before the final stage of hardening (to facilitate the removal of cement); the valgus position must remain unchanged until full polymerization. Excess cement is removed with a curette, again taking care not to move the prosthesis. It is essential to observe the following:

1. During the final stages of polymerization, the first and second assistants must remain immobile, since any motion of the limb may change the orientation of the prosthesis within the medullary canal. Maximum adduction of the leg in the cross-leg position must be retained also.
2. Avoid scratching the femoral head if it is unprotected by a plastic cover.
3. Avoid changes of orientation during the removal of the holder.
4. Cement should be tested for hardness locally, at the neck level, before attempting reduction of the prosthesis.
5. The prosthesis must not be pushed into a varus position during the polymerization phase.
6. Excess force on the "pusher" is unnecessary, even harmful, since it may change the "version" of the prosthesis.
7. The position of the vertical wires (one anterior, one posterior, or both posterior to the prosthesis) must remain undisturbed.
8. All cement must be curetted away from the trochanteric bed before hardening. The holder may be detached just before final hardening of the cement. This author does not detach the holder from the prosthesis until cement is fully polymerized.

Reduction

Attempt reduction only after achieving absolute hemostasis and removing all cement debris from the wound, particularly in the socket region.

The wound is now copiously irrigated. Cement particles and devitalized portions of muscle (usually found in the posterior aspect of the wound) are removed. Posterior capsular bleeding should be checked and controlled before reattachment of the greater trochanter.

The range of motion and stability are tested at this point, and the surgeon must ascertain that the two components are in a satisfactory relationship relative to each other. The hip must be stable before reattachment of the greater trochanter. Ideally, the orientation of the components relative to each other should be exactly the same as that noted before the cementing of the femoral component (see Chapter 15).

PHASE VII: REATTACHING THE TROCHANTER, INSERTING DEEP DRAINS, REPAIRING THE FASCIA, AND WOUND CLOSURE
Reattaching the Trochanter

Before reattaching the trochanter, release the capsule and short rotators as needed to relieve undue tension of the abductors while the trochanter is sealed against its site of detachment on the femur. A slight displacement is advisable (see Chapter 6), but no more than 1 cm lateral and distal. The vertical and cruciate wiring systems are independently tightened to fix the trochanter.

Tightening the Doubled Vertical Wire

The two ends of vertical wire (doubled) and the posterior end of the medial wires must be passed through the capsule and tendinous portion of the abductors over the greater trochanter before the trochanter is opposed against the shaft of the femur.

Proceed with the following steps:

1. Insert an awl (6 mm) at a midpoint on top of the trochanter (from lateral to medial) to create a groove to lodge the vertical wires close to the bone after they are tightened.
2. Insert a wire passer from a lateral to a medial direction and pass the two ends of the vertical wire from a medial to a lateral direction.
3. Pass the posterior end of the medial wire through the groove in a medial to lateral direction (Charnley described passing this wire after tightening the vertical wires.)
4. Manually rotate the trochanter backward (because the trochanter has a tendency to rotate in a forward direction), and hold it in place in the desired position. "Peg" it down using the sharp awl (see Figs. 18-25 and 18-26).
5. Tighten the vertical wire first. Pass the two ends of the vertical wire through the loop of the same wire (on the lateral side of the femur). Tighten the vertical wire with the wire tightener.

Note the following details:

- The vertical wire is located centrally on the trochanter. Reroute this wire if necessary.
- Make the loop horizontal to ease wire passing before tightening the wire.
- Make sure that the posterior end of the medial wire is free and not kinked.
- Avoid overtightening the vertical wire, which may fracture the trochanter.
- Use a punch and mallet to secure the cancellous surface of the trochanter to its mating surface on the femur.
- Apply a ⅓ to ½ turn to the wire tightener to compensate for possible laxity in the wire. Twist the wire while traction is applied to the wire tightener (see Fig. 18-27).
- Cut the twisted wire, leaving a 1-cm length, and hammer the ends against the shaft using a punch.

Tightening the Cruciate Wire System

The cruciate wire system is formed by the medial and lateral wires, which are independent from the vertical wire. Proceed with the following steps:

1. Pass the anterior end of the medial wire through the hole previously made through the abductors on the top of the trochanter for the vertical wire. This wire must be passed in a medial to lateral direction. Cross the medial wire ends, then bring the posterior end of the lateral wire to lie between the two medial wires. Twist the medial wires at the midpoint of the trochanter. This twist forms the "pulley" that completes the cruciform system when the two ends of the lateral wires are tightened. Finally, pass the posterior end of the lateral wire through the hole made for the vertical wire, and tighten the two ends of the same wire in front of the femur (see Fig. 18-28). NOTE: To pass the posterior and anterior medial wires, use the same track as the vertical wire.
2. Place a narrow awl proximal to the "cross-over" of the medial wires to prevent overtightening, which would cause the pulley to disappear into the abductor muscle.

3. Observe the effectiveness of the cruciate system as it is tightened. Avoid overtightening the wires.
4. Use a small Richardson retractor to retract the anterior border of the gluteus medius and minimus. Externally rotate the hip for up to 30 degrees to facilitate twisting the lateral wire.
5. Leave a 2-cm-long tail of twisted medial wire. Bend and drive the end of the twisted tail into a hole drilled into the greater trochanter. Avoid leaving projecting wire ends because this often can cause painful bursitis postoperatively.

Supplemental Methods for Trochanteric Fixation

Charnley advocated supplemental fixation of the trochanter, which can also be achieved by using a staple clamp (see Fig. 18-28). This was introduced to maximize the fixation of the greater trochanter.[3] The stable clamp is an optional supplement to any wire technique the surgeon may choose. When properly applied, this apparatus prevents forward and backward motion of the trochanter during flexion and extension of the hip. The staple clamp in Fig. 18-28 is demonstrated in conjunction with a cruciform method of fixation of the trochanter. It should be noted that before reattaching the greater trochanter, a groove is created to accommodate the screw portion of the staple clamp. The wires are tightened before tightening the staple clamp. The excess length of the screw is cut off by a double-action wire cutter when fixation is completed. As indicated previously, the staple clamp may also be used with a standard double-wire method or with a double vertical wire.

This author found that the technique for applying the trochanteric clamp is rather complicated. The clamp is rather bulky and frequently causes bursitis and discomfort postoperatively. Removal of the staple clamp is also difficult at times. This author does not use the staple clamp routinely.

Inserting Drains

Insert two medium-sized Hemovac drains into the joint space between the gluteus medius and minimus and the tensor fascia femoris muscle (see Chapter 15).

Closure of Fascia

Repair fascia thoroughly with No. 1 Teftek to achieve a perfect watertight closure. The first assistant retracts the proximal corner of the wound; the hip is placed in some flexion to provide maximum visibility of the proximal fascia. Fascia closure begins proximally and proceeds distally. Avoid inadvertent inclusion of the drains in the closure. Place the sutures at a modest distance from the fascial edge, thereby causing the edges to overlap when the sutures are tied. Abduct the hip at closure to enhance the stability of the hip and relax the fascia, easing closure.

Fat Closure

Clean the fat layer using No. 1 nylon; the full thickness of the skin and fat are brought together with five stitches, passing the needle on either side from within the wound outward (see Chapter 15). A second pair of Hemovac drains is placed deep in the subcutaneous tissue to prevent hematoma formation in both very obese and extremely thin individuals.

Skin Closure and Application of Dressing

Before tightening the retention sutures, the skin is meticulously closed with three equally spaced No. 3-0 Dermalon or nylon mattress stitches. The retention sutures are then tightened. For more details see Chapter 15.

Application of Antiembolic Stockings and Abduction Splint

While the patient is still under anesthesia, apply elastic bandages (that is, Ace bandages or antiembolic stockings) and an abduction splint. Transfer from the operating room table to the bed is supervised by the surgeon and first assistant, special care being taken to avoid dislocating the hip while the patient is still under the muscle-relaxing effect of anesthesia.

SUMMARY OF ESSENTIALS

- Place the patient on the operating table in the supine position with the ipsilateral arm at a right angle to the body while the patient is brought to the edge of the table toward the surgeon's side. The surgeon sits while performing the operation.

- Make a 20- to 25-cm incision along the femur extending headwards, and incline the incision posteriorly with the proximal end of the incision 2.5 cm posterior to the imaginary midline of the femur. Make the proximal limit of the incision 2.5 cm on a perpendicular line through the anterosuperior iliac spine. Insulate the skin edges with skin towels held in place with Moynihan clamps. Saturate the skin towels with Betadine.

- Incise the fat and fascia centered over the greater trochanter but inclined posteriorly to expose the deeper structures. Open the fascia sharply. Avoid cutting into the underlying vastus lateralis distally and the gluteus maximus proximally. Mobilize the fascia from the underlying tissue by blunt dissection using the thumb and fingers, then apply the self-retaining retractor. Place the Charnley initial incision retractor carefully at the trochanteric level, which will allow the wound to be opened in a diamond shape with equal exposure proximally and distally to the trochanter. Incise the fascia lata (iliotibial band) posteriorly, or detach a portion of the gluteus maximus insertion to the femur to enhance exposure as needed.

- Position the leg in external rotation. Expose the anterior capsule before arthrotomy using a retractor proximally to retract the abductor muscles and another retractor distally and medially to retract the tensor fascia femoris. Perform the arthrotomy of the hip along the inferior margin of the neck of the femur using an electrocautery knife.

- Detach the greater trochanter by inserting a cholecystectomy clamp intraarticularly to retrieve the Gigli's saw, and detach the greater trochanter with the superior capsule attached to it. Be careful to avoid damaging the sciatic nerve or fracturing the trochanter while the Gigli's saw is passed medially to the trochanter. An optimal size and shape of the trochanter are essential to the success of subsequent reattachment.

- Complete the capsulotomy posteriorly before dislocating the hip without external rotation.

- Using the Gigli's saw, amputate the head of the femur at the appropriate level as indicated by radiographic template. Maximize the exposure of the acetabulum by using Charnley east-west and north-south retractors to retract the trochanter, the upper femur, and the capsule of the joint to expose the acetabulum. Careless placement of the proximal jaw of the east-west retractor into an osteoporotic trochanter or erroneous placement of the retractor distally on the femur can cause fractures. Enhance the anterior exposure by placing a Hohmann's retractor against the anterior lip of the acetabulum. Excise the labrum and the remnants of ligamentum teres and fat pad from the nonarticulating portion of the acetabulum.

- Prepare the acetabulum by drilling a 12.5-mm hole after marking the correct site. The drill hole will guide the deepening and expanding reamers for orientation during acetabular preparation. Drill the pilot hole at a 30- to 45-degree angle for a high socket position and at a 90-degree angle for a low position. Deepening and expanding are carried out using Charnley deepening and expanding reamers.

- Estimate the appropriate size of the socket based on the size of the acetabulum and the method of preparation. Trim a pressure-injection cup clipped to the cup-holder with correct orientation. Make sure that the posterior wall of the cup is oriented appropriately on the cup-holder. The rim of the cup must fit the margin of the acetabulum to produce effective pressurization of the cement and orientation of the cup.

- Make two or three 12.5-mm anchor holes in the direction of the ilium, ischium, and pubis. Also use several 6-mm anchor holes in addition to the large 12.5-mm anchor holes as needed to produce maximum anchorage for the cement. Use a wire mesh restrictor to prevent cement flow into the pelvis. Remove all the debris by brushing and irrigating the acetabulum before inserting the cement. Use hydrogen peroxide to prevent clotting of blood within the small cavities of bone. Introduce the cement using a pressurization device.

- The previously rehearsed position of the cup must be reproduced after cementing the acetabular cup. The cup must fully penetrate into the acetabulum with the rim in complete contact with the bone. No hammering via the pusher onto the cup face is necessary. Disengage the cup-holder relatively early, and hold the superior lobe of the cup against the bone with your thumb. After removing the excess cement and osteophytes, copious irrigation of the wound should be routine.

- Begin preparing the femur by delivering the stump of the femur out of the depth of the wound after removing the east-west, north-south, and Hohmann's retractors. Deliver the upper femur out of the wound by placing the ipsilateral femur across the table and by performing adequate soft tissue release as necessary. Enhance the view of the upper femur by using a posterior retractor to lever the femur out of the wound depth. Remove the bony bridge between the bed of the trochanter and the neck of the femur before inserting the T-handled canal finder. The canal finder must be placed in a valgus orientation to avoid penetrating the lateral cortex. A rotary reamer is ideal to expand the upper femur to accommodate a large-caliber stem and the flange of the Cobra prosthesis. Make sure that the tapered reamer and broaches are directed in a slightly valgus orientation without anteversion or retroversion. This can be best assessed when the extremity is in the cross-leg position, using the transcondylar line of the femur as a reference. As when orienting the cup, no anteversion of either of the components is allowed. When the neck of the femur is anteverted, an anteversion of the femoral component of up to 5 or 10 degrees may be permissible. After inserting the stem, check the range of motion and perform a "pull test" (separation of the two components by traction). Test for stability of the joint in extreme ranges of motion. When the hip is unstable, discover the cause; make an appropriate adjustment to the neck length or reorientate either or both components as needed.

- Final preparation of the upper femur includes gentle curettage of the medial aspect of the neck, brushing and irrigation of the bone, followed by insertion of wires to the upper end of the femur for subsequent reattachment of the greater trochanter. A double longitudinal wire and two independent (medial and lateral) wires are used to form a 6-point fixation for the trochanter. Test the insertion of the stem just before inserting the cement.

- An unimpeded insertion of cement and stem is essential. Isolate the neck of the femur so that it is not contaminated with blood when the cement is inserted. Use cement in a high-viscosity form (doughy). Use double-thumb pressure to introduce and pressurize cement during insertion. Avoid contaminating the cement with blood, especially when the cement is inserted over the medial aspect of the neck of the femur. The stem should be held by a holder in the rehearsal position. Insert the stem while the knee is held firmly by the second assistant and the tibia is perpendicular to the floor. The surgeon must be able to reproduce the precementing orientation of the stem after inserting the cement and stem. Do not hammer the prosthesis into the medullary canal, and avoid any movement after inserting the stem fully into the canal. Irrigate the bone copiously before reducing the joint. Excess cement must be removed. Ensure the stability of the joint after cementing the femoral component and before reattaching the trochanter.

- Reattach the trochanter after it is located in its bed, in a true anatomical position. Release the joint capsule or short rotators as required. To reattach the trochanter, the vertical wires are passed over the top of the trochanter at a midpoint and passed through the loop of the same wire over the lateral side of the femur. The medial wires form a pulley. The lateral wire ends pass through it, forming four points of fixation. In short, the vertical and cruciate systems allow for a 6-point fixation of the trochanter. After twisting the wires, bury the ends to avoid irritation and bursitis.

- Close the deep fascia first after inserting a deep drain. Suture the fat with retention sutures, followed by skin closure. Apply a dressing, elastic bandages, and an abduction splint (see Chapter 15).

APPENDIX
Instrument Trays for Low-Friction Arthroplasty*

Charnley Low-Friction Arthroplasty (Prewrapped) Instruments as Sequentially Delivered to the Operating Enclosure (see Fig. 18-30)

Tray 1. Skin Incision

5	Mayo towel clips with ball-guarded points
1	Lane's dissecting forceps
1	Knife handle with blade
18	Moynihan skin-towel clips
6	Heavy rubber bands for skin-towel clips
1	Diathermy forceps (Richies)
2	Long diathermy leads
1	Diathermy-cutting needle
1	Clips for diathermy leads
1	Sucker
1	Sucker tubing

} All retained on table until end of Tray 6.

Tray 2. Exposure of Acetabulum

1	Knife handle with blade
1	Lane's dissecting forceps
1	Mayo's straight scissors (6½ inch)
2	Kocher's artery forceps (8 inch)
1	Durham retractor
†1	Morris retractor
1	Cholecystectomy forceps
1	Langenbech sharp bone hook
1	Chisel (½ inch)
1	Mallet
2	Gigli's saws with pair of handles
†1	Initial incision retractor
1	Weight and chain
1	Watson-Jones gouge
†1	Serrated and angulated femur lever

} Retained on table until end of Tray 6.

Tray 3. Cementing Hip Socket

1	Long knife handle with blade
2	Kocher's forceps
†1	Nail retractor and introducer
1	Hohmann's retractor
†1	Hohmann's retractor angulated 45 degrees
†1	Small weight and chain for use with 45 degree-angulated Hohmann's retractor
†1	Horizontal retractor
†1	Retractor screw-jack
†2	Double-handled Volkmann spoons (large and small)
†1	Serrated ring curette, double-handled
1	Mallet
†1	Socket size gauges
†1	12.5-mm pilot hole drill with centering disc

†1	Deepening reamer
†1	Expanding reamer
†1	Heavy brace handle
†1	6-mm drill with collar
†1	Rotary acetabulum nylon brush
†1	Cement restrictor and introducer
†1	Self-ejecting socket holder
†1	Socket pusher
†1	Socket trimming scissors with serrated blades

Tray 4. Preparation of Femur—Test Reduction

1	Trotter's bone rongeur
†1	Taper reamer with T handle
†2	Rotary tape femoral reamers, brace-driven (large and small)
†1	Heavy brace handle
1	Ollier retractor
2	Kocher's forceps (8 inch)
1	Chisel (1 inch)
1	Mallet
†1	Femoral prosthesis holder (hold over to next tray)
†1	Set of test prostheses

(If neck-length jig is used it is introduced at end of this stage, as are additional tools. The neck-length jig makes the set of test prostheses redundant.)

Tray 5. Wires in Femur: Cement Femoral Prosthesis

1	Lane's dissecting forceps
1	Mayo scissors
2	Kocher's artery forceps (8 inch)
1	Ollier retractor
1	Chisel (½ inch)
1	Mallet
†1	Long-handled small curette
1	Short Volkmann spoon
†6	Wire-holding forceps
†1	Set of wires 18 swg, 1 double, 2 single
1	Narrow bone rongeur (6 mm)
†1	Trochanter staple bolt length measuring device
†1	3.2 mm drill and drill stock
†1	Femoral prosthesis holder (held over from previous tray)
†1	Small fish-tailed wire pusher

---

*From Charnley J: *Low-friction arthroplasty of the hip: theory and practice,* New York, 1979, Springer-Verlag.
†Supplied by Charles F. Thackeray and arranged by the staff at Wrightington Hospital.

Tray 6. Reattachment of Trochanter

2   Kocher's forceps (8 inch)
1   Mayo scissors
2   Ollier retractors
1   Chisel (1 inch)
1   Mallet
†1 Trochanter-holding forceps
†1 Wire passer (¼ circle)
†1 Narrow bone awl
†1 Large bone awl
†1 Trochanter staple-bolt forceps
†1 Trochanter staple-bolt anterior holding device
†1 Wire tightener
†1 Wire-cutting forceps

†1 Heavy trochanter punch
†1 Small, fish-tailed wire punch
†1 Bolt cropper (12 inch)
†1 Fine-toothed metal file

Tray 7. Wound Closure

2   Needle holders
1   Mayo scissors
2   Dissecting forceps (5¾ inch and 7 inch)
1   Ollier retractor
7   Hemostats (for fat suture)
1   Packet 12 suture buttons (aluminum)
1   Packet 12 plastic foam-pressure pads
3   Drainage tubes with trocars
†1 Button crusher

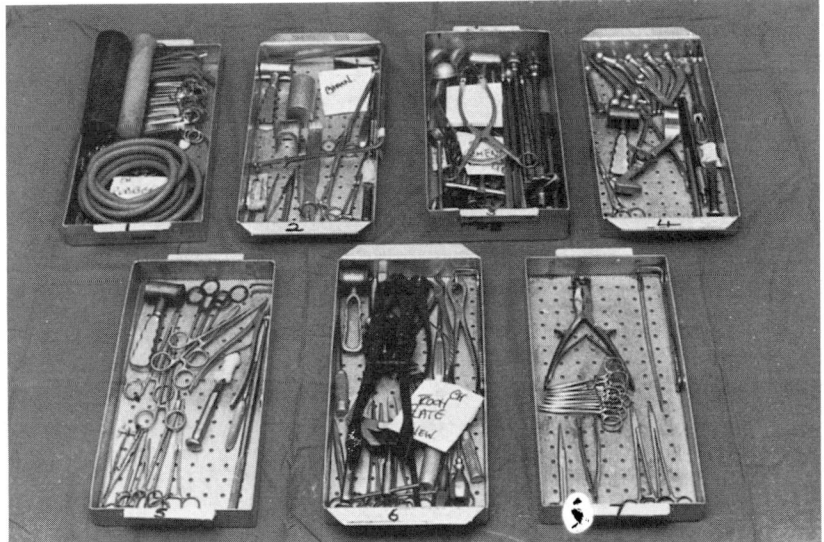

Fig. 18-30. The seven trays containing the instruments for individual, progressive phases of the operation. (From Charnley J: *Low-friction arthroplasty of the hip: theory and practice,* New York, 1979, Springer-Verlag.)

REFERENCES

1. **Charnley J:** *Personal communication.*
2. **Charnley J:** *Operative technique of low-friction arthroplasty of the hip joint,* Internal publication no. 6, 2nd revision, Centre for Hip Surgery, England, 1971, Wrightington Hospital.
3. **Charnley J:** *Total hip replacement, low-friction technique,* slide-tape presentation by Professor Sir John Charnley, C.B.E., F.R.S., F.R.C.S., Courtesy of Chas. F. Thackeray, Ltd., 1977.
4. **Charnley J:** *Low-friction arthroplasty of the hip: theory and practice,* New York, 1979, Springer-Verlag.

See Chapters 5, Acrylic Cement: Properties and Application; 15, Principles Common to all Surgical Approaches; 24, Conversion of Failed Previous Surgery; and 32, Dislocation and Instability for additional information.

CHAPTER NINETEEN

Transstrochanteric Approach (Author's Method)

- This is an operation of many details, every and all of which must be respected. Modifications are justifiable only if they can objectively improve the quality of the results.
  N.E.

PHASE I: POSITIONING, PREPARATION, AND DRAPING

Throughout the procedure the patient is in a supine position and the surgeon seated. For details on positioning, preparation, and draping for the supine position, see Chapter 15 and Fig. 19-1.

Seven trays of instruments (Chapter 19 appendix, Fig. 19-39) are delivered to the enclosure sequentially. This system of instruments facilitates the work and saves time.

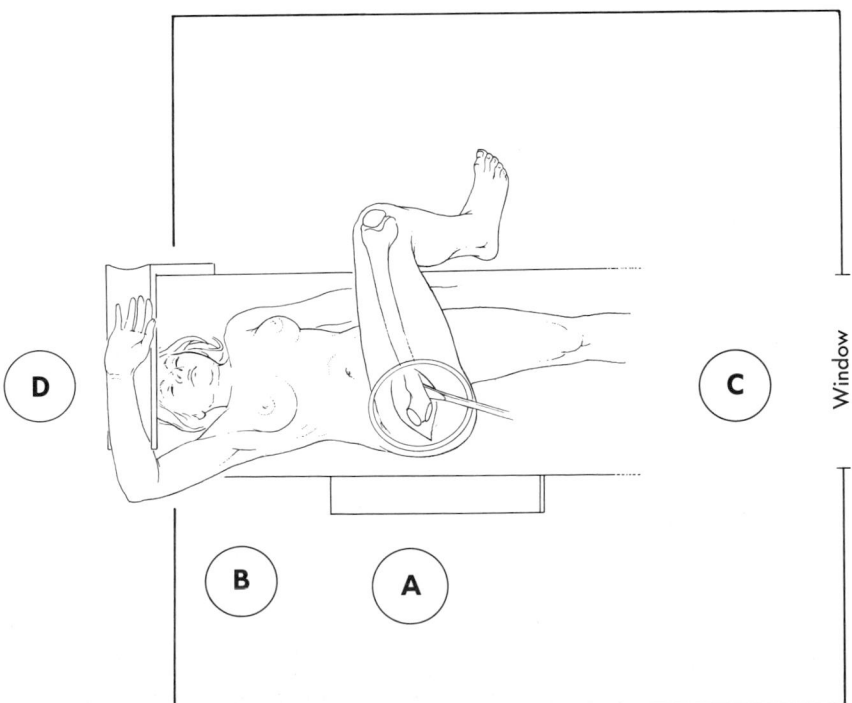

Fig. 19-1. General view of the operating room enclosure. Positions of patients, operating table, and personnel and their relationship to the operating and instrument tables. *A,* The surgeon. *B,* First assistant. *C,* Scrub nurse. *D,* Anesthesiologist. When available, a technician may also be present on the opposite side of the table from the surgeon.

PHASE II: SURGICAL EXPOSURE, LEG LENGTH MEASUREMENTS, AND BIPLANAR OSTEOTOMY
Skin Incision

The distal portion of the skin incision used here is similar to the one used by Charnley and is located along the anterior border of the femur. The proximal limb of the incision is curved while it is inclined posteriorly toward the posterosuperior iliac spine (Fig. 19-2). It is extended proximally to the level of the anterosuperior spine for approximately 2 to 4 cm. Skin towels are applied to the skin edge in a manner similar to Charnley's technique.

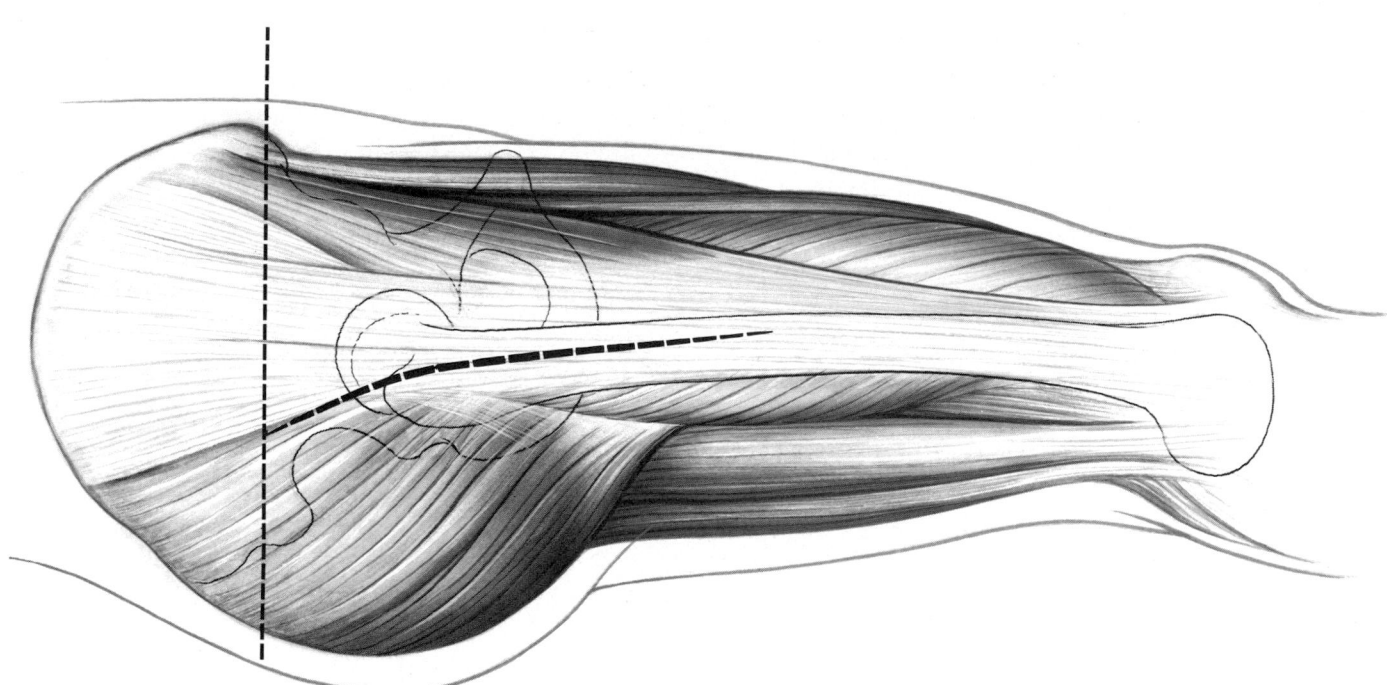

Fig. 19-2. Placement of the incision is determined by the following landmarks: (1) the anterosuperior iliac spine, which determines the proximal end of the incision, (2) the vastus lateralis ridge, which determines the center portion of the incision, (3) the anterior aspect of the shaft of the femur, which indicates the line of the distal limb of the incision. The proximal limb of the incision begins at the level of the tip of the greater trochanter, extended proximally to the level of the anterosuperior spine and inclined posterially for approximately 2.5 cm. The distal limb of the incision is parallel to the shaft of the femur beginning at the level of the tip of the greater trochanter.

Fascial Incision

Place the hip in a position of 20 degrees of flexion and 10 degrees of adduction to facilitate placing the fascial incision in the appropriate location. Take care to avoid cutting into the underlying vastus lateralis distally and the gluteus maximus proximally. Make the fascial incision by splitting the iliotibial band at its midportion distally first. The fascial incision is made along the line of incision. Avoid cutting into the fibers of the tensor fascia femoris muscle. Insert a finger into the distal opening of the fascial incision to identify the site of insertion of this muscle to the iliotibial band (Fig. 19-3). Then continue incising the fascia from the tip of the trochanter toward the posterosuperior iliac spine along the length of the skin incision.

Depending on the patient's fat thickness, select a standard or large blade, and attach it to the ring (over the flat) of an octomerous retractor. The posterior blade must be located at the center of the flat on the ring and applied to the fascia just proximal to the insertion of the gluteus maximus to the linea aspra of the femur (Figs. 19-4 and 19-5). Open the fascia by advancing the triple lead screw attached to the anterior fascial member. Note that the most effective way to retract the fascia is by placing the fascial members at the midlength of the opening to keep the wound maximally exposed in a diamond shape. Tighten the fascial member firmly to produce a wide opening of the surgical field (Fig. 19-4, *B*).

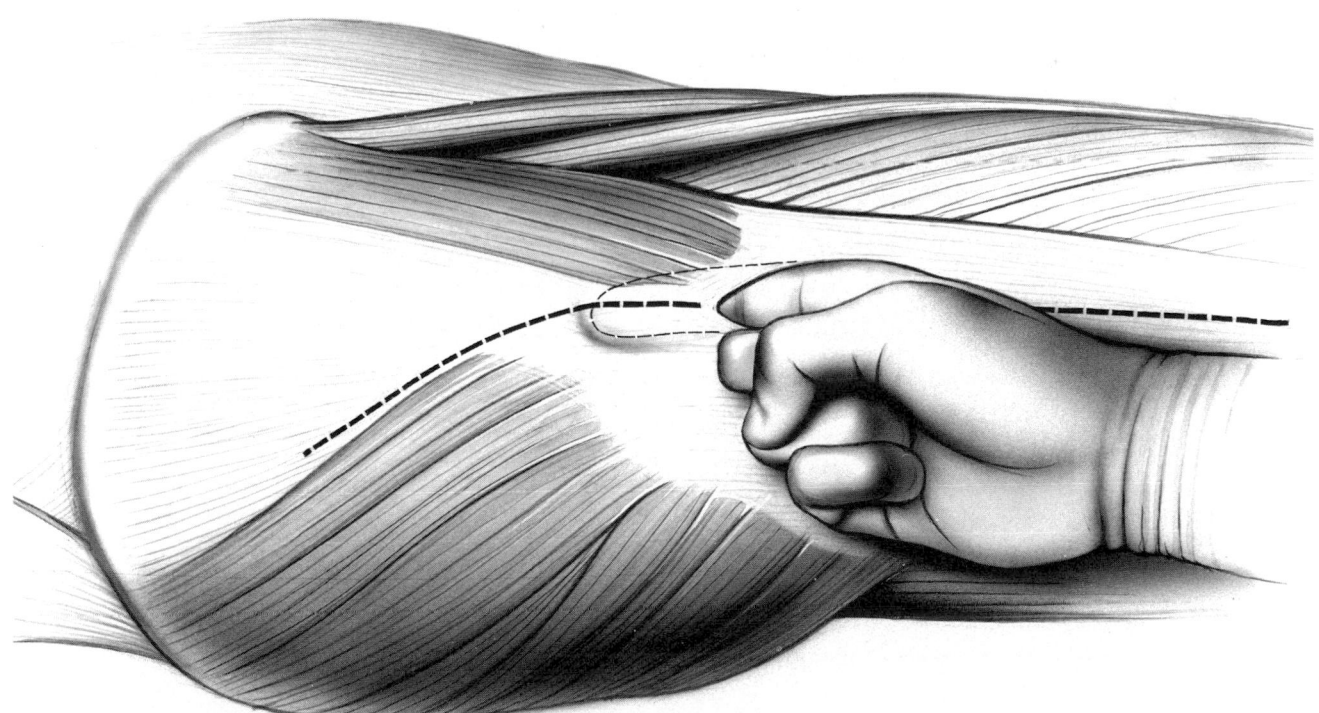

Fig. 19-3. Fascial incision is made along the line of the skin incision. An opening is first made distally along the line of incision and parallel to the shaft of the femur. Place an index finger into the opening of the fascia to verify the location of the tensor fascia femoris muscle. Fascial incision should remain posterior to its insertion to iliotibial tract while the incision is inclined posterially. Open the aponeurosis of the gluteus maximus sharply, and split the gluteus maximus muscle proximally. (Redrawn from Eftekhar NS: Total hip replacement: low-friction arthroplasty. In Evarts CM, editor: *Surgery of the musculoskeletal system,* New York, 1983, Churchill Livingstone.)

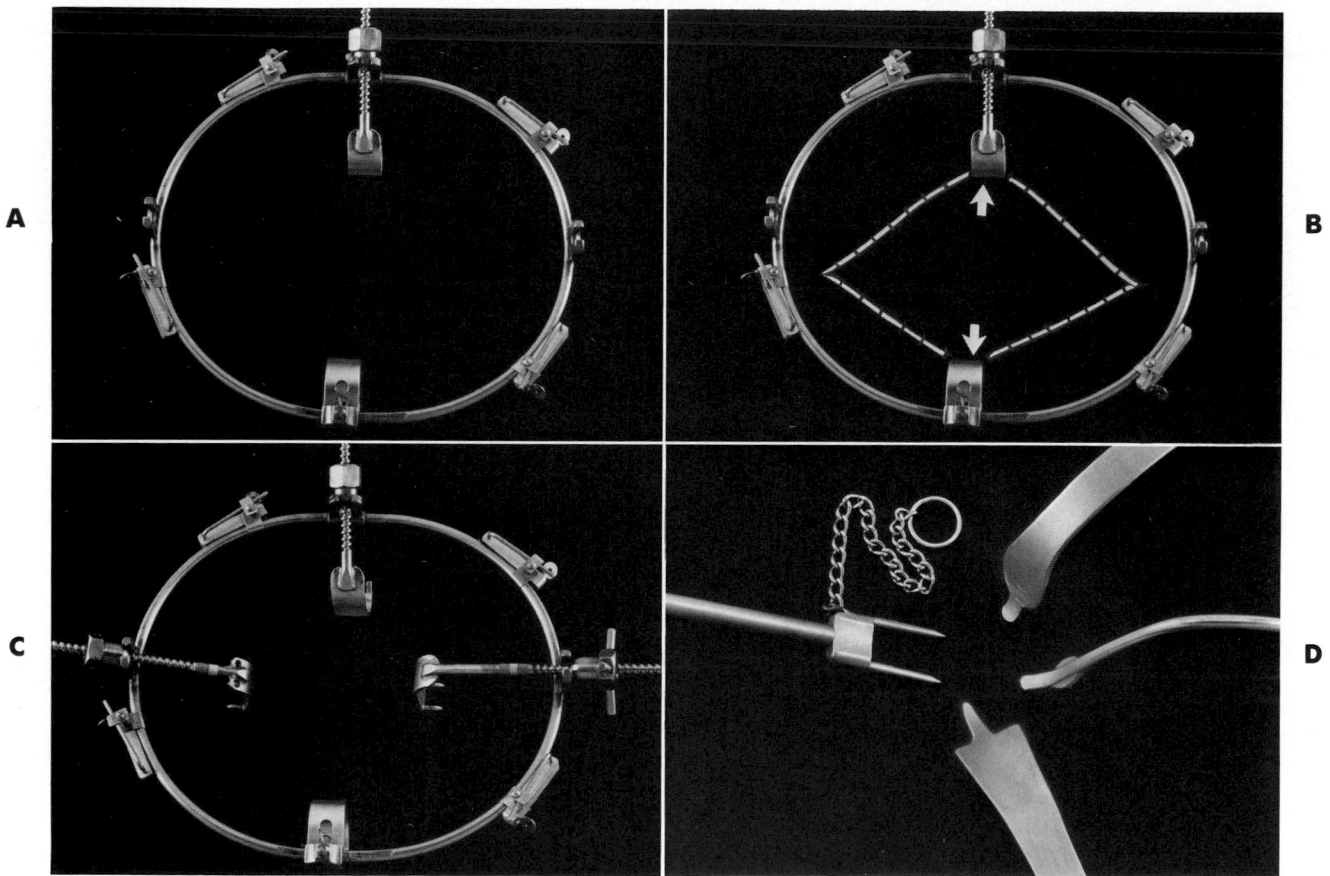

Fig. 19-4. A, Octomerous retractor (designed by the author): the ring and the fascial members *(top and bottom)*. **B,** The fascial members are centered as the wound remains open in a diamond shape. **C,** The trochanteric and femoral members *(right and left)* carry their quick-advancing triple-lead screw mechanisms. Four pairs of adjustable clips were designed to attach the acetabular retractors to the ring. **D,** The acetabular members of the octomerous retractor. The tips are specially designed to accommodate the ilium, the ischium, and the intracortoloid notch. The four acetabular members are the iliopubic (anterior acetabular, *top*), ischioliac (posterior acetabular, *bottom*), cotyloid (inferior acetabular, *right*), and iliac (superior acetabular member, *left*) or acetabular staple. Chain attached to staple is designed to remind surgeon to remove it after fixing the cup.

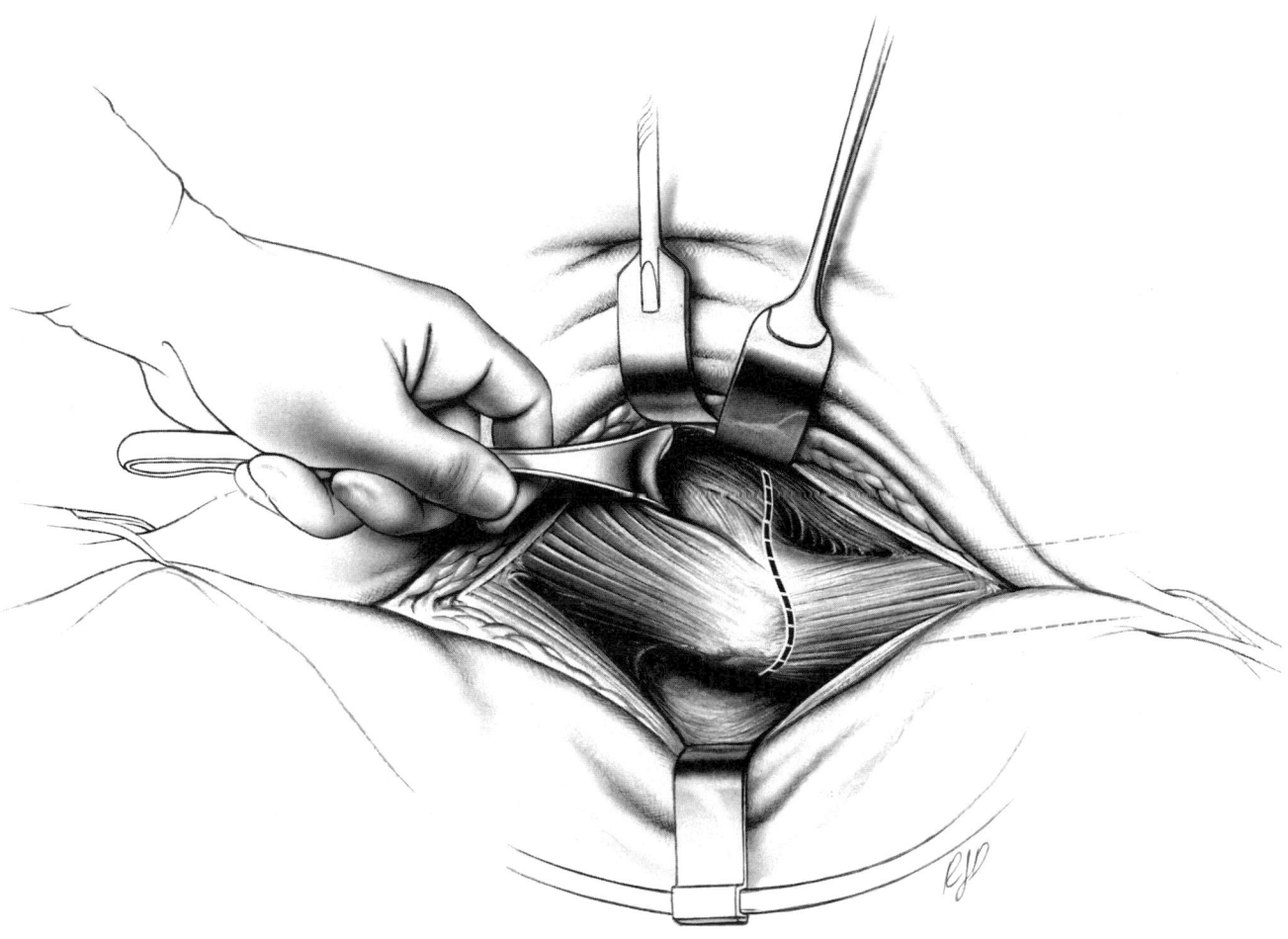

Fig. 19-5. Exposure of the anterior capsule: note the site of arthrotomy on the capsule at the level of the vastus lateralis ridge and somewhat inferior to the neck of the femur. Before arthrotomy, the entire anterior capsule must be exposed by placing a Richardson retractor proximally and a Hibbs retractor medially.

Arthrotomy and Detachment of Vastus Origin

Place the femur in 10 degrees of abduction, flexion, and external rotation. Open the interval between the gluteus medius and minimus laterally and the tensor fascia femoris medially. Maintain the exposure using deep retractors such as a Richardson to retract the glutei and a Hibbs or Durham to retract the tensor fascia femoris (see Fig. 19-5). Perform an arthrotomy along the inferior border of the neck using an electric knife. Insert a curved-tip clamp such as a cholecystectomy clamp into the joint space. Use the clamp as a target at which the osteotome will be aimed (Fig. 19-6). Detach the vastus lateralis origin, and strip it off the bone 2 cm from the vastus tubercle. Control bleeders.

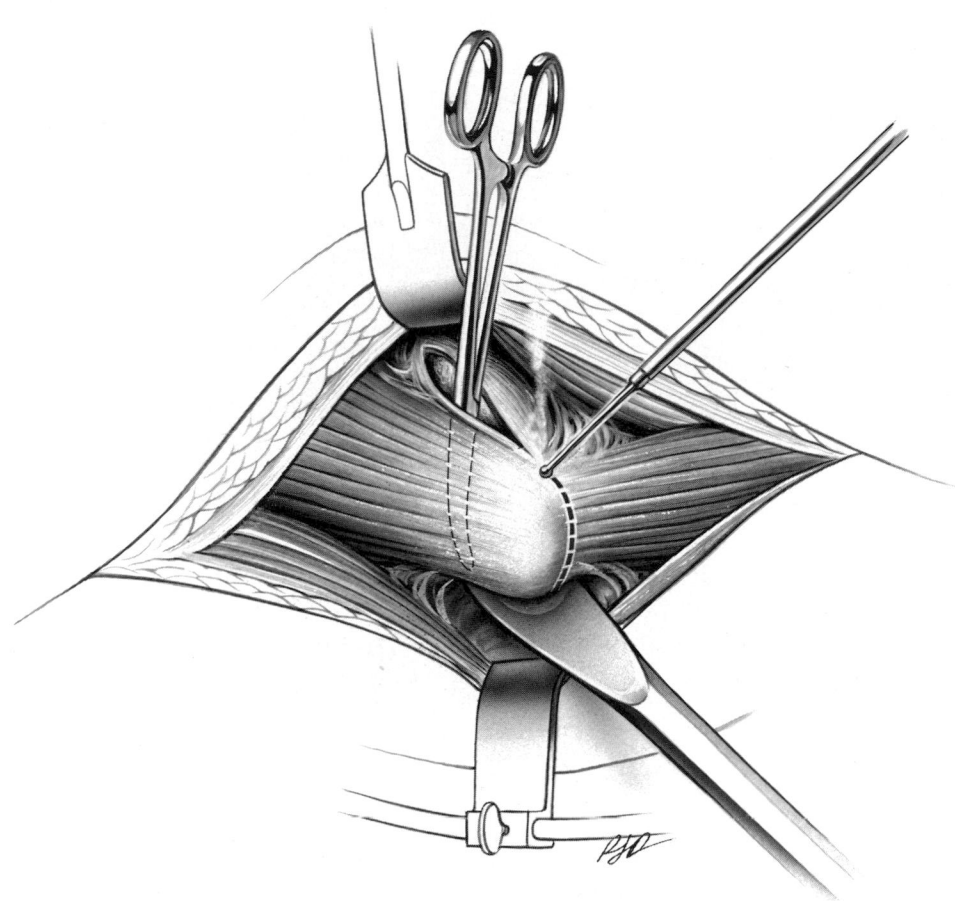

Fig. 19-6. Insert a cholecystectomy clamp over the superior aspect of the neck of the femur medial to the greater trochanter and through the posterior capsule while a Watson-Jones gouge protects the sciatic nerve. Complete the incision along the lateral aspect of the femur along the vastus lateralis ridge.

Osteotomy of the Trochanter

Successful reattachment of the trochanter and rapid healing ocurs when:

1. A large surface contact is achieved between the trochanter and its bed.
2. Flexion/extension motion of the hip does not interfere with stability of initial fixation.
3. The initial fixation includes impaction of the trochanter against its bed.

These criteria can be met if the surgeon does the following:

1. Creates an optimal size and shape of the trochanter (preferably a biplanar).
2. Creates good interlock between the trochanter and the femur with maximal initial stability.
3. Removes undue tension from abductors by capsular and short rotator releases and by avoiding overlengthening the leg.
4. Maintains the fixation by a satisfactory wiring technique and occasionally by additional support (brace or cast) to achieve union.

Performing Biplanar Osteotomy

This method produces the best results when only slight (no more than 1 cm) advancement of the trochanter is required.

1. Place the hip in 5 to 10 degrees abduction and 5 to 10 degrees internal rotation.
2. Place a flat-ended instrument such as a Watson-Jones gauge behind the trochanter to protect the sciatic nerve.
3. Use a biplanar osteotome (designed by the author) or a thin-bladed saw to osteotomize the trochanter (see Fig. 19-6).
4. Begin the osteotomy at the vastus tubercle, and finish it at the site of insertion of the cholecystectomy clamp (Figs. 19-7 and 19-8).

Note that when the surgeon plans to transfer the greater trochanter distally (more than 1 cm), the trochanter osteotomy should be made in one plane, using a flat osteotome or a reciprocating saw. Insert a cholecystectomy forceps through the opening in the capsule into the joint, and direct the osteotome or the saw toward the clamp. It is important to complete the osteotomy before separating it from the femur to avoid fracturing the trochanter.

Before attempting dislocation, retract the trochanter cephalad via its capsular attachment using a Morris or Hibbs retractor.

- Release the posterior capsule and piriformis as indicated.
- Avoid fracturing the trochanter by retracting it through the capsule. Never place the retractor on bone.
- Control posterior bleeders and the vessels accompanying the piriformis tendon (see Chapter 18).
- Measure the leg length between two fixed points, one on the pelvis and one on the femur, before dislocating the hip.

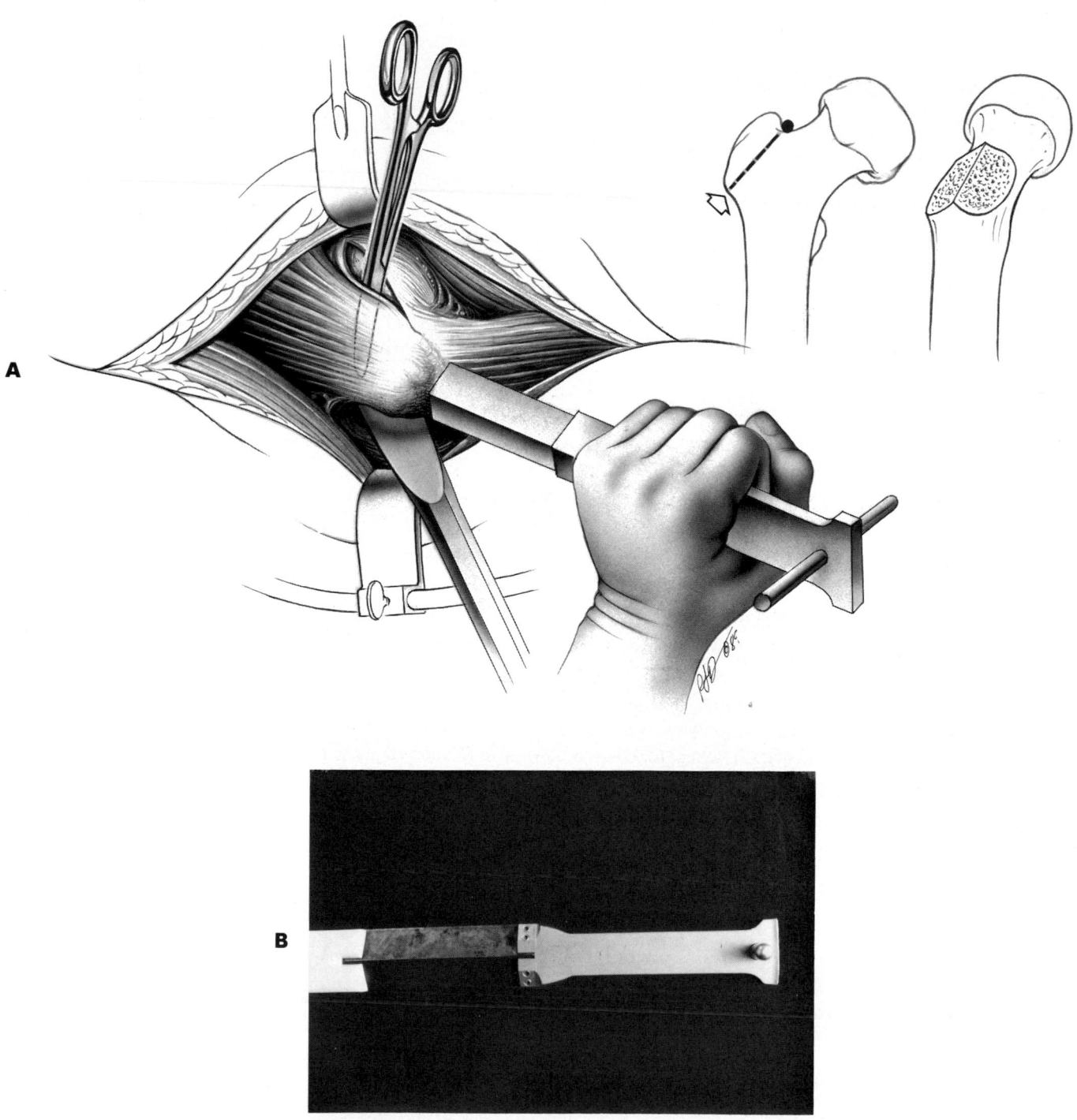

Fig. 19-7. A, The level of osteotomy of the greater trochanter is easily identified because it begins exactly at the vastus lateralis ridge. The greater trochanter must be thick enough to avoid fracture. The two planes must be symmetrical in width at the completion of osteotomy. **B,** Biplanar osteotome designed by the author.

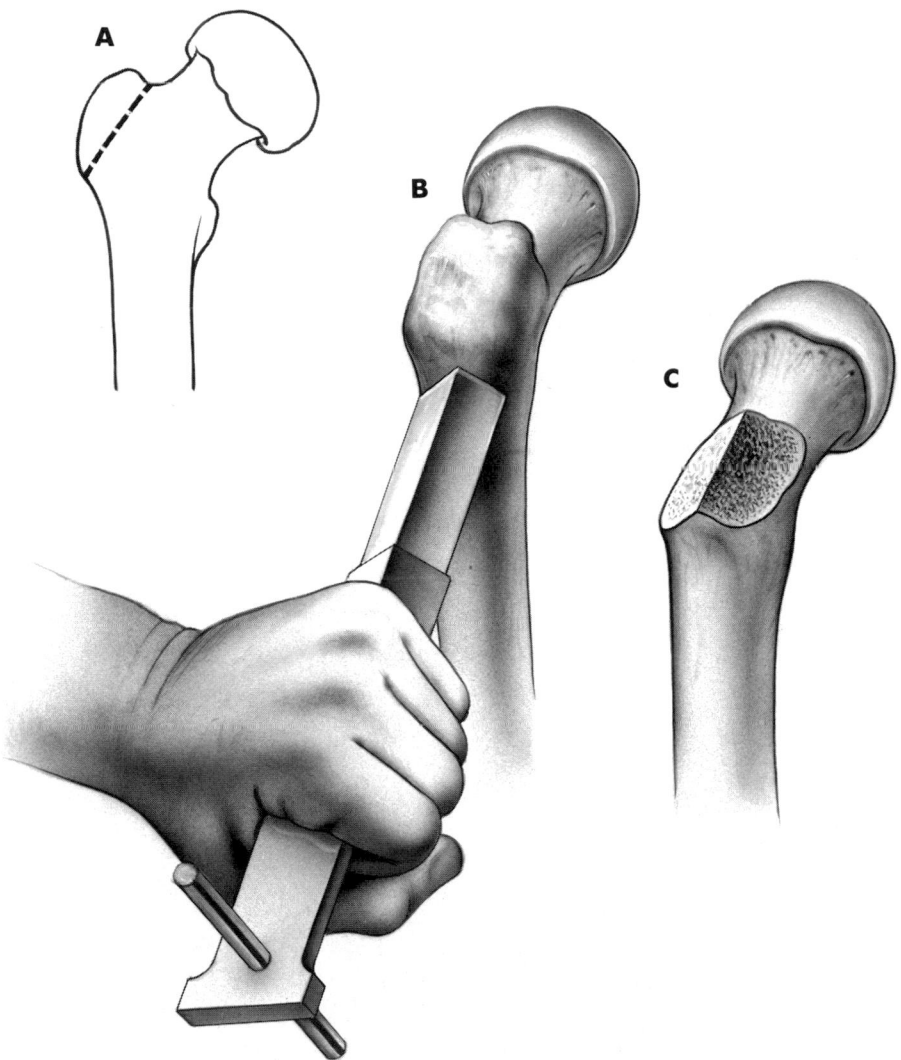

Fig. 19-8. A, Biplanar osteotomy begins at the trochanteric ridge and ends at the junction of the trochanter and the femoral neck. **B,** The osteotome must be placed to cut the bone with equal thickness anteriorly and posteriorly. **C,** The bed of the trochanter. The large surface of this site and the mechanical stability of this type of osteotomy should enhance the bony union.

PHASE III: DISLOCATING THE HIP, AMPUTATING THE HEAD, AND APPLYING THE TROCHANTERIC AND FEMORAL MEMBERS OF THE OCTOMEROUS RETRACTOR

Dislocate the hip by adduction (without rotation) while the trochanter is being retracted cephalad. Place the femur across the table, and remove the head using a Gigli's or reciprocating saw as described in Chapters 15 and 18. Fig. 19-9 demonstrates the planes of the section of the neck—the desired level of sectioning is determined by preoperative templating. Insert the trochanteric and femoral members of the octomerous retractor as follows:

- Release the inferior capsule as needed to displace the femur. Also release the superior capsule as needed to promote trochanteric mobilization.
- Place the femur across the table by adducting the hip. Place the jaws of the trochanteric and femoral retractors against the respective bones to retract the trochanter cephalad and the femur caudad via the flat part of the claws (Fig. 19-10).
- Advance the triple lead screw of these retractors simultaneously and alternately to produce and share a balanced tension.
- Visualize the acetabular rim by inserting the four acetabular retractors into the acetabular periphery in the following order: first the anterior (iliopubic), next the posterior (ilioischial), and third the inferior (intercolyloid) (Figs. 19-11 to 19-13). Insert the fourth member of the retractor, the acetabular staple. Begin the insertion in a headward direction, and drive it in until the handle reaches a plane perpendicular to the body axis (parallel to the trans-axis of the pelvis) (Fig. 19-14). Note that a constricting and thickened capsule may make it difficult to insert the periacetabular retractors. Perform a capsulotomy at the three preferred sites (safe zones), anterosuperiorly, posterosuperiorly, and inferiorly (see Fig. 19-10).

Text continued on p. 882.

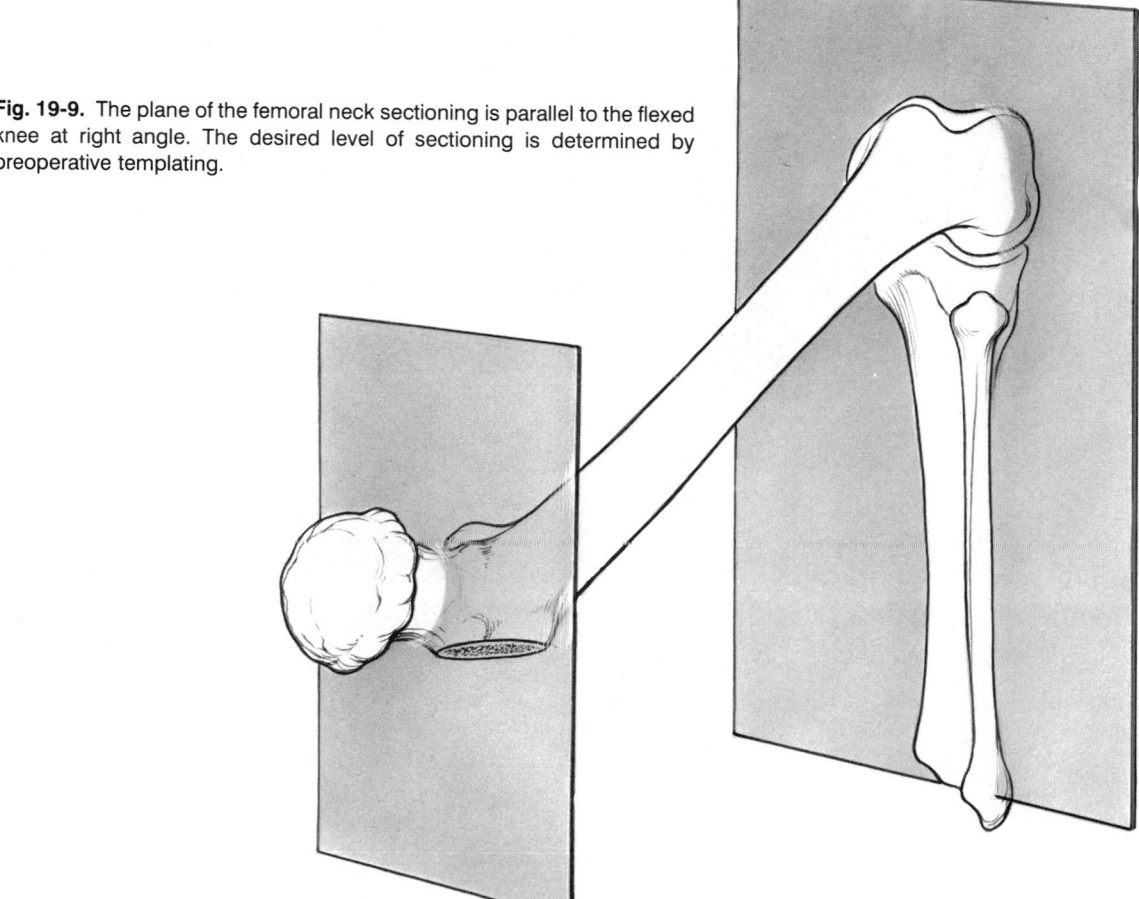

Fig. 19-9. The plane of the femoral neck sectioning is parallel to the flexed knee at right angle. The desired level of sectioning is determined by preoperative templating.

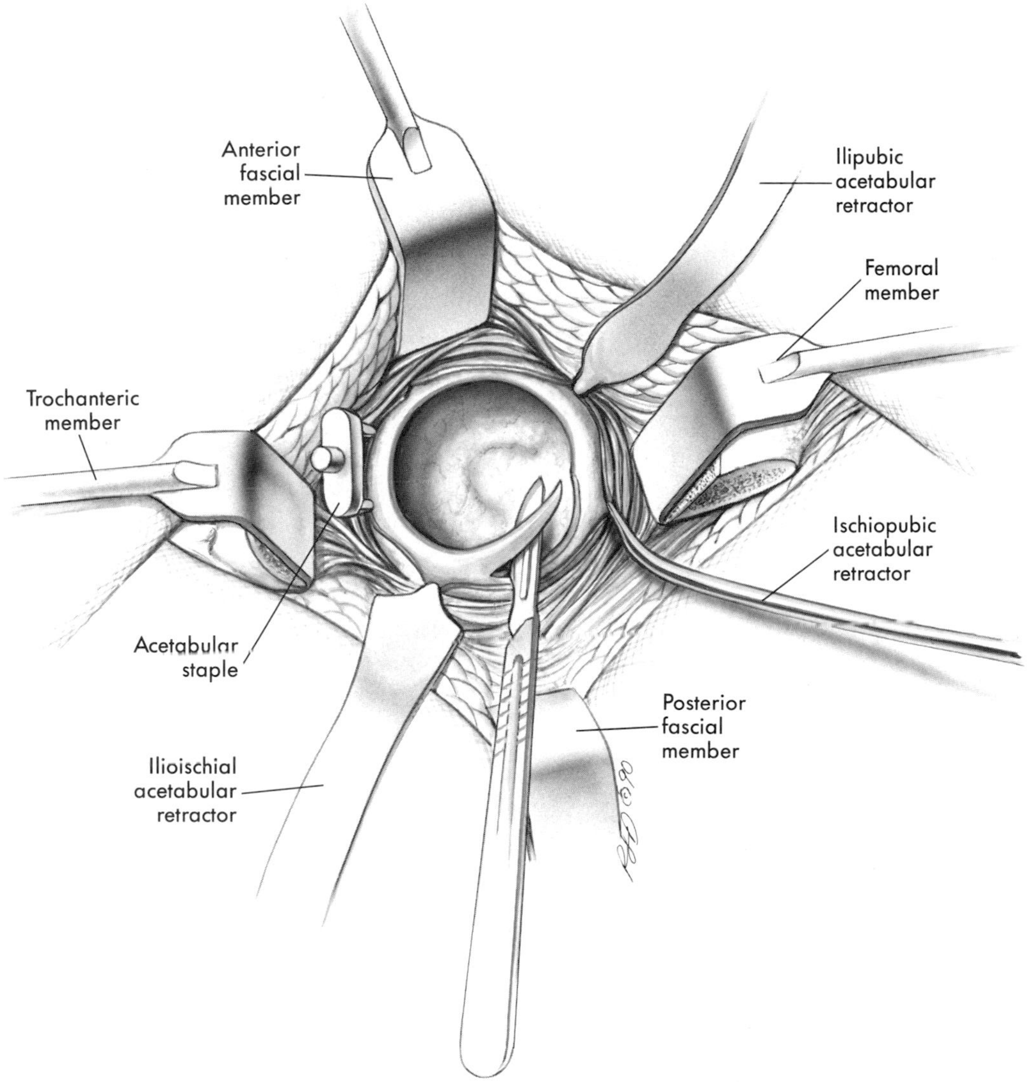

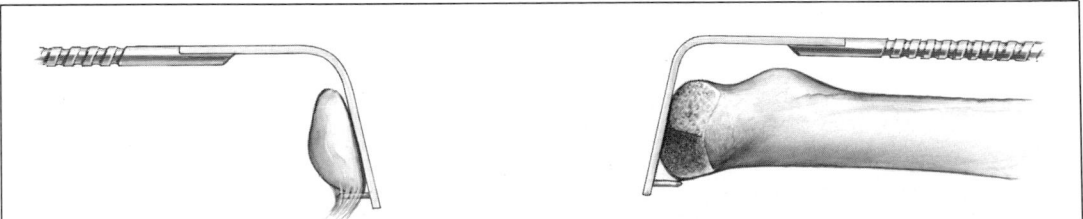

Fig. 19-10. Octomerous (eight-member) retractor in place, producing an excellent view of the acetabulum. The acetabular labrum is being excised. Inset shows the exact placement of the trochanteric and femoral members of the octomerous retractor.

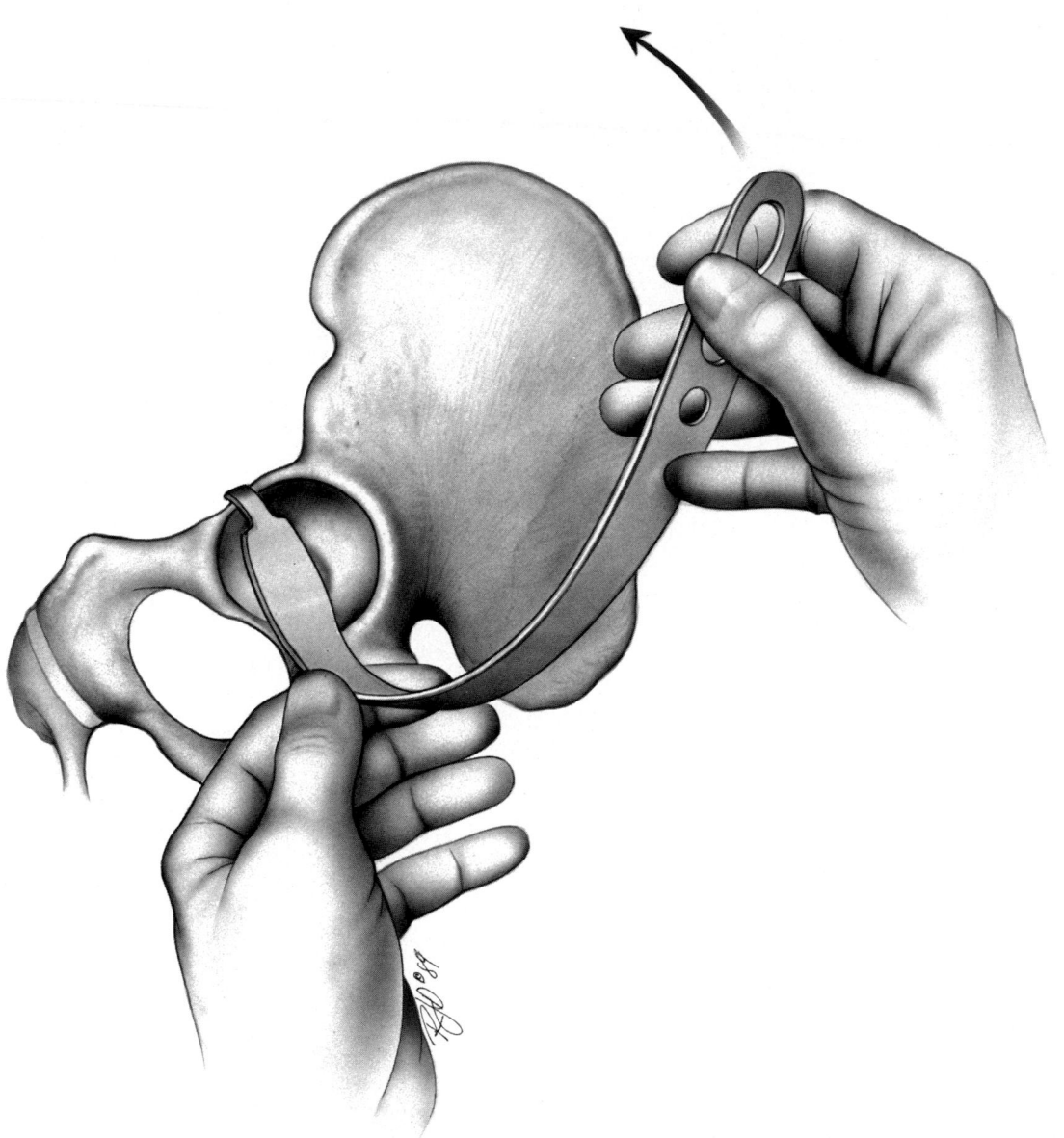

Fig. 19-11. The anterior (iliopubic) retractor is inserted from a posterior to an anterior direction as the tip is being engaged onto the bone (inside the joint capsule).

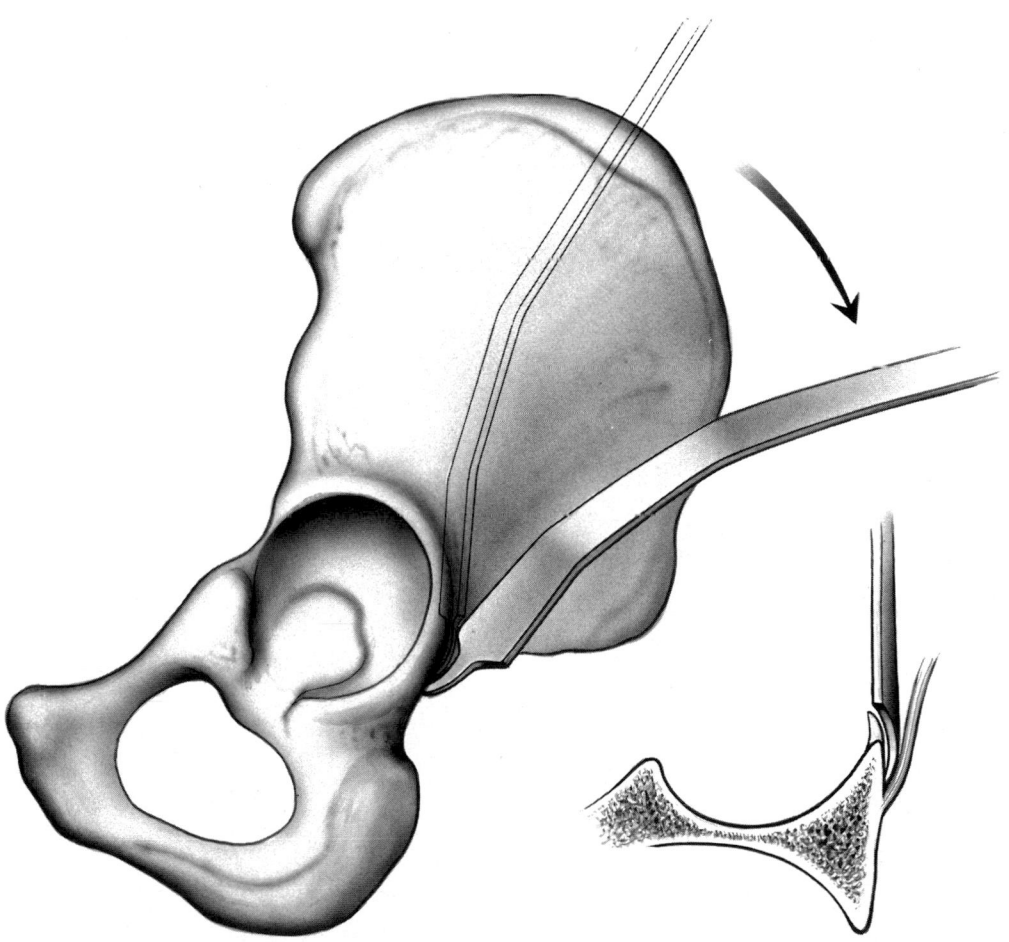

Fig. 19-12. The posterior acetabular retractor is inserted as it is engaged to the bone intracapsullarly and is inserted from an anterior to a posterior direction.

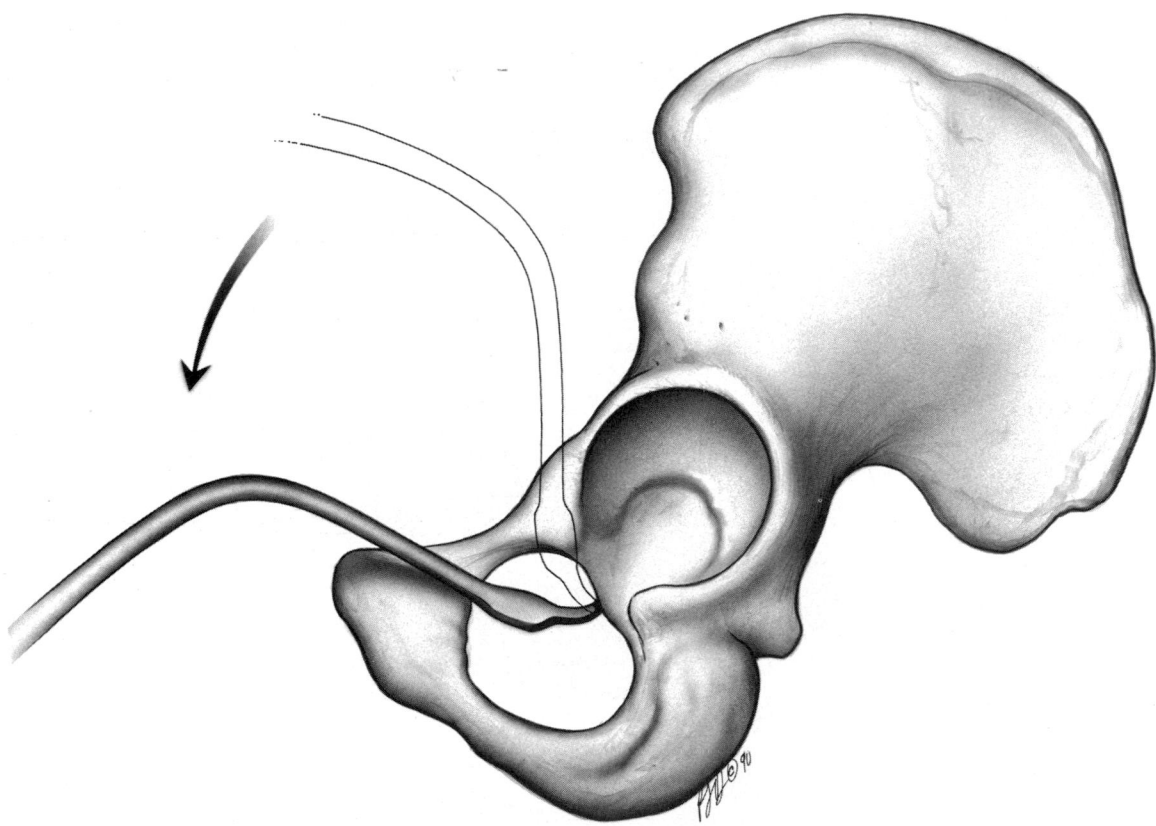

Fig. 19-13. The inferior (ischiopubic) retractor is engaged onto the bone from a cephalad to a caudad position. This retractor is placed beneath the transverse ligament.

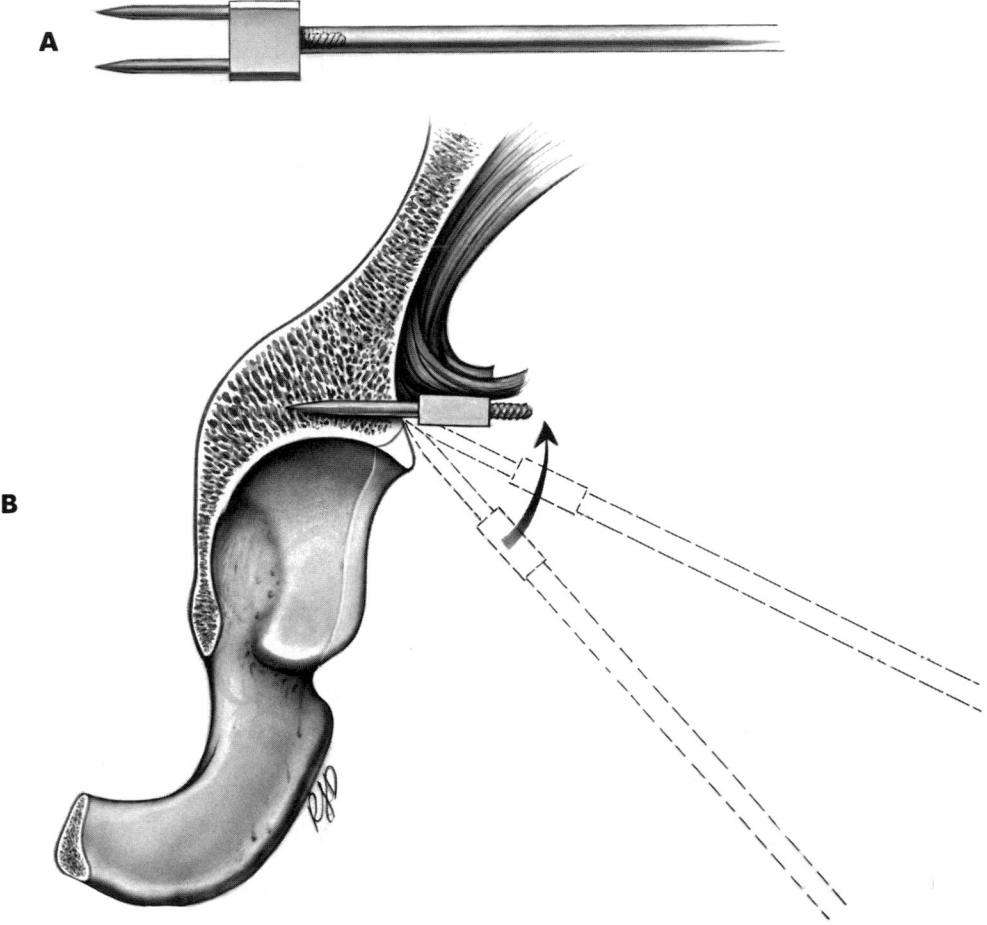

Fig. 19-14. The acetabular staple retractor is inserted. To drive the acetabular staple, **A,** attach the holder to the staple, and drive it at a sharp angle in relation to the transaxis of the pelvis. The handle of the holder is brought up toward the patient's head as it becomes parallel to the transaxis of the pelvis. It is then driven into the pelvis approximately 2 cm proximal to the lip of the acetabulum.

PHASE IV: ACETABULAR EXPOSURE, PREPARATION, AND FIXATION OF THE ACETABULAR COMPONENTS
Maximizing Exposure

An unimpeded visualization of the periphery of the acetabular margin (rim) is a prerequisite for preparing and fixating the socket. Note the following details:

- Perform adequate capsulotomy anterosuperiorly, posterosuperiorly, and inferiorly before retracting the trochanter and femur.
- Make sure the claws of the trochanteric and femoral members are adequately engaged onto the flat surfaces of the respective bones.
- Retract the femur and the trochanter by turning the knobs of the triple lead screws slowly, ensuring a shared tension on the trochanter and the femur while the knobs are being alternately advanced.
- Avoid forceful retraction by trochanteric and femoral members because the trochanter and femur may facture.
- Excise the labrum (see Fig. 19-10).

Preparing the Acetabulum

Select the site of the acetabular fixation based on the pathological morphology of the acetabulum as confirmed by x-ray. Choose the method for fixation, and follow the instructions on fixation of the cup given in Chapter 15. Preserve subchondral bone during preparation of the acetabulum.

This author's preferred method for preparation and cup fixation is as follows:

- In-situ preparation. Use debris-retaining reamers (without spigot) in a predetermined direction to remove bone cartilage to create a concentric cavity (Fig. 19-15). Such preparation is suitable for a cemented or cementless cup.
- Preparation in a lowered position. Use a long drill (6 mm outer diameter) and the author's acetabular gauge drill guide. Drill the medial wall of the acetabulum in a lowered position (Figs. 19-16 and 19-17).
- Gauging the acetabulum for size. As a rule, the last reamer used is a good guide for sizing a cementless cup because the size of the cup should correspond to the size of the last reamer. In cementing the socket, insert the trimmed cup into the acetabulum, and test it for size and coverage by bone before inserting the cement. For details, see Chapter 15. Fig. 19-18, *A* and *B*, illustrates gauging for a cemented cup using the author's cup gauge and cup holder with detachable plate (Fig. 19-18, *C* and *D*). Accurate positioning of the cup (in relation to the pelvis) requires that the patient be in a supine position. Sandbags should not be placed under the patient's buttock (Fig. 19-18, *E*). The plane of anteversion is determined by the position of the cup holder as shown in Fig. 19-18, *F*.
- For trimming the flanged cup, see Chapter 15.
- For drilling multiple anchor holes, see Chapter 15. Fig. 19-19 demonstrates drilling multiple holes (6 mm outer diameter) 1 cm deep using the author's method.
- For fixation of the cup without cement, see Chapter 15.

Text continued on p. 890.

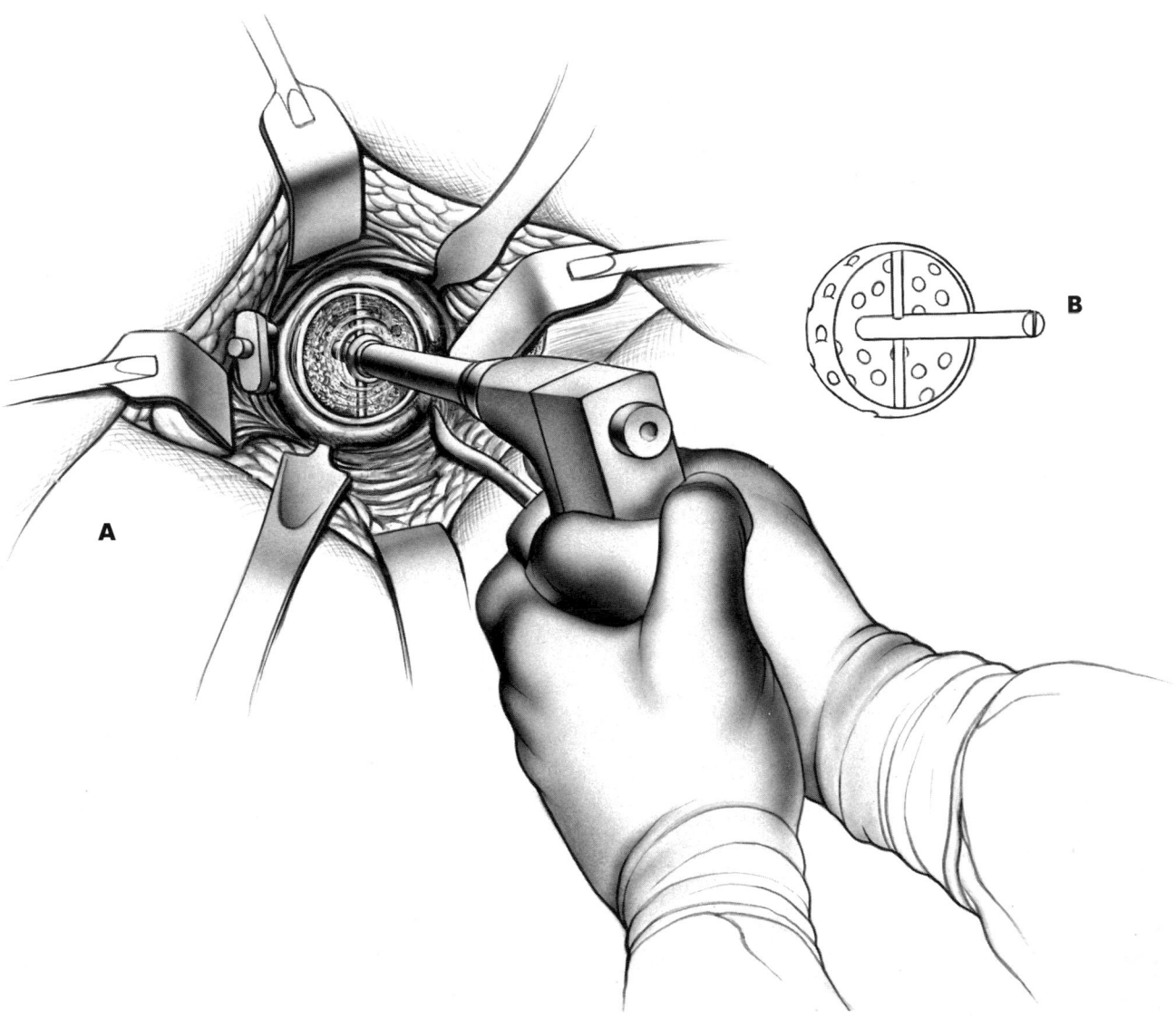

Fig. 19-15. A, Acetabular reamer with its spigot engaged. **B,** Debris-retaining reamer. Note that excellent exposure of the acetabulum must be obtained by adjusting the members of the octomerous retractor. An in-situ preparation requires the appropriate angle for reamer insertion because a concentric reaming is preferred. (From Eftekhar NS: Total hip replacement: low-friction arthroplasty. In Evarts CM, editor: *Surgery of the musculoskeletal system,* New York, 1983, Churchill Livingstone.)

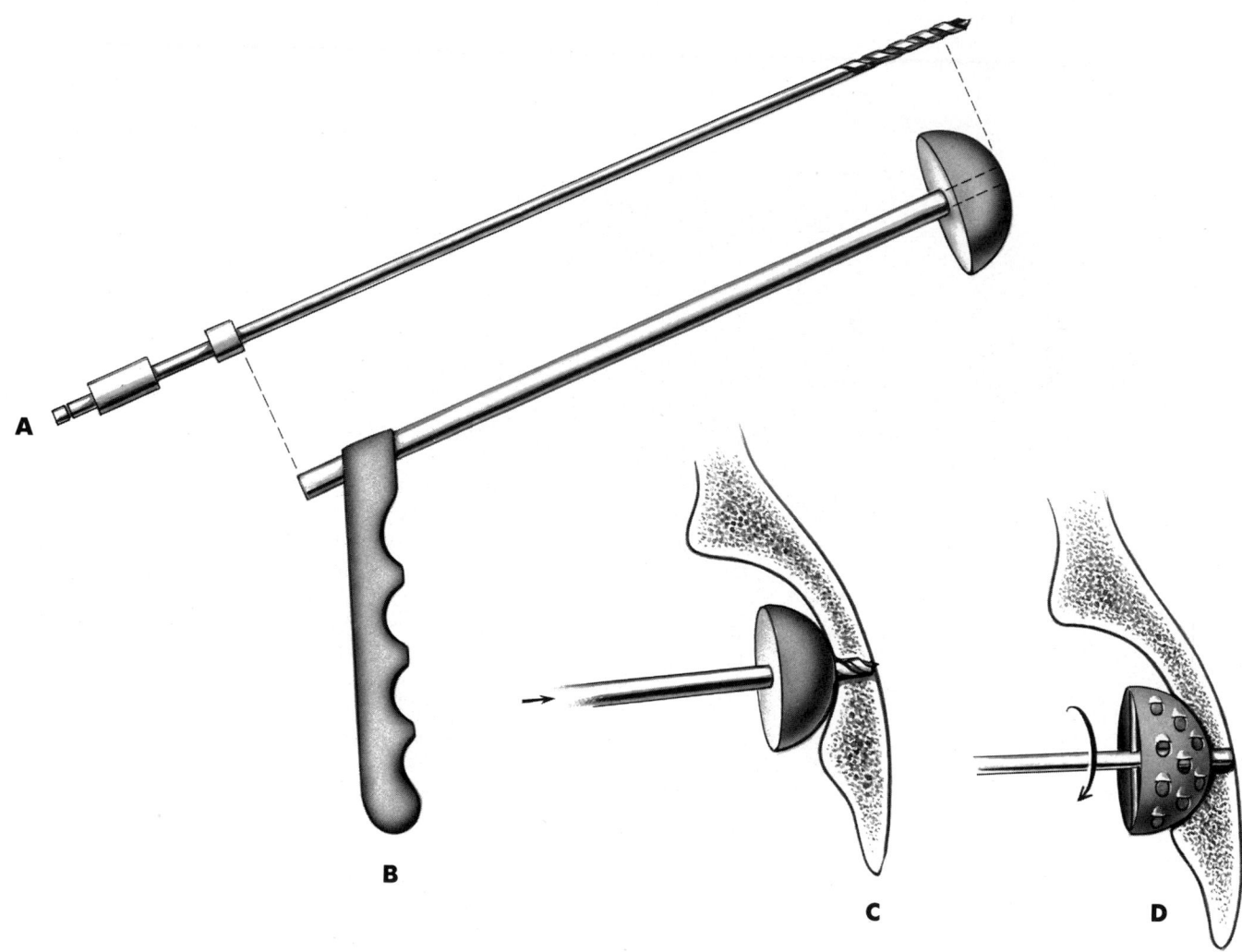

Fig. 19-16. A, Drill. **B,** Acetabular gauge—drill guide. **C,** Lowering the socket site. **D,** Reaming at a lowered level. Note lowering of the socket site to the original site of the true acetabulum. The spigotted reamers will be located at a lowered site on the acetabulum. (From Eftekhar NS: Total hip replacement: low-friction arthroplasty. In Evarts CM, editor: *Surgery of the musculoskeletal system,* New York, 1983, Churchill Livingstone.)

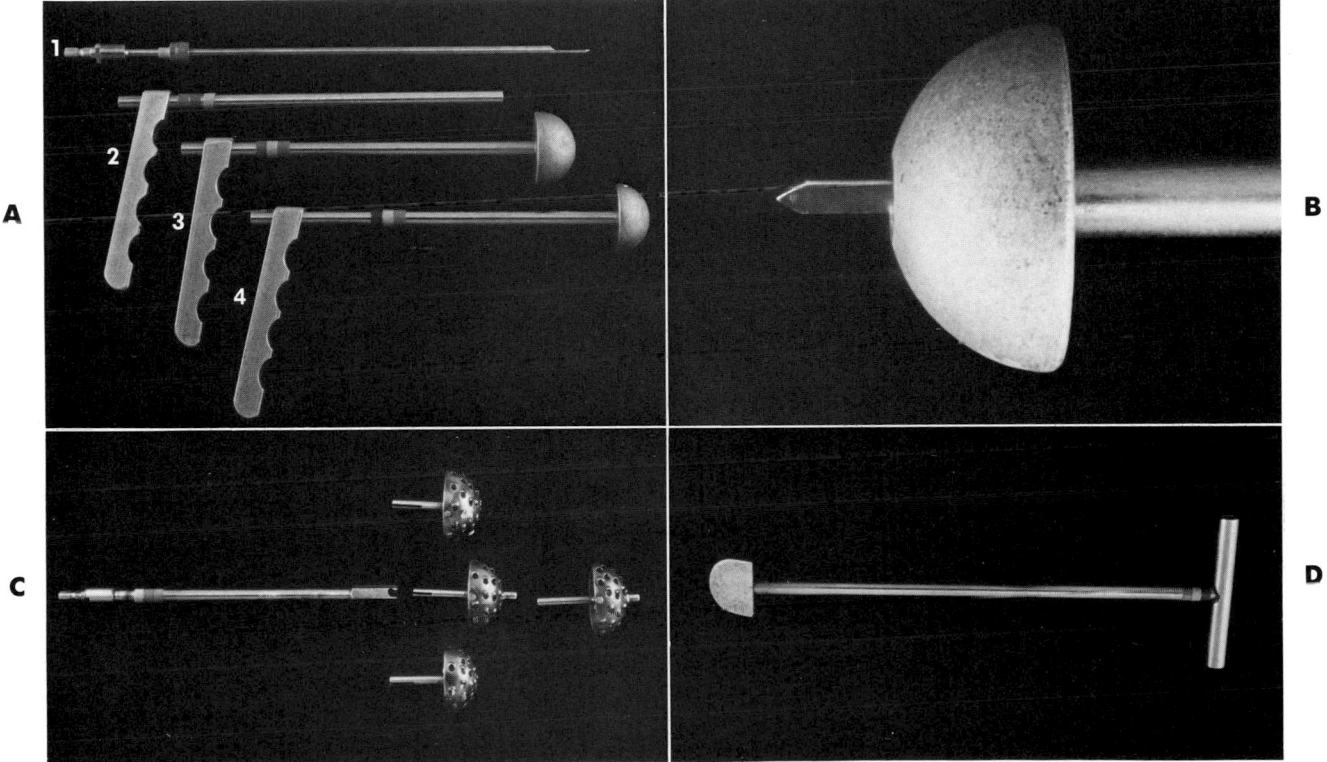

Fig. 19-17. The following instruments are designed to prepare the acetabulum in-situ and in a lowered position: **A,** **(1)** Centralizing drill (6 mm outer diameter), **(2)** Drill guide, **(3)** Acetabular gauge–drill guide, large, **(4)** Acetabular gauge–drill guide, small. **B,** Acetabular gauge–drill guide and drill, assembled. **C,** Two sizes of acetabular reamers, with and without spigots. The universal drive shaft fits all reamers. **D,** Acetabular scraper with detachable blade (designed by the author). (**A, B,** and **C** from Eftekhar NS: Total hip replacement: low-friction arthroplasty. In Evarts CM, editor: *Surgery of the musculoskeletal system,* New York, 1983, Churchill Livingstone.)

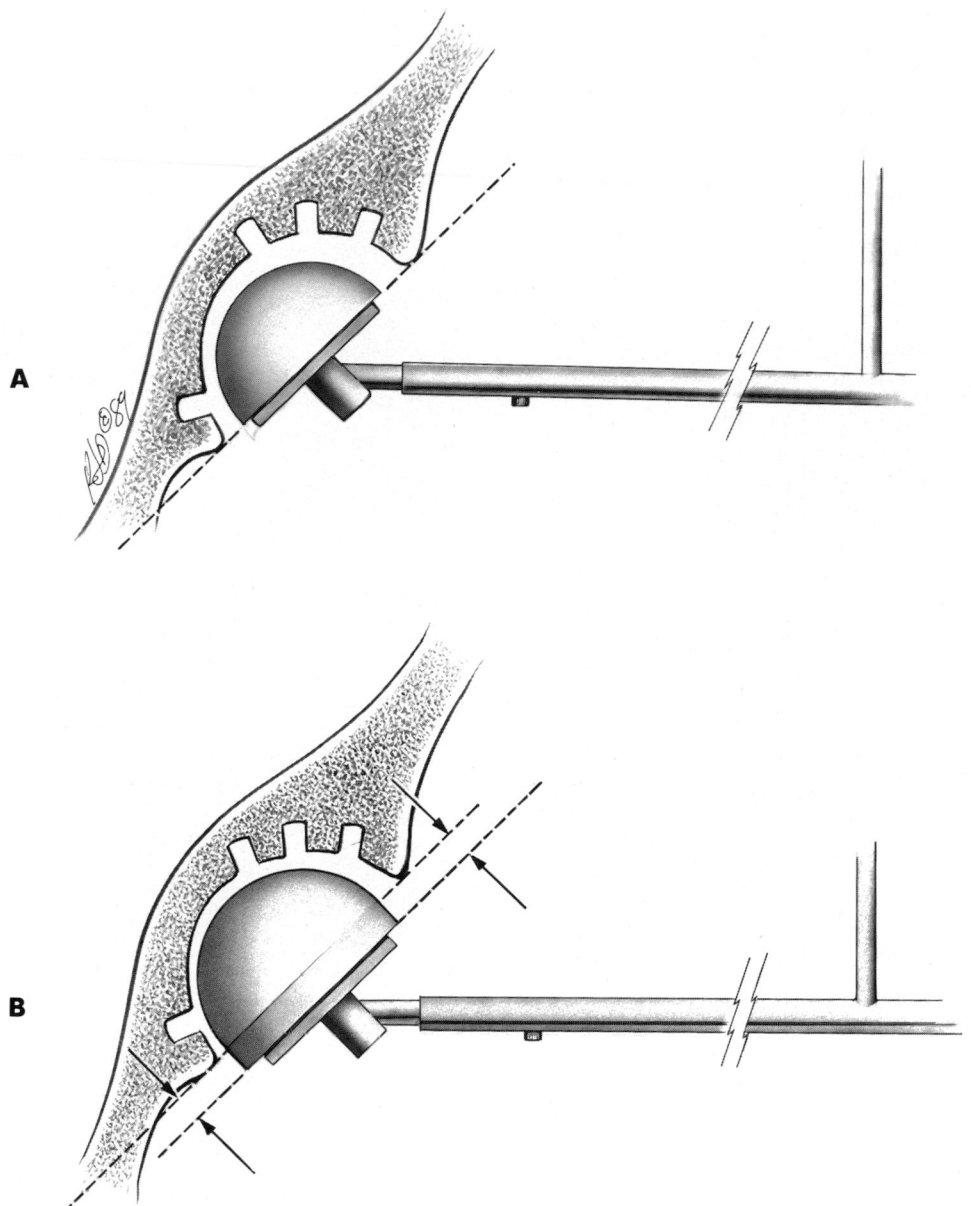

Fig. 19-18. Acetabular gauging for size and bony coverage (containment) using author's cup-holder design with gauging cup. **A,** Small cup (40 mm outer diameter) attached to the holder. **B,** Large cup (44 mm outer diameter). NOTE: Inadequate bony coverage *(distance between dotted lines)* caused by the greater outer diameter cup; the prepared acetabular cavity is identical in **A** and **B.** For this size acetabulum the smaller cup is preferred because the cup is well covered by bone.

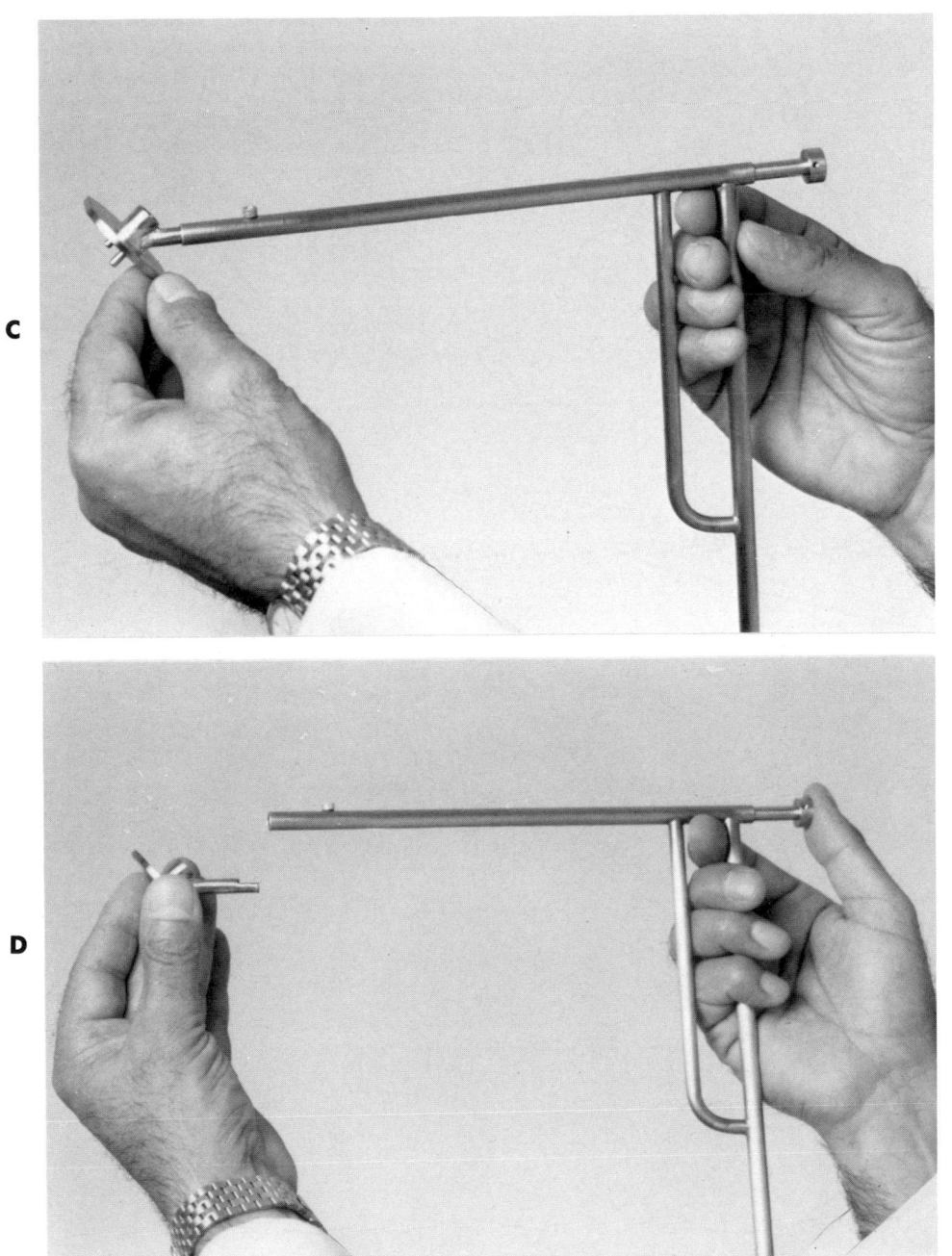

Fig. 19-18—cont'd. C, The cup holder with a detachable plate designed by the author. **D,** Note that the thumb release button detaches the plate from the aligning handle of the instrument.

Continued.

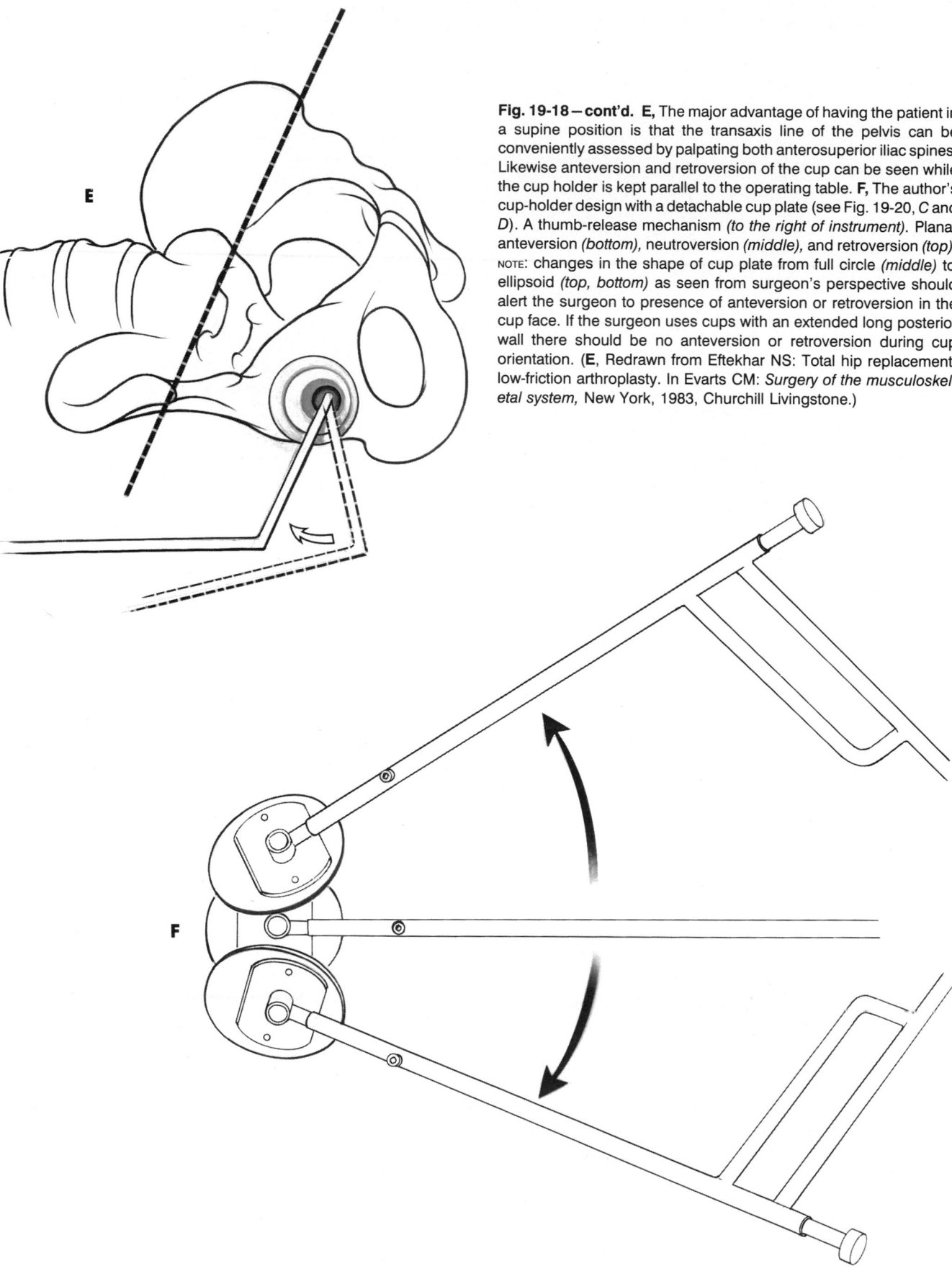

Fig. 19-18—cont'd. E, The major advantage of having the patient in a supine position is that the transaxis line of the pelvis can be conveniently assessed by palpating both anterosuperior iliac spines. Likewise anteversion and retroversion of the cup can be seen while the cup holder is kept parallel to the operating table. **F,** The author's cup-holder design with a detachable cup plate (see Fig. 19-20, C and D). A thumb-release mechanism *(to the right of instrument)*. Planar anteversion *(bottom)*, neutroversion *(middle)*, and retroversion *(top)*. NOTE: changes in the shape of cup plate from full circle *(middle)* to ellipsoid *(top, bottom)* as seen from surgeon's perspective should alert the surgeon to presence of anteversion or retroversion in the cup face. If the surgeon uses cups with an extended long posterior wall there should be no anteversion or retroversion during cup orientation. (**E,** Redrawn from Eftekhar NS: Total hip replacement: low-friction arthroplasty. In Evarts CM: *Surgery of the musculoskeletal system,* New York, 1983, Churchill Livingstone.)

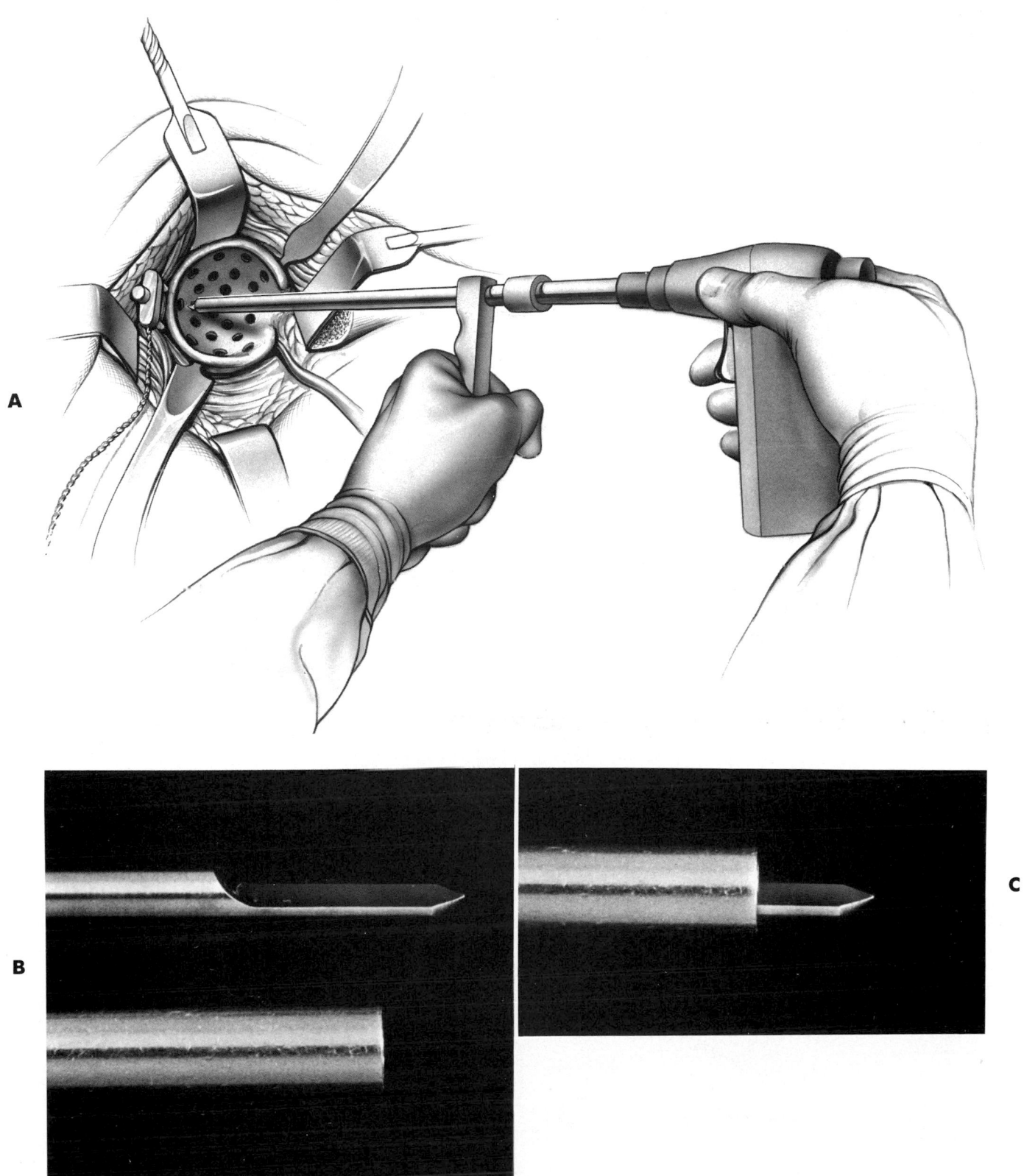

Fig. 19-19. A, Multiple holes are drilled throughout the weight-bearing portion of the acetabulum. These holes are 6 mm in diameter and must penetrate through the subchondral bone and be evenly distributed throughout the acetabulum. **B,** The cutting end of a 6-mm long drill. **C,** Author's drill and guide assembled. NOTE: the guide (sleeve) prevents more than 1-cm penetration of the drill. (From Eftekhar NS: Total hip replacement: low-friction arthroplasty. In Evarts CM, editor: *Surgery of the musculoskeletal system,* New York, 1983, Churchill Livingstone.)

Fixation of the Cup with Cement (Author's Method)

This author uses a "pressurization assembly" (attached to the octomerous retractor) to insert the cement and the cup for improved fixation and control of bleeding pressure in the acetabulum while the cement is being polymerized (Fig. 19-20). It is well recognized that (1) bleeding pressure is deleterious to cement fixation;[1] (2) a steady and continuous pressure is needed to resist bleeding pressure from bone; (3) a sustained manual pressure with a pusher cannot be reliably achieved; and (4) the patient's movements or the surgeon's inadvertent "jolts" may jeopardize cement fixation toward the end stage of cement polymerization.

The pressurization assembly is a multijointed mechanical device with variable axes that may be attached to the octomerous retractor for (1) pressurization of cement via its flanged cup, and (2) maintenance of pressure onto the cemented socket while cement is polymerized. Rehearse cup positioning and the use of a pressurization rod pusher as follows:

- Attach the pressurization assembly to the octomerous retractor loop with two holes and thumb screws to stabilize the vertical rods (Fig. 19-20, *A* to *C*). Position it between 2 o'clock and 5 o'clock for the right and between 8 o'clock and 10 o'clock for the left hip (Fig. 19-21).
- Stabilize the horizontal bar (via two thumb screws), and center the spring-loaded pressurization rod.
- Position the spring-loaded pressurization rod against the depression (cavity) on the cup holder plate attached to the trimmed cup (Fig. 19-21, *C* and *D*).
- Depress the pressurization rod button to compress the spring, thus exerting pressure on the cup. Tighten the pressurization rod thumb screws to maintain the pressurization rod in the compressed position.

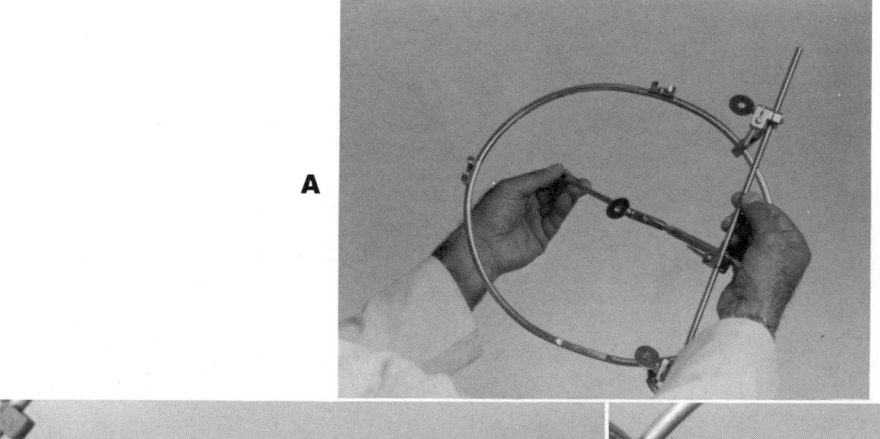

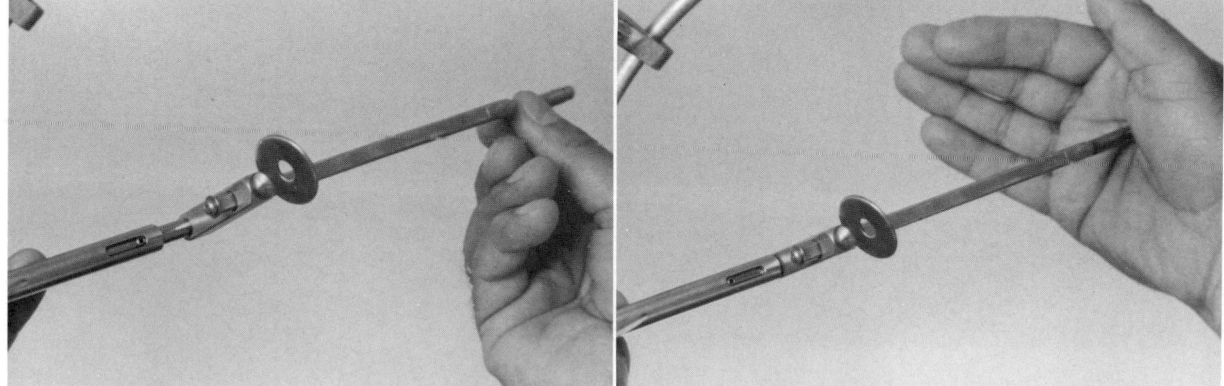

Fig. 19-20. A, The pressurization assembly is shown attached to the octomerous retractor ring via its attachment clips. **B,** The spring-loaded "pusher" of the assembly in extended position. **C,** The spring-loaded pusher in closed position exerting pressure to the palm for demonstration.

Technique for Cementing

Before inserting the cement, the socket must be tested and the assembly adjusted to maintain the cup in a stable position when the surgeon's hands are off the cup holder. There should be no impediment to delivering the cement or cup attached to the cup holder plate. Anchor holes must be clean and the entire acetabular bed free of soft tissue. Repeat irrigation and brushing as needed. Use a hydrogen peroxide-soaked sponge to pack the acetabular cavity before inserting the cement.

To insert cement, do the following:

1. Form it into a short sausage shape, and insert it into the acetabulum.
2. Insert the cup attached to the cup holder with its detachable cup holding plate. Press the pressurization rod against the cup holder plate, and tighten the thumb screws (after maximum pressure has been exerted to the spring) to maintain the pressure. The spring exerts approximately 25 lb/in^2 pressure to the face of the cup.
3. Detach the cup-holder "aligning rod" from the face of the cup holder plate by depressing its release button.
4. Remove excess cement before polymerization. Check for any remaining cement after removing the assembly from the octomerous retractor ring.

Some practical details are as follows:

1. Deliver the cement, pressurization disc, and socket (attached to the removable plate and holder) speedily to discourage bleeding behind the cement after removing the hydrogen peroxide pack from the acetabulum.
2. Make sure that the cup inserted into the acetabulum (with cement) has the identical orientation that it did at rehearsal without cement.
3. Remove the cement from the periphery of the acetabulum with a curette (after final positioning of the socket) as soon as possible. However, a straight, narrow osteotome can remove polymerized cement at a later stage (see Chapter 15).
4. Avoid inadvertent excessive proximal positioning of the socket holder resulting in an open angle (less than 40 degrees). Do not correct this error by changing the cup position into a horizontal position because this creates a space between the weight-bearing portion of the acetabulum and the cement. It is best to remove the cement and the cup at once and reintroduce a new batch of cement in the cup (after cleaning the acetabular cavity and the cup). Allow no more than 5 degrees of anteversion if the cup has a long posterior wall. Allow 15 to 20 degrees of anterversion using a cup without an extended posterior wall.
5. Avoid unchecked flow of cement into the soft tissues anteriorly or into the obturator foramen. It may cause nerve palsy.
6. Do not allow the cement to harden around the holder because it may prevent its disengagement from the cup.
7. Irrigate and remove all bone and cement particles from the wound.
8. Excise remaining osteophytes as needed to prevent impingement and dislocation (see Chapter 15).
9. Remove the acetabular retractors, including the acetabular staples.
10. Place a clean sponge into the acetabular area to prevent debris from entering the wound during the femoral preparation.

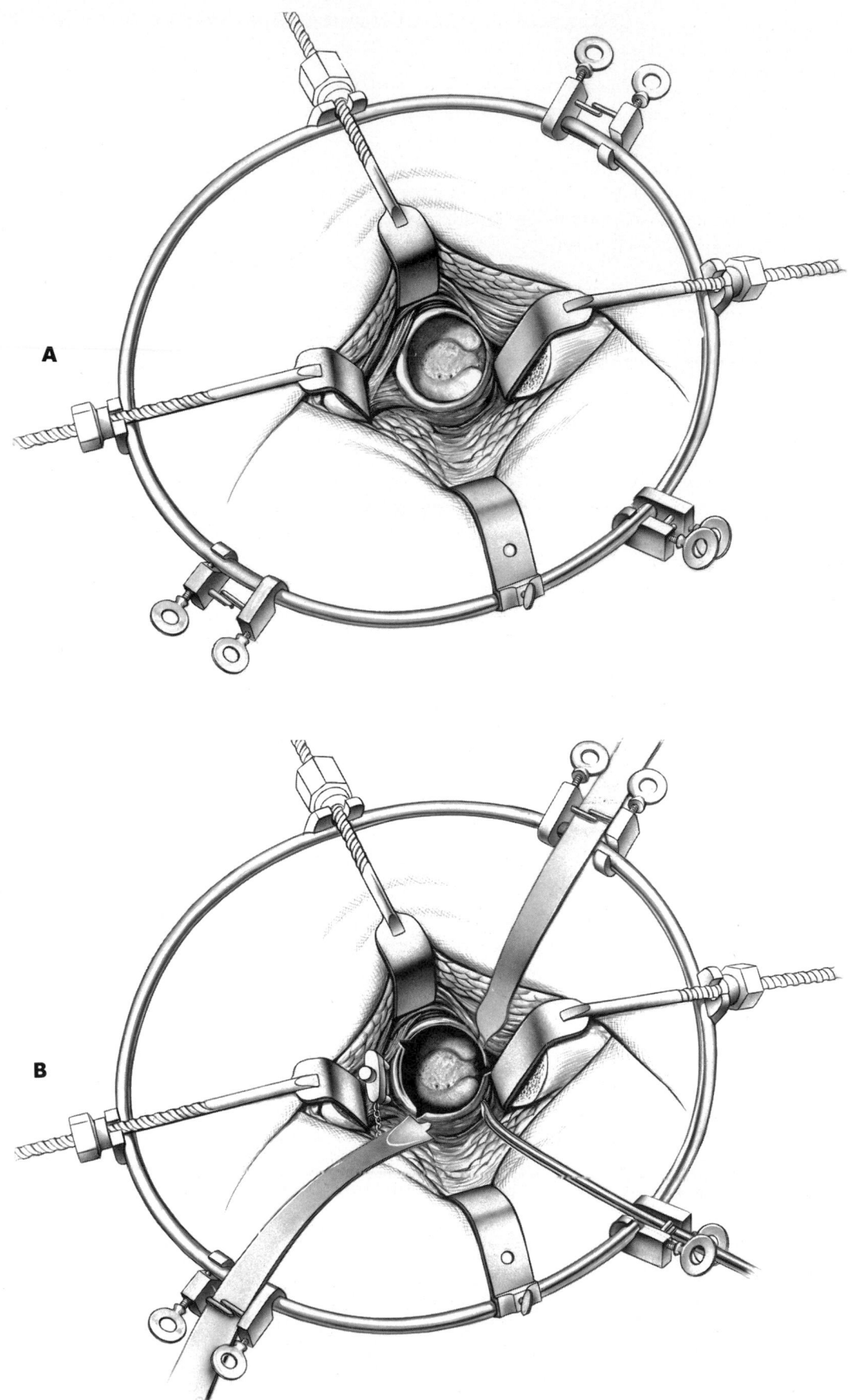

Fig. 19-21. See legend on opposite page.

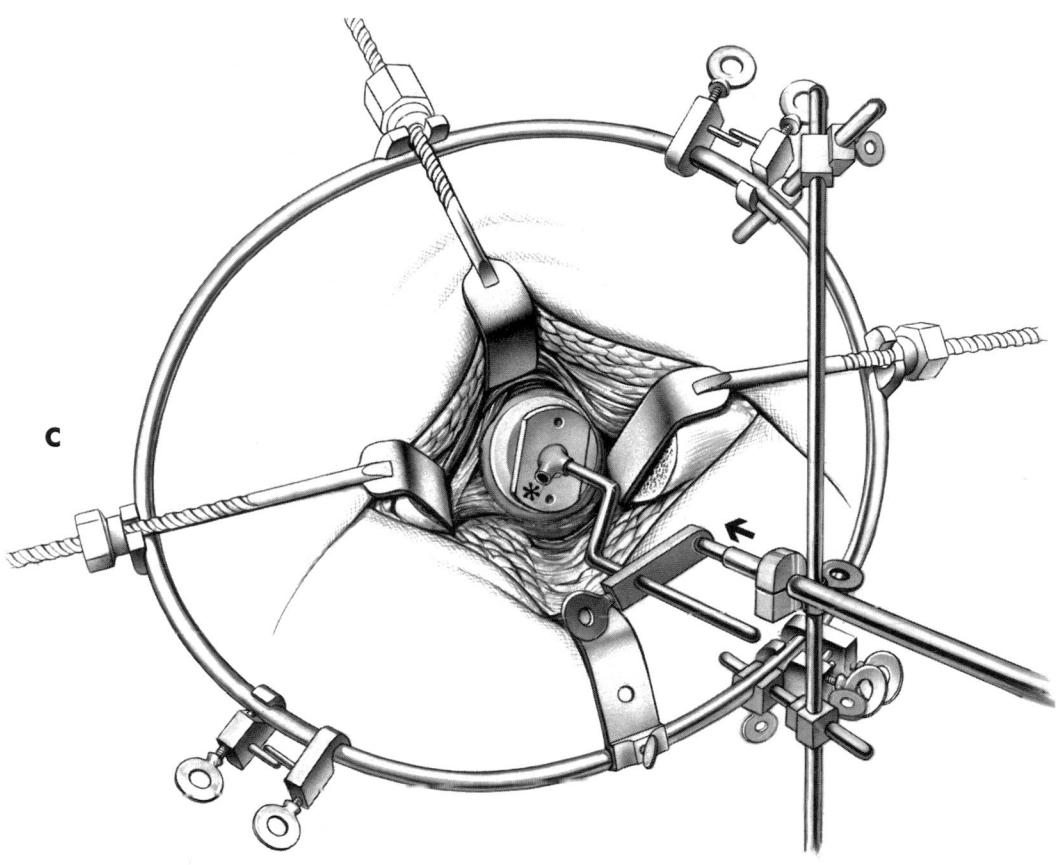

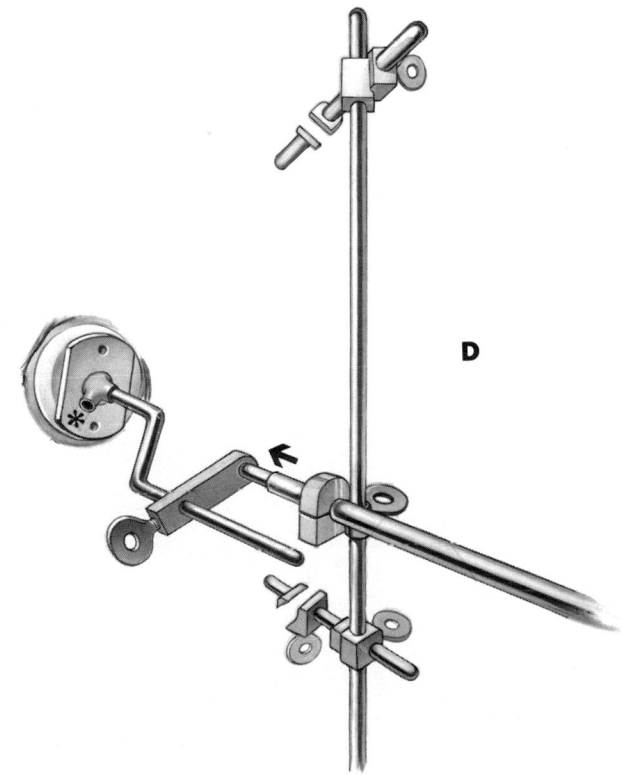

Fig. 19-21. A, The octomerous retractor; the anterior *(top)* and posterior *(bottom)* fascial blades retracting the fascia; the acetabulum is viewed at the center of the wound; the wound is opened in a "diamond" shape. NOTE: the trochanteric *(left)* and femoral retractors are applied to the trochanteric and femoral neck, respectively. **B,** The four acetabular retractors; the anterior iliopubic, posterior ilioischial, and inferior ischiopubic retractors are shown as they are individually held against the ring while retracting away the periacetabular capsule and other tissues. **C,** Pressurization assembly is fixed to the ring as it carries the pusher with its spring-loaded mechanism. Depression on the cup-holder plate is for attachment of the aligning rod of the cup holder (asterisk) and is the site of the cup holder being removed. NOTE: The surgeon's hand is off the cup holder and the cup as the spring-loaded pusher mechanically exerts pressure onto the face of the cup. **D,** The pressurization assembly (without the octomerous retractor). Note the spring-loaded pusher *(next to arrow)* and adjustable offset of the pusher with adjustable length to bypass the stump of the femur thus pressuring the cement in a direct line at 45 degrees angle to the transaxis of the pelvis.

PHASE V: FEMORAL PREPARATION, SELECTION OF FEMORAL COMPONENT, AND TEST REDUCTION FOR STABILITY AND LENGTH
Mobilizing the Upper Femur

Complete mobilization of the upper femur by releasing the short rotators and contracted capsule as described in Chapter 18 so that the leg can be placed across the table without effort. Trochanteric osteotomy facilitates the preparation and cementing of the femoral component. It provides unimpeded access to the end of the femur while preparing and inserting the cement and prosthesis (Fig. 19-22). It allows mobilization of the upper femur in hips with flexion and adduction deformity with marked stiffness. This is particularly important in large-boned men with hyperproductive osteoarthritis who also exhibit shortening of the limb. In mobilizing and "freeing up" the upper femur, a complete capsular release and iliopsoas tenotomy can be accompanied safely. This allows the leg to assume a cross-legged position with the transcondylar line of the knee exhibited as a point of reference for proper orientation of the femoral component. It also lessens the hazards of intraoperative fractures of the femur in severely deformed hips and osteoporotic femora. Finally it allows good access to the top of the femur for pressurization and insertion of a large-caliber stem in the appropriate direction and without impediment. For removal of cement in revision surgery, see Chapter 25.

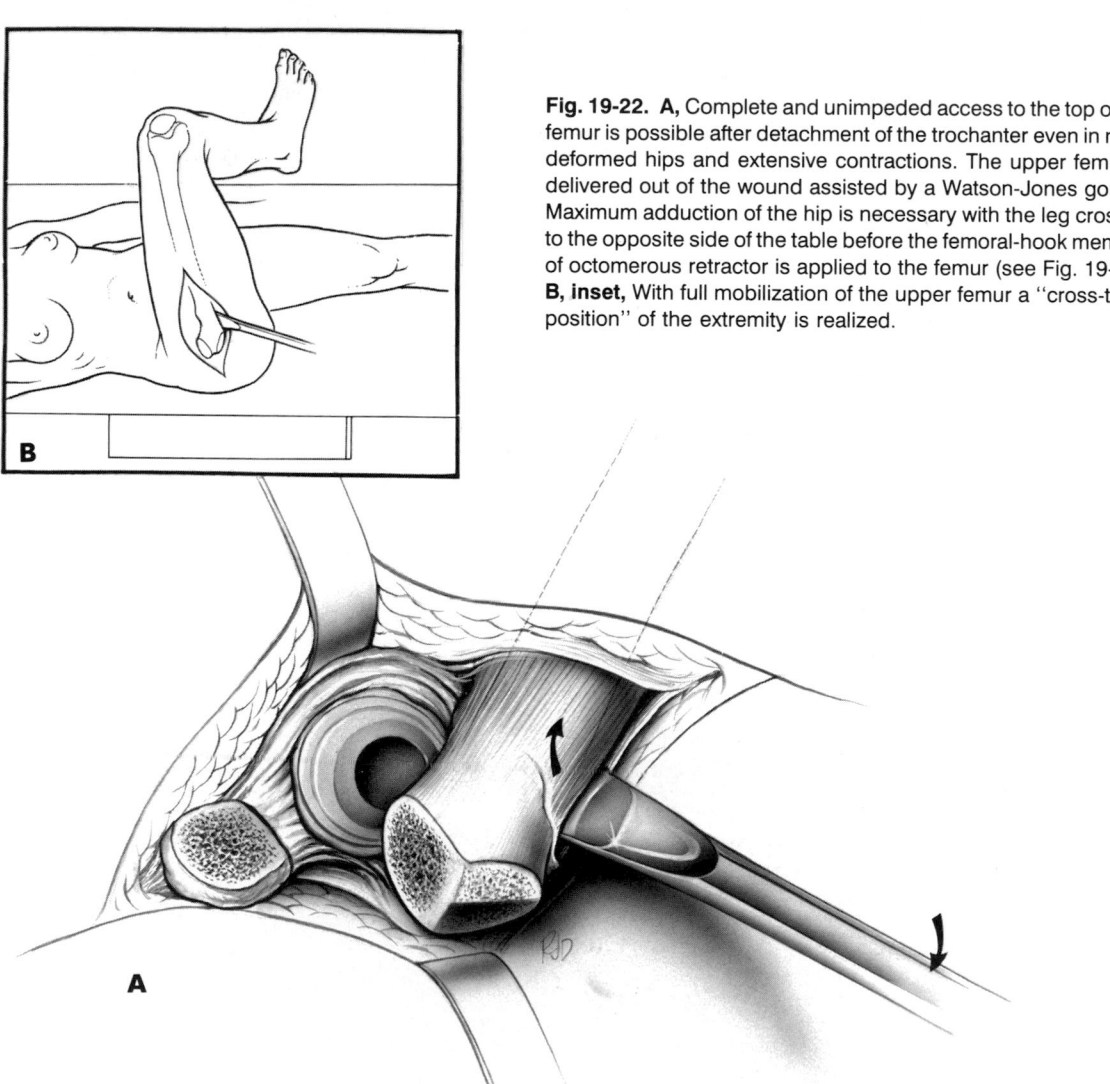

Fig. 19-22. A, Complete and unimpeded access to the top of the femur is possible after detachment of the trochanter even in most deformed hips and extensive contractions. The upper femur is delivered out of the wound assisted by a Watson-Jones gouge. Maximum adduction of the hip is necessary with the leg crossed to the opposite side of the table before the femoral-hook member of octomerous retractor is applied to the femur (see Fig. 19-23). **B, inset,** With full mobilization of the upper femur a "cross-table position" of the extremity is realized.

Preparing the Canal

The canal is prepared differently for cemented and uncemented prostheses (see Chapter 15). For cemented stems observe the following:

- Remove the femoral member of the octomerous retractor (the claw), and replace it with the femoral-hook retractor (Fig. 19-23).
- Insert the tapered T-handled canal finder at the junction of the site of the osteotomized trochanter and the neck (the site of removed bony ridge) (Figs. 19-24 and 19-25, A).
- Enlarge the medullary cavity by using tapered rotary reamers (blunt tip, available in two sizes) (see Chapter 16). (Fig. 19-25, D).
- Be sure the prepared canal is large enough to accept the largest-caliber stem without undue damage (Fig. 19-25, B). The stem should be positioned in a neutral orientation (no varus or valgus and no more than 5 to 10 degrees of anteversion). One should always allow for at least 3 to 4 mm of cement thickness in addition to centering the stem within the shaft without any exaggerated valgus or any varus alignment.
- Use a long-handled curette (Volkmann's spoon) to remove loose cancellous bone and marrow from medial neck and calcar region and the level of distal and lateral corresponding to the stem tip level.
- Use supplemental curved broaches if preferred to ream bone along the lateral and proximal femur to ensure the centralization of the proximal stem within the canal.

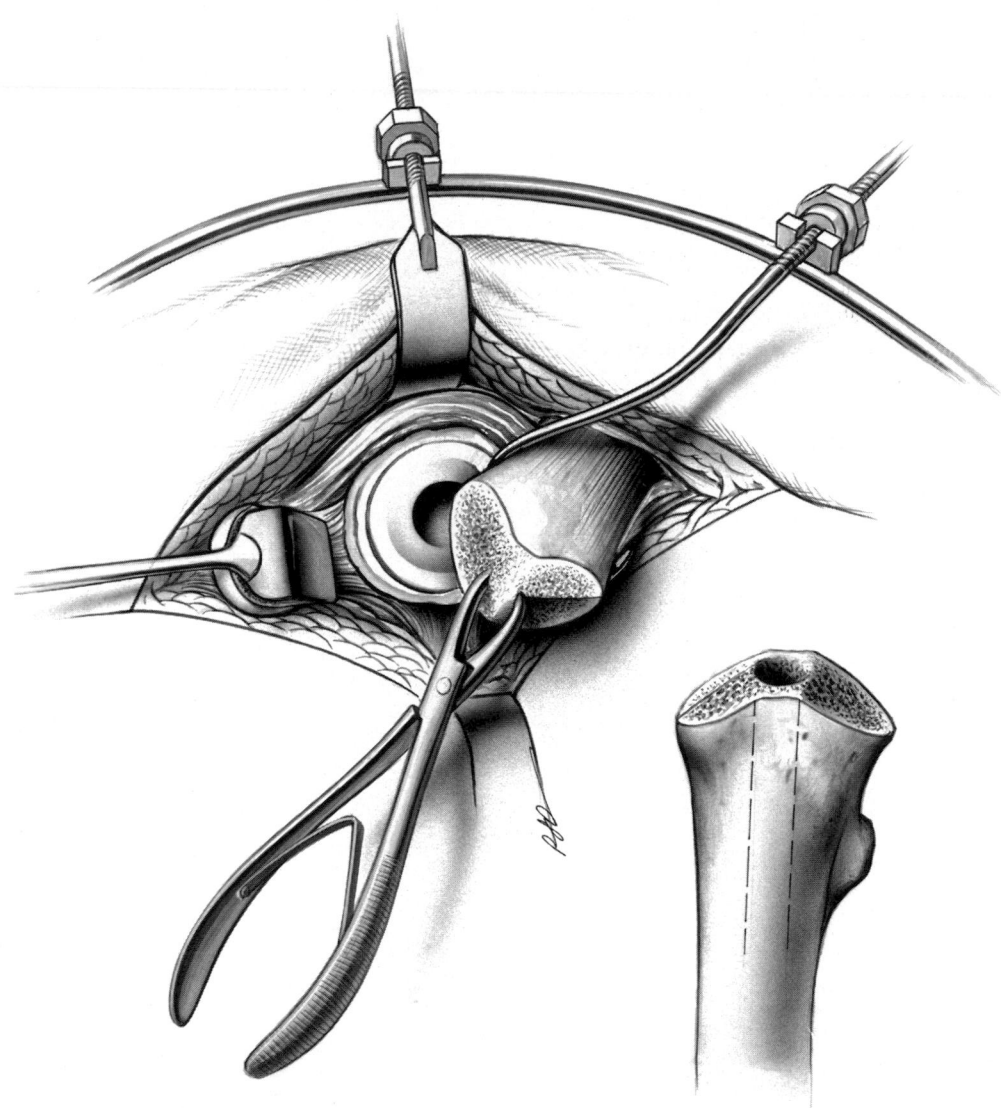

Fig. 19-23. To facilitate entry to the femur while remaining centered in the shaft, a rongeur is used to remove the cortical bridge between the trochanteric bed and the sectioned neck. Note that the femoral-hook member of the octomerous retractor helps deliver the femoral stump out of the wound. **Inset,** The cavity can be prepared in a straight line when the starting point is correct.

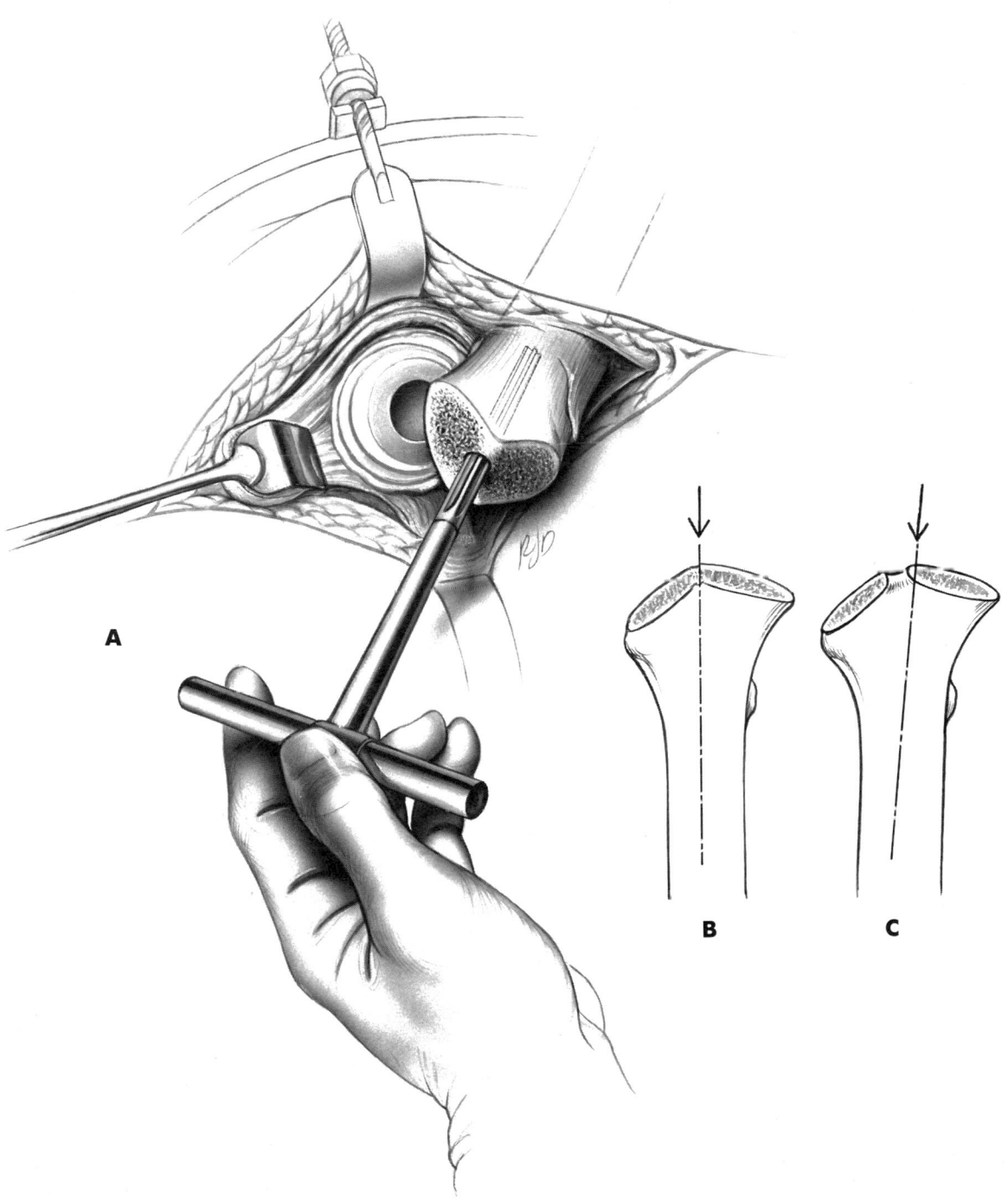

Fig. 19-24. A, The medullary canal is opened with tapered pin T-handled reamer. Initially the tapered reamer is inserted at the junction of the cut surfaces of the trochanter and the neck. The direction is in slight valgus, but generally the center of the femoral shaft must be observed. To remain centered within the medullary canal, the bed of the trochanter is encroached. The tapered pin reamer enters somewhat posterior to the cut surface of the neck and is aimed toward the patella. **B,** The correct, and **C,** incorrect directions of tapered reamer.

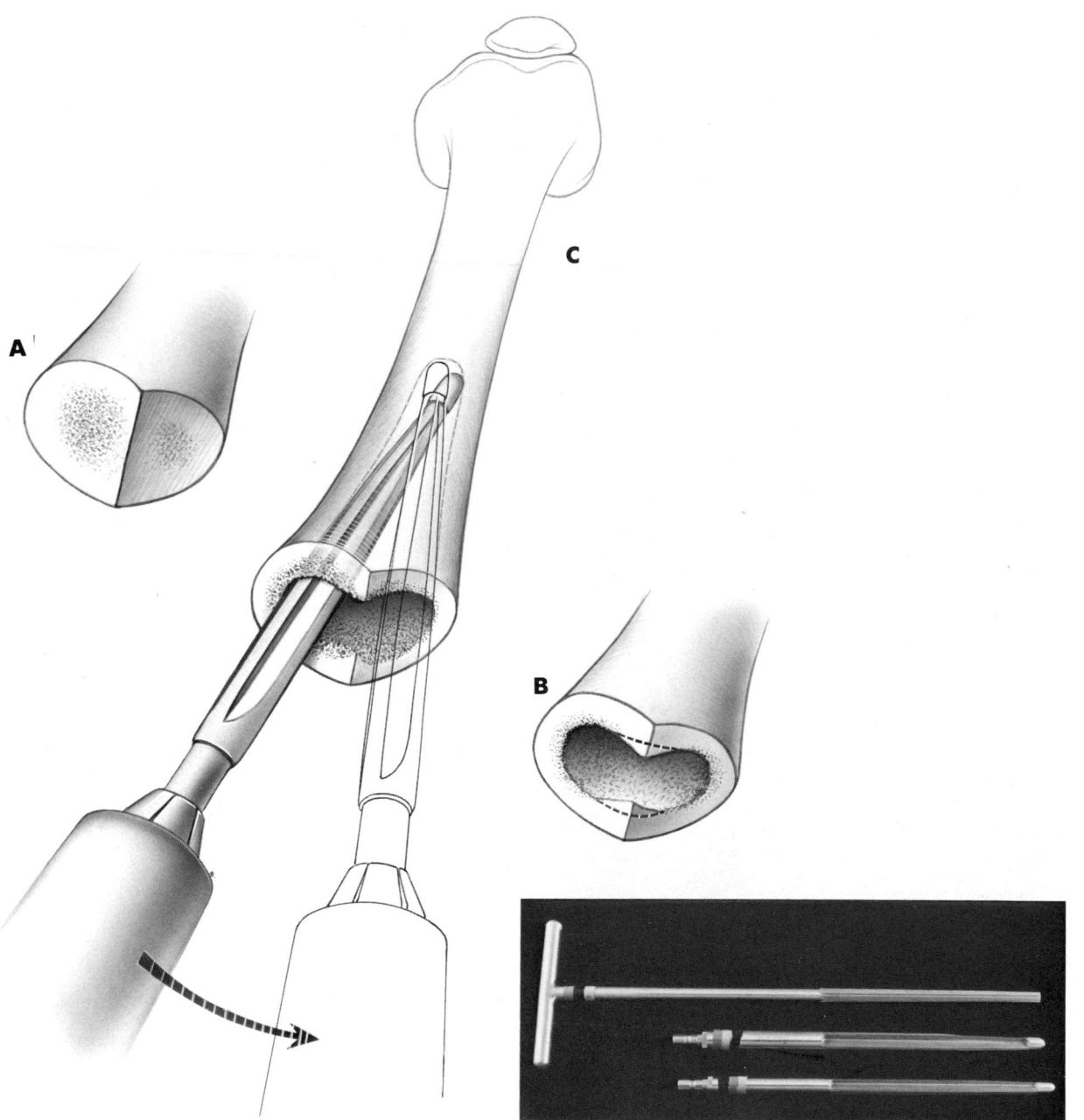

Fig. 19-25. Medullary canal is best opened by a Charnley T-handled tapered reamer (canal finder) at the junction of the femoral neck and trochanteric bed. **A,** The tapered reamer can be centered within the canal aiming at the patella. The use of a tapered rotary reamer (blunt tip) prevents accidental perforation of the femoral shaft. The tapered reamer is operated in low speed and shifted from medial to lateral. **B,** The upper femur is enlarged to allow insertion of the provisional prosthesis, which must be loose within the medullary canal to allow space for the cement. **C,** Mediolateral shift of the drill handle removed bone in respective areas of the upper femur. Note that the reamer must be withdrawn for about half its length before it can effectively remove bone from the top of the femur (encroachment onto the trochanter bed has been exaggerated for demonstration). **D,** Three key instruments in preparing the medullary canal include Charnley T-handled reamer (canal finder) top. Small and large tapered reamers are used with air-driven power tools. These reamers (designed by the author) incorporate a blunt tip for safety to avoid perforating the shaft of the femur when used eccentrically in the medullary canal. (From Eftekhar NS: Total hip replacement: low-friction arthroplasty. In Evarts CM, editor: *Surgery of the musculoskeletal system,* New York, 1983, Churchill Livingstone.)

Centralization of Stem

As stated previously and discussed in Chapter 6, the cemented stem should ideally be inserted centrally into the medullary canal.

Proximal Centralization

The author's technique for centering the stem in the medullary canal proximally and distally is as follows:

- Select a test femoral prostheses of appropriate size (depending on the size of medullary cavity), and adjust its attached thumb screw to locate the proximal stem centrally in the canal (Fig. 19-26, *A*).
- Insert a locating pin (attached to a short chain) to stabilize the stem while it is being reduced into the acetabular cup for a test rehearsal (Fig. 19-26, *B* to *D*).
- Remove the test trial stem, leaving the locating pin behind.

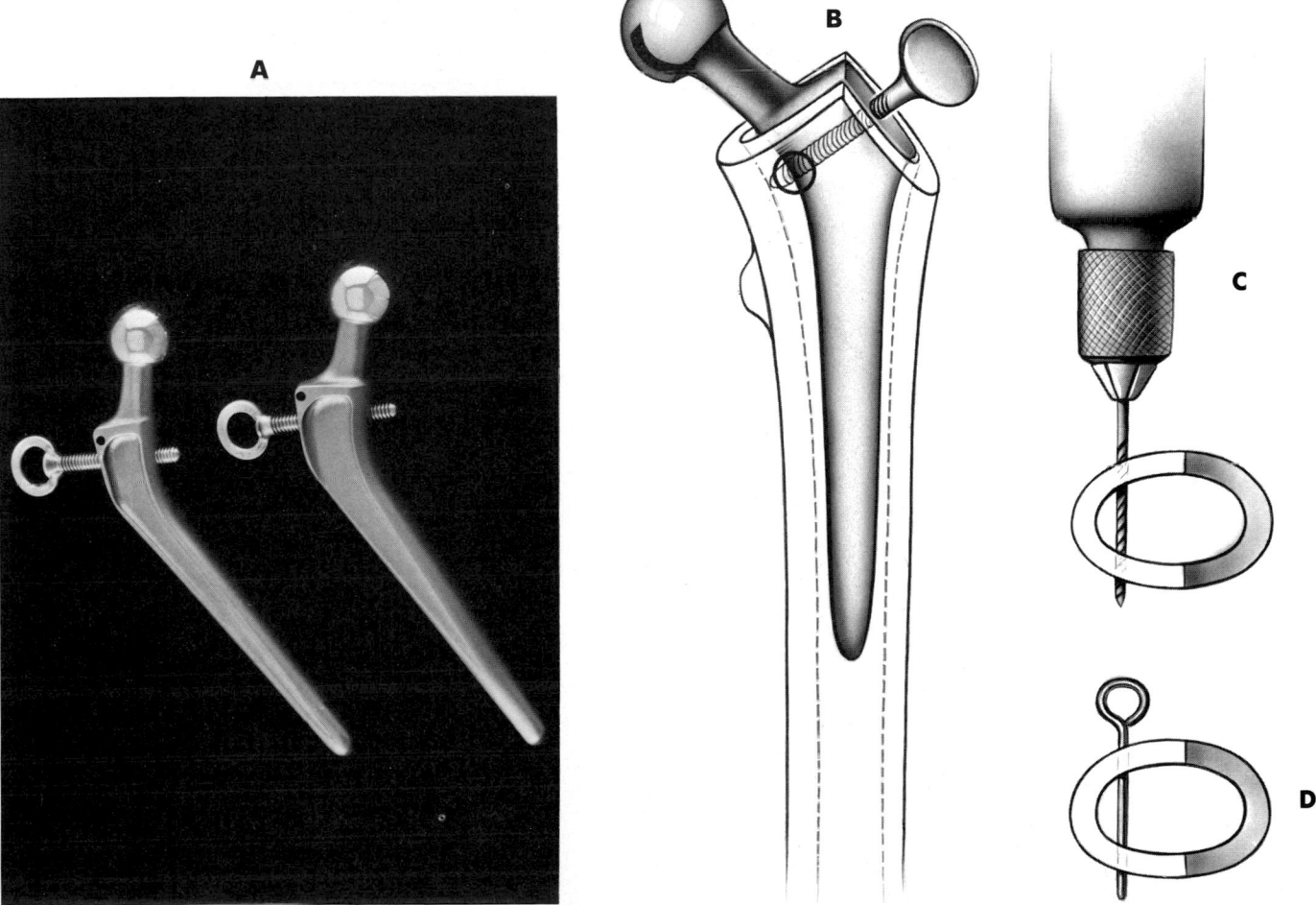

Fig. 19-26. A, Two test trial prostheses (provisionals) for medium and large stems of the biomechanical prostheses. Proximal centralization is accomplished by turning the thumb screw of the provisional prosthesis clockwise until centralization is achieved. **B,** Proximal centralization is accomplished by a provisional prosthesis carrying a thumb screw. The thumb screw is turned clockwise after insertion of the stem to centralize the upper end of the prosthesis within the upper end of the femur. Once a satisfactory position is achieved, the hip joint is reduced to determine the length of the neck and the stability of the joint. **C, D,** A locating pin is inserted at the most proximal level of the cut surface of the neck, from the anterior to posterior surface of the femoral neck as close as possible to the medial surface of the proximal stem. This is accomplished by drilling a 2.5-mm outer-diameter drill bit. **D,** A 2-mm locating pin through the drill hole is used to keep the prosthesis from drifting into a medial direction. (From Eftekhar NS: Total hip replacement: low-friction arthroplasty. In Evarts CM, editor: *Surgery of the musculoskeletal system,* New York, 1983, Churchill Livingstone.)

Distal Centralization

Centralize the stem in the medullary canal distally using a centralization plug, delivered via an appropriately sized delivering tube (four sizes are available) (Fig. 19-27, *A*) as follows:

- Insert the desirable plug into the appropriate sized delivery tube, and insert the tube to the marking on the instrument (Fig. 19-27, *B* to *E*).
- Eject the plug by the plunger to deliver it to the appropriate level.
- Reinsert the test prosthesis, which will automatically be centered in the canal proximally by the locating pin and distally by the centralization plug (Fig. 19-28).

Reduction and Rehearsal for Stability and Length

Place the hip joint through a full range of motion, and ensure stability and proper leg length (see Chapter 15).

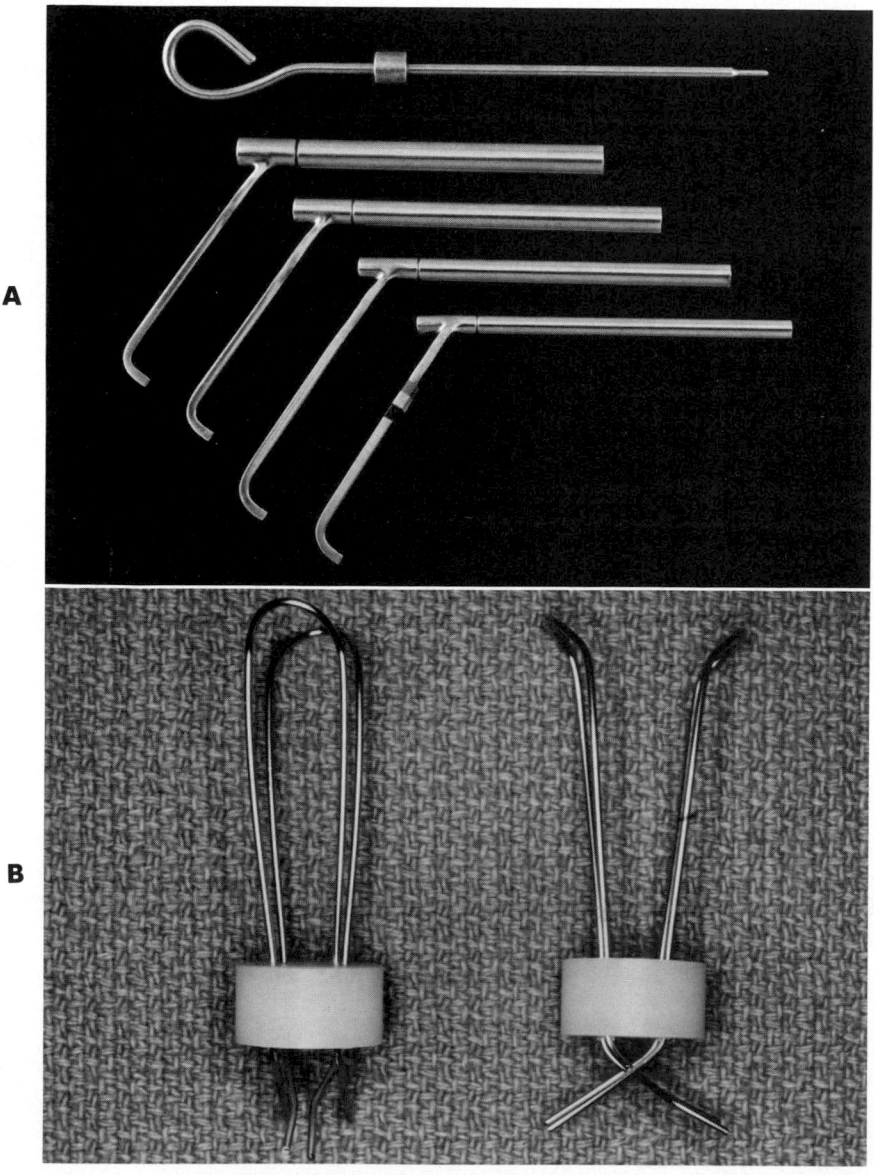

Fig. 19-27. A, Four sizes of delivery tubes for the intramedullary centralization plug. The plunger is shown at the top. **B,** Centralization plug, designed by the author, has three portions: the "arms," "body," and "legs." The arms allow entry of the tip of the stem, the body plugs the medullary canal, and the legs prevent the plug from distal migration.

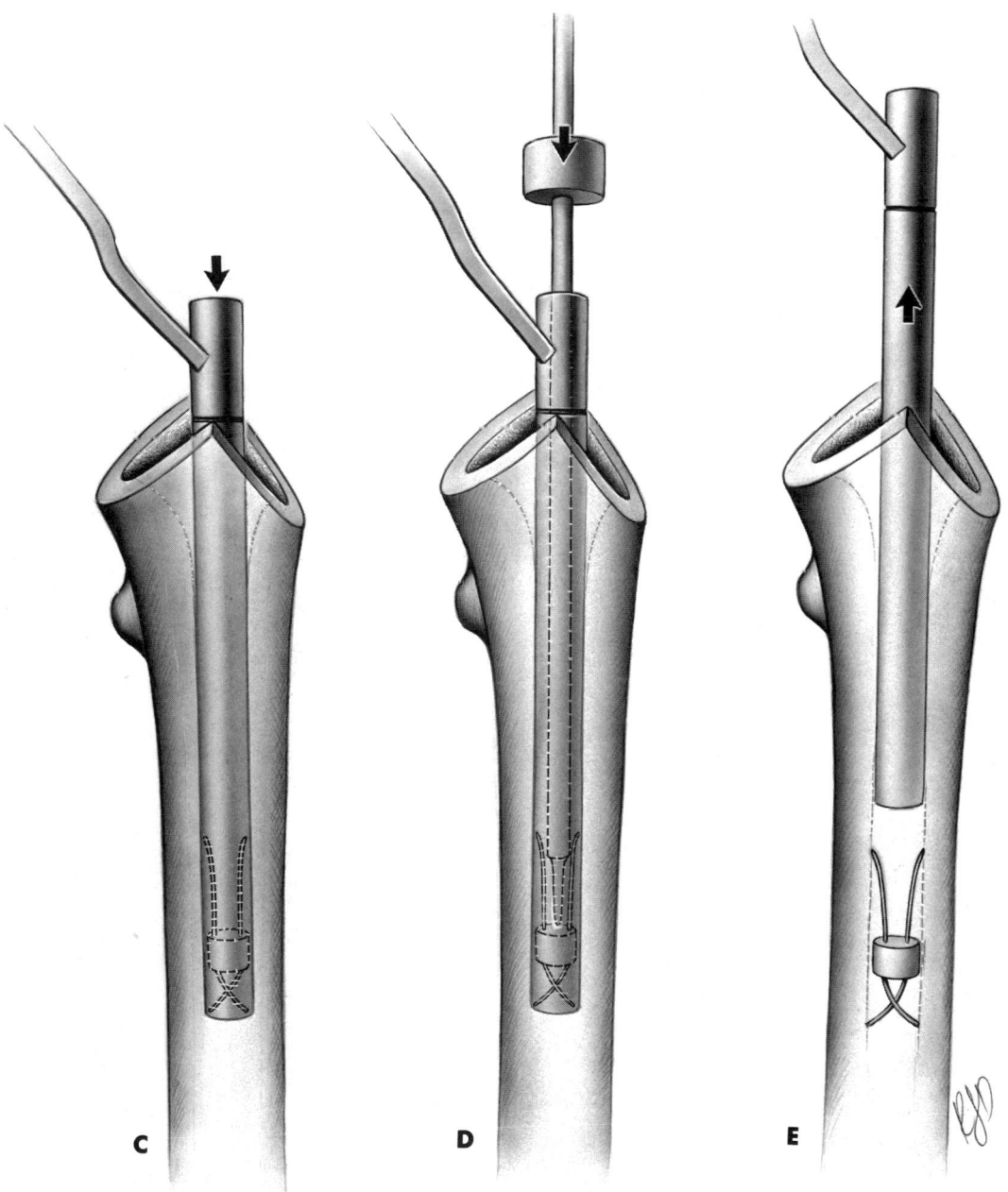

C   D   E

Fig. 19-27—cont'd. C through **E,** The delivery tube is inserted into the femoral canal to the appropriate level. Then the plunger is inserted via the proximal opening of the tube to deliver the plug into the canal. The tube is removed, leaving the centralizing plug behind. NOTE: the size of tube selected determines the appropriate size plug. (From Eftekhar NS: Total hip replacement: low-friction arthroplasty. In Evarts CM, editor: *Surgery of the musculoskeletal system,* New York, 1983, Churchill Livingstone.)

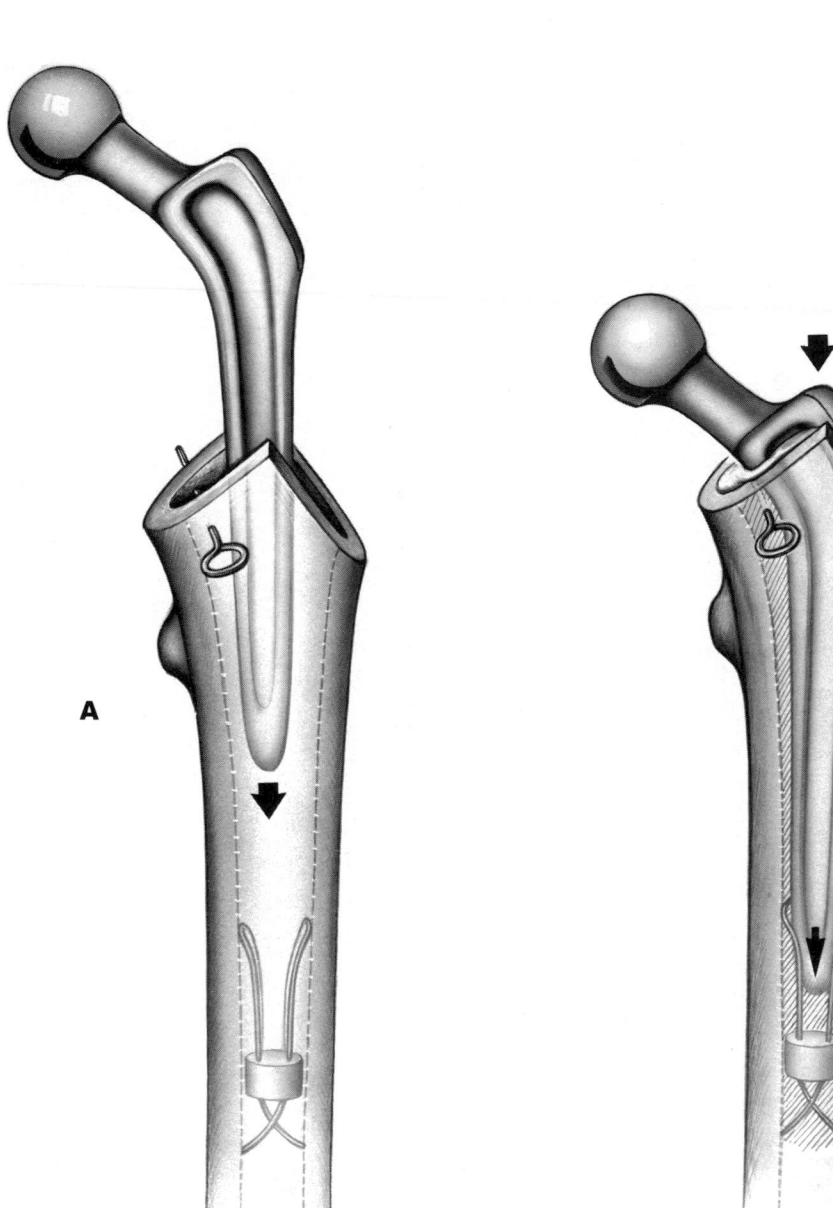

Fig. 19-28. A, The actual prosthesis is now inserted with the locating pin and the centralizing plug in place. The hip is then reduced. This ensures that the position of the prosthesis is ideal and that by distal centralization the orientation of the stem remains acceptable. **B,** With the locating pin in place and the centralizing plug already delivered, the cement and stem are inserted without concern to the varus or valgus position, but the stem is pushed against the locating pin. Obviously, the prosthesis cannot be put into a varus position because of the presence of the locating pin. The locating pin is removed only after full polymerization of the cement. The chain attached to the locating pin is a reminder that the pin must be removed before reducing the hip. The locating pin is removed by an alternate counterclockwise and clockwise repetitive motion and is pulled by the handle. (From Eftekhar NS: Total hip replacement: low-friction arthroplasty. In Evarts CM, editor: *Surgery of the musculoskeletal system,* New York, 1983, Churchill Livingstone.)

PHASE VI: INSERTING WIRES, PACKING AND INSERTING CEMENT, AND INSERTING THE STEM

Before inserting the cement, observe the following:

- Position the femur across the table using the femoral-hook member of the octomerous retractor.
- Irrigate the femur, and use a rotary brush to remove debris, fatty marrow, and clots.
- Remove sharp spicules that might tear the glove when inserting the cement.
- Rehearse the stem (actual prosthesis) held by the holder. Make sure that full insertion is possible and that the stem remains centered while it fully penetrates the canal.

Inserting Wires to Reattach the Trochanter

The method of inserting wires is identical to that described in Chapter 18. Note that drilling for double vertical wire (the lateral aspect of the femur) must be done 2 to 3 cm distal to the trochanteric ridge if a modest advancement of the trochanter on the shaft of the femur is anticipated. The two transverse drill holes for medial and lateral wires must be through the cortex to avoid injury to the trochanteric bed. The medial wire should be pushed (within the medullary cavity) against the lateral wall of the femoral cortex while the medial and lateral wire holes are drilled anteroposteriorly through the cortex of the femur. Separate and place the vertical wires, one anteriorly and the other posteriorly, in the femur while they emerge from the medullary canal of the femur. Make a small notch in the opening of the neck to locate them. Insert the trial prosthesis, making sure that insertion of the stem is easy and that the wires are not misplaced and do not prevent the stem from being fully inserted.

Packing and Inserting Cement

Insert 3- or 4-mm suction tubing into the canal while hydrogen-peroxide-soaked ribbon gauze is inserted into the medullary canal (see Chapter 15).

Insert cement when it no longer adheres to the surgeon's glove. Use the double-thumb-pressure technique as described in Chapter 15. Avoid mixing cement with blood while it is being inserted. Remove the venting tube when the canal is filled, then add more cement (without tubing).

Inserting the Stem

Firmly attach the prosthesis to the holder, and insert the stem into the cement mass in a straight line with the femur. The holder designed by the author is lightweight and protects the femoral head prosthesis (Fig. 19-29). It should be detached only after the cement is fully polymerized. Allow no more than 5 to 10 degrees of anteversion to accommodate the natural anteversion of the femoral neck. Insert the stem; observe the details described for cement insertion in Chapter 15. Reduce the hip, and test for stability because it must be stable before the trochanter is reattached (see Chapters 15 and 18).

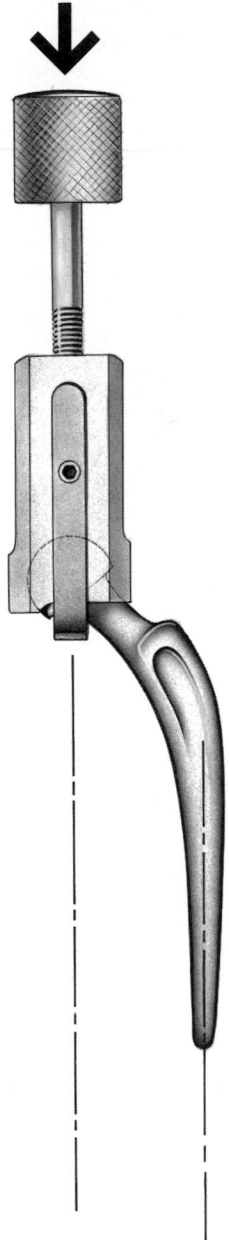

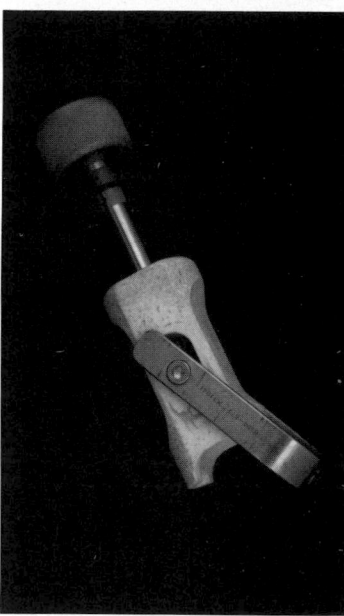

Fig. 19-29. Femoral holder (designed by the author) produces a positive hold on the prosthesis. Its small size and light weight allow the surgeon to control the direction of the stem and maintain the holder on the stem while the cement is being fully polymerized.

PHASE VII: REATTACHING THE TROCHANTER, REPAIRING THE VASTUS LATERALIS, AND FASCIA AND WOUND CLOSURE

Reattaching the trochanter by two independent systems, a vertical and a cruciate system following Charnley's technique, is this author's preferred method (see Chapter 18).

Reattaching a Biplanar Osteotomized Trochanter

Release the capsule or piriformis to advance the trochanter and allow reattachment without tension. Pass the vertical and the posterior ends of the medial wires as described in Chapter 18.

- Place the hip in neutral rotation and without abduction/adduction.
- Position the two planes of the V-shaped trochanter against the bed of the detached trochanter.
- A perfect fit of the trochanter is important to achieve stability. Rotate the trochanter as needed to fit onto its bed. The trochanter may be advanced up to 1 cm along the proximal-distal length of the bed.
- Maintain the reduction using an awl. The vertical wire ends are now passed through the loop of the same wire on the shaft of the femur. Apply a wire tightener, and secure the trochanter. Use a curved-end impactor to impact the trochanter against its bed, and retighten it further to pick up the slack (caused by impaction of bone). Do not overtighten this wire because it may fracture the trochanter. Now bring the posterior and anterior ends of the medial wires to form a pulley on top of the trochanter, and form the cruciate arrangement described in Chapter 18.
- Attach the vastus lateralis to the gluteus medius using 3 to 4 nonabsorbable sutures.

Alternative Method of Trochanteric Reattachment

In certain cases, such as revision surgery or when there are severe anatomical deformities of the trochanter, abductors, or the femur, it may be advantageous to transpose the trochanter to a new site on the femur, that is, over the vastus ridge or distal to it. When the surgeon decides to transfer the trochanter, he or she must osteotomize the trochanter in a single plane (Fig. 19-30) and modify wiring technique because the cruciform wiring technique is unsuitable (see Chapter 18). This author finds that a modified insertion of double vertical and one or two transverse wires is most effective. The technique is as follows:

1. Drill a hole 2½ to 3 cm distal to the trochanteric ridge where the osteotomy of the trochanter was carried out, and bring the two ends of the vertical wire through the shaft of the femur. Bring this wire laterally close to the trochanteric bed.
2. Pass a single horizontal wire circumferentially around the femur proximal to the lesser trochanter. When the neck of the femur is absent or short, drill a hole through the bone of the lesser (front to back) trochanter to engage wire to the bone. To facilitate the passage of the wire, use a Charnley wire passer (Fig. 19-31), which is passed under muscle fibers of the vastus lateralis and inserted as close as possible to the posterior aspect of the femur. Repeat this maneuver to pass the wire in front of the femur (Fig. 19-32).

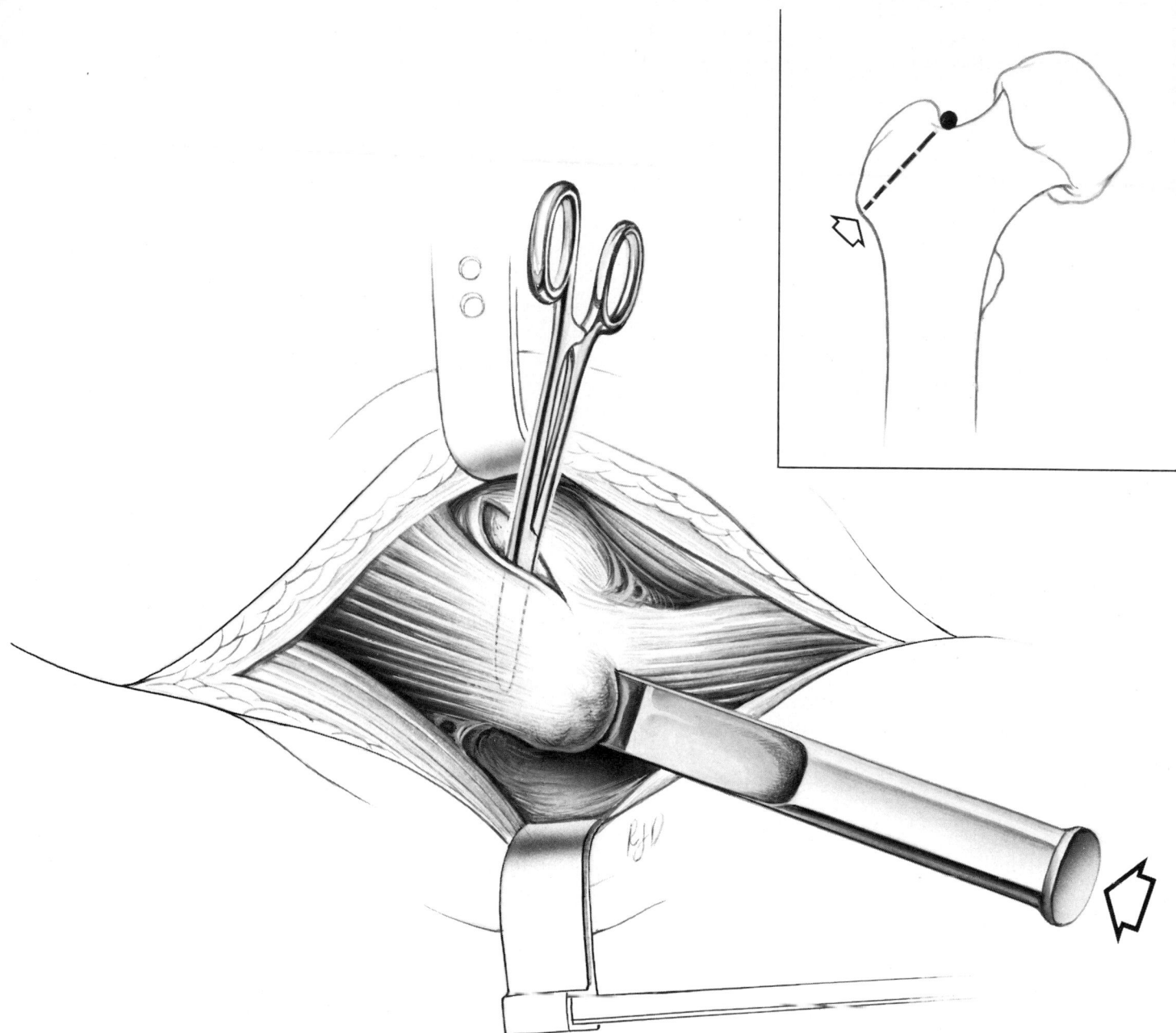

Fig. 19-30. When the surgeon plans to transfer the trochanter to an advanced position, a flat osteotomy is preferred; broad, thin osteotome may be used. Cholecystectomy forceps are forced through the capsule into the joint to point direction of osteotome, which is at junction of inner aspect of greater trochanter and neck of the femur. This point of reference is maintained by first assistant as target for osteotome to reach. Inset illustrates starting point *(arrow)* and target for osteotome.

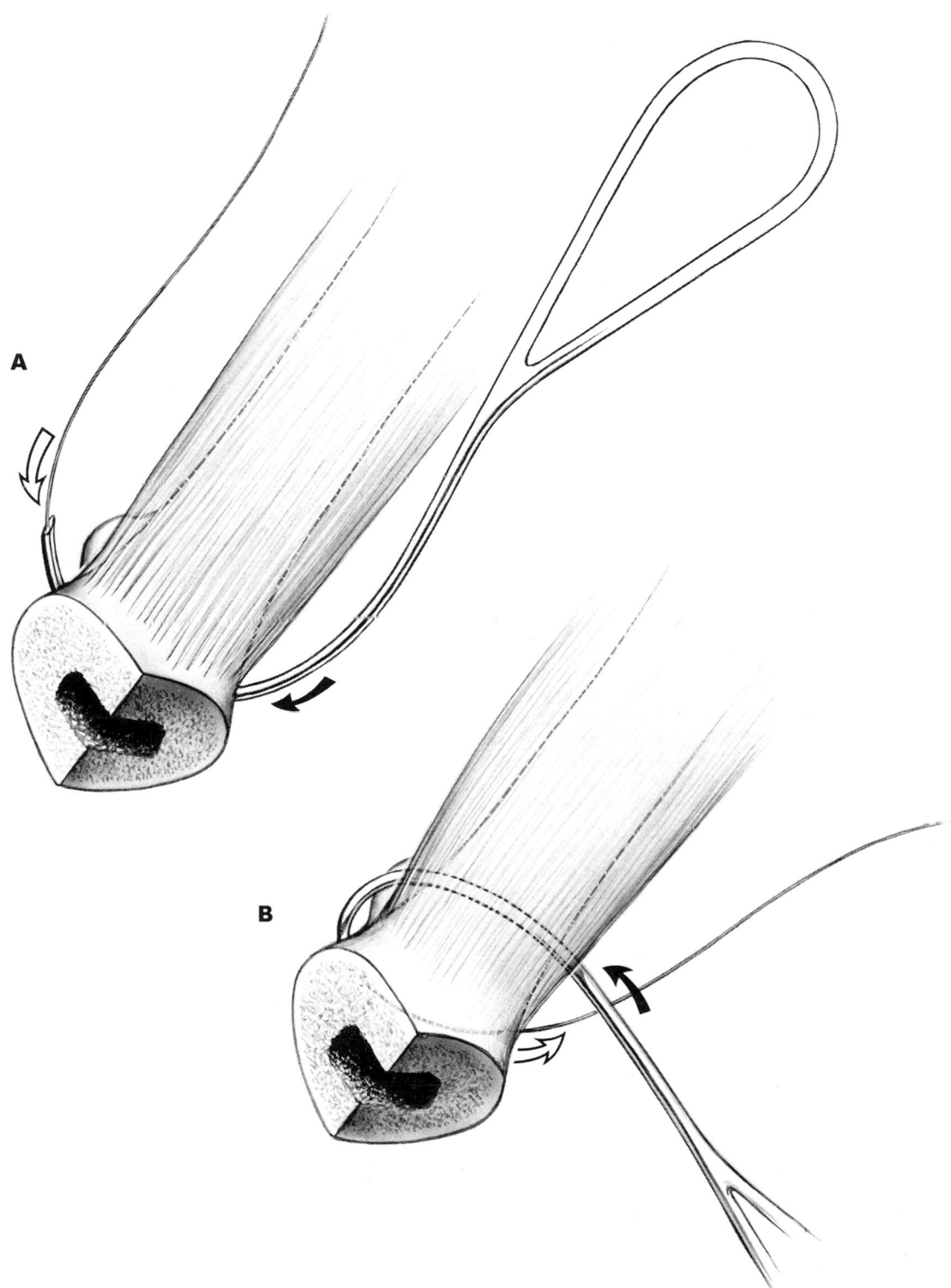

Fig. 19-31. An alternative method of wire fixation to femur is used when the upper femur is defective. Wire passer is used to pass horizontal wire. It is first inserted under muscle fibers of vastus lateralis and inserted as close to posterior aspect of femur as possible and revealed medially just above the lesser trochanter. **A,** Wire is about to be drawn from the medial to the lateral side of the femur. **B,** Wire passer is again inserted but this time in front of the femur to recover second end of loop of wire.

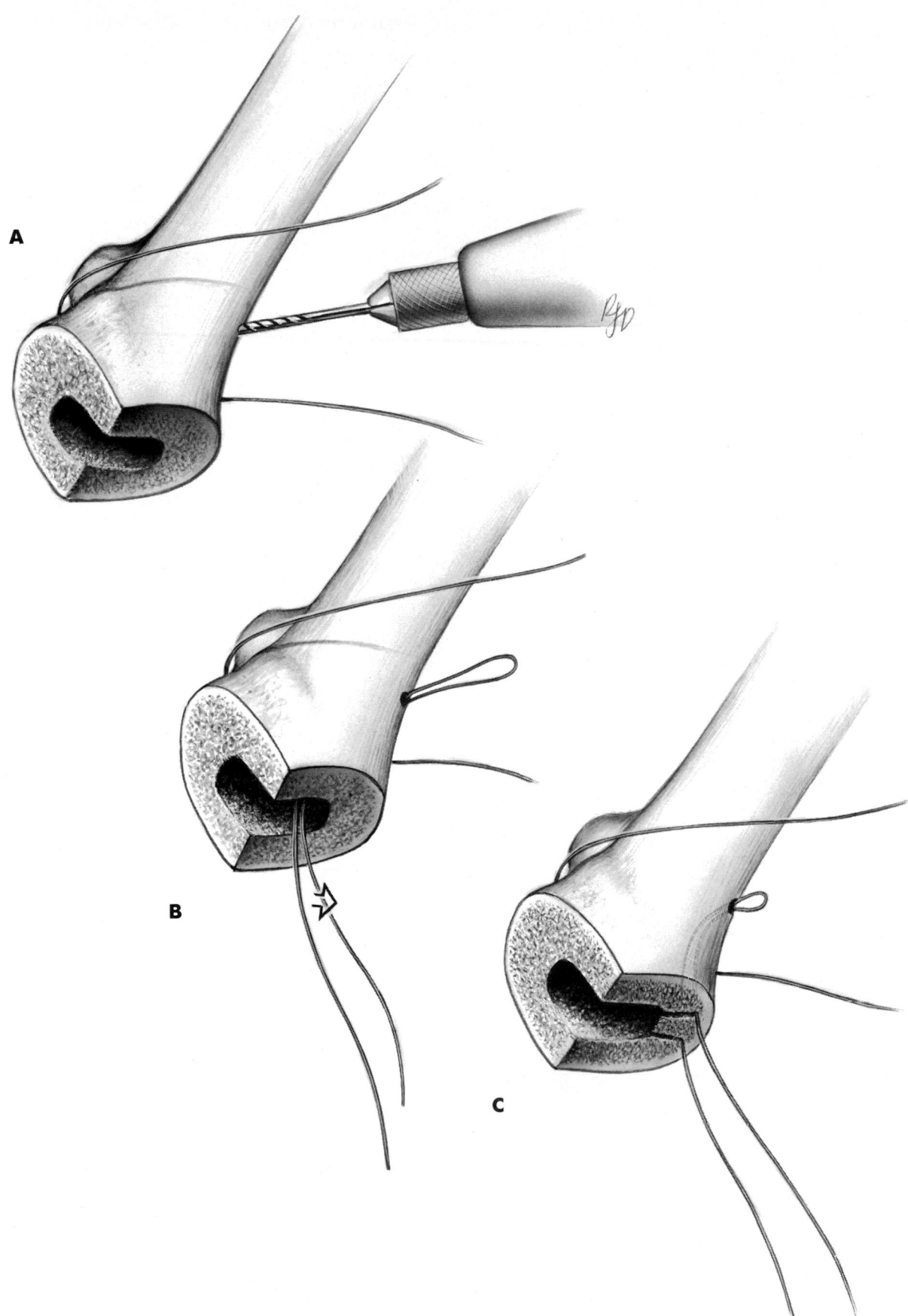

Fig. 19-32. Vertical wire, doubled, is passed through the hole made in the lateral aspect of the femur. **A,** Lateral surface of the shaft of the femur is presented to the surgeon, and a drill hole is made for vertical wire. Hole is at midlateral position on the femur, 2.5 cm distal to the vastus lateralis ridge. **B,** Vertical wire is passed through the hole on the lateral side of the shaft of the femur and emerges through the opening of the end of the neck and finally, **C,** positioned temporarily close to the outer cortex of the femur.

Reattaching a Single-Plane Osteotomy (Interlocking Technique)

Before reattaching the greater trochanter, the following steps must be completed: (1) Place the hip in some degree of adduction to create a space between the trochanter and the upper end of the femur. (2) Identify the vertical and transverse wires, assess the location and direction of the abductor muscle fibers, the greater trochanteric axis, and their relationship to the midlateral cortex of the femur. Determine the desired position of the greater trochanter against the femoral shaft. Divide the piriformis tendon if there is a fixed external rotation deformity. Release of the piriformis (short rotator) often allows the trochanter to rotate forward along its longitudinal axis (Fig. 19-33). Excess forward displacement of the trochanter should be avoided since it reduces the coaptation. (3) Apply a sharp bone hook just proximal to the greater trochanter at the insertion of the abductor tendon and pull the trochanter distally to assess the amount of displacement possible. (4) The hip is then brought to neutral position, and the site most suitable for trochanteric attachment is determined. Ideally, the center of the trochanter should lie at the level of the vastus ridge, requiring no more than 5 or 10 degrees abduction of the hip and no more than a moderate degree of tension on the abductor mechanism (see Fig. 19-33). If the greater trochanter cannot be brought distally to the level of the ridge, the lateral posterior and superior capsule or short rotators can be detached from the greater trochanter at the site of their insertion. If this maneuver is necessary, bleeders must be looked for and controlled.

Passage of Wires

The two vertical wires (identified by dark-handled clamps) are passed through the tendon of the abductors as close as possible to the greater trochanter. This can be accomplished by using a wire passer or directly by straightening the end of the wire and pushing it through the soft tissues using the wire-holding forceps. The anterior and posterior ends of the doubled vertical wire must be kept approximately 1 cm apart to distribute the forces over the top of the greater trochanter (Fig. 19-34). Care is taken to avoid puncturing one's gloves (by not touching the tips of the wires while they are passed through the abductor tendon). The black-handled clamps are reapplied to the ends of the vertical wires once they are recovered.

The trochanteric holding forceps are now applied, holding the trochanter in its optimal orientation and against the vastus ridge as if it were to be fixed in position. This enables the surgeon to drill the holes through the trochanter in the proper orientation. A line drawn between these two holes should be perpendicular to the longitudinal axis of the trochanter. The trochanteric clamp is held firmly by the first assistant while the surgeon drills two holes using a 2-mm drill point. The wires are passed from within outwards, identified, and grasped by wire clamps (see Fig. 19-34). In doing so, three minor details must be observed: (1) the distal 2 to 3 cm at the ends of the wires should be straightened out to ease their passage through the drilled holes; (2) care must be taken with an osteoporotic trochanter so that it is not fragmented by the trochanteric clamp; and (3) the ends of the wires are identified and held by silver-handled clamps to prevent perforation of the gloves.

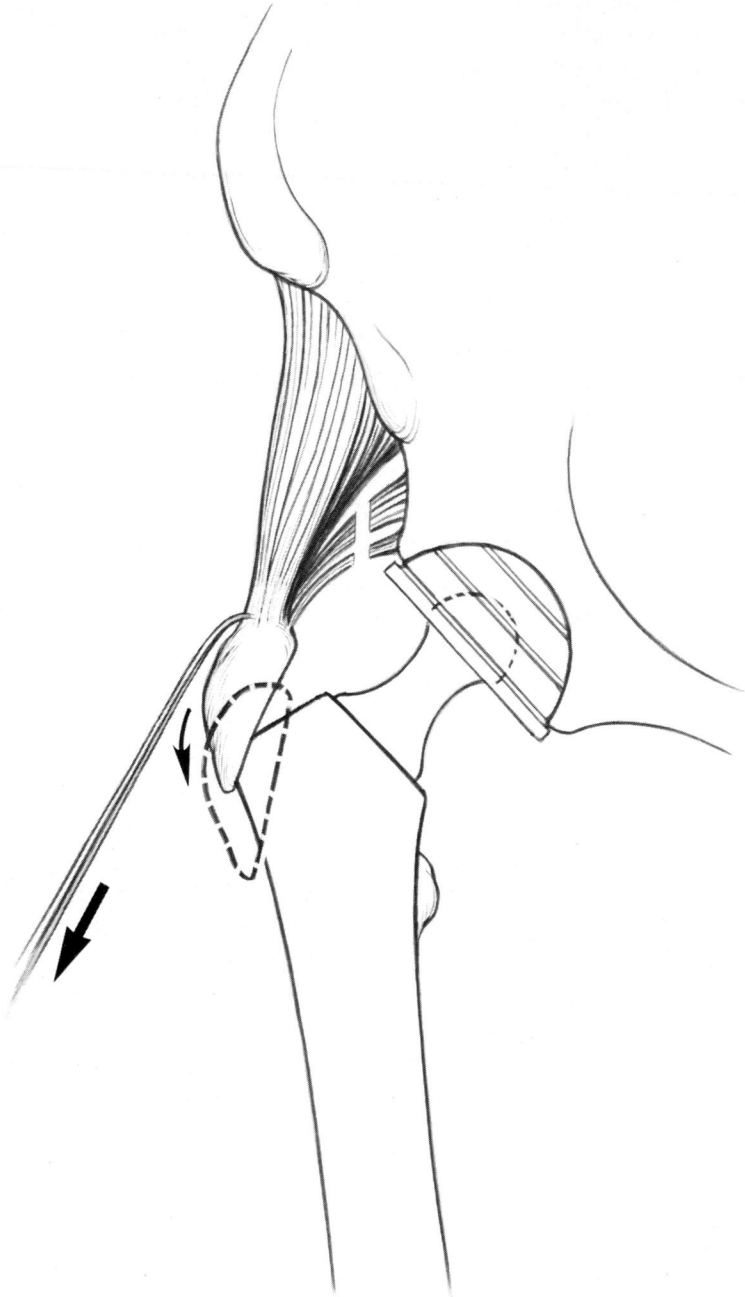

Fig. 19-33. Assessing amount of greater trochanter distal displacement. Hook is engaged onto outer aspect of trochanter, and hip is brought to a few degrees of abduction. Release of short rotators and superior capsule may be needed if trochanter does not conveniently reach level of vastus lateralis ridge.

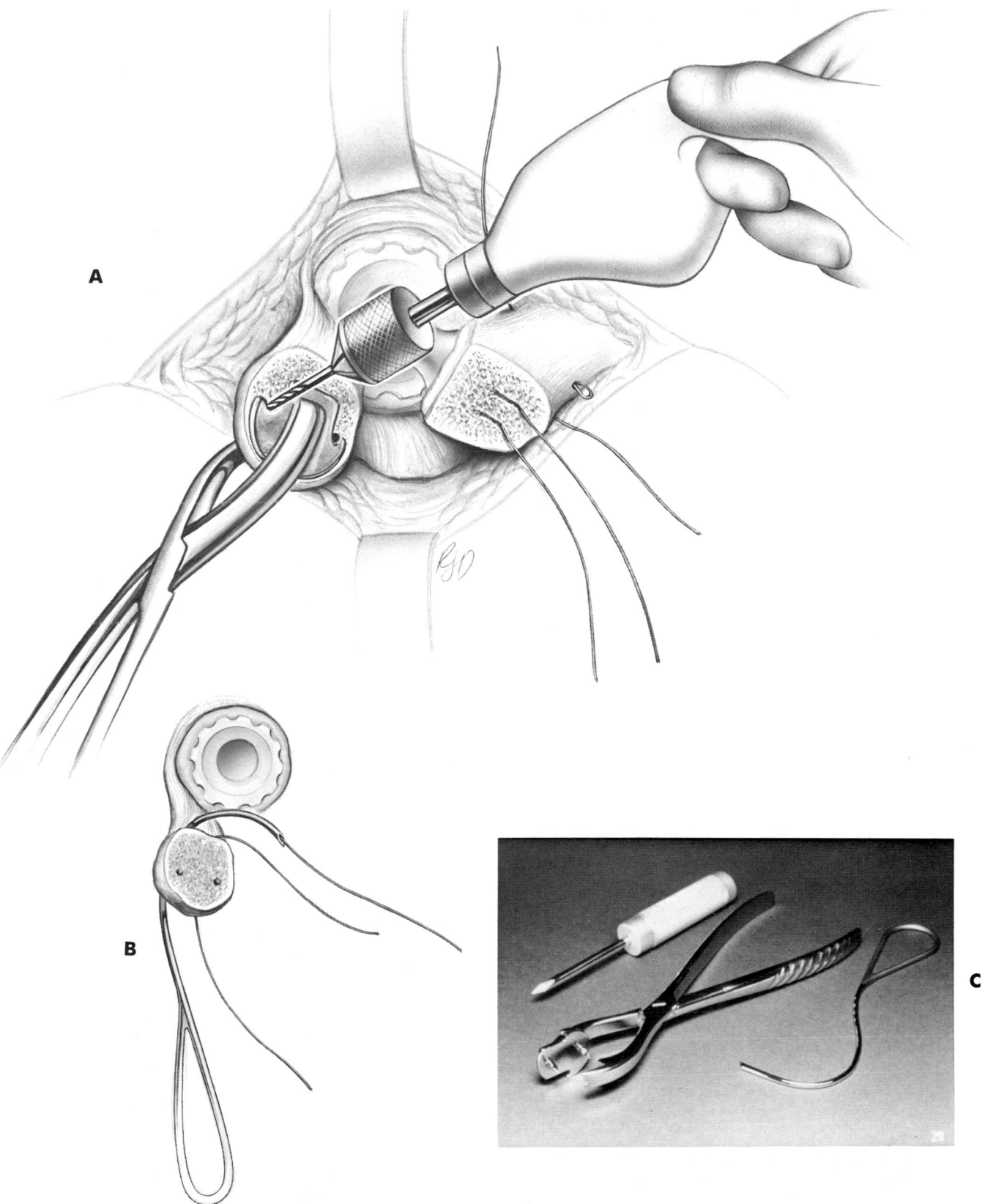

Fig. 19-34. A, Drill holes are being made to pass transverse wires. Trochanter is held in suitable position by trochanteric clamp. NOTE: position of doubled vertical wire and transverse wire. **B,** Wire passer has been pushed through abductor tendon just above trochanter, keeping as close to bone as possible. Two ends of vertical (double) wire are being inserted into wire passer to pull them through abductor tendon above trochanter. **C,** Essential instruments for passing trochanteric wires include a 6-mm awl, trochanteric forceps, and a wire passer. The sharp awl is introduced from lateral and superior surface of the trochanter toward the acetabulum to facilitate insertion of the wire passer, as close to bone as possible.

Interlocking of Trochanter

Before tightening the wires, determine where the greater trochanter will be interlocked. The site of the eminence is determined by holding the trochanter at the desired site. The anterior and posterior aspects of the shaft of the femur are then bevelled in this area at the level of the vastus lateralis ridge, leaving a pyramid-shaped prominence (Fig. 19-35, *B*). Hollow out the cancellous surface of the greater trochanter using a 12.5 mm gouge (Fig. 19-35, *A*), taking care not to disturb the transverse wires while the bone is being removed. The pyramid-shaped prominence created in the region of the vastus ridge is now inserted into this hollowed-out area, achieving a mechanical interlocking. Full penetration of the prominence into the trochanter must be achieved before attempting to tighten the wires. This maximizes the bony contact necessary for rapid union; it also provides a bed for the trochanter away from exposed cement and prevents forward and backward motion of the trochanter, the cause of early fatigue fracture failure of the wires.

Before tightening the wires the surgeon must make sure that (1) the limb is in neutral position while the trochanter is fitted onto the eminence; (2) the prominence and the hollowed trochanter fit together snugly without excessive abduction of the extremity; (3) no kinks or loose loops of wire are present, especially medial to the shaft and proximal to the trochanter; and (4) the femoral prosthesis is located within the socket, determined by placing the index finger along the neck of the prosthesis reaching the junction of the head and the socket.

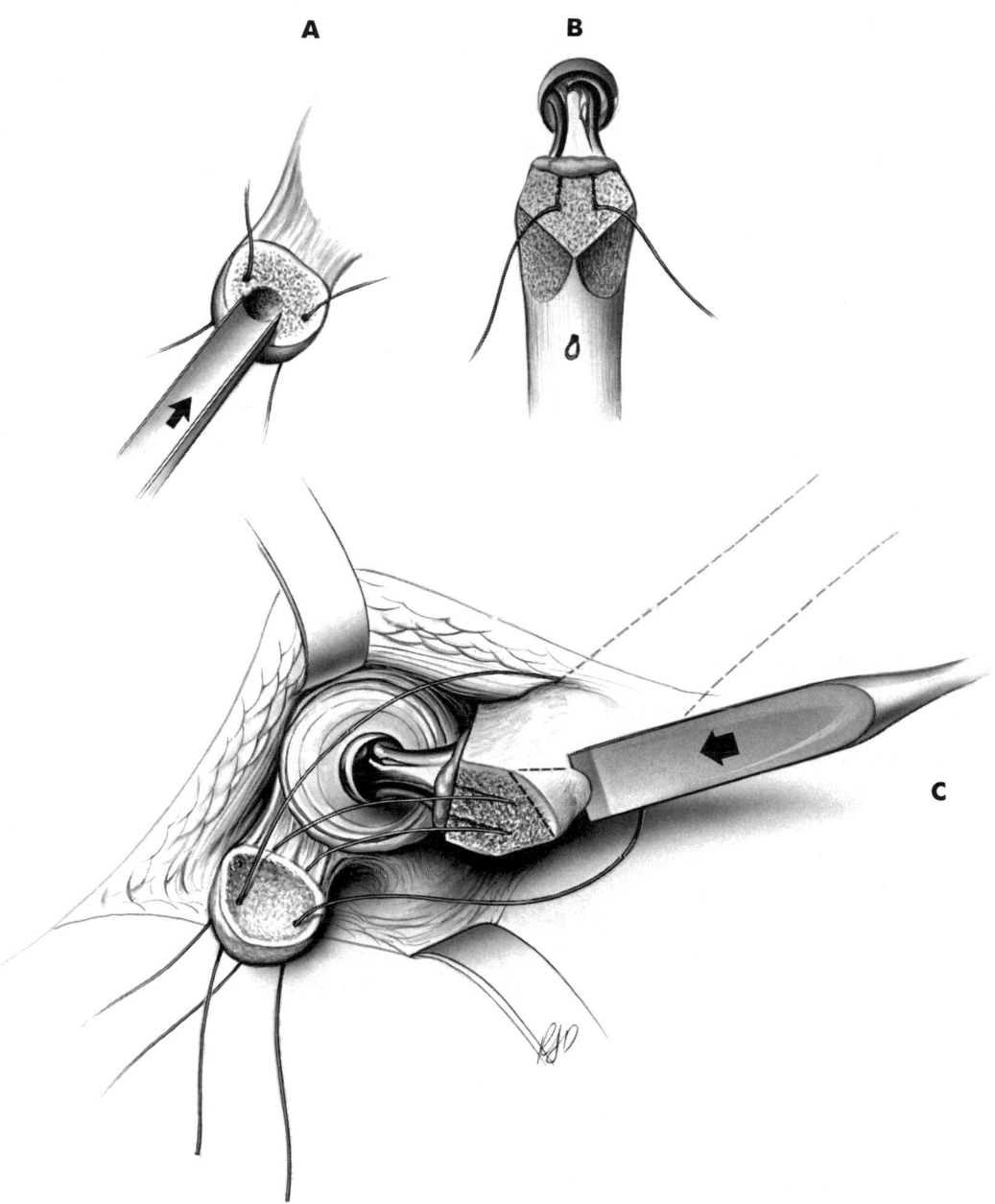

Fig. 19-35. Interlocking technique after single-plane (flat) osteotomy of the trochanter. **A,** General view of both wires passed and in position after disengagement of trochanter-holding forceps. NOTE: osteotome is beveling anterior aspect of shaft of femur at area of vastus lateralis ridge. Similar beveling is done posteriorly. **B,** Pyramid-shaped prominence created in region of vastus lateralis ridge. NOTE: location of vertical wire loop in relation to prominence. **C,** Hollowing of cancellous surface of greater trochanter by ½-inch gouge.

Tightening of Wires

The longitudinal and transverse wires are preferably tightened simultaneously using two wire tighteners, but it may be done in sequence. After identifying the anterior and posterior transverse wire ends, a single overhanded throw is made tying them over the outer aspect of the trochanter (Fig. 19-36). The wires are gripped in the jaws of the tightener (after being crossed over each other) and fully tightened. An occasional pull on the bow during the tightening eliminates any residual laxity (looseness) in the wire, but at the same time care must be taken not to pull the femoral prosthesis out of the socket. Place the vertical wires over the lateral aspect of the greater trochanter; the second assistant pulls them distally while the transverse wires are tightened (Fig. 19-37). A gentle hammering via the trochanter impacts against the shaft provides for a "snug" coaptation. Apply a second wire tightener to the vertical wires (which have been passed in the opposite direction) through the loop of the vertical wire (see Fig. 19-36).

A slight loosening of the transverse loop may take place as the result of a subsequent distal shaft of the trochanter, which will be rectified by further tightening of the transverse loop (via the first tightener). This alternate tightening may be repeated until a firm fixation is accomplished.

Note that when distal movement of the trochanter has taken place (while tightening the vertical wires) and firm contact between the trochanter and the shaft is apparent, further tightening may damage (split) the trochanter; care must be taken therefore not to overtighten the wires. The end longitudinal wires are then twisted upon themselves, turned, cut short, and buried in the soft tissues. If the trochanter has been ideally reattached by the method described, it should be in the desired position relative to the shaft (centered over the ridge) and exhibit no forward or backward motion in relation to the shaft of the femur when tested at surgery. Do not use a wire tightener that spreads widely such as a Kirschner bow because it may cause tissue damage.

Common Sources of Failure

Too small a trochanter makes interlocking difficult or impossible. On the other hand, too large a trochanter containing the ridge renders the creation of the prominence impossible. The wires may be damaged by the clamps and weakened by careless handling. If the wires are passed through the substance of the abductor tendon carelessly, the abductor muscle may be damaged, or the surgeon's gloves may be punctured.

The transverse wires may be ripped out of the trochanteric drill holes and through the substance of the trochanter if they are carelessly pulled while bringing the trochanter down upon the shaft. If the limb is not continuously held in neutral rotation during the tightening of the wires, the trochanter may be fixed excessively anteriorly or posteriorly. If the longitudinal wires are placed too far posterior or too far anterior to the longitudinal axis of the trochanter, the trochanter may rotate when the wires are tightened. The transverse wire must not be tightened over the greater trochanter before pulling the loop snugly against the medial side of the femur shaft. Excessive tightening of the longitudinal wires may fracture the trochanter, especially if the bone is osteoporotic. The trochanter may escape between the longitudinal wires (because of the pull of the abductors) if the wires are placed too far apart. Twisting the wrong wire ends (for example, one end of the transverse to the vertical) leads to failure of trochanteric fixation.

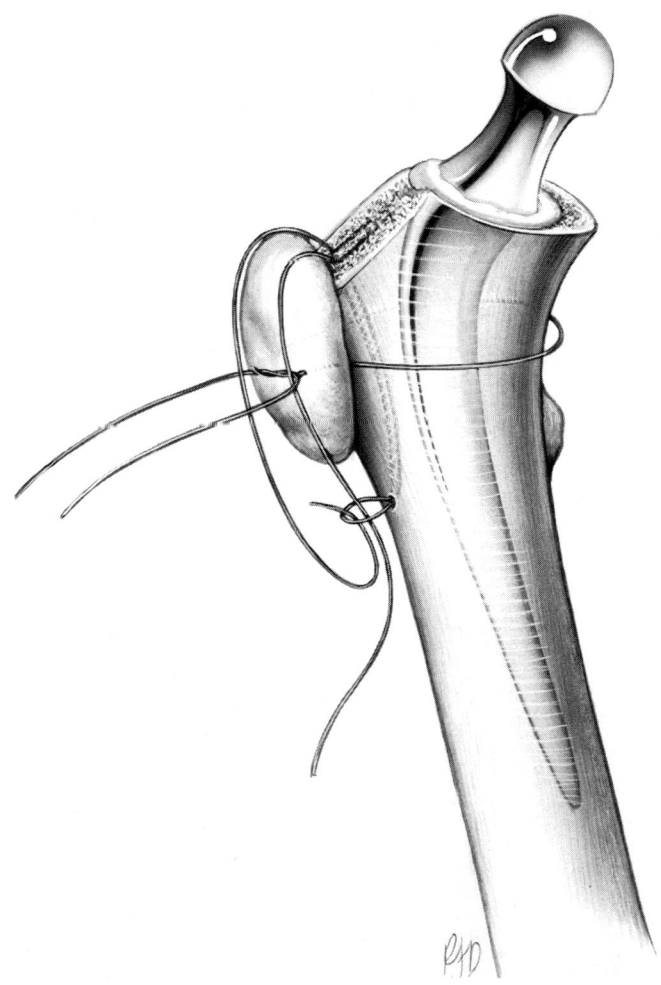

Fig. 19-36. General view of wires just before tightening. Trochanter is in an advanced position and held by traction on double wire. Ends of transverse wire have been passed through trochanter and tied. Vertical wire ends are passed over trochanter and in and out of loop of same wire.

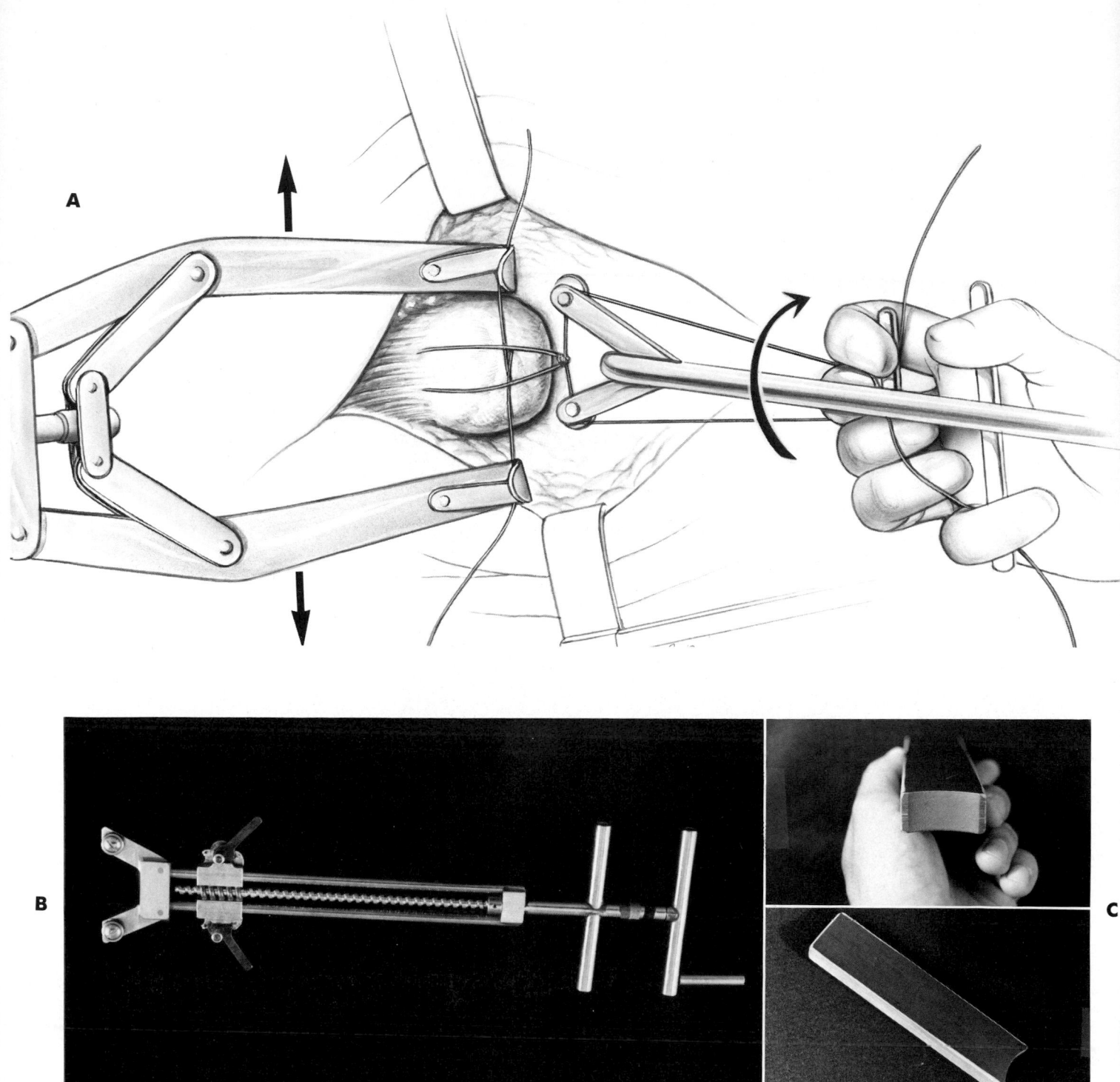

Fig. 19-37. A, Having tightened half-knot in transverse wire by tightener (Kirschner bow, *left*), vertical wire passed through loop is being tightened by second wire tightener. Distal movement of trochanter as result of tightening of vertical wire now may loosen transverse wire, which is corrected by further tightening. This alternate tightening of wires allows perfect adjustment. Final maneuver includes twisting both vertical and transverse wire ends. Author uses two wire tighteners of own design *(right),* which have the major advantage of not spreading apart while the wires are tightened, a feature required when working in a limited space. **B,** Wire tightener designed by the author. The pulling mechanism of this wire tightener is facilitated by a trip lead quick-advancing screw mechanism. **C,** Trochanteric impactor (designed by the author) is used to "coin" the trochanter against its bed. Two or three gentle hammer blows onto the impactor provide further stability for the trochanter by interdigitation of cancellous surfaces.

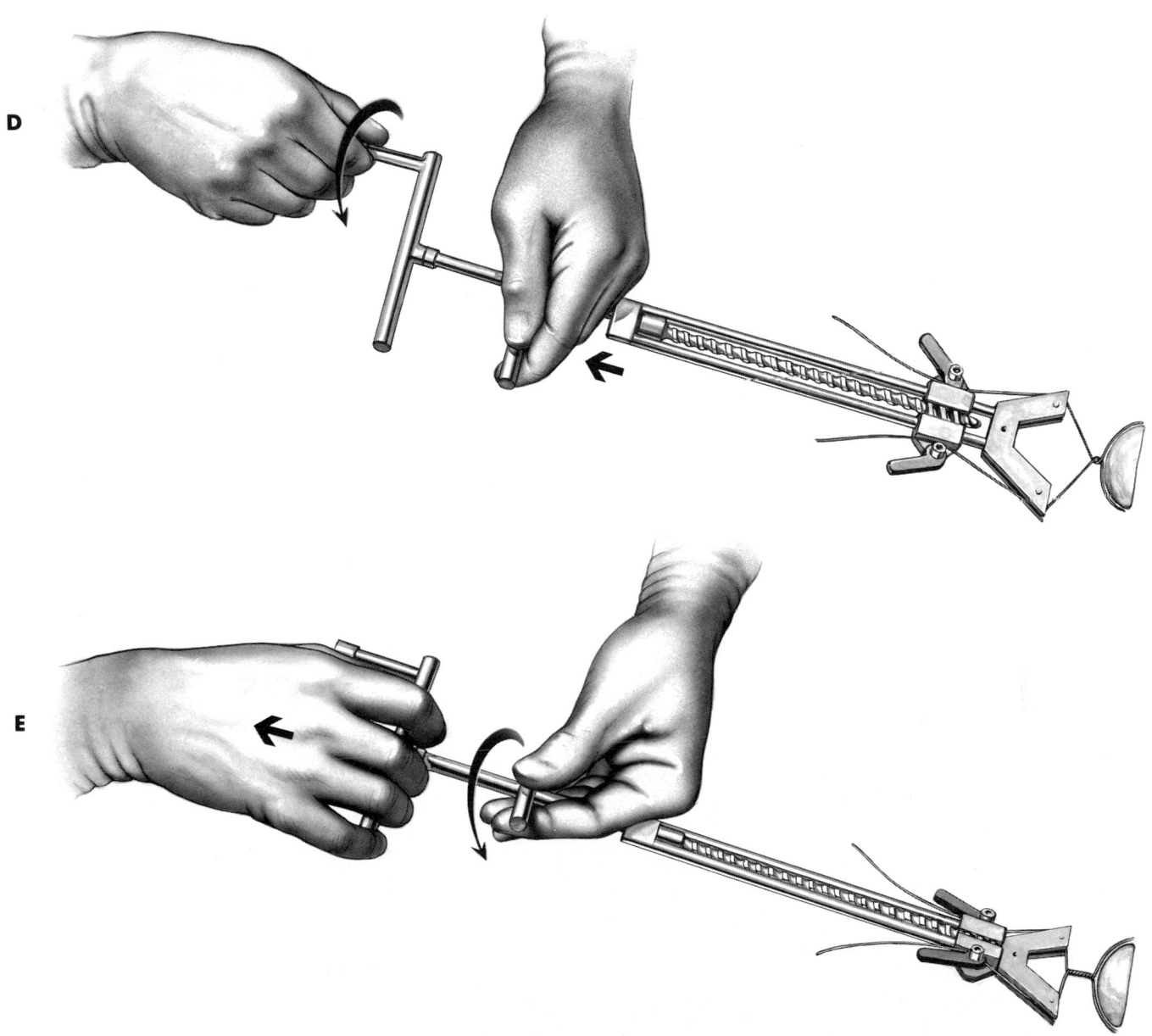

Fig. 19-37—cont'd. D, Operation of wire tightener: Step 1: Tightening. Wires clamped in the cam and pulled by the surgeon's left hand *(straight arrow)*. Further tightening by clockwise twisting of the handle *(right hand, curved arrow)*. **E,** Step 2: Twisting. Tension is maintained on the lower bar *(straight arrow)* while it is twisted counterclockwise. This mechanism allows twisting while wire is being advanced to make the tail. (**B** from Eftekhar NS: Total hip replacement: low-friction arthroplasty. In Evarts CM, editor: *Surgery of the musculoskeletal system,* New York, 1983, Churchill Livingstone.)

Repair of Vastus Lateralis Cuff

After the wires have been tightened, bring the detached proximal end of the musculotendinous vastus lateralis "cuff" over the wires, and suture it to the abductor tendon and aponeurosis. Nonabsorbable suture material is used. After this is done, the wires are no longer visible (Fig. 19-38). This can successfully be achieved if the cuff has been well developed at the time of its detachment from the shaft. A good closure of wires will prevent development of bursitis around the exposed wires.

Insertion of Hemovac Drains

Two medium-sized Hemovac drains are placed along the space between the vastus lateralis and the deep fascia. The two ends are brought out through the skin away from the incision; one drain is placed next to the arthroplasty anteriorly, the other is placed posteriorly. Both are then connected to the suction tubing temporarily to avoid clotting during the completion of wound closure. To avoid communication between the deep and superficial layers of the wound, the drains must not be brought through the opening in the tensor fascia femoris.

The octomerous retractor is now removed, and wound closure begins.

Wound Closure

Begin wound closure after the wound is irrigated copiously using a jet lavage. Use retention sutures and carry out skin closure as detailed in Chapter 15.

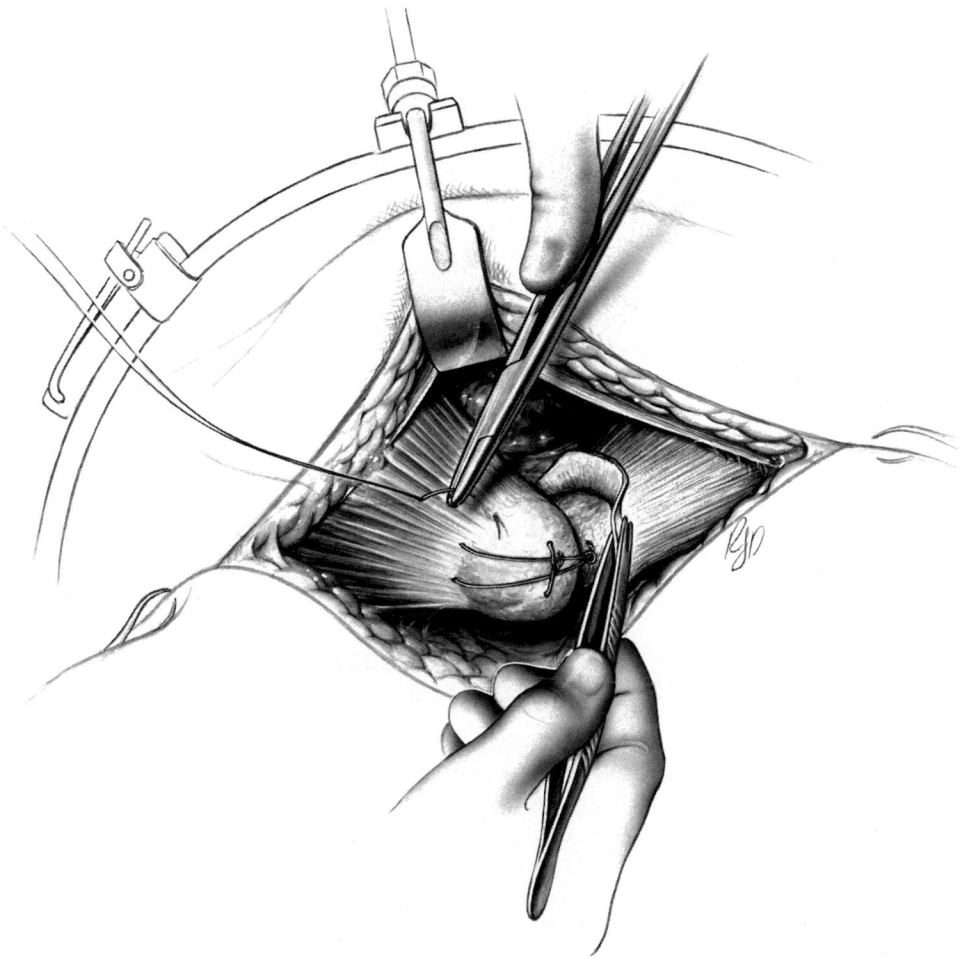

Fig. 19-38. Musculotendinous cuff of vastus lateralis is reattached to cover wires over trochanter.

SUMMARY OF ESSENTIALS

- The incision is along the shaft of the femur extending proximally and posteriorly to allow access to the femur and the acetabulum. The fascia is incised along the line of incision. The inclination of the incision proximally and posteriorly must extend for 2 to 4 cm proximal to the level of the anterosuperior spine.

- Maximize the exposure by mobilizing the fascia before applying the fascial members of the octomerous retractor.

- The key instrument for this approach, the octomerous retractor, is designed to facilitate complete exposure of the acetabulum and delivery of the upper femur. This allows the surgeon to perform the arthroplasty procedure with minimum assistance. Adjustment and readjustment of the members of this eight-member retractor are necessary to provide a safe and effective hip exposure. It is essential that the surgeon be familiar with the instrument before application in the operating room. Training on a cadaver is recommended.

- The retractor's main frame consists of a stainless steel loop, 300 cm in diameter, with three hemispherical receptors to receive the fascial and trochanteric and femoral members of the retractor. The acetabular members of the retractor (four in number) produce retraction of the tissue anteriorly, posteriorly, medially, and superiorly.

- Perform a biplaner osteotomy of the trochanter using a planar biplane osteotome. A curved clamp placed intracapsularly is used to guide the direction of the osteotomy starting over the vastus lateralis ridge.

- Perform a capsulotomy, and reflect the greater trochanter in a headward direction. Control the bleeders while the hip is maximally adducted and internally rotated, making sure that the sciatic nerve is protected throughout this step.

- Dislocate the hip by adduction (without rotation), and remove the femoral head at a level previously determined and estimated by a radiographic template. If dislocation is not possible, transect the neck in situ, and remove the head in a retrograde fashion.

- Exposure of the periphery of the acetabulum is essential. Begin by inserting the trochanteric and femoral members of the octomerous retractor. Visualize the rim of the acetabulum before placing the acetabular retractors. Release the capsule radially as indicated to facilitate insertion of the acetabular retractors. Observe the type of acetabular pathology, and prepare the acetabulum accordingly.

- Produce a cavity large enough to accommodate the acetabular component and the cement (when it is used). Produce a cavity the exact size of the acetabular component for press-fit designs. Protect the integrity of the acetabulum by preserving the subchondral bone of the roof. Use a debris-retaining reamer to prepare a bony cavity that has full support from the ilium, ischium, and pubis and that can contain the cup and cement (when it is used).

- Locate the center of rotation of the hip joint as close to a normal and anatomical position as possible by placing the cup in a low position in the acetabulum.

- Gauge the socket for size, and select the appropriate cemented or cementless socket. When using cement, trim the flange of the socket and ensure a proper fit before insertion. Test for orientation, and make multiple cement anchor holes. Insert the cementless socket in the appropriate orientation, and fix the screws through the shell of the acetabular component. Use pressurization assembly to maintain the pressure onto the face of the cup and cement when cement is used. Remove the pressure from the face of the cup only after full polymerization of cement has occurred. Make sure to clean the acetabulum thoroughly by irrigation and packing it with hydrogen-peroxide-soaked gauze before cementing the acetabular component. For cementless cups, make sure the fit is perfect and orientation is appropriate.

- If necessary, further mobilize the upper femur by soft tissue release. Remove the cortical bridge between the trochanteric bed and the sectioned neck. Insert a tapered straight reamer to open the medullary canal. Enlarge the medullary canal with rotary reamers to accommodate a large-caliber flanged stem. For a cemented femur, remove all the loose cancellous bone from the medial aspect of the neck. Use appropriately sized broaches to insert a cementless stem. When it is used, a varus alignment or an exaggerated valgus alignment of the prosthesis must be avoided. Centralize the stem proximally and distally, the former by using a special trial prosthesis and a locating pin and the latter by delivering a centralization plug to ensure an appropriately centered stem within the shaft of the femur.

- Perform a test reduction for stability and leg length. A satisfactory reduction should include perfect stability of the hip before reattaching the trochanter with full coverage of the prosthetic head within the acetabular component. Effective neck length (patient's femoral neck and prosthetic neck length) must produce stability and equal leg length. The causes of instability must be sought and corrected before inserting the wires to reattach the greater trochanter.

- Insert a double vertical wire through the medullary canal and two single wires for two independent vertical and cruciate wiring systems. Plug the medullary canal at the appropriate level. Insert cement after brushing and irrigating the canal. Insert the stem as held by a holder in a prerehearsed direction.

- As the wires are being tightened, be sure that reduction of the trochanter into its bed is perfect.

- Interlock the trochanter over the vastus lateralis ridge. Use simultaneous tightening of the vertical and transverse wires when performing a flat osteotomy of the greater trochanter.

- During wound closure, the vastus lateralis muscle must be repaired so that it covers the wires.

REFERENCES

1. **Benjamin JB, Gie GA, Lee AJ, et al:** Cementing technique and effects of bleeding, *J Bone Joint Surg* 69[Br]:620, 1987.
2. **Charnley J:** *Low-friction arthroplasty of the hip,* New York, 1979, Springer-Verlag.
3. **Eftekhar NS:** *Principles of total hip arthroplasty,* St Louis, 1978, Mosby–Year Book.
4. **Eftekhar NS:** Total hip replacement using principles of low friction arthroplasty. In Evarts CM, editor: *Surgery of the musculoskeletal system,* New York, 1983, Churchill Livingstone.
5. **Eftekhar NS, Pawluk RJ:** The role of acetabular preparation in total hip replacement. *The Hip Society: Proceedings of scientific meeting of The Hip Society,* St Louis, 1979, Mosby–Year Book.

See Chapters 6, Biomechanics: Fixation and Loosening; 15, Principles Common to all Surgical Approaches; 18, Transtrochanteric Approach (Author's Method); and 25, Revision in Absence of Infection for additional information.

APPENDIX: INSTRUMENTS USED FOR TRANSTROCHANTERIC APPROACH TO TOTAL HIP ARTHROPLASTY

Tray #1 Skin Incision

2 Knife handles with blade	2 Long diathermy leads:
2 Lane's dissecting forceps	1 for cutting
5 Mayo towel clips, sharp	1 for diathermy
2 Mayo towel clips, dull	1 Diathermy cutting needle
18 Moynihan skin-towel clips	4 Paper clips
6 Heavy rubber bands for Moynihan clips	2 for diathermy leads
1 Diathermy forceps (Richies)	2 for stool drape
	1 Suction tip and tubing

Tray #2 Exposure of the Acetabulum

2 Knife handles
1 Lane's dissecting forceps
1 Richard (medium) retractor
1 Watson-Jones gauge
2 Hibb's retractors
  1 large
  1 small
1 Cholecystectomy clamp
1 9 inch Kocher
1 T-handle large bone hook
1 Mallet
1 Weight and chain
2 Gigli's saws with handle

1 Bi-plane osteotome and plastic tip
1 Ribbon osteotome
*1 Octomerous retractor ring and eight clips
*2 Posterior blades for octomerous retractor
  1 small
  1 large
*1 Anterior claw for octomerous retractor
*2 Claws for octomerous retractor (identical)
*1 Acetabular staple and chain
*1 Acetabular staple insertor/extractor
*4 Acetabular retractors for octomerous retractor
  (Hohmann type)
1 Charnley weight and chain

Tray #3 Acetabular Cup Fixation

1 Air power drill
1 Air power saw handle
1 Chuck adaptor
1 Acetabular gauge (wooden handle), AO
4 Debris-retaining reamers, acetabular
†2 Debris-retaining reamers, spigotted
1 Reamer holder
*1 Jacobs' chuck long-handle key
1 Acetabular brush (disposable)
1 Sharp Hohmann retractor
1 Long T-handle curette
1 Heavy cutting scissors
*1 6-mm long drill bit

*1 Long drill guide
*2 Acetabular gauge drill guides (40 mm and
  4 mm outer diameter)
2 12.5 mm drill tips
*1 Cup pusher
*1 Cup holder/ejector (2 pieces)
*1 Cup holder/ ejector for 26 mm socket
1 socket pressurization assembly
2 Bone punches
  1 small
  1 large
1 Mallet

Tray #4 Preparation of Femur Test Reduction

1 Bone rongeur (large)
1 Tapered T-handle reamer
*2 Rotary medullary reamers
1 Osteotome (wooden handle, AO), 2 cm wide
1 Mallet
1 Octomerous retractor (femoral hook)
*1 Locating pin with chain
†1 Bone block chain
†1 Bone graft cutter

†1 Bone graft insertor
4 Centralization gauges/delivery tubes
*1 Centralization ejector rod
1 Femoral brush (disposable)
2 Femoral broaches
1 Tomy bar
1 Femoral brush holder
2 Test prostheses
1 Test prostheses set (wrapped)

*Designed and manufactured in collaboration with Rudolph Gand at Columbia-Presbyterian Medical Center, New York, New York.
†Zimmer U.S.A.

Tray #5 Insertion of Wires and Femoral Component Fixation

1 Jacobs' chuck head and key
1 $\frac{7}{64}$ drill bit (sterile package)
6 Wire-holding forceps (color coded)
1 Fine plain forceps (toothless)
1 Fine narrow rongeur
1 1″ ribbon (disposable)
1 Polyvinyl suction tubing (4 mm outer diameter)

1 Long-handled curette
*1 Femoral prosthesis holder
1 Small curette (standard)
1 Mallet
1 Set wires, Ortron (2 single, 1 double)
1 Waston-Jones gauge

Tray #6 Reattachment of Trochanter

1 Knife handle and blade
1 Trochanterical holding forceps, flat
*1 Trochanterical holding forceps, biplane
1 Wire passer (½ circle)
1 Narrow bone drill

1 Large bone drill
*2 Wire tighteners
1 Wire cutter
*1 Concave end punch
1 Small Richardson retractor

*Designed and manufactured in collaboration with Rudolph Gand at Columbia-Presbyterian Medical Center, New York, New York.

Tray #7 Wound Closure

2 Needle holders
1 Mayo scissors
1 Dissecting forceps
10 Hemostats

2 Medium-sized drains (disposable)
1 Button crusher
10 Buttons (disposable)
10 Double needle-ended #1 nylon

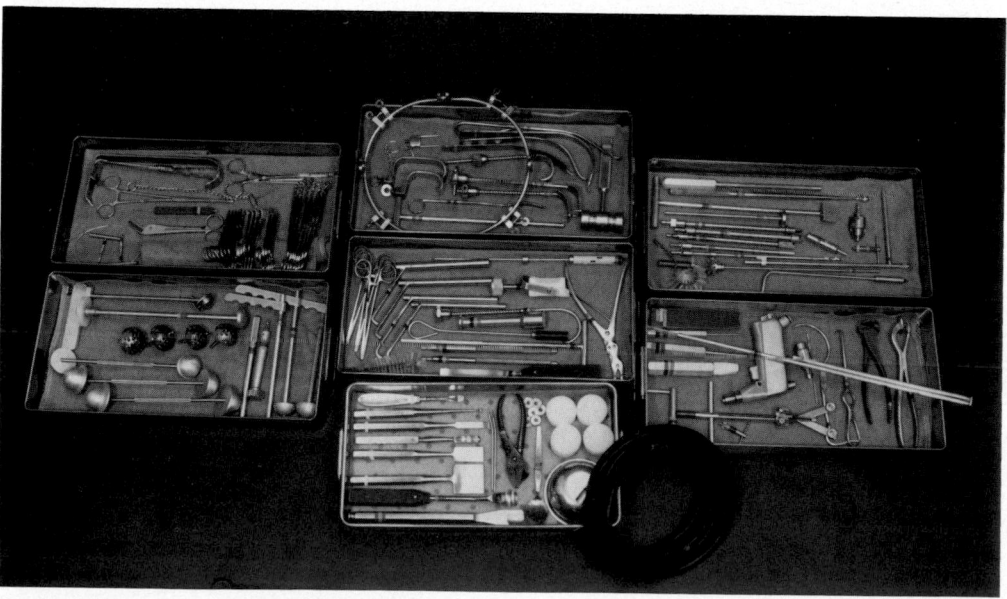

Fig. 19-39. Seven trays of instruments are delivered to the enclosure. The instruments are prewrapped and sterilized and stored next to operating room. The trays are presented to the surgeon in sequence and according to each phase of the procedure.

Index

Biplanar osteotomy—cont'd
  trochanter in—cont'd
    union rate of, 1655
Bipolar prosthesis, 1064
  avascular necrosis and, 469
  bone graft and, 618-622
  conversion of, 1128
  in pelvic discontinuity and union, 1209
  protrusio acetabuli and, 1060-1061
  recurrent dislocation and, 1543
  results with, 1398-1399
  revision surgery and, 1435
  rheumatoid arthritis and, 983
  as total hip arthroplasty alternative, 482-483
Bladder, 25, 44
  medial wall of acetabulum and, 770
  prosthesis protrusion and, 1066, 1069
Bleeding
  capsulotomy and, 825, 827
  dextran and, 409
  Gaucher's disease and, 1019
  heparin and, 408
  intramedullary, 712-714
  intrapelvic intrusion of cement and, 1169
  Paget's disease and, 1018
  perioperative, 1575-1576
  preoperative planning for, 1576
  sciatic nerve palsy and, 1558
  warfarin and, 405
Blood
  in cement, 180, 200
  for culture, 1495
  loss of
    anesthesia and, 317-318, 319
    estimation of, 322-323
    inadequate exposure and, 332
    intraoperative blood collection and, 326
    measurement of, 1575
    revision surgery and, 1416
  nonunion and, 1657
  pseudarthrosis and, 1335
Blood pressure
  acrylic cement and, 206-208
  postoperative bleeding and, 1575, 1576
Blood transfusion
  alternatives to homologous, 326-327
  arthroplasty without, 327
  autologous, 323-326
  intraoperative blood salvage and, 326
  postoperative, 594
  preoperative planning and, 322-327
  rheumatoid arthritis and, 976
  sickle cell disease and, 1021
Body-exhaust system, 360, 642
Body weight
  arthroplasty contraindications and, 433
  load reduction and, 228
  prosthesis size and, 281
Body-weight moment arm, 229-230
Boiling in bone graft antigenicity, 612
Bolts in trochanteric union, 1663-1664
Bone
  absorption of
    prosthesis collar and, 264-265
    screw-plate-bone junction and, 253
  atrophy of, 1373

Bone—cont'd
  cancellous; see Cancellous bone
  cement and
    circulation in, 79-81
    interface of, 90, 203-205
  curettage of, 711
  defects of; see Bone defects
  disorders of; see Bone disorders
  ectopic formation of; see Ectopic bone formation
  fixation strength and, 203
  immunogenicity of, 610
  implant bonding and, 9
  load and, 25-26
  loss of
    corticocancellous, 1246
    repeated surgery and, 1162
    resection pseudarthrosis and, 1333-1334
    revision surgery and, 1436
  metastatic lesion of, 1079
  mineral content changes in, 82-83
  mounting of, 240
  necrosis of, 83
    implantation and, 78
    reaming and, 80
    screw-plate-bone junction and, 253
  preparation of
    ankylosing spondylitis and, 1010
    conversion surgery and, 1111
    Identifit prosthesis and, 530, 531
    juvenile rheumatoid arthritis and, 989
    Paget's disease and, 1018
    preoperative planning for, 328
    revision surgery and, 1171-1172
    transtrochanteric approach in, by author's method, 882-889
  radionuclide imaging of, 1488-1489
  remodeling of; see Bone remodeling
  resorption of
    polyethylene wear debris and, 128
    porous-coated stem and, 96
    stem failure and, 294
  revision surgery and, 1284, 1424-1425
  stem fracture and, 297-298
  tumors of; see Tumor
Bone banking, 613-615, 617
Bone block in congenital dysplasia and dislocation, 947-952
Bone chips, 620
  cavitary defects and, 1201, 1202
  congenital dysplasia and dislocation and, 947, 948
  floor defect and, 1199
  hemispherical graft and, 1206
  impaction of, 1055
  preparation of, 1172
Bone defects
  acetabular classification of, 1191-1207
    cavitary defects in, 1200, 1201, 1202, 1203
    combination segmental and cavitary defects in, 1201, 1204, 1205-1206
    enlarged acetabulum in, 1191
    pelvic discontinuity and nonunion in, 1201-1207, 1208-1213
    segmental and defect fractures in, 1207
    segmental deficiencies in, 1191-1201
  femoral, 1227-1235, 1236, 1237
    cement fixation in, 1233-1235
    management of, 1229-1233
Bone disorders, 969-1031
  ankylosing spondylitis in, 1000-1010